Applied Veterinary Histology

Applied Veterinary Histology

William J. Banks, Ph.D., D.V.M.

Professor, Department of Anatomy
College of Veterinary Medicine and Biomedical Sciences
Colorado State University
Fort Collins, Colorado

Illustrated by:
Biomedical Media
College of Veterinary Medicine
and Biomedical Sciences
Colorado State University

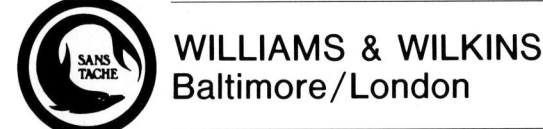

WILLIAMS & WILKINS
Baltimore/London

Library of Congress Cataloging in Publication Data

Formerly *Histology and Comparative Organology: A Text-Atlas*

Banks, William J.
    Applied veterinary histology.

    Edition for 1974 published under title: Histology and comparative organology: a
text-atlas

    Includes index.
    1. Veterinary histology. I. Title. [DNLM: 1. Anatomy, Veterinary. 2. Histology.
SF747.3 B218a]
SF761.B32   636.089′1018   80-22672
ISBN 0-683-00410-7

Composed and printed at the
Waverly Press, Inc.
Mt. Royal and Guilford Aves.
Baltimore, MD 21202, U.S.A.

DEDICATED TO
BRENDA, VICTORIA
AND KRISTIN
whose love, patience,
understanding and encouragement
made this book possible.

DEDICATED TO
BRENDA, VICTORIA
AND KRISTIN
whose love, patience,
understanding and encouragement
made this book possible.

Preface

The original edition of this textbook, *Histology and Comparative Organology: A Text-Atlas*, was an attempt to present the elements of histology that are applicable to veterinary medicine. Structure and function, integrated throughout the text, were presented in a succinct format. This parochial and concise approach, although affording a foundation in microanatomic organization, did not consider the application and relevancy of histology to clinical endeavors. Similarly, functional considerations were limited in scope. In confidence that histology is a fundamental and relevant component of medical education, the revision of the original text was undertaken to broaden the scope and utility of the book.

The elements of histology have been retained in a concise format but have been expanded as necessary and selectively to maintain pace with the recent remarkable expansion of knowledge of microscopic structure. The histophysiology of cells, tissues and organs has been expanded and broadened but remains integrated with structural considerations. Numerous examples of the applicability of histology and histophysiology to medicine and surgery have been interwoven throughout the text. The principles of renewal and repair of all tissues and most organs have been included with the microanatomic and physiologic considerations. The text has been thoroughly revised, rewritten and updated to present an applied approach to histology for veterinary medical students.

The basic organization of the book is unchanged. The text, now divided into five sections, proceeds from principles of histology to cytology, histology, organology and exfoliative cytology. The first section consists of three new chapters that are designed to give the student a perspective of the scope of histology as a basic medical science, an appreciation of the methods of histology and insights into the interpretation of the methods of histology and insights into the interpretation of histologic specimens. The chapter on cytology, which comprises the second section, has been expanded to include the chemical, physical and biologic properties of cells. A concerted attempt has been made to correlate the ultrastructural features of cells to those features visible with light microscopy, thus bridging the "conceptual gap" between ultrastructural cytology and histology. Section III presents the basic tissues. The morphology has been updated, while the histophysiology has been expanded to afford the student a better appreciation of the role of the basic tissues in the structural and functional complexity of the animal body. The majority of the text is devoted to comparative organology. An introductory chapter on organology presents the organizational schemes that characterize tubular and parenchymatous organs. Subsequent chapters present the morphologic features of specific and/or unique organs that characterize the major domestic species, including carnivores, herbivores and birds. Histophysiology is expanded and integrated with the morphology of each of the organs. The last section in the text consists of a chapter on clinical cytology. The normal exfoliative cytology of various organs, tissues and body cavities is compared and contrasted with abnormalities associated with these structures.

The new approach of this textbook has been influenced by the author's experience in teaching functional anatomy to first- second- and third-year veterinary students. The constructive comments of these students, relating to veterinary histology in general and the original edition of the textbook specifically, have had a profound impact upon the revision process. Similarly, the comments of colleagues and reviewers have been influential. All have expressed the desirability and need for a text that integrates histologic and functional properties as well as demonstrating the applied significance of these principles. This text is an attempt to satisfy that need and is consistent with the author's educational philosophy.

Visual aids are essential components of the armamentarium of the effective teaching histologist. Because the text is replete with illustrative materials, it should serve as a valuable teaching and learning aid. The textual material is complemented by 883 black and white figures. Although the majority of the original light and electron micrographs have been retained, many have been replaced, improved or supplemented with new micrographs. Electron micrographs of selected tissues and freeze-fractured specimens, as well as some scanning electron micrographs of selected organs, have been added to clarify or complement specific presentations of certain structures. Over 240 medical illustrations, diagrams and flow charts complement the micrographs and text. Additionally, eight color plates have been added to assist the learning process. All of the illustrative materials should serve to improve the comprehension of structural and functional principles.

This text is not intended to be a definitive tome for the rapidly expanding, vast and dynamic field of veterinary histology. Rather, it is envisioned as a positive step in the integration of histologic and physiologic principles that are applicable to veterinary medicine and surgery.

William J Banks
Fort Collins, Colorado

Acknowledgments

The author is indebted to numerous individuals who have contributed directly or indirectly to this book.

Mrs. R. Colter of the Histology Preparation Laboratory, Department of Anatomy, Colorado State University, was most helpful. She was always willing to obtain, prepare or retrieve specimens that eventually were incorporated into the book. The assistance of Mr. D. Dunham and Mr. W. Kuenning of the University Electron Microscopy Training Center, Colorado State University was appreciated.

The review of specific chapters by Drs. W. M. Aufderheide (Department of Pathology), G. F. Grauer (Department of Clinical Sciences), D. C. Lueker (Department of Microbiology), M. A. Thrall (Department of Pathology) and L. Wilke (Department of Physiology and Biophysics) of Colorado State University was appreciated. Their expertise and enthusiasm for their subject areas and their willingness to review specific chapters were most helpful. The suggestions of Dr. R. D. Frandson during the formative stages of the revision process were extremely valuable.

The micrographs, negatives or samples supplied by Drs. M. Carry, C. J. Connell, D. L. Eisenbrandt, J. J. England, G. P. Epling, R. A. Kainer, D. E. Kelly, J. W. Newbrey, H. O. Nornes, R. W. Norrdin, J. E. Rash, J. Storz, M. A. Thrall, W. Todd and Ms. A. M. Sheppard were most helpful. The permission granted by other authors and publishing companies to use selected micrographs from copyrighted materials was appreciated.

The staff of the Department of Radiology, Veterinary Teaching Hospital, Colorado State University, was most helpful. A special thanks to Dr. J. Lebel, Staff Radiologist, for his friendship and assistance during the formative stages of the revision process.

The typing by my sister, Eileen K. Banks, and Mrs. Elaine Winn was most helpful and appreciated. Their timely assistance reduced the mounds of written and rough-typed copy into a manageable work load for the primary typist. The bulk of the typing was accomplished by my able, conscientious, organized and extremely patient wife, Brenda F. Banks. Her ability to interpret cryptic syntax, decipher editorial and scientific hieroglyphics, organize the tumultuous progression of events and culminate with an impeccable final copy seems inconceivable. But she did it, all the time maintaining a smile despite the adversity. It is impossible to express my appreciation adequately.

The willingness of Dr. M. A. Thrall, Assistant Professor of Pathology and Clinical Pathologist, Veterinary Teaching Hospital, Colorado State University, to participate in the writing of this text was most appreciated. Her authoritative chapter, *Introduction to Clinical Cytology*, is a useful addition to the textbook.

The expert assistance of the staff of Biomedical Media, College of Veterinary Medicine and Biomedical Sciences, Colorado State University, was of inestimable value during the revision process. Their patience with the author, their ability to translate obscure ideas into reality, their enthusiasm for their art and their professional expertise made the project enjoyable. The author is grateful to Mr. T. O. McCracken, Director and Affiliate Faculty Member, Department of Anatomy, and his able staff: J. Daughterty, M. L. Kessel, K. Jee, P. Jones, L. Schuler and C. Turner. All of the medical illustrations, diagrams and flow charts are the result of the efforts of these talented and gracious individuals. Additionally, the assistance of J. Sugimoto and C. Blackwell was most appreciated.

Four individuals deserve special recognition of their efforts. They read the entire manuscript, offered many helpful suggestions and were a source of encouragement and support. Their diverse perspectives afforded the author valuable insights. Mr. D. Beezley. Ph.D. candidate in the Department of Anatomy, Colorado State University, spent many hours with the author discussing various aspects of the manuscript. Dr. J. J. England, Assistant Professor of Microbiology and Staff Virologist, Diagnostic Laboratory, Veterinary Teaching Hospital, Colorado State University, offered many suggestions that proved to be useful. The critical comments of Ms. H. C. Strout, Senior Veterinary Student at Colorado State University, were most helpful in generating an improved manuscript. Dr. R. A. Kainer, Professor of Anatomy, spent many hours with the author. His critical comments and hours of intense discussion were valuable and appreciated. To these colleagues and special friends, my sincerest gratitude is expressed.

The completion of this project would not have been possible without the patience, support, encouragement and understanding of my spouse, Brenda, and our children, Victoria and Kristin.

The able assistance of the staff of the Williams & Wilkins Co. was most helpful and made the project enjoyable and gratifying. The author is indebted to the original editor for this project, Ms. S. A. Finnegan, currently Vice President and Editor-in-Chief, whose patience and encouragement precipitated the revision process. Early in the revision process, Ms. N. C. Tyler, Editor for Veterinary Medicine, assumed responsibility for the project. In the fine tradition of her predecessor, Ms. Tyler immediately embarked upon her responsibilities with professional expertise and enthusiasm. Her invaluable assistance throughout the project was appreciated greatly.

To my numerous students and colleagues, from whom I have learned so much, my sincerest appreciation is expressed.

William J. Banks
Fort Collins, Colorado

Contents

SECTION IV: COMPARATIVE ORGANOLOGY

Chapter 19 Digestive System **373**

Chapter 20 Urinary System **424**

Chapter 21 Respiratory System **439**

Chapter 22 Endocrine System **456**

Chapter 23 Male Reproductive System **477**

Chapter 24 Female Reproductive System **494**

SECTION V:
EXFOLIATIVE CYTOLOGY

List of Color Illustrations

(appears following Chapter 12)

SECTION I:

GENERAL PRINCIPLES OF HISTOLOGY

1: Insights into Histology

Introduction

As a new discipline is approached, it is often difficult to place the knowledge to be acquired into the proper perspective. Questions concerning the nature, scope, depth and relevance of such information often arise, and certainly, these questions are justifiable. The intent of the following short discourse is to answer a number of them.

The ultimate goal for the student of the biomedical sciences is an understanding of the organism in health and disease. The living organism is the sum of its constituent parts and so much more; thus, the study of constituent parts is essential to gain some insights about the whole organism. Histology is one of those relevant biomedical disciplines that affords insights through an in-depth approach to the structure and function of the constituent parts.

Classically, *anatomy* is that branch of biomedical science that deals with the external and internal structure of the organism. Although classically considered to be a descriptive science exclusively, the objectives of this discipline are multiple. Descriptions of basic architectural patterns are fundamental to the discipline, as is an understanding of functional relationships and mechanisms. It is customary and didactically expedient to subdivide the science of anatomy into subdisciplines based upon the nature of the component parts and the methods by which they are studied. Accordingly, *gross anatomy* includes all those structural features which are studied by direct visual inspection, palpation and/or dissection, while *histology* encompasses the study of structures that are not visible to the unaided eye.

If the student were to consult a medical dictionary, then he (she) would find that the terms *histology* and *microscopic anatomy* are synonyms. Unfortunately, the synonymous definition of these terms gives little insight into the evolution of this anatomic subdiscipline. Although it began as a simple descriptive science of subgross anatomic organization, histology has evolved into a hybridization of anatomy, physiology, chemistry and physics. Whereas the classic definition of histology implies a purely descriptive science, the modern histology, microscopic anatomy, is a sophisticated science concerned with tissue structure and function from a broad and multidisciplinary approach.

Organology is the study of the structure and function of the numerous and varied component organs of an animal. Although studies of these organs may be approached from different perspectives, organs are studied commonly with a microscope. Thus, this branch of science falls within the purview of histology. *Comparative organology* emphasizes the organizational and functional differences and/or similarities of organs between and among various groupings of animals. This approach is essential for the student of Veterinary Medicine.

The expansion of any discipline, histology notwithstanding, is linked inexorably with the technical achievements of many disciplines. Advances in physics and engineering led sequentially to the development of varied light optical microscopes, the transmission and scanning electron microscopes and other sophisticated optical instruments used in histology. The transmission and scanning electron microscopes are the tools of *ultrastructural cytology*, an area of study encompassed by histology. Similarly, insights from inorganic chemistry and biochemistry have been applied to cells and tissues. Histology, then, includes *histochemistry* and *cytochemistry*. Numerous other disciplines have contributed various approaches: autoradiography, fluorescence techniques, immunocytochemistry and culture techniques. These varied approaches require some type of microscope for observation. Importantly, these are some of the tools of modern histology.

Historical Perspective

The evolution of this science into modern histology is an exciting and complex story that encompasses many years of man's recorded history. It includes numerous and diverse applications of physical science, as well as the insights and impetus of many biologists. Although the following is not intended to be a complete historical sketch, hopefully, it will put the science of histology into proper historical perspective and demonstrate the interdependency of many disciplines.

As early as 2000 BC, the Egyptians recognized the magnifying properties of curved surfaces and were able to refine and polish stones into magnifying lenses. This information spread along the Mediterranean Sea to the Greeks and Romans. Alhazan, an Arabian physicist (1000 AD) demonstrated a basic understanding of the principles of optics and described how portions of curved surfaces functioned as simple magnifiers.

Before the Renaissance and the revival of scientific and intellectual inquiry in Europe, a noteworthy but unheralded contribution was made by Roger Bacon (1276). He conducted numerous experiments with lenses and referred to the use of convergent lenses as a simple microscope. This discovery occurred approximately 300 years before the historical recognition of the development of the first compound microscope. The development of the compound microscope was linked intimately with varied experiments and was credited to the Dutch Janssen brothers (1590). Their accomplishment was duplicated by Galileo (1610) and Robert Hooke (1665). By present day standards these instruments were quite primitive, but numerous and significant contributions were made notwithstanding their shortcomings. To list all the contributions and the contributors in chronologic order is beyond the scope of this presentation; however, the following is applicable directly to the development of histology.

Many contributors—most noteworthy were Grew, Malpighi, Hooke, Swammerdam and Leeuwenhoek—expanded our knowledge through numerous and varied observations of microscopic structure and microorganisms through the beginning of the 18th century. Although inquiry continued through the 18th century, the most notable contributions were by van Haller and Wolff. By the beginning of the 19th century the accumulation of knowledge from intensive observation had set the stage for the blossoming of the microscopic sciences.

Bichat's (1802) published observations of tissues and the introduction of the term histology by Mayer (1819) helped to establish this discipline as an important part of medical inquiry. The pronouncement of the *cell theory* by Schleiden (1838) and Schwann (1839) was additional impetus to expanding knowledge. Shortly thereafter, Henle (1841) wrote a comprehensive treatise on human histology. Subsequently, Virchow (1863) applied the cell theory to the human organism and described various categories of specialized cells. His statement that human disease resulted from fundamental changes in the constituent cells was a significant application of the cell theory. These insights form the foundation of modern medicine.

The progress in histology was neither uniform nor explosive. Although curious individuals supplied the impetus for inquiry, their advances were and still are dependent upon technological progress in other disciplines. An understanding of optical principles and the ability to transform these principles into precise optical instruments was central to the development of the discipline. Histology, therefore, was the primary beneficiary of significant theoretical and practical applications from physics. By the beginning of the 19th century the basic properties of light and lenses were understood sufficiently to improve and refine light optical systems. Amici's (1827) ability to grind lenses resulted in precision optical instruments, while Abbe's (1877) formulation of a theory of microscopic vision set forth a mathematical basis for improvements that were predicated upon a definition of resolution and the role of diffraction in image formation. The refinements that resulted in these instruments led to continual contributions to histology.

Despite these advances, one question needed further clarification. What, if any, are the similarities and/or differences between living cells and tissues and those "artifacts" seen with the bright-field microscope? This was, and still is, a reasonable question to ask. It demonstrated a significant insight about the response of cells and tissues to potentially harsh treatment—fixation, dehydration, embedding, sectioning, staining and mounting. This question could not be broached until 1932. In that year Zernicke introduced the phase-contrast microscope. His contribution permitted scientists to observe living cells and tissues. This most notable of contributions, probably one of the most significant contributions to biology, permitted the demonstration of remarkable similarity between "living entities" and the "constant artifacts" which resulted from the harsh preparatory techniques of conventional histology.

The 1930's were good years for histologists. Despite the significance of the previous contributions, other branches of physics finally intersected the developing course of histology and opened phenomenal vistas. In the 19th century numerous physicists were gaining insights into magnetism, electricity, Gaussian dioptrics, atomic structure and quantum mechanics. Their understanding of the properties and behavior of electrons in magnetic fields set the stage for the development of the electron microscope. Knoll and Ruska (1931), interested in observing cathodic emitters, built a dual lens electron microscope and showed the instrument at a German science fair. Five days before the showing, Rudenberg applied for a German patent for an electron microscope. Similar instruments were constructed in other parts of the world shortly after the initial unveiling by Knoll and Ruska. In 1934, the first electron micrographs of a biologic specimen were taken by Marton of the Free University of Brussels. By 1941, the electron microscope was being applied to various structural studies in biology. The continuing techno-logic advances of the 1940's and 1950's converted these primitive microscopes into sophisticated instruments in the 1960's. During this decade, too, the scanning electron microscope became available commercially. In just 30 short years the scope of histology was expanded by technology which had increased greatly the resolving power (TEM) and depth of field (SEM) of optical instruments applicable to histologic studies.

Today, the technology still advances and histologists are still the beneficiaries. X-ray spectroscopy, long the exclusive purview of the physical sciences, is available to the biologist. Both wave dispersive (electron probe) and energy dispersive x-ray analytic electron microscopes are being applied to quantitative and qualitative elemental analyses of biologic specimens. Modern histology will continue to grow and flourish as man's technologic insights are expanded and applied to this discipline.

Tissues—The Elements Of Organization

The term histology was derived from the Greek terms, *histos* (web) and *logos* (study), and means the study of tissues. The etymologic derivation of the English word *tissue* is from the French *tissu*, which means *texture* or *weave*. This word was introduced into the medical sciences by the French gross anatomist and physician, Marie F. X. Bichat, in the late 18th century. As a result of his detailed gross dissections, he became fascinated by the various textures and weaves of those structures he had dissected. His observations resulted in the publication of a book in which he described more than 20 different tissues. It is interesting to note that this brilliant anatomist, considered by most as the Father of Histology, did not use a microscope to found this discipline. Shortly after his death at the turn of the 19th century, the term histology was coined.

The original concept of 20 tissues comprising the body was useful in establishing the discipline. Today, most histologists recognize four basic tissue types with each type consisting of a number of subtypes. Some histologists, believing that the uniqueness of adipose tissue warrants a separate classification as a tissue, support the concept of five basic tissues. All of the diverse organs of the body result from the unique aggregation, association and interdependence of these basic types. The tissues, then, are the building blocks upon which the organs are constructed in a logical, orderly and consistent manner. A thorough understanding of the tissues, their morphology and function, is essential for a comprehensive grasp of organ structure and function. Just as the organism is the sum of its organ components, so are the organs the sum of their tissue components. Similarly and logically, the tissues of the body are the endproduct of their cellular and extracellular compo-nents. This logic can be extended to a more basic level, because the cells and extracellular products are the result of their biochemical components.

A logical approach to histology is one that progresses from the biochemistry to the cells and tissues and ends with a study of the organs. Most students will have been exposed to biochemistry and cytology by this stage of their scientific growth and development. It is essential, therefore, to discuss the next order of organization—the tissues.

A tissue is defined as *a group of more or less similar cells and their extracellular products that perform a specific function or a spectrum of related functions.* This is a workable definition, but it does present some problems. In some tissues the cells may be identical. In others, they may be quite dissimilar. In either case, however, it is their functional relationship which unifies. Some tissues are characterized by scant amounts of extracellular materials, while others have tremendous amounts of these materials. Again, their functional relationships satisfy the definition. Extremes in structural and functional characteristics still satisfy the basic definition. Any artificial scheme of grouping biologic entities is prone to interpretive problems, because *man classifies, nature doesn't.*

The *basic* or *simple tissues* of the body are: epithelia, connective tissues, muscular tissues, nervous tissues and perhaps adipose tissue. These are the components of all the organs of the body. Although the basic tissues will be covered in detail in Section 3, it is appropriate to put them in perspective now.

The first of these basic tissues is the *epithelium* (*epi*—upon, *thele*—nipple). Epithelia cover all of the external body surfaces and all of the internal tubes of the body and form glands. Most of the epithelial tissues are derived from the *ectoderm* (the external covering) and the *endoderm* (the internal covering); however, some epithelia are derived from the *mesoderm* of the embryo.

Characteristically, epithelial tissues have a high cellular density. The cells, usually quite similar and sometimes identical, are the predominant feature. Little extracellular material is associated with these cells.

Protection is one of the prime functions of these tissues, but it is just one of a multiplicity of vital functions performed. There are numerous morphologic modifications to epithelia that permit this functional diversity. The nature of the epidermis of the skin affords protection from mechanical, bacterial and dessicative damage, whereas the selective absorptive properties of the intestines afford protection against the absorption of microorganisms, toxins and other potentially toxic materials. Similarly, various materials (microorganisms, particulate matter, debris) are transported along epithelial surfaces by the action of cilia. Such modifications of the epithelia of the respiratory system also afford protection to the organism.

Secretory activity is a major function of epithelia. Special glandular modifications of epithelia comprise vital functional adaptations. Sebaceous glands of the skin elaborate an oily material which softens the hairshafts and keeps the skin pliable and impermeable to the movement of various materials in either direction. Mucous glands of various types secrete a viscous material which serves to moisten and lubricate many of the internal tubes of the body. Other glands elaborate materials such as saliva and digestive juices.

Many types of epithelial cells perform essential absorptive functions. Examples would include the cells of the respiratory, gastrointestinal and urinary systems. Essential digested materials are absorbed by the gastrointestinal epithelium. Oxygen passes through the lining epithelium of the lung, whereas essential metabolites are absorbed by the tubular lining cells of the kidney.

Because the epithelial tissues are in contact with the animal's external environment (even the contents of internal tubes are external to the organism), much information concerning this environment can be sensed by these cells. Therefore, sensory functions are important homeostatic adaptations. These include cellular sensory modifications of the skin, gustatory organs, olfactory epithelium and others.

Lastly, the gonads are composed of epithelial cells whose function is the perpetuation of the species.

The foregoing discussion establishes that epithelial cells perform a diversity of functions. It will become apparent in Section 3 that there are corresponding morphologic adaptations that permit this functional diversity.

The *connective tissues*, derivatives of the mesoderm, comprise one of the most diverse groups of the basic tissues. Although they are well-named on the basis of their connective and binding properties, they subserve a variety of other functions. A partial list of these varied functions includes support, protection, mobility, insulation, thermoregulation, energy storage, repair and nutrition.

Characteristically, connective tissues consist of groups of cells, in some cases quite dissimilar, that are separated by large quantities of extracellular material, most of which is secreted by the constituent cells. These extracellular materials (*intercellular substance*) consist of various fibers and other biochemical compounds that impart specific structural and functional characteristics to these tissues. This intercellular material is suited ideally to the binding and connecting properties of some of these tissues. Similarly, the dense intercellular materials of cartilage and bone suit them ideally for their primary functions of support and mobility. Adipose tissue is a unique tissue which subserves protective, insulative, thermoregulatory and metabolic functions. Blood, with its varied formed elements and plasma, is a unique connective tissue which affects, directly or indirectly, every cell of the body. The nutritive and defensive functions of this tissue are of vital importance to the organism.

The *muscular tissues* are derived from the mesoderm also. The cells of these tissues are modified uniquely for contraction. The movement of materials through the internal tubes of the body is accomplished primarily by smooth muscle. This movement includes the expression and transport of glandular secretions, the peristaltic movement of food through the digestive tract and the movement of blood through the vascular system. The movement or translocation of the organism within its environment is a function of the skeletal muscle of the body. The continuous movement of blood within the vascular system is the function of the cardiac muscle mass. The continuous demands made upon this organ are phenomenal. That it responds successfully for so long is even more remarkable. Throughout the course of the 70-year human life span the heart will have beaten approximately 2.58×10^9 times and will have pumped about 1.84×10^8 liters of blood.

Nervous tissue is derived from ectoderm and includes components of the brain, spinal cord and peripheral nerves. This tissue is organized uniquely to receive, transmit, integrate and associate various stimuli from the animal's external and internal environment. The essence of these combined activities is the initiation of a response that maintains the well-being of the organism.

The basic tissues, then, are the building blocks of a more complex organizational heirarchy—the organs. A comprehensive understanding of these tissue components is not only essential but simplifies the study of comparative organology.

2: Methods of Histology

Introduction

The technologic progress in various areas of science affords the histologist a multiplicity of approaches for the study of cells and tissues. The type of information desired usually dictates the suitability of one approach over another or a combination of approaches. The maximal information that is attainable with any particular technical approach requires a complete familiarity with the technique, an understanding of the nature and limitations of the informational output and a comprehensive appreciation of its advantages and disadvantages. The following is an attempt to acquaint the student with the diversity of techniques that are available to examine living cells, dead cells and components of cells. Any combination of these methods may be components of a comprehensive approach to histologic problem solving.

The direct observation of living cells and tissues may be achieved in a variety of ways. *Cell culture* is one of the most widely used of these techniques. The discovery of antibiotics has made this approach almost a matter of simple routine. Culturing techniques permit the continual observation, manipulation and testing of explanted cells without any jeopardy to the donor (Figs. 2.1, 2.2). This approach has afforded valuable information about cellular differentiation, cellular transformation, cytogenetics, cellular metabolism, cell-to-cell interactions, host/parasite relationships and numerous other fascinating biologic processes. Of special interest to medicine is the indispensible function of cell culture in diagnostic virology (Figs. 2.3, 2.4), vaccine development and vaccine production.

An adjunct to direct observation is the implantation of *transparent viewing chambers* and the *exteriorization and transillumination* of organs and tissues. Although the exteriorization technique imposes a limited time frame for observation, valuable insights concerning microcirculation and the response of various tissues and organs to chemotherapeutic agents has been obtained. The implantation of transparent viewing chambers permits an extended period of observation. By implanting various cells into animals in this manner significant insights have been gained concerning neovascularization, cellular differentiation and movement, and other vital processes. The anterior chamber of the eye, by virtue of the transparent cornea, is a naturally-occurring viewing chamber that is utilized in this approach to biologic inquiry.

The selective uptake of *vital* and *supravital stains* has added appreciably to our understanding of the function of some cells, cellular organelles and inclusions, and extracellular matrix materials. These stains have such low toxicity that they may be injected into a living organism (vital) or applied to living cells extirpated from the organism (supravital).

Oxytetracycline, a broad spectrum antibiotic, may be used as a vital stain also. At therapeutic dosages it is selectively deposited at all surfaces upon which bone and similar tissues are being formed (Figs. 2.5, 2.6). Through carefully timed serial administration of the drug, valuable insights concerning rates of bone formation have been obtained.

Lithium carmine and trypan blue are vital dyes that have been utilized to study the phenomenon of phagocytosis. These dyes are selectively phagocytized by certain protective cells of the body.

Janus green B and neutral red are supravital stains that are used to study mitochondria and lysosomes.

The separation and purification of subcellular fractions through *differential centrifugation* and *density gradient centrifugation* have proved to be invaluable aids for the study of biochemical and metabolic phenomena.

The simplest method for the direct observation of living cells is to remove them from the organism, place them on a slide and examine them with a *phase-contrast microscope* (Fig. 3.4) or *dark-field* microscope.

Living cells and tissues are difficult to examine microscopically because they are relatively transparent and thick. The indices of refraction of cellular constituents are sufficiently similar to preclude easy identification and differentiation of them. Therefore, superimposition artifacts and excessive absorption of light limits the amount of useful and reliable information that can be obtained from them. These problems are reduced when thin sections of tissues are obtained, stained and examined. Such an ap-

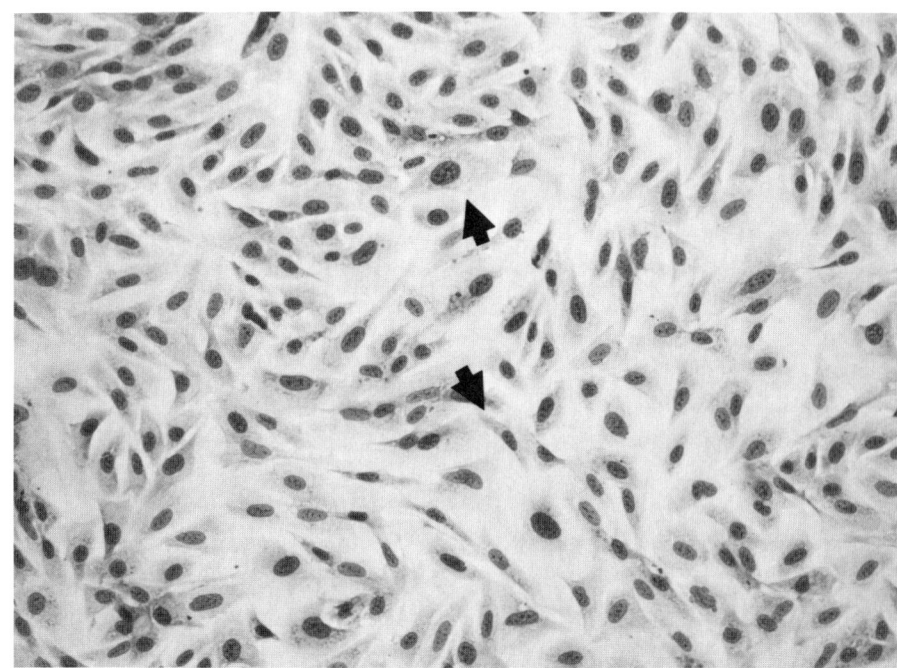

Fig. 2.1 A low power micrograph of a monolayer of normal bovine fetal spleen cells. Contact inhibition results in the formation of a monolayer of stellate- and spindle-shaped cells (*arrows*). ×40 (Giemsa stain). (Courtesy of H. Storz). All light micrographs are labeled as the magnification with the microscope before photographic enlarging. All electron micrographs are labeled as total magnification, including photographic enlarging.

proach requires excessive handling and processing of tissues. However, it is the standard approach to histologic examination.

Tissues and cells for microscopic examination are usually killed by careful fixation to minimize alterations of in vivo morphology. Subsequent processing ends with the tissues being embedded in a material that facilitates thin sectioning. Although a variety of techniques is used, the most commonly utilized procedure is the paraffin technique.

The Paraffin Technique

This technical approach to the preparation of samples for histologic examination is a simple and reliable procedure. Although modification of cells and tissues does occur as a result of the treatments encompassed by this technique, the end results are reliable and permit inferences to the in vivo situation. Unquestionably, it is the most common technique used for the preparation of specimens for histology courses, diagnostic histopathology and morphologic research at the light microscopic level.

The discussion is not intended to give the student expertise in this subject; specialized textbooks and courses are available which afford an in-depth approach to the subject. The student should understand the technique, the rationale for each of the steps, the limitations and advantages of this approach, and its usefulness in academic and diagnostic endeavors.

Acquisition. The acquisition of the sample is probably the most critical step in the process. It requires that the histologist knows gross anatomy; a sample of the mandibular salivary gland is of little value if the sample desired was the mandibular lymph

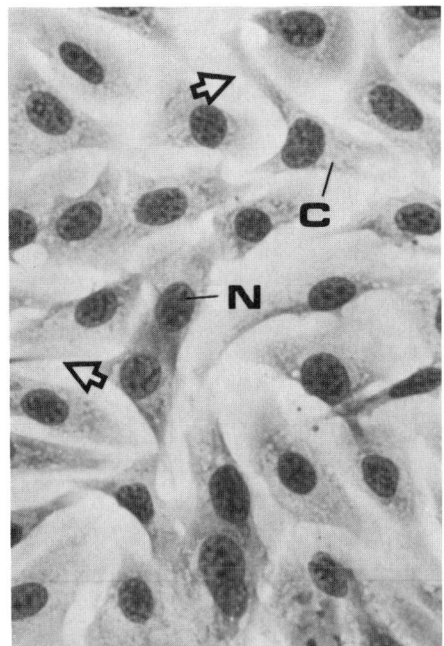

Fig. 2.2 A medium power micrograph of a monolayer of normal bovine fetal spleen cells. The nuclei (N) are vesicular and the foamy and granular cytoplasm (C) has processes (*open arrows*) that impart a stellate or spindle appearance. ×100. (Giemsa stain). (Courtesy of H. Storz).

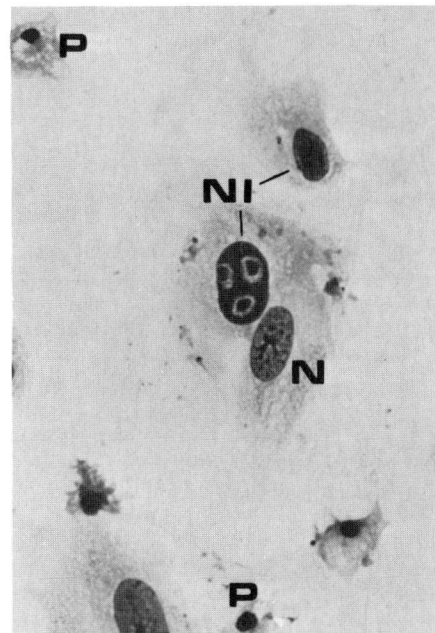

Fig. 2.4 A medium power micrograph of a monolayer of bovine fetal spleen cells 48 hours postinfection with a parvovirus. Pyknotic nuclei (P), normal nuclei (N) and nuclei with inclusion bodies (NI) are apparent. Note the altered cell shapes. Compare with Figure 2.2. ×100 (Giemsa stain). (Courtesy of H. Storz).

node. Once the desired sample is identified, it must be obtained with as little trauma as possible. Living tissues are fragile entities the morphology of which changes with excessive handling and poor extirpation techniques. A "tissue conscience" is as important to the histologist as it is to the surgeon. The use of dull and dirty scalpels or scissors and excessive pressure or traction applied with thumb forceps during sampling can induce drastic alterations to the components.

Most cells and tissues begin to undergo degenerative changes as soon as they are separated from their ideal microenvironment. This process of autolytic change can be minimized by reducing the amount of time that tissues are out of their normal environment. Tissues must be removed rapidly and deftly; they should reach the fixative in the shortest time possible.

Fixation. Chemical fixation is a process in which various chemical agents are applied to histologic specimens for the primary purpose of stopping *postmortem autolysis*. These agents denature protein and inactivate the enzymes through which autolytic changes are mediated. Generally, the action of fixatives is sufficiently broad to react with most of the biochemical components of the cells. The frequently used chemical fixatives are formaldehyde, glutaraldehyde, paraformaldehyde, ethyl alcohol, acetic acid, picric acid, potassium dichromate, mercuric chloride, chromic acid and osmic acid. Each has specific properties that result in various advantages and disadvantages of use.

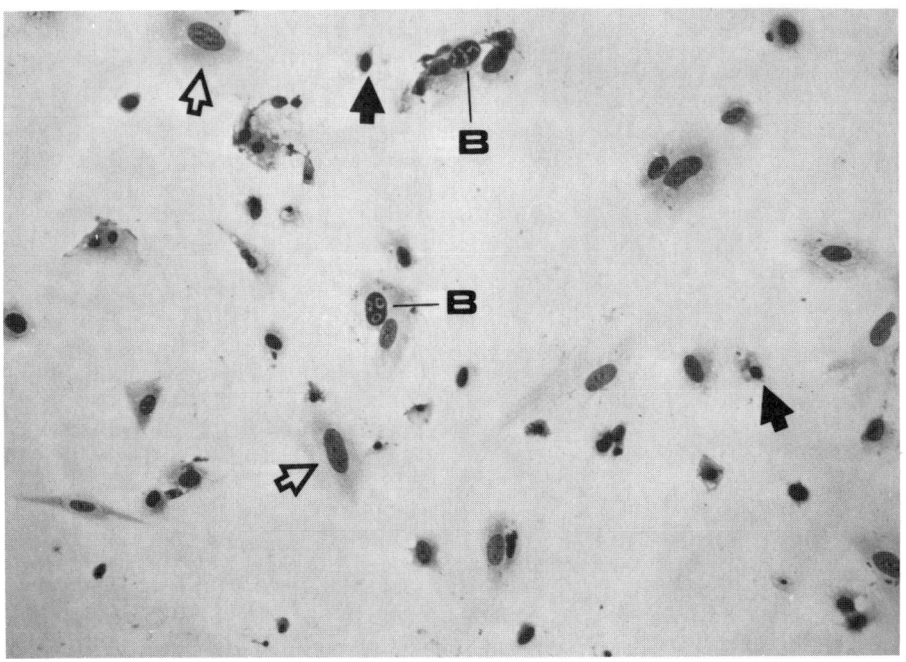

Fig. 2.3 A low power micrograph of a monolayer of bovine fetal spleen cells 48 hours postinfection with a parvovirus. The cells have been altered from the infection. The even distribution of cells as a monolayer is not apparent. Most of the cells are round and have withdrawn their cytoplasmic processes. Some nuclei are normal (*open arrows*), whereas others are pyknotic (*solid arrows*). Some cells contain nuclear inclusion bodies (B). ×40 (Giemsa stain). (Courtesy of H. Storz).

Chemical fixatives have various properties that must be considered in relation to the purpose for which the sample is obtained. Some chemical agents are *coagula-tive fixatives*. They induce changes in cells similar to those that occur when heat is applied to an egg. The conformation of macromolecules is altered markedly by such coagulative fixatives as ethanol and methanol. Others are described as *additive fixatives*. These types of fixatives achieve fixation by chemically reacting with the biochemical components of the cell. They do not induce the marked morphologic changes characteristic of the other broad category of fixatives. The aldehydes (formaldehyde, paraformaldehyde and glutaraldehyde) are additive fixatives that can be used in histologic studies. *A 10% solution of neutral-buffered formalin is one of the most commonly employed fixatives.* It consists of 10 volumes of commercial formalin (40% formaldehyde in water) and 90 volumes of phosphate-buffered water.

The action of most fixatives is multiple: 1) prevent postmortem autolysis, 2) facilitate sectioning of the tissues by hardening them, 3) enhance staining by acting as a mordant, 4) minimize the leaching of many constituents that results from subsequent processing, 5) stabilize structural components in near in vivo conditions, and 6) protect the histologist through their antiseptic properties.

Once the sample of tissue has been removed, it should be immersed in fixative immediately. Trimming of the block of tissue in fixative should result in a sample that is only a few millimeters thick. This permits thorough penetration (and fixation) of the entire sample. The most ideal ratio of fixative volume to tissue volume is about 30:1.

The actual time required for complete fixation to occur varies with the diffusion properties of the fixative, the concentration of the fixative and the density of the tissue. Most formaldehyde fixation is achieved within a 24-hour period.

Dehydration and Clearing. A variety of substances are used for this portion of the procedure. If paraffin or a similar substance is to be infiltrated into a sample to permit sectioning, then "something" must first be removed. That "something" is the 75% water that occurs in most tissues. After the extensive washing in water that functions to remove excess fixative, the sample is dehydrated as a preparatory stage to embedding.

Many *dehydrating agents* are used (ethanol, butanol, dioxane, isopropanol), but the most commonly used agent is ethanol. Tissue samples are subjected to increasing concentrations of alcohol until total dehydration is achieved with absolute ethanol. The use of this substance requires that the samples be processed through a clearing substance. Commonly employed *clearing agents* are xylene, toluene and benzene. Although clearing agents clear opacities from dehydrated tissues and make them transparent, this result is incidental to the function of these agents. Generally, dehydrating and embedding agents are not miscible in each other. Clearing agents are substances that are miscible in dehydrating and embedding agents; thus, the clearing agent replaces the dehydrating fluid and the

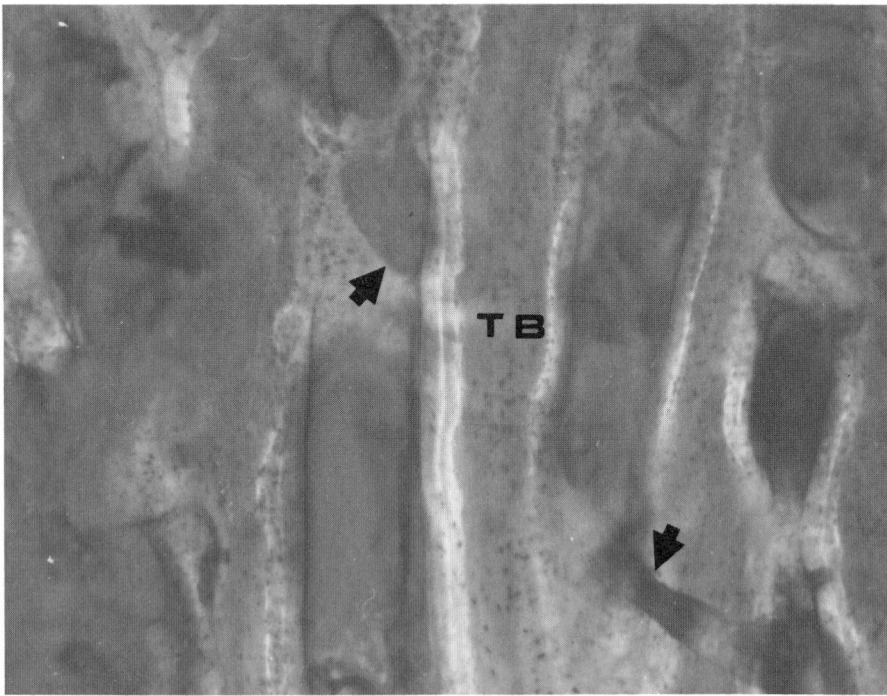

Fig. 2.5   A 50 μm section of trabecular bone from an equine third carpal bone undergoing fracture repair. Tetracycline at therapeutic levels (5 mg/#) was administered at 10-day intervals and the sample was obtained 20 days after the initial injection. Two bright bands of fluorescence within the trabecular bone (TB) indicate the amount of bone formed during the 10-day interim. *Solid arrows* are for orientation and comparison with Figure 2.6. ×40 (oxytetracycline labeled, fluorescence microscopy).

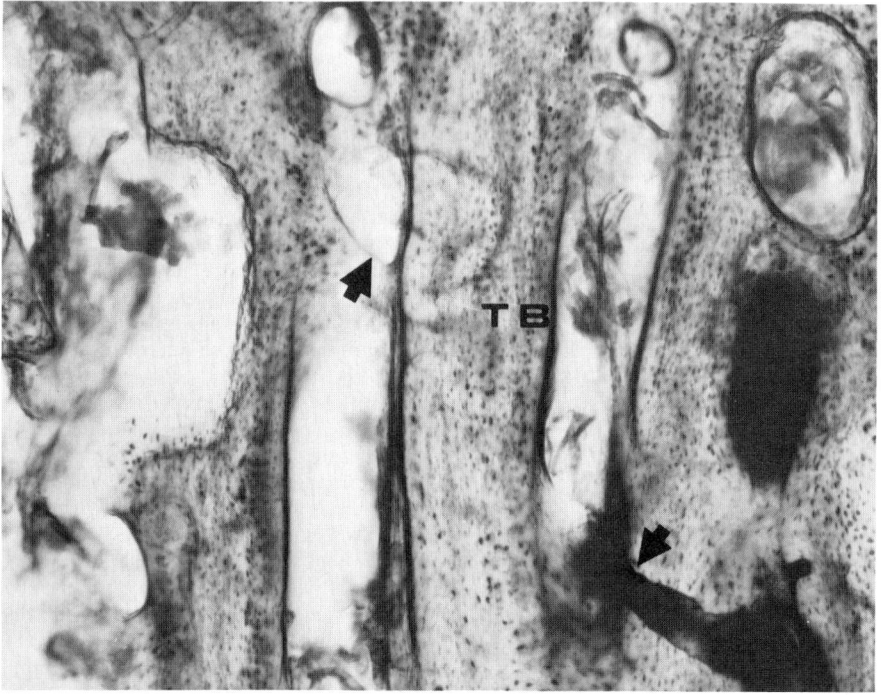

Fig. 2.6   A bright-field micrograph of the same tissue field in Fig. 2.5. The coupling of fluorescence and bright-field microscopy affords valuable insights about the morphologic and dynamic changes that accompany fracture repair. ×40.

embedding agent replaces the clearing substance.

Coincidentally, when calcified tissues are processed by this technique the decalcification of the tissues occurs immediately after fixation but before dehydration.

Embedding. This step is the one that ultimately permits the specimen to be sectioned sufficiently thin to allow microscopic examination. The cleared specimens are processed through solutions containing increasing concentrations of paraffin. Infiltration may be enhanced through the use of vacuum. The pure embedding reagents must be kept at their melting points (50–68°C) throughout the infiltration process, but the heat required to maintain the melted paraffin may induce some morphologic changes. These can be minimized by using soft paraffin (50–52°C), but thin sections are hard to achieve. The hard paraffin (60–68°C) causes more heat damage but facilitates thin sectioning. Generally, the most important consideration is the use of soft paraffin for soft tissues and hard paraffin for hard tissues.

The infiltrated samples are placed into molds, surrounded with paraffin and cooled. These blocks are then ready for sectioning.

Sectioning. After the paraffin has hardened, the molds are removed and the blocks are trimmed to expose the embedded tissue. They are then mounted on a *microtome* and thin shavings (*sections*) are removed from the cutting surface. The tendency of these sections to form a ribbon, the trailing edge of one section adhering to the leading edge of the subsequent section, facilitates the collection of the samples. Because some compression is associated with the sectioning process, ribbons may be floated on a warm water bath, stretched and picked up on slides. Alternatively, portions of the ribbons may be put on slides and the slides are then placed on a warming table.

The development of precision cutting instruments, microtomes, was a significant step in technologic advances affecting histology. The *rotary microtome* permits the precision cutting of thin sections in 1 micrometer (micron) increments. Most sections for routine histologic examination are cut between 5–7 micrometers.

Staining and Mounting. The section and/or sections of paraffin-embedded materials affixed to glass slides simplify the remaining steps of staining and mounting. Most stains that are used for histology are soluble in water or alcohol; therefore, the paraffin must be removed before staining. The reverse order of the previous procedures is used. The sections are cleared to remove the embedding medium and carried through decreasing concentrations of alcohol to allow rehydration, if necessary. Then the slides with their adherent sections are stained. Once again they are dehydrated, cleared and subsequently covered with a mounting

medium that is miscible with the clearing agent. A coverslip is applied to produce a permanent preparation.

Principles of Staining

Most observations of histologic sections are achieved with a bright field microscope. As mentioned previously, the optical densities of cellular and tissue components are sufficiently similar that detailed study is impossible without some sort of optical enhancement. Stains are one way to accomplish this enhancement. Myriads of stains and stain combinations are available and are used in the histology laboratory (Plate I). Their reactivity with cells and tissues is variable. Some stains are very selective, having a high specificity for certain cellular and/or tissue components. Alizarin red S and oxytetracycline are examples of stains that have a specificity for sites at which bone matrix is being formed. Other stains are available for the selective staining of cellular components (mitochondria, Golgi apparatus) and extracellular materials (reticular fibers, elastic fibers, collagenous fibers). Some stains are not selective and generally stain cellular and extracellular tissue components. Hematoxylin (H) and eosin (E) are examples of general stains that are used frequently in histology. Various stains of selected organs and tissues are included in Plate I.

Stains are especially useful, and the information obtained is maximized when the mechanism which governs their staining properties is understood. Unfortunately, the detailed chemical reactions for all stains is not understood. Numerous diversified stains exist for which the staining mechanisms are known. These afford the histologist the additional advantage of chemical insights to cells and tissues.

Most of the stains used in histology are salts which dissociate in water. They are described as *acid stains* or *basic stains*. If the coloring component is in the acidic radical, then the stain is designated an acid stain. If the coloring component is in the basic radical, then the stain is designated a basic stain.

The efficacy of acidic and basic stains is predicated upon the distribution of anionic and cationic charges that are generally associated with proteins and complex proteins (lipoproteins, glycoproteins) in cells and tissues. The net charge on these substances is a function of the total number and nature of their ionizable radicals and the pH of their environment. Proteins are true *ampholytes*, substances which are capable of acting like acids and bases depending upon the pH of the microenvironment.

Within cells and tissues these differentially charged molecules express different affinities for the charged groups of the dyes. Basic cellular components react with acid

stains (*neutralization*). The basic components of the cells and tissues are *acidophilic*; they have an affinity for the acid dyes. Acidic components of these entities react with basic stains. These components are *basophilic*; they have an affinity for the basic dyes.

This is the mechanism characteristic of the commonly used H and E staining combination. The basic dye, hematoxylin, is applied first and is followed by the acidic dye, eosin. Hematoxylin imparts a bluish purple color to acidic components such as chromatin, ergastoplasm and some cellular secretions. Eosin imparts a pink to red color to basic components such as cytoplasm, and numerous extracellular products.

The *modified Romanowsky stains* are useful dye combinations that contain methylene blue and eosin. Methylene blue is readily oxidized to form azure dyes. Combinations of methylene blue and the azure dyes (azure A, azure B, azure C) are referred to as *polychromed methylene blue*. This combination of basic dyes is characterized by a broad staining range of acidic components. Eosin is the acidic counterstain. This combination of stains is used commonly to study peripheral blood smears and bone marrow samples (Plate VI).

The *periodic acid-Schiff* (PAS) reaction is a commonly employed and useful tool for histologic studies. The procedure involves two steps to achieve the characteristic reactivity. The first reaction involves the oxidation of α-amino alcohols and/or 1,2 glycol groups to aldehydes by periodic acid. These aldehydes are then subjected to the Schiff reagent. The Schiff reagent consists of basic fuchsin which has been decolorized from its original red-violet color by the addition of sulfurous acid. The subsequent reaction of the aldehydes with the reagent forms a complex which restores the magenta color. Hematoxylin is the usual counterstain. Many carbohydrates and carbohydrate-protein complexes give a positive reaction with PAS. Among those substances that are reactive are glycosaminoglycans, mucoproteins, glycoproteins, glycogen, secretory products of many cells, cartilage matrix and many others (Plate I.12).

The selective use of stains is an important aspect of histologic inquiry. The differential staining properties of many cellular and tissue components permit easy identification as well as affording the opportunity to gain insights about their biochemical properties.

Selected Preparation Techniques

The amount and kind of information that can be obtained in histologic studies is limited only by the number of approaches that can be utilized. If structural relationships are the only concern, then the paraffin technique is a useful method. However, it has numerous shortcomings related to the fixation employed, subsequent processing, and the time required to complete the procedure. Numerous technical approaches are available which, when employed, provide a variety of different information. Some tissues and some endeavors lend themselves to these various approaches, while the type of information desired may dictate a specific technical approach.

Cytologic Studies. This approach to histology is useful when tissue architecture is a minimal concern. It simply involves obtaining some cells, smearing them on a slide, fixing them, staining them and conducting the examination (Plates VII, VIII). The peripheral blood is commonly examined in this manner (Plates VI, VII). The technique, however, is adaptable to any body orifice from which cells are shed routinely. Vaginal and/or cervical smears, conjunctival scrapings, tracheal washes and analyses of urinary sediment are useful techniques that offer insights about the organs from which the samples were obtained. Cerebrospinal fluid taps, impression smears and needle biopsies of organs are useful methods. Similarly, aspirates of the contents of coelomic spaces, organs and swellings of the body are invaluable aids in morphologic and diagnostic endeavors. Clinical cytology is covered in-depth in Chapter 26.

Freezing Techniques. A concern for the alteration of morphology and function that may result from fixation and subsequent processing has been a strong impetus for the use of freezing techniques. Also, frozen sections may be processed very rapidly for examination. Biopsy samples obtained during surgery are usually prepared by this technique.

The *freeze drying technique* is one in which freshly extirpated samples are frozen to liquid nitrogen temperatures ($-170°C$) while under vacuum. The sublimation of water that results negates the necessity of fixation, dehydration and clearing. Samples are embedded, sectioned and stained. Of special interest is the ability to conduct chemical studies on such tissues. Valuable insights concerning the localization and activity of many enzymes have been obtained. Importantly, tissues prepared by this technique have fewer artifacts than those prepared by conventional chemical fixation.

Samples prepared by the *frozen section technique* afford advantages similar to the previously described technique; however, some damage occurs in the sample due to ice crystal formation and section thinness is limited. Tissue samples are frozen rapidly to $-40°C$ and are cut with an apparatus that maintains this temperature. This device, a *cryotome*, is a rotary microtome contained within a closed environment.

Histochemistry and Cytochemistry. These techniques are attempts by histologists to localize and characterize biochemical compounds within intact cells and tissues that biochemists readily characterize in test tubes. The procedures range from simple to complex, but the principle which governs this technology is simple. If a biochemical constituent can be complexed with a stain to enhance its visualization, then it lends itself to study. Naturally, the precision of the visualization and interpretation is a function of the specificity of the staining reaction, the localization and stability of the component being studied, and the degree to which the substance being examined is altered by processing techniques.

The chemical constituents of cells and tissues can be examined by histochemical and cytochemical methodologies: carbohydrates, fats, proteins, enzymes, minerals. The following examples demonstrate the scope of such studies.

The PAS technique is a simple histochemical procedure. Unfortunately, PAS reacts with many sugar-containing compounds. However, if glycogen were of interest, then PAS could be useful if coupled with a procedure to remove glycogen. Glycogen stains magenta with the PAS reagent. Confirmation of the presence of this substance can be obtained by first subjecting sections to α-amylase and then using PAS. A simple comparison between amylase-digested samples and those samples stained only with PAS permits reasonable inferences about the presence and/or absence of this substance in cells.

Alcian blue (Plate I.8), toluidine blue and aldehyde fuchsin are useful stains for the demonstration of different types of *mucosubstances* (sugar-containing substances).

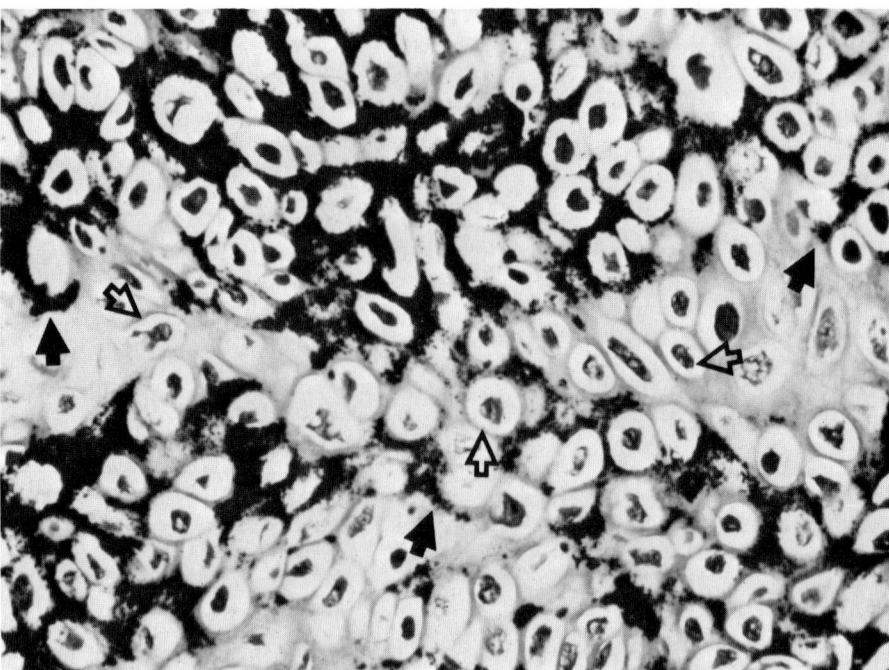

Fig. 2.7 A section of developing cervine antler. The antler contains cartilage with chondrocytes (*open arrows*) surrounded by the matrix which they secrete. Mineralization of the cartilage (*solid arrows*) occurs before bone formation. The individual foci of mineralization (*solid arrows*) coalesce (*dark-staining areas*). ×80 (von Kossa stain).

Many substances secreted by cells contain these materials (some hormones, cartilage matrix, connective tissue and bone matrix, mucin). Identification of these materials in sections offers valuable insights about the composition and distribution of these entities.

The ability to stain bone mineral was mentioned previously. Oxytetracycline, alizarin red-S and the von Kossa stain are useful stains for the demonstration of this material (Fig. 2.7) (Plate I.10).

Valuable insights concerning the distribution, localization and activity of enzymes within cells have resulted from the ability to capture, stabilize and subsequently stain the reaction products of many enzymatic reactions. The techniques utilized for these studies are diversified, but some are predicated upon the following principle:

$$AB \xrightarrow{E} A + B \xrightarrow{C} BC\downarrow$$

Substrate AB is acted upon by enzyme E to yield products A and B. Product B is complexed with agent C to produce an insoluble and colored precipitate. One of the first histochemical studies was that conducted on alkaline phosphatase by Gomori and Takamatsu independently. It is classic and demonstrates the generalized principle. Thin sections of tissue were incubated with a phosphorylated compound (glycerophosphate) and calcium. The enzyme (phosphatase) cleaved the phosphate that was captured by the calcium as a clear precipitate. The insoluble calcium phosphate was converted to a colored precipitate (cobalt sulphide) by reacting the sections with cobalt nitrate and ammonium sulfide sequentially. Modern technology has resulted in numerous refinements to the technique that have increased specificity and improved localization.

Variations of this approach are applicable to other enzyme systems such as: hydrolases, oxidoreductases, esterases, peptidases and others. Such approaches have added appreciably to the general understanding of cellular biochemistry and its relationship to morphology.

The term *histochemistry* is confined generally to studies conducted at the light microscopic level of investigation, whereas *cytochemistry* is applicable to electron microscopic endeavors; however, the terms may be used synonymously. In enzyme studies, the effects of chemical fixation and the denaturation of enzymes is an important consideration. Freezing techniques and/or moderate chemical fixation are used. Electron microscopic studies of cytochemical phenomena require additionally that the trapped endproducts are electron dense in order for visualization and localization to occur (Fig. 2.8).

Autoradiography. This technique is useful for histologic studies of dynamic cellular processes. Sections of tissues are incubated with substances that have radioactive labels. Most generally these markers are soft β-emitters. The sections are then coated with a photographic emulsion which is exposed by the radiation. The latent image in the photographic emulsion is developed routinely. Staining of the sections allows the visualization of the silver grains superimposed upon the section (Fig. 2.9). Because the silver grains are black and electron dense, these specimens may be examined with light or electron microscopes. Insights concerning cellular synthesis, secretion and mitosis have resulted from this methodology.

Immunocytochemistry. This technique is useful at the light and electron microscopic levels of investigation for the identification and localization of potentially antigenic substances (proteins, polysaccharides). A purified extract of the desired substance is prepared and injected as an *antigen* (Ag) into another animal. The animal develops an immune response and *antibodies* (Ab) are produced. The antibodies are subsequently isolated and purified. The nature of

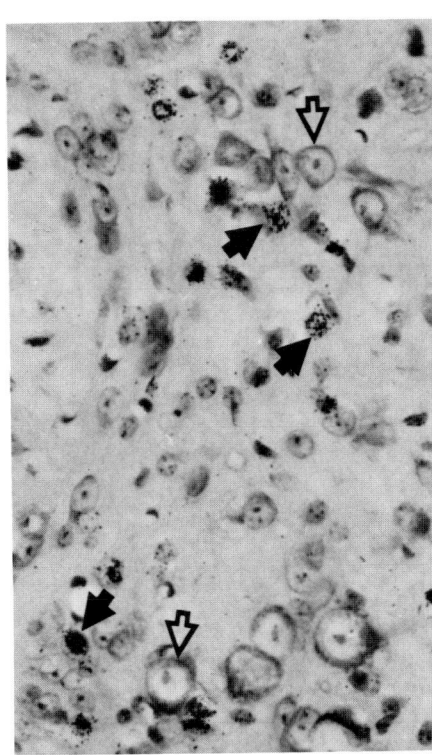

Fig. 2.9 An autoradiograph of the substantia gelatinosa of the developing spinal cord of a mouse. The nuclei of some neurons (*open arrows*) are unlabeled, whereas the nuclei of other neurons (*solid arrows*) are labeled with tritiated thymidine. The silver grains are positioned over the labeled nuclei. ×100. (Courtesy of M. Carry and H. O. Nornes).

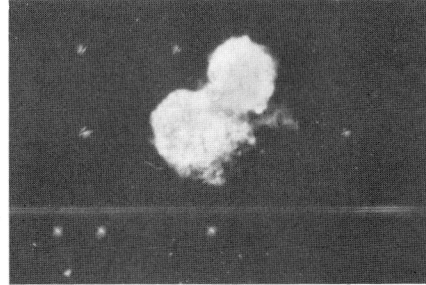

Fig. 2.10 Direct fluorescent antibody reaction of bovine lung cells for IBR virus. Both cells are positive for the virus as evidenced by the bright fluorescence associated with them. ×400. (Courtesy of J. J. England).

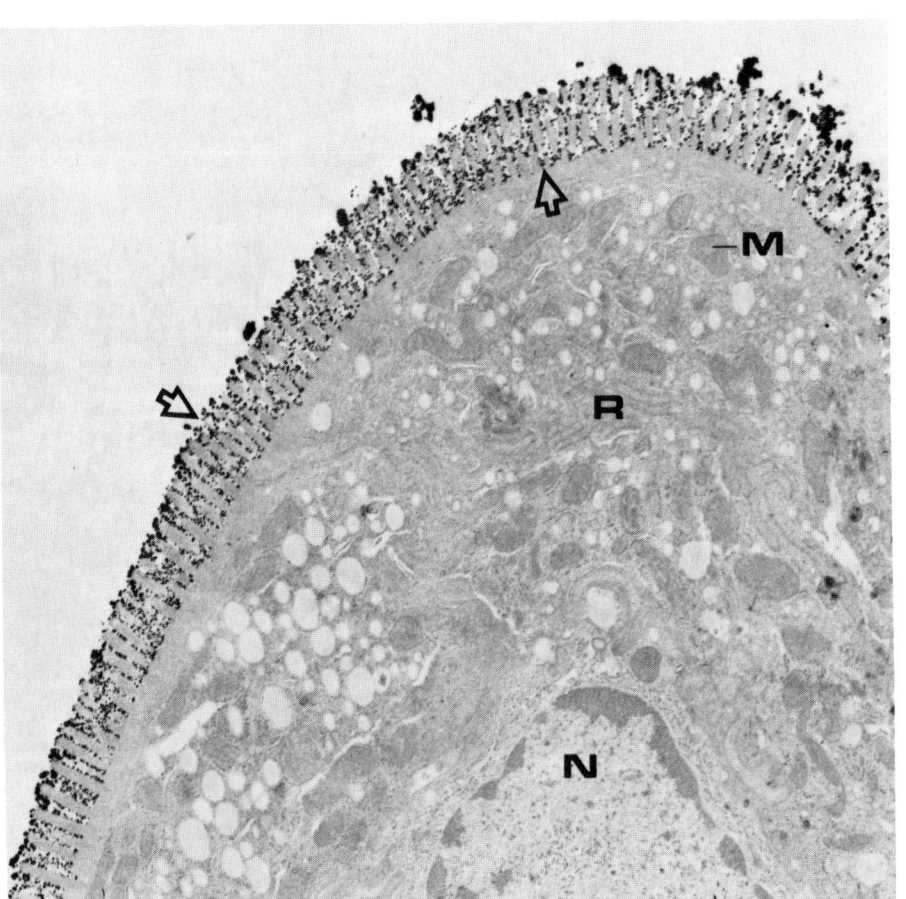

Fig. 2.8 An electron micrograph of a mouse intestinal lining cell. The dense granules (*open arrows*) associated with the microvilli represent reaction foci for the enzyme alkaline phosphatase. M, mitochondria; R, rough endoplasmic reticulum; N, nucleus. ×6,000 (modified Gomori technique).

subsequent treatment is determined by the nature of the specific immunochemical technique utilized. In the *direct fluorescent antibody technique* a fluorescent dye, usually fluorescein isothiocyanate (FITC), is complexed with the antibody. The Ab-FITC is allowed to interact with the specimen. Subsequent washing removes all of the reagent except that which has formed an Ag-Ab-FITC complex. Examination with an ultraviolet light source demonstrates fluorescence and localization of the antigen (Fig. 2.10). In the *indirect fluorescent antibody technique* an additional step is required to produce an *antiglobulin* (An) to the originally-produced antibody. The fluorescent tag is attached to the antiglobulin. The sample is incubated as described previously with a resultant Ag-Ab-An-FITC complex being formed. This technique has the advantage of increasing the intensity and sensitivity of the reaction by allowing more complexes to form.

The markers used in this technique are not confined to fluorescent dyes. The enzyme *peroxidase* may be conjugated to the antibody or to the antiglobulin. The visualization of the reactive complex is achieved by the histochemical demonstration of peroxidase activity. Similarly, *ferritin* may be complexed with the antibody or antiglobulin. Ferritin contains 23% iron, is electron dense and permits visualization of the reaction with the electron microscope.

Investigations employing these techniques are not confined to substances considered to be classic antigens. Although this approach is a useful diagnostic tool for microbial agents, numerous histologic entities may be used as antigens. These include substances such as pituitary hormones, hypothalamic releasing factors, specific immunoglobulins and others. Any substance of the body capable of inducing a humoral antibody response in another animal may be localized via this technology.

Transmission Electron Microscopy. The preparation of biologic materials for electron microscopy is similar to those procedures described for the paraffin technique. Fixation, dehydration and clearing, embedding, sectioning and staining are necessary supportive processes.

The sample must be acquired as atraumatically as possible. Any careless handling and/or introduction of contamination during this phase is readily observable at the levels of magnification used. Techniques of fixation, usually achieved with aldehydes (paraformaldehyde, glutaraldehyde) and/or osmic acid, must be excellent and are usually achieved at 4°C. Dehydration is similar to light microscopic preparations. Clearing agents are used in the manner described previously to permit the embedding of specimens in plastics. Plastic embedding, the precision of the cutting instruments and the use of glass or diamond knives facilitate the acquisition of very thin specimens (300–600 Å thick). Thin sections are essential to allow the electron beam to pass through the specimen. If specimens are too thin, then insufficient scatter occurs, whereas excessively thick specimens absorb too much of the electron beam. Heavy metal stains (osmic acid, lead, uranium) are used to stain selectively cellular and extracellular constituents. These heavy metals, dispersed differentially throughout the specimen, account for the differential scattering of the electron beam and subsequent image formation (Fig. 2.11).

During the sectioning process, 1–2 μm sections of tissue are often examined for

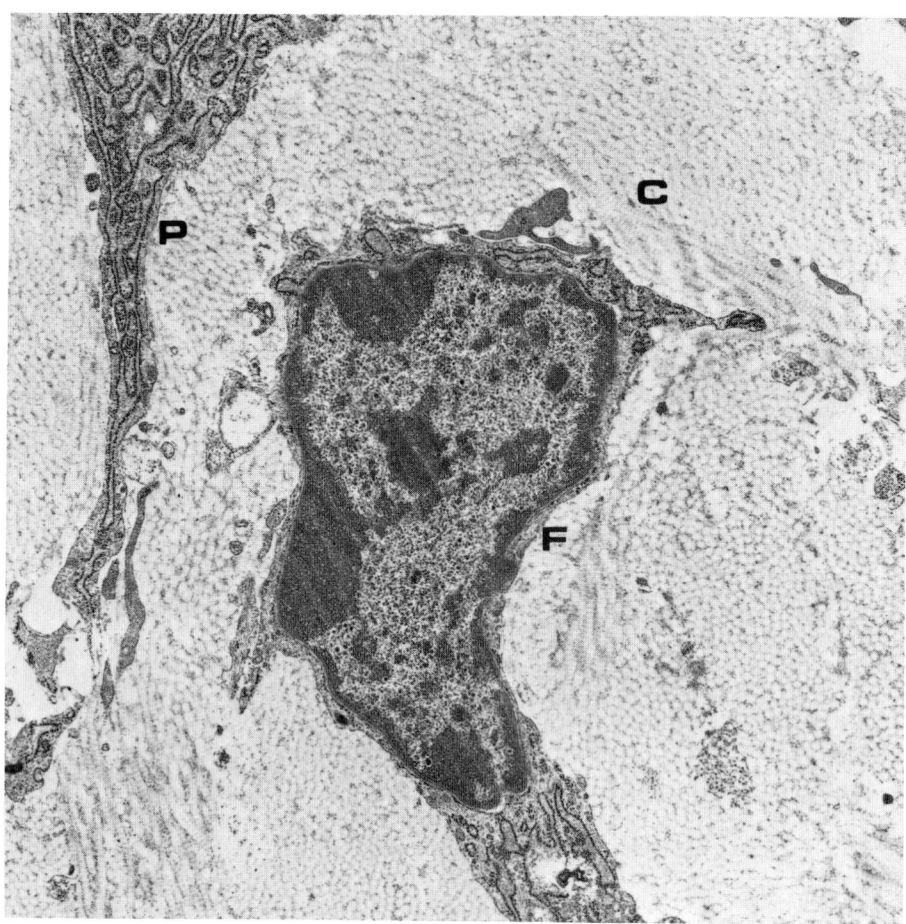

Fig. 2.11   An electron micrograph of a section of cervine dermis. The fibroblast (F) is surrounded by collagen (C) cut in longitudinal and cross section. P, cytoplasmic process of another fibroblast. ×6,000.

purposes of orientation. These thick sections are useful for histologic study (Fig. 2.12).

Scanning Electron Microscopy. The preparation techniques for this type of microscopy are similar to those of transmission electron microscopy; however, sectioning and staining are not required. Specimens utilized in this technique are those which afford a natural or artificially-induced surface. Specimens are acquired, fixed and dried by *critical point drying* techniques to minimize surface tension distortion of their three-dimensional surface topography. They are then coated with a conductor, usually gold, which will backscatter secondary electrons to a collector. Such specimens require minimal treatment, yet they afford phenomenal insights into three-dimensional morphologic relationships (see Chapter 13, Fig. 13.8).

Freeze Fracturing. This technical approach utilizes the rapid freezing of samples with liquid nitrogen and bypasses the need for chemical fixation and dehydration. Frozen samples are mounted to plates within a special apparatus. The plates are moved slightly and the specimen is fractured. Metals, which are vaporized from a heated source, coat the fractured surfaces and form ultrathin metallic replicas of the fracture-induced surfaces.

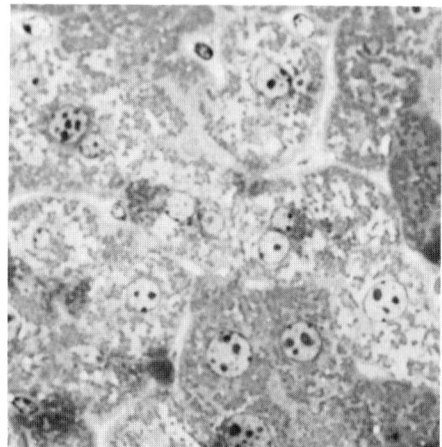

Fig. 2.12   A light micrograph of a plastic-embedded, 1 μm section of murine liver. ×160. (Toluidine blue). (Courtesy of D. Dunham).

The metallic replicas are removed from the fractured tissues and are used as the sample that is examined with the transmission electron microscope. This technique affords high resolution insights into the architecture of real and induced surfaces—plasmalemma, cytomembranes, organelles and inclusions (Fig. 2.13).

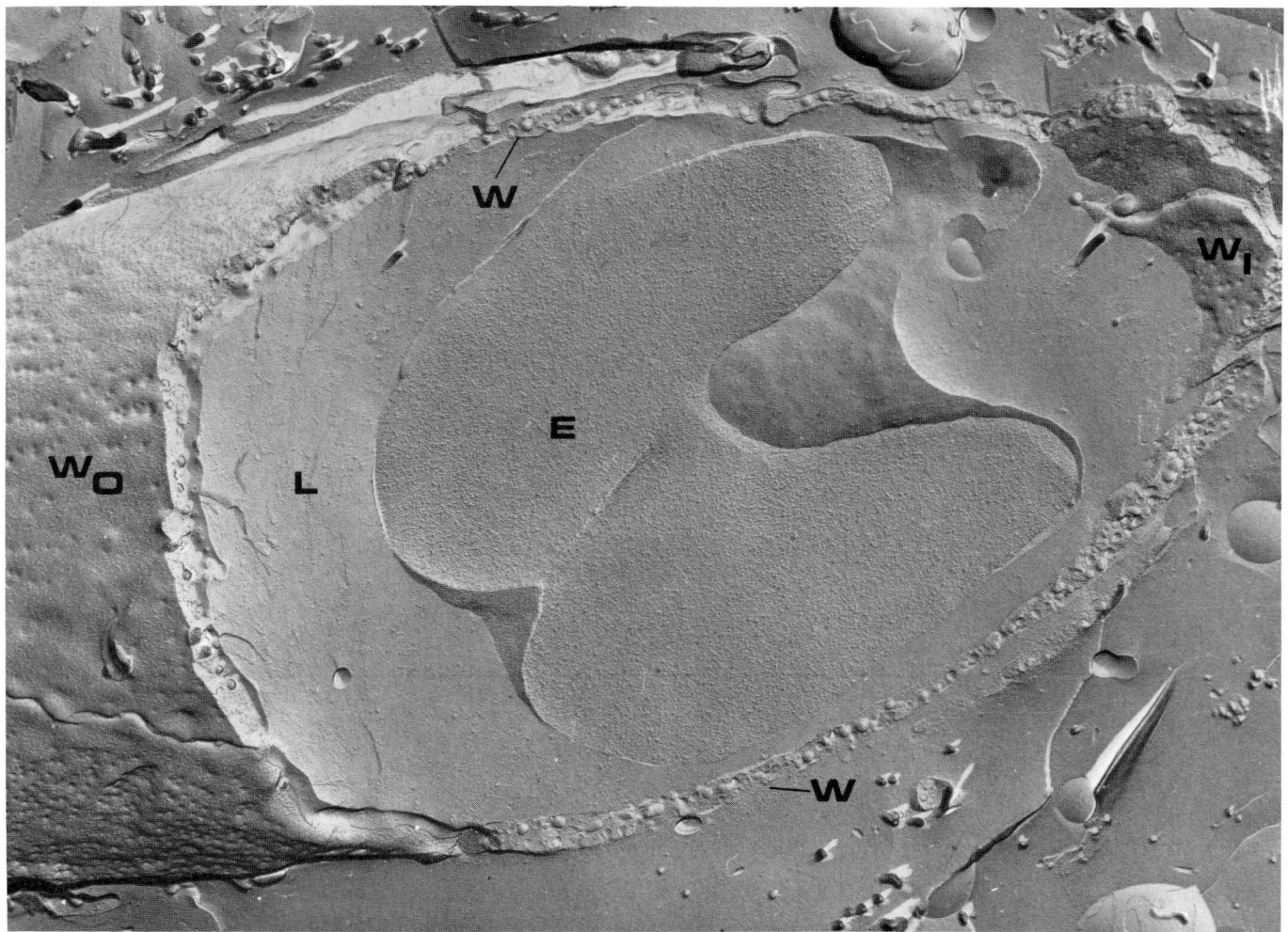

Fig. 2.13   An electron micrograph of a freeze-fractured capillary. An erythrocyte (E) occupies the lumen (L) of the capillary. The wall of the capillary has been fractured in longitudinal (W) and cross section. The inner (W_i) and outer (W_0) surfaces of the capillary wall are apparent. ×20,500. (Courtesy of J. E. Rash).

References

Baker, J. R.: *Cytological Techniques: The Principles Underlying Routine Methods.* 5th edition, John Wiley and Sons, Inc., New York, 1966.

Davenport, H. A.: *Histological and Histochemical Technics.* W. B. Saunders, Philadelphia, 1960.

Gahan, P. B.: *Autoradiography for Biologists.* Academic Press, New York, 1972.

Gomori, G.: *Microscopic Histochemistry: Principles and Practice.* The University of Chicago Press, Chicago, 1952.

Hayat, M. A.: *Basic Electron Microscopy Techniques.* Van Nostrand Reinhold Company, New York, 1972.

Hayat, M. A.: *Principles and Techniques of Scanning Electron Microscopy: Biological Applications.* Vol. I, Van Nostrand Reinhold Co., New York, 1974.

Hearle, J. W. S., Sparrow, J. T. and Cross, P. M.: *The Use of the Scanning Electron Microscope.* Pergamon Press, New York, 1972.

Humason, G. L.: *Animal Tissue Techniques.* 3rd edition, W. H. Freeman and Company, San Francisco, 1972.

Koehler, J. K. (ed.): *Advanced Techniques in Biological Electron Microscopy.* Spinger-Verlag, New York, 1973.

Koss, L. G.: *Diagnostic Cytology and Its Histopathologic Bases.* 2nd edition, J. B. Lippincott Co., Philadelphia, 1968.

Lillie, R. D.: *H. J. Conn's Biological Stains.* 9th edition, Williams & Wilkins Co., Baltimore, 1977.

Pearse, A. G. E.: *Histochemistry: Theoretical and Applied.* Vols. I and II, 3rd edition, Williams & Wilkins Co., Baltimore, 1968.

Pease, D. C.: *Histological Techniques for Electron Microscopy.* 2nd edition, Academic Press, New York, 1964.

Wischnitzer, S.: *Introduction to Electron Microscopy.* 2nd edition, Pergamon Press, New York, 1970.

3: Microscopy and Interpretation

Introduction

The approach to the study of histology not only requires an appreciation of preparation techniques but an understanding of the numerous ways by which cells and tissues may be examined. Both aspects dictate and/or limit the type of information that can be obtained. Preparation and examination is complemented by the ability to interpret what is observed. The histologist, therefore, must combine these three facets of study to obtain a comprehensive understanding of structure and function.

Microscopy

The beginning study of microscopic structure, for most individuals, is an excursion into the realm of entities whose dimensions and relationships are difficult to visualize. Most individuals can conceptualize those animate and inanimate objects that are familiar parts of daily existence. The word "chair" immediately evokes an image and an association of that image with functional relationships. Similarly, conventional methods of measurement are applied easily to familiar objects.

The new student of histology is confronted with the interesting challenges of being able to conceptualize this new realm of structure and to appreciate the functional and dimensional relationships of the histologic components of the organism. The accompanying table and figure present dimensional considerations, whereas the remainder of the text is devoted to the interpretive challenges (Table 3.1, Fig. 3.1).

The effective and efficient use of any instrument requires an understanding of its principles of operation, its advantages and limitations. This most certainly applies to the primary tool of the histologist—the microscope.

The ability of the microscope to magnify objects is an important consideration in its usefulness to histology; however, the ability to display points that are approximated closely to each other as separate images is the most significant consideration. The display of closely spaced objects as separate images is the *resolving power* of a lens or lens system. It is defined mathematically as $R = .61 \lambda/NA$. The resolving power (R in Å) is determined by the wave length (λ in Å) of the illuminating source and the numerical aperture (NA) of the objective lens.

TABLE 3.1
Linear Measurements

Unit	Abbreviation	Relationships
Centimeter	cm	$1\,cm = 10^1 mm,\ 10^4 \mu m,\ 10^7 nm,\ 10^8 \text{Å}$
Millimeter	mm	$1\,mm = 10^{-1} cm,\ 10^3 \mu m,\ 10^6 nm,\ 10^7 \text{Å}$
Micrometer (micron)	μm	$1\,\mu m = 10^{-4} cm,\ 10^{-3} mm,\ 10^3 nm,\ 10^4 \text{Å}$
Nanometer (millimicron)	nm	$1\,nm = 10^{-7} cm,\ 10^{-6} mm,\ 10^{-3} \mu m,\ 10^1 \text{Å}$
Angstrom	Å	$1\,\text{Å} = 10^{-8} cm,\ 10^{-7} mm,\ 10^{-4} \mu m,\ 10^{-1} nm$

The numerical aperture for a lens, $n \sin \alpha$, is the refractive index (n) multiplied by the sine of the half angle formed between the specimen and the maximal opening of the lens and is a description of the light gathering properties of the lens. Wave lengths of about 5000Å are used commonly in light microscopes, whereas the numerical aperture of good oil-immersion objective lenses is about 1.4. The resolving power for this system would be approximately 2200Å. Any components closer than 2200Å would not be seen as separate objects. A reasonable estimate of the theoretical resolving power of an optical system is $\lambda/2$.

Other factors also have an effect upon resolution and image quality. *Spherical aberration*, the inability of a curved surface to bring monochromatic light to a single focus, can affect resolution. Similarly, *chromatic aberration*, the manifestation of multiple focal points based upon the differential refraction of polychromatic light, can affect image quality. Generally, these aberrations are not significant in good light-optical systems because the lenses are corrected for them.

Bright-Field Microscopy. The bright-field microscope is the instrument most commonly used in histology (Fig. 3.2). The limit of resolution of the compound microscope is approximately 2200Å. A significant advantage to the microscopist using this type of microscope is the ability to distinguish structural detail based upon the differential light absorption of stained components. Because of the transparency of living tissues, stained sections are necessary for maximal effectiveness of this type of microscopy.

The resolution of bright-field microscopy can be increased by using an illumination source with a shorter wavelength. Wave-

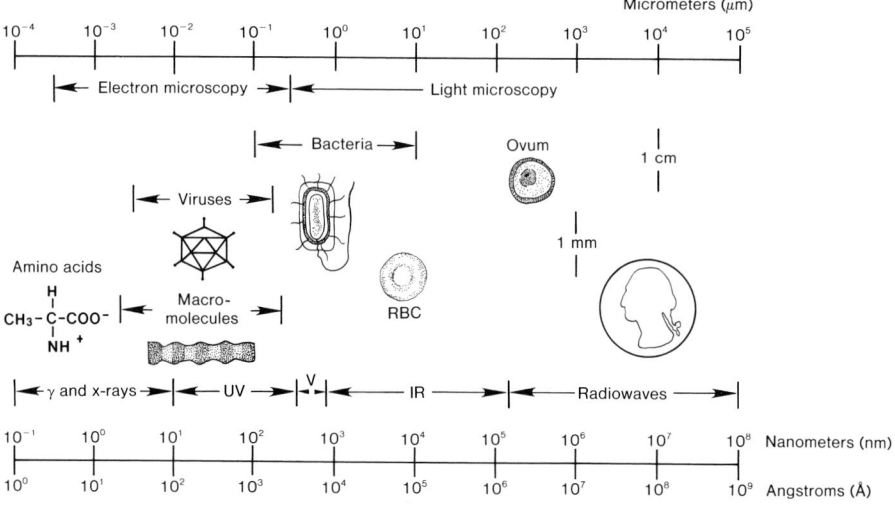

Fig. 3.1 Scalar relationships and relative sizes of biologic and nonbiologic entities. All light micrographs are labeled as the magnification with the microscope before photographic enlarging. All electron micrographs are labeled as total magnification, including photographic enlarging.

niques must be employed. Also, these wavelengths are damaging to living specimens. The primary application of this type of microscopy is in microspectrophotometry as an adjunct to histochemical studies.

Fluorescence Microscopy. This is a form of visible light microscopy in which an ultraviolet emitter is used as the light source. This monochromatic light serves as an excitatory illumination source to molecules that absorb the light and re-emit wavelengths in the visible range of the spectrum

(Plate I.10). Barrier filters prevent the shorter wavelengths from reaching the retina. This is the type of microscopy used in the fluorescent antibody techniques described previously.

Dark-Field Microscopy. This type of microscopy is achieved by slightly modifying a bright-field microscope. The usual condenser is replaced by one that causes light to strike the image at an oblique angle without any direct illumination reaching the objective lens. That light which does reach the

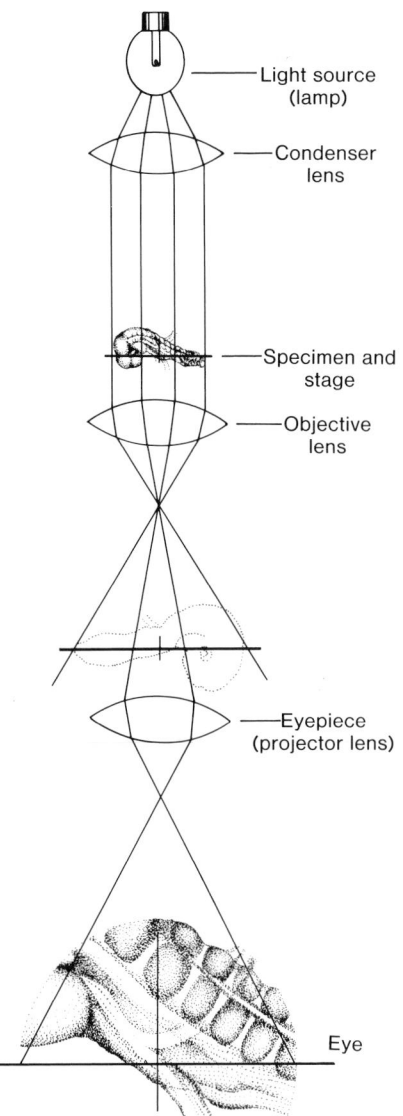

Fig. 3.2 Diagram of the optical pathway in a bright-field microscope. The light source passes through glass lenses and the specimen before forming an image within the eye on the retina. Compare with Figure 3.7.

lengths shorter than 4000Å are not transmitted through glass lenses; therefore, the ultimate limitation to resolution with this microscope is a function of lens characteristics, not wavelength.

Ultraviolet Microscopy. This type of microscope utilizes an ultraviolet radiation source which emits radiation with wavelengths between 1000 and 3000Å. An estimate of resolution is between 500 and 1500Å. Quartz lenses are necessary to allow this short wave radiation to enter the optical system. Initially, this type of microscopy would seem to offer the advantage of increased resolution. Unfortunately, significant disadvantages prevent its routine use. Ultraviolet radiation cannot be seen and is damaging to the retina; therefore, photographic tech-

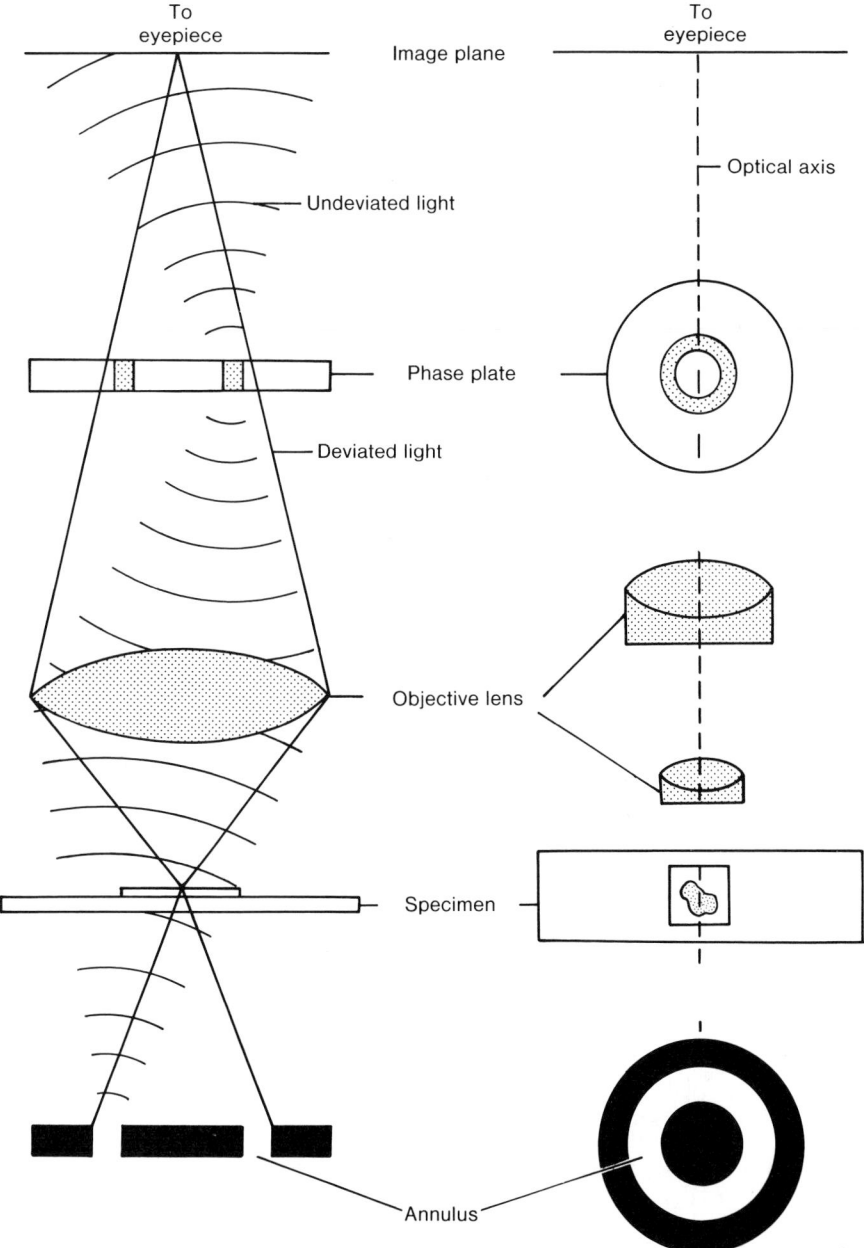

Fig. 3.3 Diagram of the optical pathway and primary constituents of a phase-contrast microscope. The annulus and phase plate are the unique components of the microscope. The annulus presents an annular ring of light to the objective lens, thus separating the undeviated and deviated light rays from each other. The phase plate, built into the back focal plane of the objective lens, retards the central (undeviated) beam by $\frac{1}{4}\lambda$ and absorbs about 75% of this central light. The retardation is manifested as interference at the image plane and accounts for the contrast enhancement.

objective lens results from the scattering of light which occurs at the boundaries (interfaces) between components with different refractive indices. Cells and other tissue components appear bright against a dark background. The limits of resolution are similar to the bright-field microscope. Darkfield microscopes enable the microscopist to examine living, unstained specimens.

Phase-Contrast and Interference Microscopy. The phase-contrast microscope is a modified conventional microscope which requires a special condenser (Zernike condenser) and a phase plate positioned behind the objective lens. The alignment of optical components is achieved with a focusing telescope. As mentioned previously, living and/or unstained biologic materials are transparent; therefore, it is difficult to observe structural detail in these specimens. As these types of specimens are transilluminated, the various constituents will transmit phase altered light as a function of their slightly different refractive indices and thicknesses. This phase altered (deviated) light interacts with the normophasic (undeviated) light to produce an image. The image created through constructive and destructive interference results in an alteration of intensity that is visible. The essence of the phase-contrast microscope, therefore, is the conversion of undetectable phase differences to amplitude differences that are visible to the human retina (Fig. 3.3). It is especially useful for the study of living and unstained specimens (Fig. 3.4).

The interference microscope utilizes the same principles as the phase-contrast microscope, but the former has more precision and is useful in density determinations. The dry mass and refractive indices of cells and tissues may be determined with this precision instrument.

The same principles govern the Nomarski interference phase microscope. Its singlemost advantage is the three-dimensional imaging of cells and tissues (Figs. 3.5, 3.6).

Polarizing Microscopy. Many substances that are contained within or are products of cells have a highly ordered molecular organization. When a beam of polarized light is passed through such substances, the transmitted light is split into two rays that are perpendicular to each other. An *ordinary ray* follows the laws of refraction, while the *extraordinary ray* undergoes a velocity change. This phenomenon is called *birefringence*; i.e., the property of having more than one refractive index dependent upon the plane of polarized light vibration relative to the molecular orientation. Such substances are *anisotropic*. Substances that possess a single refractive index independent of the plane of polarized light vibration are *isotropic*.

This type of microscope is simply a bright-field microscope to which a polarizer and an analyzer has been added with the specimen located between them. It is useful in studying such cellular components as the A (anisotropic) and I (isotropic) bands of muscle, and the orderly nature of bone (Fig. 3.7).

Transmission Electron Microscopy (TEM). Abbe's prediction of the necessity of shorter wavelengths for the improvement of reso-

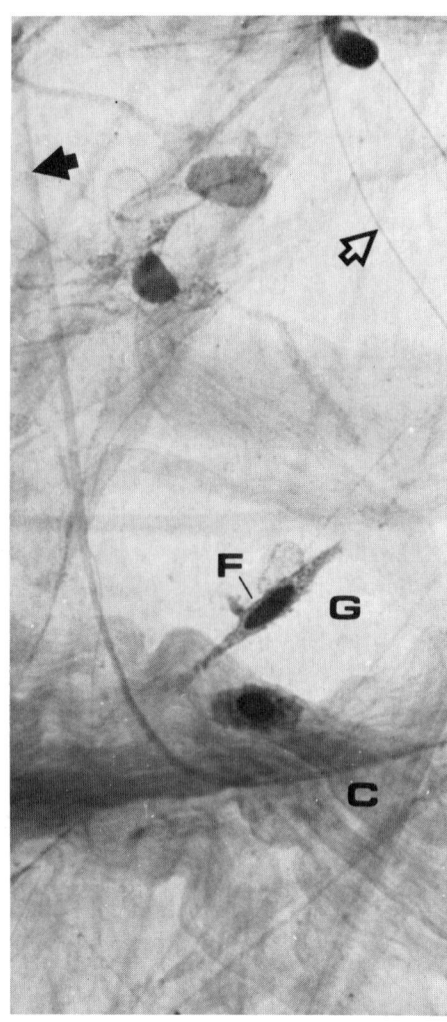

Fig. 3.5 Bright-field micrograph of a stretch preparation of loose connective tissue. F, fibroblast; *Solid arrow*, collagenous fiber; *Open arrow*, elastic fiber; C, mass of collagenous fibers; G, ground substance. Compare with Figure 3.6. X160.

lution (R = .61 λ/NA) was fulfilled upon development of the TEM. Although the general principles which govern light optical systems are applicable to the electron microscope, these instruments possess a number of unique features and characteristics because of the nature of the illumination source—the electron (Fig. 3.8). The massive inverted column of the TEM consists of a source of electrons, a means of accelerating electrons, electromagnetic lenses to control them, a vacuum system and an image translation system.

The light source is a triode in which the heated tungsten filament (*cathode*) is the source of electrons. Electrons are accelerated away from the cathode by the high potential of the *anode plate*, while the *grid* (*gun cap*) controls the amount of electron flow. The wavelength of the electrons is a function of the accelerating voltage, as expressed by de Broglie as $\lambda = 12.3/\sqrt{V}$. The wavelength at 50,000 volts would be 0.05Å,

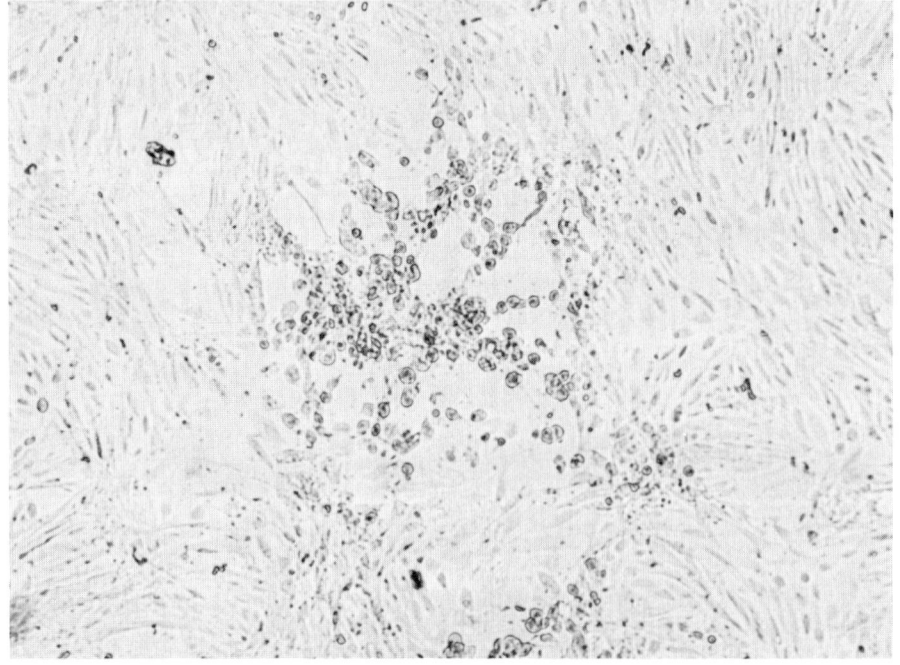

Fig. 3.4 Phase contrast micrograph of bovine embryonic lung cells in culture. The culture was infected with IBR virus particles. The clumped cells in the center of the field are undergoing cytopathic effects as a consequence of the viral infection. X16. (Courtesy of J. J. England).

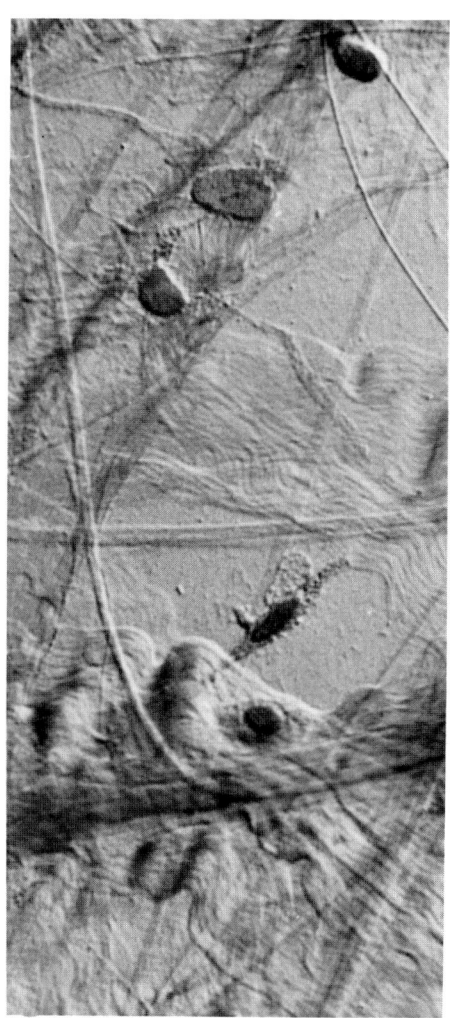

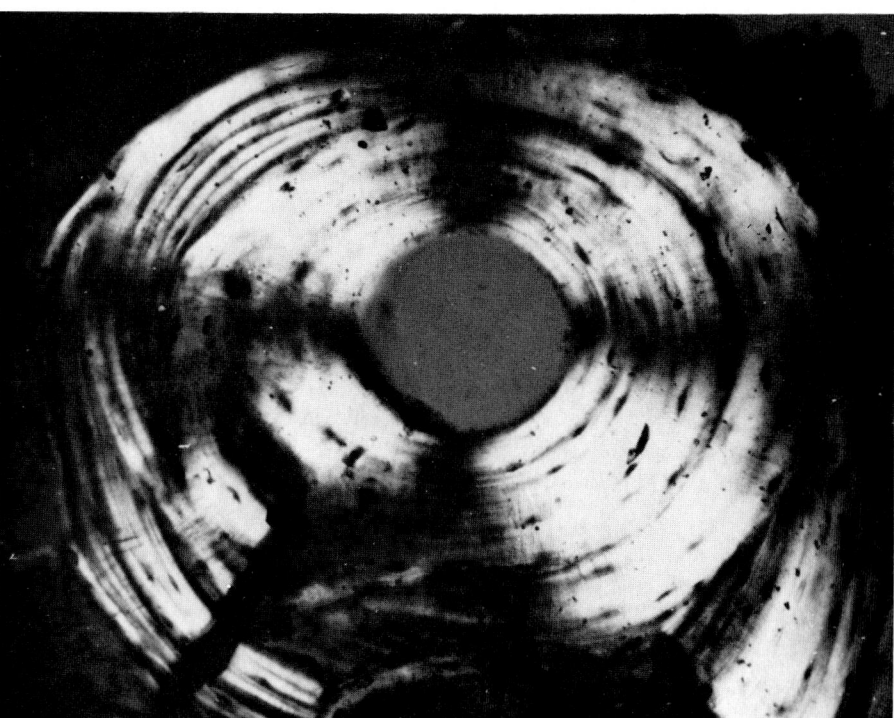

Fig. 3.7   A canine osteon of bone photographed with polarizing microscopy. The four light bands radiating from the center of the osteon are indicative of the anisotrophic properties of lamellar bone. X40.

Fig. 3.6   Nomarski interference phase micrograph of the same tissue field as that of Figure 3.5. The three-dimensional relief is a distinct advantage of this type of optical system. X160.

while at 100,000 volts it would be 0.04Å. A theoretical approximation of resolution (λ/2) would be 0.025Å and 0.02Å, respectively, or a 110,000 fold improvement over conventional optical systems. Practically, this has not been achieved because of the imperfection (spherical aberration) of the lenses used. Most modern TEM's permit 3–5Å resolution, but the nature of most biologic specimens limits the average routine resolution to 10–15Å.

Electromagnetic lenses control the path of the electrons through the condenser, objective and projector lenses to a phosphorescent viewing screen. The invisible electrons strike the fluorescent screen, and light in the visible spectrum is emitted; the beam is converted to a visible image. Photographs are used routinely to study morphology revealed by the TEM.

Because the mean free path of electrons in air is small, all of these events must occur within a vacuum.

The nature of the illuminating beam requires that the specimens are thin (< 1000Å) and stained with materials sufficiently dense to scatter electrons. The "depleted" beam which is projected to the viewing screen, in all simplicity, can be considered a shadow of the specimen.

The penetration power of an electron beam is proportional to the accelerating voltage. This knowledge was the impetus for the development of a high voltage transmission electron microscope (HVTEM). A number of advantages are associated with this development. The increased penetration of a 1,000,000 volt (1 MEV) beam permits the use of 1 micron sections. These thick sections facilitate stereopair production that allows microscopists to reconstruct three-dimensional models of cellular components. Because a 1 MEV beam imparts less energy to the cells through which it passes than lower voltages, living specimens have been observed. Spherical aberration should be reduced in 1 MEV microscopes and higher resolution should be achieved.

Scanning Electron Microscopy (SEM). The optical system of the SEM is simpler than that of a TEM and its principles of operation are different (Fig. 3.9). The SEM consists of an electron source (cathode, grid and anode), condenser lens and objective lens. The beam is focused onto the surface of a coated specimen; however, the beam is not stationary. A scan generator moves the beam across the surface of the specimen in an orderly manner—a raster pattern. The scan generator also synchronizes the raster pattern of a cathode ray tube (CRT) with that of the beam raster. Electrons are backscattered off the surface of the specimen and picked up by an electron collector. The synchronized scan of the beam raster with that of the CRT permits a point for point display of the backscattered electrons on the CRT. The various angles of the specimen determine, point for point, the number of electrons that will reach the collector. This accounts for the variable intensity on the display screen. Magnification in this microscope is a function of the CRT raster scan length divided by the beam raster scan length. Because the CRT scan is constant, the progressive decrease in beam raster scan length results in an increased magnification.

The SEM does not replace the TEM. The biggest advantage of the SEM is its depth of field. This permits the display of three-dimensional images. While the resolution of the SEM is in the 75Å–100Å range, the information gained from this instrument complements that gained from the TEM.

Interpretation

The interpretive skills required of the histologist are numerous and varied. The approach to interpretation demands a comprehensive appreciation of the limitations and advantages of the varied preparatory techniques that may be employed. If an histologist were interested in observing and/or staining various lipid components of cells, then the paraffin technique would probably be of little value. Many lipids are soluble in the chemicals (alcohol, xylene, chloroform) used for processing tissues by this method-

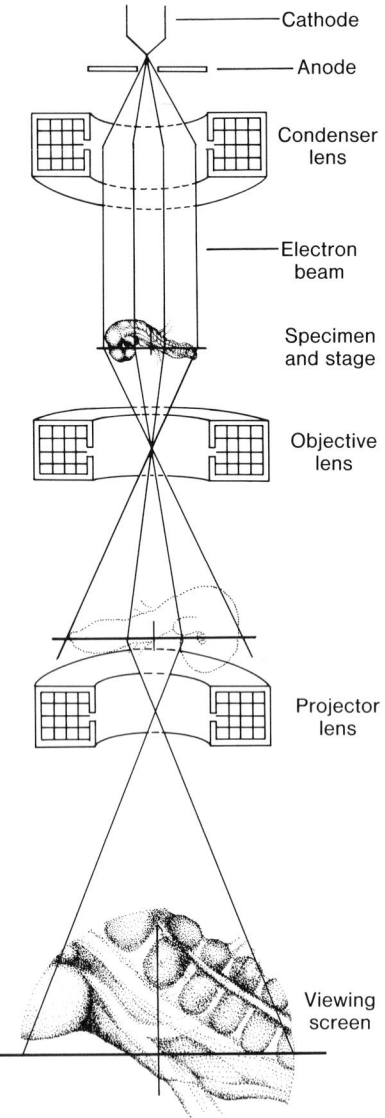

Fig. 3.8 Diagram of the electron pathway in a transmission electron microscope. The illumination source emits electrons which are refracted by magnetic lenses. Whereas the optical components are the same as a compound microscope, the TEM is many times larger than its bright-field counterpart. Compare with Figure 3.2.

microscopes is necessary and advantageous for the solution of histologic problems.

Notwithstanding the significance of the previously discussed factors, the most important aspect of interpretive skills is an understanding of structure. This understanding must be sufficiently comprehensive to enable the histologist to translate the two-dimensional and static structural and functional representations of sections into the three-dimensional and dynamic relationships that characterize the living organism. The remainder of this discussion is directed toward the skills requisite for the examination and interpretation of histologic sections prepared by the paraffin technique.

Examination of the Specimen. Most histo-

logic studies are initiated at the time the sample is obtained. The histologist knows the organ from which the sample was obtained and probably noted its gross structural features (normal or abnormal). By the time the sample is examined there may be little need to wonder about its origin. The study of histology without benefit of gross anatomic integration creates an artificial didactic situation, especially during examinations, that requires the student histologist to rely upon microscopic features to identify cells, tissues and organs.

The initial step in the examination of sections, whether in the teaching or research lab, does not begin with the microscope. All sections of known or unknown origin are

ology. Similarly, accurate indications of glycogen content are difficult to obtain if cells and tissues are exposed routinely to water during processing. Free glycogen molecules, being water soluble, are leached out of the tissues during processing. A consideration of the type of fixation is important to the enzyme histochemist, because complete or partial denaturation of proteins will affect enzyme catalysis dramatically.

Similarly, the type of microscope chosen to examine tissues is linked to the preparation processes required. Also, the type of information that can be obtained from a specified type of microscopy is limited. In many instances, the use of different types of

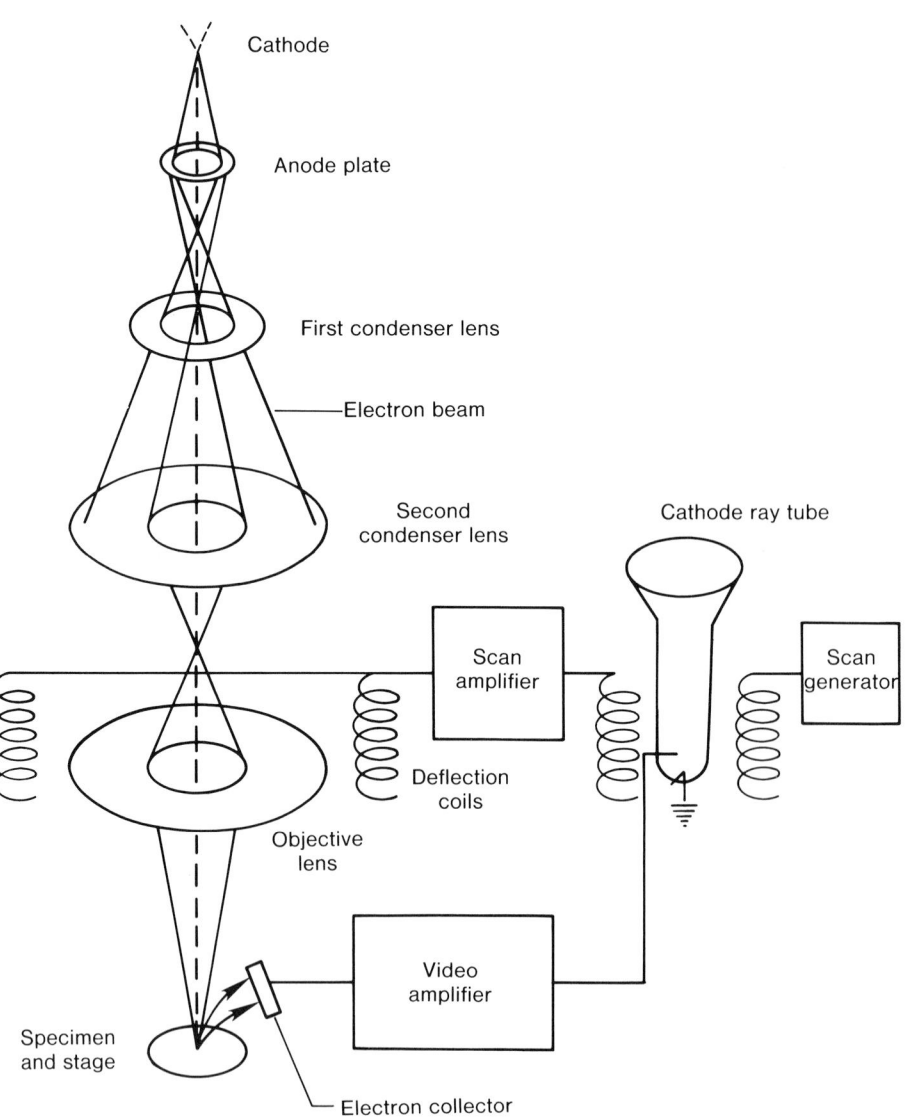

Fig. 3.9 A schematic diagram of a scanning electron microscope. The electrons pass through the column to the objective lens. The objective lens focuses the electron beam on the specimen. The deflection coils move the beam back and forth over the specimen. The detector picks up backscattered electrons. The signal is converted to an image on a cathode ray tube. Micrographs are obtained by photographing the display face of the cathode ray tube.

best examined first with the naked eye. Many features of histologic structure are evident through the use of this cursory yet effective first step. The distribution of staining properties (basophilia, acidophilia), the presence or absence of hollow spaces (lumina) and other architectural features may serve to direct examination to certain areas of the section. Moreover, such an examination, if conducted carefully, limits the number of interpretive possibilities that exist.

The tendency "to want to see more" by going directly to the highest magnification usually results in a lack of orientation. Each incremental increase in magnification is always accompanied by a progressively narrower field of vision. It is best to progress through each stage of magnification noting the specific architectural features, cellular components, extracellular materials, etc. Through this approach the microscopist, literally, gets more and more information about less and less tissue. A routine examination often culminates with use of the oil-immersion lens.

Color and Morphology. The use of stains in histology has been and will continue to be a valuable aspect of this type of inquiry. Much of our current knowledge of this subject is related, directly or indirectly, to an understanding of staining mechanisms and the distribution of these chemicals in cells and tissues. To ignore that certain cells or tissues have specific characteristics with certain stains would be ridiculous. To draw conclusions that all cytoplasm is pink and all nuclei are blue would be just as ridiculous. That may be true with H and E, but these are not the only basic and acidic stains available to histologists.

The most important features to learn about cells and tissues initially are their morphologic characteristics. If morphology is learned, understood and appreciated, then the color really doesn't matter; color should be an aid to learning and study, not a crutch. Electron micrographs are an important part of the study of histology; they are black and white. The sooner the student can learn to rely on morphology independent of tinctorial properties, the sooner the student will make the transition from histology, per se, to ultrastructural cytology. This text will assist in that transition. The judicious use of color in the text is intended as an aid to study.

Sectioning and Morphology. Numerous and fascinating challenges await the student when the examination of sections is initiated. These challenges have been the same for every microscopist since the science began. Hopefully, the combined insights of histologists over years of inquiry will preclude the necessity of the student's "rediscovering the histologic wheel when attempting to build his (her) biologic cart."

The first challenge is to realize that the fixed, processed, stained and sectioned piece of the body truly represents a reasonable sample of body constituents. The structural and functional relationships that are visible on the slide are, in fact, a captured moment in the life of the organism or a part of the organism. The cells and tissues may not have had the exact same structural or functional characteristics the moment before section acquistion nor the moment later, if the life of that sample had progressed beyond the sampling point. The sample, however, is representative; therefore, reasonable inferences about the organism and/or its constituent parts can be made. The combined wisdom of histologists since the days of Bichat permits this positive statement.

The second challenge, somewhat similar to the first relates to the reliability of a section of tissue. Does a section of tissue from the spleen, liver, kidney, lung or any other organ truly represent the entire organ? Admittedly, the student is forced to accept on faith, or conduct extensive self inquiry, that the sample does represent something from within the organism. But does a section of tissue, approximately 1 inch square by 5–7 microns thick really represent the entire organ? The student could tediously construct three-dimensional models from serial sections or he (she) could accept on faith that such samples really do represent the entire organ. In fact, histologists through the years have conducted (and are still conducting) these types of studies. All the student need do is accept that samples of such small dimensions are representative and then proceed mentally to convert these biplanar and static samples into three-dimensional and dynamic pictures.

The last challenge is the necessity and ability of converting biplanar sections into a three-dimensional whole. Such a transition is necessary. Scientists don't work with sections for the sake of the sections. They are simply an expeditious way of gaining insights about the constituent parts, and thus the organism, without examining every milligram of the organism. The ability to convert these images is a function of familiarity and exposure. Additionally, the combined knowledge of histology is helpful.

Those items with which we are most familiar in our everyday existence are easily conceptualized. Again, the word "chair" evokes a mental image of a chair without much difficulty. What, however, is the mental image of a chair if a person were shown this item in various planes of section (view)? The drafting student may have the advantage. Being familiar with top, side and front views (sections), this student might construct the orthographic projection (three-dimensional image) quite readily. Others of us may take longer but end at the same point— a three-dimensional image of a chair. In many instances in histology, however, the student must be prepared to think three-dimensionally from a single point of view or plane of section. A section normal to the long axis of pancake-shaped or flattened cells gives misleading information about cell shape (Fig. 3.10). In both instances, the third dimension must be considered.

The correlation of three-dimensional structure with biplanar representations of familiar items is useful. The first slice perpendicular to the long axis of a hard-boiled egg rarely causes concern about the absence of a yolk. Progressive sectioning eventually results in demonstrating the yolk in subsequent planes of section. Progressive sectioning, also, will "lose" the yolk. The three-dimensional relationship of the yolk to the white accounts for its sectioned structure. Similar problems are encountered in sections of tissues. Although all cells have nuclei, not all of the nuclei will be encountered in a single section (plane) of a given tissue (Fig. 3.10). The student can be as confident about the presence of a nucleus as he (she) was about the presence of a yolk. Importantly, misinterpretations of three-dimensional structure and components can occur with sectioning of an egg. Similar misinterpretations can occur in histology. The following considerations help to minimize such interpretive errors: familiarity with that which is sectioned, increasing the number of sections and faith in the accumulated knowledge of histology relating to three-dimensional structure.

The tissue components of many organs are disposed generally in a pattern that affords various architectural subdivisions. The section of the familiar lemon demonstrates aptly the alteration of appearance associated with a specific slice or section of this fruit (Fig. 3.11). Sections of organs also will appear differently as a function of the plane of section. The student must be aware of these different representations when slides are being examined.

Some organs of the body are arranged as solid tubular structures. Often they are sectioned in various planes that vary from simple longitudinal or cross sections. Their representation is best compared with different planes of section of a coaxial cable (Fig. 3.12). The altered appearance of the cable, especially in the oblique section, gives the misleading impression of discontinuity between the components.

Many organs of the body are arranged three-dimensionally as elongated, hollow tubular structures (Fig. 3.13). The accompanying diagram demonstrates that such structures may assume various shapes in section. These shapes, if not carefully examined and interpreted, can give false impressions of the real nature of these structural entities.

Histologic Artifacts. There is no doubt that processing tissues for histologic examination induces many changes in cells and tissues. The student must learn to distinguish between changes that are constant and predictable and those alterations that result from capricious handling and/or processing of samples—*artifacts*.

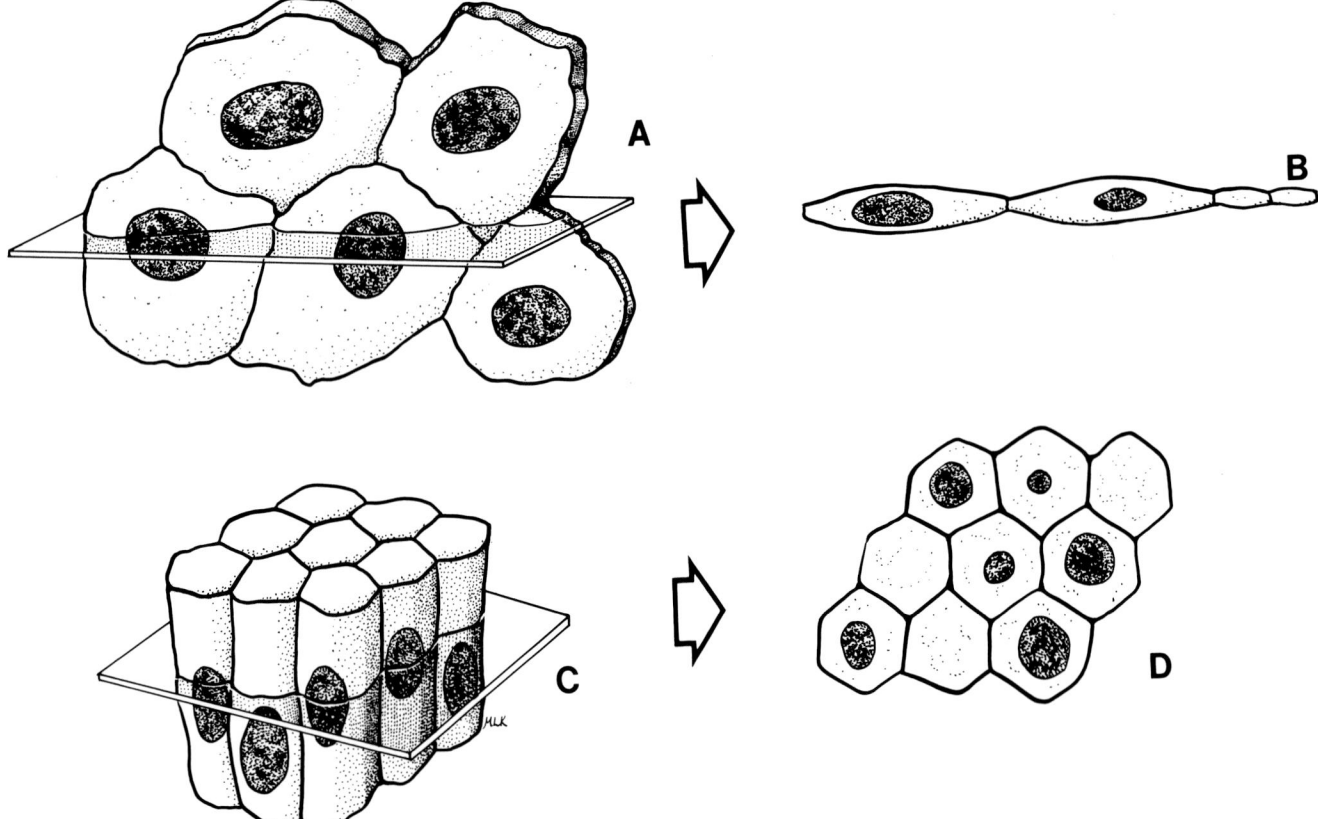

Fig. 3.10   The apparent alteration of cell shape with different views. *A*. The flattened or pancake-shaped cells appear round in surface view. *B*. After sectioning in a plane perpendicular to the surface, the cells appear flattened and elongated. The cells are a variable length, the nuclei are different sizes, and two of the cells appear to be devoid of nuclei. *C*. Some cells appear as columns when viewed from the side. *D*. After sectioning in a plane parallel to the surface, the cells appear more like those in *A* than *C*. Whereas their hexagonal shape is obvious in section, it would not have been obvious in a true side view. The uniform cells now appear to have nuclei of different sizes, and some cells appear to be devoid of nuclei.

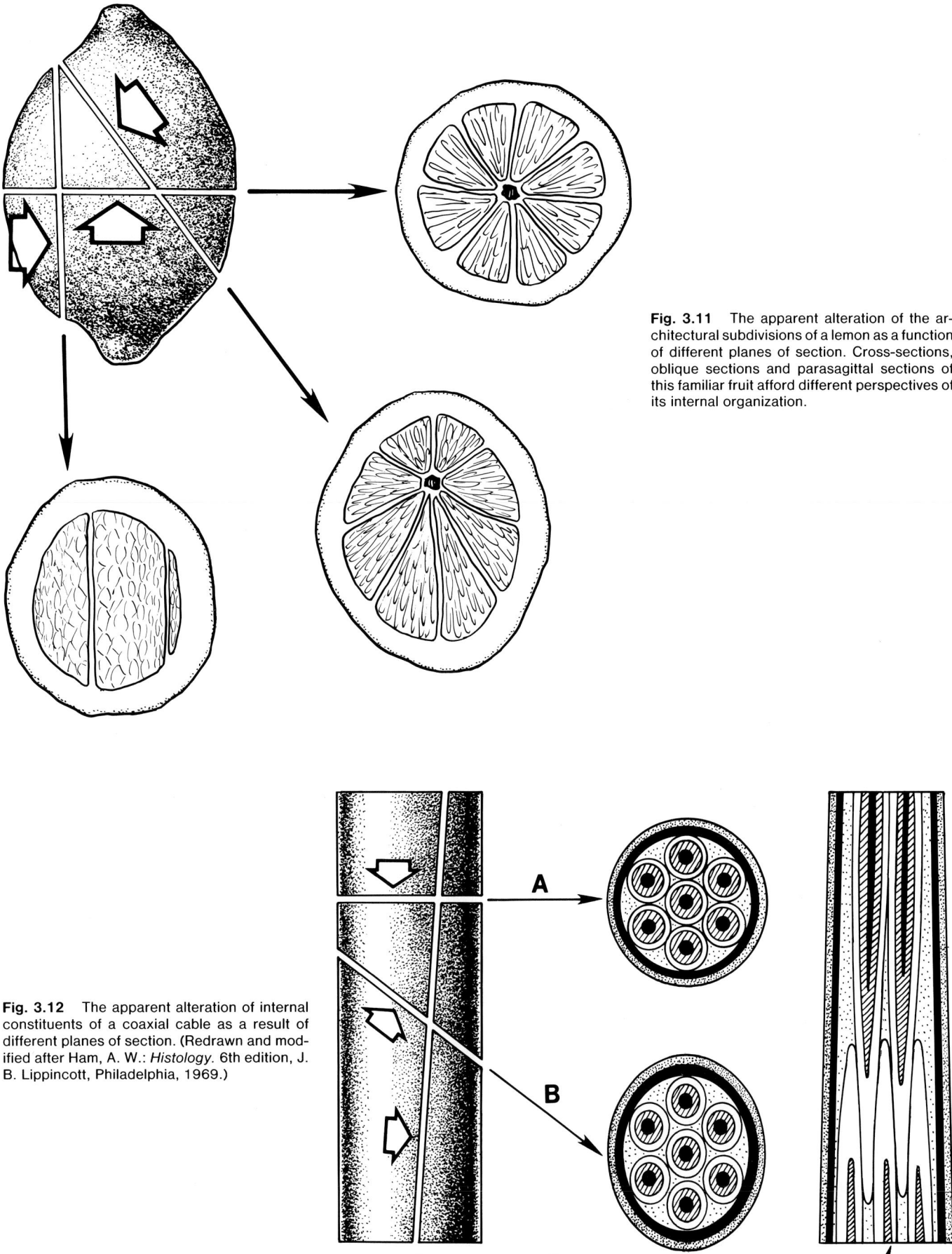

Fig. 3.11   The apparent alteration of the architectural subdivisions of a lemon as a function of different planes of section. Cross-sections, oblique sections and parasagittal sections of this familiar fruit afford different perspectives of its internal organization.

Fig. 3.12   The apparent alteration of internal constituents of a coaxial cable as a result of different planes of section. (Redrawn and modified after Ham, A. W.: *Histology.* 6th edition, J. B. Lippincott, Philadelphia, 1969.)

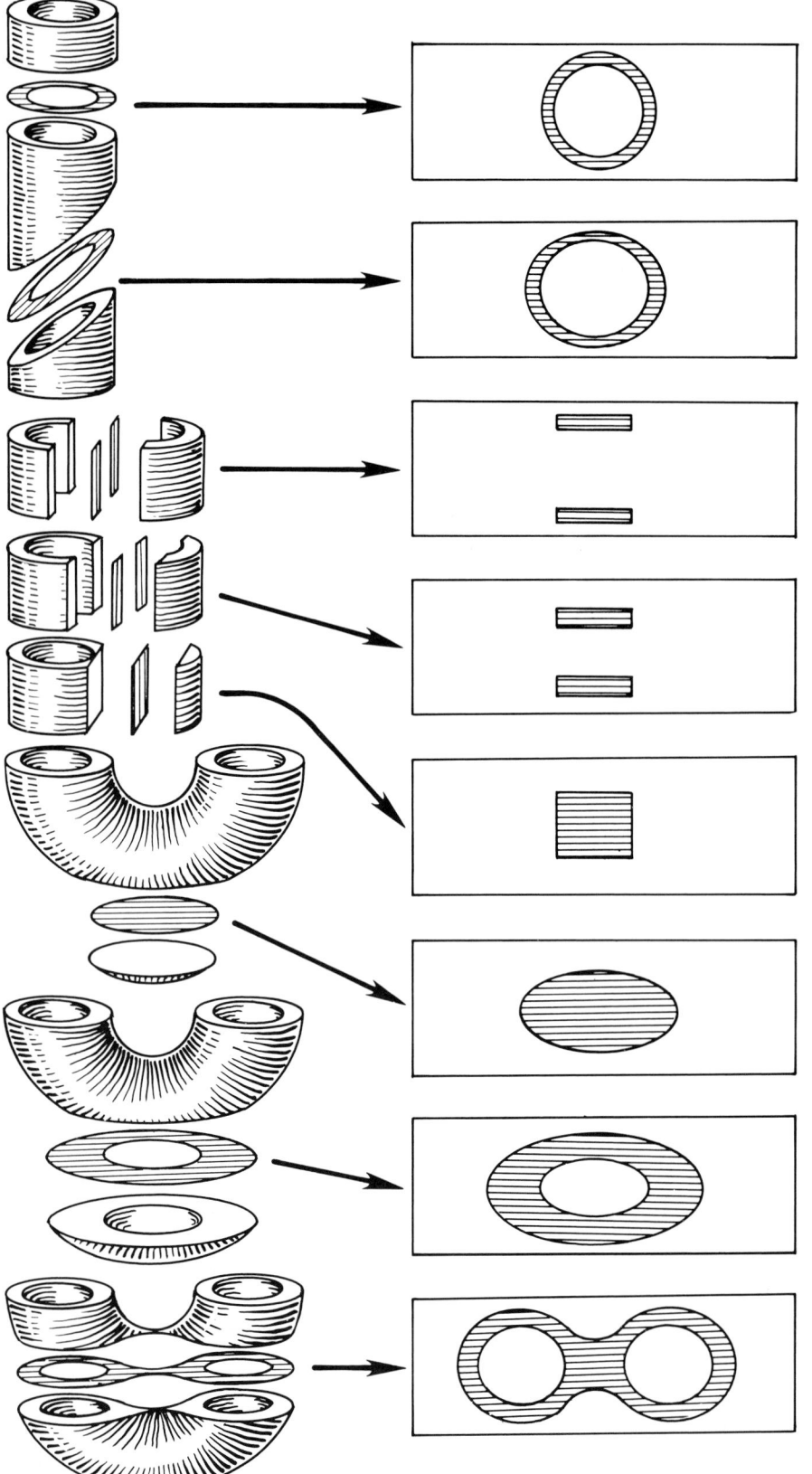

Excessive shrinkage and/or swelling can alter the biplanar relationships of tissue components. Incomplete embedding often results in the complete loss of an area of a tissue during the sectioning process. Incomplete removal of the stain can be manifested as an excessive tissue precipitate. Improper knife angles during sectioning can impart a wavy (alternating thick and thin) characteristic to the tissue. The thick portion will appear more dense because of superimposition artifacts. Similarly, poorly sharpened knives will nick and scratch the paraffin block during sectioning. If the section is not stretched onto the slide, then folds or wrinkles will become apparent. Excessive stretching of the paraffin section can distort spatial relationships, too.

Most of the aforementioned are recognized easily once noted. All that remains is to embark upon the "study of constant artifacts"—histology.

References

Brachet, J. and Mirsky, A. E.: *The Cell: Biochemistry, Physiology and Morphology.* Vol. I, Academic Press, New York, 1959.

Bullivant, S.: Freeze-etching and freeze-fracturing. *In*: Koehler, J. (ed.), *Advanced Techniques in Biological Electron Microscopy*, pp. 66–112. Springer-Verlag, New York, 1973.

Causey, G.: *Electron Microscopy: A Textbook for Students of Medicine and Biology.* Williams & Wilkins Company, Baltimore, 1962.

Cosslett, V. E.: *Modern Microscopy or Seeing the Very Small.* Cornell University Press, Ithaca, 1968.

Elias, H.: Three-dimensional structure identified from single sections. *Science*, 174:993, 1971.

Elias, H. and Pauly, J. E.: *Human Microanatomy.* 3rd edition, F. A. Davis Company, Philadelphia, 1971.

Grivet, P.: *Electron Optics.* Vols. I and II, 2nd edition, Pergamon Press, New York, 1972.

Hall, T., Echlin, P. and Kaufmann, R.: *Microprobe Analysis as Applied to Cells and Tissues.* Academic Press, New York, 1974.

Hayat, M. A.: *Principles and Techniques of Scanning Electron Microscopy: Biological Applications.* Vol. 1, Van Nostrand Reinhold Company, New York, 1974.

Needham, G. H.: *The Practical Use of the Microscope Including Photomicrography.* Charles C Thomas Co., Springfield, 1958.

Pollister, A. W. (editor): *Physical Techniques in Biological Research*, 2nd edition, Vol. III, Academic Press, New York, 1966–1969.

Sjostrand, F. S.: *Electron Microscopy of Cells and Tissues: Instrumentation and Techniques.* Vol. I. Academic Press, New York, 1967.

Weibel, E. R.: Stereological principles for morphometry in electron microscopic cytology. *In*: Bourne, G. H., et al. (ed.), *International Review of Cytology*, pp. 235–302, 1969.

Wischnitzer, S.: *Introduction to Electron Microscopy.* 2nd edition, Pergamon Press, New York, 1970.

Woldseth, R.: *X-Ray Energy Spectrometry.* Kevex Corporation, Burlingame, 1973.

Wren, L. A.: *Understanding and Using the Phase Microscope.* Unitron Instrument Co., Newton Highlands, Mass., 1963.

Fig. 3.13   The appearance of a hollow structure in various planes of section. (Redrawn and modified after Ham, A. W.: *Histology.* 6th edition, J. B. Lippincott, Philadelphia, 1969).

SECTION II:
CYTOLOGY

4: Cytology

Chemical And Physical Properties

Protoplasm. The cell, as the basic unit of metazoan organization, is a complex aggregation of chemicals which interact in numerous and varied ways to manifest properties routinely ascribed to living entities. This aggregation, *protoplasm*, is one of the most complex physicochemical substances known to man. It is a regulated, integrated, dynamic, balanced and maintained accumulation of biochemical substances, salts and water. An understanding of protoplasm requires an understanding of its molecular components. Although the molecular components of protoplasm vary, some generalizations are possible. This diversity of components is the basis for cellular variability.

Water constitutes approximately 75% of the protoplasmic mass and occurs in two forms—*bound water* and *free water*. Bound water constitutes less than 10% of the total water and is intimately involved in the structural integrity of the chemical components. Free water is that which is involved actively in protoplasmic processes. It is also the solvent in which all of the miscible substances are dissolved, as well as the phase throughout which other substances are suspended. This suspension of particles imparts colloidal properties to protoplasm.

A *colloid* is an aggregate of atoms or molecules that is dissolved in but separated from the solvent phase and contains particles of a size sufficient to prevent their passing through a semipermeable membrane. Upon evaporation of the solvent, the colloid remains as an amorphous and sticky residue. Proteins possess colloidal properties and may exist in protoplasm as *sols* or *gels*. Sols are colloidal suspensions which have fluid-like properties, whereas gels are semisolid; both, however, are viscous, having gelatinous or mucinous characteristics. Commercial gelatin undergoes a sol/gel transformation during a temperature-dependent "hardening" phase that is a reasonable example of this property in cells. Protoplasmic proteins, as sols and/or gels, account for many of the significant structural and morphological properties ascribed to cells.

Crystalloids are substances, which when dissolved in the solvent (water), pass through semipermeable membranes and diffract light upon evaporation of the solvent. Important crystalloids include glucose and numerous ions. Potassium is the primary protoplasmic cation, whereas phosphate, bi-carbonate and sulfate are the primary protoplasmic anions. Sodium and chloride are the primary extraprotoplasmic ions.

Nucleic acids, proteins, carbohydrates and lipids are the most commonly occurring biochemical substances of the protoplasm. These can occur as *macromolecules* which are composed of smaller monomeric subunits.

Compartmentalization. The boundary layer between the protoplasm and its surrounding environment is the *plasma membrane*. This membrane, itself a modification of the protoplasm, circumscribes the protoplasmic mass, defines the limits of this living entity, and imparts important characteristics to it. Another structure, the *nucleus*, is membrane-bound within the protoplasm and contains protoplasm which is called *nucleoplasm* or *karyoplasm*. The cytoplasm is that portion of the protoplasm between the nucleus and the *cell membrane (plasmalemma)*. A cell consists of these three components—plasma membrane, cytoplasm and nucleus.

The plasma membrane and nuclear membrane are complex structures whose biochemical components impart gel characteristics. Proteins are significant contributors to this important characteristic. As *hydrophilic* (water-loving) *colloids*, proteins permit the movement of crystalloids and water to and from the cell, as well as between the two major compartments of the cell—nucleus and cytoplasm. Furthermore, lipid components of membranes permit the movement of lipid-soluble substances through them.

The cell consists of numerous aggregations of macromolecules which compartmentalize it and effectively divide it into regions characterized by specific form and function. These compartments are the *organelles*, which consist of cytomembranes and specific proteins (enzymes) or nucleic acids. Organelles permit the separate yet integrated conduct of essential metabolic processes, as well as those special functions for which the cell is modified. The remainder of the protoplasm, the *cytoplasmic* and *nuclear matrix*, consists of the fluid phase within which is contained all of the dissolved substances, including proteins as sols, which are essential to the cell and its metabolism.

Nucleic Acids and Nucleotides. Nucleic acids are considered the repository of information essential for life. They contain the genetic information and serve as blueprints for the synthesis of the most important products of cells—proteins.

The nucleic acids are macromolecules which consist of repeating monomeric units, *nucleotides*. Nucleotides are composed of a *pentose sugar, phosphoric acid* and a *nitrogenous base*. The nitrogenous bases are either a *purine (adenine, guanine)* or *pyrimidine (cytosine, thymine, uracil)*.

Based upon the constituent sugar, nucleic acids are classified into two groups. *Deoxyribonucleic acid (DNA)* contains the sugar *deoxyribose*, whereas *ribonucleic acid (RNA)* contains the sugar *ribose*. The bases which occur in DNA are adenine, cytosine, guanine and thymine; whereas, in RNA uracil replaces thymine.

Although DNA is primarily the nucleic acid of the nucleus, small quantities of DNA occur as circular forms in mitochondria. RNA, however, occurs in both, especially the cytoplasm. Both nucleic acids are complexed with proteins to form *nucleoproteins*.

As the repository of genetic information within the nucleus, the quantity of DNA is a constant. This quantity must double before mitosis to insure that the daughter cells receive the species-specific amount. Similarly, this amount must be halved in the gametes (via meiosis) to insure that the species-specific amount is restored as a result of fertilization.

Different types of RNA have been identified in cells. *Ribosomal RNA (rRNA)* comprises approximately 85% of the cytoplasmic RNA and is complexed with protein as *ribonucleoprotein. Messenger RNA (mRNA)*, which is *encoded (transcribed)* by a single strand of DNA, carries the sequencing information for protein synthesis to the ribosomes and attaches to rRNA. *Transfer RNA (tRNA)* complexes with cytoplasmic amino acids and carries them to mRNA to effect the synthesis of proteins (*translation*).

The acidic nature of these compounds generally assures that they will stain with a basic dye. Many of the basophilic components of cells contain nucleic acids; however, not all cellular basophilia is attributable to these substances. Moreover, the basic nature of some proteins with which nucleic acids are associated will impart an acidophilia. The nucleolus of cells is a good example. Specific histochemical tests are available for DNA (Fuelgen stain) and RNA (ribonuclease).

Although nucleotides are essential components of nucleic acids, not all nucleotides are confined to these macromolecules. *Adenosine triphosphate (ATP)* is a high energy storage compound that releases energy for cellular processes when a phosphate bond is broken and the compound is converted to *adenosine diphosphate (ADP)*. The conversion process, ADP$\rightleftharpoons$ATP, is the means of energy storage and release upon demand.

Cyclic adenosine monophosphate (cAMP) is an important free nucleotide and is considered a second messenger within the cell. Upon stimulation of specific receptors on cell membranes, *adenyl cyclase* activity increases and causes an increased formation of cAMP from ATP. The increased levels of cAMP stimulate enzymatic reactions. Also, studies of cAMP in bacteria have demonstrated that this compound may be a factor in gene regulation.

Proteins. Proteins, as the primary structural and functional components of cells, are essential for the architectural and metabolic integrity of living systems. These are macromolecules which are composed of repeating amino acid units joined covalently. This *peptide linkage* is formed by the carboxyl group (−COOH) of one amino acid being joined to the amino group (−NH$_2$) of another amino acid with the extrusion of one molecule of water. The particular sequence of amino acids in a protein is called the *primary structure*. If the number of amino acids produces a molecular weight greater than 10,000 then the molecule is a protein; less than 10,000 it is a *polypeptide*.

The regular, coiled conformation of peptide chains represents the *secondary structure*. This is especially the characteristic of the α-helix of fibrous proteins. Some peptides, however, are sufficiently folded to impart a globular configuration referred to as the *tertiary structure*. The *quarternary structure* results from the association of a number of globular and/or fibrous proteins. The fibrous proteins of cells include fibrinogen, myosin and tropocollagen. The globular proteins are the biologically most active substances. These include the enzymes, some hormones and the structural proteins of membranes.

Proteins occur as *simple (native)* or *conjugated* proteins. Simple proteins yield only amino acids upon hydrolysis, whereas conjugated proteins yield amino acids and nonproteinaceous prosthetic groups. Examples of simple proteins include the albumins, globulins and histones. The numerous and diverse types of conjugated proteins are classified generally on the type of prosthetic group. *Nucleoproteins* are those macromolecules which consist of a nucleic acid and protein. *Chromoproteins* contain a metal which imparts pigmentation to the protein. Hemoglobin is a good example. *Glycoproteins* or *mucoproteins* are proteins which contain a carbohydrate prosthetic group. Examples are mucin and the organic matrices of cartilage and bone. *Lipoproteins* are characterized by a lipid prosthetic group. The

components of cellular membranes are common examples of these macromolecules. *Phosphoproteins* contain a phosphorus prosthetic group; milk casein is an example.

As true *ampholytes*, proteins are capable of acting as acids or bases, depending upon the pH of their environment. Therefore, they will stain with the conventional acidic and basic stains used in histology. These large, nondiffusible and charged colloids are stabilized with most fixatives in such a way as to permit visualization (staining) with minimal denaturation (alteration to their tertiary structure).

Carbohydrates. Many carbohydrates are important to the cell. These compounds are classified as *monosaccharides, oligosaccharides* and *polysaccharides*. Monosaccharides conform to the formula $(CH_2O)_n$. The pentose sugars (n = 5) are characterized by ribose and deoxyribose. Their significance in nucleic acids was discussed previously. Glucose, fructose and galactose are hexose sugars (n = 6). The monosaccharides are important because they serve as immediate sources of energy (glucose) and as the building blocks of more complex orders of molecular organization. These polymers may consist of unaltered monosaccharides, amino sugars, uronic acids or a combination of these monomers. *Amino sugars* are characterized by the replacement of one of the hydroxyl groups with a primary amine. Such a replacement on glucose results in glucosamine. The oxidation of the hydroxyl group in the C_6 position results in a *uronic acid*. If the monosaccharide were glucose, then glucuronic acid would result. These forms of the monosaccharides occur in many polysaccharides: chondroitin sulfates of cartilage matrix, matrix components of loose connective tissue (hyaluronic acid) and the anticoagulant heparin.

The union of two monosaccharides via a glycosidic linkage results in the formation of a specific form of oligosaccharide—a *disaccharide*. Examples are maltose and sucrose. Progressive addition of monomeric units results in the formation of longer chain saccharides. Arbitrarily, a chain of 10 or more monosaccharides is called a polysaccharide.

Glycogen is one of the most important intracellular polysaccharides. It is the storage form of energy for the cell. Other polysaccharides that are important are hyaluronic acid, heparin, sialic acid, chondroitin sulfates, dermatan sulfate and keratan sulfate. Many polysaccharides, beside those listed, occur as prosthetic groups of conjugated proteins. These complexes, referred to as mucoproteins or glycoproteins, are more simply called *mucosubstances (proteoglycans)*. Distinction of the polysaccharides is often made on the basis of the presence or absence of acid groups. Accordingly, some are *acid mucopolysaccharides (acid mucosubstances)* and *neutral mucopolysaccharides (neutral mucosubstances)*.

Most carbohydrates can be stained for visualization with the microscope. (Glucose, however, is difficult to demonstrate by routine techniques because it is highly water soluble. The use of PAS and special staining techniques for glycogen were discussed in Chapter 2.) Histochemical methods are available for the demonstration of mucosubstances. These methods are complex but are effective when used diligently. *Metachromasia* is an important staining property of acid mucosubstances. This phenomenon, although not completely understood, is defined as a shift of color from that of the original dye to a new color following the formation of the stain-tissue complex. Many stains possess this characteristic. Aldehyde fuchsin is one of the stains used commonly. Unfortunately, metachromatic staining fades with time. Alcian blue is an effective stain for demonstrating metachromasia without the problem of fading.

Lipids. Lipids comprise a heterogeneous group of compounds which subserve a variety of functions. *Neutral fats* are esters of fatty acids and glycerol which are stored within cells as sources of high energy. Hydrolysis of fats yields the previously esterified components. The fatty acids may undergo β-oxidation with the acetyl groups (2-carbon chains) becoming activated as acetyl-CoA. Acetyl-CoA, then, can enter the tricarboxylic acid cycle (TCA cycle) by condensing with oxaloacetic acid. Fatty acid metabolism is an important source of activated acetate to drive the TCA cycle.

Phospholipids are fats in which one of the fatty acids has been replaced by a phosphoric acid and a nitrogen-containing compound, such as choline, ethanolamine or serine. Lecithin, cephalin and sphingomyelin are examples, respectively. These compounds, with structural proteins, are important constituents of cellular membranes and the myelin sheath. Because these compounds are characterized by polar (hydrophilic) and nonpolar (hydrophobic) ends, they are an effective means of achieving chemical and physical compartmentalization of the cell.

Sterols comprise a group of lipids which have the basic structure of the cyclopentanoperhydrophenanthrene ring. Cholesterol may be considered the prototype compound. Cholesterol, itself, is an important component of cell membranes. Many sterols function as hormones. These include estrogen, testosterone, progesterone, glucocorticoids and mineralocorticoids.

A large group of lipids is complexed with sugars as *glycolipids*. These are the cerebrosides and gangliosides which are essential components of cell membranes.

Waxes are similar to the neutral fats, except they consist of longer chain fatty acids. They are cellular products which serve protective functions.

Lipids can be demonstrated in a histologic sample; however, lipid solvents must be avoided. The paraffin technique, therefore, is of little value. Commonly employed lipid dyes are osmium tetroxide and the Sudan stains.

Biologic Properties

The unique aggregation of the previously-described molecular components imparts the varied properties to protoplasm that are ascribed to living entities. Whereas free-living unicellular organisms are required to be totally self-contained and conduct all living processes, the metazoan organism is a complex array of numerous cells that are dependent upon one another for a variety of functions. Significantly, these cells are not only interdependent but interact in such a way as to maintain an ideal internal environment in which all constituent cells may flourish. This interdependence or *division of labor* requires that some cells perform specific functions beyond those simply essential for survival. The following properties are characteristic of cells:

Metabolism is a process that is basic to all cells. It is the sum of all chemical reactions that occur within the cell. Reactions resulting in the synthesis of new molecular components that are essential for growth, maintenance and repair are termed *anabolic*. Those reactions that result in the degradation of cellular components or products with a release of energy are termed *catabolic*. *Internal respiration*, or the chemical utilization of foodstuffs for the production of energy, is the classic example of catabolism. Whereas catabolism is an energy-producing process, anabolism is an energy-requiring process. Not all cells are characterized by the same metabolic activity or requirements. Although all cells must produce energy, different pathways may be utilized. Oxidative pathways (TCA cycle) are essential for the cells of the brain, whereas skeletal muscle cells can function for some time in an oxygen-deprived environment. Similarly, some cells are highly modified for the synthesis and secretion of proteins (hepatocytes, plasma cells, fibroblasts), while others are modified for the storage and secretion of lipids (adipocytes, spongiocytes). The basis for the similarities and differences is found in the molecular constituents of the protoplasm.

Irritability is that property of cells enabling them to respond to stimuli in their environment. It is this property of reactivity to stimuli that accounts for the biologic behavior of cells. The contraction of muscle cells, the secretions of glands and the generation of nerve impulses are basic reactions predicated upon irritability. A unique aspect of irritability is that of *conductivity*. This is the special property of some cells (nerve, muscle) to transmit waves of excitation along their cell membranes. It is a special form of information transmission.

A special form of the reactivity of cells is that manifested as *contractility*. Most cells are capable of changing shape, but muscle cells are uniquely adapted to change shape by shortening along their long axes. This characteristic enables them to accomplish work.

Endocytotic and exocytotic processes are essential for the *homeostasis* of all cells. *Endocytosis* is that process characterized by materials gaining access to the cell. Some fluids and components thereof may diffuse through the plasmalemma. Other fluids may gain entry via vacuoles formed in the cell membrane that eventually are "pinched-off" within the cytoplasm. These events are characteristic of *pinocytosis*. The engulfment and uptake of particulate matter is a special form of endocytosis called *phagocytosis*. The exit of materials from the cell is *exocytosis*. The egress from the cell of the waste products of metabolic processes is termed *excretion*, whereas the movement out of the cell of special products synthesized by it is termed *secretion*.

Growth, maintenance and *reproduction* of the protoplasm are universal characteristics. New molecular components are constantly added, while others are replaced continually. A normal cell, however, is incapable of continuous and unchecked growth. Most cells are spheroids; they are unable to support their increasing volumes because of the limitation imposed by their surface areas. The attainment of this critical mass is generally a stimulus for mitosis. Not all cells retain the capacity to divide; some, however, retain a high mitotic potential.

General Morphologic Characteristics

The division of labor and specialization that characterizes the component cells of metazoans results in functionally diverse and interdependent cellular populations. This specialization is so precise that functional inferences can be made from structure alone; the converse is true also. Despite the degree of specialization, most cells have characteristics in common (Fig. 4.1). The morphologic diversity of cells is the basis for the subsequent discussion. Various morphologic characteristics are demonstrated in Plate II.

Cellular Shape. The shape of an animal cell is often described as spheroidal; this is a misleading and poor generalization. Specialization has a profound influence on cell shape. Cellular contact and pressure, as well as the inherent ability to alter shape, are determinants of morphological configuration. Thus, a cell may be round (Fig. 4.2),

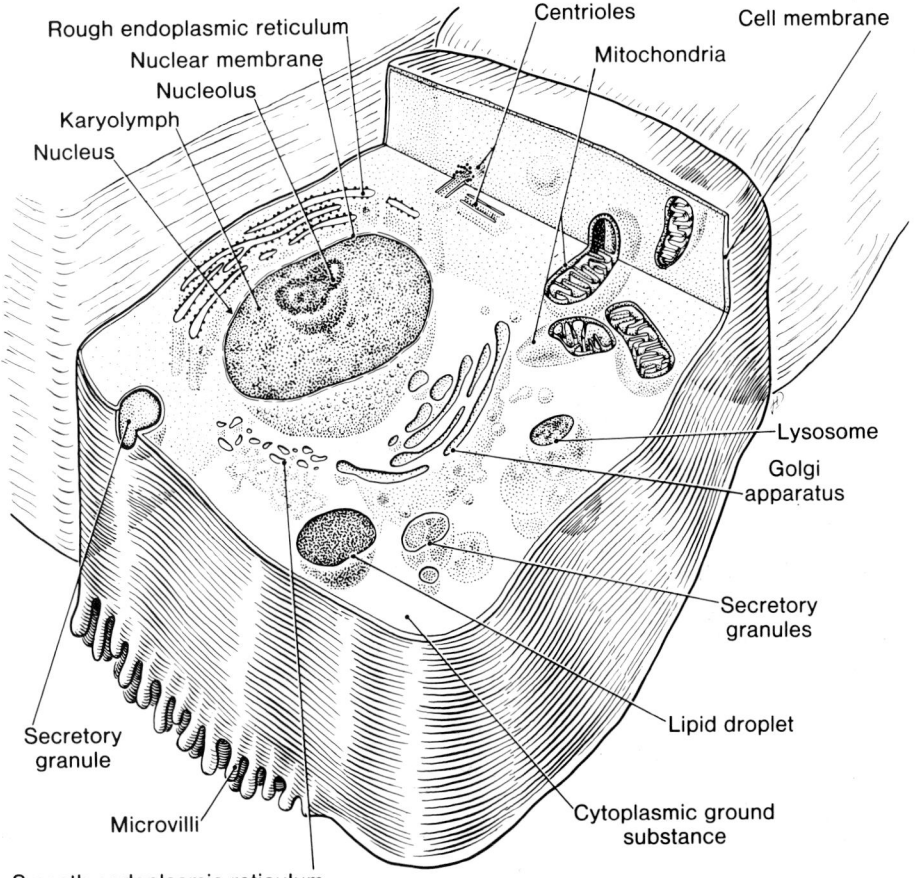

Fig. 4.1 Schematic diagram of a typical cell. The major cellular components are included and labeled.

Rough endoplasmic reticulum
Nuclear membrane
Nucleolus
Karyolymph
Nucleus
Centrioles
Cell membrane
Mitochondria
Lysosome
Golgi apparatus
Secretory granules
Lipid droplet
Secretory granule
Microvilli
Cytoplasmic ground substance
Smooth endoplasmic reticulum

stellate (Fig. 4.3), spindle-shaped (Fig. 4.4), elongated (Fig. 4.5), columnar (Fig. 4.6), squamous (Fig. 4.7), cuboidal (Fig. 4.8) and myriad other shapes. Some cells may progress through a number of these shapes before a definitive shape is attained. Also, cellular shape is influenced in such a way as to indicate the type and amount of specific functional activity taking place within the cell.

Cellular Structure. Despite the diversity of cellular shape, the constituent organelles generally are positioned spatially in an organized and predictable manner. The nuclei of round, spheroidal, cuboidal or spindle-shaped cells are usually rounded and located centrally (Fig. 4.2). Other shapes may characterize the nuclei of round cells (Fig. 4.9). The nuclei become ovoid and oriented parallel to the long axis as cells become elongated (Figs. 4.10, 4.11). Nuclear position and shape may be correlated with the position of other organelles, as well as with the shape of the cell.

The Golgi apparatus is located generally in a juxtanuclear position, while the position of other organelles (rough endoplasmic reticulum, smooth endoplasmic reticulum, mitochondria) and inclusions (secretory droplets, fat) will vary with the specific cell type considered. The numbers and types of organelles and inclusions are a function of degree and type of specialization also.

Most notably, many cells (especially epithelial cells) are spatially polarized (Fig. 4.12). The nuclei of such cells are usually positioned eccentrically, and there is a corresponding orderly spatial relationship of other organelles and inclusions. Such organizational patterns are usually associated with secretory activity.

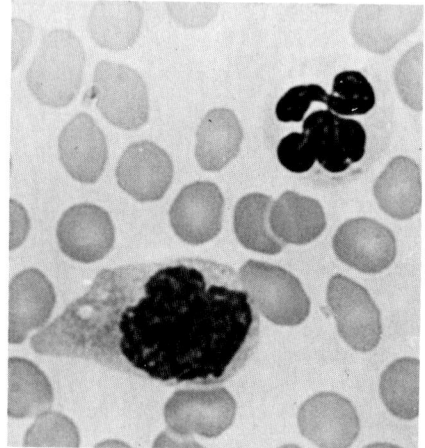

Fig. 4.2 Round cells. The large round cells are feline leukocytes. The cell with the lobulated nucleus (*top*) is spheroidal. The cell with the round nucleus (*bottom*) is elongated slightly. The background cells are erythrocytes devoid of nuclei. X400. All light micrographs are labeled as the magnification with the microscope before photographic enlarging. All electron micrographs are labeled as total magnification, including photographic enlarging.

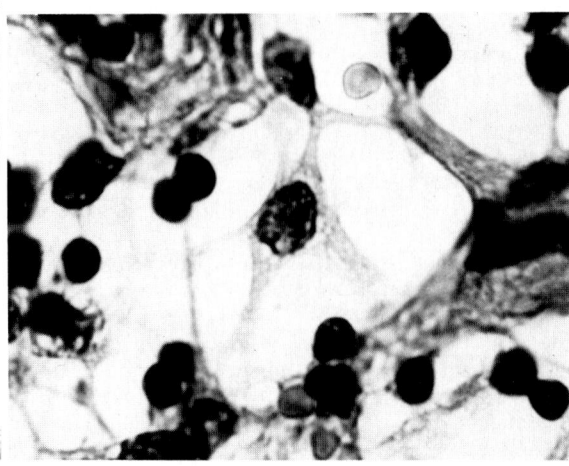

Fig. 4.3 Stellate Cell. A reticular cell from a canine lymph node is in the center of the field. The elongated cytoplasmic processes impart a star-shaped appearance. X160.

In certain types of cells, mitochondria assume positions in intimate contact with foldings of the plasma membrane. Such associations are generally indicative of active transport and the movement of high volumes of fluid.

Cellular Size. Cells vary not only among the various groups of animals (*interspecific*) but even within the body of a specified organism (*intraspecific*). There is no correlation, however, between the size of the organism and the size of its cells; i.e., the cells of the horse will not be significantly larger than the cells of the dog. Some cells are *macroscopic* (visible with the unaided eye), whereas others have a wide range of *microscopic sizes* (visible only with the aided eye). The *perikaryon* of a microgliocyte may be a few micrometers in diameter; the red blood corpuscle (RBC) ranges from 4–7 μm in diameter depending on the species, while the ovum may be as large as 300 μm in diameter. (Incidentally, because RBC's will appear in most sections examined, they can serve as a built-in micrometer.) The length of a striated muscle cell may be in inches, although the length of a nerve cell extending from the ventral horn of the spinal cord to the tip of an appendage may be several feet long. Even within the narrow limits of microscopic observation, a wide diversity of size may exist in at least one dimension. Giant cells, such as the megakaryocytes, are appreciably larger than developing red blood corpuscles (Fig. 4.13). Similarly, striated muscle cells are much larger than the fibroblasts associated with them. Generally, most mammalian cells will range between 10 and 30 μm.

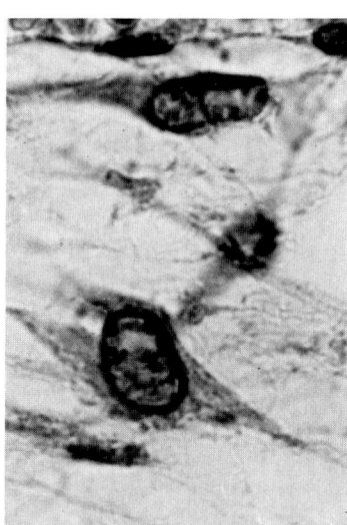

Fig. 4.4 Spindle-shaped cells. The elongated and flattened cells are mesenchymal cells from a sample of bovine loose connective tissue. These cells may appear stellate in a different plane of section. X400.

Nucleus

The nucleus, as a constantly occurring and required component of most cells, is responsible for the control and mediation of numerous cellular activities. The information necessary for the control of cellular activity is encoded in the DNA macromolecules. This information is the basis for all generalized cellular form and function, because all nuclei contain the same genetic information. The unique features of specialized cells is a manifestation of the differential utilization of this genetic information by the repression or derepression of specific gene loci. Some functional correlations with nuclear morphology are possible. The most distinguishable of these are the morphologic criteria associated with a dividing (*mitotic*) and nondividing (*intermitotic, interphase* or *vegetative*) cell. Because the greatest number of cells encountered in the body will be performing vegetative functions, the interphase nucleus will be discussed first. The features of the mitotic nucleus will be discussed subsequently.

In the interphase nucleus, four distinct components may be identified: *nuclear membrane, karyolymph, chromatin* and *nucleolus* (Fig. 4.14).

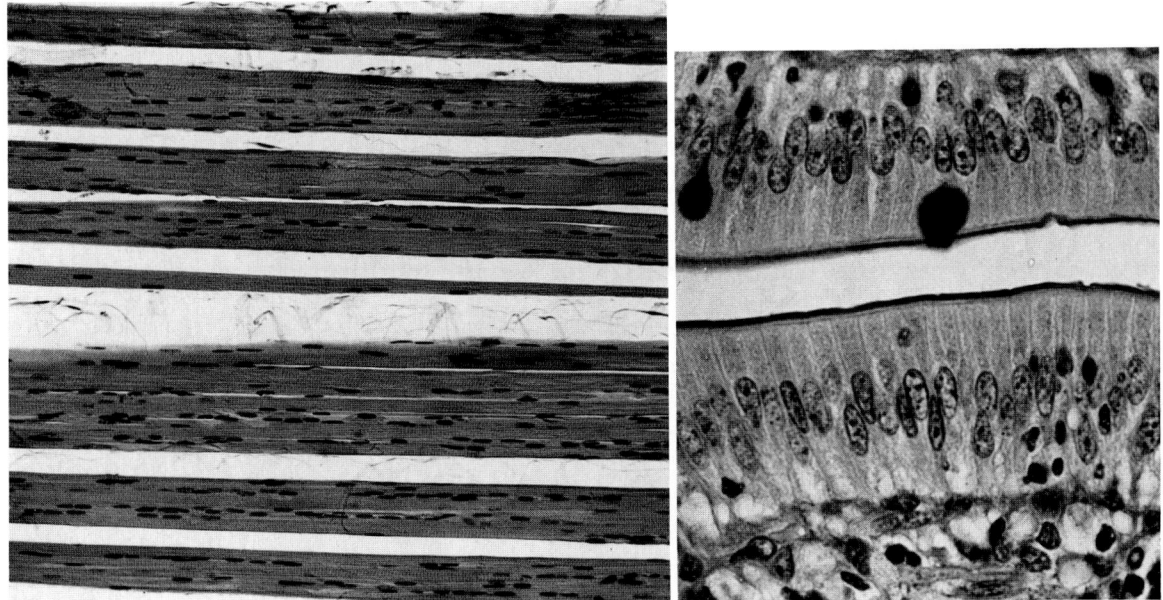

Fig. 4.5   Elongated Cells. The elongated multinucleated cells are skeletal muscle cells. X40.

Fig. 4.6   Columnar cells. These lining cells are longer than they are wide. Compare this micrograph with the drawing of columnar cells in Figure 3.10. X160.

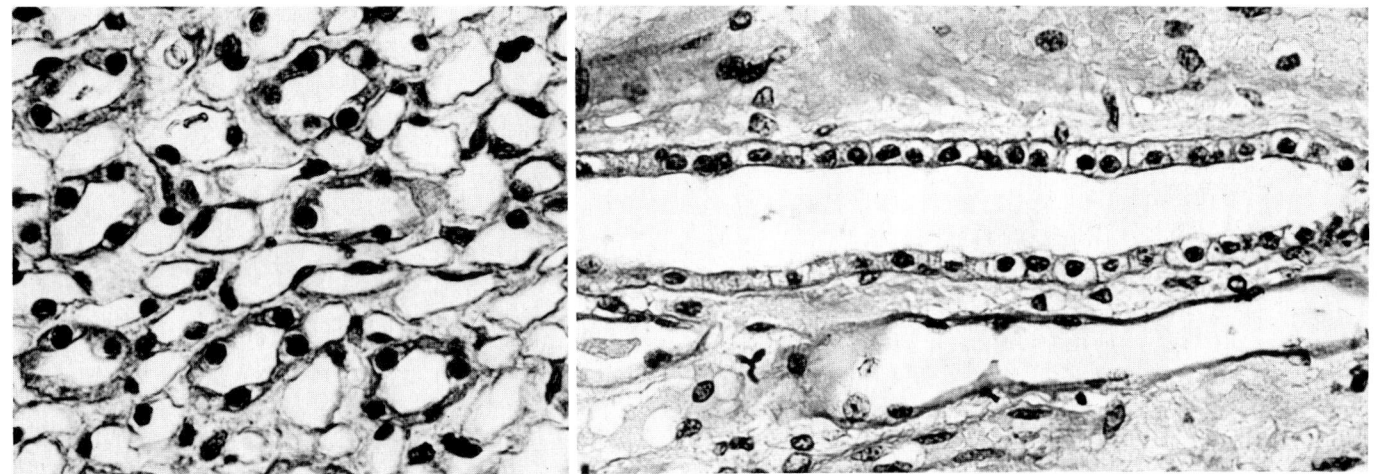

Fig. 4.7   Squamous cells of the tubules of a canine kidney. The tubules are lined by flattened cells with a prominent nucleus. The cytoplasm appears as thin rims of dark-staining material. X160.

Fig. 4.8   Cuboidal cells. The cuboidal cells line the lumen of a tubule from the canine kidney. Appearing as squares in biplanar sections, the cells have a cuboidal shape in three dimensions. X100.

Number. Most often a cell will be mononucleated (Figs. 4.2–4.4, 4.6, 4.8–4.10). Some, however, may be *binucleated*, while others may be *multinucleated* (Fig. 4.15). Other extremes may range from enucleation, as in the mammalian erythrocyte (Figs. 4.2, 4.9) and certain cells of the lens, to the case of the spermatozoon, in which the bulk of the cell is composed of a nucleus.

Shape. Nuclear morphology varies with the shape of the cell. Round to oval cells usually possess a similarly shaped nucleus (Figs. 4.3, 4.8, 4.9). Elongated cells usually possess an elongated nucleus (Figs. 4.5, 4.6, 4.10, 4.11). Others however, may possess nuclei that are crescent-shaped or lobulated (Figs. 4.2, 4.9).

Position. The position of nuclei within cells is variable. They may be central, paracentral or eccentrically-positioned. However, specific cell types are characterized generally by similarly or identically positioned nuclei. Definite spatial relationships are identifiable between the nucleus, cytoplasmic organelles and inclusions. These are apparent especially when a cell has a distinct polarity (Fig. 4.12). Cells that accumulate large quantities of inclusions or secretory products (adipose cells, goblet cells) may have nuclei that are flattened against the margin of the cell.

It is important to remember that the position of the nucleus within a cell may not be apparent in all planes of section. The nucleus may be above or below the plane of section.

In some cells, the nucleus may be the only dominant feature (Fig. 4.4). Stellate or squamous cells may possess small quantities of cytoplasm that are difficult to resolve with light microscopy (Fig. 4.7). Lining cells (endothelium) of blood vessels and lymph vessels, lining cells of certain kidney tubules and the alveolar lining cells of the lung may give the impression of having a large nucleus and little else.

Nuclear Envelope. A darkly basophilic (blue-staining with hematoxylin) line of demarcation between the nucleus and sur-

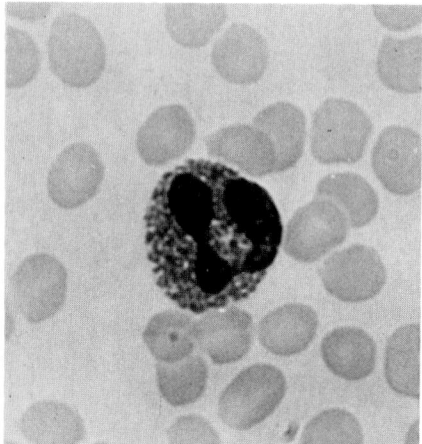

Fig. 4.9 A round cell with a lobulated nucleus. The nuclear configuration is typical of this feline eosinophil. X400.

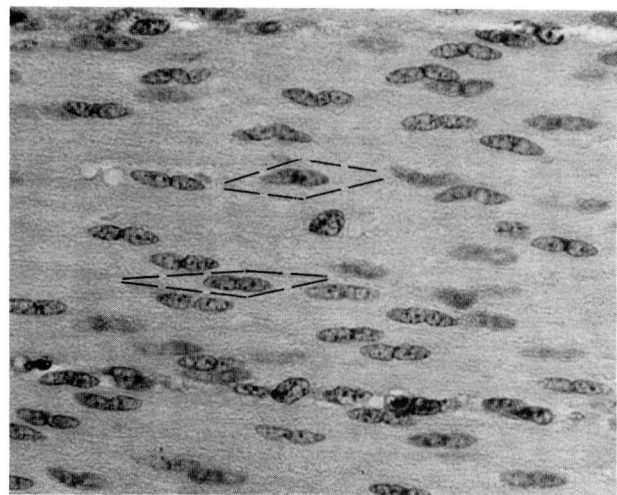

Fig. 4.11 Smooth muscle cells from the intestine of a dog. The approximate margins of the cells are indicated by *dashed lines*. The elongated nuclei are oriented along the long axes of the cells. X160.

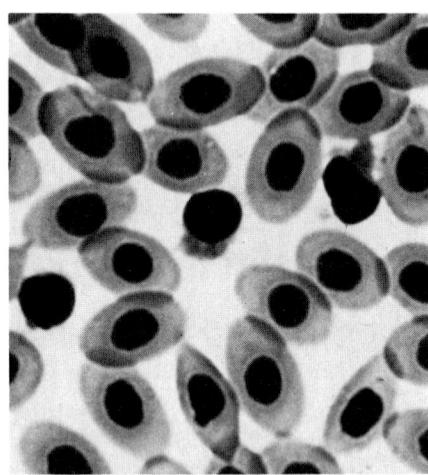

Fig. 4.10 Avian erythrocytes. The slightly elongated cells contain elongated nuclei oriented parallel to the long axis of the cells. X400. Compare with Figure 4.6.

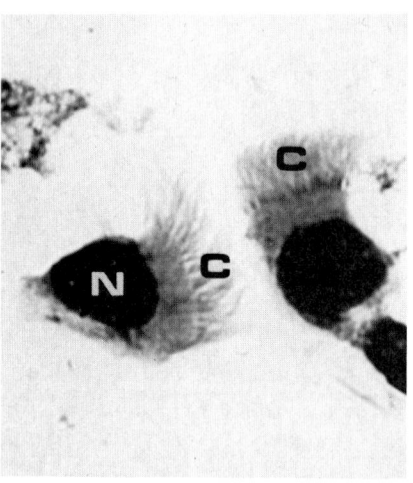

Fig. 4.12 Polarized cells. These ciliated cells were exfoliated from the epithelial lining of the trachea. The nuclei (N) are displaced basally. The apical borders have cilia (C). Polarization of cellular components, as evidenced by basal displacement of the nuclei, is a typical epithelial characteristic. X160.

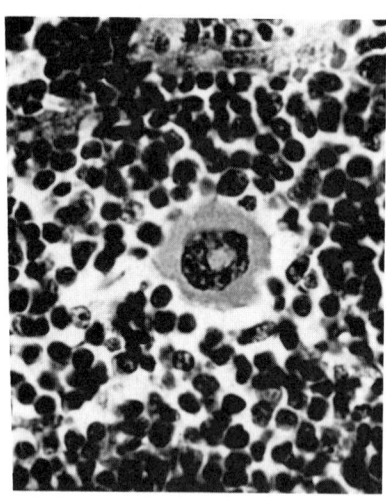

Fig. 4.13 A megakaryocyte and other cells of the bone marrow. The megakaryocyte in the center of the field is many times larger than the cells surrounding it. X100.

rounding cytoplasm is apparent in light microscopic sections (Figs. 4.2, 4.3, 4.4). This limiting membrane represents a condensation of nuclear and cytoplasmic components, as well as stain, on either side of the *nuclear membrane* or *nuclear envelope*. The electron microscope (Fig. 4.16) reveals two membranes comprising the nuclear envelope, the *inner* and *outer nuclear membranes*. Each of these measures approximately 7.5 nm and they are separated from each other by a *perinuclear space* or *cisterna* that varies from 40 to 70 nm wide. The perinuclear space, and thus the outer nuclear membrane, is continuous with profiles of the rough endoplasmic reticulum (Fig. 4.17). *Ribonucleic protein* or *ribosomes* are often attached to the outer nuclear membrane. The intimate relationship of rough endoplasmic reticular profiles to the nuclear membrane is especially apparent near the termination of mitosis. Rough endoplasmic

reticulum forms the nuclear envelope. The inner nuclear membrane is sometimes associated with filaments that form a *fibrous lamina* along its nuclear (inner) margin. The nuclear envelope is not a continuous, uninterrupted, structural entity. Rather, the inner and outer nuclear membranes are continuous and reflected at certain points. Points of discontinuity or fusions between the inner and outer membranes are manifested as openings or *nuclear pores* (Fig. 4.18). The nuclear pores are approximately 70 nm in diameter. When sectioning perpendicular to the nuclear membrane is accomplished, they appear to be covered by a septum or diaphragm that is thinner than the membranes that limit the pore (Fig. 4.16). On face view, these structures have a

more complex architecture than is visible in the perpendicular plane (Fig. 4.18). Filamentous material appears to contribute to a centrally-positioned *annulus*. This morphology is indicative of open communication between the nucleus and cytoplasm. Unfortunately, little is known of the biochemical composition and physiologic properties of this complex. The degree of architectural organization, however, implies that nuclear pores may form a highly selective and specialized complex for the passage of materials between the nucleus and cytoplasm.

Nuclear Matrix. The aforementioned limiting membrane encloses the *matrix of the nucleus*. This *nuclear sap* or *karyolymph* is the soluble phase of nuclear material. With the information gained from electron micrographs it is apparent that it is more than simply a fluid material. Accordingly, the

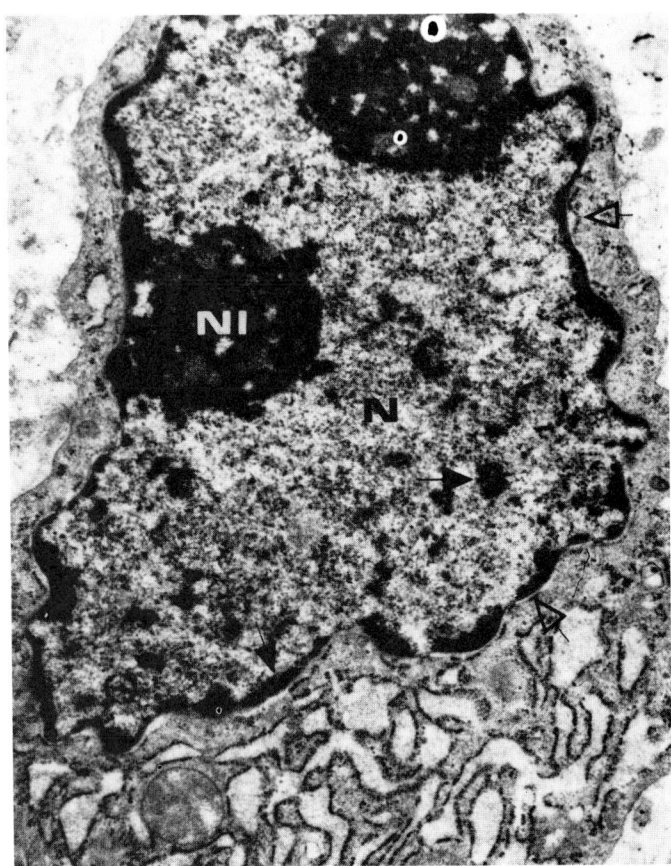

thetic activity of a cell. The more heterochromatin, the less active is the cell; the more euchromatin, the greater will be the potential protein synthesis (Figs. 4.14, 4.19).

Some of the hetereochromatin is distinguishable as a *Barr body*. These bodies consist of a condensation of one of the X chromosomes. The female of a species contains two X chromosomes; one is condensed, inactive and visible as a Barr body. The other one is active in metabolic processes and part of the euchromatin of the nucleus. Because the male contains one Y and one X chromosome, it is assumed that the X chromosome remains active during interphase. The presence of a Barr body in normal circumstances identifies the cell as a female (Plate VI. 23).

Nucleolus. The *nucleolus*, or "little nucleus," is a prominently staining, highly refractive, smooth-surfaced body found in the nucleus (Fig. 4.19). It may occur singly or there may be more than one. It is readily identifiable in those cells involved in protein synthesis. Also, it is a characteristic of blastoid and malignant cells.

Fig. 4.14 An electron micrograph of a fibroblast of loose connective tissue. The nucleus (N) contains two nucleoli (NI). Heterochromatin (*solid arrows*) is interspersed with euchromatin. The nuclear envelope (*open arrows*) surrounds the nucleus. The condensation of heterochromatin along the peripheral margin of the nucleus precludes the visualization of the inner nuclear membrane at this magnification. X16,000.

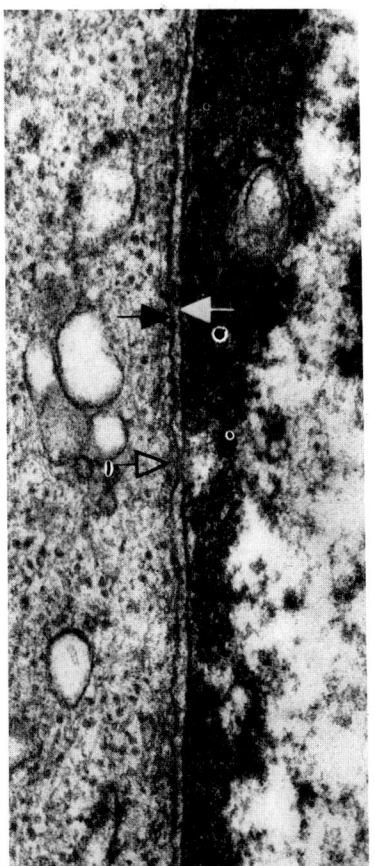

Fig. 4.16 An electron micrograph of the nuclear membrane of a fibroblast. The outer nuclear membrane (*black arrow*) is separated from the inner nuclear membrane (*white arrow*) by the nuclear cistern. Heterochromatin obliterates portions of the inner nuclear membrane. A nuclear pore (*open arrow*) is apparent. X52,000.

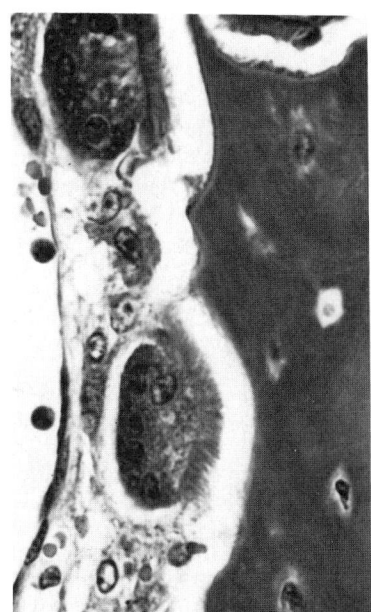

Fig. 4.15 Multinucleated cells of bone. The osteoclasts contain a variable number of nuclei. X100.

terms *nuclear matrix* and *nuclear ground substance* have been proposed to describe it more precisely.

Chromatin. *Chromatin* is contained within the confines of the nuclear envelope and is suspended in the nuclear matrix. The term, chromatin, is actually used to describe any area in the nucleus suspected of containing *deoxyribonucleic acid* (DNA) and its bound protein. Different types of chromatic material are recognizable during the interphase. *Heterochromatin* is that chromatin which is deeply stained with basic dyes and is condensed (Figs. 4.12, 4.14). It is metabolically inert. *Euchromatin* stains lightly, is dispersed and is the metabolically active form of DNA (Figs. 4.14, 4.19). Various ratios of heterochromatin/euchromatin will appreciably alter the appearance of a nucleus from *condensed* (much heterochromatin) to *open* or *vesicular* (little heterochromatin). These nuclear features are aids for the identification of specific cell types. In some instances, the spatial distribution of one to the other is a diagnostic feature of some cell types. Most significantly, the amount of euchromatin is an indicator of the potential protein-syn-

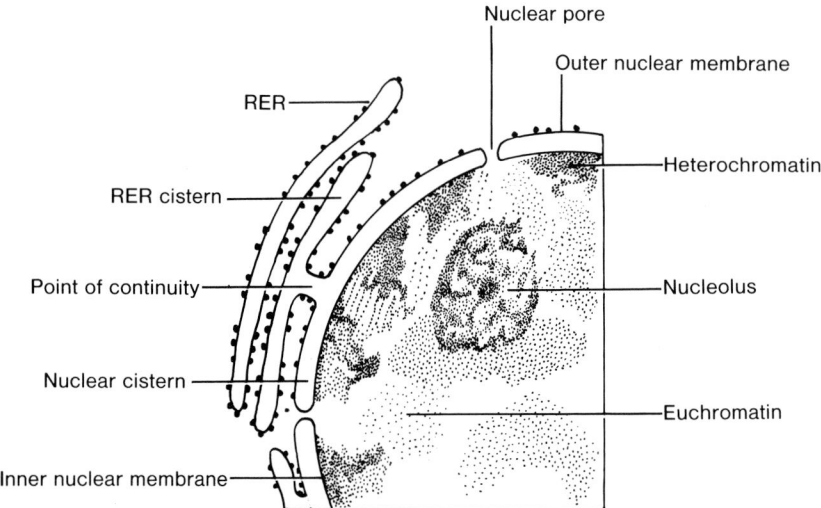

Fig. 4.17 A schematic representation of a portion of the nucleus and rough endoplasmic reticulum (RER) as visualized with the electron microscope. The perinuclear space or cistern is continuous with the cistern of the RER. Ribosomes are attached to the outer nuclear membrane.

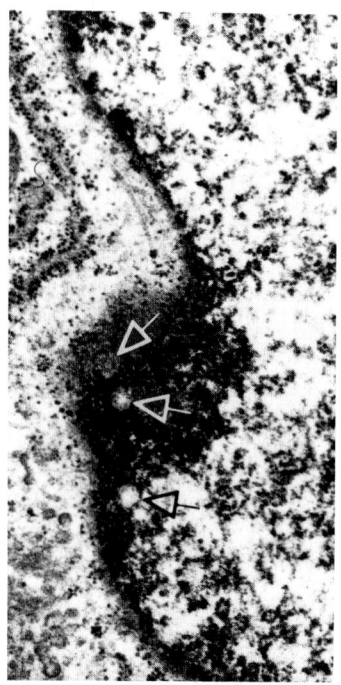

Fig. 4.18 An electron micrograph of the face view of a nuclear membrane. The nuclear pores (*open arrows*) are not simple openings between the nucleus and cytoplasm. An annulus (*upper arrow*) and particulate matter (*middle arrow*) characterize the apertures. X23,000.

Examination of electron micrographs reveals that this structure is a discrete body that is not membrane-bound (Fig. 4.20). It occurs freely in the nucleus or may be attached to the inner nuclear membrane. It is composed of filamentous (*pars fibrosa*) and granular (*pars granulosa*) materials, both of which contain RNA. Chromatin material surrounds or extends into the nucleolus. This *nucleolus-associated chromatin* represents specific areas on specific chromosomes called *nucleolus organizers*.

The filamentous and granular components form thread-like and anastomotic strands called the *nucleolonema* (Fig. 4.20). Densely packed filaments form a centrally-positioned and rounded mass called the *pars amorpha*. Both sets of terms, pars fibrosa/pars granulosa and nucleolonema/pars amorpha, are applicable to this structure. The latter set of terms, however, is more descriptive of the morphologic features.

The nucleolus is the center for the synthesis of rRNA. The ribosomal subunits may be formed in the pars fibrosa, mature in the pars granulosa and subsequently assembled into functional ribosomes in the cytoplasm.

Because this structure contains high concentrations of RNA, basophilic staining characteristics can be anticipated. Various functional states of the cell, however, may cause an acidophilia. These staining properties are dependent upon the relative amounts of RNA and acidic/basic proteins that are present.

Cytoplasm

General Characteristics. The cytoplasm, which is composed of numerous biochemical and morphologic entities, is present (in varying amounts) in all living cells. The types, kinds and numbers of morphologically and biochemically identifiable components are responsible for the specializations that contribute to histologic identification.

The bulk of the cytoplasm, or *ground substance*, is an admixture of water, protein, carbohydrates, organic salts and inorganic salts. The physical characteristics of the cytoplasm are in a constant state of flux. Thus sol-gel properties are apparent. Although this is not generally apparent in somatic cells, some cells (egg cells, amoeboid cells) possess a clear, peripheral *ectoplasm* and an internal, granular *endoplasm*. The former is

more viscous (gel-like) and relatively free of organelles compared to the more fluid, granular (sol-like) and organelle-rich endoplasm.

The cytoplasm of mature somatic cells is generally *acidophilic*; however, it may be totally or focally *basophilic*, as well as totally or focally *chromophobic* or *neutrophilic*. These staining characteristics contribute to the overall light microscopic appearance of a cell, enabling the microscopist to identify numerous cell types. Numerous cytoplasmic components contribute to the general characteristics of a cell. Among these are the organelles, vacuoles, granules, crystals, droplets, amount and distribution of cytoplasm, amount and distribution of organelles and inclusions. The size, shape, location and number of nuclei, as well as the distribution of chromatin contained therein, are additional aids to the cellular morphologist.

Plasma Membrane, Glycocalyx and Cytomembranes. The *plasma membrane* (*plasmalemma, cell membrane*) encloses the entire cytoplasm and is that portion of the cell exposed to the extracellular environment. It is approximately 8.0 nm thick. Because the limit of resolution of the white light microscope is approximately 200 nm, it is impossible for the plasmalemma to be resolved. Despite this, *cellular limits* are discernible within the aforementioned limits of resolution. This is due to a condensation of structural protein, addition of stain and the condensation of contiguous materials at the interfaces, as well as the presence of a *cell coat*. The plasma membrane is not seen with light microscopy, but the cell limit does define the peripheral extent of the cell.

Despite the ability of the electron microscope to resolve the plasmalemma, no concise and definitive structure has been determined for this entity. It appears as a trilaminar structure composed of two *osmiophilic* bands separated by an *osmiophobic* band (Fig. 4.21). Each band is approximately 2.5 nm wide. This is supposed to correspond to a sandwich-like relationship in which two layers of protein are laid upon a layer of lipid (protein-lipid-protein). This structural design comprised the unit membrane concept and was supposed to be applicable to the structural configuration and biochemical composition of all membrane systems. Too many variations, structurally and chemically, have been observed (Fig. 4.22).

Various approaches have contributed to current knowledge of membrane structure—electron microscopy, physiology, biochemistry, physics, immunocytochemistry and freeze-fracture techniques. All seem to confirm that the most reasonable representation of membranes is the lipid-globular protein mosaic model (Fig. 4.23). The basic model is a bimolecular leaflet of phospholipids with their hydrophilic (polar) groups directed outward and their hydrophobic (nonpolar) groups directed inward. Proteins are

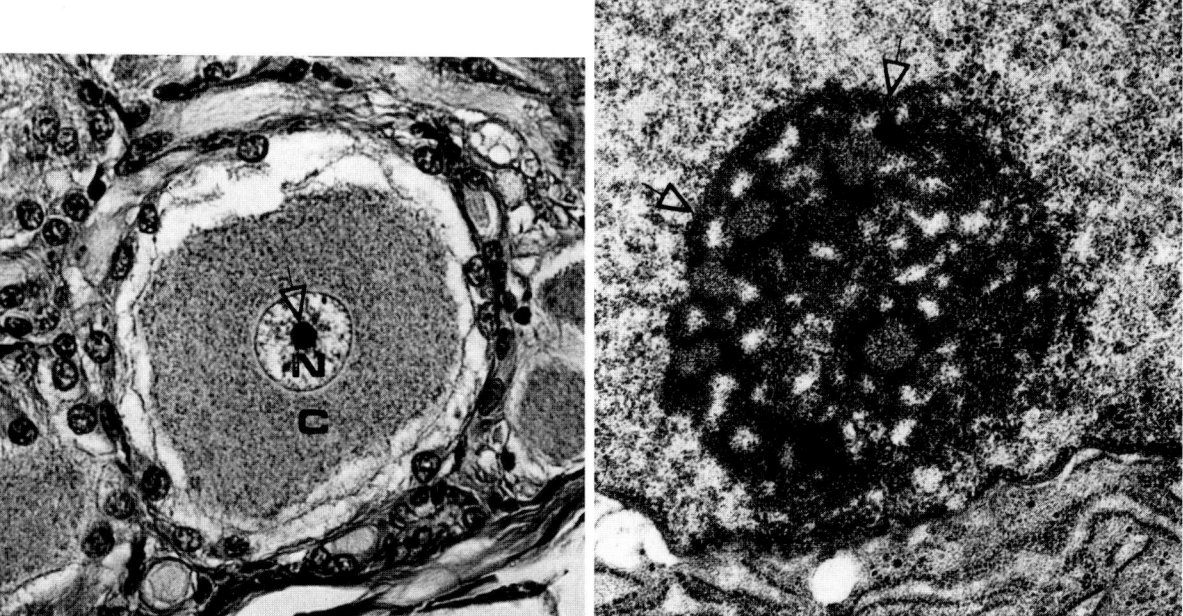

Fig. 4.19 A ganglion cell. The cytoplasm (C) contains a vesicular nucleus (N) in which euchromatic material predominates. A prominent nucleolus (*arrow*) is present. X100.

Fig. 4.20 An electron micrograph of a nucleolus. The nucleolonema (*arrows*) is the prominent feature of this section. X25,000.

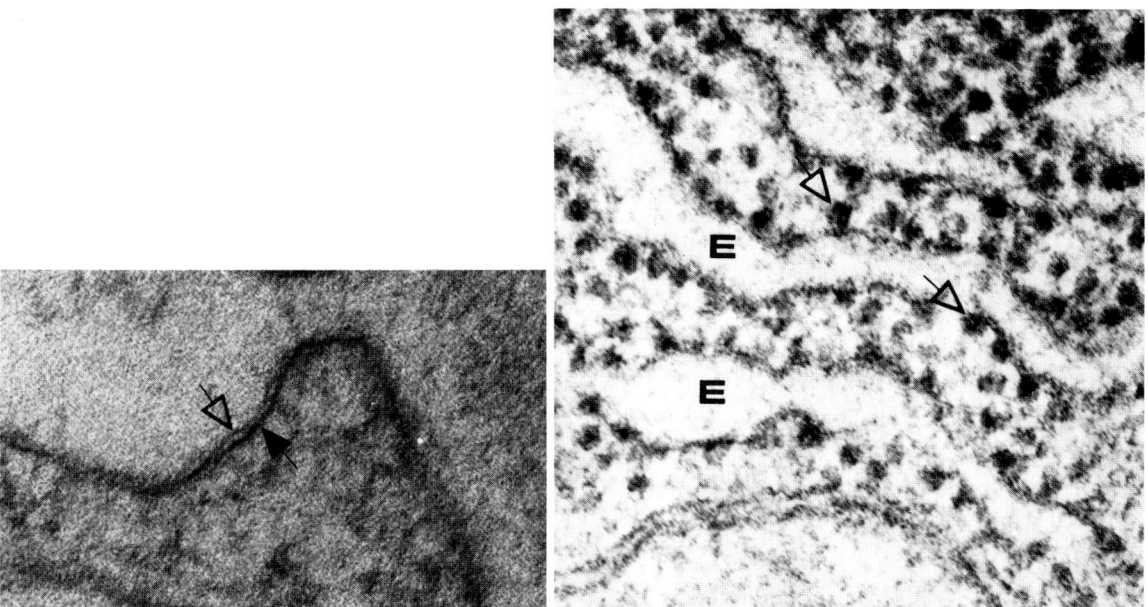

Fig. 4.21 Trilaminar plasma membrane. The outer, thinner lamina (*open arrow*) is separated by a translucent space from the inner, thicker lamina (*solid arrow*). X215,000.

Fig. 4.22 Globular cytoplasmic membranes. The cisterns (E) of the granular endoplasmic reticulum are membrane-bound and studded with ribosomes (*open arrows*). The trilaminar appearance is not evident. Rather, the membrane components appear to be globular. X156,000.

embedded within the lipid bilayer and project variously from either surface. Polysaccharides project from the outer surface. These are attached to proteins (glycoproteins) and lipids (glycolipids). The positions of the protein constituents are not constant. Instead, the changing properties and protein constituents (enzymes, receptor sites, antigenic sites, permeability sites) impart a fluid nature (fluid mosaic model) that appears to correspond to dynamic physiologic activities. The hydrophilic, globular proteins can account for the selective permeability of certain water-soluble substances and may function as pores, whereas the lipid components explain the relative ease of passage of lipid-soluble substances.

Continued research is essential to determine the precise morphologic, physiologic and biochemical nature of this structure. Continued refinement of the various models will lead ultimately to a greater understanding of cell membranes, those structures essential for many of the properties ascribed to cells.

The periphery of the plasma membrane is covered by a layer of material which is

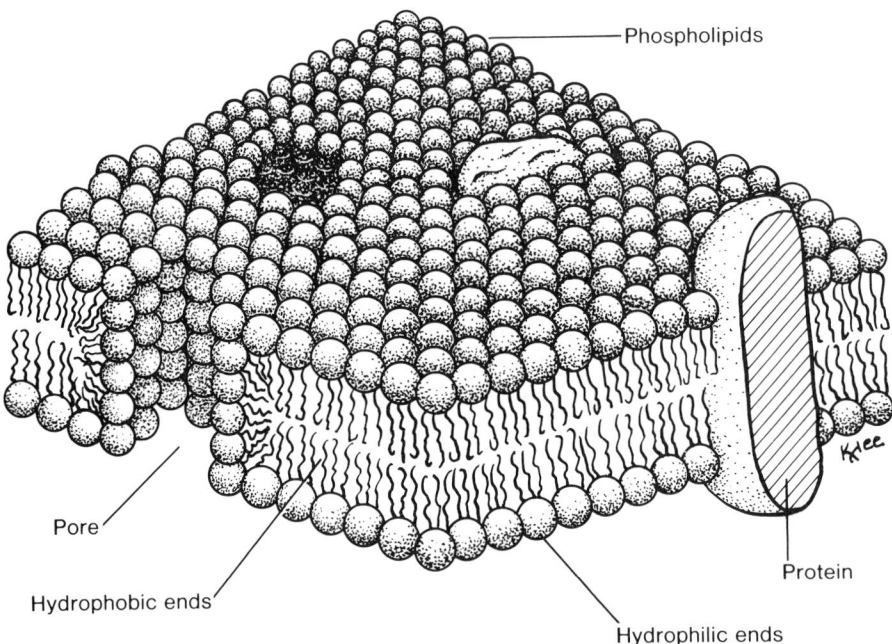

Phospholipids

Pore

Hydrophobic ends

Hydrophilic ends

Protein

Fig. 4.23 Schematic diagram of the mosaic model of membrane structure. Proteins are embedded within a sea of lipids. Pores probably represent the cores of proteins through which certain water-soluble constituents move rapidly. Carbohydrates, not depicted, are attached to protein and lipid components of the membrane.

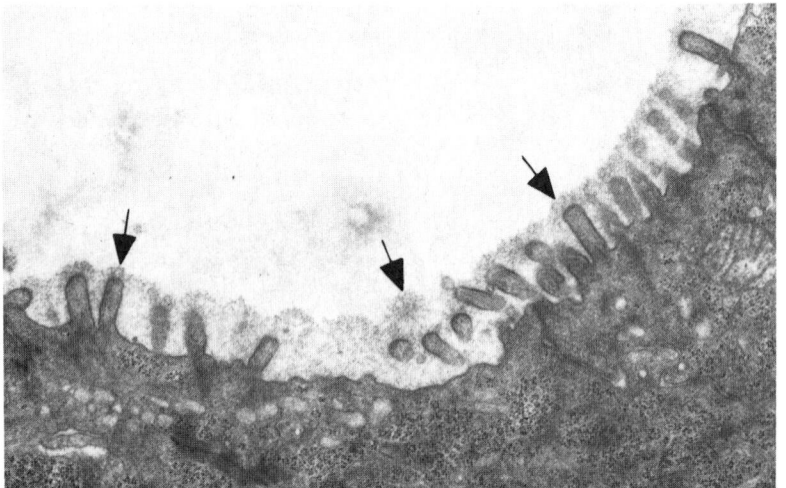

Fig. 4.24 An electron micrograph of the glycocalyx. The glycocalyx (*arrows*) covers the microvilli and apical surface of these mouse intestinal cells. X14,000. (Courtesy of A. M. Sheppard.)

rich in carbohydrates. The *glycocalyx* (*cell coat*) probably occurs on all cells and is well-developed on some. It appears as "fuzzy" material with the electron microscope (Fig. 4.24). The glycocalyx is attached to and is intimately integrated into the structural components of the plasmalemma as glycoproteins (*proteoglycans*) and glycolipids. The predominant polysaccharide is *sialic acid*. This imparts a negative charge through the ionization of its acidic groups. The polysaccharides of the cell coat account for its positive reaction with PAS (Fig. 4.25).

The characteristics of the cell coat are not uniform on all cells. Its morphology varies

with the free, lateral or basal surfaces of some cells, especially epithelial cells.

The functions of this cellular component are variable and significant. *Cellular recognition* may be achieved between cells based upon specific biochemical components contained within it. Cells in cultural monolayers maintain this relationship by *contact inhibition*. Cell-to-cell *adhesion* and attachment to associated connective tissue is achieved through this cellular component. *Absorption* of some materials involves the glycocalyx. Finally, *antigenicity* is associated with it.

Lipid and protein constituents, as described for the fluid mosaic model of the

plasmalemma, occur in the cytomembranes that are components of the organelles.

Ribosomes and Granular Endoplasmic Reticulum. The cytoplasm of many cells possesses either a total or focal basophilia which is referred to as the *ergastoplasm*. These areas contain high quantities of RNA and protein, *ribonucleoprotein* (*RNP*). Although tRNA and mRNA are present in the cytoplasm, the primary contributor to this staining property is ribosomal RNA. *Ribosomes* are small granules in the cytoplasm which consist of approximately 60% RNA and 40% protein. These structures occur in the cytoplasm as single units, *free ribosomes*, or as multiple units, *polyribosomes* or *polysomes* (Fig. 4.26). The free ribosomes and polysomes of the cytoplasm are responsible for the synthesis of protein for intracellular use. These free granules are characteristic features of differentiating and growing cells. They are the means by which these cells increase their quantity of structural and functional proteins.

An extensive network of tubules, flattened vesicles and cisternae extends throughout the cytoplasm of many cells. When ribosomes and polysomes are attached to this network (reticulum), the organelle is called the *granular* (*rough*) *endoplasmic reticulum* (Figs. 4.22, 4.26, 4.27). (Recall that this organelle is also continuous with the outer nuclear membrane.) In many cells, this organelle is scattered randomly throughout the cytoplasm. The distribution of this organelle in the plasma cell imparts a total cytoplasmic basophilia. In others, its distribution is associated with cellular polarity. The pancreatic acinar cell is an example of a cell characterized by a basally-positioned basophilia due to the polarized position of rough endoplasmic reticulum (Fig. 4.28). The proteins synthesized by the ribosomes of the rough endoplasmic reticulum (*RER*) are primarily for extracellular use. Examples include the humoral antibodies (immunoglobulins) produced by plasma cells and the digestive enzyme precursors secreted by the pancreatic acinar cells.

The type, quantity and distribution of ribosomes and RER afford valuable insights into cytoplasmic function. Nuclear and nucleolar morphology provide reasonable indications about cytoplasmic and cellular activity. A cell with a vesicular nucleus, prominent nucleolus and cytoplasmic basophilia can be expected to have a high potential for protein synthesis.

The details of the mechanisms of protein synthesis, intracellular transport and secretion are fascinating parts of cellular activities. Insights concerning these processes are the culmination of the combined efforts of histologists and biochemists using varied experimental methodologies. The process of protein synthesis is summarized graphically in Figure 4.29. The ribosome consists of subunits of *rRNA* which are synthesized in the nucleolus, transported to and subsequently assembled in the cytoplasm. The two *subunits* of unequal size form a groove at their point of contact. A slender strand of mRNA is believed to attach to the ribosomes at this groove. The *transcription* of the mRNA occurs on the euchromatic DNA and requires the enzyme *RNA polymerase.*

The messenger leaves the nucleus encoded with the proper information relating to amino acid sequence. This information (*codon*) results from various triplet combinations of the bases. Transfer RNA is synthesized in the nucleus and is active in the cytoplasm. There is a specific *tRNA* for each of the naturally-occurring amino acids. Specific amino acids are transferred from the cytoplasmic pool to the appropriate tRNA by the activity of a specific *aminoacyl-tRNA-synthetase*. The tRNA essentially consists of two specific functional sites. One is specific for the proper amino acid and the other is specific for the codon of mRNA. Complementary base sequencing on the tRNA accounts for the base pairing with the mRNA. Attachment of the tRNA to an *initiator codon* of mRNA initiates polypeptide synthesis. The tRNA is subsequently released from the messenger and the ribosome moves along the mRNA. Another tRNA is then ready to read the next mRNA codon. Released tRNA is available for the transfer of another specific amino acid, whereas the released ribosomes are available for repeated nonspecific utilization. The specificity for the protein resides in the mRNA. This assembly process of amino acids into polypeptides is called *translation.* Assembly is a rapid process; some experimental data indicate approximately 10 msec per amino acid.

The length of the mRNA determines the number of ribosomes associated with it and thus the length of the polypeptide chain. The protein products of free polysomes are destined for intracellular use. Protein synthesis destined for secretion occurs on the RER. The proteins gain access to the tubules or cisterns of the RER and are translocated to the Golgi apparatus and emerge as *condensing vacuoles* which are converted to *secretory granules.*

Agranular Endoplasmic Reticulum. The *smooth (agranular) endoplasmic reticulum* is not as extensive as its granular counterpart, except in certain types of cells. The smooth, anastomosing, tubular profiles do not have ribosomes associated with their membranes (Fig. 4.30). These profiles are similar to and often indistinguishable from the Golgi profiles. Functionally, they are associated with glycogen metabolism and synthesis, lipid metabolism, ion concentration and distribution and detoxification of certain substances. They are found in large quantities in cells in which ion balance is essential in maintaining electrical potential and in liver cells. The latter play an important role in glycogen metabolism and the detoxification of various substances.

Golgi Apparatus. The *Golgi apparatus* or *Golgi complex* is an organelle which may be visualized with light microscopy. Special stains such as silver or osmium can be used to impregnate or stain the organelle as a positive image. It appears as a network of tubules and vacuoles scattered throughout the cell, sometimes in more than one focus, or is juxtaposed to the nucleus and confined to a discrete area (Fig. 4.31). With routine staining (H and E), however, an extensive Golgi complex appears as a negative image

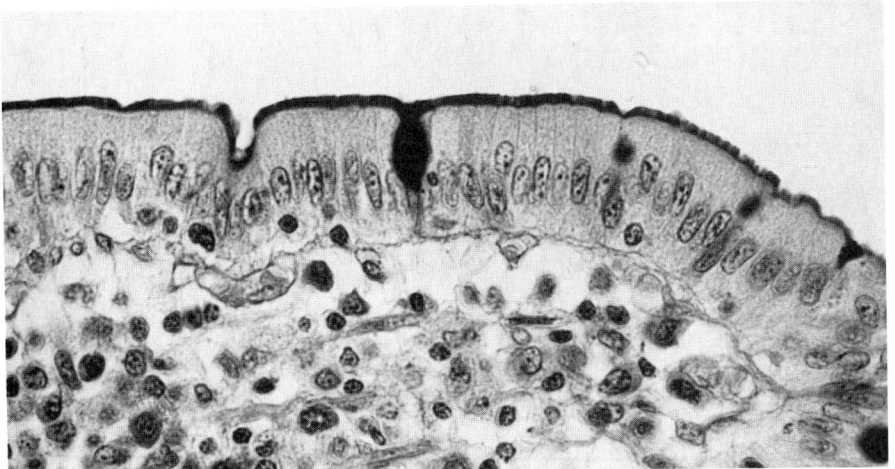

Fig. 4.25 The glycocalyx as visualized with light microscopy and special staining. The apical, striated border of these intestinal lining cells is covered by a dark-staining glycocalyx. X160 (PAS).

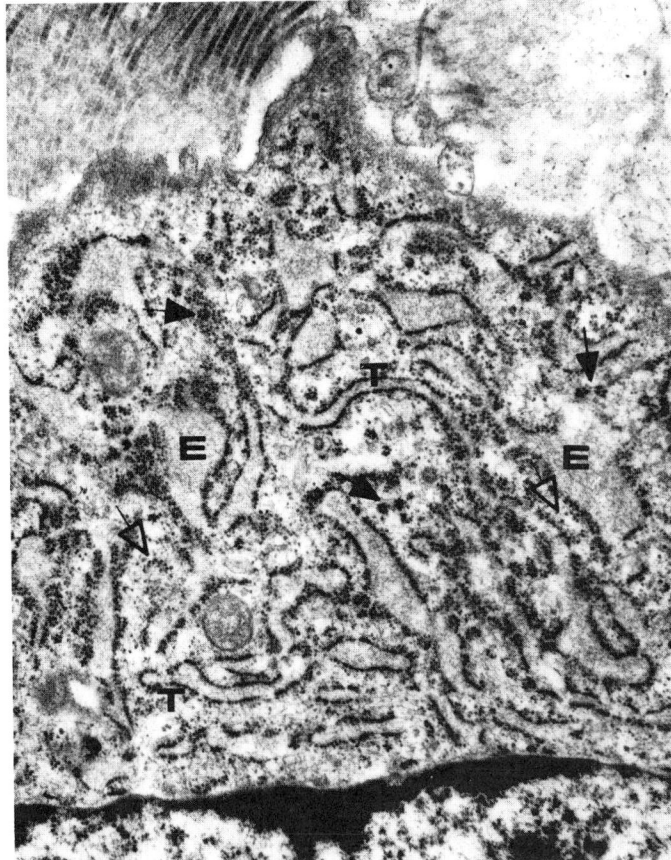

Fig. 4.26 An electron micrograph of a fiber-forming cell. The cytoplasm contains numerous profiles of granular endoplasmic reticulum. Some are tubular (T) while some are cisterns (E). Ribosomes (*open arrows*) and polyribosomes (*solid arrows*) are abundant. X20,000.

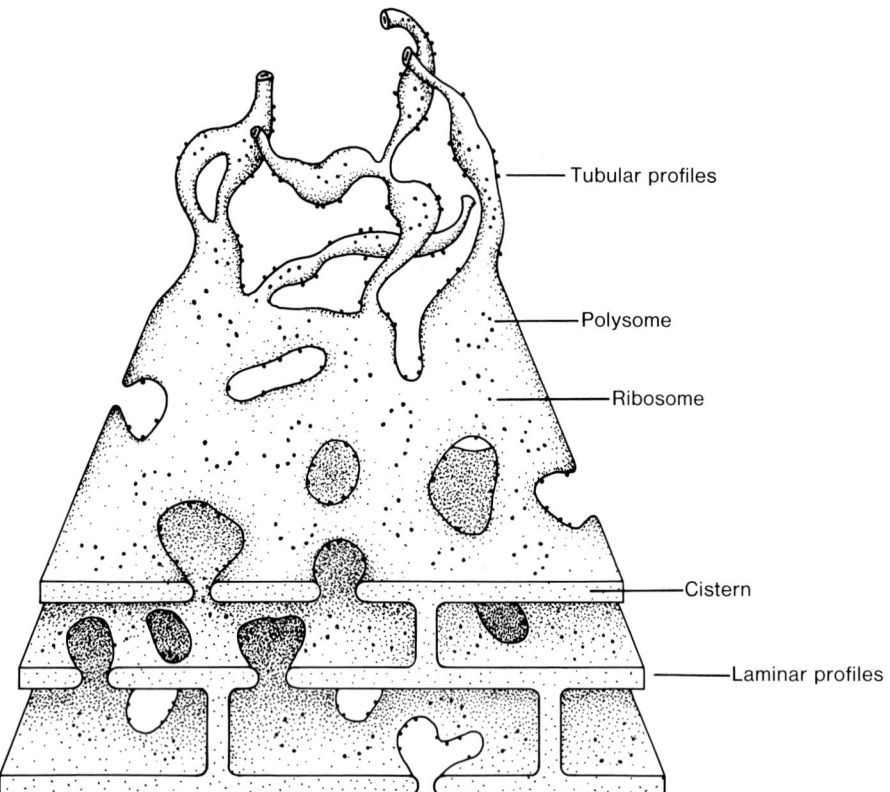

Fig. 4.27 Schematic representation of the rough endoplasmic reticulum. The anastomotic plates and tubules may be scattered randomly or placed in an orderly fashion throughout the cytoplasm.

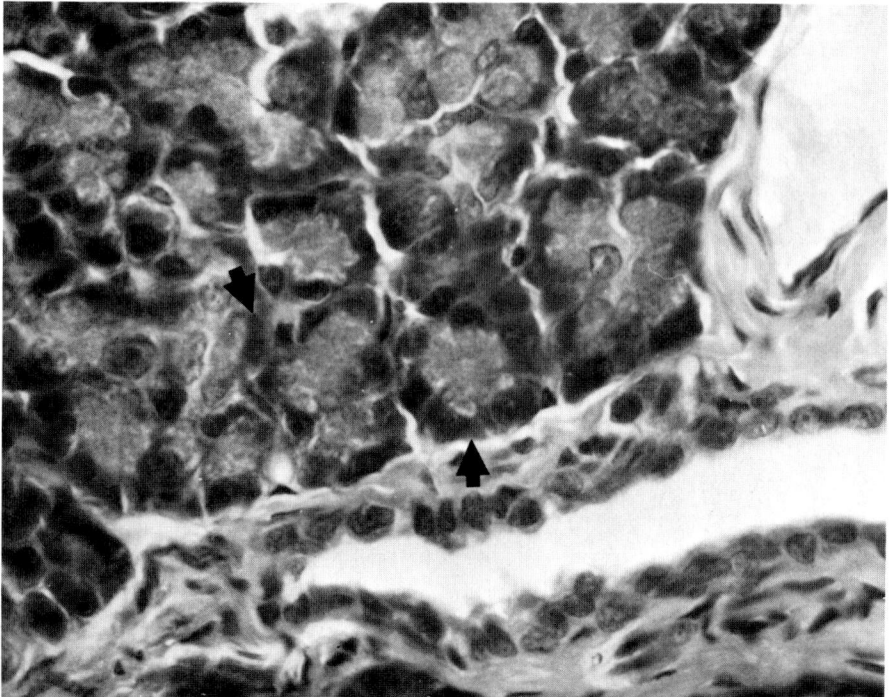

Fig. 4.28 Ergastoplasm of pancreatic acinar cells. The apical margins of the cells are light-staining (acidophilic). The basal portions (*arrows*) are dark-staining (basophilic). The pancreatic acinar cells are polarized cells. X40.

because of its chromophobic staining properties. In those cells in which polarity is apparent, such as epithelial cells, the position of the Golgi apparatus reflects this polarization; it is supranuclear, located be-tween the nucleus and the apical or luminal surface of the cell (Fig. 4.31).

Electron microscopy has contributed significantly to an understanding of the morphology of this organelle (Fig. 4.32). The Golgi apparatus consists of a parallel array of smooth-surfaced membranes that are disposed as flattened saccules. These saccules have dilated cisternae at their peripheral margins. The entire complex assumes a semi-ilunar configuration in this zone of cytoplasm reserved exclusively for the Golgi apparatus. The *convex face* is called the *immature* or *formative surface* because of its association and ultimate fusion with *transfer vesicles* from the RER. Numerous fenestrations characterize this surface. The *concave face, mature face*, is associated intimately with numerous *secretory vesicles* in various stages of condensation and maturation (Fig. 4.33).

The Golgi apparatus was considered to be functionally uniform because of the uniformity of its membrane morphology. But special staining and histochemical techniques have demonstrated a distinct polarity. A few saccules of the immature face stain with osmium tetroxide and contain *transferases* for sugars. The saccules of the mature face do not stain with osmium and contain the enzyme *thiamine pyrophosphatase* (*TPP*). The function of TPP is unknown. Hydrolytic enzymes are associated with the middle saccules. Also, different types of secretory granules may be formed on the inner (concave) and outer (convex) face. This experimental evidence is interpreted as being indicative of functional specialization within the complex.

The membranes of the Golgi stack are in a constant state of flux. "New membrane" is added constantly by the incorporation of transfer vesicles and "old membrane" is lost at the mature face through secretory vesicles. Exocytotic processes involve membrane-bound vesicles derived from the Golgi apparatus being incorporated into the plasmalemma. The translocation of membranes from the immature face through the Golgi stack to the surface of the mature face ultimately contributes to the plasmalemma and the glycocalyx.

Beside the significance of the Golgi apparatus in the dynamic turnover of the cell membrane, it is significant in the alteration and packaging of secretory units for intracellular and extracellular use. Protein transferred to the stack is condensed, probably at the expense of water, and sugars may be added. The complex is also responsible for the synthesis of polysaccharides, as well as the formation of mucosubstances in those cells characterized by these types of secretory products. Additionally, the Golgi complex is important in the formation of lysosomes.

Mitochondria. At the light microscopic level, *mitochondria* appear as threads or granules with various staining techniques. Special staining techniques, however, stain them specifically; e.g., the supravital stain, Janus green B. Their shape is quite varied; even within a specific cell type they are extremely pleomorphic, ranging from round

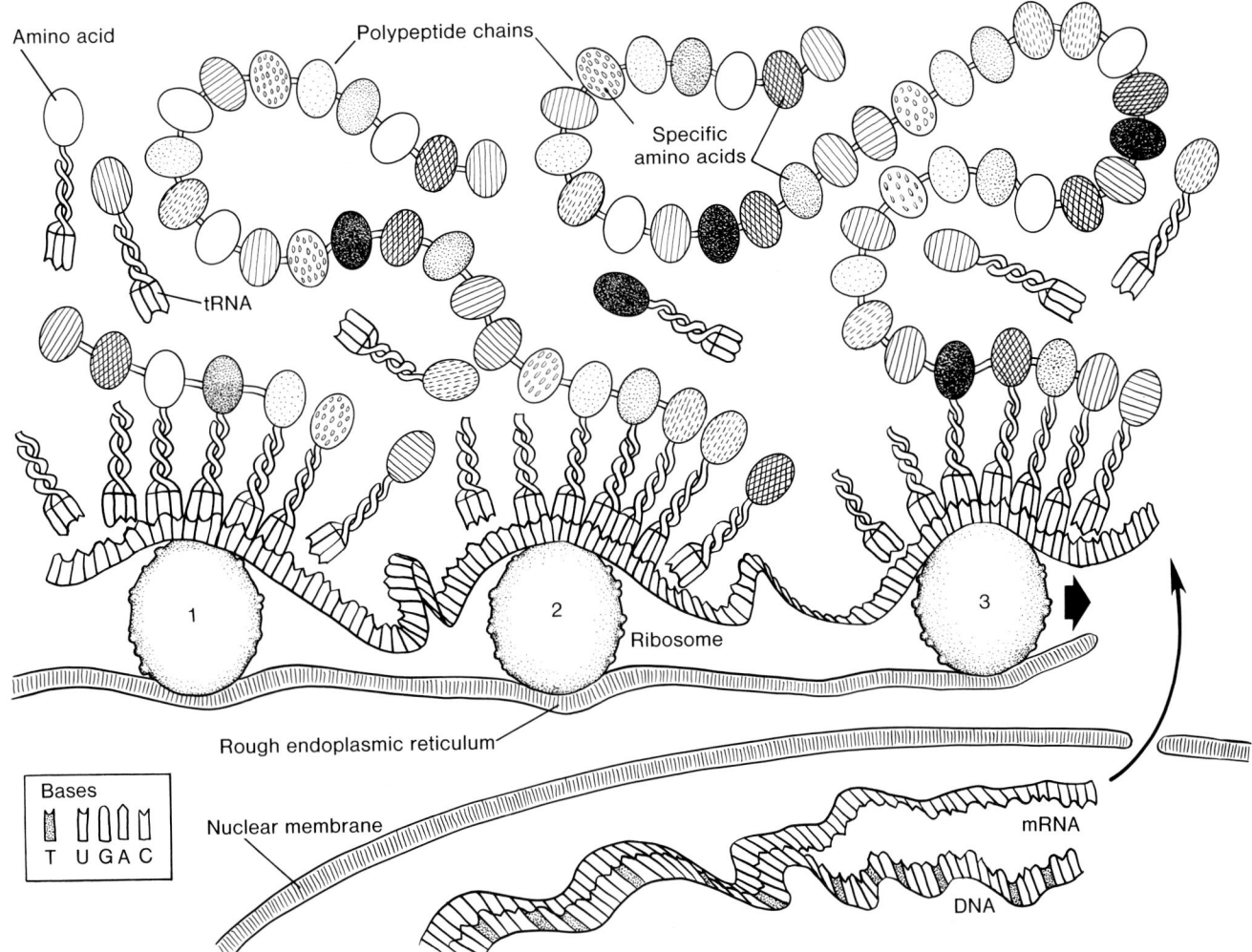

Fig. 4.29   Schematic representation of protein synthesis upon the ribosomes of the granular endoplasmic reticulum. After transcription of mRNA upon DNA within the nucleus, the messenger enters the cytoplasm and becomes attached to ribosomes. The mRNA fits in the groove between the two subunits of the ribosome. The activation of specific tRNA occurs after its linkage to the appropriate amino acid in the cytoplasm. The nature of the message, codon, of the mRNA determines which tRNA attaches at the codon site, and therefore which amino acid is utilized in the sequence. As the ribosomes move along the mRNA, the tRNA molecules with attached amino acids translate the code and the appropriate amino acids are deposited in the proper sequence for a specific protein. The tRNA molecules are released and available to attach to other free amino acids. The length of the mRNA determines the number of amino acids in the chain; the length of the mRNA determines the distance traversed by the ribosomes and thus the length of the protein that is assembled. Each ribosome is responsible for the synthesis of a complete chain of amino acids. As the ribosomes move from point 1 to point 3, the chain lengthens. Upon reaching the end of the mRNA at point 3, the ribosome is released, the amino acid chain is freed and the ribosome is available to attach to another mRNA. The bases involved in the codon include uracil (U), adenine (A), cytosine (C) and guanine (G). Thymine (T) occurs in DNA.

to oval or from elongated to filamentous. The number of mitochondria in a cell varies with the energy requirements of the cell. The size of mitochondria is also quite varied. Although most may be 2–3 μm long, they may exceed a length of 10 μm.

At the electron microscopic level, mitochondria are demonstrable as a double-membrane system (Fig. 4.34). The *outer mitochondrial membrane* has a smooth contour, is approximately 7.0 nm thick and defines the peripheral limits of the organelle. The *inner mitochondrial membrane* is approximately 8.0 nm thick and is modified into platelike or tubular folds (*cristae mitochondriales*). The cristae are separated by a *mitochondrial matrix* which is homogeneous and finely granular but of varying density.

Electron-dense granules, *mitochondrial granules*, occur within the matrix (Fig. 4.35).

In vitro studies have determined that mitochondria are capable of changing shape. A change in shape or conformation has been linked with *coupled* or *uncoupled oxidative phosphorylation*. The *orthodox conformation* is associated with coupled oxidative phosphorylation and is represented morphologically by the "typical" picture of mitochondria (Fig. 4.34). The *condensed conformation* is associated with an uncoupled oxidative phosphorylation and is represented by mitochondria with enlarged cristae and a condensed mitochondrial matrix (Fig. 4.36).

The inner mitochondrial membrane and mitochondrial matrix contain all the enzymes of the citric acid cycle and those

involved in oxidative phosphorylation, as well as those involved in fatty acid oxidation. The primary role of mitochondria, therefore, is the production of energy. Mitochondria, however, also contain DNA and RNA. They therefore possess some genetic and protein-synthetic potential. As such, they are capable of replication, although the exact method (budding or division) is yet to be determined.

Lysosomes. *Lysosomes* are membrane-bound particles that are rich in *hydrolytic enzymes*. There is no single description applicable to these particles. They are represented morphologically by numerous shapes and sizes. Except in a few instances, the histochemical demonstration of specific hydrolases (*acid phosphatase, arylsulfatase*) is

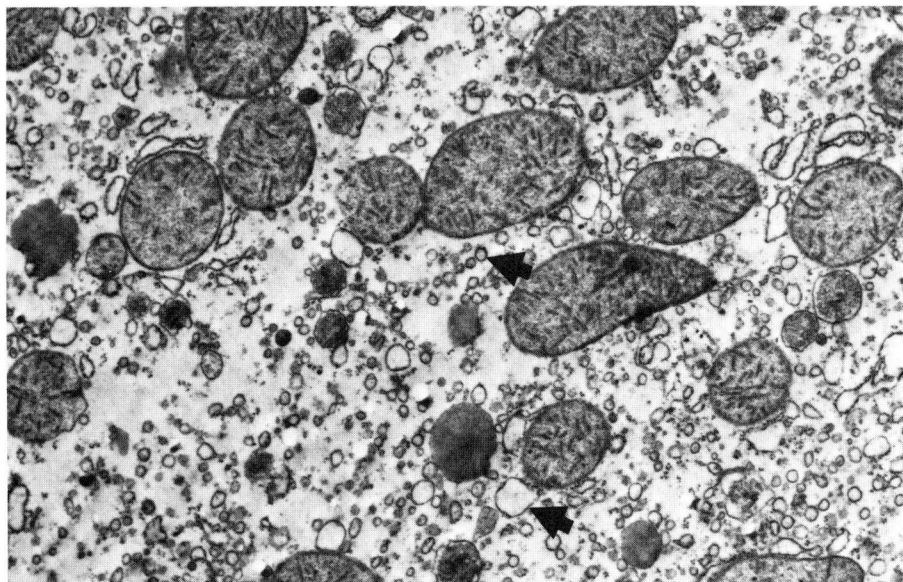

Fig. 4.30 An electron micrograph of smooth endoplasmic reticulum of an hepatocyte. Although the cell has been ruptured, the tubular profiles (*arrows*) of the organelle are obvious. Mitochondria and rough endoplasmic reticulum are present also. X11,400.

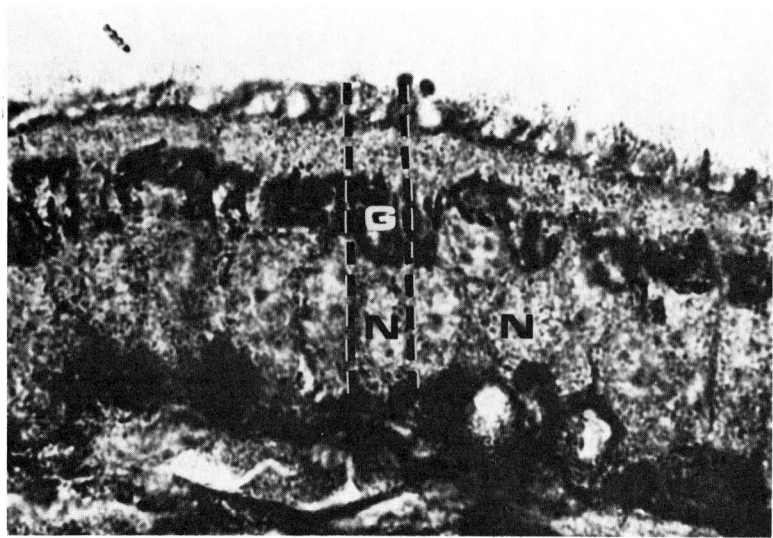

Fig. 4.31 Golgi apparatus of lining cells of the ductus epididymidis. The approximate lateral limits of one cell are defined by *dashed lines*. The nucleus (N) is positioned basally, while the silver-impregnated Golgi apparatus (G) is supranuclear. X400 (silver stain).

necessary for the absolute identification of these organelles. At the light microscopic level, the specific granules of basophils, eosinophils and neutrophils are representative of lysosomes and clearly demonstrate the range of structure and staining properties associated with these particles (Fig. 4.37).

Although the concept of lysosomes was initially derived from biochemical investigations, electron microscopic studies have added appreciably to an understanding of their structure and relationship to cell function. Lysosomes are particles in various stages of formation, maturation and activity. This continuum is represented by particles of varying morphologic configuration.

The adjoining scheme represents the relationship of lysosomal particles in various stages of activity (Fig. 4.38). Vacuoles bud from the Golgi complex and are transformed into *dense bodies* (*primary lysosomes, inactive lysosomes*). The fate of these primary lysosomes is dependent upon the subsequent activity with which they are associated. Two distinct types of activity are associated with lysosomes, *endocytosis* and *autophagocytosis*. Endocytotic activity may be further subdivided into *phagocytosis* or *pinocytosis*.

In *phagocytosis*, particulate matter is engulfed by the cell in the form of membrane-bound vesicles (*phagosomes*). The union of

a primary lysosome with a phagosome produces a *secondary* or *active lysosome*, often referred to as a *phagolysosome*. Upon completion of the digestive activity of this newly formed structure, or during an arrest in the activity, a resulting *residual body* is formed. The latter, upon completion of the digestive function, is extruded from the cell.

In *pinocytosis*, fluid material is engulfed by the cell in *pinocytotic vesicles*. These vesicles fuse with primary lysosomes, but their integrity is not lost; i.e., they appear within a dense body as vesicles. At this point, the primary lysosome and engulfed pinocytotic vesicles are referred to as a *multivesicular body*. After the completion of the digestive process, it is assumed that the multivesicular body is converted to a primary lysosome for future functioning or, as in the case of phagocytosis, a residual body is formed.

In *autophagocytosis*, a sequence of events occurs that is similar but not identical to that associated with phagocytosis. Various organelles, as well as insoluble portions of cytoplasm, tend to degenerate or become functionless. These are represented as *foci of cytoplasmic degeneration*. These degenerative or functionless cytoplasmic components are engulfed by primary lysosomes and are referred to as *autophagic vacuoles* or *cytolysosomes*. The fate of cytolysosomes is similar to the fate of phagolysosomes.

Numerous other terminologies have been applied to lysosomes. It should be clear that the complexity and diversity of lysosomal function accounts for the heterogeneity of these particles. The significance of lysosomes in cellular function cannot be overstated. They are extremely important organelles. Not only are they responsible for routine digestive properties of cells, but they are also important organelles through which protective functions of cells are mediated. They are responsible for protecting cells, and hence the body, against foreign materials, and also for destroying cells. These organelles account for *autolytic processes*. Under normal conditions, routine cellular death (*necrobiosis*) is mediated through autolysosomal function (*autolysis*). In pathological conditions, lysosomes can account for abnormal cell death (*necrosis*) via autolytic processes as well.

Centrioles, Basal Bodies and Annulate Lamellae. The *centrioles* of resting cells are two small bodies contained within an area of gelatinous material referred to as the *centrosphere*. Although these bodies are usually inconspicuous in resting cells, special staining techniques can be utilized to demonstrate them at the light microscopic level.

The two small dots or bodies shown by the light microscope are resolved with the electron microscope as cylindrical units which are 150 nm in diameter and approximately 500 nm long (Fig. 4.39). They are oriented perpendicular to each other. Each cylinder is composed of nine groups of three tubules. Although cylindrical, the nine groups of tubules are oriented eccentrically to each other. Fibrous material connects the terminal tubules of each group to the terminal tubules of adjacent groups. Also, fibrous material connects the peripherally located groups to the center of the centriole. Ideal sections and good resolution are requisite to demonstrate this fibrillar substructure.

Centrioles play a significant role in the mitotic process, at which time they duplicate themselves and are associated with the microtubules of the spindle apparatus. A dense cytoplasmic region adjacent to the centrioles within the centrosphere has been associated with microtubule formation. This dense region has been implicated as either a *microtubular subunit aggregation center* or a *subunit synthesizing center*. The functional relationship of this dense region to the centrioles is not clear.

The basal bodies are structurally similar to the centrioles. The former are structurally associated with cilia and are responsible for the formation of cilia.

Annulate lamellae are stacks of membranes that seem identical to the nuclear envelope, even to the presence of pore-like structures. They are found commonly in the cytoplasm of certain gametes. Their function is unknown.

Microbodies. *Microbodies* or *peroxisomes* are spherical or ovoid organelles that are smaller than mitochondria. Special staining techniques are required for their demonstration at the light microscopic level. They can be identified on the basis of the presence of the following enzymes: uricase, catalase and *d*-amino oxidase. Some investigators have proposed that they are developing mitochondria (not widely accepted), whereas others claim that they are related to lysosomes. It appears as though they are specific organelles, the specific function of which is yet to be elucidated.

At the electron microscopic level of examination, microbodies are bound by a single membrane that encloses a matrix, the granularity and homogeneity of which have been compared to the mitochondrial matrix. A central density, core or crystalloid particle may be present within the matrix. The size, shape and nature of these particles, as well as the presence or absence of same, is species-dependent. These organelles, most commonly with a diameter of 300–600 nm, are closely associated with smooth endoplasmic reticular profiles and are believed by some investigators to be derived from this organelle. Cells with altered lipid metabolism have an increased number of peroxisomes.

Microbodies have been identified in liver cells, the epithelial lining cells of the proximal convoluted tubules of the kidney, macrophages and other cell types. They are, however, of variable occurrence in other cells of various animals.

Microtubules. *Microtubules* occur in a variety of cells and subserve various functions. Except in the case of the mitotic spindle apparatus, microtubules are difficult to identify at the light microscopic level. Even then, they appear as fibers rather than being resolved as tubules.

With the electron microscope, they are resolved as tubules with an outside diameter of 20–26 nm and a wall 5–7.0 nm thick (Fig. 4.40). Microtubules are composed of a protein which is similar to the actin of muscle cells. This protein is called *tubulin*. Microtubules are found scattered throughout the cytoplasm of many cell types, as well as being preferentially distributed throughout the cytoplasm in certain cells. It is believed that they are significant contributors to the maintenance of cell shape; thus, they may be considered a part of the cytoplasmic skeleton. They are found in cilia, in flagella and in the manchette of spermatids. They are significant, therefore, in the development of motility associated with these structures. Also, they are longitudinally oriented along the axoplasm of neurons, wherein

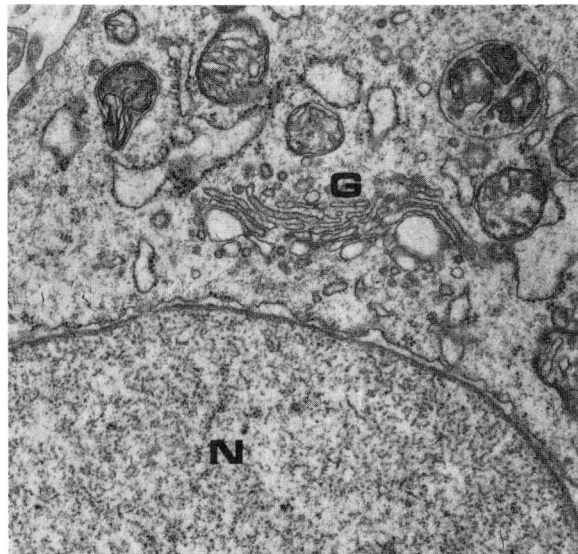

Fig. 4.32 An electron micrograph of the Golgi apparatus. The Golgi apparatus (G) is positioned close to the nucleus (N). X20,000.

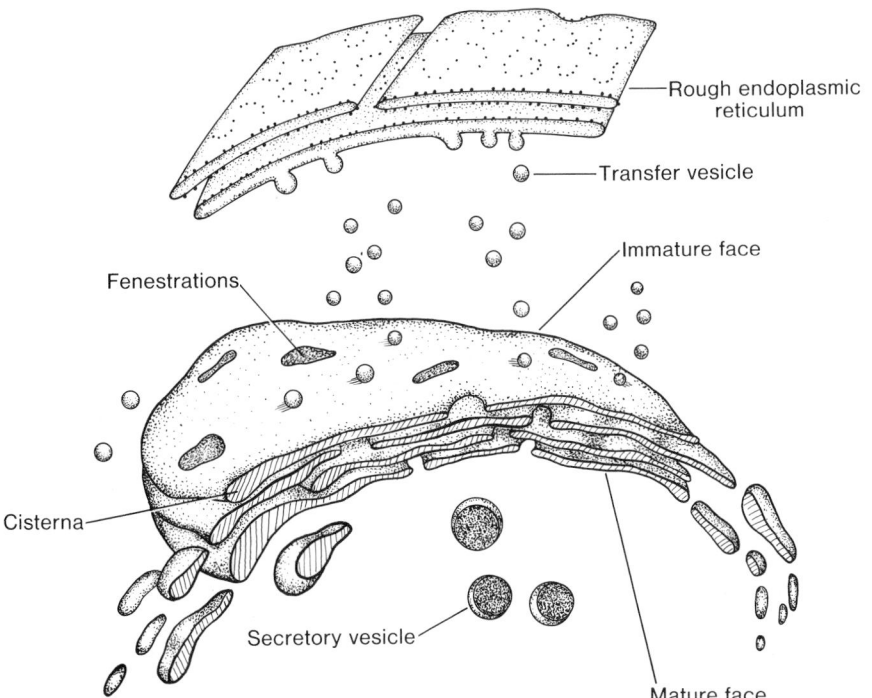

Fig. 4.33 Diagram of the Golgi apparatus and its relationship to the rough endoplasmic reticulum. Transfer vesicles bud from the RER and fuse with the immature face. Materials enter the stack at the immature face, traverse the stack and emerge as presecretory vesicles. The vesicles mature into secretory vesicles.

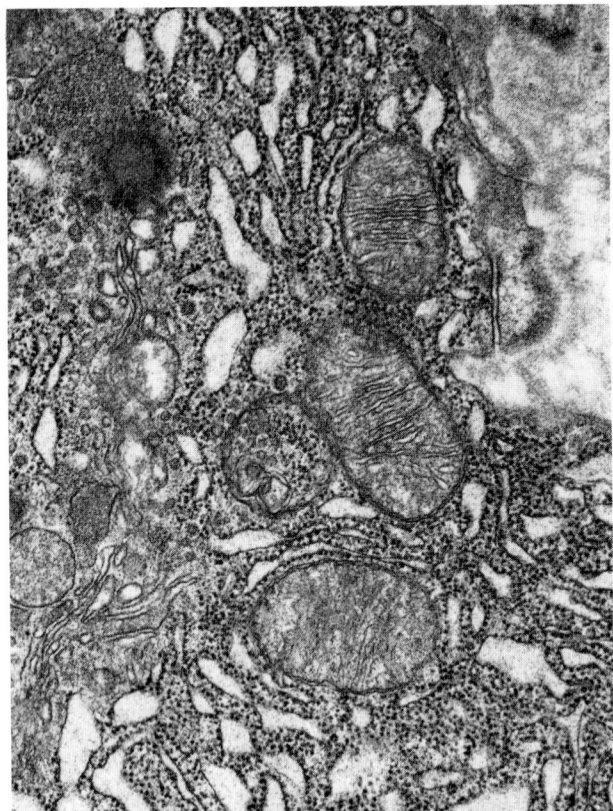

Fig. 4.34   Typical mitochondria. The mitochondria are in the orthodox conformation. The cristae are prominent, whereas the mitochondrial matrix is dense. X27,000.

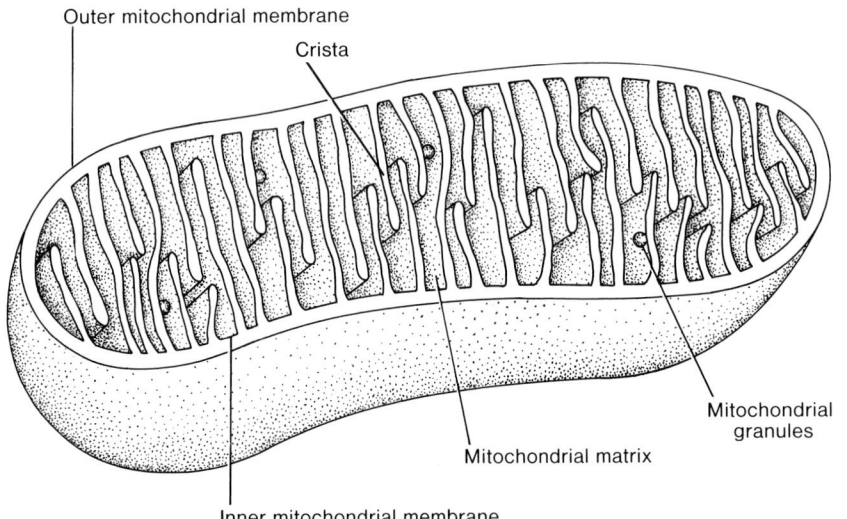

Fig. 4.35   Diagram of a typical mitochondrion.

they serve as a transport medium for various secretory products.

Filaments and Fibrils. *Cytofilaments* or *tonofilaments* are scattered throughout the cytoplasm and constitute the *cell web* (Fig. 4.41). These cytoplasmic components are 4–5.0 nm thick and are of variable lengths. They serve as supportive or skeletal components of the cytoplasm. Although individually beyond the limits of resolution with the light microscope, they are resolved when they are grouped together as *tonofibrils*. These tonofibrils constitute the *terminal web* of some cells and are associated with plasmalemmal modifications utilized in cellular attachments.

In those cells modified for contractile functions (smooth muscle, skeletal muscle, cardiac muscle, myoepithelial cells), filaments with contractile properties are either randomly dispersed throughout the cytoplasm or are oriented into highly organized contractile units. These *myofilaments* are divisible into two distinct subgroups. *Myosin myofilaments* are approximately 10 nm in diameter, whereas *actin myofilaments* are about 6.0 nm in diameter. Although not resolved as individual units at the light microscopic level, they are observable as larger *myofibrils*.

Secretory Inclusions. The secretory products of cells are varied and include such products as enzymes, acids, proteins and mucus. In some instances, the morphology of a given cell may be altered significantly through its involvement in a specific secretory function or through the accumulation of its secretory products. In other instances, the synthesis and/or elaboration of a secretory product is not accompanied by a change in cellular morphology. Specific examples of the aforementioned conditions follow in subsequent chapters. A few general examples will serve to illustrate cellular secretory activity.

The morphologic configurations of the secretory products are as diverse as the products themselves. Lysosomes, as secretory products for intracellular use, have already been described. *Zymogen* granules, membrane-bound packets of enzyme precursors for extracellular use, typify many protein-secreting cells. As in the case of the pancreatic acinar cell, these secretory products appear as granules in a subluminal position. The granules are derived from the mature face of the Golgi complex, mature as they move toward the lumen and are individually secreted at the apical cell surface (Fig. 4.42).

Some cells that secrete *mucoid substances* (mucus) are characterized, as in the case of the *goblet cell* depicted (Fig. 4.43), by a very foamy cytoplasm. The cytoplasm is basophilic and the nucleus is displaced basally. The foamy appearance is attributed to the packets of mucous precursor material contained within the cytoplasm (Plate II. 9).

The secretion of lipid material is normally associated with cells that possess a foamy but acidophilic cytoplasm. In these cases, however, the foamy appearance is a result of lipids having been leached from the cytoplasm. Cells from the cortex of the adrenal gland exemplify this type of secretory inclusion product (Fig. 4.44) (Plate II. 3).

As mentioned previously, other cells secrete various products that are not visible at the light microscopic level. Among these are the numerous cells of connective tissues. They secrete mucopolysaccharides and proteins without any definitive, routine light microscopic evidence of this activity.

In some cells, a watery or *serous* secretion is accompanied by attendant alterations at the secretory surface. However, the accumulation of light microscopically visible products is not evident. The serous cells of some glands, characterized as cells with a finely granular and acidophilic cytoplasm and centrally or paracentrally located nuclei, exemplify another variation in cellular

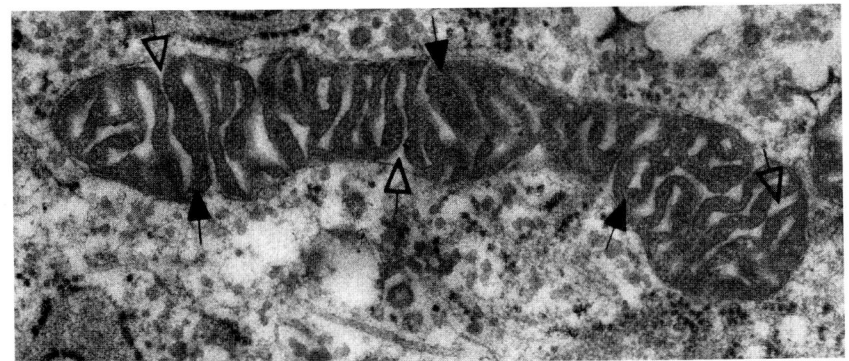

Fig. 4.36 An electron micrograph of a mitochondrion in the condensed conformation. The cristae (*open arrows*) are separated from each other by a condensed matrix (*solid arrows*). X48,000.

from the cytoplasm by the fat solvents used routinely in the preparatory techniques. Special handling and staining techniques are necessary for the demonstration of lipids. At the electron microscopic level, lipid inclusions appear as osmiophilic bodies of varying density (Fig. 4.48). The degree of dark staining (uptake of osmium) is a function of the lipid composition of the droplet. Although they appear to be membrane-bound, they actually occur free in the cytoplasm. The precipitation of osmium at the lipid-cytoplasmic interface may be misinterpreted as a membrane. In specific instances, however, triglycerides in intestinal lining cells are membrane-bound.

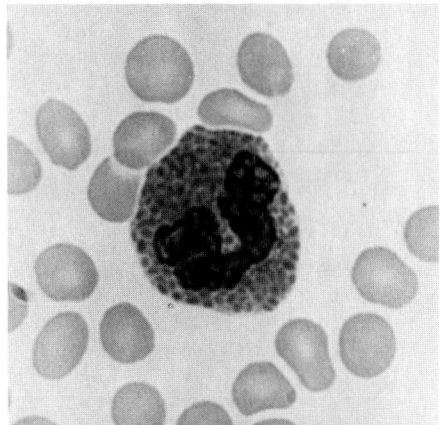

Fig. 4.37 A feline basophil. The small, specific granules scattered throughout the cell are lysosomes. X400.

secretory activity and resulting products (Fig. 4.45) (Plate II. 8).

Cellular secretory methods and products are discussed in Chapter 5.

Nutritive Inclusions. Most cells possess the ability to store various products that subserve a nutritive function. The most common of these that are readily visible at the light microscopic level are *glycogen* and *lipids*. Glycogen is especially apparent in the liver, skeletal muscle and cells of cartilage. A carmine stain is used specifically to identify glycogen, but the use of PAS and diastase is also an acceptable demonstration method. At the electron microscopic level, glycogen may appear as single particles which range from 15.0–30.0 nm in diameter with an irregular outline (*beta particles*) (Fig. 4.46). Accumulations in the form of *rosettes* (*alpha particles*) are also demonstrable (Fig. 4.47).

Lipid droplets within cells represent the storage of triglycerides. Various cells store these lipids to varying degrees. The ultimate storage of lipids is manifested in fat cells. The large vacuities do not represent lipids, rather the foci from which they were leached

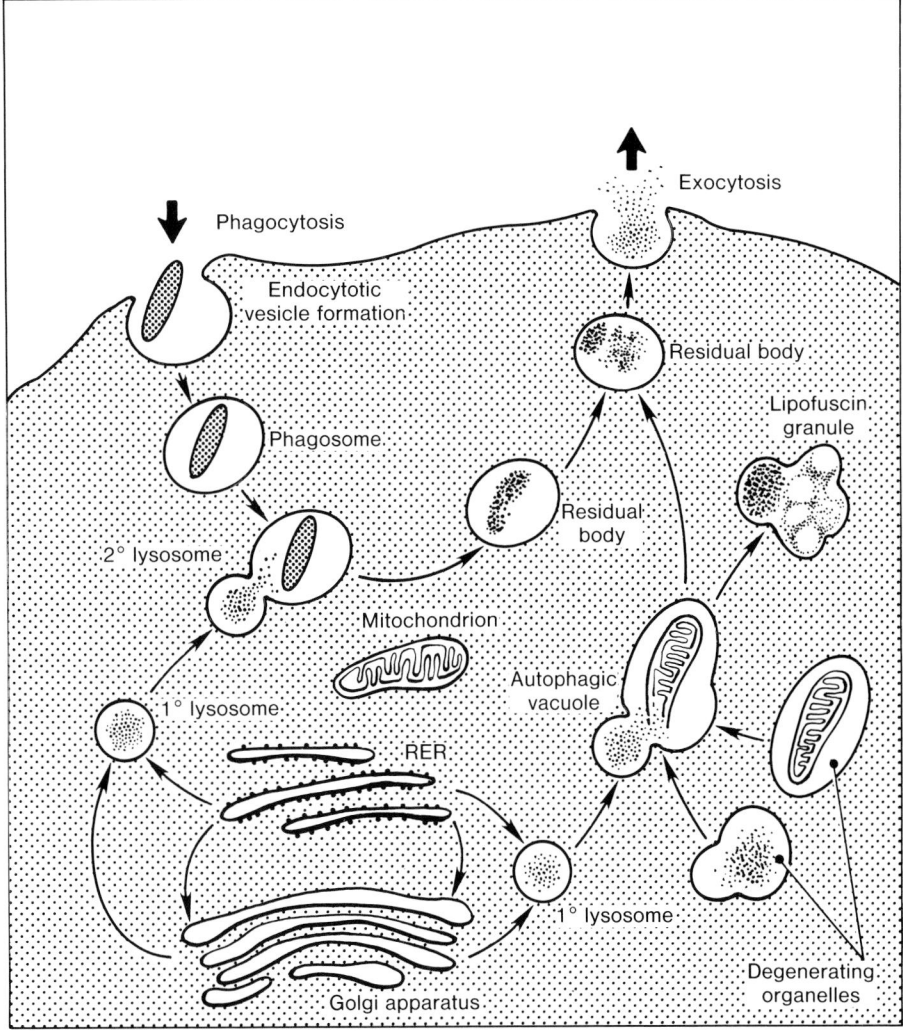

Fig. 4.38 Diagram of lysosomal activity during phagocytosis and autophagocytosis. Particulate matter engulfed by the cell in endocytotic vesicles enters the cytoplasm within phagosomes. Primary lysosomes produced by the Golgi apparatus and/or the RER fuse with the phagosomes to form activated or secondary lysosomes. The digestion of the particulate matter culminates in the formation of a residual body that may be retained within the cell or extruded by exocytosis. Foci of degenerating organelles may be engulfed initially by membranes of the RER. Fusion with primary lysosomes forms autophagic vacuoles (secondary lysosomes). Residual bodies and/or lipofuscin granules result from autophagocytosis.

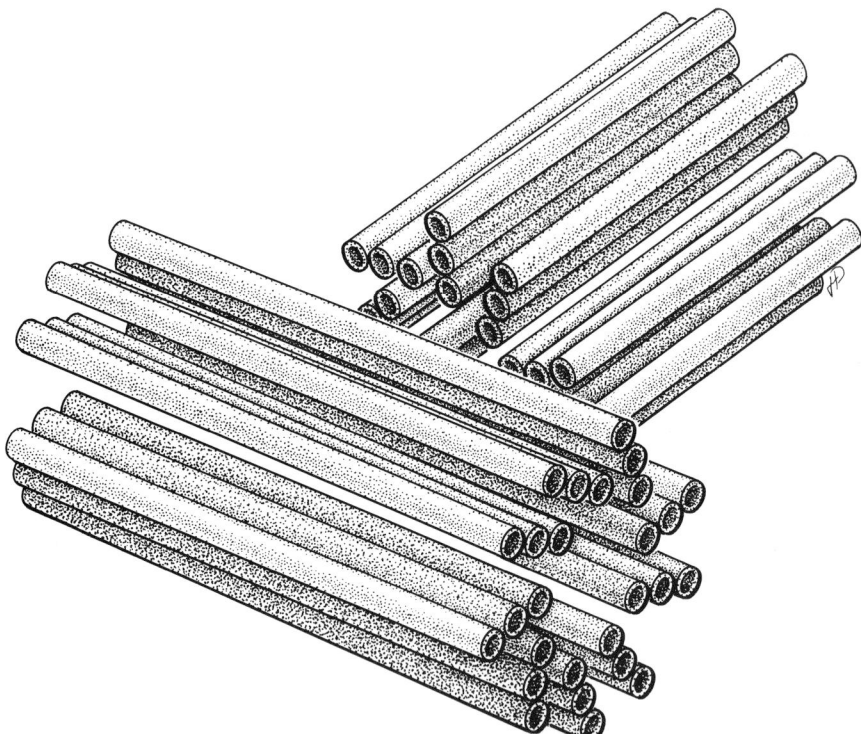

Fig. 4.39 Diagram of centrioles. Centrioles are paired structures that are oriented perpendicular to each other. Each component consists of nine groups of three tubules.

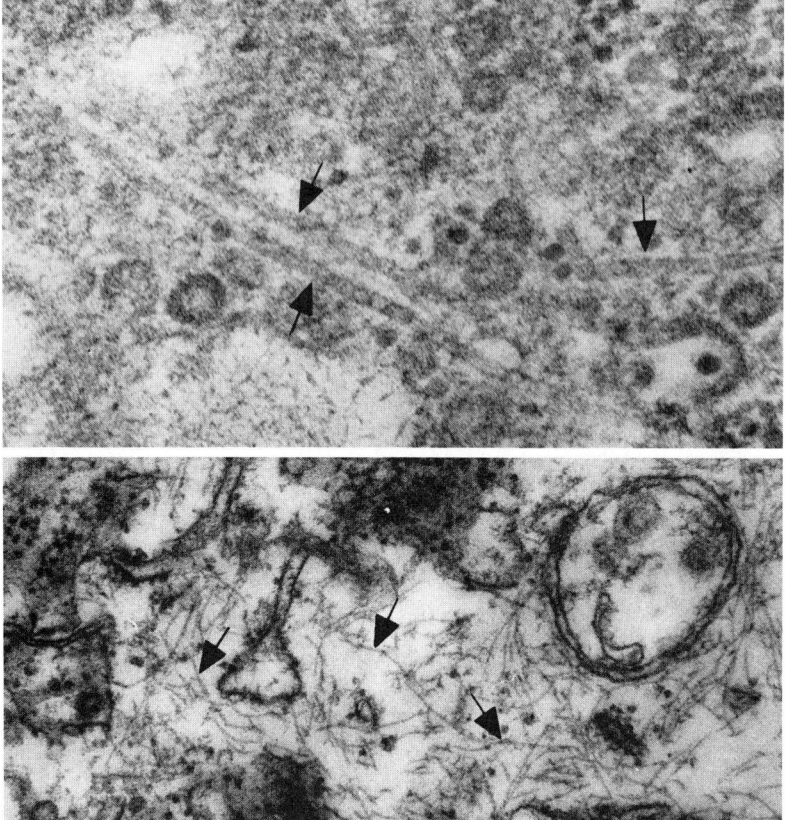

Fig. 4.40 An electron micrograph of microtubules. The microtubules (*arrows*) are scattered throughout the cytoplasm. The distribution of microtubules is very specific and/or organized in some cells. X94,000.

Fig. 4.41 An electron micrograph of cytofilaments. The cell was ruptured during processing. Because much of the normal cytoplasmic matrix was lost, the cytofilaments (*arrows*) are observed easily. X52,000.

Miscellaneous Inclusions. Numerous types of other inclusions occur within a large variety of cells. The most notable of these are the *pigment granules.*

Melanin is the brown pigment responsible for that coloration in a variety of foci scattered throughout the body. It is produced in *melanocytes* and is transferred to *melanophores.*

Lipofuscin is a gold-brown pigment, the origin of which has been debated. Current thought is that this pigment occurs in residual bodies as a terminal inclusion of lysosomal activity. These residual bodies are heterogeneous inclusions that may contain vacuoles, lipid droplets and matrix materials, as well as lipofuscin. The accumulation of this pigment progresses with age; thus, it is often referred to as the "wear and tear" pigment. Altered cellular function is generally associated with its accumulation in nerve cells and cardiac muscle cells.

Hemosiderin is a red-brown pigment resulting from the degradation of hemoglobin. It is involved in the mechanism whereby iron is recycled in the body. Although this pigment can be found in numerous intracellular and extracellular foci throughout the body, it is especially prominent in the phagocytes of the spleen.

Numerous crystalline inclusions occur in a variety of cell types. These will be discussed in subsequent chapters.

Cell Division

Cell Cycle. The necessity of adding new cells to the body during prenatal and postnatal growth phases should be apparent. However, the addition of new cells to the somatic complement does not cease with the termination of growth. Rather, the *replacement* of old or dead cells with new ones is a constant but variable occurrence. Some cells, as those of the skin, are replaced at regular intervals; others, such as the muscle cells of the heart, are not replaced. Generally, however, the body has the means to replace most cells. Besides the ability to replace worn out cells, one other criterion must be satisfied; i.e., *the ability to replace a given cell with an identical cell.* The mechanism responsible for this faithful replication is *mitosis.*

This built-in replacement mechanism implies that cell lives are finite. This, of course, is true, but the longevity of a cell is variable and specific for different cell types. Within the framework of a finite existence for various cell types, a definitive *cell cycle* can be defined. The cell cycle is defined as the passage of a cell through the interphase and mitosis, whereas the *generation time* is the time period required to complete one cycle (Fig. 4.49).

Although routine histological staining techniques allow only for the recognition of interphase and mitotic cells, autoradiographic techniques add valuable insights

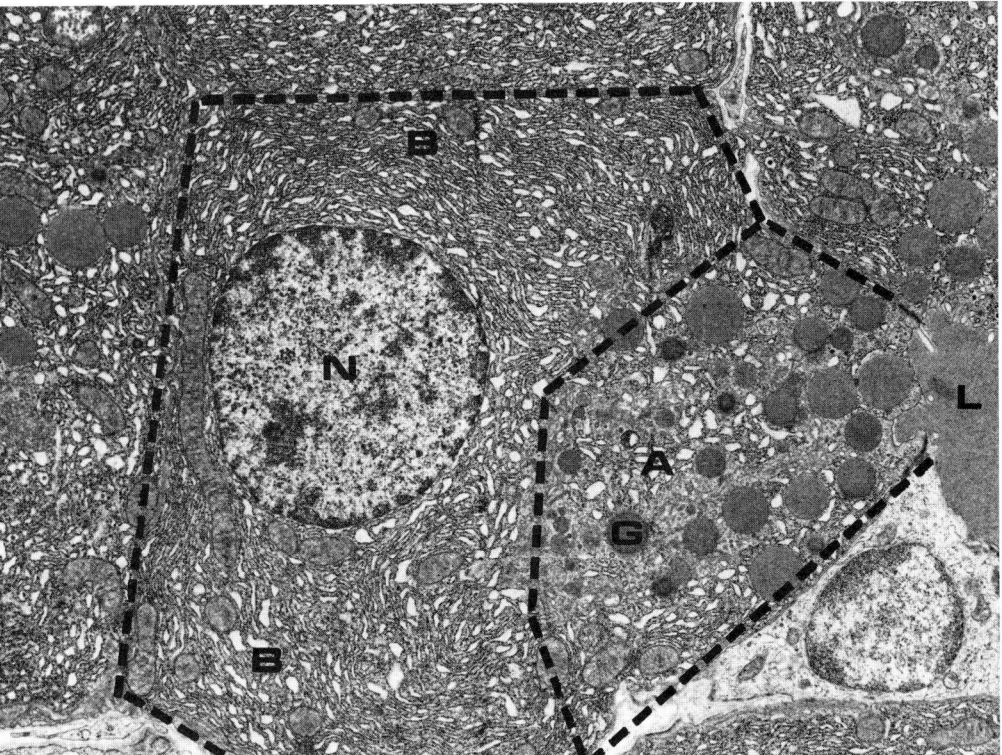

Fig. 4.42 An electron micrograph of pancreatic acinar cells. The approximate limits of one cell (*outer dashed line*) are indicated. The apex (A) of the cell borders the lumen (L). The apex (*inner dashed line*) contains numerous zymogen granules (G). The basal portion (B) contains the nucleus (N), granular endoplasmic reticulum and mitochondria. X7,000.

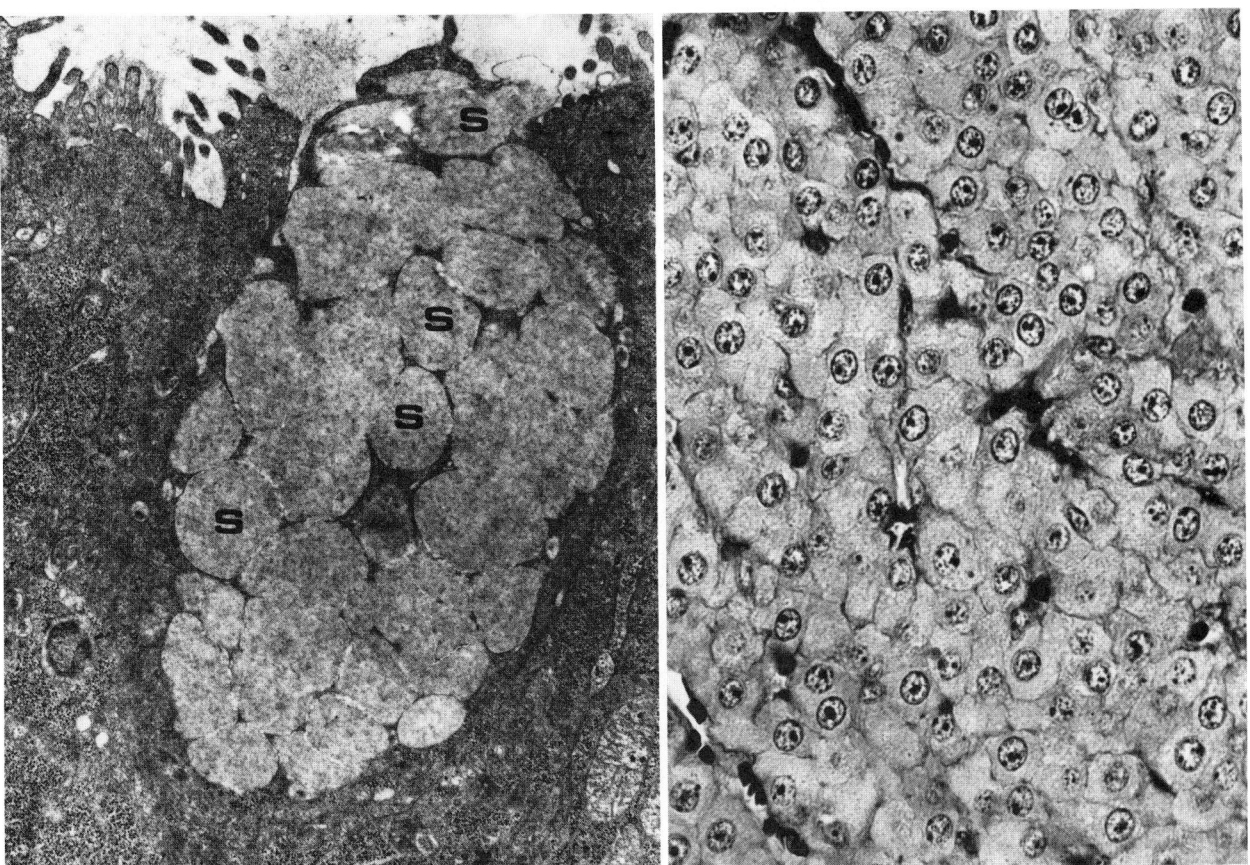

Fig. 4.43 An electron micrograph of a goblet cell from the epithelial lining of a mouse intestine. The cytoplasm has been displaced peripherally by the numerous secretory droplets (*S*). The nucleus is not in the plane of section. Compare with Figure 5.19. X14,000. (Courtesy of A. M. Sheppard.)

Fig. 4.44 Lipid-containing cells from the adrenal cortex. The pyramidal cells have a foamy appearance due to their lipid content. Whereas the lipids were removed from the cells during processing, the spaces that remain actually impart the foamy appearance. X160.

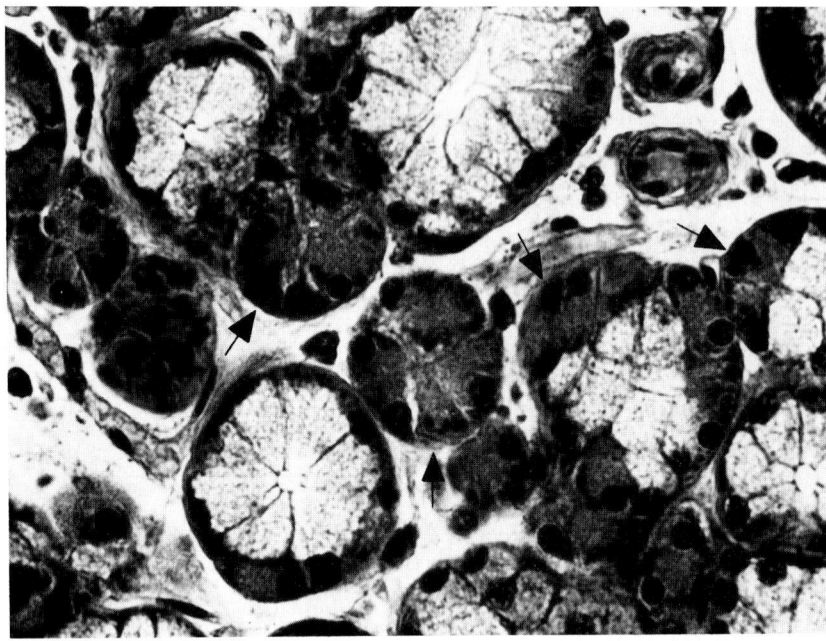

Fig. 4.45   Serous cells from a salivary gland. The dark cells (*arrows*) are the serous cells. The light-staining, pyramidal-shaped cells are mucous cells. X160.

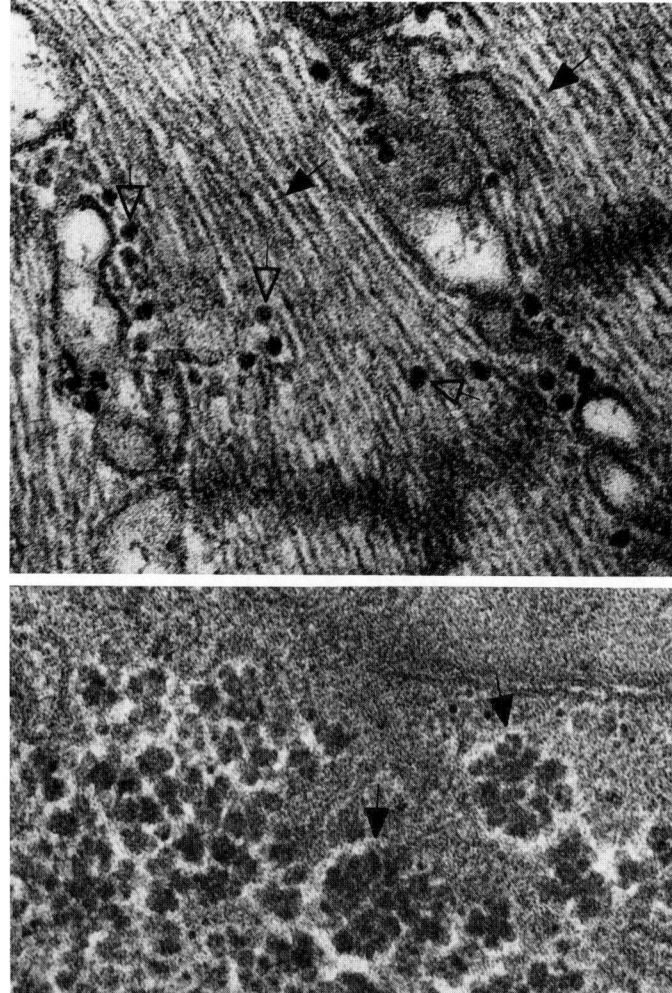

Fig. 4.46   An electron micrograph of glycogen particles. The beta particles (*open arrows*) are scattered among the myofilaments (*solid arrows*) of a striated muscle cell. X51,000.
Fig. 4.47   An electron micrograph of glycogen particles. *Arrows*, alpha particles. X133,000.

relative to other stages of activity during the cell cycle. Through the use of tritiated thymidine (a DNA precursor), subdivisions of the interphase are apparent. The *preduplication* or *presynthetic phase* (G_1) represents the period before the uptake of the labeled thymidine. This phase may be referred to as the *vegetative phase*. It is the stage during which time the cell will conduct its routine functions. Also, if the cell has a potential for mitosis, it is during this stage that the metabolites necessary to support mitosis will be accumulated. Most of the cells or accumulation of cells examined in histology will be in this stage.

The *duplication phase* (S) is the stage during which time DNA replication takes place, as evidenced by the nuclear uptake of the labeled thymidine. Not all the chromatic material is labeled (or duplicated) simultaneously. *Telomeric* (near the chromosome ends) replication occurs before *centromeric* (near the middle of chromosomes) replication. The end result, however, is the duplication of the chromosomes and a doubling of the DNA complement.

The *postduplication phase* (*postsynthetic phase*) is the G_2 stage. The naming of this phase refers only to the termination of DNA replication. Much synthetic, and therefore duplicative, activity characterizes this stage. The synthesis of histones, as well as that of RNA, occurs in this stage.

The interphase of the cell cycle is an extremely active phase responsible for a variety of cellular functions and events: increase in the total mass of a cell, increase in nuclear and nucleolar mass, duplication of chromatic material, synthesis of RNA and proteins and the conduction of routine cellular functions. In comparison with the interphase, the mitotic phase of the cell cycle is extremely short.

Much valuable information concerning the cell cycle has been obtained from studies of cultured cells, especially synchronized cell cultures. Cells in these types of systems grow rapidly and have a rapid doubling time. This type of growth is encountered rarely in the cells of the adult body. The G_1 phase may be protracted in somatic cells. Such protracted phases of vegetative activity are referred to by some authors as the G_0.

Differentiation and Mitotic Potential. During early stages of embryonic and fetal growth, most of the cells of the body have a high potential for division as well as the potential to become a variety of cells. As development ensues, the *differentiation* of varied cell populations is apparent. A consequence of this *specialization* (differentiation) is the *reduction or loss of cell potentiality* and a *reduction or loss of reproductive capacity* (*mitotic potential*).

Generally, highly specialized cells possess a low capacity for or an inability to duplicate themselves. Neurons (Fig. 4.19) and cardiac muscle cells are examples of these.

Specialized cell populations usually have specific cells associated with them from

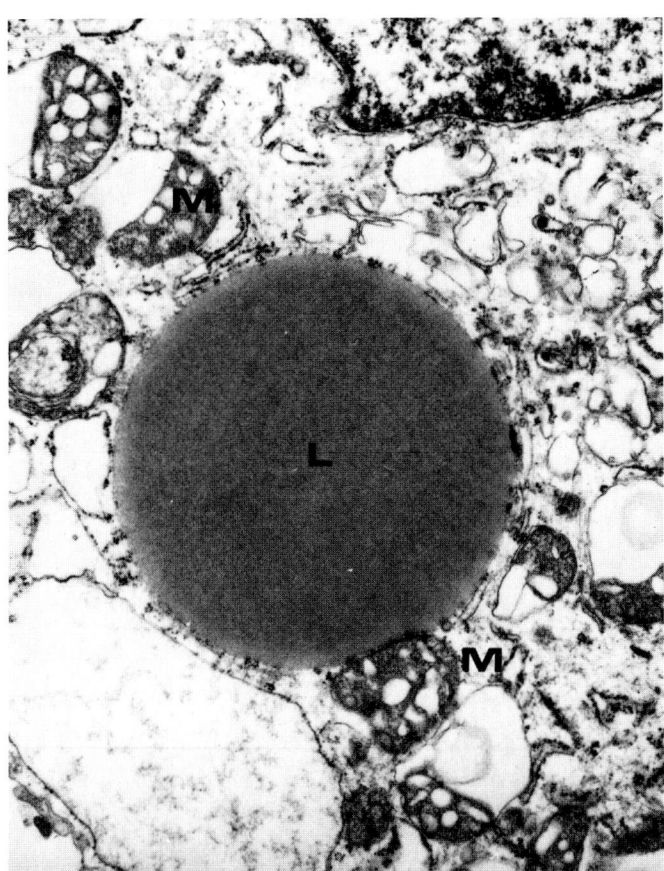

Fig. 4.48 An electron micrograph of lipid droplets from a tumor cell. The lipid droplet (L) is not membrane-bound. Condensed mitochondria (M) are present also. X20,000.

The *mesenchymal cell* of the body represents a cell similar to the aforementioned. It is a stem cell. However, this cell possesses a high potentiality and reproductive capacity. It is an undifferentiated cell capable of specializing into a variety of cell types: muscle cells, bone cells, cartilage cells, blood cells, etc. It is scattered throughout the body in association with numerous cell populations wherein it retains this ability for mitosis and multiple expression. It is especially apparent around small blood vessels in the *perivascular space*. It is a stellate or fusiform cell with a scant cytoplasm and a large, vesicular nucleus. Its ultrastructural features conform to the relationships discussed regarding euchromatin, ribosomes, polyribosomes and granular endoplasmic reticulum.

Some cells, despite their high degree of differentiation, still retain a high reproductive capacity under certain conditions. One example of this apparent paradox is the *hepatocyte*. The cells of the liver, after an injury, become highly mitotic.

In order to maintain the reproductive capacity described, the dividing cells will commit one cell to the differentiated state and retain the other in an undifferentiated condition for future division.

Divisional Sequence. The continuum of the divisional process has been arbitrarily divided into five stages: *interphase, prophase, metaphase, anaphase* and *telophase*. The last four stages actually comprise *mitosis*; however, the significance of the interphase can-

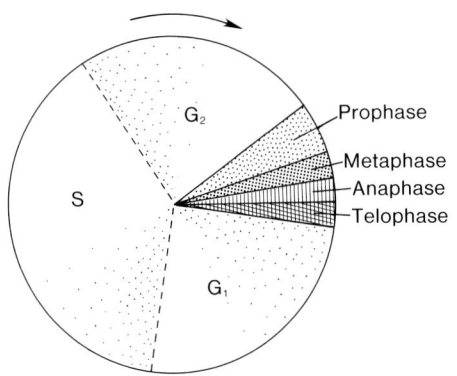

Fig. 4.49 Diagram of the cell cycle. The generation time of mammalian cells is variable but may average about 20 hours. The mitotic phase is the shortest, approximately 2 hours. The S phase is the longest, about 7 hours. Specific generation times characterize specific cells of the body.

which other members of their population arise. These are referred to generally as *stem cells*. The basal layer of cells of the epidermis (stem cell or germinative cell layer) is an example of a residual cell population within a community of specific cells that retains the ability to replace cells lost from the skin. These cells are capable only of forming "epidermal" cells. Other examples will be included in subsequent sections.

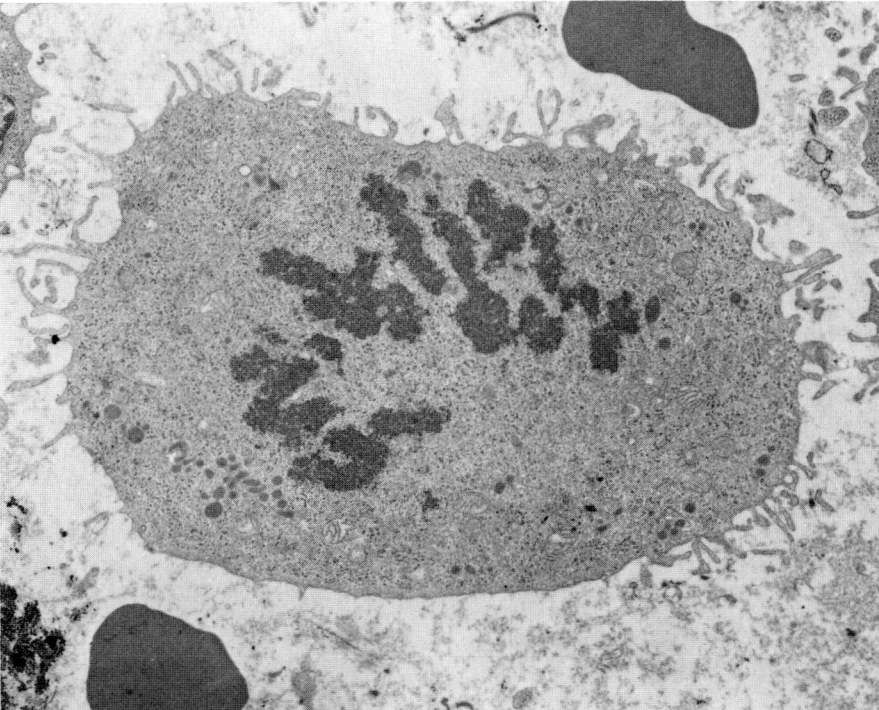

Fig. 4.50 An electron micrograph of a dividing mesenchymal cell from the connective tissue space. The cell is in prophase. The chromosomes are condensed, the nuclear membrane has disintegrated, but spindle fibers are not evident. The mesenchymal cell has a high mitotic potential. X2,000.

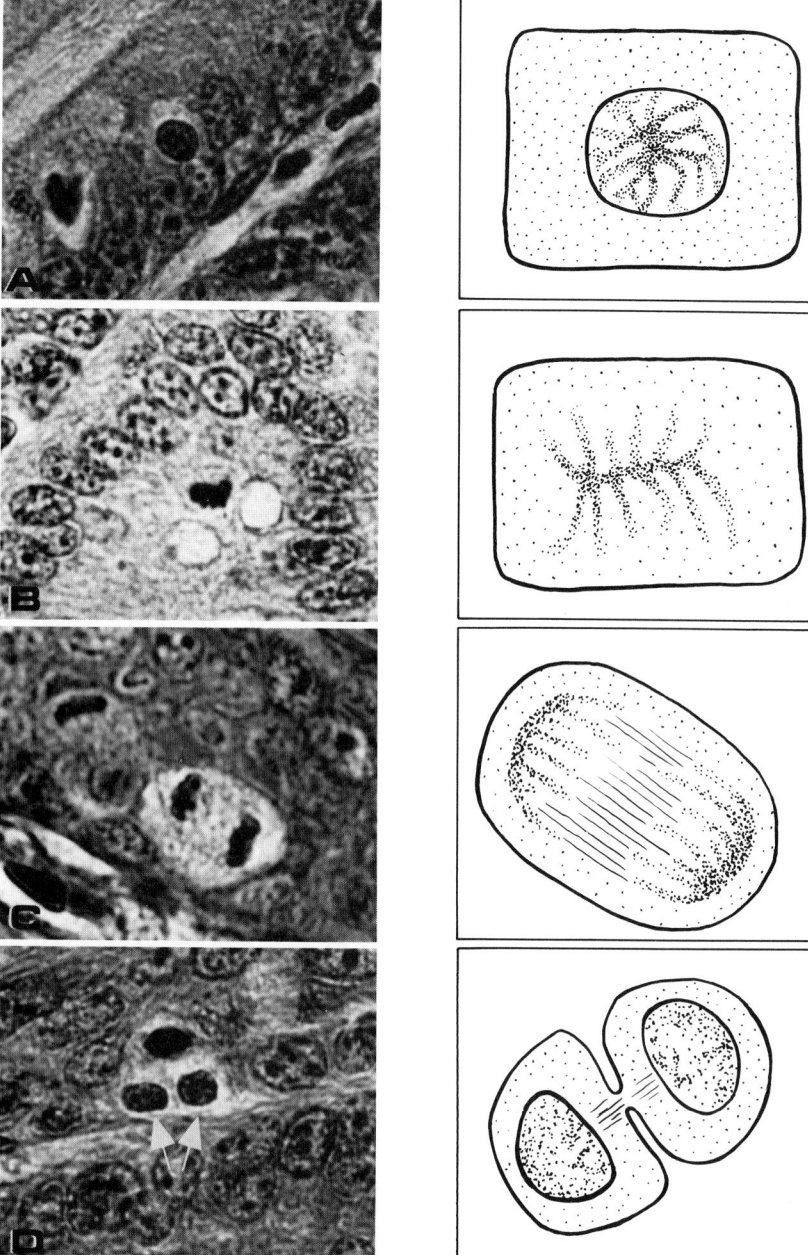

Fig. 4.51 Mitosis of the lining cells of an intestinal crypt. The prophase (A) is initiated and the chromosomes migrate to the equitorial plane during metaphase (B). During the anaphase (C), the chromosomes migrate toward the poles. During telophase (D), daughter cells (*arrows*) are formed. The cell above the daughter cells has entered prophase.

Fig. 4.52 Diagram of phases of mitosis. The diagram matches the events in Figure 4.51. The daughter cells remain connected for a short time via the midbody.

With the splitting of the two chromatids at the centromere, daughter chromosomes begin to migrate to the opposite cellular poles. These events mark the initiation of the *anaphase* (Figs. 4.51, 4.52). Thus, the anaphase is characterized by the initiation of *karyokinesis*.

The reconstitution of the nuclear membrane marks the initiation of the *telophase* (Figs. 4.51, 4.52). The chromosomes become dispersed while the nucleus enlarges. *Cytokinesis*, initiated peripheral to the equatorial plane, is completed and two identical daughter cells result.

References

General References

Bloom, W. and Fawcett, D. W.: *A Textbook of Histology*. 9th ed. W. B. Saunders, Philadelphia, 1968.

Brachet, J. and Mirsky, A. E.: *The Cell: Biochemistry, Physiology and Morphology*. 6 Vols. Academic Press, New York, 1959–1964.

Bresnick, E. and Schwartz, A.: *Functional Dynamics of the Cell*. Academic Press, New York, 1968.

DeRobertis, E. D. P., Nowinski, W. W. and Saez, F. A.: *Cell Biology*. 4th ed. W. B. Saunders, Philadelphia, 1965.

DuPraw, E. J.: *Cell and Molecular Biology*. Academic Press, New York, 1968.

Fawcett, D. W.: *An Atlas of Fine Structure: The Cell, Its Organelles and Inclusions*. W. B. Saunders, Philadelphia, 1967.

Ham, A. W.: *Histology*. 6th ed. Lippincott, Philadelphia, 1969.

Lentz, T. L.: *Cell Fine Structure: An Atlas of Drawings of Whole-Cell Structure*. W. B. Saunders, Philadelphia, 1971.

Matthews, J. L. and Martin, J. H.: *Atlas of Human Histology and Ultrastructure*. Lea and Febiger, Philadelphia, 1971.

Porter, K. R. and Bonneville, M. A.: *Fine Structure of Cells and Tissues*. 3rd ed. Lea and Febiger, Philadelphia, 1968.

Sandborn, E. B.: *Cells and Tissues by Light and Electron Microscopy*. 2 Vols. Academic Press, New York, 1970.

Nucleus

Bennett, H. S.: Fine structure of cell nucleus. chromosomes, nucleoli and membrane. Rev. Mod. Phys. *31*:297, 1959.

Dalton, A. J. and Haguenau, F.: *Ultrastructure in Biological Systems: The Nucleus*. Vol. 3. Academic Press, New York, 1968.

Monneron, A. and Bernard, W.: Fine structural organization of the interphase nucleus in some mammalian cells. J. Ultrastruct. Res. *27*:266, 1969.

Moses, N. J.: Studies on nuclei using correlated cytochemical, light and electron microscopic techniques. J. Biophys. Biochem. Cytol. *2*:397, 1956.

Wischnitzer, S.: The submicroscopic morphology of the interphase nucleus. Inter. Rev. Cytol. *34*:1, 1973.

Nuclear Envelope

Abelson, H. T. and Smith, G. H.: Nuclear pores: The pore-annulus relationship in thin section. J. Ultrastruct. Res. *30*:558, 1970.

Barnes, B. G. and Davis, J. M.: The structure of nuclear pores in mammalian tissues. J. Ultrastruct. Res. *3*:131, 1959.

Franke, W.: Isolated nuclear membranes. J. Cell Biol. *31*:619, 1966.

Franke, W. and Kartenbeck, J.: Structure of nuclear membranes isolated from brain cells. Experientia. *25*:396, 1969.

Kessel, R. G.: Fine structure of the pore-annulus complex in the nuclear envelope and the annulate lamellae of germ cells. Z. Zellforsch. *94*:441, 1969.

Wiener, J., Spiro, D. and Lowenstein, W. R.: Ultrastructure and permeability of nuclear membranes. J. Cell Biol. *27*:107, 1965.

the centrioles move toward opposite poles of the cell. *Spindle fibers*, composed of microtubles, are apparent between the migrating centrospheres.

During the *metaphase* (Figs. 4.51, 4.52), the chromosomes migrate toward and align themselves along the *equatorial plane* of the cell. Microtubules attach themselves to the *centromere* and each chromosome is composed of two *chromatids* attached at the centromere. The alignment along the equatorial plane is random and *homologous chromosomes* do *not* align themselves one next to the other as pairs. This is an important distinction between *mitosis* and *meiosis*.

not be neglected and has been elaborated upon previously.

During the *prophase* (Figs. 4.50, 4.51), the chromatic material undergoes a progressive condensation which culminates with the chromosomes becoming distinct entities in late prophase. During the latter part of prophase the nuclear membrane disintegrates. At the same time, the nucleolus disappears. In the cytoplasm, the *centrosphere* divides, each part containing a pair of *centrioles*, and

Yoo, B. Y. and Bayley, S. T.: The structure of pores in isolated pea nuclei. J. Ultrastruct. Res. *18:*651, 1967.

Chromatin

Barr, M. L.: The significance of the sex chromatin. Int. Rev. Cytol. *19:*35, 1966.

Bujard, H.: Electron microscopy of single stranded DNA. J. Molec. Biol. *49:*125, 1970.

Dales, S.: A study of the fine structure of mammalian somatic chromosomes. Exp. Cell Res. *19:*577, 1960.

Osgood, E. E., Jenkins, D. P., Brooks, R. and Lawson, R. K.: Electron micrographic studies of the expanded and uncoiled chromosomes from human leukocytes. Ann. N. Y. Acad. Sci. *113:*717, 1963.

Priest, J. H. and Shikes, R. H.: Distribution of labeled chromatin. J. Cell Biol. *47:*99, 1970.

Watson, J. D. *Molecular Biology of the Gene.* W. A. Benjamin, Inc., New York, 1965.

Nucleolus

Bernhard, W. and Granboulan, N.: Electron microscopy of the nucleolus in vertebrate cells. In *Ultrastructure in Biological: The Nucleus,* edited by A. J. Dalton and F. Haguenau. Vol. 3. Academic Press, New York, p. 81, 1968.

Vincent, V. S. and Miller, O. J., Jr. (eds.): The nucleolus, its structure and function. Nat. Cancer Inst. Monogr. *23:* 1965.

Cellular Membranes

Bolis, L. and Pethica, B. A.: *Membrane Models and the Formation of Biological Membranes.* North Holland Publishing, Amsterdam, 1968.

Dalton, A. J. and Haguenau, F. (eds.): *Ultrastructure in Biological Systems: The Membranes.* Vol. 4. Academic Press, New York, 1968.

Davson, H.: Growth of the concept of the paucimolecular membrane. Circulation *26:*1022, 1962.

Finean, J. B.: The molecular organization of cell membranes. Progr. Biophys. *16:*143, 1966.

Hendler, R. W.: Biological membrane ultrastructure. Physiol. Rev. *51:*66, 1971.

Korn, E. D.: Structure of biological membranes. Science *153:*1492, 1966.

Robertson, J. D.: The ultrastructure of cell membranes and their derivatives. Biochem. Soc. Sympos. *16:*3, 1959.

Rothman, J. E. and Lenard, J.: Membrane asymetry. Science. *195:*743, 1977.

Singer, S. J. and Nicolson, G. L.: The fluid mosaic model of the structure of cell membranes. Science. *175:*720, 1972.

Sjostrand, F. S.: A comparison of plasma membranes, cytomembranes and mitochondrial membrane elements with respect to ultrastructural features. J. Ultrastruct. Res. *9:*561, 1961.

Sjostrand, F. S.: A new repeat structural element of mitochondrial and certain cytoplasmic membranes. Nature *199:*1262, 1963.

Vanderkooi, G. and Green, D. E.: New insights into biological membrane structure. Bioscience *21:*409, 1971.

Ribosomes and Granular Endoplasmic Reticulum

Alfrey, V. G.: Nuclear ribosomes, messenger RNA and protein synthesis. Exp. Cell Res. *9:*183, 1963.

Haguenau, F.: The ergastoplasm: Its history, ultrastructure and biochemistry. Int. Rev. Cytol. *7:*425, 1958.

Palade, G. E.: A small particulate component of the cytoplasm. J. Biophys. Biochem. Cytol. *1:*59, 1955.

Porter, K. R.: Observations on a submicroscopic basophilic component of the cytoplasm. J. Exp. Med. *97:*727, 1953.

Palade, G.: Intracellular aspects of the process of protein synthesis. Science. *189:*347, 1975.

Rich, A.: Polyribosomes. Sci. Amer. *209:*44, 1963.

Spirin, A. S. and Gavrilova, L. P.: *The Ribosome.* Springer-Verlag, New York, 1969.

Agranular Endoplasmic Reticulum

Christensen, A. K.: Fine structure of testicular interstitial cells in the guinea pig. J. Cell Biol. *26:*911, 1965.

Christensen, A. K. and Fawcett, D. W.: The fine structure of the interstitial cells of the mouse testis. Amer. J. Anat. *118:*551, 1966.

Ito, S.: The endoplasmic reticulum of gastric parietal cells. J. Biophys. Biochem. Cytol. *11:*333, 1961.

Remmer, H. and Merker, H. J.: Effects of drugs on the formation of smooth endoplasmic reticulum and drug metabolizing enzymes. Ann. N. Y. Acad. Sci. *123:*79, 1965.

Golgi Complex

Beams, H. W. and Kessel, R. G.: The Golgi apparatus: Structure and function. Int. Rev. Cytol. *23:*209, 1968.

Berlin, J. D.: The localization of acid mucopolysaccharides in the Golgi complex of intestinal goblet cells. J. Cell Biol. *32:*760, 1967.

Caro, L. G. and Palade, G. E.: Protein synthesis, storage and discharge in the pancreatic exocrine cell. An autoradiographic study. J. Cell Biol. *20:*473, 1964.

Hodge, A. J., McLeon, S. D. and Mercer, F. V.: A possible mechanism for the morphogenesis of lamellar systems in plant cells. J. Biophys. Biochem. Cytol. *2:*597, 1956.

Jamieson, J. D. and Palade, G. E.: Intracellular transport of secretory proteins in the pancreatic exocrine cell. I. Role of the peripheral elements of the Golgi complex. J. Cell Biol. *34:*597, 1967.

Neutra, M. and Leblond, C. P.: Synthesis of the carbohydrate of mucus in the Golgi complex as shown by electron microscope radioautography of goblet cells from rats injected with glucose-H^3. J. Cell Biol. *30:*119, 1966.

Neutra, M. and Leblond, C. P.: The Golgi apparatus. Sci. Am. *220:*100, 1969.

Mitochondria

Ashwell, M. and Work, T.: The biogenesis of mitochondria. Ann. Rev. Biochem. *39:*251, 1970.

Claude, A. and Fullom, E. F.: Electron microscopic study of isolated mitochondria. J. Exp. Med. *81:*51, 1945.

Fernandez-Moran, H., Oda, T., Blair, P. V. and Green, D. E.: A macromolecular repeating unit of mitochondrial structure and function. J. Cell Biol. *22:*63, 1964.

Green, D. E. and Young, J. H.: Energy transduction in membrane systems. Amer. Sci. *59:*92, 1971.

Hackenbrock, C. R.: Ultrastructural basis for metabolically-linked mechanical activity in mitochondria. I. Reversible ultrastructural changes in metabolic steady state in isolated liver mitochondria. J. Cell Biol. *30:*269, 1966.

Hackenbrock, C. R.: Ultrastructural basis for metabolically-linked mechanical activity in mitochondria. II. Electron transport-linked ultrastructural transformations in mitochondria. J. Cell Biol. *37:*345, 1968.

Hall, D. and Palmer, J.: Mitochondrial research today. Nature *221:*717, 1969.

Lehninger, A. L.: *The Mitochondrion.* Benjamin, New York, 1964.

Munn, E. A.: *The Structure of Mitochondria.* Academic Press, New York, 1974.

Wagner, P.: Genetics and phenogenetics of mitochondria. Science *163:*1026, 1969.

Weber, N. E. and Blair, P. V.: Ultrastructural studies of beef heart mitochondria. I. Effects of adenosine diphosphate on mitochondrial morphology. Biochem. Biophys. Res. Commun. *36:*987, 1969.

Lysosomes

DeDuve, C.: Lysosomes. Sci. Amer. *208:*5, 1963.

Gahan, P. B.: Histochemistry of lysosomes. Int. Rev. Cytol. *21:*1, 1967.

Gordon, G. B., Miller, L. R. and Bensch, K. G.: Studies on the intracellular digestive process in mammalian tissue culture cells. J. Cell Biol. *25:*41, 1965.

Novikoff, A. B., Essner, E. and Quintana, N.: Golgi apparatus and lysosomes. Fed. Proc. *23:*1010, 1964.

Centrioles and Basal Bodies

Randall, J. and Hopkins, J. M.: Studies on cilia, basal bodies and some related organelles. II. Problems of genesis. Proc. Linnean Soc. London *174:*37, 1963.

Szollosi, D.: Centrioles, centriolar satellites and spindle fibers. Anat. Rec. *148:*343, 1964.

Wolfe, J.: Basal body fine structure and chemistry. Adv. Cell Mol. Biol. *2:*151, 1972.

Yamada, E.: Some observations on the fine structure of the centriole in the mitotic cell. Kurume Med. J. *5:* 36, 1958.

Microbodies

Hruban, Z. and Rechcigl, M., Jr.: Microbodies and Related Particles: Morphology, Biochemistry, and Physiology. Int. Rev. Cytol. Suppl. I. Academic Press, New York, 1969.

Microtubules, Filaments and Fibrils

Behnke, O.: Studies on isolated microtubules. Evidence for a clear space component. Cytobiol. *11:*366, 1975.

Brody, I.: The ultrastructure of the tonofilaments in the keratinization process. J. Ultrastruct. Res. *4:*265, 1960.

Huxley, H. E.: Electron microscopic studies in the structure of natural and synthetic protein filaments from striated muscle. J. Molec. Biol. *7:*281, 1963.

Inoué, S. and Stephens, R. E. (ed.): *Molecules and Cell Movement.* Raven Press, New York, 1975.

Ledbetter, M. C. and Porter, K. R.: Morphology of microtubules of plant cells. Science *144:*872, 1964.

Sandborn, E., Koen, P. F., McNabb, J. D. and Moore, G.: Cytoplasmic microtubules in mammalian cells. J. Ultrastruct. Res. *11:*123, 1964.

Slautterback, D. B.: Cytoplasmic microtubules. I. Hydra. J. Cell Biol. *18:*367, 1963.

Inclusions

Billingham, R. E. and Silvers, W. K.: The melanocytes of mammals. Quart. Rev. Biol. *35:*1, 1960.

Bjorkerud, S.: The isolation of lipofuscin granules from bovine cardiac muscle. J. Ultrastruct. Res. *5:*5, 1963.

Napolitano, L.: The differentiation of white adipose cells. An electron microscope study. J. Cell Biol. *18:*663, 1963.

Revel, J. P.: Electron microscopy of glycogen. J. Histochem. Cytochem. *12:*104, 1964.

Cell Division

Flemming, W.: Contributions to the knowledge of the cell and its vital processes. J. Cell Biol. *25:*3, 1965. (A translation of the 1880 work.)

Mazia, D.: How cells divide. Sci. Amer. *105:*101, 1961.

Mazia, D.: Fibrillar structure in mitotic apparatus. In *Formation of Cell Organelles,* edited by K. B. Warren. Academic Press, New York, 1967.

SECTION III:

HISTOLOGY

5: Epithelia

General Characteristics

Form. Epithelial tissues consist of aggregations of cells that cover or line the surfaces of the body and/or organs. Epithelia are composed generally of similar cells, or cells closely related structurally or functionally. They are in intimate contact with each other with little *intercellular substance* between them; therefore these tissues have a *high cellular density.* Their close contact forms an effective barrier between the underlying connective tissue and the external environment or the environment characteristic of the tubular contents of the organ of which they are a part.

One margin of the cell is free, in contact with the environment (external or internal), and is termed the *apical* or *luminal border.* The *basal border* contacts the underlying connective tissue, while the *lateral surface* affords contact between adjacent cells. These cells possess apical/basal modifications that generally impart a distinct *cellular polarity.* Although cellular polarity is not a feature unique to epithelial cells, this characteristic is well-developed in them and their constituent organelles reflect this polarity.

Epithelia are separated from the connective tissue by a *basement membrane.* Epithelial tissues are avascular and are dependent upon the underlying connective tissue for the movement of metabolites and waste products.

The apical, lateral and basal borders of epithelial cells have numerous modifications: *microvilli, kinocilia, stereocilia, desmosomes, basal lamina* and various *junctional alterations.* Not all of these modifications are unique to epithelial cells, but they occur with sufficient frequency to be described as epithelial characteristics. (See Surface Specializations of Epithelia.)

Functional Correlates. Epithelial cells are modified sufficiently to subserve numerous and varied functions that are essential to the organism. *Protection* from various insults—mechanical, bacterial, desiccative, ultraviolet radiational—is an important function and is achieved in various ways by these tissues. The body is protected from the aforementioned insults by virtue of its thickened and pigmented epithelial covering—the epidermis. The lining of the body tubes (digestive, respiratory and genitourinary systems) are subjected to mechanical injury, bacterial invasion and other insults to these surfaces. The effects of these challenges are minimized by the lining epithelium. *Transport* of particulate matter along epithelial surfaces affords protection and is achieved by ciliary action along the apical borders of lining cells.

Secretion of various materials is an indispensable epithelial function. Waxy secretions of epithelial cells lubricate the covering epithelium and its associated structures—hairs and feathers. Also, secretions of epithelial cells moisten and protect lining epithelia. Other cells elaborate voluminous quantities of a watery secretion. During a 24-hour period, the secretory cells of the salivary glands of herbivores may secrete 10–15 gallons of this watery product. Some secretory cells assist with *excretory functions.* Certain cells of the urinary and integumentary epithelia are involved in the elaboration of urine and sweat. In some animals, the formation of sweat subserves a significant role in *thermoregulation.* In the dairy cow, specific epithelial cells of the udder are responsible for the formation of 50–100 pounds of milk per day. As such, these cells perform an important adjunctive function to *reproduction.* Some epithelial cells are modified to synthesize and secrete digestive enzyme precursors, essential elements for the nutritional well-being of the organism. All of these examples of secretion characterize cells which elaborate their products onto a lining or covering epithelium. These are the cells of the *exocrine glands* or the *glands of external secretion.*

Absorption of various materials through the epithelial cells of the lungs, gastrointestinal tract and kidney tubules also represents another physiologic modification of epithelia. The selective uptake of various substances and the exclusion of others indicate that this function is highly selective and specific.

Whereas the secondary association of nerve fibers with epithelial cells and the skin imparts a sensory function to this covering, other epithelial cells are modified specifically as *sensory receptors.* Olfactory, gustatory and auditory sensations are mediated through such cells.

Certain cells of epithelial origin which have secondarily lost their associations with lining epithelia are important mediators of *internal communication.* These cells elaborate the hormones of the body and are components of the *endocrine glands* or the *glands of internal secretion.*

Other epithelial cells, such as those that line the vascular and lymphatic systems, insure that *functional exchange* occurs between the blood and lymphatic channels and the rest of the somatic (body) cells. Other similarly shaped cells line the body cavities (coelomic spaces) and facilitate the movement of the visceral organs over smooth and lubricated surfaces.

Lastly, specific cells are reserved for the perpetuation of the species. These epithelial cells of the gonads perform the important *reproductive function.*

Not all epithelial cells perform all the aforementioned functions. Some of them, however, perform a variety of these functions simultaneously. Most importantly, the lining cells of epithelia form an effective barrier or interface that prevents the free outward movement of vital tissue fluid components while preventing the ingress of certain materials to the underlying fluid compartment. This is accomplished while exerting a selective influence on the ingress and egress of various substances. Some epithelial cells are more effective barriers than others; others characteristically permit some leakage across the lining.

Origin of Epithelia. During the early course of development, the embryo differentiates into three distinct germ layers—*ectoderm, mesoderm* and *endoderm.* The outer covering (ectoderm) is separated from the inner lining (endoderm) by an intermediate packing layer, the mesoderm. Most of the epithelia are derivatives of the ectoderm and endoderm; a few are derived from mesoderm.

Diverse epithelial structures result from the development and differentiation of the ectoderm. The epithelium of the skin (epidermis) and its derivatives (hair, feathers, claws, hooves, horns, combs, wattles) are formed from the ectoderm. Invagination of the epidermis into the associated mesoderm results in the formation of sweat glands, sebaceous glands, mammary glands and hair (feather) follicles. The ectoderm also differentiates into the epithelium of the nasal cavity; paranasal sinuses and part of the buccal cavity; the terminal portions of the digestive tract and genitourinary system; dental laminae; Rathke's pouch and the adenohypophysis; the lens of the eye, conjunctiva and the outer layer of the tympanic membrane; organs responsible for auditory, olfactory and gustatory sensations; cells of the central and peripheral nervous systems and iridial musculature. Early in development, all of these derivatives are typically epithelial in character. Only the cells of the nervous system and iridial musculature secondarily lose their epithelial characteristics.

51

The endoderm differentiates into numerous and diverse epithelial derivatives that line the inner aspect of the developing organism. This simple endodermal lining is characterized by numerous invaginations into the associated mesoderm. Among the epithelial derivatives of the endoderm are the lining of the digestive tract, except its initial and terminal portions; the parenchyma of the liver, pancreas and other digestive glands; the glands of internal secretion (thyroid, parathyroid, adrenal cortex); thymus; trachea and lungs; urinary bladder, accessory sex glands and portions of the sex organs; portions of the oropharynx, nasopharynx, pharyngotympanic tube, middle ear cavity and the inner lining of the tympanic membrane. With the exception of the thymus, the other endodermal derivatives retain their epithelial characteristics throughout adulthood.

The mesoderm differentiates into the remaining tissues and organs of the body, including the adrenal cortex and part of the kidney. Additionally, this layer forms two kinds of epithelial cells. During the process of coelomic space formation, the mesoderm splits and becomes lined by flattened cells which originate from the mesoderm and have epithelial characteristics. These cells, because of their unique origin and position, are called *mesothelium*. The cells line the peritoneal, pericardial and pleural cavities. Also, the differentiation of the lining cells of the heart, arteries, veins, capillaries and lymphatics occurs from the mesoderm. These lining cells are referred to as *endothelium*.

The *mesectoderm* consists of mesenchyme derived from neural crest cells. These primitive cells give rise to many cell types. One type, *mesenchymal epithelium*, lines certain spaces of the body. Mesenchymal epithelial cells comprise the leptomeninges (pia mater and arachnoid membrane), perilymphatic lining of the ear and the iridial lining.

Unique Relationships. Epithelial tissues are avascular. They are dependent totally upon the underlying connective tissue for all of their nutrients. Similarly, waste products pass into this space for removal by the component vessels. This functional dependency upon the connective tissue is a requirement of all tissues. For those tissues that are "embedded within" or "surrounded by" the connective tissue space, the dependent relationship is less obvious than that noted in epithelia. Any separation of epithelia from the underlying connective tissue may have disastrous effects upon the integrity of this cellular boundary. The significance of this relationship is recognized by the use of a collective term that includes the epithelium and its associated connective tissue—*membrane* or *epithelial membrane*. These membranes have different properties in different foci in the body. The integument is a membrane that consists of a thickened layer of epithelial cells with an underlying dermis (fibrous connective tissue). This particular architecture permits mobility, expansion and contraction while insuring an intimate and continuous association between the two constituents. Similarly, moistened membranes (serous membranes, mucous membranes) have epithelial and connective tissue components. They are discussed in Chapter 13.

The intimate relationship described for epithelia and their underlying connective tissues requires some sort of "glue" to hold them together. This is achieved by the *basement membrane*. This structure varies in thickness but is usually visible with the light microscope. Although it is difficult to visualize with routine H and E, it is demonstrable with silver stains and PAS. It is a consistent modification associated with the basal border of epithelial cells. See *Basal Border Modifications* for a more complete discussion.

As mentioned previously, not all epithelial cells retain those characteristics which typify this tissue. The *glands of internal secretion (endocrine glands)* secondarily lose their association with a surface lining. Their basal surfaces, however, are still associated with the connective tissue. Thyroid lining cells form unique relationships in which these cells lose their original association with a surface but secondarily acquire a lumen for the temporary storage of their secretory products. These follicles or hollow spheres of cells maintain their apical/basal relationships. Other glands (parathyroids, adrenal cortex, adenohypophysis, liver) are composed of cords or clumps of cells. The epithelial nature of these cells may seem obscure. In the liver, however, careful examination with the electron microscope confirms their epithelial characteristics. The epithelial components of the thymus, which are derivatives of the endodermal lining of the pharyngeal pouches, form a cellular network (reticulum) that obscures their epithelial nature. These cells are called *epithelial-reticular cells*.

Classification. The classification and naming of epithelial tissues is based on two criteria: the number of cells layered upon each other and the predominant or surface cell shape (Fig. 5.1). An epithelial lining is either *simple* (one cell layer), *stratified* (more than one cell layer), *pseudostratified* (one cell layer appearing as more than one) or *transitional* (layers subject to change).

Simple epithelia are named according to the predominant cell type accordingly: *squamous, cuboidal, columnar* or *pseudostratified*. Stratified epithelia, however, are named on the basis of the shape of the apical or luminal cell type accordingly: *squamous, cuboidal* or *columnar*. Although current indications are that transitional epithelium actually represents a pseudostratified condition, it is worthy of special consideration because it is capable of varying the number of layers that are apparent. Some authors, however, may also refer to it as a stratified cuboidal epithelium.

Simple Epithelia

Simple Squamous Epithelium. This type of tissue is characterized by extremely thin cells, the cytoplasm of which is barely visible with light microscopy (Fig. 5.2). Often there is a prominent bulge into the free surface at the location of the nucleus. The cytoplasm is expansive, and nuclei are generally quite a distance from each other. In many instances the cytoplasm, although expansive, is thin and gives the appearance of being absent. However, electron micrographs verify its presence and nature (Fig. 5.3). In surface view the cells composing this tissue are polygons, but they appear spindle-shaped when cut perpendicular to the free surface or basal surface.

This morphology is suited ideally for the transport of materials across a diminished cytoplasmic mass. Pinocytotic activity, as evidenced by the presence of caveolae and pinocytotic vesicles, is confirmed with electron micrographs (Fig. 5.50). The endothelial lining of blood vessels permits the movement of fluids, crystalloids and some colloids. The lining comprises the functional exchange mechanism between the intravascular and extravascular space. Similarly, this type of epithelium in the lung contributes to the blood-air boundary and facilitates the exchange of oxygen and carbon dioxide. Thin segments of the loop of Henle in the kidney are involved in fluid exchange. The mesothelium of the coelomic spaces permits the passage of tissue fluid into the body cavities, as well as serving as a smooth surface for the movement of organs.

OCCURRENCE: Lining of coelomic spaces (mesothelium); lining of cardiovascular and lymphatic systems (endothelium); functional lining of lung; small ducts of numerous glands; specific portions of kidney tubules and Bowman's capsule; membranous labyrinth of the inner ear.

Simple Cuboidal Epithelium. The general shapes of the cells of this type of tissue are described as cubes. In actuality, they appear as squares in sections perpendicular to the apical border (Fig. 5.4). From surface views they may appear as squares or hexagons. Nuclei are usually *central* or *paracentral* in position. Lateral cell borders may or may not be distinct. Naming of this tissue is sometimes difficult, because there is a continuum of cellular conformation from squamous to columnar. Some histologists will use modifiers such as "high cuboidal" or "low columnar."

This type of epithelium is associated generally with secretion and absorption. Some of these cells may comprise nonsecretory or nonabsorptive linings of tubules.

OCCURRENCE: Secretory and duct portions of numerous glands; certain tubules of the kidney;

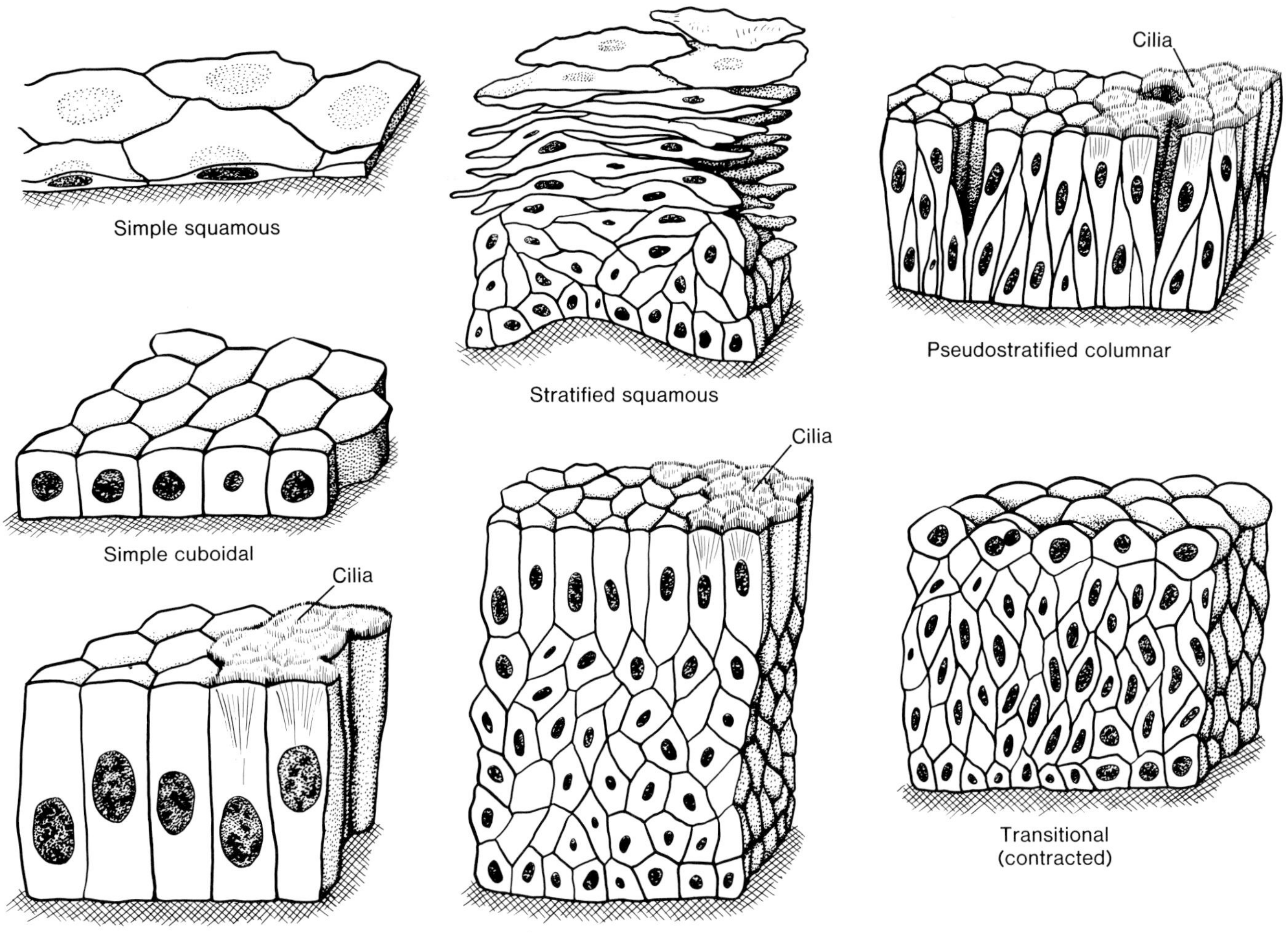

Simple squamous

Stratified squamous

Cilia

Pseudostratified columnar

Simple cuboidal

Cilia

Cilia

Simple columnar

Stratified columnar

Transitional
(contracted)

Fig. 5.1 Diagram of types of epithelium. Simple, stratified, pseudostratified and transitional epithelia are shown in relation to their underlying connective tissue. Simple cuboidal, simple columnar, stratified columnar and pseudostratified columnar epithelia may be ciliated.

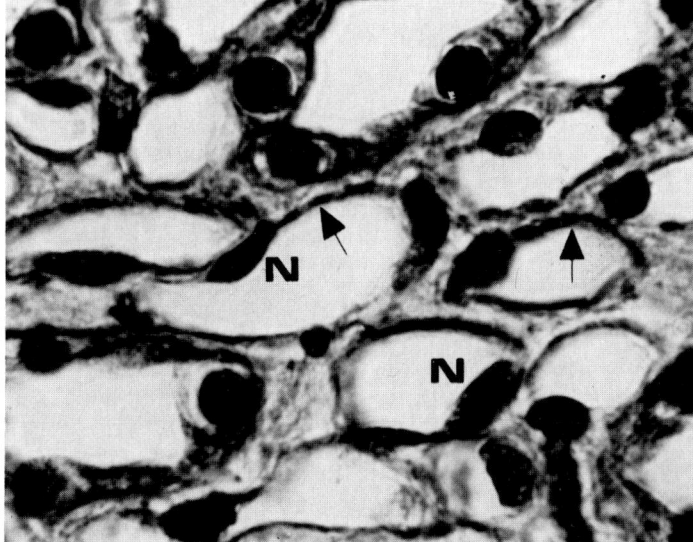

Fig. 5.2 Simple squamous epithelial lining of canine kidney tubules. The dark nuclei (N) are the obvious components of the cell. The cytoplasm, which is barely visible (*arrows*), appears as a thin rim or cytoplasmic process. The lining cells are actually pancake-shaped cells that are folded upon themselves and adjacent cells as a tube. X160. All light micrographs are labeled as the magnification with the microscope before photographic enlarging. All electron micrographs are labeled as total magnification, including photographic enlarging.

specific portions of the respiratory tree; surfaces of the lens and iris; surface epithelium of the ovary; specific tubules of the testis; pigmented epithelium of the retina (Plate III.1).

Simple Columnar Epithelium. The basic morphologic feature of this tissue is that the cells are taller than they are wide (Fig. 5.5). The nuclei, similarly, are elongated and generally displaced toward the basal border. There is, therefore, a distinct cellular polarity. Usually the nuclei will form a distinct row; occasionally they may form two rows due to a crowding of cells.

This type of morphology is associated typically with secretory processes. Most of the exocrine glands of the body are composed of these types of cells. Another important process is that of absorption. Various apical border modifications suit them ideally for these functions.

OCCURRENCE: Lining of glandular stomach, small and large intestine; middle portions of the respiratory tree; lining of the uterus and uterine tubes; lining of the secretory and conducting portion of many glands; lining of the cholecyst (Plates III.2, III.3, III.4).

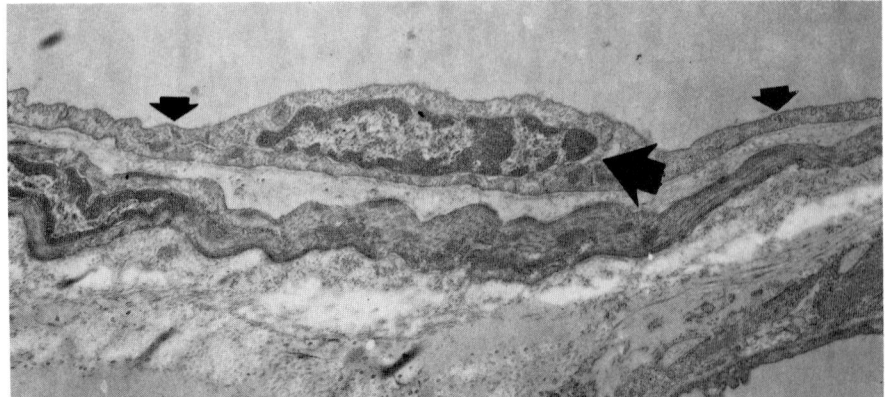

Fig. 5.3 An electron micrograph of a simple squamous epithelial lining cell of a pulmonary alveolus. The nucleus (*large arrow*) protrudes into the lumen. The attenuated lateral projections of cytoplasm (*small arrows*) comprise the major lining component of the alveolus through which gaseous exchange occurs. X120,000. (Courtesy of G. P. Epling)

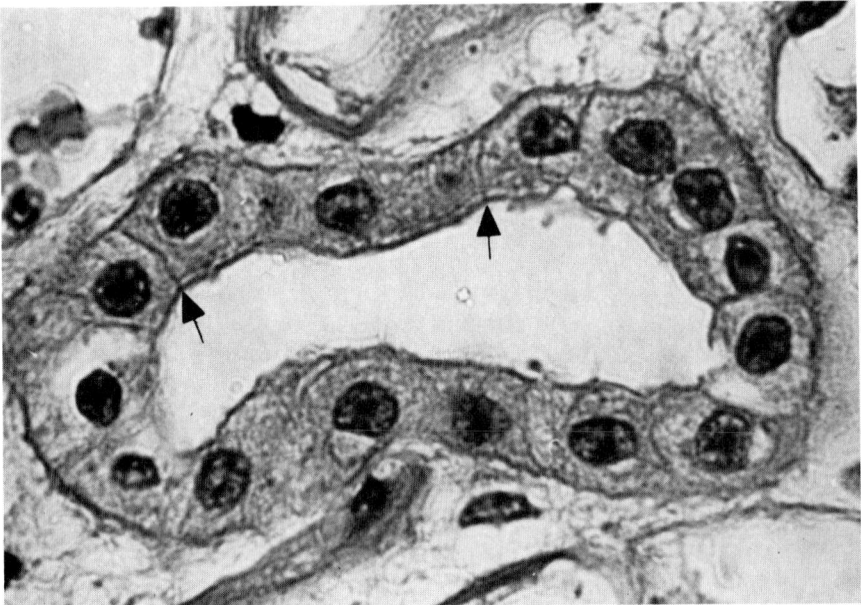

Fig. 5.4 Cuboidal epithelial lining of a collecting tubule from the equine kidney. The nuclei occur within a homogeneous cytoplasm. The cellular limits of some cells are apparent (*arrows*). Although these cells appear as squares in biplanar sections, they are actually cubic structures when viewed three dimensionally. X320.

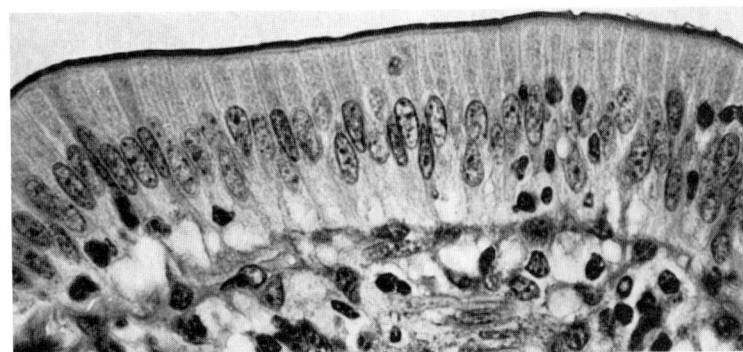

Fig. 5.5 Columnar cells from the duodenum of a bird. The elongated and basally positioned nuclei accentuate the cellular polarity. Compare with Figure 3.10. The lining cells depicted are absorptive cells. X320.

Pseudostratified Epithelium. All of the cells of this type of epithelium reside on the basement membrane. Not all of them, however, reach the free surface. Only the columnar cell component reaches the luminal surface. In section this epithelial type appears to be overcrowded with cells (Figs. 5.6, 5.40). The basal and middle part of the lining is congested with the nuclei of the three cell types that comprise this epithelium—basal cells, fusiform cells and columnar cells. A fourth type of cell, a *goblet cell*, is present in certain loci. Surface modifications, *cilia*, are often found on the luminal surfaces of the columnar cells. This epithelial type is most precisely referred to as *pseudostratified columnar* or *pseudostratified ciliated columnar epithelium.*

This epithelium is most often confused with simple columnar epithelium that has been cut on a plane oblique to the surface (Fig. 5.7). However, careful examination of the sections will show that, even in an oblique plane, simple columnar epithelium does not possess the degree of nuclear congestion mentioned previously.

The primary function of this type of epithelium is to serve as a lining of certain tubular organs. Significant alterations to their apical surfaces, cilia, afford a protective function. Numerous goblet cells, single-celled mucous glands, supply a viscous protective layer. Particulate matter contained within the mucous layer is moved by the cilia toward the exterior. The mucus and cilia comprise an important protective mechanism called the *mucociliary apparatus.*

OCCURRENCE: Lining of upper respiratory tract, lining of specific regions of urogenital system; ducts of glands at points of transition between simple and stratified epithelium (Plate III.7).

Stratified Epithelia

Stratified Squamous Epithelium. Characterized by many cellular layers which are derived from a single basal layer, this type of epithelium is found where protection of the underlying tissues is an important functional consideration (Fig. 5.8). The thickness of this tissue type may vary from quite thin to exceedingly thick.

The basal layer of cells (*stratum basale*) consists of a single layer of cuboidal or columnar cells which are extremely basophilic due to the extensive ergastoplasm (Fig. 5.9). As the name implies, this cell layer resides on the basement membrane and is partially responsible for giving rise to subsequent cellular components.

The cells of the *stratum spinosum* are lighter in staining affinity than those of the basal layer and are progressively more flattened toward the luminal surface. Shrinking of cells by processing techniques demonstrates intercellular spaces in which numerous cellular processes from adjacent cells are in contact with one another (Fig. 5.10). These processes (*spines* or *prickles*) are not actually intercellular bridges but represent two cellular processes joined by a *desmosome*. This configuration is responsible for the naming of this layer as *spinous cell layer* or *prickle cell layer*.

Together, the *stratum basale* and the *stratum spinosum* are referred to as the *stratum germinativum* or *Malpighian layer*. Mitoses within the germinal layer are responsible for the replacement of cells lost at the luminal surface.

The *stratum granulosum*, depending upon the specific location of the epithelium, may be several cell layers thick or may be totally absent. The granularity of the spindle cells of this layer is attributable to the basophilic *keratohyalin* granules (Fig. 5.11). These are precursor substances to *keratin*. Degenerative changes in the cells, as evidenced by pyknotic nuclei, are also characteristic of the cells of this layer.

The cells of the *stratum lucidum* are extremely flattened, pale-staining or slightly acidophilic. This layer, which is of variable occurrence, represents dead or dying cells. Nuclei are either indistinct or missing and the cytoplasm is agranular. Occasionally, granules of *eleidin* are present. The closely packed cells of this region may be several layers thick.

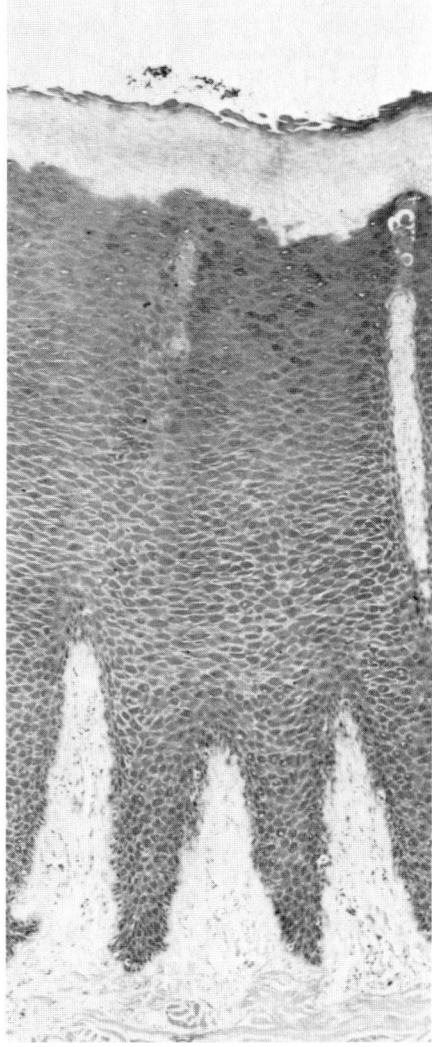

Fig. 5.8 Stratified squamous epithelium of the canine muzzle. The epithelium, intimately associated with the underlying connective tissue, is highly cornified (*light-staining material at the top of the field*). X25.

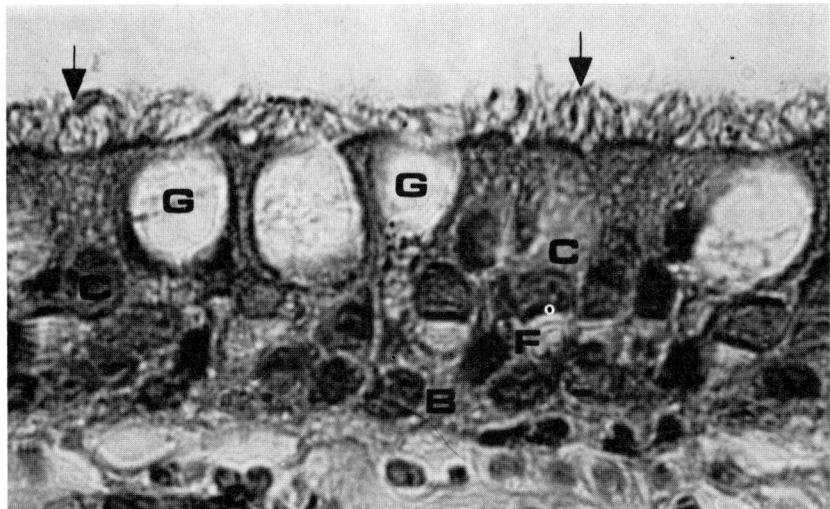

Fig. 5.6 Pseudostratified ciliated columnar epithelial cells of the ovine trachea. All cells of the lining contact the basement membrane, but not all cells reach the luminal surface. Compare with Figure 5.1. The "stratification" is evident because of the arrangement of the nuclei of basal (B), fusiform (F) and columnar cells (C). Cilia (*arrows*) occur along the luminal border. Goblet cells (G) are present. X320.

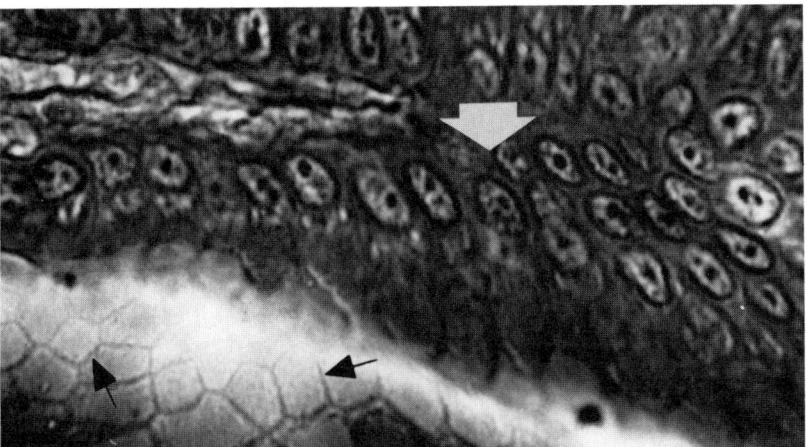

Fig. 5.7 Oblique section of simple columnar epithelium from the duodenum of a bird. The cells to the left of the *white arrow*, cut normal to their longitudinal axes, appear as typical simple columnar cells. Those to the right of the *white arrow*, cut obliquely to their longitudinal axes, give the impression of stratification. This occurs because of the obliquity of the section and the unevenness of nuclear location within the cell. *Solid arrows*, cross sections of the same cells. Note the uneven registration of nuclei in Figure 5.5. X320.

The *stratum corneum* (Fig. 5.12) is a well-developed layer of closely packed, dead cells in those regions typified by a high degree of *keratinization* (footpads). The remainder of the skin is less keratinized, but this stratum is still present. The cells which are being sloughed comprise a *stratum disjunctum*. Lesser degrees of keratinization or a total absence thereof are characteristic of the entrance and exit of the digestive tube, as well as portions along its length (esophagus, nonglandular portions of the ruminant stomach).

In those stratified squamous epithelia that are either minimally keratinized or nonkeratinized, not all of the aforementioned layers are distinguishable (Fig. 5.13). The *basal layer* is usually the only distinct layer. The remaining layers are sometimes referred to as *parabasal*, *intermediate* and *superficial*.

Stratified squamous epithelium, in most locations, is a thick epithelial membrane.

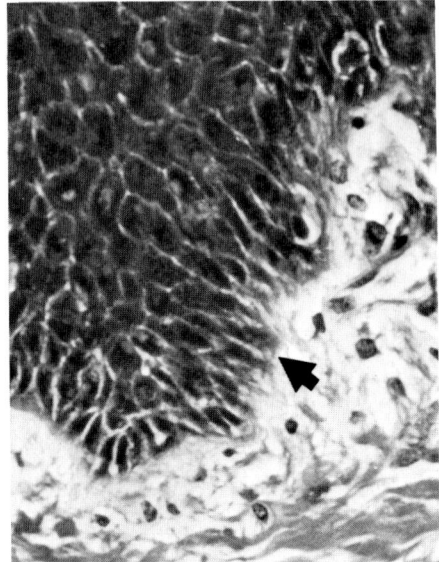

Fig. 5.9 The stratum basale (*arrow*) of the stratified squamous epithelium of the canine muzzle. X400.

The interface between the basal cell layer and the associated connective tissue presents numerous interdigitations. This particular morphologic relationship affords a large surface area for diffusion, as well as a large area for adhesion.

The protective function of this tissue is manifested in varied ways. The keratinized layer protects against dessicative and mechanical damage. The significance of this function is best considered in the epidermis. Even those epithelia that are not keratinized, or only minimally keratinized, afford protection from mechanical damage. The dental pad of ruminants also permits mastication with minimal damage from the abrasive action of foodstuffs. The upper digestive tract of ruminants is protected from the abrasiveness of roughened foodstuffs by this epithelium. Significantly, this epithelium also serves an absorptive function in ruminants. Volatile fatty acids (acetic, butyric and propionic), which are essential components of ruminant metabolism, are absorbed from the forestomachs through stratified squamous epithelium.

OCCURRENCE (*keratinized*): General body surface; buccal cavity; anal region; ruminant forestomach (Plate III.5).

OCCURRENCE (*nonkeratinized*): Vestibular region of respiratory system; oral, esophageal and anal portions of digestive system; cornea of eye; conjunctiva; portions of the male and female urogenital systems (Plate III.6).

Stratified Cuboidal Epithelium. This epithelium consists of two layers of cells (Fig. 5.14). The basal layer consists of polygonal cells responsible for the regeneration of lost cells. The superficial or luminal layer is occupied by cuboidal cells. Although this epithelium is characteristic of a few loci, it

is encountered frequently in areas of transition from simple to stratified epithelia. Some authors refer to transitional epithelium as stratified cuboidal.

OCCURRENCE: Specific portions of genital system; ducts of various glands, zones of transition between simple and stratified epithelia.

Stratified Columnar Epithelium. This tissue may consist of two, three or more layers of

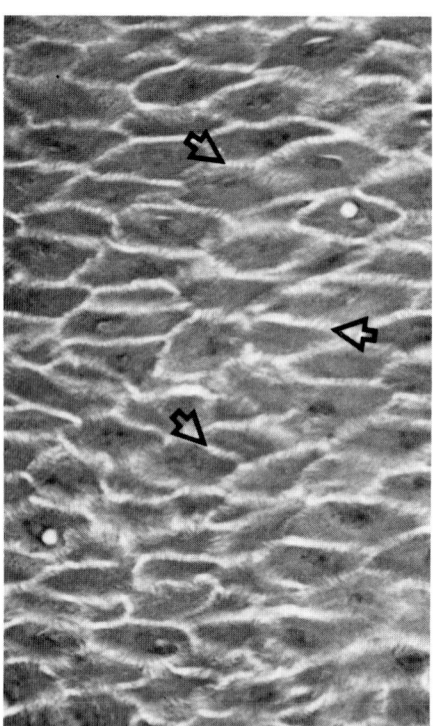

Fig. 5.10 The stratum spinosum of stratified squamous epithelium of the canine muzzle. Spinous processes (*arrows*) between cells are apparent. X400.

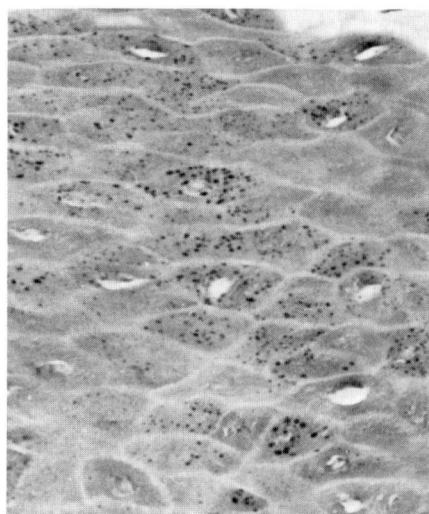

Fig. 5.11. Stratified squamous epithelim of the canine muzzle. The stratum granulosum occurs at the junction of the stratum corneum or stratum lucidum. X400.

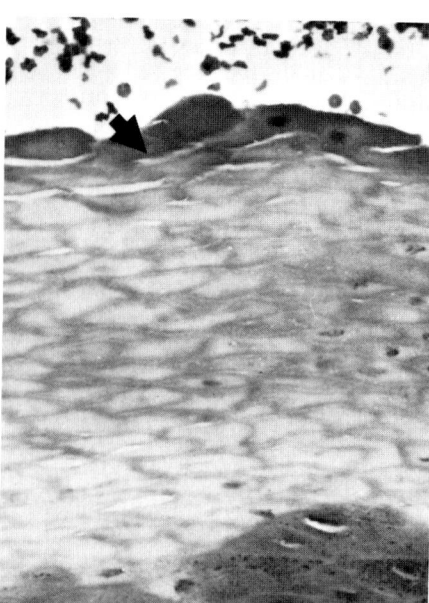

Fig. 5.12 The stratum corneum and stratum disjunctum (*arrow*) of stratified squamous epithelium of the canine muzzle. X400.

cells (Fig. 5.15). The basal and luminal cells are sometimes separated from each other by intermediate cell types. The basal cells are normally cuboidal; the intermediate, polygonal; the apical cells, columnar. This tissue is sometimes difficult to distinguish from pseudostratified epithelium.

Stratified cuboidal and columnar epithelia are presumed to serve only a lining function. Their interdigitation between the simple epithelia of glands and the stratified or pseudostratified epithelia of lining surfaces affords a gradual transition from one type to the other.

OCCURRENCE: Points of transition between columnar or pseudostratified and stratified epithelium; portions of the upper respiratory tract; ducts of some glands.

Transitional Epithelium

Transitional Epithelium. This tissue is normally considered a stratified type. However, a recent study has indicated that it may be pseudostratified. Whichever is the case, it still deserves special attention because of its ability to change shape as a result of the pressure applied on it from the luminal surface. Because it is associated only with the urogenital system, it is sometimes referred to as *urothelium*.

In the relaxed state, it may consist of as many as 6 or 7 layers (Fig. 5.16). The basal cells are very small and assume a polyhedral configuration. The cells of the intermediate region are polyhedral or pear-shaped. The cells at the luminal border are cuboidal and their apical borders bulge into the lumen.

During distention, the thickness of the epithelium is markedly reduced (Fig. 5.17). As few as two or three layers may be appar-

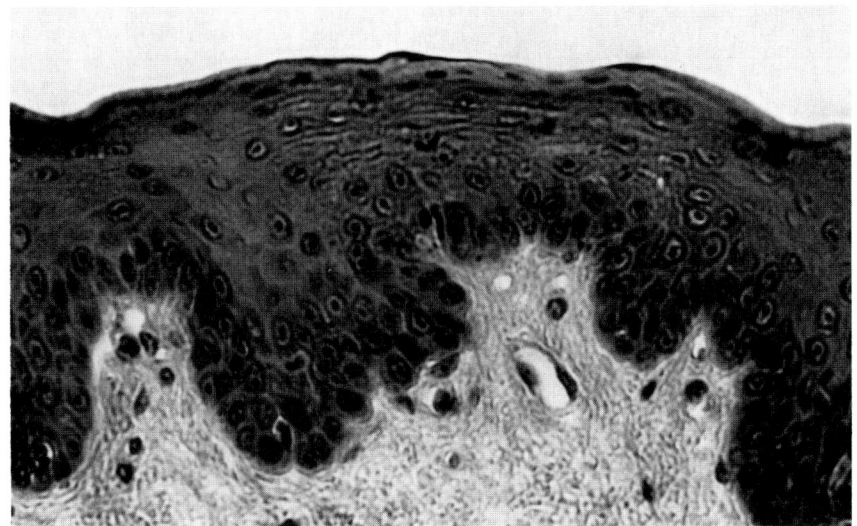

Fig. 5.13 Nonkeratinized stratified squamous epithelium from the feline buccal cavity. X125.

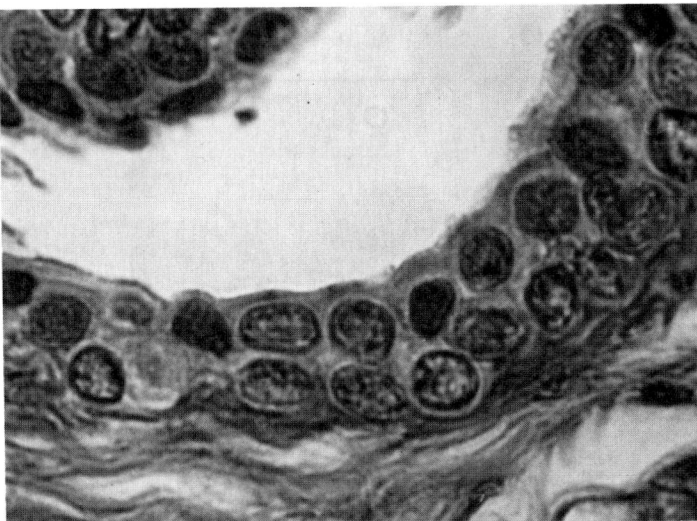

Fig. 5.14 Bistratified cuboidal epithelium of a duct from a feline salivary gland. X400.

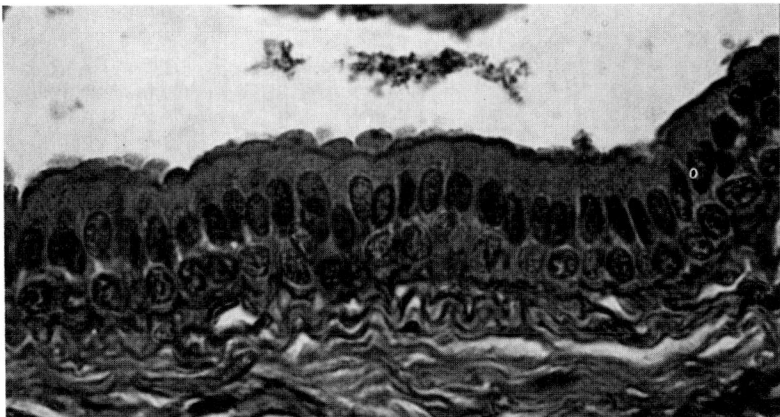

Fig. 5.15 Bistratified columnar epithelium of a duct from a feline salivary gland. X400.

ent. In a state of distention, this tissue is sometimes mistaken for stratified squamous epithelium.

This epithelium functions as a lining that is capable of accommodating to the stretching that results from an increased luminal volume. More importantly, it is an effective barrier to the movement of water. Urothelium prevents the movement of water from the connective tissue space to the luminal space occupied by the hypertonic urine.

OCCURRENCE: Lining of specific regions of the urinary system.

Glandular Epithelia

General Features and Classification. Although epithelia are primarily lining tissues, a significant function of these tissues is associated with the ability of single cells and propulations of cells to produce a variety of products for extracellular use. Modifications of these surface linings are manifested in a variety of ways to accomplish a diversity of secretory functions. Not only are epithelia modified morphologically to accomplish secretory activity, but there are various mechanisms utilized as well. Also, the relationship of glandular tissue to surrounding tissue is varied. Accordingly, there are numerous ways by which glandular tissue may be classified:

1. Number of cells comprising the gland
   a. Unicellular
   b. Multicellular
2. Relationship to lining and surrounding tissue
   a. Exocrine
   b. Endocrine
3. Configuration of multicellular glands
   a. Simple
   b. Compound
4. Method of elaboration
   a. Apocrine
   b. Merocrine
   c. Holocrine
5. Type of secretory product
   a. Serous
   b. Mucous
   c. Miscellaneous

Because "Man classifies and nature doesn't," there are numerous examples that do not fit perfectly into any one of the classifications. However, an awareness of the organization of glandular tissue through these varied classifications will serve to give insights into this specialized function of epithelial tissues.

Number of Cells in a Gland. Glands are either *unicellular* or *multicellular*.

Unicellular glands are simply specialized cells that are scattered throughout an epithelial lining. Although there are varied modifications, the most common and representative unicellular gland is the goblet cell (Fig. 5.6). It is scattered commonly throughout the respiratory and digestive systems and occasionally in the urinary system

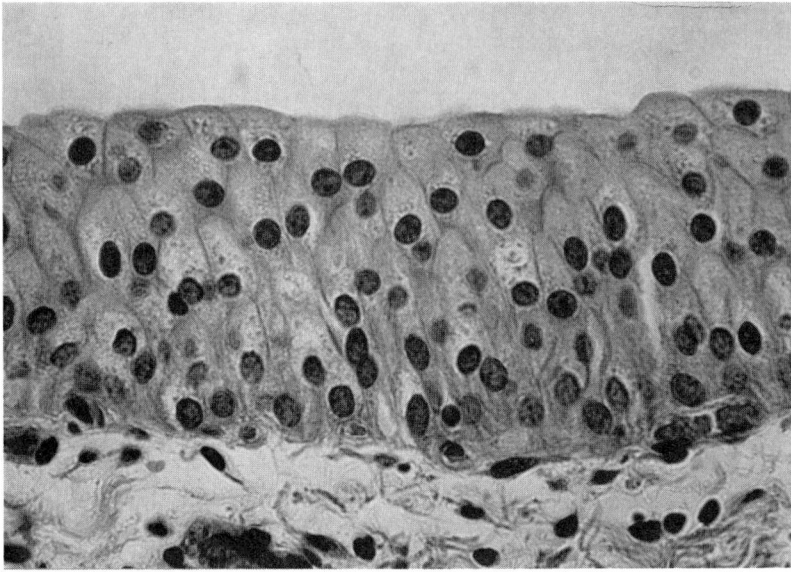

Fig. 5.16 Relaxed (contracted) transitional epithelium of the bovine bladder. X160.

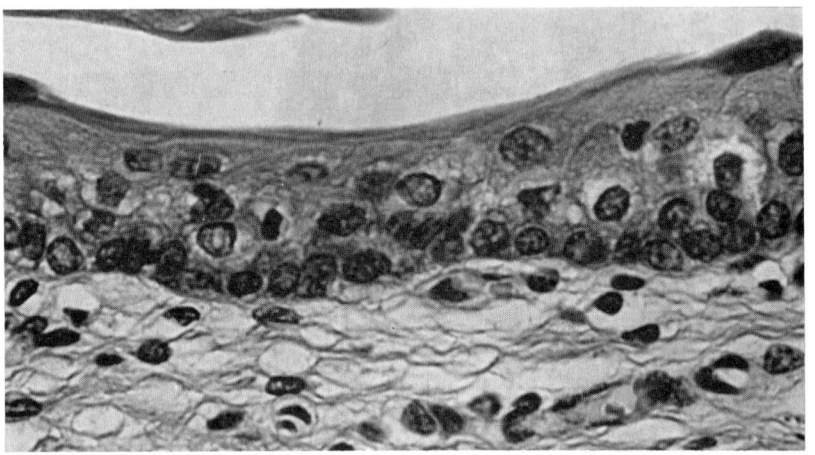

Fig. 5.17 Distended (stretched) transitional epithelium of the canine bladder. Compare with Figures 5.1 and 5.16. X160.

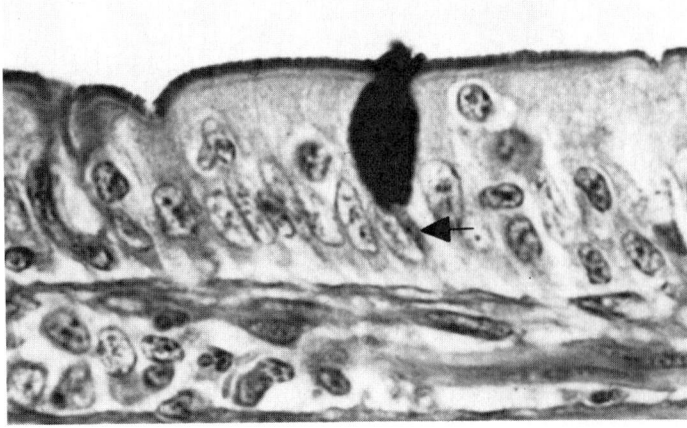

Fig. 5.18 Goblet cell within the lining epithelium of the feline jejunum. The bulk of the goblet cell (*dark mass*) contains premucin. The nucleus (*arrow*) is displaced basally. Note the extrusion of the secretory product upon the apical border of the cells. Compare with Figure 5.6. X250. (Alcian blue and PAS).

(Plates III.3, III.4). Until active, it cannot be distinguished from other columnar cells with which it is associated. When activity commences, droplets appear in the cytoplasm and eventually accumulate until the entire apical and middle portion of the cell is filled and swollen with the *premucin* droplets (Figs. 5.18, 5.19). These impart a foamy and basophilic appearance to the cytoplasm. The remainder of the cytoplasm and nucleus is displaced to the narrow basal region of the cell. Expulsion of the mucoid substances may be explosive or gradual. If explosive, the cell returns to a columnar configuration from which state the process will resume. If gradual, the continuing process does not alter the configuration of the cell.

Multicellular glands are quite diversified. Entire sheets of epithelia may perform a secretory function as in the lining of the glandular stomach. Intraepithelial glands, which are rare, represent accumulations of specialized secretory cells within an epithelial lining (Fig. 5.20). The glands occur in the lining of the upper respiratory system and male genital system. The greatest diversity of form and function is represented by those multicellular glands that assume an extraepithelial relationship to the epithelial lining. This type of gland represents most of those encountered in the body. Their true relationship to the epithelial lining is sometimes obscured by the morphologic complexity they assume and the plane of section during observation. Their relationship to the lining is best understood by examining their developmental process (Fig. 5.21). Specific loci within the epithelial lining retain the potential for mitosis. The mitotic process is directed in such a way that a cord of cells invaginates into the underlying connective tissue space. These cells, however, do *not* actually invade the space but are separated from it by the basement membrane. A tube develops within the cord while the remainder of the cells continue to proliferate and are subsequently converted to secretory cells. The secretory cells as a unit are referred to as an *adenomere*. The tube connecting the adenomere to the epithelial surface is the duct of the gland. In some instances, portions of the duct may also become secretory. Further modifications to this basic scheme for extraepithelial glands will be discussed subsequently.

Relationship to Lining and Surrounding Tissue. In the previous example of the formation of an extraepithelial gland, the persistence of the duct establishes that the gland will be of the *exocrine* variety. The growth of the adenomere and associated ducts is not limited to the simple example which has been cited. Rather, very elaborate duct and secretory conformations may develop. Whether a simple or complex arrangement, all these glandular types possess the common characteristic of cellular secretions being deposited into a system of ducts that will eventually open at an epithelial surface.

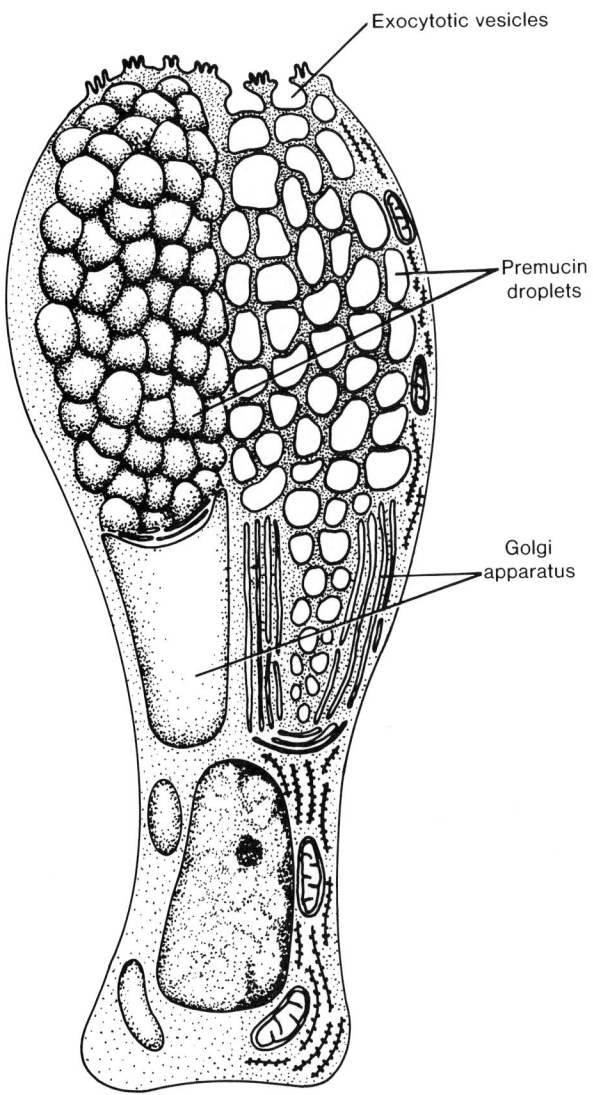

Exocytotic vesicles

Premucin droplets

Golgi apparatus

Fig. 5.19 Biplanar and three-dimensional diagram of a goblet cell. The premucin droplets occupy the bulk of the cytoplasmic volume and displace cytoplasmic components peripherally and basally. Premucin droplets fuse with the apical plasmalemma as exocytotic vesicles depositing the mucinogen at the cell surface.

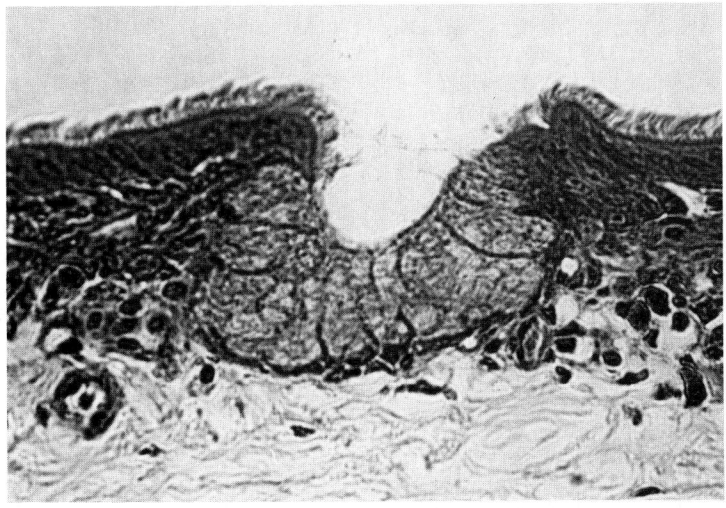

Fig. 5.20 Intraepithelial gland from the avian respiratory mucosa. X200.

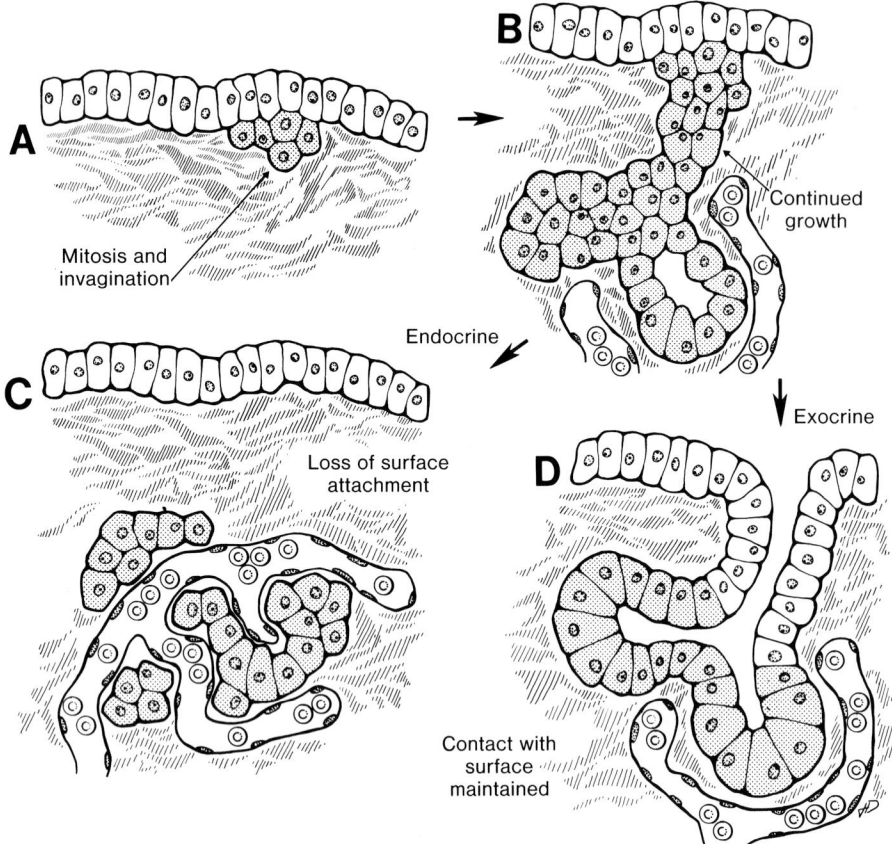

Fig. 5.21 Diagram of the development of exocrine and endocrine glands. Mitotic activity of the lining cells results in an invagination of the epithelium into the connective tissue (A). Continued mitotic activity and growth establishes a mass of cells attached to the surface (B). The disintegration of the surface attachment isolates the cord or clumps of cells in close association with capillaries as endocrine glands (C). The persistant attachment of the cells to the surface and the formation of a lumen establishes the exocrine glands (D).

the duct system which connects to the surface upon which the gland empties its secretion. It is the largest of the ducts. Most glands are subdivided into smaller units called lobes. *Lobar ducts* drain the secretory products of lobes and are connected to the excretory ducts. The large continuations of the lobar ducts within a lobe are referred to as *intralobar ducts*. Smaller subdivisional units of lobes are called lobules. Lobules are drained by *lobular ducts*. The continuation of the lobular duct within a lobule is called the *intralobular duct*. This duct is continuous with the secretory portion of the gland. This is a simple scheme for naming ductal components of glands. Also, blood-vascular patterns of certain organs are named according to this scheme. (Refer to Chapter 13 for an in-depth discussion of the organization of parenchymatous organs).

There are numerous examples of simple and compound glands associated with organs or structured as entire organs. These will be described as encountered in subsequent sections.

Method of Elaboration. Not all of the secretory cells of the body elaborate their products in a manner identical to one another.

In contrast to the aforementioned type, some glands lose their connection to an epithelial surface (Fig. 5.21). In such cases, the adenomere does not assume a tubular configuration. Rather, the secretory cells arrange themselves as cords or clumps of cells and deposit their secretory products into the adjacent connective tissue space. These are *endocrine* or ductless glands of the body (glands of internal secretion).

Some glands may be both exocrine and endocrine. The pancreas and liver are examples. These will be described with the endocrine and digestive systems, respectively.

Configuration of Multicellular Glands. Various configurations are assumed by multicellular glands in extraepithelial positions. In a single section of these glands the three-dimensional relationships can only be inferred. The following classification is based on serial sections and three-dimensional reconstructions of them. For this reason diagrams have been used. In the subsequent sections on organology the student should refer back to this classification to appreciate fully the relationship of specific glandular tissue to the organs with which they may be associated. Multicellular exocrine glands may be either *simple* or *compound.* This classification is based upon the simplicity or

complexity of the duct system associated with the secretory portions of the gland. The *secretory endpieces* (*adenomeres*) may be *tubular* (a hollow cylinder), *alveolar* (globular or pear-shaped) or *tubuloalveolar* (combination) (Fig. 5.22).

In a *simple gland*, the adenomere deposits its products into an unbranched duct. The adenomeres may be *straight tubular* as are the intestinal glands (Fig. 5.23), *coiled tubular* as are the sweat glands (Figs. 5.24, 5.25) or *alveolar*. The adenomeres may be branched and still deposit their products into a single duct system (Fig. 5.26). In these instances, they are referred to as *branched tubular* as in the submucosal glands of the intestine (Fig. 5.26) or *branched alveolar* as in the sebaceous glands (Fig. 5.27). The terms *alveolar* and *acinar* are often used synonymously.

In *compound* glands there are numerous subdivisions of the duct system and a variety of adenomeres (Fig. 5.28). They may be *compound tubular* as in some of the salivary glands, *compound acinar* as in the pancreas or *compound tubuloalveolar* as in some of the salivary glands and the mammary gland.

The subdivisions of the duct system of these compound glands are based on the organizational pattern of the gland (Fig. 5.29). The *excretory duct* is that portion of

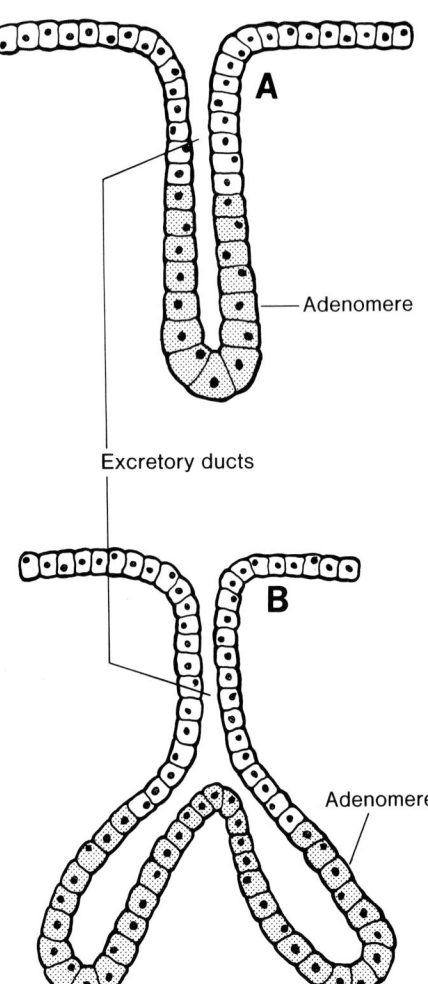

Fig. 5.22 Diagram of tubular glands. The adenomeres may be straight (A) or branched (B) tubules.

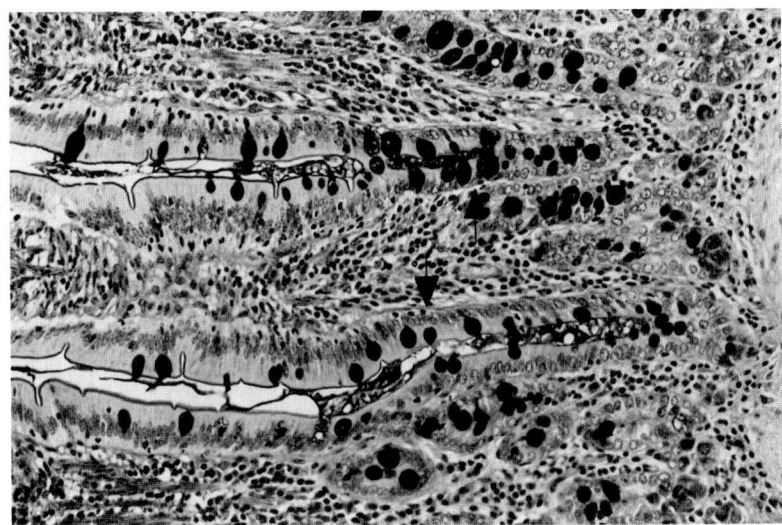

Fig. 5.23.   Straight tubular glands from the equine duodenum. X40. (Alcian blue and PAS).

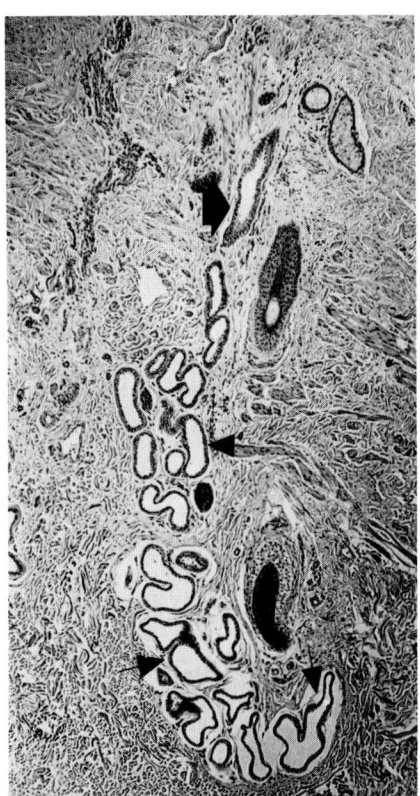

Fig. 5.24   Coiled tubular sweat glands (*small arrows*) from the ovine skin. Its tortuous configuration is responsible for the discontinuities apparent in section. The excretory duct (*large arrow*) eventually connects the adenomere to the surface. X9.

Three secretory methods are recognized: *merocrine, apocrine* and *holocrine*. This classification is based upon the amount the cell actually contributes to the secretory end product.

In the *merocrine* method of elaboration,

the cell contributes nothing more than the actual product it has produced. The membrane surrounding the secretory droplet fuses with the plasma membrane and thus opens the product to the extracellular space (Figs. 5.18, 4.42, 4.43). None of the cytoplasmic components along the secretory surface is lost, except the secretory product itself. This method is typical of most of the glands of the body (Fig. 5.30).

In the *apocrine* method of secretion, the secretory product and a portion of the cytoplasm along the secretory surface are lost

as the secretory end product. Characteristically, blebs or bulges along the secretory surface may be recognized during this process (Fig. 5.31). The extent of the cytoplasmic contribution in this method has been questioned recently. This method is typical of most of the sweat glands of domestic species, some of the sweat glands of man and some products of the mammary gland. (Plate III.8).

The *holocrine* method is characterized by the entire glandular epithelial cell becoming the secretory product. This unique secretory method, although not encountered commonly, has important functional significance. Because cells are lost continually by this method, glandular function would cease if cellular replacement were not accomplished. The continued function of holocrine glands is assured by the presence of a copious supply of stem cells. Typically, mitotic activity of these cells is characterized by one of the daughter cells being committed to glandular secretion while the other daughter cell retains its primitive stem cell characteristics for future mitosis. (Importantly, this type of daughter cell relationship is characteristic of all cellular replacement activity. It is just obvious with this method of secretion.)

In sebaceous glands, the stem cells are located at the periphery of the alveolus along the basement membrane (Fig. 5.32). Mitotic activity of these cells forces cells into the interior of the adenomere at which time they begin to accumulate their lipid secretory product. The cells undergo necrobiosis

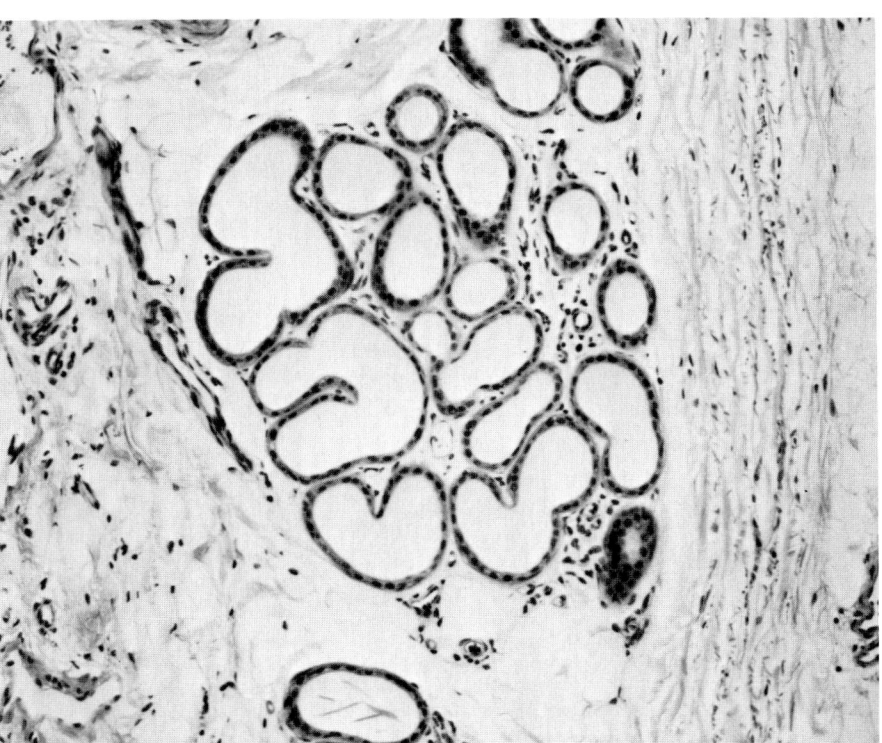

Fig. 5.25   Adenomere of a coiled tubular sweat gland of ovine skin. X40.

and become the secretory product (Plate III.9).

The sebaceous glands represent the classic example of the holocrine method of secretion. Other organs, the gonads and hematopietic organs, elaborate cells which become the "secretory products" of these glands. The ovary and seminiferous tubules elaborate germ cells that are shed from the body (Fig. 5.33). Also, the hematopietic tissues of the body produce blood cells that are "secreted" into the vascular spaces.

These examples represent two different extremes in holocrine secretion. But, there are two unifying characteristics: cells are modified and shed from the body to subserve specific functions; the continued function of these organs requires a supply of stem cells.

Types of Secretory Units. The varied secretory products of the body require that many different cells are involved. Of this vast diversity, two distinct types of secretory cells are recognized: *serous* and *mucous cells*. Besides a cellular morphologic basis for recognition, the secretory products of these two cell types are different. The serous cells secrete a clear, watery type of fluid which may contain enzymes, while the mucous cells produce a more viscous fluid which is rich in mucoid materials. Not all secretory cells can be included in this classification. Rather, the cells of many secretory units associated with the digestive, reproductive and respiratory systems conform to this classification. It is especially applicable to the salivary glands.

In *serous exocrine glands*, the serous cell is the predominant secretory unit. It is a wedge-shaped or pear-shaped cell which may possess a finely granular, acidophilic cytoplasm (Fig. 5.34). A distinct polarity may be apparent; the apical portion of the cell is acidophilic, while the basal portion is basophilic due to the accumulation of ergastoplasm (pancreatic acinar cell). The rounded nucleus is either central or para-

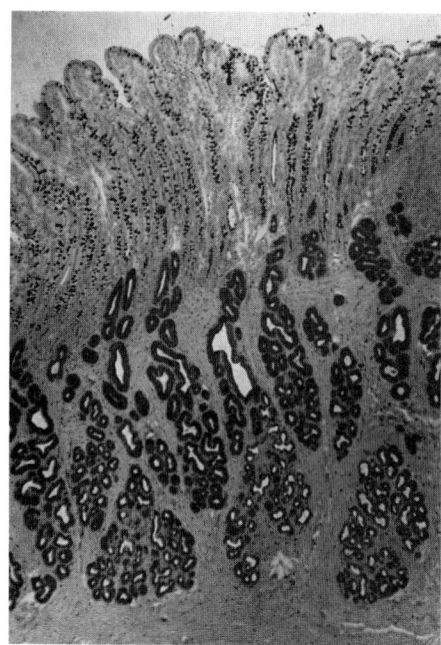

Fig. 5.26 Submucosal glands of the canine duodenum. The branched tubular glands are stained dark. X8 (Alcian blue and PAS).

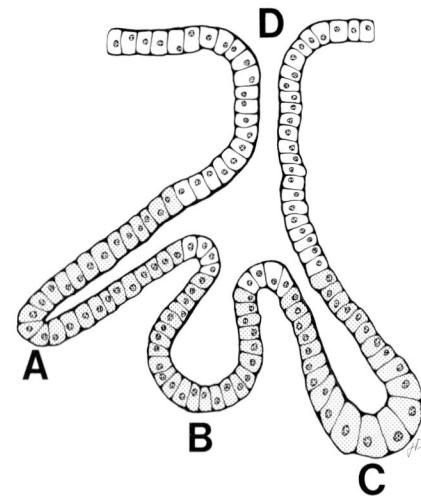

Fig. 5.28 Diagram of the configurations of the adenomeres of compound glands. Tubular (A), acinar (B) or tubuloalveolar (C) adenomeres open into a branched duct system (D).

central in position. The lateral margins of the cells usually are indistinct.

Entire adenomeres may be composed of these cells. These adenomeres may assume a tubular, alveolar or tubuloalveolar configuration.

In *mucous exocrine glands* the predominant secretory unit is the mucous cell. It is a pear-shaped cell with a foamy and basophilic cytoplasm (Fig. 5.35). A marked polarity is apparent; i.e., the hyperchromatic, flattened nucleus is situated against the basal margin of the cell. This cell is similar to the goblet cell described previously (Plate III.10).

Entire adenomeres may be composed exclusively of these cells. These units may assume a tubular or alveolar configuration.

Mixed glands may be composed of these two cell types in various arrangements (Plate III.11) (Fig. 5.36). An entire gland may possess separate serous and mucous adenomeres (Fig. 5.37). Serous and mucous cells may be intermingled with each other and discharge their products on the luminal surface (Fig. 5.38). *Serous demilunes* may be attached to a mucous adenomere (Fig. 5.39). In this instance, small canals (*secretory canaliculi*) connect the serous cells with the luminal surface (Fig. 5.36).

Special Epithelia

At certain loci, epithelial tissues are modified to perform highly specialized functions. Among these epithelial tissues are *ciliated epithelium, neuroepithelium, pigmented epithelium* and *myoepithelium*.

Ciliated Epithelium. Cilia are slender, cytoplasmic processes of the luminal surfaces of cells. Cilia are modified either for movement of materials along a sheet of epithelium or

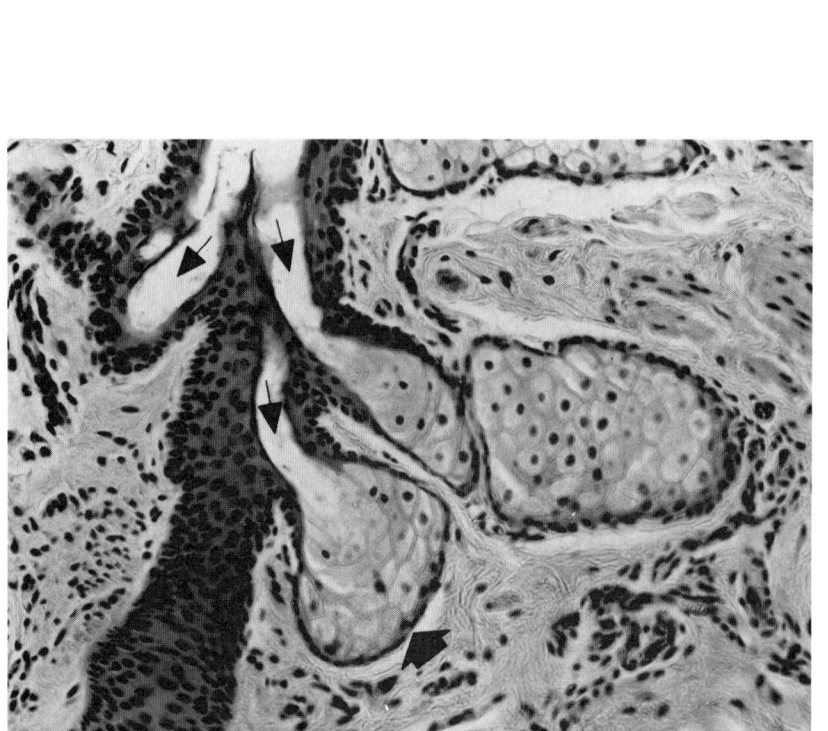

Fig. 5.27 Alveolar gland from ovine skin. The sebaceous glands are branched alveolar glands. The ducts (*small arrows*) are continuous with the alveolar adenomeres (*large arrow*). X50.

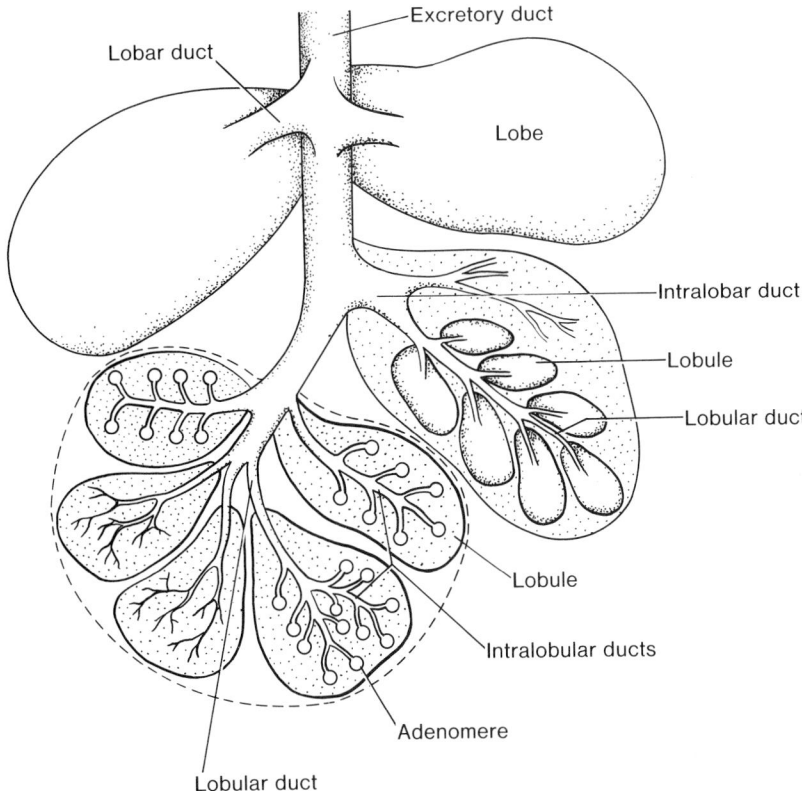

Fig. 5.29 Diagram of the subdivisions of a compound gland. One lobe (*dashed line*) is enlarged to show the intralobular relationships. The flow of secretory products is adenomere—intralobular duct—lobular duct—intralobar duct—lobar duct—excretory duct.

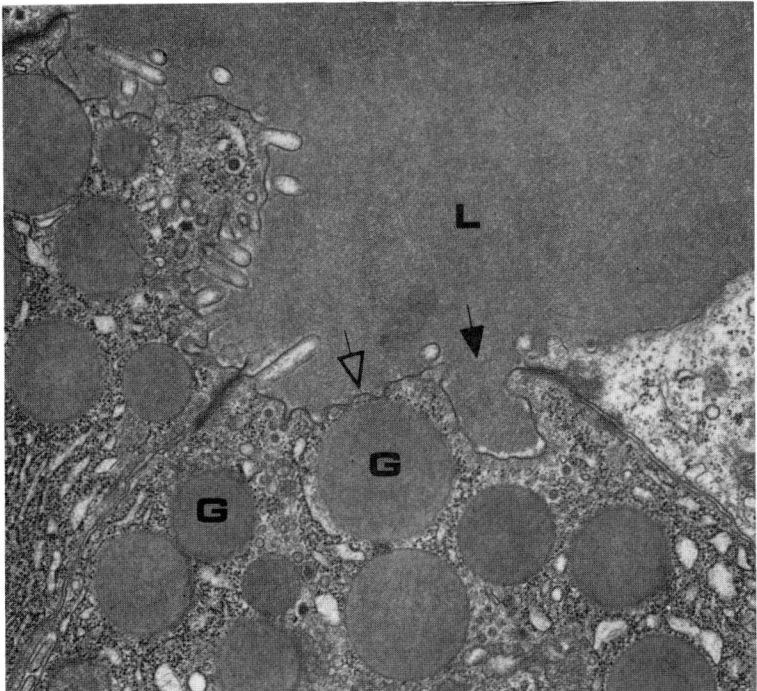

Fig. 5.30 An electron micrograph of the luminal border of pancreatic acinar cells. The lumen (L) is filled with secretory material from the zymogen granules (G). A granule (*solid arrow*) may have fused with the cell membrane, while another granule (*open arrow*) is about to fuse with the cell membrane. X22,000.

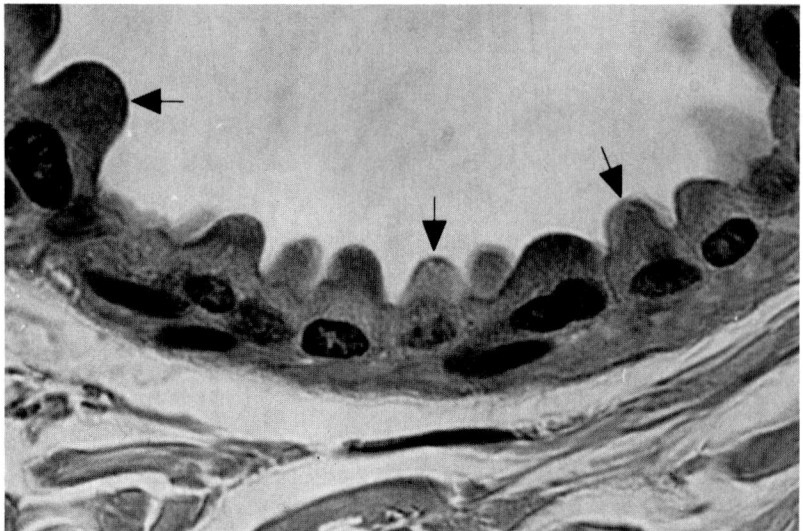

Fig. 5.31. Apocine tubular sweat glands of the ovine skin. The apical blebs (*arrows*) indicate the apocrine method of secretion. X500.

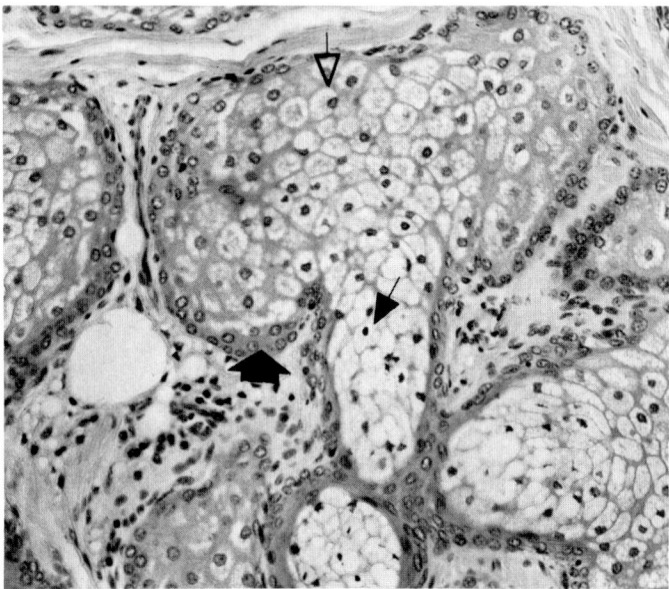

Fig. 5.32. Sebaceous glands of the ovine orbital sinus. The peripheral cells (*large solid arrow*) are the stem cells for the adenomere. The cells accumulate lipids (*open arrow*), the nuclei become pyknotic (*small solid arrow*) and the cells die. X50.

for the facilitation of secretory activity. They are referred to as *kinocilia* and *stereocilia*, respectively.

Kinocilia are highly structured, cytoplasmic processes which are usually associated with cells of pseudostratified columnar or simple columnar epithelia (Fig. 5.6). Isolated cells within the epithelial sheet or the majority of cells within the epithelial sheet may be ciliated. Kinociliated cells occur in the respiratory tract and the male and female genital system.

Stereocilia are long, unstructured, branched, protoplasmic structures from the luminal surface of cells which increase surface area for secretory activity (Fig. 5.40).

They occur on the pseudostratified columnar cells of the ductus epididymidis of the male genital system.

Neuroepithelium. Certain cells of epithelial sheets are modified to receive and transmit sensory information. These cells are associated with organs modified to receive optic, olfactory, gustatory, auditory and kinesthetic sensations. Although these cells may transmit information to the central nervous system by different means, they are similar in that all of them perceive stimuli through typical or modified cilia. *Support cells* (*sustentacular cells*) are normally associated with these sensory cells. The hair cells of the spiral organ of the ear and of the semicir-

cular canals are examples of these modified epithelial cells.

Pigmented Epithelium. Various cells of the body typically possess various types of pigments. In one instance, however, an entire sheet of epithelium, the pigmented epithelium of the retina of the eye (Fig. 5.41), is modified to contain large quantities of melanin.

Myoepithelium. *Myoepithelial cells* or *basket cells* are specialized epithelial cells associated with the adenomeres of most exocrine glands of the body. They are spindle cells which surround the secretory endpieces (Fig. 5.42). Although of epithelial origin, they contain myofibrils, are contractile and are responsible for the expression of secretory products into ducts. They are associated with salivary glands, sweat glands, mammary glands and others.

Endothelium. As simple squamous epithelial cells, these lining cells are modified uniquely for the transport of materials between the vascular space and the connective tissue space. They are capable of mitosis and phagocytosis.

Mesothelium. This simple squamous epithelium retains mitotic, phagocytic activity and primitive mesenchymal cell characteristics. They are capable of differentiating into fibroblasts. The integrity of the contents of the coelomic spaces is dependent upon the selective permeability of these cells. The reactivity of these cells is an important aspect of surgical intervention which involves the pericardial, pleural or peritoneal cavities.

Epithelial-Reticular Cells. These cells are the epithelial components of the thymus gland. Their morphologic features were discussed previously and will be discussed in-depth in a subsequent section. They form a cellular reticulum which may be a significant contributor to the thymic-blood barrier.

Cells of Endocrine Organs. These cells, uniquely modified to elaborate their protein or steroid secretory products (*hormones*) into the blood, assume varied morphologic configurations. They are discussed in-depth with the endocrine organs.

Surface Specializations of Epithelia

Cell-to-Cell Modifications. The lateral surfaces of epithelial cells are modified variously for different functions. These surfaces are modified to hold cells together, serve as diffusion barriers, facilitate diffusion between component epithelial cells and permit intercellular communication. The lateral surface modifications include alterations of the glycocalyx, lateral plasma membranes and filamentous components of the cytoplasm. Although lateral surface modifications have been recognized and described for some time, a detailed understanding of the morphology and function of these structural alterations had to await modern histologic methodology (electron microscopy and freeze-fracture techniques).

The attachment points of epithelial cells to each other are visible with the light microscope. This apicolateral alteration of cell surfaces was called the *terminal bar*. It appears as a continuous and collar-like alteration around the entire cell. With the electron microscope, this modification is seen as a complex of different structural alterations that occurs at the junction between adjacent cells. Thus, the name *junctional complex* is applied more appropriately to this structure. The discrete units of junctional complexes may comprise continuous modifications along contiguous cell surfaces. Such bands of alteration are confined to distinct zones; thus, they are described as zonular (L. small

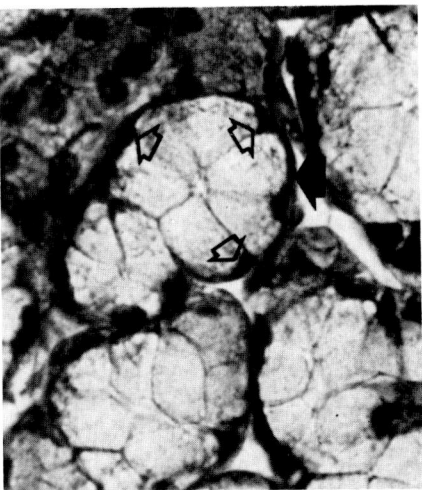

Fig. 5.35 Mucous cells of a mucous adenomere from a salivary gland (*solid arrow*). The cells are pyramidal, the cytoplasm is foamy and the flattened nuclei (*open arrows*) are basally positioned. X160.

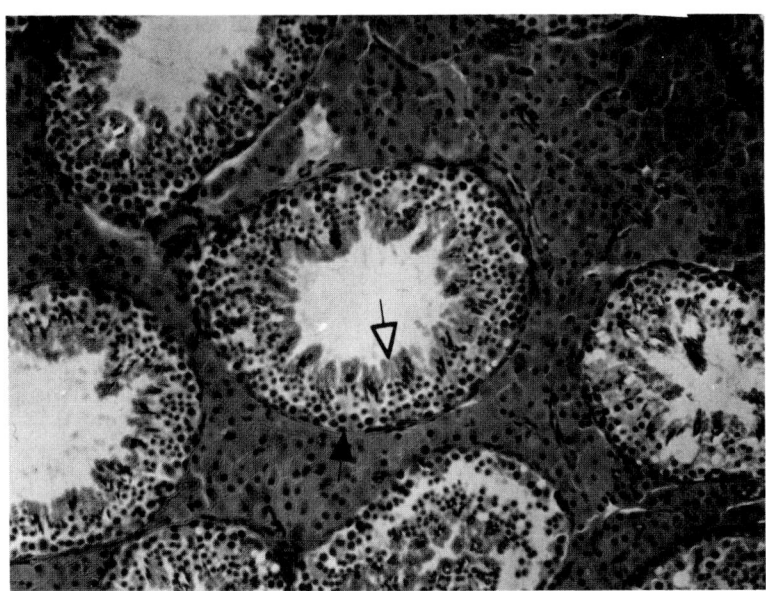

Fig. 5.33 Seminiferous tubules of the porcine testis. The germinal cells (*solid arrow*) differentiate into spermatozoa (*open arrow*) that become the "secretory product" of the tubules. X40.

zone). Others may be disposed as discrete patches or spots of alteration which are described as "spot welds" along contiguous surfaces. They are referred to as macular (L. a spot) alterations. Junctional complexes (Fig. 5.43) may consist of the following discrete components: *tight junction* (*zonula occludens*), *intermediate junction* (*zonula adherens*), *desmosome* (*macula adherens*) and *gap junctions* (*nexus, close junction, communicating junction*).

The *tight junction* (Fig. 5.44) is the most commonly encountered component of junctional complexes. The outer and dense laminae of contiguous cell membranes are fused as one with a resultant obliteration of intercellular space. Cytoplasmic condensation may be apparent on either side of the junction. When this type of junction is well-developed, the epithelium forms an effective barrier between the luminal and connective tissue spaces. The movement of extracellular materials is facilitated when these junctions are not well-developed. The impermeability and/or leakiness of an epithelium is related to this lateral plasmalemmal modification.

The *intermediate junction* (Fig. 5.44) is usually associated with a tight junction and is characterized by the juxtaposition of adjacent cell membranes. They are not fused but are separated by a 15-nm space which is filled with a polysaccharide adhesive material. These junctions, too, extend around the apicolateral portions of the cell. The adjacent cytoplasmic condensations contain numerous cytoplasmic filaments which are continuous with the cytofilaments of the *terminal web*. These intermediate junctions seem to be the anchoring point for the cytofilaments. These cytofilaments, believed to consist of contractile proteins (*actin* and *myosin*), extend into the terminal portions

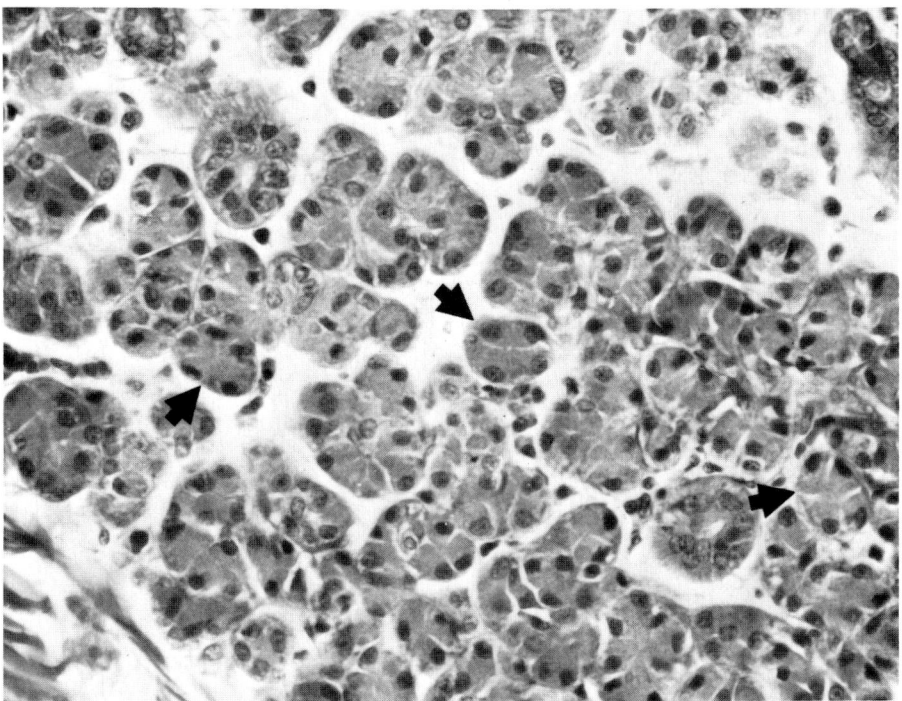

Fig. 5.34 Serous cells of an adenomere from a salivary gland. The serous cells (*arrows*) are pyramidal cells with round paracentrally positioned nuclei. The dark cytoplasm is granular and acidophilic. X160.

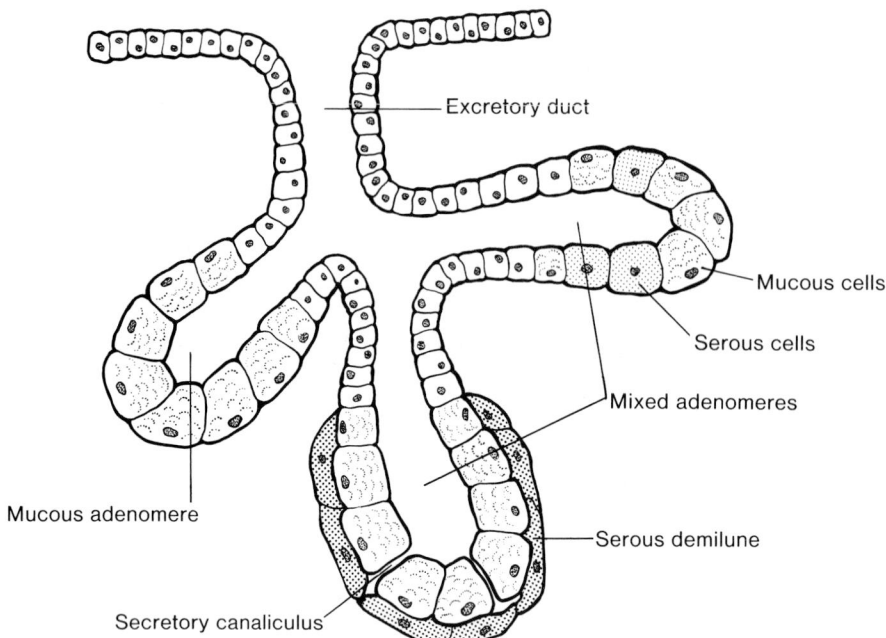

Fig. 5.36.   Diagram of adenomeres of a salivary gland. The adenomeres may be mucous, serous or mixed. Mucous adenomeres may have serous demilunes in association with them. Serous and mucous cells may be intermingled within an adenomere.

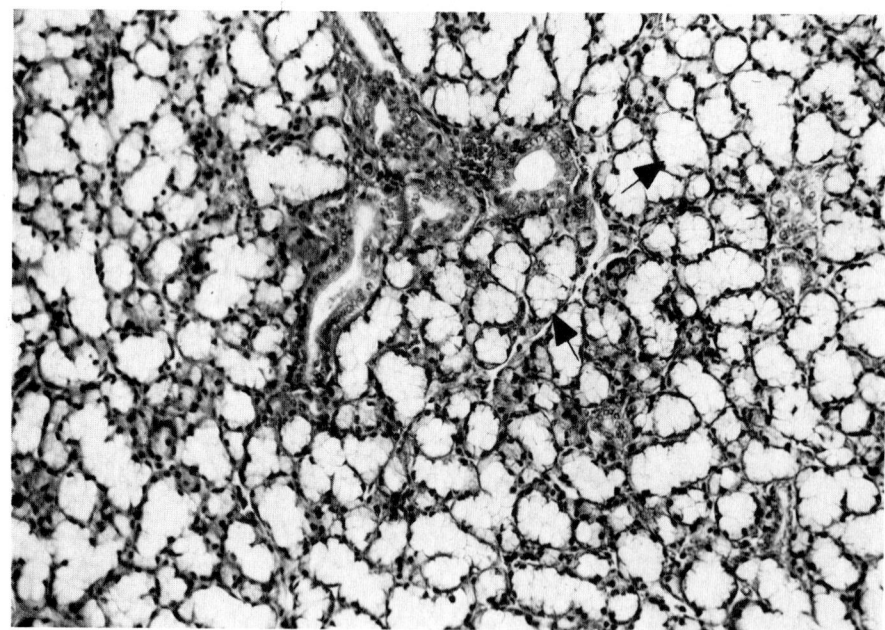

Fig. 5.37   Canine salivary gland. The mucous adenomeres (*arrows*) comprise the bulk of the gland. X40.

of microvilli. Cytofilaments may account for the characteristic shape of many cell types.

The *desmosomes* (Gr. bond + body) do not encircle the cell totally but are scattered along the cell margins at discrete locations. They can be considered analogous to "spot welds" between cells (Fig. 5.44). Moreover, they are not confined to junctional complexes. The cytoplasmic margin of each contributing cell membrane is coated by a dense material in which tonofilaments are embedded. These tonofilaments originate in the cytoplasm, form loops in the dense material

associated with the demosomes and return to the cytoplasm. Demosomes, therefore, may play a significant role in the cytoskeletal architecture of the cell. A space of 25 nm between adjacent cell membranes is typical and a dense intermediate line may be apparent in this intercellular space. The presence of a sialic acid-rich material indicates that this is a modification of the glycocalyx for cellular adhesion.

The *gap junction* appears similar to the tight junction but is separated by a 20-nm intercellular space. Tracer and freeze-frac-

ture studies have added appreciably to an understanding of these junctions. Face views demonstrate that these areas are composed of an orderly array of hexagonal subunits. These hexagonal subunits appear to consist of contiguous proteins which extend through the cell membranes and are in contact with each other. These junctions, therefore, may serve as an ionic bridge between contiguous cells. Nexi are not confined to epithelial cells. They occur between smooth and cardiac muscle cells and are associated with the transfer of excitatory stimuli from cell to cell. These junctions in epithelial cells may be the basis of intercellular communications that could account for the coordinated activities of epithelial membranes.

All of these junctions may be part of a junctional complex, but it is not uncommon to observe them as separate entities.

The remaining 15–nm space between cells is occupied by the glycocalyx. The glycocalyx, as well as the aforementioned junctional alterations, are coupled with cellular interdigitations (Fig. 5.45) to insure maximum cellular adhesion. The type and extent of these lateral cell margin modifications permit the selective passage of small and large molecules as well as the passage of cells in certain instances.

Basal Border Modifications. The primary modifications associated with the basal border of epithelial cells are: *basal lamina, basal invaginations, caveolae* and *pinocytotic vesicles*, and *hemidesmosomes.*

All epithelial tissues, except in a few specific instances, are separated from the underlying or surrounding connective tissue by a boundary layer called the *basement membrane.* It is readily demonstrable with periodic acid-Schiff (PAS) staining or silver impregnation, but it is not observable with routine hematoxylin and eosin staining (Figs. 5.46, 5.47).

The ultrastructural detail of the basement membrane has been elucidated with the electron microscope (Fig. 5.48). The light microscopic entity actually includes the basal cell membrane, amorphous cell coat, some dense material and associated connective tissue fibrils. Some dense material (50–70 nm wide) underlies the basal cell membrane and closely follows the contour of this membrane. This dense band of the *basal lamina* is homogeneous and contains a fine feltwork of filaments which project into the underlying connective tissue space as well as into the 40-nm space between the dense band and epithelial cell membrane. This light-staining zone of the basal lamina represents the cell coat.

Although the basal lamina has been considered a condensation product of the connective tissue space, current immunological evidence indicates that it may be of epithelial origin. Whatever its origin, the basal lamina is a structure significant in adhesion and filtration.

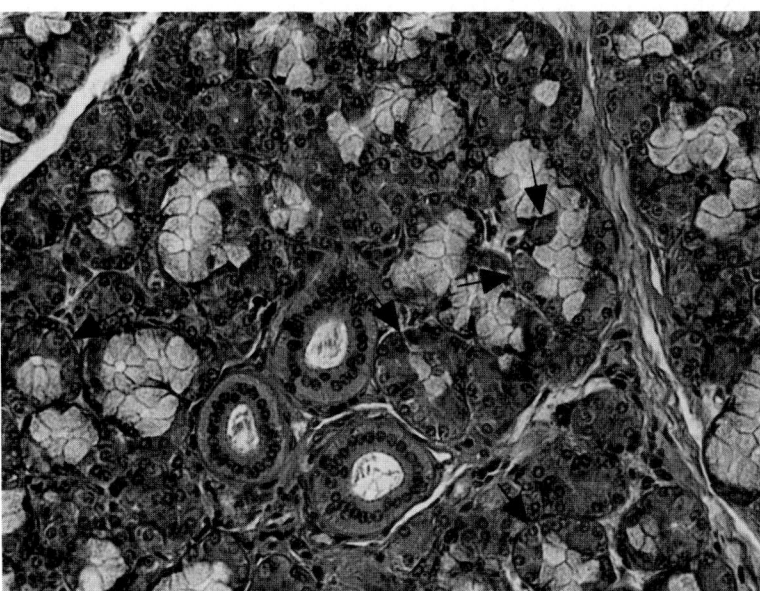

Fig. 5.38 Porcine salivary gland. *Arrows* indicate areas within adenomeres in which serous cells are intermingled among mucous cells. X63.

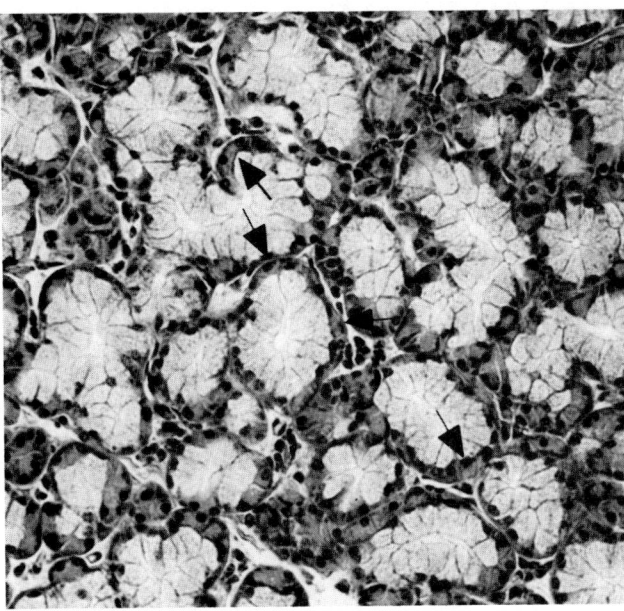

Fig. 5.39 Equine salivary gland. The serous cells (*arrows*) are disposed as demilunes around the mucous adenomeres. X63.

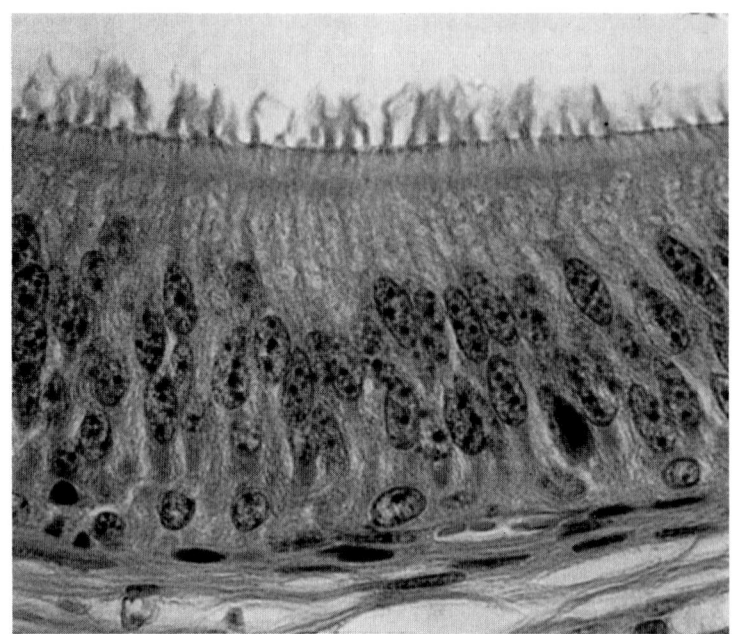

Fig. 5.40 Stereocilia of the equine ductus epididymidis. X200. (See Figure 5.58 also).

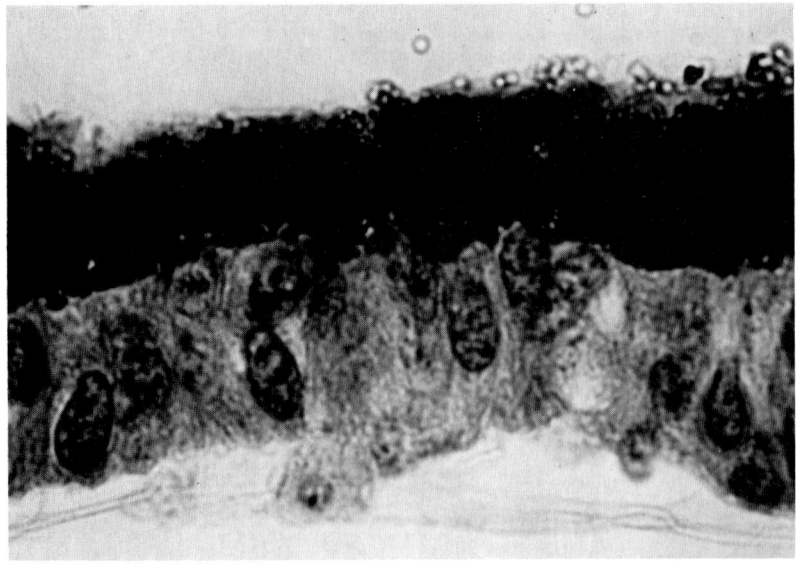

Fig. 5.41 Nonneural portion of the feline retina. The pigment epithelium at the *top* of the micrograph is obscured by the pigment. The columnar cells in the *lower* part of the micrograph comprise a separate layer. X320.

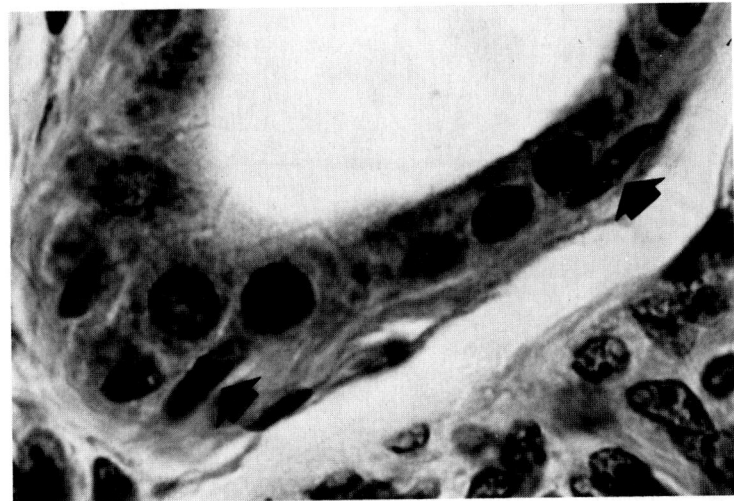

Fig. 5.42   Secretory endpiece of a bovine sweat gland. *Arrows*, myoepithelial cells. X320.

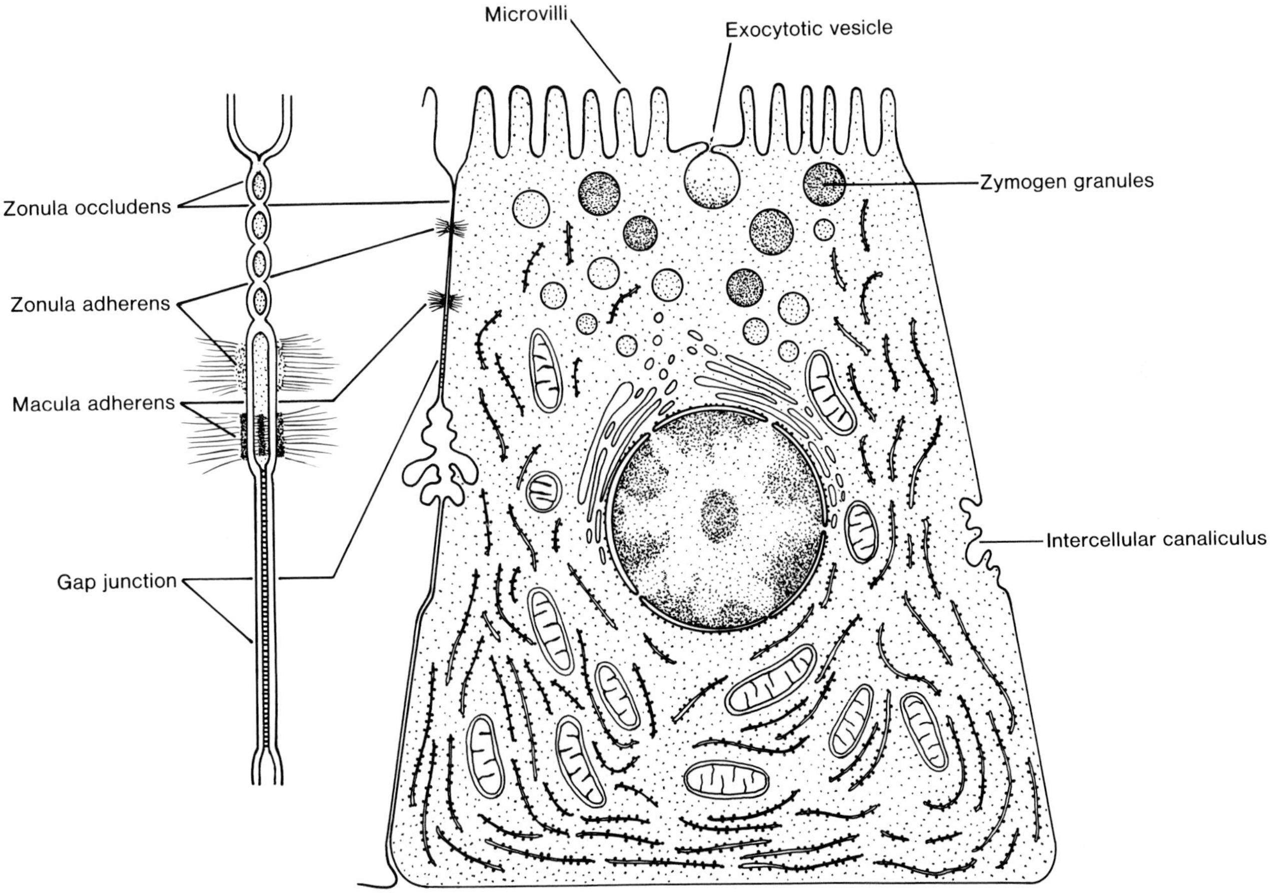

Microvilli

Exocytotic vesicle

Zymogen granules

Zonula occludens

Zonula adherens

Macula adherens

Intercellular canaliculus

Gap junction

Fig. 5.43   Drawing of a secretory cell as visualized with the electron microscope. Apical and lateral cell membrane modifications are illustrated. (Redrawn and modified from Bloom, W. and Fawcett, D. W.: *A Textbook of Histology*, 10th edition, W. B. Saunders, Philadelphia, 1975).

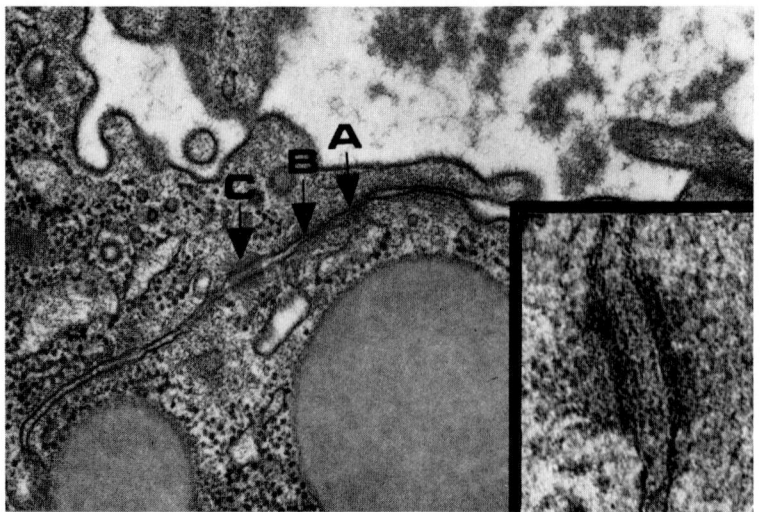

Fig. 5.44 An electron micrograph of junctional complexes between pancreatic acinar cells. The tight junction (A), intermediate junction (B) and desmosome (C) are indicated. X41,000. *Inset:* High magnification of a desmosome. X146,000.

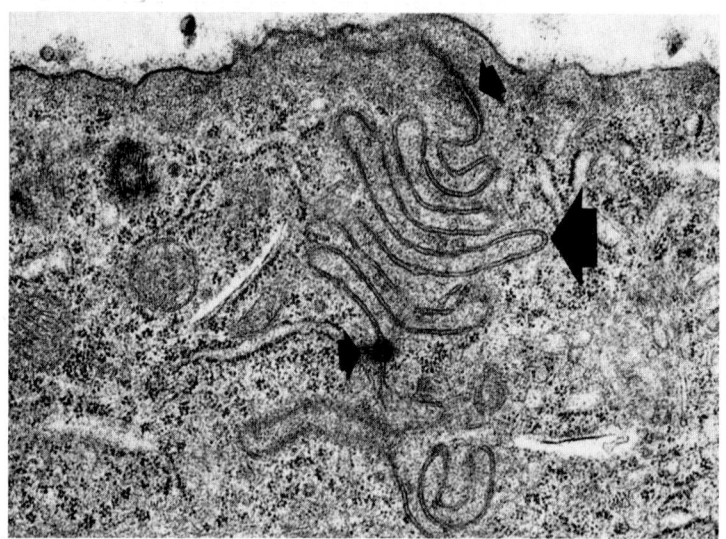

Fig. 5.45 An electron micrograph of lateral surface modifications between adjacent intestinal lining cells of a mouse. Lateral interdigitations (*large arrow*) are apparent. Near the apical cell surface, an intermediate junction is visible at the *small arrow*. A desmosome is visible in the middle of the micrograph at the *small arrow*. X25,000. (Courtesy of A. M. Sheppard).

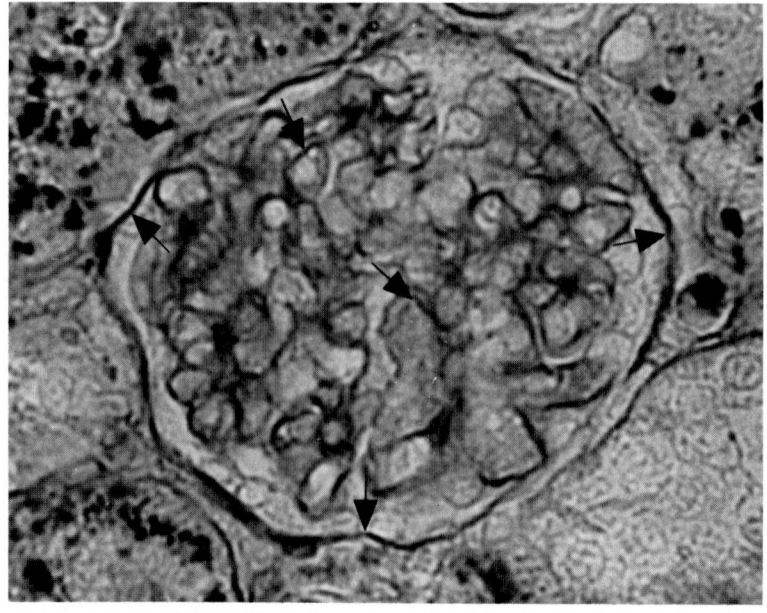

Fig. 5.46 Glomerulus of a canine kidney stained with PAS. The basement membrane (*arrows*) is defined clearly. Compare with Figure 5.47. X250.

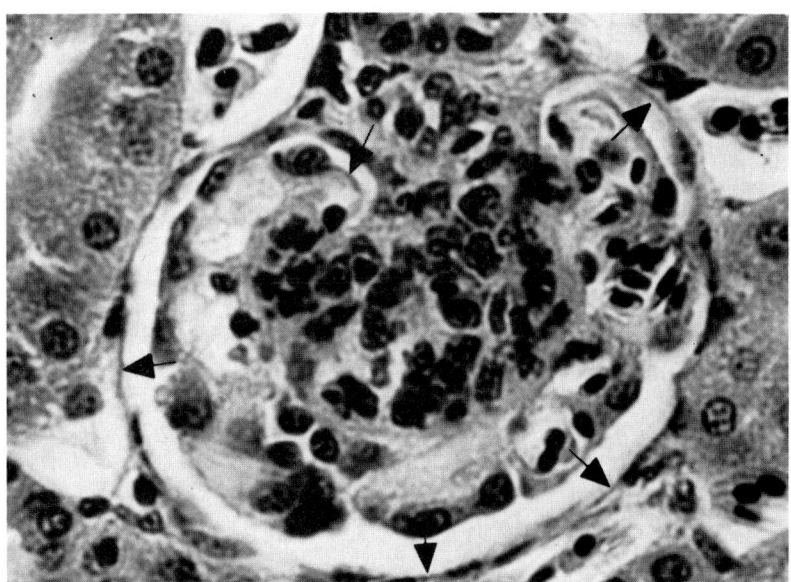

Fig. 5.47   Glomerulus of a canine kidney stained with H and E. The cellular limits (*arrows*) are visible, but the basement membrane is not apparent. Compare with Figure 5.46. X250.

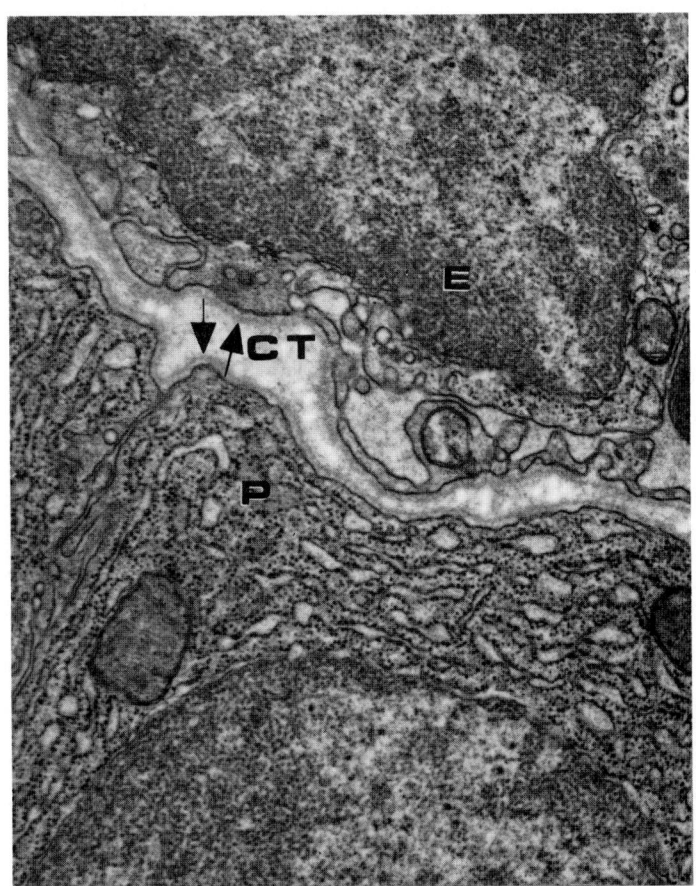

Fig. 5.48   An electron micrograph of pancreatic acinar cells, associated connective tissue and capillary endothelium. The pancreatic acinar cell (P) and the endothelial cell (E) are bounded by individual basal laminae (*arrows*). The intervening space is connective tissue (CT). X25,000.

The terms basement membrane and basal lamina are not synonymous. One is a light microscopic term, while the other is derived from electron microscopy. Importantly, the basement membrane of light microscopy includes the basal cell membrane, basal lamina (dark and light zones) and associated connective tissue fibers.

The basal cell membranes may be regularly contoured or may possess numerous infoldings (Fig. 5.49). The latter modification is especially apparent in cells involved

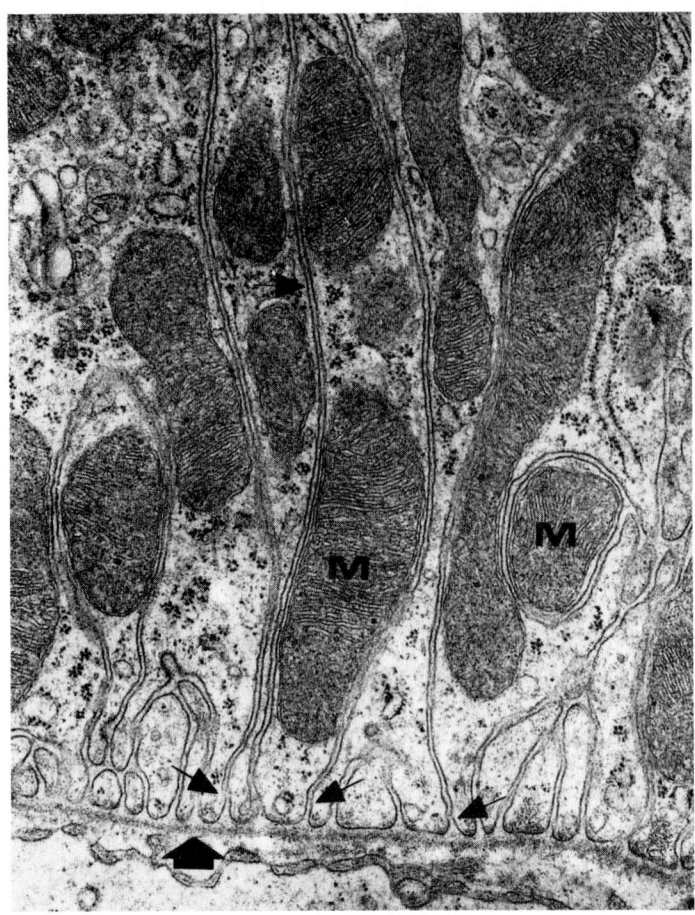

Fig. 5.49   An electron micrograph of a lining cell of the proximal convoluted tubule of a canine kidney. Numerous basal cell membrane infoldings are evident (*small arrows*). Mitochondria (M) are contained within the cytoplasm between the membranes. The basal lamina (*large arrow*) is apparent. X18,000.

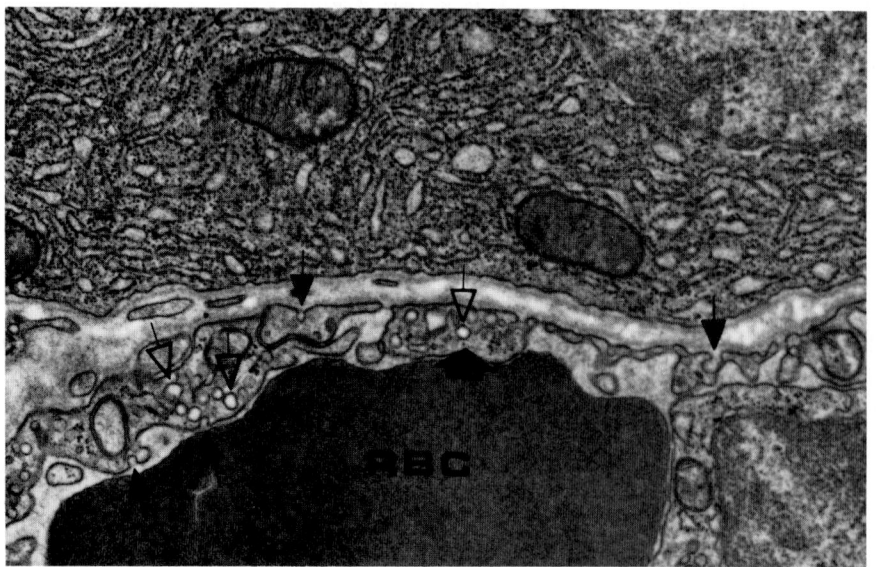

Fig. 5.50   An electron micrograph of a capillary. An erythrocyte (RBC) is bounded by capillary endothelium (*large solid arrow*). Pinocytotic vesicles (*open arrows*) and caveolae (*solid arrows*) are apparent. X18,000. Compare with Figure 5.51.

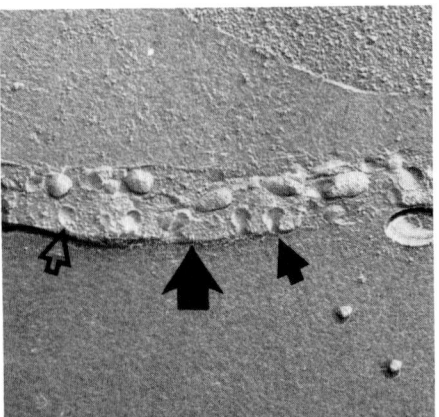

Fig. 5.51   An electron micrograph of a freeze-fractured capillary. The capillary endothelium (*large arrow*) contains pinocytotic vesicles (*open arrow*) and caveolae (*solid arrow*). X43,000. Compare with Figure 5.50. (Courtesy of J. E. Rash).

in transport activities. In either case, small bulblike invaginations of the cell membrane (*caveolae*) exist (Fig. 5.50). These pinch off from the membrane and form *pinocytotic vesicles* (Fig. 5.50). These two structures rep-

resent mechanisms for *endocytotic* and/or *exocytotic* activity (Fig. 5.51).

Hemidesmosomes (*half-desmosomes*) are sometimes encountered along the basal cell membrane (Fig. 5.52). As the name implies,

these structures are identical to one-half of a desmosome, with one exception. Fine filaments traverse the light zone perpendicular to the desmosome and are continuous with the dense zone of the basal lamina.

Apical Border Modifications. The primary apical border modifications of epithelia are:

microvilli, caveolae, pinocytotic vesicles and *cilia.*

Microvilli occur on the surfaces of most cells. They are extremely variable in size, distribution and organization. Their prime function is to increase the absorbing surface area of a cell. Microvilli achieve their highest degree of development in epithelia. They are slender, cylindrical cellular processes

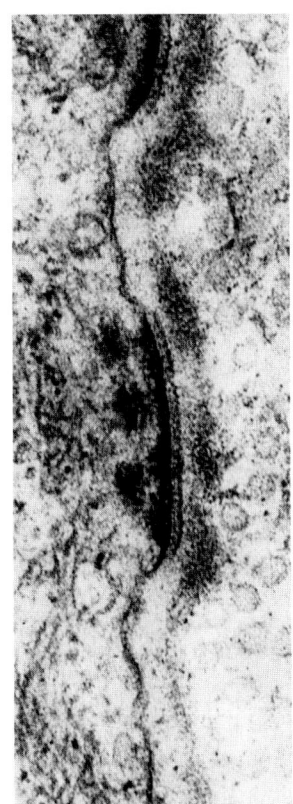

Fig. 5.52 An electron micrograph of the basal border of an intestinal lining cell of a mouse. A hemidesmosome is visible in the center of the field. X91,000.

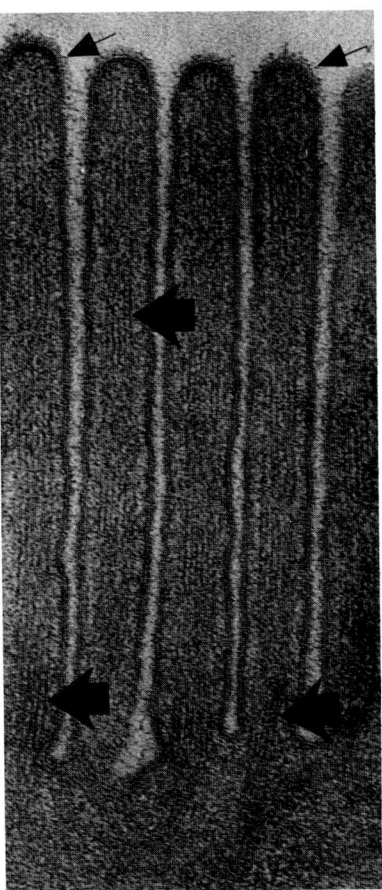

Fig. 5.54 An electron micrograph of the striated border of the intestinal lining cells of a mouse. The microvilli are arranged in an orderly manner, are covered by a glycocalyx (*small arrows*) and contain cytofilaments (*large arrows*). X70,000.

which are oriented perpendicular to the apical, free or luminal surface.

Microvilli of intestinal epithelial cells are highly ordered structures on the free borders which form a *striated border* or *brush border* (Fig. 5.53). These processes are 1 to 1.5 μm long and approximately 0.1 μm in diameter. They are juxtaposed to each other in a parallel arrangement (Fig. 5.54). The cores of the microvilli are composed of cytofilaments which extend down to the ectoplasm in which the terminal web is located. The cytofilaments of the microvilli are connected to those of the terminal web.

Certain lining cells of the kidney also possess a marked development of microvilli on their apical borders. These, however, are not in as orderly an arrangement as those described previously (Fig. 5.55). In the past, this arrangement was referred to as a *brush border*, whereas the highly ordered array was called a *striated border.* Now these terms are used synonymously, because both represent modifications to increase the cell surface. The surface coat or glycocalyx associated with microvilli is prominent.

Cilia are typical apical modifications of specialized epithelial cells (Figs. 5.6, 5.20, 5.40). These structures, however, are not confined to epithelial cells. *Kinocilia* or motile cellular processes may be as long as 10 μm with a diameter of approximately 0.2 μm (Fig. 5.56). These long, cylindrical and tapered processes contain microtubules embedded within a matrix and are covered by the plasma membrane. A central pair of tubules is surrounded by nine doublets of tubules (Fig. 5.57). These tubular structures are connected by fine cytofilaments. At the point of union between the cilium and the

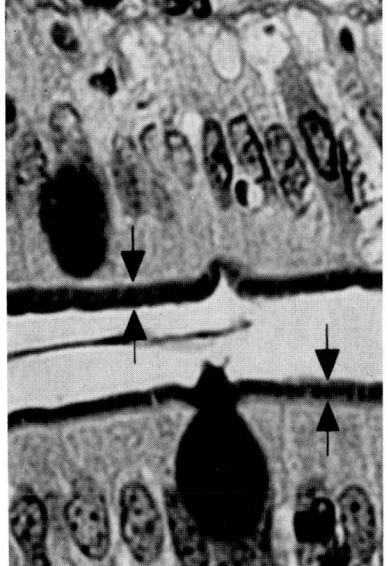

Fig. 5.53 Striated border of lining cells of the equine jejunum (*arrows*). X250 (Alcian blue and PAS).

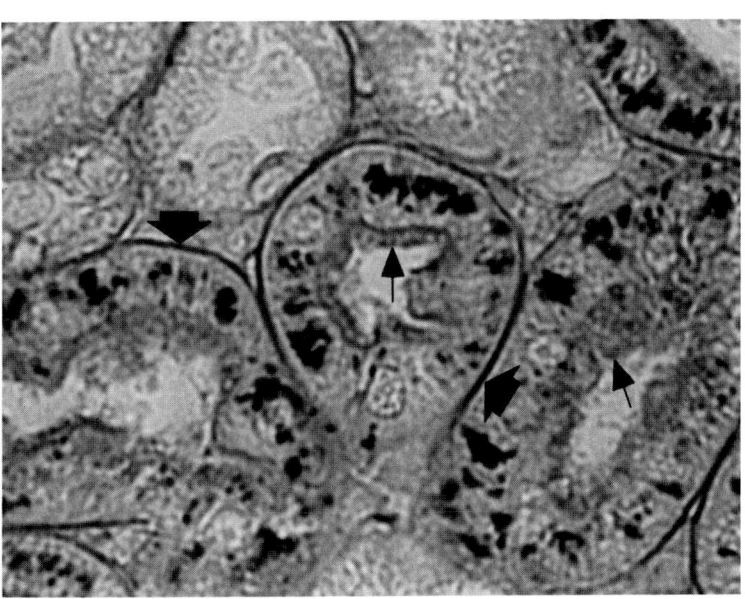

Fig. 5.55 Brush borders (*small arrows*) of the lining cells of the proximal convoluted tubules of a canine kidney. The basement membranes also are defined clearly (*large arrows*). X250 (toluidine blue and PAS).

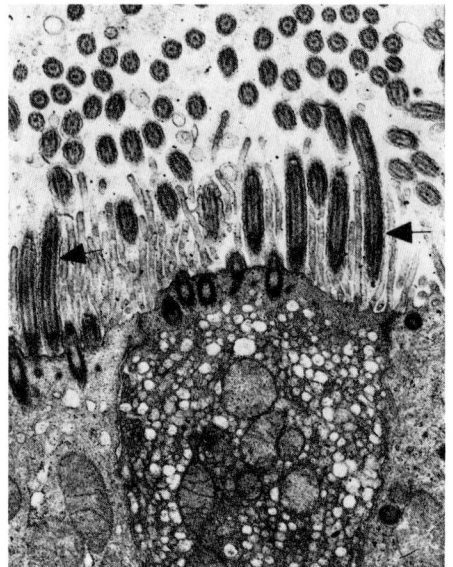

Fig. 5.56 An electron micrograph of ciliated cells from the trachea of a mouse. *Arrows*, cilia. X8,000.

cell, the central pair of tubules terminates above a *basal plate*, while the peripheral pairs of tubules gain another tubule and are converted to nine sets of triplets of the basal body.

Stereocilia do not possess this complex organizational pattern (Fig. 5.58). They may be considered extremely long and branched microvilli.

The *caveolae* and *pinocytotic vesicles* of the apical border are similar in structure and function to those structures associated with the basal border (Figs. 5.50, 5.51).

Regeneration and Repair of Epithelia

Epithelial tissues, in most locations, are subjected to harsh environments that result in cells being damaged and lost. Notwithstanding this factor, the lives of epithelial cells are finite and therefore epithelial membranes require renewal and replacement of lost components. In most instances, this need is satisfied by the presence of undifferentiated stem cells being included in the epithelial membrane. Various epithelial membranes accomplish this activity in different ways.

Simple epithelial membranes that are composed of squamous, cuboidal and columnar cells that are not highly differentiated for secretory and/or absorptive functions retain a high mitotic potential. These cells serve as their own stem cells. This applies to typical epithelial lining cells as well as endothelial and mesothelial cells.

In those epithelial membranes which are lined by columnar cells that are differentiated and specialized for absorptive or secretory functions (stomach, intestines), the

specialization is accompanied by an attendant reduction in mitotic potential. Such cellular membranes are dependent upon stem cells for cellular replacement. The location

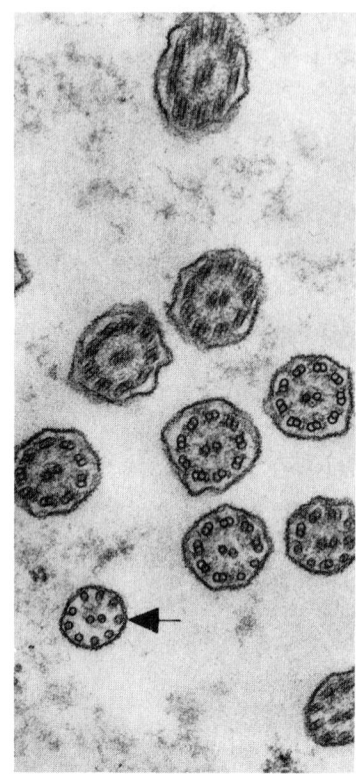

Fig. 5.57 An electron micrograph of cross-sections of cilia. The doublet and central pairs of microtubules are apparent. The configuration of the peripheral microtubules is altered at the tip of the cilium (arrow). X44,000.

of the stem cells in these simple epithelia varies. In the small intestine, epithelial lining cells of the villi are lost at the tips of these surface modifications. The stem cells are located some distance away from this locus in the depths of the intestinal crypts. Mitotic activity is characteristic of the crypts and the daughter cells migrate along the glandular epithelium of the crypts, up the lateral shoulders of the villi and are shed at the apices of the villi.

The basal cells of stratified epithelia are the stem cells of these membranes. The basal and fusiform cells of pseudostratified columnar epithelia are capable of differentiating into lining cells and goblet cells. Similar relationships are assumed to occur in the replacement of transitional epithelium.

The replacement of lost cells in stratified squamous epithelia is a necessity, because cells are shed constantly at the surface. Replacement through mitotic activity is the function of the stratum basale and stratum spinosum. Wound repair of the epidermis and underlying connective tissue (dermis) has been studied extensively. The nature of this process depends upon the nature and extent of the injury. After disruption of the epidermis, epidermal cells from the basal layers along the wound margin demonstrate ameboid activity and migrate to initiate coverage of the exposed connective tissue. Mitotic activity of these and contiguous germinal cells then occurs. Within 48 hours, the underlying connective tissue is covered by these proliferative cells. This activity occurs beneath the scab. Proliferation continues, the epithelium is restored and the scab of cellular and vascular debris is lifted from the replaced epidermis by 7 days. Attendant

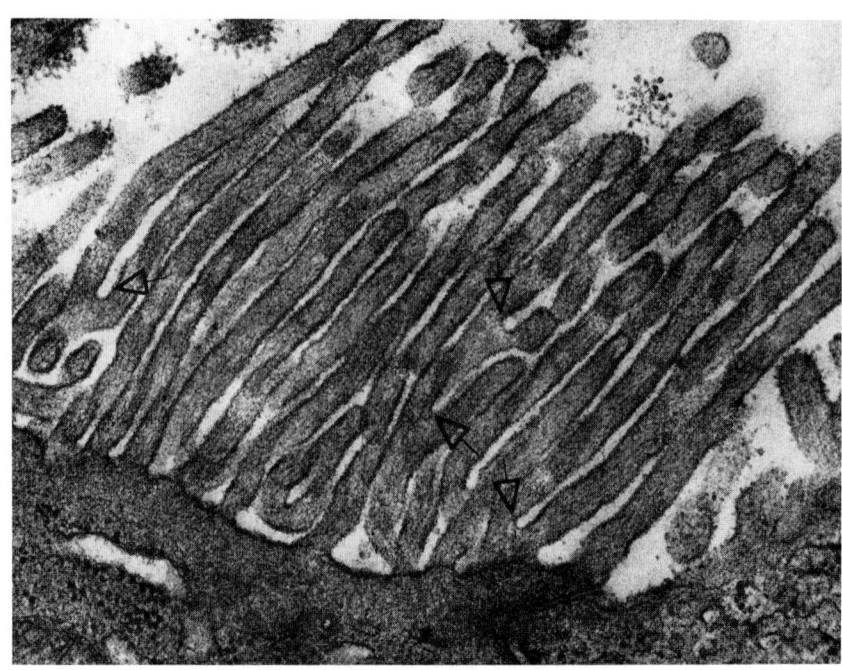

Fig. 5.58 An electron micrograph of stereocilia of the lining cells of the trachea of a mouse. The stereocilia are branched (*arrows*) and lack the internal organization of kinocilia. X46,000.

changes in the associated connective tissue are discussed in Chapter 18.

References

Epithelium

Brody, I.: The keratinization of epidermal cells of normal guinea pig skin revealed by electron microscopy. J. Ultrastruct. Res. *2:*482, 1959.

Dunn, J. S.: The fine structure of the absorptive epithelial cells of the developing small intestine of the rat. J. Anat. *101:*57, 1967.

Fawcett, D. W.: *An Atlas of Fine Structure.* W. B. Saunders, Philadelphia, 1965.

Hackemann, M., Grubb, C. and Hill, K. R.: The ultrastructure of normal squamous epithelium of the human cervix uteri. J. Ultrastruct. Res. *22:*443, 1968.

Hicks, R. M.: The fine structure of the transitional epithelium of rat ureter. J. Cell Biol. *26:*25, 1965.

Matthews, J. L. and Martin, J. H.: *Atlas of Human Histology and Ultrastructure.* Lea and Febiger, Philadelphia, 1971.

Porter, K. R. and Bonnevile, M. A.: *Fine Structure of Cells and Tissues.* 4th edition, Lea and Febiger, Philadelphia, 1973.

Zelickson, A. S.: *Ultrastructure of Normal and Abnormal Skin.* Lea and Febiger, Philadelphia, 1967.

Glandular Epithelium

Bullough, W. S. and Ebling, F. J.: Cell replacement in the epidermis and sebaceous glands of the mouse. J. Anat. *86:*29, 1952.

Ekholm, R. and Edlund, Y.: Ultrastructure of the human exocrine pancreas. J. Ultrastruct. Res. *2:*453, 1959.

Gabe, M. and Arvy, L. Gland Cells. *In:* Brachet, J. and Mirsky, A. E. (editors), *The Cell: Biochemistry, Physiology, Morphology,* Vol. V, pp. 1–88. Academic Press, New York, 1961.

Junqueria, L. C. and Hirsh, G. C.: Cell Secretion: A study of pancreas and salivary glands. Inter. Rev. Cytol. *5:*323, 1956.

Parks, H. F.: Morphological study of the extrusion of secretory materials by the parotid glands of mouse and rat. J. Ultrastruct. Res. *6:*449, 1962.

Scott, B. L. and Pease, D. C.: Electron microscopy of the salivary and lacrimal glands of the rat. Amer. J. Anat. *104:*115, 1959.

Special Epithelia

Arstila, A. and Wersall, J.: The ultrastructure of the olfactory epithelium of the guinea pig. Acta Otolaryng. Stockholm *64:*187, 1967.

Edwards, E. and Duntley, S.: The pigments and color of living skin. Amer. J. Anat. *65:*1, 1939.

Fitzpatrick, T. B. and Szabo, G.: The melanocyte; cytology and cytochemistry. J. Invest. Derm. *32:*197, 1959.

Frisch, D.: Ultrastructure of mouse olfactory mucosa. Amer. J. Anat. *121:*87, 1967.

Lundquist, P. G., Kimura, R. and Wersall, J.: Ultrastructural organization of the epithelial lining in the endolymphatic duct and sac in the guinea pig. Acta Otolaryng. Stockholm *57:*65, 1963.

Rhodin, J. and Dulhan, T.: Electron microscopy of the tracheal ciliated mucosa in rat. Z. Zellforsch. *44:*345, 1956.

Travill, A. A. and Hill, M. F.: Histochemical demonstration of myoepithelial cell activity. Quart. J. Exp. Physiol. *48:*423, 1963.

Surface Specializations

Barber, V. C. and Boyde, A.: Scanning electron microscopic studies of cilia. Z. Zellforsch. *84:*269, 1968.

Claude, P. and Goodenough, D. A.: Fracture faces of zonulae occludentes from "tight" and "leaky" epithelia. J. Cell Biol. *58:*390, 1973.

Curtis, A. S. G.: Cell contact and adhesion. Biol. Rev. *37:*82, 1962.

Farquhar, M. G. and Palade, G. E.: Junctional complexes in various epithelia. J. Cell Biol. *17:*375, 1963.

Fawcett, D. W.: Physiologically significant specializations of the cell surface. Circulation *26:*1105, 1962.

Fawcett, D. W.: Surface specializations of absorbing cells. J. Histochem. Cytochem. *13:*75, 1965.

Fawcett, D. W. and Porter, K. R.: A study of the fine structure of ciliated epithelia. J. Morph. *94:*221, 1954.

Goodenough, D. A.: The structure and permeability of isolated hepatocyte gap junctions. Cold Spring Harbor Symp. *40:*37, 1975.

Granger, B. and Baker, R. F.: Electron microscope investigation of the striated border of intestinal epithelium. Anat. Rec. *107:*423, 1950.

Hashimoto, K., Gross, B. G. and Lever, W. F.: Electron microscopic study of apocrine secretion. J. Invest. Derm. *46:*378, 1966.

Ito, S.: The surface coat of enteric microvilli. J. Cell Biol. *27:*475, 1965.

Kelly, D.: Fine structure of desmosomes, hemidesmosomes and an adepidermal globular layer in developing newt epidermis. J. Cell Biol. *28:*51, 1966.

Kurtz, S. M. and Feldman, J. D.: Experimental studies on the formation of the glomerular basement membrane. J. Ultrastruct. Res. *6:*19, 1962.

Pierce, G. B., Jr., Midgley, A. R., Jr. and Sri Ram, J.: The histogenesis of basement membranes. J. Exp. Med. *117:*339, 1963.

Satir, P.: Cilia. Sci. Amer. *204:*61, 1961.

Sorokin, S. D.: Reconstruction of centriole formation and ciliogenesis in mammalian lungs. J. Cell Sci. *3:*207, 1968.

Susi, F. R., Belt, W. D. and Kelly, J. W.: Fine structure of fibrillar complexes associated with the basement membrane in human oral mucosa. J. Cell Biol. *34:*686, 1967.

Repair and Regeneration

Hunt, T. K. and Van Winkle, Jr., W. (ed). *Fundamentals of Wound Management in Surgery - Wound Healing: Normal Repair.* Chirurgecom, Inc., South Plainfield, New Jersey, 1976.

Leblond, C. P. and Walker, B. E.: Renewal of cell populations. Physiol. Rev. *36:*255, 1956.

Odland, G. F. and Ross, R.: Human wound repair. I. Epidermal regeneration. J. Cell Biol. *39:*135, 1968.

Peacock, Jr., E. E. and Van Winkle, Jr., W.: *Surgery and Biology of Wound Repair.* W. B. Saunders, Philadelphia, 1970.

Ross, R. and Odland, G. F.: Human wound repair. II. Inflammatory cells, epithelial-mesenchymal interactions and fibrogenesis. J. Cell Biol. *39:*152, 1968.

Weiss, P.: The biological foundations of wound repair. The Harvey Lectures, *55:*13, 1961.

6: Proper Connective Tissues and Adipose Tissue

General Characteristics

Form and Function. Connective tissues, as a group comprising one of the basic tissue types, are derived from the mesoderm. This group is composed of various subtypes of diverse tissues that, despite their differences, share many characteristics. These tissues consist of heterogeneous populations of cells that are separated from each other by copious amounts of *extracellular material* (*intercellular substance*), most of which is secreted by the constituent cells. The fibrous and amorphous components comprise the connective tissue *matrix*. The fibers may impart a feltwork or weave-like consistency to the matrix. The *ground substance* is the amorphous component and consists of *mucopolysaccharides* (*glycosaminoglycans*). These substances fill in the spaces around the fibers and cells which together then form a three-dimensional framework that serves to connect and support other tissues and organs. The relative amount of the cells and matrix components of connective tissues varies throughout the organism in response to structural and functional needs. For this reason, precise definitions, descriptions and the classification of connective tissues are difficult. In many instances they appear as a gradual continuum of components that blend into each other. Classification schemes, however, have been devised (Fig. 6.1). They are useful because they give recognition to distinctive types in the spectrum of overlapping characteristics and afford an orderliness to this broad category of tissues.

Connective tissues, depending upon the cell population and type of matrix, serve numerous and multiple functions. By virtue of their fibrous components they *connect* one tissue or organ to another. Also, they are the means through which organs are *suspended* from the walls of the body. Various connective tissues *insulate* organs from mechanical damage. These tissues are responsible for the form of organs and the body. They are an important line of *defense* because numerous protective cells are part of their cellular population. The connective tissues serve a *nutritive* function as well. Not only do vascular beds have to traverse connective tissues to reach other tissues, but metabolites also move through the connective tissue space to reach individual cells. *Heat regulation, water metabolism* and *food storage* are also important functions. In conjunction with other tissues they aid in the *support* and *locomotion* of the body. Some connective tissues also play an important role in *repair* and *regeneration*.

Origin of Connective Tissue. All of the connective tissues are derivatives of mesoderm. This compartment of mesenchyme begins early in development as a well-defined, well-delineated and continuous space bounded by the ectoderm peripherally and the endoderm internally. The connective tissue compartment consists initially of mesenchymal cells, a fine meshwork of collagenous fibers and ground substance. Many tissues develop within this space. The *mesenchymal cell* is the stem cell for all mesodermal derivatives, including all of the cells of the connective tissues (Fig. 6.2). These mesenchymal cell derivatives comprise the heterogeneous population of cells that occurs in these tissues and accounts for their unique properties.

Progress in development is characterized by the continuous and progressive "invasion" of the connective tissue compartment by invagination of cells from the ectoderm and endoderm. Also, continuous development of cavities within the mesoderm (celomic spaces), the differentiation of vascular elements (endothelium) and the differentiation of muscles and supportive tissues all tend to infringe upon this compartment. The net result is that the connective tissue compartment is converted into a tortuous, irregular and apparently discontinuous array of spaces that are interspersed among all of the other components that have "invaded into" or developed within the compartment.

The gradual and continuous infringement of other tissues upon the connective tissue compartment results in an irregularly-shaped connective tissue space (Fig. 6.3). The general impression of this space is that it is discontinuous and is interspersed secondarily among the other tissue components with which it is associated. Nothing is further from the actual reality of the relationship. Those elements which invaginate into or are developed within the connective tissue never actually gain access to the connective tissue compartment. They are separated from it by the ever-present basal lamina, which is visible with the electron microscope. The relationship is similar to attempting to gain access to the air-filled space of a balloon by pushing a finger into it. The finger never gains access to the space but is always covered by the peripheral margin of the balloon. The basal lamina is analogous to the peripheral margin of the balloon. (N.B.: This is the same type of relationship that the organs of the body have with the celomic spaces. Organs may infringe upon the celomic spaces but never actually gain access to them because of the everpresent mesothelial lining).

The presence of a basement membrane (light microscopic structure) and basal lamina (electron microscopic structure) was discussed in detail with epithelial tissues. As ectodermal and endodermal derivatives infringe upon the connective tissue compartment, they essentially "push" the basal lamina in front of them. Even those elements, nonconnective tissue, which develop within the mesenchyme secondarily develop a basal lamina. Whereas the concept of a basal lamina was presented previously as an interface between epithelial and connective tissues, it is now appropriate to broaden the concept. *The basal lamina separates all connective tissues from nonconnective tissues.*

In its broadest sense, the basal lamina may be considered the peripheral limit of the connective tissue compartment. Cells of connective and supportive tissues are devoid of a basal lamina. Some minor exceptions to this generalization will be discussed with other organs, but one major exception causes a classification dilemma. Because all nonconnective tissues are covered by and separated from the connective tissue space by a basal lamina, what then is the proper classification of adipose tissue? Adipose tissue generally occurs in intimate association with the proper connective tissues. Isolated populations of fat cells or entire sheets, as adipose tissue, occur "in" the connective tissue compartment. Yet, these cells are covered by a basal lamina. Classically, adipose tissue was considered a connective tissue. The presence of a basal lamina, however, precludes its inclusion with these tissues. Also, adipose tissue is highly cellular with little intercellular matrix. As with muscle, adipose tissue may be considered a separate and distinct tissue. It may be useful to consider that there are five basic tissue types and give adipose tissue its assumed "rightful" place among the classification scheme. But, "man classifies and nature doesn't."

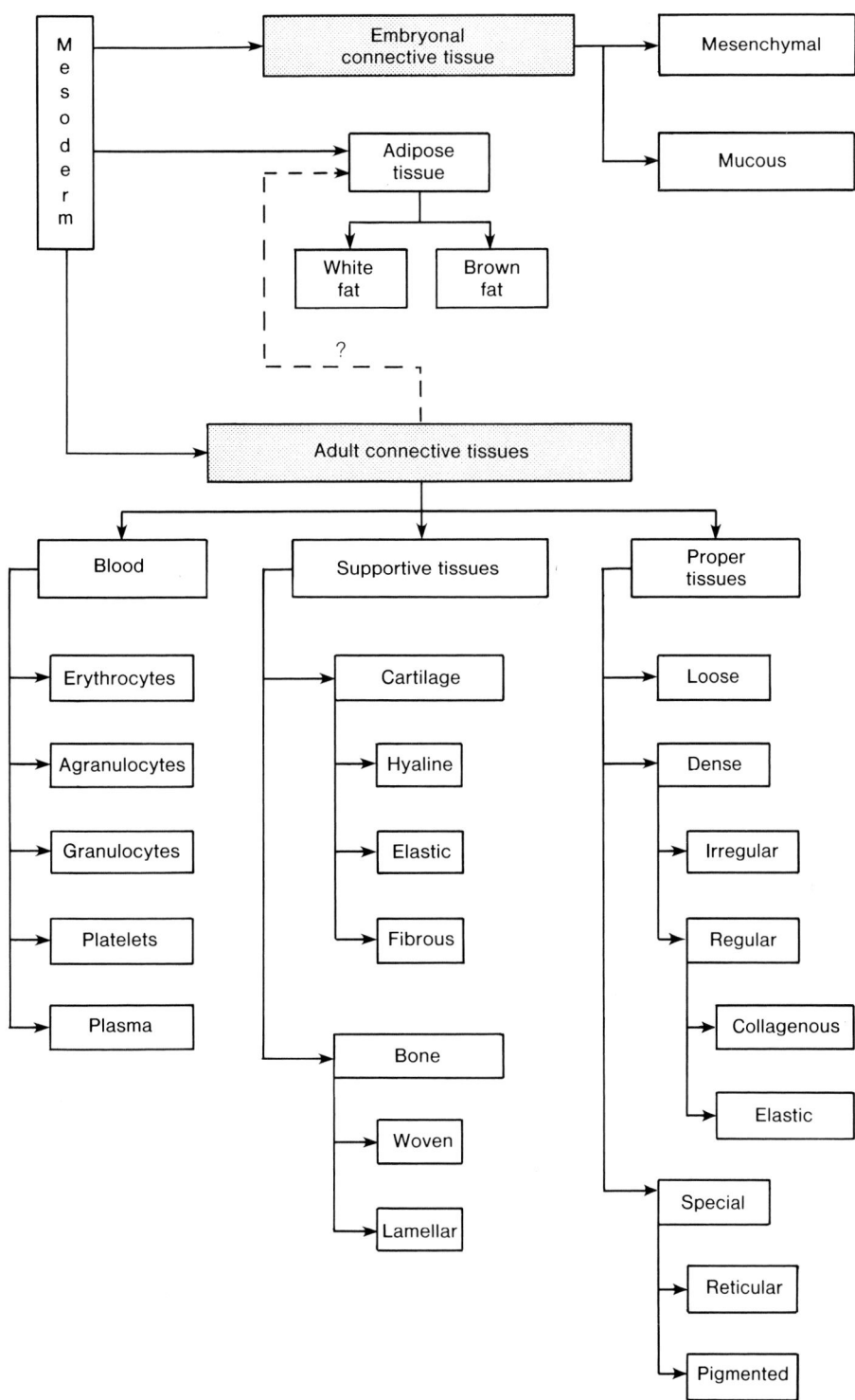

Fig. 6.1 Organizational scheme of connective tissue. All light micrographs are labeled as the magnification with the microscope before photographic enlarging. All electron micrographs are labeled as total magnification, including photographic enlarging.

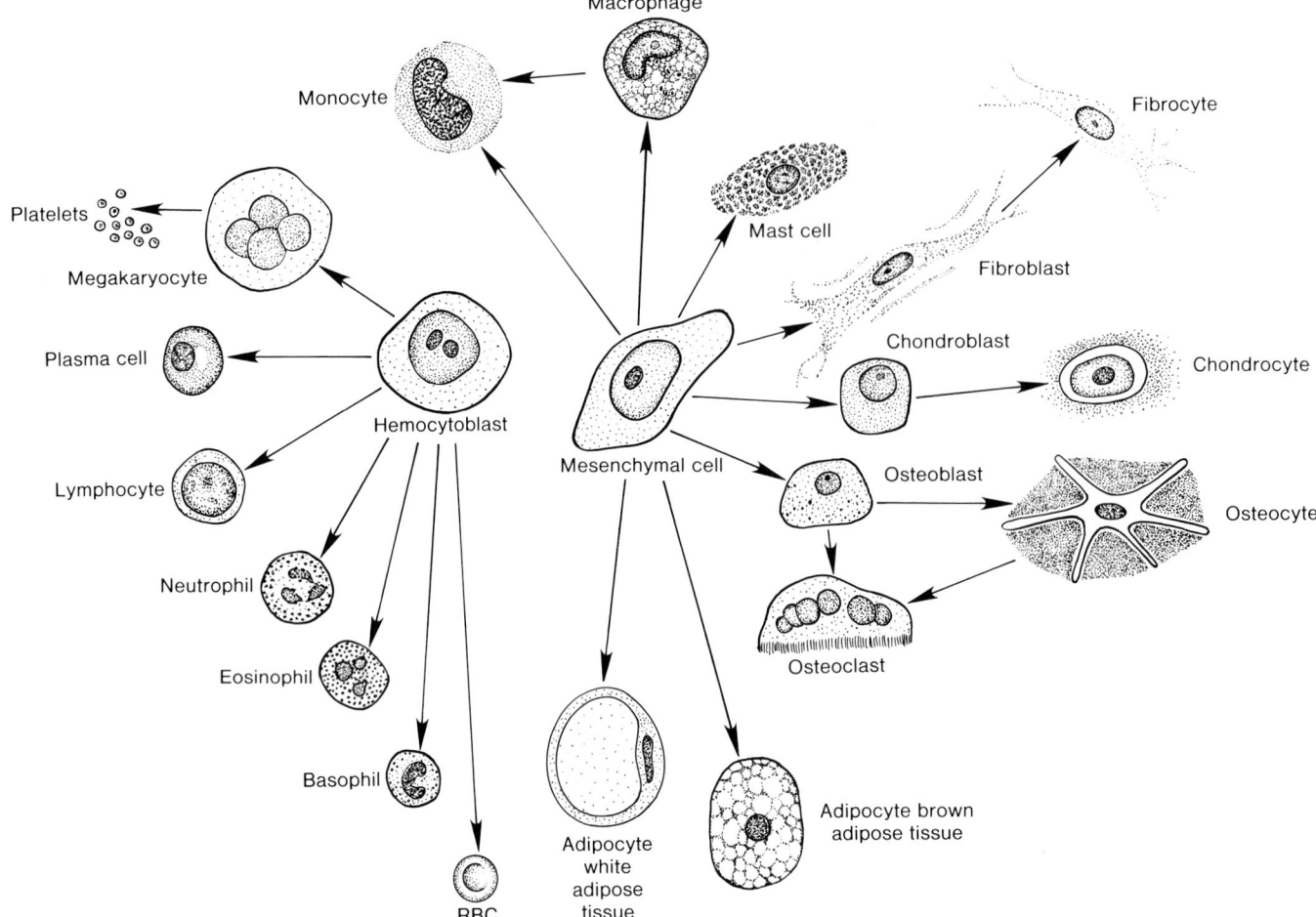

Fig. 6.2 Connective tissue cell derivatives from the mesenchymal cell. The precise relationship between closely related cells is not intended. Detailed relationships among these cells is discussed in subsequent chapters.

Whatever the ultimate classification of this tissue, it is more important at this point to recognize that this metabolically active tissue subserves valuable functions for the organism.

Unique Relationships. The unique relationship of the connective tissue compartment, basal lamina and epithelial tissues was discussed previously. Because the connective tissue compartment is intimately associated with all tissues, the significance of this relationship must be extended to include them as well.

All metabolites that are carried by the vascular system must leave the capillaries, cross the basal lamina, traverse the connective tissue compartment and cross the basal lamina again before being picked up by epithelial cells. Similarly, waste products of metabolism follow the reverse sequence from the epithelial cells back to the vascular beds. This applies equally to other tissues, whether they are of epithelial origin or not. Connective tissue cells, however, are bathed continuously by the fluids (*connective tissue fluid*) that account for this two-way flow pattern. This fluid, also referred to as *extracellular fluid (ECF)*, comprises a vast extra-

cellular fluid compartment. The peripheral limits of the ECF compartment correspond to the limits of the connective tissue space as delimited by the basal lamina. Importantly, the integrity of epithelial barriers is essential for the maintenance and turnover of the ECF.

The ECF is in a constant state of flux. Fluids with essential metabolic components leave the arterial side of the capillary bed, enter the connective tissue space and eventually reach all of the cells of the body. These same fluids, depleted of their metabolites and replaced by metabolic waste products and by-products, are returned to the circulation via the venous side of the capillary bed and lymphatic capillaries. This percolation of fluids occurs through the matrix, fibrous and amorphous, of the connective tissue compartment.

This region is also one of the important "battlegrounds" of the body. It is the compartment within which the organism mounts numerous specific (humoral antibodies, cell-mediated immunity) and nonspecific immune responses (phagocytosis). Resident populations of cells (histiocytes and mast cells) and transient populations of cells

(neutrophils, eosinophils, plasma cells) all contribute to the protective significance of this compartment.

The proper connective tissues of the body affect, directly or indirectly, all of the constituent cells, tissues and organs of the metazoan organism.

Classification. Despite the problems associated with a definitive classification scheme, the relationship outlined in Fig. 6.1 are useful. Four criteria are used primarily for the classification of connective tissues:

1. predominant cell type or types
2. type of fibrous components of the matrix
3. number of fibers in a unit area of the matrix
4. orderliness of the matrix components

The two broad categories of connective tissues are the embryonal and adult connective tissues.

Extracellular Components

Fibers. Three types of fibers are characteristic of connective tissues: *collagenous, reticular* and *elastic* fibers. They occur in varying quantity, organization and combination in these tissues. These fibers, in combination with the ground substance, impart the varied physical characteristics associated with connective tissues.

These fibers are secreted by the various cells of the connective tissue. They are the *neutral mucosubstances (glycoproteins)* that characterize these tissues.

Collagenous fibers, the secretory products of *fibroblasts,* are the most numerous of the fibers encountered in connective tissues. In light microscopic sections stained with hematoxylin and eosin (H and E) they appear as pink-staining, wavy bundles of indefinite length with a diameter of between 1 and 12 μm (Fig. 6.4). In most connective tissues they are oriented in random directions; thus, these fibers may be cut in cross-section, longitudinally or diagonally. In stretch preparations their length, thickness and random orientation are more apparent (Fig. 6.5).

With the electron microscope and appropriate staining, a light and dark banding is observed. One light and dark band represents a 64-nm period. This periodicity is repeated along the entire length of the collagenous fiber (Fig. 6.6). The collagenous fibers of both light and electron microscopy are composed of smaller units. The basic unit of collagen is the *tropocollagen* molecule. This macromolecule is composed of three proteins that are entwined about each other in a helical array along their entire 280-nm length. Tropocollagen is approximately 1.5 nm wide. This molecule is synthesized by the cell and secreted into the extracellular environment.

Current evidence indicates that the synthesis of collagen precursors is similar to the synthesis of other proteins (Fig. 6.7). Translation occurs on the ribosomes of the rough endoplasmic reticulum and results in the synthesis of polypeptide chains that consist of approximately 250 amino acids. Three polypeptides become associated with each other as a nonorderly array called *pro-alpha chains.* These chains traverse the RER and reach the Golgi apparatus. Within the Golgi stack *glycosylation* occurs (sugars are added) and an orderly helical arrangement is achieved. These molecules are longer than the typical tropocollagen molecules encountered outside the cell. They are called *procollagen* molecules. The tailpieces on these molecules may inhibit spontaneous intracellular polymerization. Procollagen is transported to the cell surface within the secretory vesicles. At or near the surface, a *procollagen peptidase* removes the tailpieces and tropocollagen results. Once outside the cell, numerous tropocollagen molecules polymerize into larger units. However, this is not random. Rather, they align themselves in such a way as to overlap each other by approximately one-quarter of their length (Fig. 6.8). This accounts for the periodicity. Tropocollagen molecules polymerize to form *microfibrils* less than 40 nm in diameter. Further polymerization of bundles of microfibrils forms *fibrils* (approximately 0.5 μm in diameter) that are visible with the light microscope. Bundles of fibrils form the characteristic *fibers* of light microscopy. Although these fibers stretch minimally, they impart tremendous tensile properties to those tissues in which they are characteristic.

The *reticular fibers* of light microscopy are difficult to demonstrate with routine staining. As such, they are indistinguishable from collagen. Reticular fibers are readily demonstrable with special staining. They are easily observed with silver staining techniques (Fig. 6.9). Because of their ability to be stained with silver, they are referred to as *argyrophilic.* Unfortunately, the electron microscope has never satisfactorily demonstrated reticular fibers. Rather, reticular fibers are observed as small fibrils or *microfibrils of collagen.* It appears that reticular fibers are actually collagenous fibers that have undergone minimal polymerization. This reduced polymerization with its associated reduced availability of reactive groups may account for the argyrophilia associated with reticular fibers.

The *elastic fibers* of light microscopy are not easily demonstrated with routine staining. With H and E, however, the discerning eye will note that the elastic fibers stain a brighter pink than collagen. With special

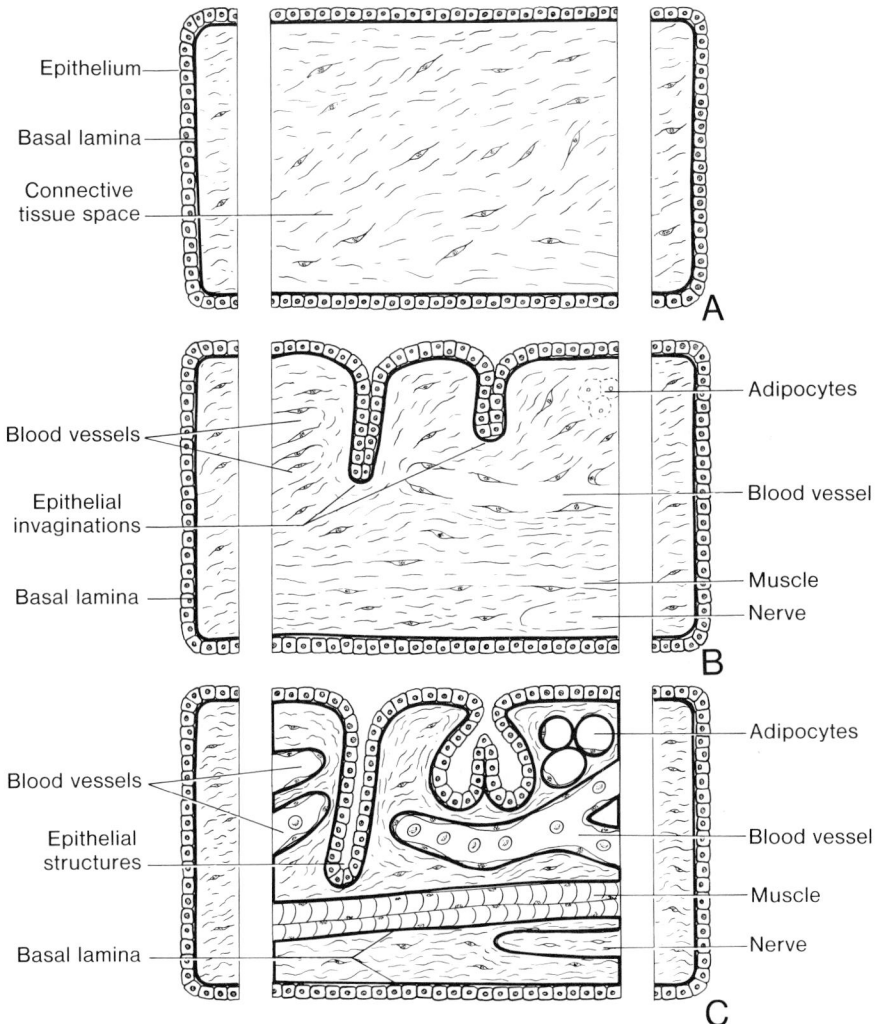

Fig. 6.3 Schematic representation of the connective tissue space and basal lamina. Although the connective tissue space, as defined by the peripherally positioned basal lamina, is a single, vast, continuous space, it is represented as a discontinuous space in these diagrams to imply its vastness. A single closed compartment in a diagram does not do justice to it. A. Early in development, the connective tissue space may be visualized as a compartment that consists exclusively of connective tissue components—mesenchymal cells, fibroblasts, fibers and amorphous matrix materials. The boundary of the compartment is defined by the basal lamina (*dark black line*). B. As development progresses, various cells differentiate within or invade into the compartment. C. Complete development of components associated intimately with the connective tissue has been achieved. Although the connective tissue compartment has been reduced in volume and has become very irregular, its integrity is still maintained. Nothing has gained access to the compartment. The basal lamina still separates connective tissue components from nonconnective tissue components.

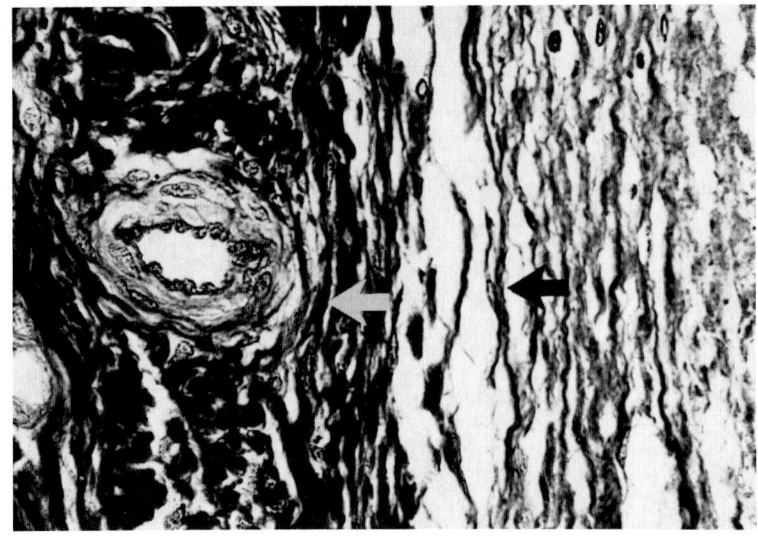

Fig. 6.4 Collagenous fibers of the capsule of the adrenal gland. Coarse fibers (*white arrow*) and fine fibers (*black arrow*) comprise the capsule. X160 (Azan).

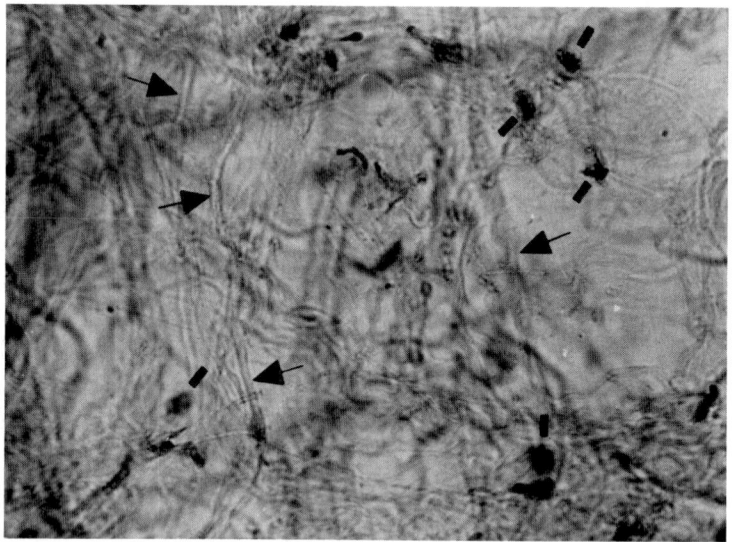

Fig. 6.5 Stretch preparation of connective tissue from the subcutis of a mouse. The collagenous fibers (*arrows*) are oriented randomly. The cells (*bars*) are out of the plane of focus. X160.

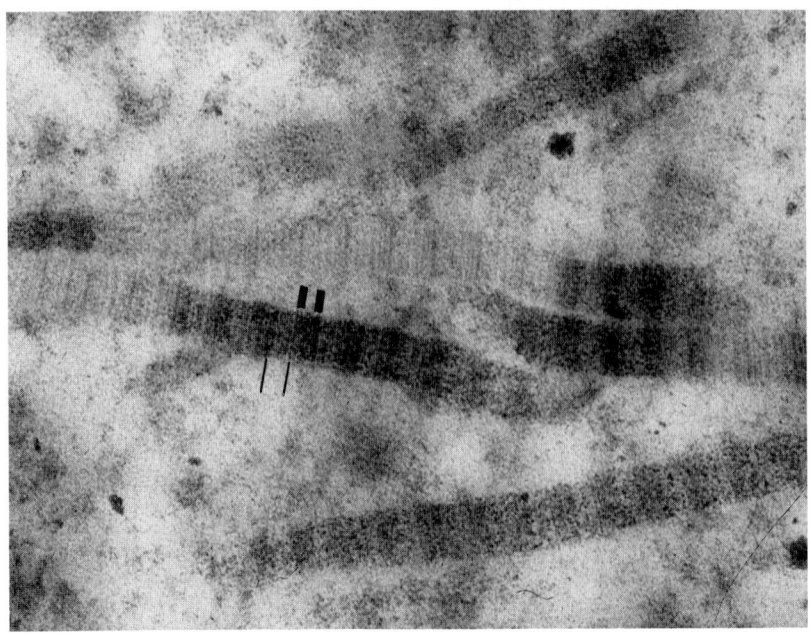

Fig. 6.6 An electron micrograph of sectioned collagen. The periodic banding is obvious. The dark band (*thick bars*) and light band (*thin bars*) comprise the typical 64-nm period of collagen. X94,000.

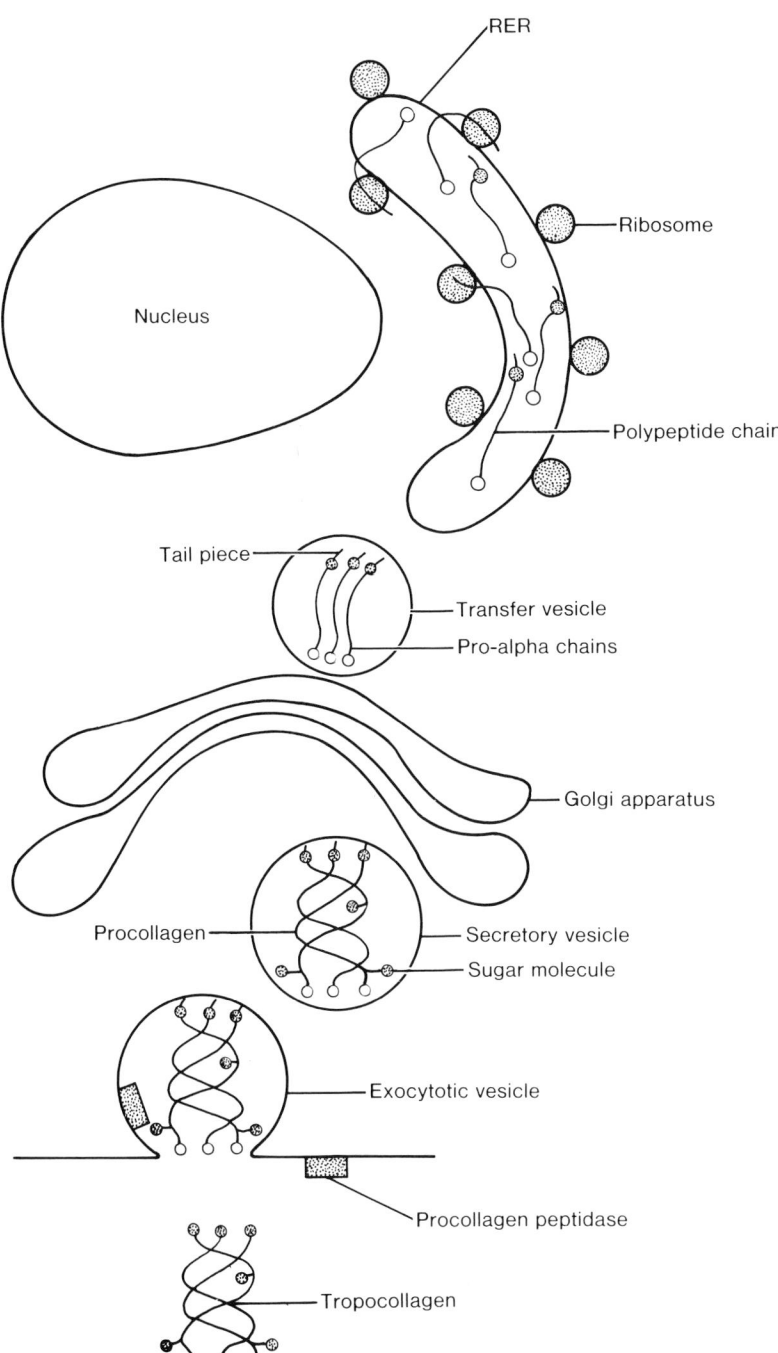

Fig. 6.7 Synthesis and secretion of tropocollagen. The synthesis of tropocollagen is similar to the synthesis of other proteins. The mRNA for collagen is formed within the nucleus by transcription. The mRNA enters the cytoplasm and attaches to the ribosomes of the rough endoplasmic reticulum (RER). Translation results in the formation of polypeptide chains. Hydroxylation of proline and lysine occurs on the ribosome during translation. The polypeptides gain access to the cisterns of the RER during translation and become associated as pro-alpha chains. Transfer vesicles are incorporated into the immature face of the Golgi apparatus. Glycosylation within the Golgi stack results in the formation of ordered procollagen molecules. The procollagen molecules leave the mature face of the Golgi apparatus within secretory vesicles. The secretory vesicles fuse with the plasma membrane as exocytotic vesicles. A procollagen peptidase, located either within the secretory vesicles or on the cell membrane, cleaves the tailpiece resulting in the secretion of tropocollagen. (Redrawn and modified from Hunt, T. K. and Van Winkle, Jr., W.: *Fundamentals of Wound Management in Surgery-Wound Healing: Normal Repair.* Chirurgecom, Inc., South Plainfield, New Jersey, 1976).

At the electron microscopic level, elastic fibers are represented as amorphous, electron-dense material with darker peripheral fringes (Fig. 6.13). They do not have any periodic cross-banding.

Ground Substance. The fibrous and cellular components of connective tissues are surrounded by and embedded within an amorphous material that comprises the *ground substance*. The components of this substance are secreted by the characteristic cells of these tissues. The ground substance is a viscous material in the gel form that binds great quantities of water. This bound water is the medium through which the movement of metabolites and waste products must occur. The ground substance and ECF, although considered as separate entities, are, in fact, inseparable.

The ground substance, composed of components that are highly water-soluble, is observed rarely with routine preparation techniques. Special care (freezing) must be taken to preserve this material for staining. The spaces observed between fibers and cells are the spaces that were occupied by this material in vivo. In cartilage and bone, however, the ground substance is preserved readily by routine preparatory methods.

The ground substance of connective tissues consist of mucopolysaccharides. These substances are referred to currently as *glycosaminoglycans.* (Any polysaccharide which contains an amino sugar is now called a glycosaminoglycan.) The glycosaminoglycans are either sulfated (*acidic mucosubstances*) or nonsulfated (*neutral mucosubstances*). *Hyaluronic acid, chondroitin-4-sulfate, chondroitin-6-sulfate, dermatan sulfate, keratan sulfate* and *heparin* are the major mucopolysaccharides of the connective tissues (Fig. 6.14). These biochemical substances are conjugated to proteins (collagen, noncollagenous proteins) to form *protein-polysaccharide complexes (proteoglycans)* within which the cells and fibrous components are suspended. Variation in the amount and type of proteoglycans in the ground substance is sufficient to alter the characteristics of the connective tissues.

Hyaluronic acid is a viscous substance that occurs in loose connective tissue, synovial fluid and vitreous humor. Its capacity to bind water contributes significantly to the delicate balance of ECF that exists within the connective tissue space. Hyaluronic acid is also significant in resisting the spread of invasive materials and microorganisms within the connective tissue compartment. Certain bacteria facilitate their movement through this compartment by secreting the enzyme *hyaluronidase.* Similarly, certain injectables are spread more easily throughout this compartment when accompanied by the injection of this enzyme. Hyaluronidase is known as the "spreading factor."

Heparin is a highly sulfated compound that is secreted by the mast cells of the connective tissue compartment. It is an effective anticoagulant in vivo and in vitro.

staining techniques, they are easily observed as long, thin or wavy fibers (Fig. 6.10). In stretch preparations they are not only more refractile than collagenous and reticular fibers, but they are observed as long, thin, branched, straight fibers. If they are broken, they are wavy fibers with a corkscrew appearance (Figs. 6.11, 6.12).

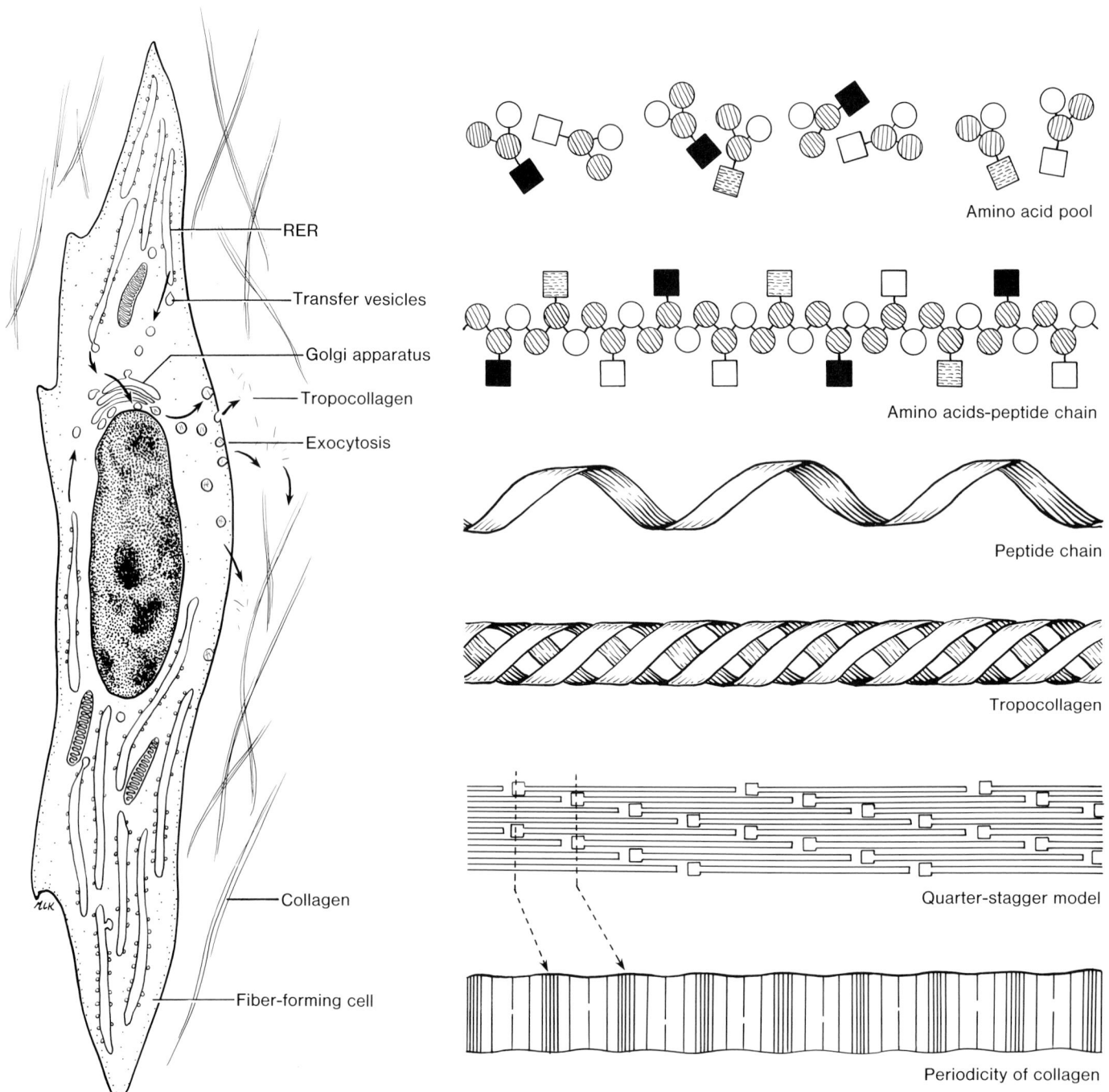

RER

Transfer vesicles

Golgi apparatus

Tropocollagen

Exocytosis

Collagen

Fiber-forming cell

Amino acid pool

Amino acids-peptide chain

Peptide chain

Tropocollagen

Quarter-stagger model

Periodicity of collagen

Fig. 6.8 Synthesis, secretion and polymerization of tropocollagen. Glycine, proline and lysine comprise the majority of amino acids incorporated into tropocollagen. Hydroxyproline is a specific marker of collagen, because it does not occur in other biochemical substances in significant amounts. The amino acids are sequenced during translation to produce typical polypeptide chains. Tropocollagen, the secretory product of fiber-forming cells (fibroblasts, osteoblasts, chondroblasts), polymerizes within the connective tissue compartment to form typical collagen. Whereas other models have been proposed to account for the 64-nm periodicity of collagen, the quarter-stagger model is shown. This model accounts for most of the repetitive features of collagen in relation to the 280 nm length of tropocollagen. The quarter-stagger model would be exact if the periodicity of collagen were 70 nm. Other models have been proposed to account for the discrepancy of 24 nm. Importantly, not all collagen has a 64-nm periodicity; it may range from 20–1000 nm in some tissues (Redrawn and modified but based on descriptions by J. Goss and K. R. Porter, Connective Tissue: Intracellular Macromolecules, J. and A. Churchill Ltd., London, 1964).

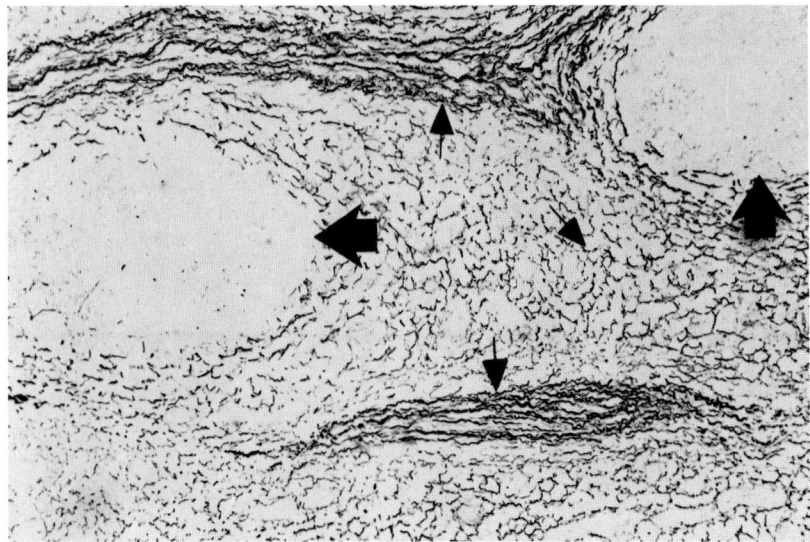

Fig. 6.9 Reticular fibers within a canine lymph node. The argyrophilic fibers (*small arrows*) are arranged in dense and loose aggregates. Areas devoid of fibers (*large arrows*) are the germinal centers of the lymph nodules within the node. X40 (Snook's reticulum stain).

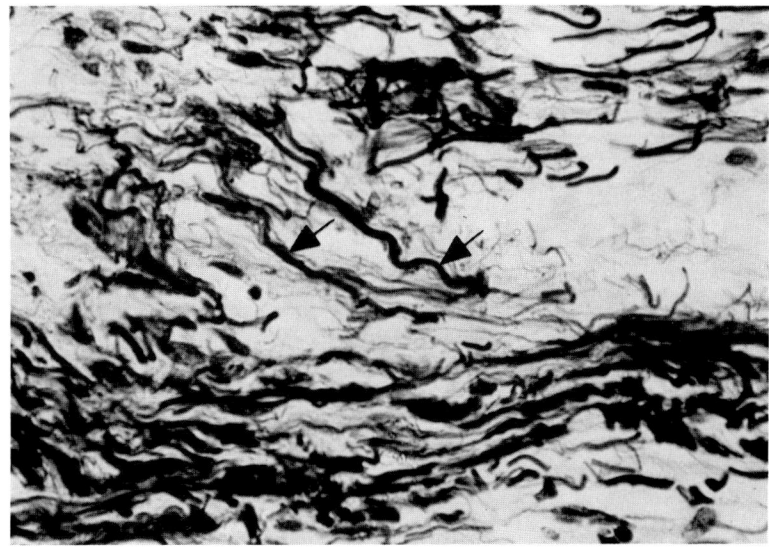

Fig. 6.10 Elastic fibers of loose connective tissue. Although the elastic fibers (*arrows*) are difficult to demonstrate with routine stains, the fibers are demonstrable with special staining techniques. X160 (Verhoeff's stain).

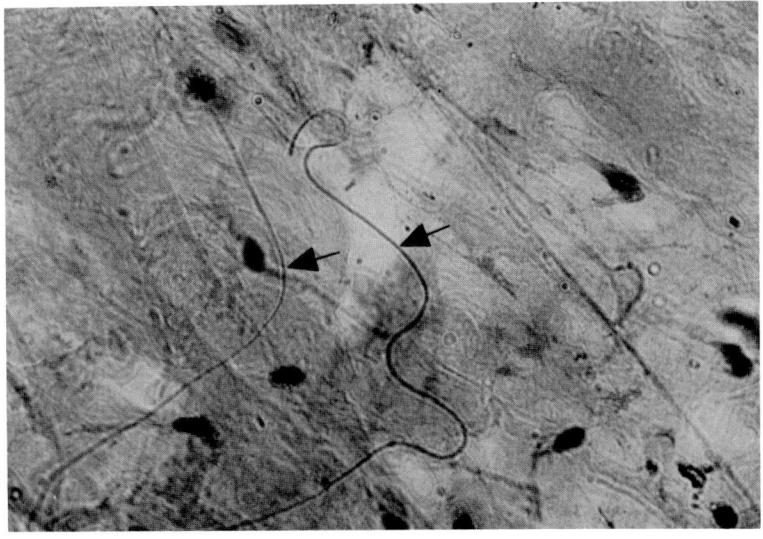

Fig. 6.11 Elastic fibers in a stretch preparation of loose connective tissue from the subcutis of a mouse. The broken elastic fibers (*arrows*) appear wavy. Other cellular and fibrous components are not in the plane of focus. X160.

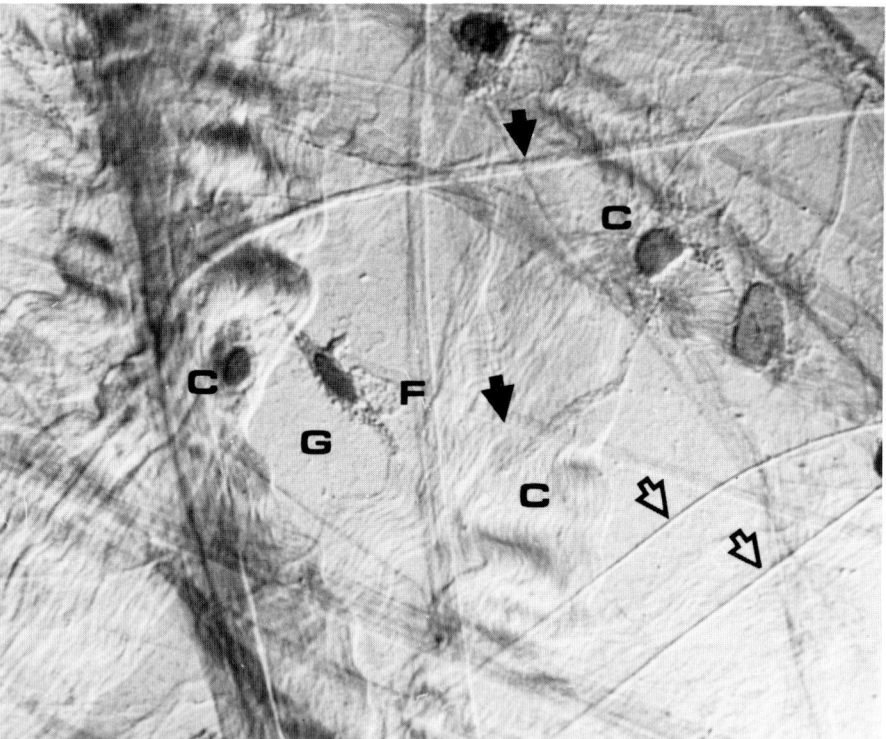

Fig. 6.12 Normarski interference contrast micrograph of the loose connective tissue of the murine subcutis. F, fibroblasts, G, ground substance; *open arrow*, elastin; *solid arrows*, collagen; C, bundles of collagenous fibers. X160.

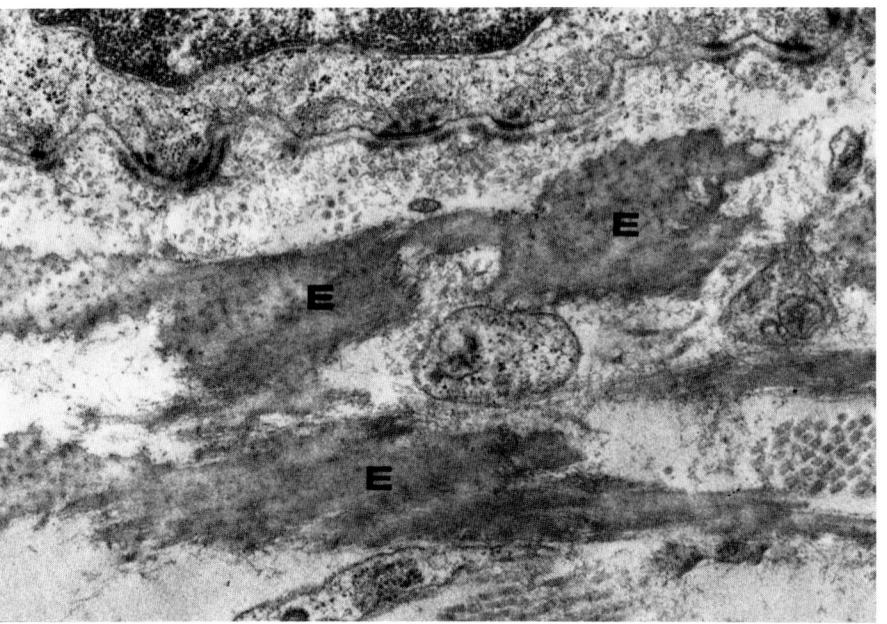

Fig. 6.13 An electron micrograph of elastic fibers. The irregularly shaped elastic fibers (E) are scattered throughout the connective tissue. X26,000.

The remaining glycosaminoglycans do not occur generally in the proper connective tissues. Chondroitin sulfates and keratan sulfate occur in cartilage, bone, cornea and the nucleus pulposus of intervertebral discs, while dermatan sulfate may be found in the ligamentum nuchae, skin and tendons. These substances usually impart an in-creased viscosity to the tissues of which they are components. These will be discussed with the appropriate tissues.

The matrix of connective tissues, then, consist of fibrous components and glycos-aminoglycans. The type and amount of each of these major components account for the various characteristics associated with these tissues. The matrix may be as pliable as the typical aerolar (loose) connective tissue, as resiliant as hyaline cartilage or as rigid as bone. In the latter instance, mineral is added to the organic matrix.

Metachromatic stains and PAS are useful for the study of matrix components of con-nective tissues. A marked metachromasia is associated with the number of sulfate groups present in the ground substance. PAS-reac-tivity is confined to the neutral mucosub-stances.

Tissue Fluid Dynamics

Ground Substance and Tissue Fluid. The unique characteristics of the connective tis-sues are attributable to the nature of the constituent glycosaminoglycans. These sub-stances, as proteoglycans, are capable of binding large quantities of water. Because dissolved substances that are essential for normal cellular function are transported through this fluid medium, the ground sub-stance and the ECF assume a transport role that is critically important to the well-being of all cells of the body. Unfortunately, rou-tine preparations of connective tissues do not demonstrate these components except as spaces between the constituent fibers and cells. Nevertheless, these spaces and the components they contained prior to pro-cessing are important.

Body Water. The total volume of water is about 65% of the total body weight. This percentage, however, is related more directly to the mass of the lean tissues of the body rather than to total body weight. Lean ani-mals contain a higher percentage of water than do obese animals. The distribution of the water volume is not equal, because tis-sues and organs of the body contain differ-ent but characteristic amounts of water (Ta-ble 6.1). Moreover, this unequal distribution of water is identified as *extracellular fluid* and *intracellular fluid* (Fig 6.15). The extra-cellular fluid comprises approximately 24% of the total fluid volume and includes the *plasma* (4%), *interstitial* or *tissue fluid* (15%) and *transcellular fluid* (5%). The transcellu-lar fluids are those that occur in the body cavities, hollow visceral organs, eye and as secretory products of various glands. The remaining 41% of the fluid compartment is intracellular. Importantly, these separate fluid compartments are exchangeable and are in a state of flux.

Vascular and Tissue Fluid Exchange. The vascular system is the means by which all required metabolites and oxygen are brought to the proximity of the cells that require them. These materials must traverse the tissue fluid. Similarly, metabolic waste products, including carbon dioxide, traverse the tissue fluid and are then transported in the blood to their appropriate sites of excre-tion (kidneys) or exchange (lungs). Al-though a basal lamina and endothelial bar-rier separate the vascular compartment from the extravascular compartment (tissue fluid compartment), these spaces may be considered a continuum on the basis of the movement of crystalloids and gases between these two fluids. These substances move down their concentration gradients (*diffusion*) randomly to or from the vascular compartment through spaces between endothelial cells or through fenestrations within endothelial cells. Pinocytotic vesicles, which may be apparent in the endothelial cells, do not account for the rapid movement of diffusible particles and water. Rather, they may assist in the transcapillary movement of macromolecules between the two fluid compartments. The selective permeability of the endothelial cells precludes, except for a minimal amount, the transport of macromolecules (proteins) across this barrier.

The Starling-Landis Concept. The random movement of crystalloids and ions across the capillary wall is augmented by *filtration*. Filtration is the movement of fluids and dissolved solutes across the capillary boundary. The movement is governed by forces that act across the capillary wall and account for the bulk translocation of fluids and solutes. These forces were first described and quantified by Starling and Landis as being a combination of hydrostatic and colloid osmotic pressures.

Vascular *hydrostatic pressure* (*HP*) is initiated by the mechanical driving force of the heart, as well as by the active and passive contributions of the mural elements of blood vessels. (The pressures used in this discussion do not characterize all tissues; however, the relative pressures are representative and serve to illustrate the principle.) Although vascular HP drops appreciably in the arterial side of the capillaries to 40 mm Hg, this

Table 6.1
Percentage of Water in Canine Tissues*

Tissue or Organ	% Water
Brain	75
Peripheral nerve	66
Liver	75
Lung	79
Cardiac muscle	78
Skeletal muscle	77
Bone	52
Skin	64
Kidney	80
Spleen	77
Connective tissue	60

* These values are averages; variations from these values occur.

exceeds the hydrostatic pressure within the tissue fluid, which is 5 mm Hg (Fig. 6.16). The *effective hydrostatic pressure* (*EHP*) in this portion of the capillary bed is 35 mm Hg, favoring the outward movement of fluids.

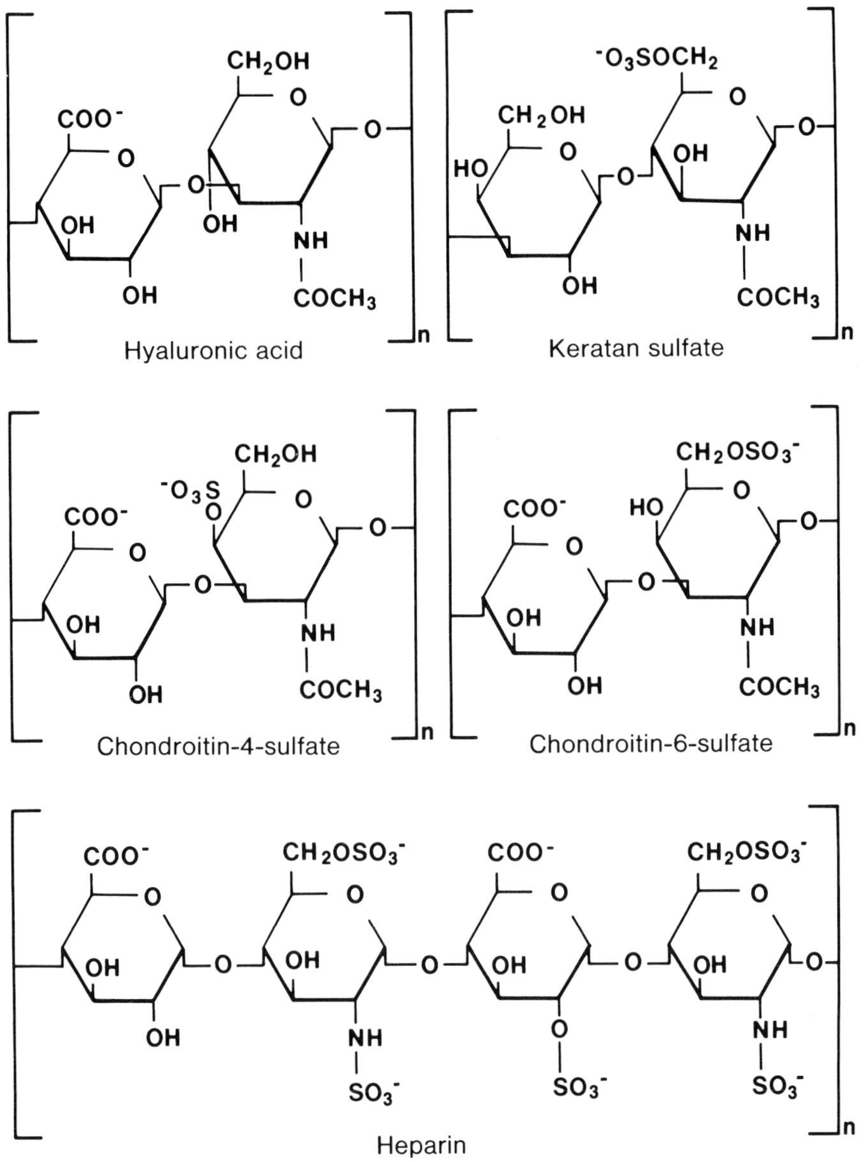

The plasma proteins, principally albumin, contribute to the *colloid osmotic pressure* (COP) of the blood. This is approximately 25 mm Hg in the arterial side of the capillary bed; the COP of the tissue fluid is approximately 3 mm Hg. The *effective COP* (ECOP) in this part of the capillary bed is 22 mm Hg, favoring the movement of water into the capillary bed. (Remember that water moves from an area of low oncotic pressure, low solute concentration, to an area of high oncotic pressure, high solute concentration, when separated by a semipermeable membrane.) The *net driving force* (EHP minus ECOP) in this part of the capillary is 13 mm Hg; therefore, the movement of fluids is normally from the capillary bed to the connective tissue compartment (Fig. 6.17).

The net outward driving force insures that fluids are "pushed" into the tissue fluid space. A gradual change in the governing parameters assures that fluid is returned to the venous side of the capillary bed (Fig. 6.16). As fluids leave the capillary bed, the HP within the capillary on the venous side is reduced to 15 mm Hg, while the tissue HP is maintained at 5 mm Hg. The EHP (10 mm Hg) of the blood of the capillary bed still favors the movement of water into the tissue fluid. The COP of the blood and tissue fluid remains constant at 25 and 3 mm Hg, respectively. The ECOP in the venous portion of the capillary is 22 mm Hg inward. A net driving force of 12 mm Hg favors the return of fluids to this portion of the capillary. So, the proteins of the blood plasma, which constantly tend to draw water into the capillary, exert this effect when the capillary hydrostatic pressure is reduced. The discrepancy between the net outward and net inward forces accounts for approximately 1% of the fluids not being returned to the capillary bed. This small amount of fluid, as well as any proteins that may have escaped into the tissue fluid is returned to the circulation via the lymphatic capillaries (Fig. 6.17).

Fig. 6.14 Chemical composition of selected glycosaminoglycans. The chain length (n) varies among these substances: hyaluronic acid, n = 2500, keratan sulfate, n = 10–20; chondroitin sulfates, n = 60; heparin, n = 15.

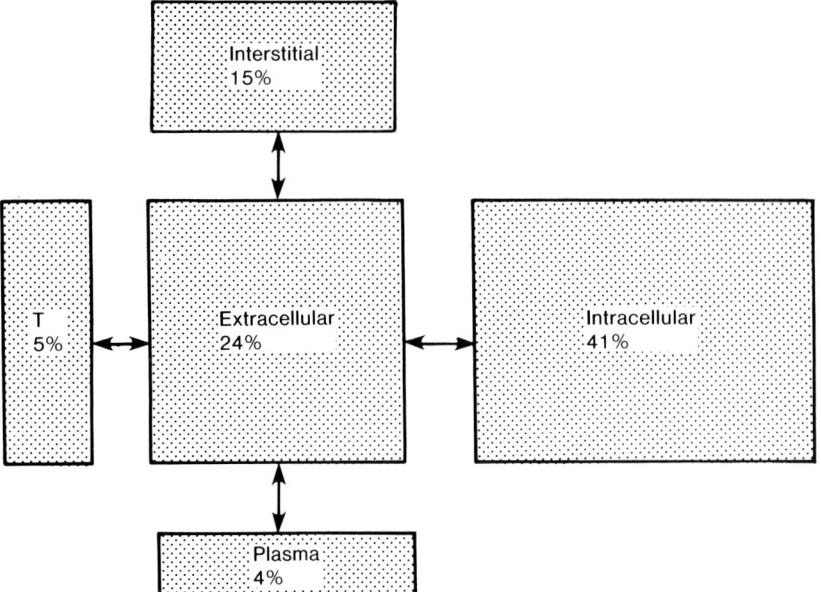

Fig. 6.15 Distribution of fluids within the animal body. The percentages are based upon water comprising 65% of body weight. The 24% extracellular fluid consists of transcellular fluids (T), plasma and interstitial fluid. The fluids move freely between all fluid compartments.

This mechanism of exchange accounts for the dynamic and continuous formation and turnover of fluids throughout the body. Although the numerical parameters vary slightly between specific loci, the relationships between HP and COP do not. Importantly, this is the mechanism that insures that the cells of the body are bathed continuously in a fluid environment conducive to their homeostasis. This mechanism is also important in the formation of urine.

Plasma, Tissue Fluid and Lymph. The *plasma* or intercellular fluid phase of the blood contains numerous and varied crystalloids as well as the plasma proteins (albumin, globulins, fibrinogen). Because the colloids do not leave the blood in any significant quantity under normal conditions, only the water and crystalloids gain access to the connective tissue space. *Tissue fluid*, then, is plasma devoid of most of its characteristic proteins. The tissue fluid that gains access to the lymphatic capillaries is called *lymph*.

Alterations to Fluid Exchange. Numerous factors can influence and alter the delicate balance that exists among the fluid components of the vascular system, lymphatic system and connective tissue compartment. Alterations (excessive water intake or loss, electrolyte imbalances, protein deficiencies, inflammation, systemic diseases) can be manifested as a localized or generalized disruption of fluid balance.

Edema, the retention and accumulation of excess tissue fluid in the connective tissue compartment, is a common manifestation of altered exchange processes. Histologically, it is manifested as an altered spatial relationship between the fibrous and cellular

components of the connective tissue compartment. Four basic mechanisms account for the excessive formation of tissue fluid; *lymph vessel obstruction, increased capillary permeability, decreased concentration of plasma proteins and venous obstruction.*

Lymph vessel obstruction (Fig. 6.18) exerts its influence upon this process in two ways. First, lymph obstruction prevents the return of tissue fluid to the circulation, resulting in a gradual and continuous increase of fluids within the connective tissue compartment. This increases the tissue fluid HP. Also, a progressive accumulation of proteins occurs in the connective tissue compartment. The proteins increase the connective tissue COP, which results in the propensity to attract and hold more water. Certain parasitic diseases and metastatic tumors may result in lymphatic obstruction. Also, solid tumors may grow around and subsequently occlude major lymphatic channels.

An increased capillary permeability (Fig. 6.19) results in the leakage of plasma into the connective tissue compartment. The increased COP due to excessive proteins in the connective tissue compartment causes an increased amount of tissue fluid. Most significantly, the blood has a decreased ability to attract water back into the capillaries. Inflammatory processes, allergic reactions, toxic substances and burns may cause edema due to increased capillary permeability.

A decreased vascular COP is associated with a decreased concentration of plasma proteins (Fig. 6.20). Such a deficiency results in a diminished ability to attract fluid into the blood from the connective tissue. Hypoproteinemia may result from liver disor-

ders, excessive protein loss in the urine, protein malnutrition, excessive protein loss through the digestive tract and parasitism.

Venous obstruction (Fig. 6.21) results in an increased capillary HP. When the HP exceeds the capillary COP, fluids are retained in the connective tissue compartment. Venous obstruction may result from congestive heart failure, inflammation of veins, increased pulmonary resistance and tight bandages. Generally, any rise in venous blood pressure can cause edema.

The real significance of the altered exchange associated with the aforementioned problems is not the swelling. The swelling expands the connective tissue compartment and may compromise the nutritional microenvironment of the cells. Diffusion distances for metabolites are increased and waste products of metabolism may accumulate. The tissue fluid compartment is able to accommodate a 30% increase in tissue fluid before altered spatial relationships of components are noted. This results from the capacity of the glycoproteins of this compartment to absorb the increased fluid.

Resident Cell Population

The cell population of any connective tissue will vary with the tissue, as well as the physiologic state of the tissue at the time of observation. Nevertheless, there are some cells of connective tissues that are encountered frequently. These may be referred to as the *resident cell population* and include *mesenchymal cells, reticular cells, fibroblasts*

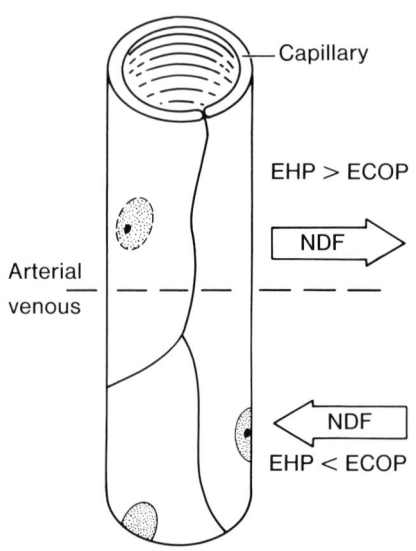

Fig. 6.16 Filtration across the capillary bed. Movement of fluids and solutes occurs on the arterial side of the capillary bed because the effective hydrostatic pressure (EHP) is greater than the effective colloid osmotic pressure in this region. The net driving force (NDF) is reversed on the venous side of the capillary bed because the ECOP is greater than the EHP in this region.

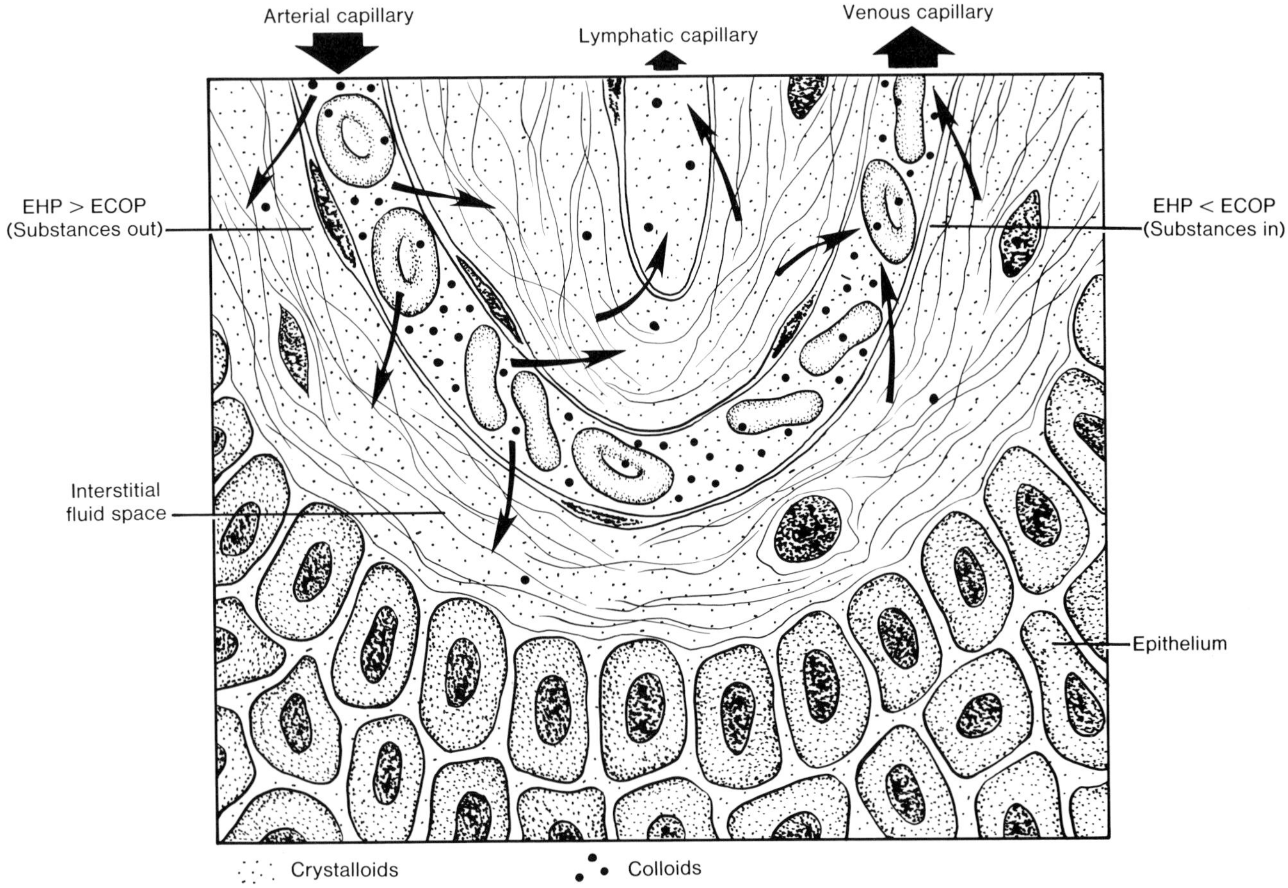

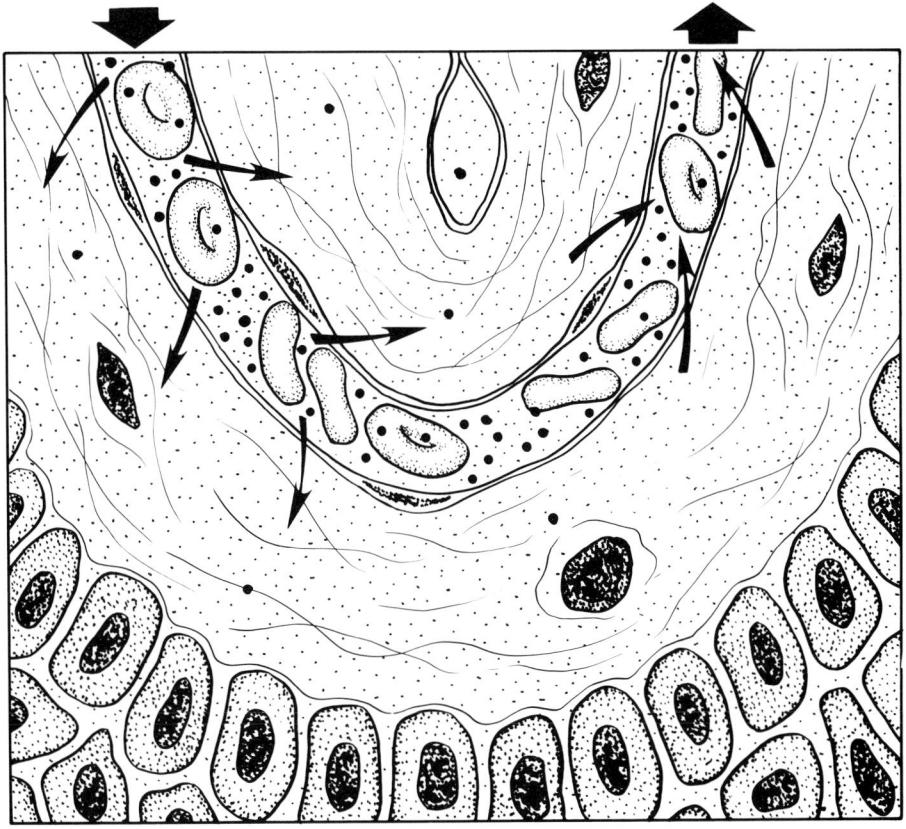

Arterial capillary

Lymphatic capillary

Venous capillary

EHP > ECOP
(Substances out)

EHP < ECOP
(Substances in)

Interstitial
fluid space

Epithelium

:·: Crystalloids   •·• Colloids

Fig. 6.17 A diagram to demonstrate the normal movement of fluids and crystalloids between the capillary bed and the fluid space (connective tissue compartment). The basal lamina is not shown but separates the connective and nonconnective tissues. Substances move into the connective tissue on the arterial side of the capillary bed and are returned to the capillary bed on the venous side. Very few colloids escape into the interstitial space. (EHP-effective hydrostatic pressure, ECOP-effective colloid osmotic pressure). The labels used for Figure 6.16 are applicable to Figures 6.17–6.20. (Figs. 6.16–6.20 were redrawn and modified from Ham, A. W.: *Histology*, 7th edition, J. B. Lippincott Company, Philadelphia, 1974).

Fig. 6.18 Altered tissue fluid formation and exchange resulting from lymphatic obstruction. Lymphatic obstruction causes excessive fluid and colloids to accumulate in the interstitial fluid space. The interstitial compartment swells and alters cellular and matrix component relationships.

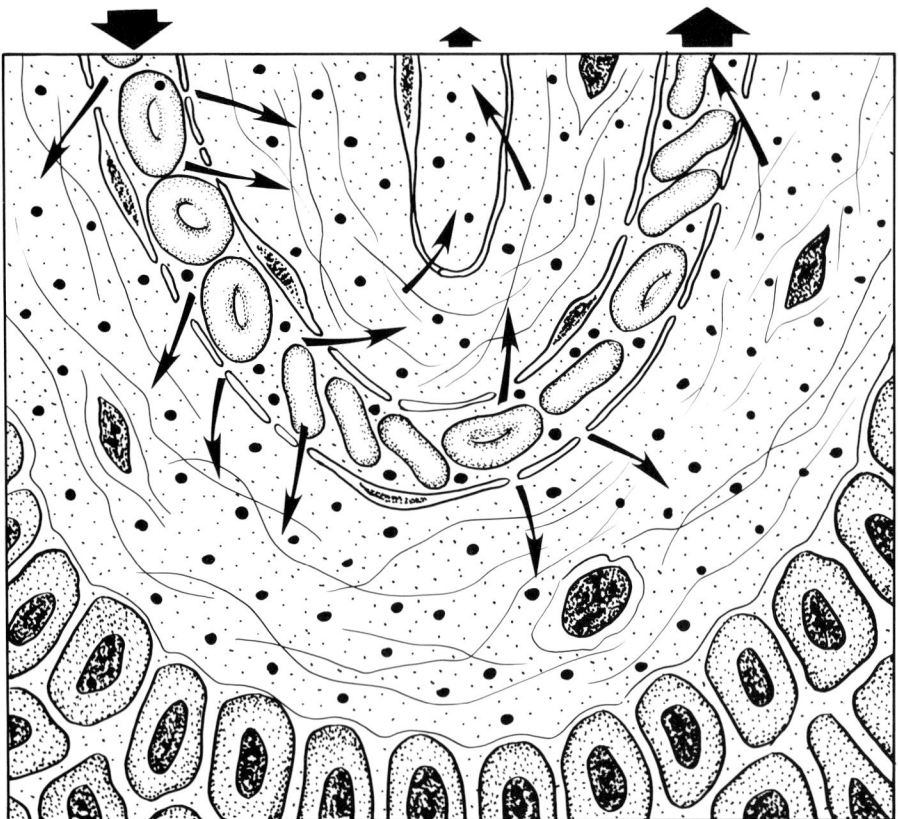

Fig. 6.19 Altered tissue fluid formation and exchange resulting from increasd capillary permeability. The movement of colloids into the interstitial space causes the space to swell.

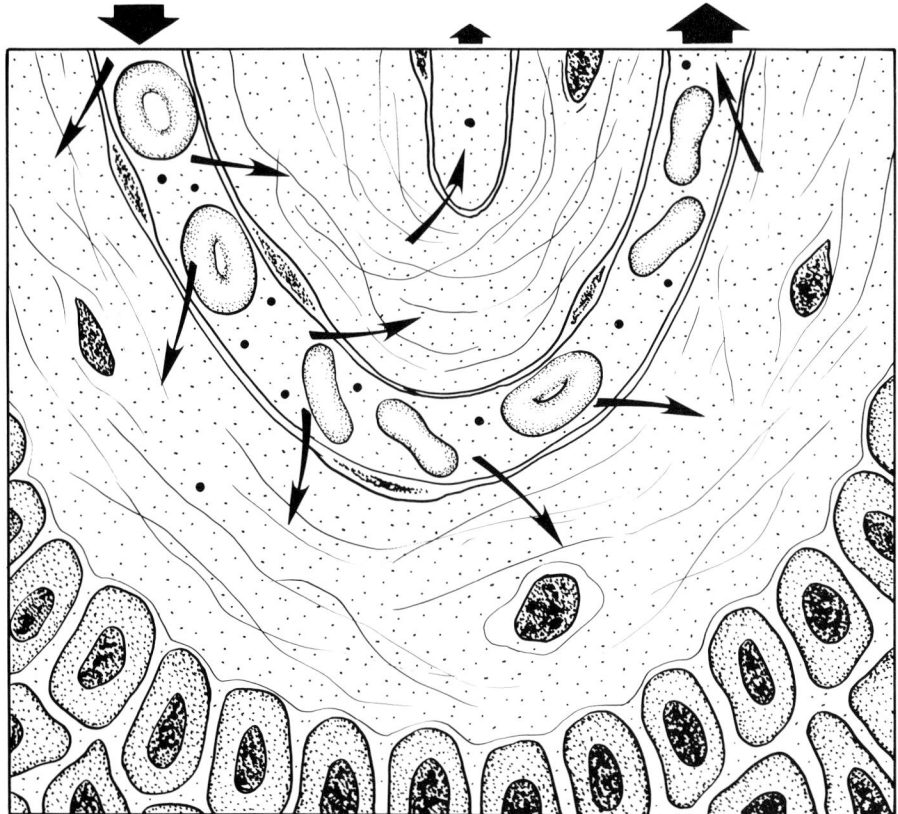

Fig. 6.20 Altered tissue fluid formation and exchange resulting from decreased vascular colloid osmotic pressure. The capillary bed has a diminished ability to attract fluids. The fluids accumulate in the interstitial space and swelling results.

(fibrocytes), *macrophages, pericytes, fat cells* and *mast cells.*

Mesenchymal Cells. The *mesenchymal cell* is the precursor of most connective tissue cells. It is a stellate or spindle cell with a high nuclear to cytoplasmic ratio. It has a large, vesicular nucleus that is rich in euchromatin (Fig. 6.22). The cytoplasm is acidophilic and scant. In most preparations the cytoplasm is indistinguishable from surrounding matrix components (Plate II.6). At the ultrastructural level, the predominant cytoplasmic organelle is the polyribosome (Fig. 6.23). The combination of prominent euchromatin and extensive free polyribosomes is indicative of the high protein synthesis potential of this cell. The protein produced, however, is for intracellular use initially. Few other organelles are apparent. Despite the presence of free polyribosomes, the cytoplasm has acidophilic staining properties. The acidophilic nature of other cytoplasmic components masks the basophilia of these particles.

Although mesenchymal cells are scattered throughout the connective tissue space, they are sometimes difficult to distinguish. They are most prominent in the perivascular area. These cells represent residual portions of the mesenchymal connective tissue from which mesodermal components are derived. The mesenchymal cells are the stem cells of these adult tissues through which replacement and repair are mediated. These cells, scattered throughout the connective tissue compartment, are probably the primary means through which *metaplasia* occurs.

Reticular Cells. The *reticular cell* is a stellate or spindle-shaped cell that occurs in myeloid tissue and lymphatic organs. It generally forms a *cellular reticulum* in association with a fibrous stroma of reticular fibers. The nucleus is round to oval and vesicular (Fig. 6.24). The cytoplasm is extensive and slightly basophilic. The cytoplasmic processes of these cells are in contact with each other and account for the typical *cellular meshwork* or *reticulum.*

The reticular cells of the body are attributed with diverse functional activities. Reticular cells, functioning like fibroblasts, form the fibrous stroma, reticular fibers, of the organs and tissues of which they are an integral part. Reticular cells have been attributed with phagocytic activity also. Light microscopic evidence supports the existence of *phagocytic reticular cells*, whereas evidence from electron microscopy refutes it. Similarly, *primitive reticular cells*, some sort of undifferentiated stem cell, are believed by some to be the stem cells for bone marrow elements and macrophages. Compelling evidence is lacking for either theory. The exact nature and potential of the reticular cell has not been defined clearly. This name, reticular cell, may encompass a single cell type that is pluripotent (unlikely) or may encompass more than a single type of cell (likely). More research is needed to clarify the questions relating to this cell.

The reticular cell occurs not only in association with reticular fibers but is the characteristic resident cell of reticular connective tissue.

Fibroblasts. The *fibroblasts*, or fiber-forming cells of connective tissues, are the most frequently encountered cells. As young cells, the fibroblasts are stellate or spindle-shaped with long cellular processes. The large oval or round nucleus is vesicular and has a prominent nucleolus (Fig. 6.25). There is an abundance of basophilic cytoplasm. This form of the cell is the active fiber-forming cell, one in which there is an abundance of granular endoplasmic reticulum and a well-developed Golgi apparatus (Fig. 6.26).

Inactive fibroblasts, sometimes referred to as *fibrocytes*, have nuclei that contain more heterochromatin than their active counterparts. Fibrocytes are spindle-shaped cells with a scant cytoplasm that is acidophilic, if it is visible. A corresponding reduction in their intracellular organelles is characteristic. Fibrocytes may, in fact, just be inactive fibroblasts. Or, they may represent cells that have a reduced synthetic potential that are concerned with the gradual and continuous replacement of matrix components. This may be a manifestation of altered activity during a different stage of their life cycle, a relationship similar to the chondroblast/chondrocyte and osteoblast/osteocyte discussed in Chapters 7 and 8.

Fibroblasts are potentially reactive cells. *Fibrosis*, the formation of fibrous connective tissue as a reaction to chronic insult, results from the activity of these cells. Similarly, repair of matrix components after injury (laceration, surgical incision, inflammation) results from the activity of these cells. Excessive quantities of fibrous connective tissue (*granulation tissue*), especially characteristic of connective tissue repair in the horse, is the end product of fibroblastic activity.

The fibroblast is responsible for the secretion of tropocollagen. Once outside the cell, tropocollagen polymerization results in the characteristic collagen. The precise role of the fibroblast in the process of polymerization and spatial orientation of the polymerized fibers has not been determined. The collagenous fibers of some tissues are oriented randomly within the matrix. In others, there is an orderly spatial arrangement. The cell may contribute to precise spatial arrangements by the orientation of protofibrils attached to their surfaces that serve as orientation and polymerization foci. Mechanical stress in the tissues, however, may serve as the basis for spatial orientation. A combination of both mechanisms may be influential.

Macrophages. *Macrophages* are also referred to as *histiocytes* and *clasmatocytes*. They are the resident phagocytic cells of the connective tissue compartment. They may be either *fixed* or *wandering*. As fixed cells they are most prominent in the pericapillary space. However, they may also be fixed

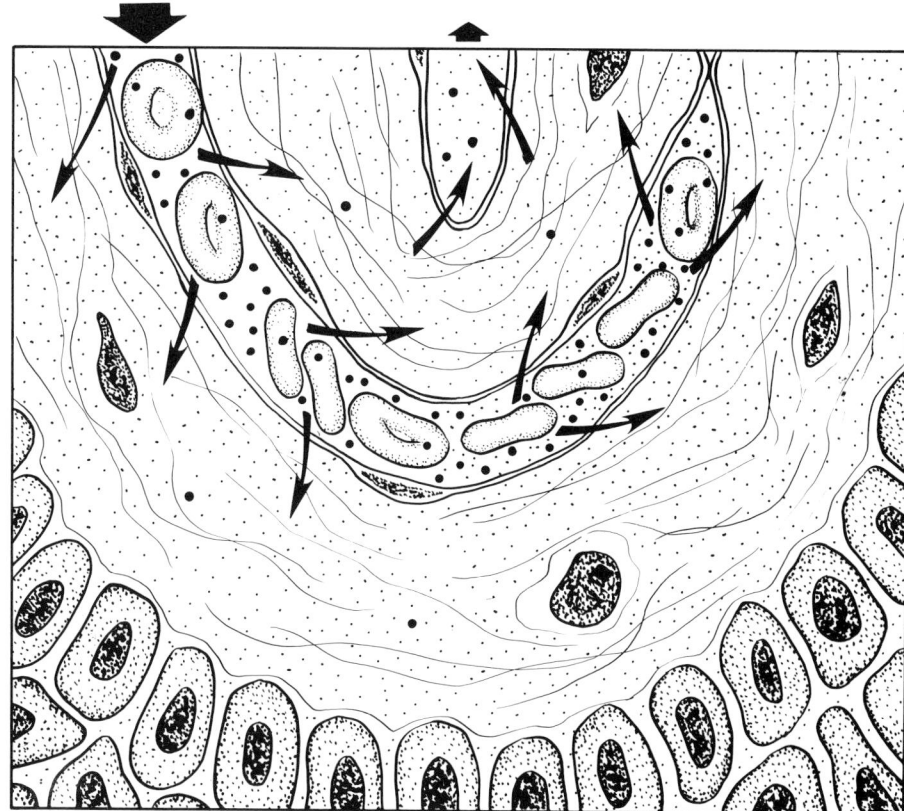

Fig. 6.21 Altered tissue fluid formation and exchange resulting from a venous obstruction. Capillary hydrostatic pressure increases and fluids are retained within the interstitial space. Swelling results.

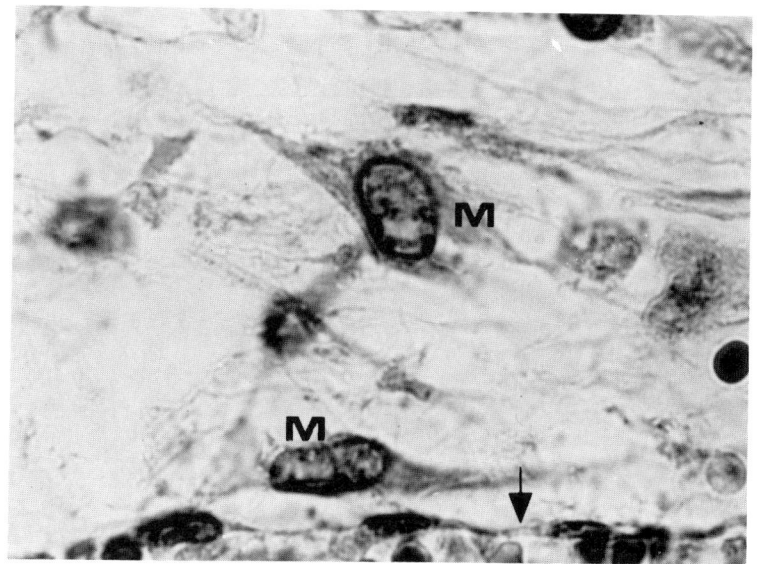

Fig. 6.22 Mesenchymal cell from the perivascular space of loose connective tissue. The mesenchymal cells (M) are typical and occur close to a capillary (*arrow*). X400.

along the length of a collagenous fiber. When activated by various stimuli they become *wandering* or *amoeboid*.

Macrophages are pleomorphic. They vary from spindle-shaped in the fixed configuration to round or oval with blunt cellular processes in the wandering stage. The nucleus of the macrophage is the key to the identification of this cell (Fig. 6.27). The nucleus is slightly smaller than the fibroblast nucleus and is darker because of the coarse heterochromatic pattern. Lastly, but most importantly, the nucleus is often indented; i.e., it is *bean-shaped* or *kidney-shaped*. Usually, the cell is polarized. The concavity or indentation of the nucleus faces the bulk of

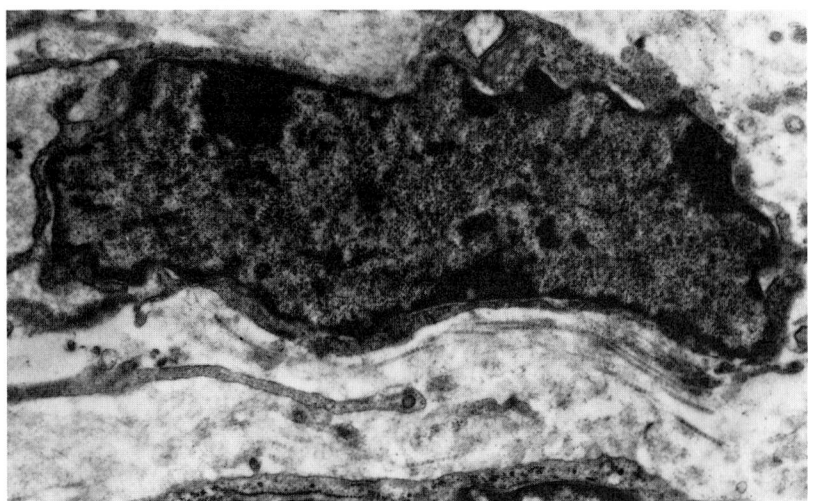

Fig. 6.23 An electron micrograph of a mesenchymal cell. The ratio of the nuclear/cytoplasmic volumes of the cell is large. X12,000.

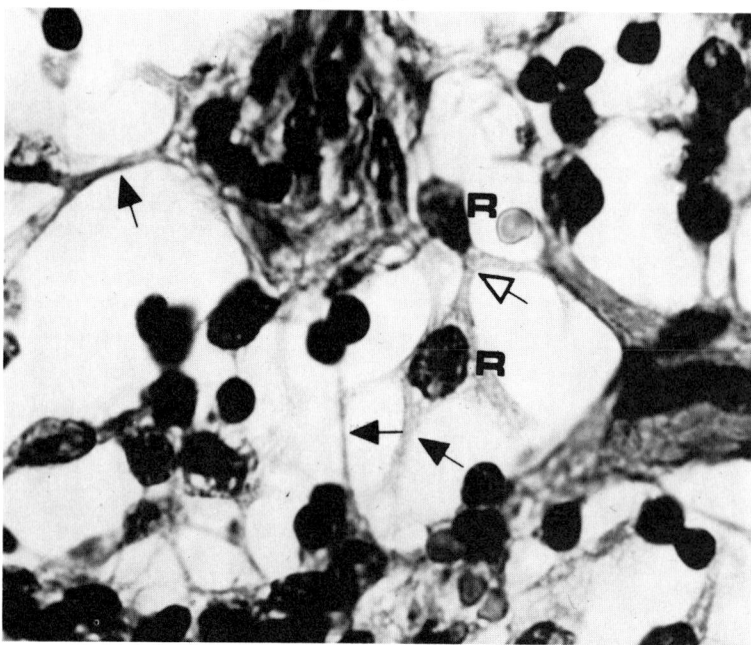

Fig. 6.24 Reticular cells of the medullary region of a canine lymph node. The reticular cells (R) extend cytoplasmic processes (*solid arrows*) that contact the cytoplasmic processes of other reticular cells forming a cellular reticulum. Points of contact between these stellate-shaped cells (*open arrow*) are apparent occasionally. X320.

Pericytes. Any cell that occurs around a capillary or small vessel may be a pericyte. Thus, macrophages, mesenchymal cells and fibroblasts, by virtue of their perivascular position, may be referred to as pericytic. However, in a more specific context, the *pericyte* is a specific cell or cell type. *Pericytes* or *cells of Rouget* are in intimate contact with the endothelial lining cells of the small vessel with which they are associated (Fig. 6.29). They are invested with a basal lamina except at the point of contact with the endothelial cell (Fig. 6.30). Some of these cells have been shown to be contractile; thus, they may control the size of the vascular lumen. Others have not been demonstrated as contractile and their function is unknown.

Mast Cells. *Mast cells* are sometimes referred to as *tissue basophils.* These cells are of variable occurrence in the connective tissue space but can be found readily along the pathway of small vessels. Usually, they occur in small clusters. These cells are of variable size and shape in different species. Generally, they are ovoid cells with a small, pale, ovoid and centrally located nucleus. The prominent feature is the presence of basophilic granules in the cytoplasm (Fig. 6.31). It is not uncommon to find these highly refractile granules surrounding the mast cell. These cells are fragile and rupture readily during preparatory techniques. The granules are also highly water-soluble; thus,

the cytoplasm. The basophilic cytoplasm may possess a juxtanuclear pale-staining region.

At the ultrastructural level, the prominent organelles in macrophages are the Golgi apparatus (in the nuclear indentation), rough endoplasmic reticulum and lysosomes (Fig. 6.28). At the light and electron microscopic level, ingested particulate material may be apparent if the cell is active.

There are multiple origins of this cell in the connective tissue compartment. Mesenchymal cells and reticular cells may give rise to this cell. The blood *monocyte* and the macrophage (histiocyte) are considered

identical cells. Within the confines of the blood vascular system (*intravascular*) this cell is referred to as a monocyte. Once it enters the connective tissue compartment (*extravascular*) it is referred to as a histiocyte or macrophage.

Macrophages are one of the prime cellular agents for defense against the invasion of particulate matter into the body. They also play a significant role in the phagocytosis and removal of cellular debris. They are important cells in the immune response, because they are involved in the processing of antigenic materials. They comprise the reticuloendothelial system.

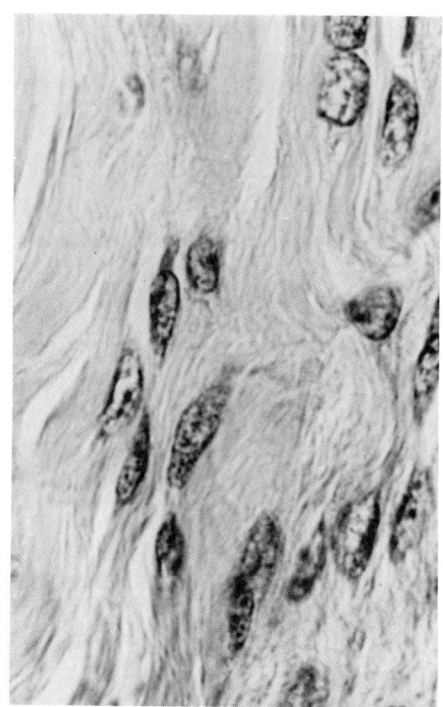

Fig. 6.25 Fibroblasts of loose connective tissue. The cytoplasm is barely visible, whereas the vesicular nuclei are apparent. Collagenous fibers are oriented randomly throughout the section. X340.

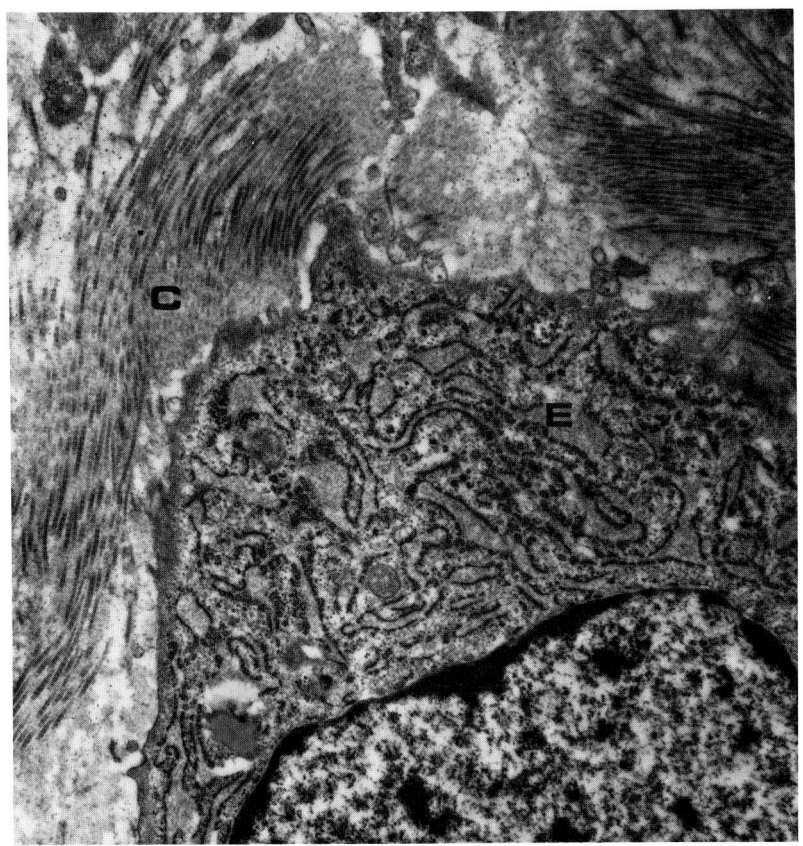

Fig. 6.26 An electron micrograph of a fibroblast. The cell contains extensive quantities of granular endoplasmic reticular profiles (E) that are filled with a granular material. Collagenous fibers (C) are present in the connective tissue space. X6,000.

they are preserved rarely by routine techniques.

The granules of mast cells contain two substances of medical significance, *heparin* and *histamine*. The mast cells of some species also contain *serotonin*. Heparin is significant as an anticoagulant. *Fibrinogen*, as well as other proteins, escape into the connective tissue. Heparin prevents fibrin formation and thus insures against the possible clotting of this substance in the local environment. Heparin also acts as a *clearing agent* on blood. Through a mechanism that is not understood, heparin is linked with *lipoprotein lipase*. The latter is responsible for clearing fat from blood plasma.

The mast cell releases many substances that are involved in allergic responses and anaphylaxis (Type I Hypersensitivity). *Histamine*, the decarboxylation product of histidine, is a vasoactive substance which dilates most capillary beds and causes an increased capillary permeability. It also causes the contraction of smooth muscle, as well as the stimulation of exocrine glands. This substance also functions to attract esoinophils. The *slow-reacting substance of anaphylaxis* (*SRS-A*) released from mast cells stimulates smooth muscle contraction and increases capillary permeability. *Eosinophilic chemotactic factor* and *platelet-activating factors* are also released by mast cells. Additionally, *kallikrein, neutrophil chemotactic factor* and *neutrophil immobilization factor* are released by mast cells as a part of the type I hypersensitivity response. The type I reaction is

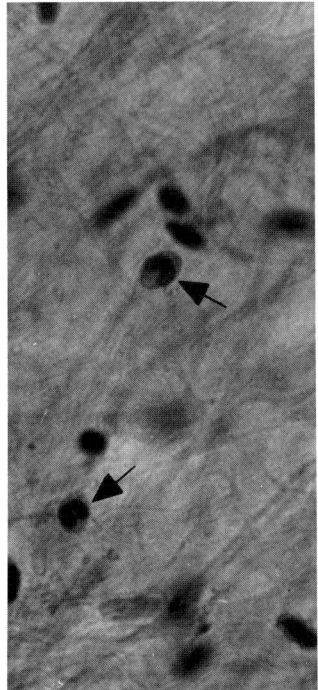

Fig. 6.27 Macrophages in a stretch preparation of loose connective tissue. The nuclei of the macrophages (*arrows*) are typical. The other cellular and matrix components are out of the plane of focus. X100.

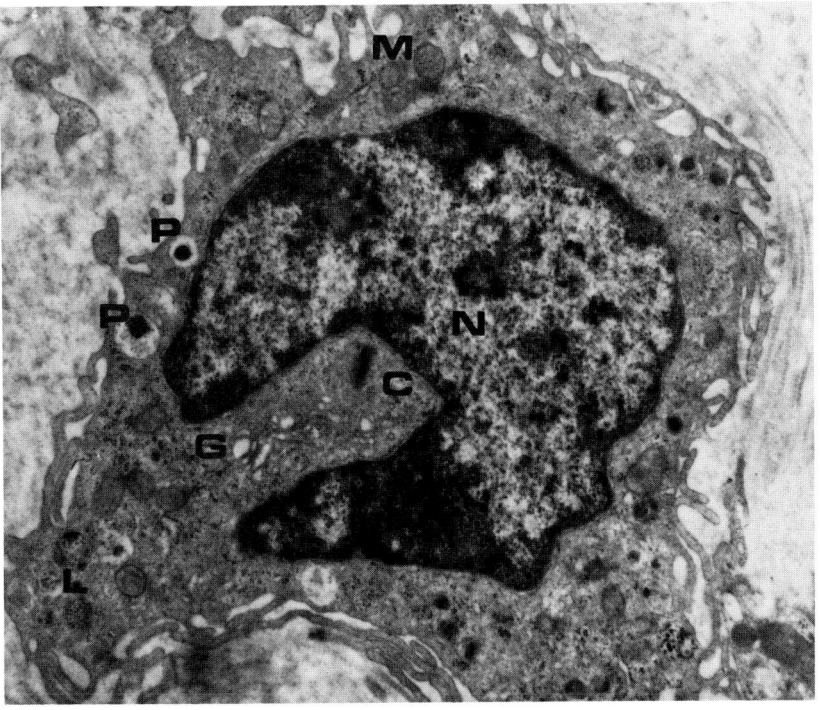

Fig. 6.28 An electron micrograph of a macrophage from loose connective tissue. The horseshoe-shaped nucleus (N) is typical. The Golgi apparatus (G) is well-developed and juxtanuclear. One of the centrioles (C) is visible. Mitochondria (M) are scattered throughout the cell. Phagosomes (P) and lysosomes (L) are typical features of active macrophages. X26,000.

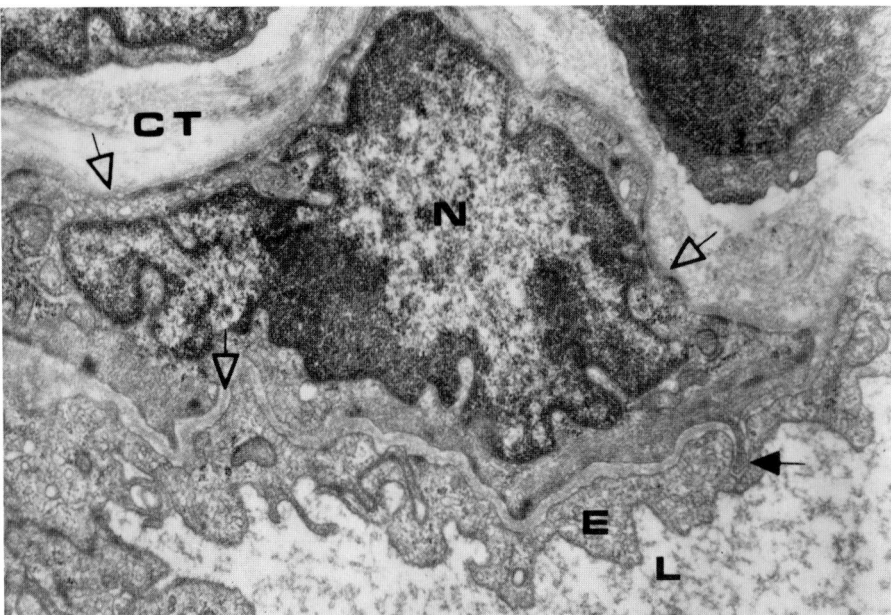

Fig. 6.29 An electron micrograph of a pericyte from a bovine lung. The nucleus (N) of the pericyte is prominent. The cell is in close association with an endothelial cell (E) which defines the lumen (L) of the capillary. The basal lamina (*open arrows*) surrounds the pericyte and separates it from the connective tissue (CT) and endothelium. The area indicated by the *solid arrow* is enlarged in Figure 6.29. X17,000. (Courtesy of G. P. Epling).

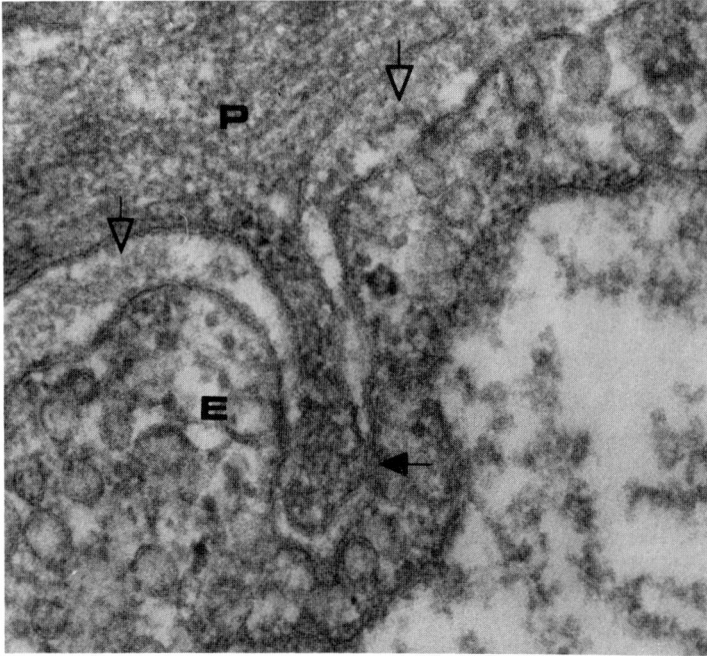

Fig. 6.30 An electron micrograph of the contact between a pericyte and an endothelial cell within the bovine lung. The pericyte (P) and endothelial cell (E) are separated by a basal lamina (*open arrows*) except at a single contact point (*solid arrow*). X125,000. (Courtesy of G. P. Epling).

discussed with the immune system (Chapter 17).

Although the mast cell is known to be derived from the mesenchymal cell, very little information is available about its cell cycle and generation time. Similarly, very little is known about the turnover and replacement of these cells, although they are assumed to be derived from mesenchymal cells in the adult also. They are sometimes referred to as tissue basophils; an unfortunate name, because the inference is that they are somehow related to the blood basophil (basophilic leukocyte). The basophil and mast cell are independent cell types.

Fat Cells. *Fat cells, adipocytes,* occur as single cells, clusters of cells or as massive sheets of cells associated with connective tissues, especially loose connective tissue. Because of their enigmatic relationship to connective tissues, these cells and adipose tissue are discussed in a subsequent section of this Chapter.

Transient Cell Population

Because the resident cell population can vary with the tissue and its physiologic state, it is reasonable to assume that similar conditions will influence the transient cell population. Most of the transient cells are protective and in some areas of connective tissue may be considered residents. However, in most instances their numbers will vary. The *transient cell population* includes *plasma cells, pigment cells, lymphocytes, monocytes, neutrophils, eosinophils* and *basophils.* Only the plasma cell and pigment cell will be discussed here; the blood cells are discussed in Chapter 10.

Plasma Cells. *Plasma cells* perform an important function in the immediate and prolonged protection of the organism against antigens. These cells synthesize and secrete large quantities of *humoral antibodies* (*immunoglobulins*) that are an important part of the specific immunologic response of the animal. These cells may be encountered in the connective tissue of any part of the organism. They generally occur in the connective tissues of those areas that are continually subject to antigenic challenge. They can be considered a part of the resident cell population of the connective tissues associated with the epithelial linings (membranes) of the gastrointestinal, genitourinary and respiratory organs.

The plasma cell is easily demonstrated by routine techniques. It is a rounded cell with a definite polarity. The basophilic cytoplasm contains the eccentrically placed and round nucleus (Fig. 6.32). The nucleus contains extensive heterochromatin which is sometimes arranged as the spokes of a wheel. A juxtanuclear, pale-staining region is often apparent. This region corresponds to the position of the well-developed Golgi apparatus. The basophilia of the cytoplasm is due to the extensive development of rough endoplasmic reticulum and free ribosomes (Fig 6.33).

Pigment Cells. This is a nondescript term for any cell that contains pigment. However, the means by which cells acquire pigment are quite different. *Melanoblasts* are cells derived from *neural crest ectoderm.* These cells migrate throughout the body and come to reside in various regions—the connective tissue associated with the skin, as well as the iris and choroid of the eye. They possess the

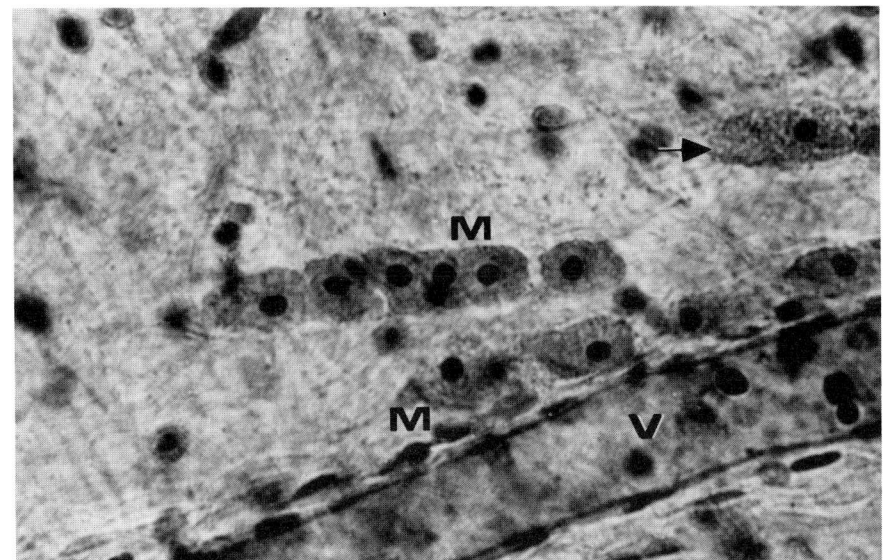

Fig. 6.31 Mast cells in a stretch preparation of murine subcutis. The mast cells (M) are aligned along a blood vessel (V). A ruptured mast cell (*arrow*) has extruded its granules into the surrounding environment. Ruptured mast cells are observed frequently in histologic preparations as a result of harsh handling during processing. ×160.

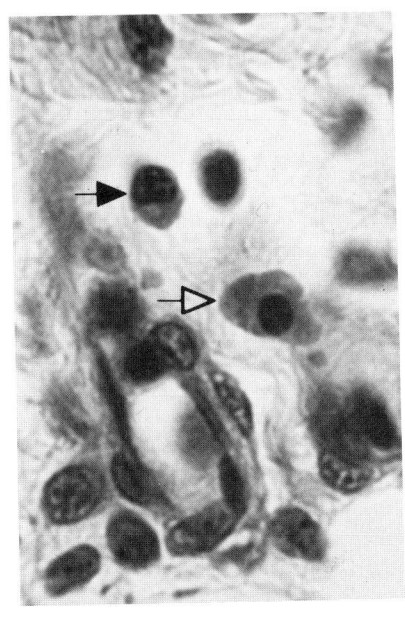

Fig. 6.32 A plasma cell of loose connective tissue. The plasma cell (*solid arrow*) is typical. Note the position of the nucleus and the negative Golgi area. A macrophage (*open arrow*) also is present. Note the differences between these cells. ×160.

potential to produce melanin but do not do so until they have achieved their place of residence. When they begin to synthesize melanin, they are termed *melanocytes* (Fig. 6.34). Melanocytes are able to invade epithelial layers and pass their pigmentation to other cells. These passive recipients of this pigment are termed *melanophores*. Melanocytes rarely occur in the connective tissue compartment. The pigmented cells of this

compartment have either passively received the pigment or have phagocytosed the pigment. Thus, they are *melanophores* or *chromatophores*.

A simple histochemical test, the *dihydroxyphenylalanine (DOPA) reaction*, is used to determine which cells are melanocytes. Only melanocytes are capable of converting DOPA into melanin because of the presence of the enzyme *tyrosinase*.

The primary function of these cells is to protect the body from excessive exposure to ultraviolet radiation. Of interest, melanoblasts and melanocytes can be involved in the formation of rapidly spreading and, therefore, potentially dangerous cancerous growths.

Embryonal Connective Tissues

Mesenchymal Connective Tissue. This typical, unspecialized mesodermal tissue of the embryo is a transitory tissue that disappears rapidly from the developing organism as differentiation occurs (Fig. 6.35). The primary constituent of this tissue is the mesenchymal cell. These stellate or fusiform cells form numerous cellular contacts and give the appearance of a *cellular reticulum*. Although the intercellular spaces are usually pale-staining and appear devoid of any material, a ground substance of mucopolysaccharides is present. Although fibers are not common in this tissue, it is not unusual to encounter delicate collagenous or reticular fibrils close to cells that are differentiating into fibroblasts. Also, mesenchymal cells are capable of producing small quantities of fibers and ground substance.

This tissue is derived from mesoderm. Most importantly, this tissue is the percursor

for other tissues, such as *proper* and *special connective tissues, cartilage, bone, blood* and *muscle*.

In the adult, the mesenchymal connective tissue is reduced to isolated and scattered foci of mesenchymal cells in those tissues derived from it.

Mucous Connective Tissue. This connective tissue is a more advanced stage of the one described previously. It is the characteristic connective tissue of the umbilical cord (but it is not confined to it), wherein it is referred to as *Wharton's jelly* (Fig. 6.36). It consists of a cellular reticulum of *fibroblasts* and a few scattered *mesenchymal cells*. The matrix is composed of mucin and contains delicate collagenous fibers. With proper fixation the ground substance will appear granular.

In the developing embryo, this connective tissue occurs in the subepidermal regions as well as the umbilical cord. In the adult it is usually the transitory tissue deposited during the repair of supportive tissues. Also, it is found normally in the comb and wattles of gallinaceous birds. It also occurs in specific portions of the lamina propria of the ruminant omasum.

Proper Connective Tissues

Areolar Connective Tissue. This tissue is often referred to as *loose* or *ordinary* connective tissue. It is the most ubiquitous of the connective tissues. It is composed of a loose array of randomly oriented *collagenous, reticular* and *elastic fibers*. Collagenous fibers, however, are the predominant extracellular formed elements. All of the cells previously described, except the reticular cell, may occur in this connective tissue. Normally, the predominant cell type is the fibroblast or fibrocyte (approximately 90%). The prevalent ground substance component is hyaluronic acid; however, some chondroitin sulfate and dermatan sulfate are also present. This combination of matrix components imparts a soft, pliable and elastic quality to the tissue (Fig. 6.37).

The accompanying photomicrograph of a stretch preparation of subcutis serves as an example of loose connective tissue (Fig. 6.38). Within the ground substance, collagenous and elastic fibers are apparent in random orientation. Reticular fibers are present but require special staining techniques for their demonstration. Numerous vessels and scattered fat cells are present. At higher magnification, all the cells mentioned may be encountered.

In section, loose connective tissue assumes a different appearance (Fig. 6.39). Nevertheless, the interlacing and randomly oriented bundles of fibers with cells scattered between is typical. In this instance the primary cell population consists of fibroblasts. Examination at higher magnification will reveal the other cells.

In a section of loose connective tissue associated with the upper digestive tract a

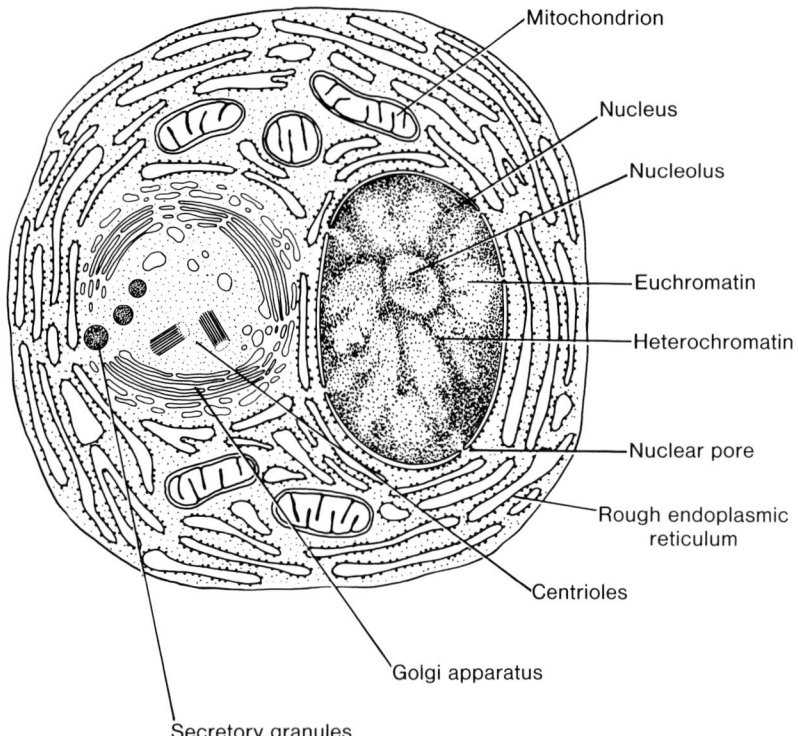

Fig. 6.33 A diagram of a plasma cell as visualized with the electron microscope. The constituent organelles are indicated. Note the spoke-wheel configuration of the chromatin, extensive rough endoplasmic reticulum and well-developed Golgi apparatus.

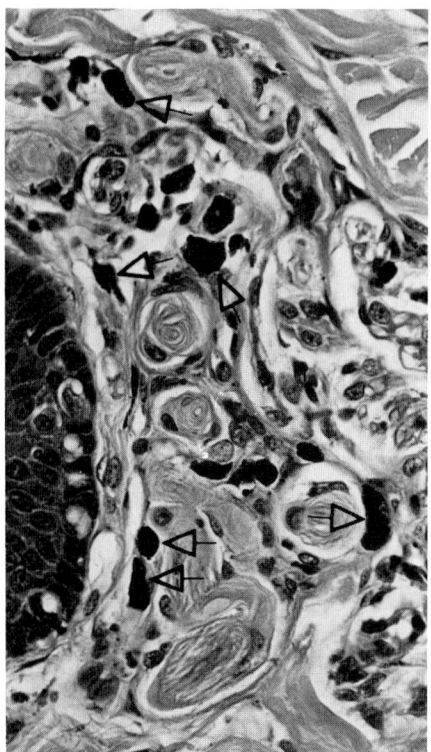

Fig. 6.34 Pigment-bearing cells (*open arrows*) of the connective tissue of the dermis. ×100.

very different appearing tissue is observed (Fig. 6.40). Although the fibers and fibroblasts are present, the predominant feature is the presence of defensive cells—lympho-

cytes, plasma cells and macrophages. This appearance is typical in this and similar regions that are subjected to constant insult. The previous example of this tissue (Fig. 6.39) would appear similar in response to an insult (Plate IV. 2).

MORPHOLOGIC FEATURES:
1. A fine network of collagenous, reticular and elastic fibers loosely arranged in random array.
2. The predominance of collagenous fibers and fibroblasts.
3. The large number of cells and few fibrous components.
4. The variation of cellular constituents with location and physiology.

OCCURRENCE: Subepithelial connective tissue, mesenteries, between muscles and nerves, components of most organs (Plate IV. 1).

Dense White Fibrous Connective Tissue—Irregular. This connective tissue, most often abbreviated as *DWFCT*, is closely related to areolar connective tissue. Admittedly, there are gradations between the two extremes of loose and dense. Primarily, DWFCT differs quantitatively from loose connective tissue.

In section (Fig. 6.41) thick, wavy collagenous fibers predominate. Reticular and elastic fibers, however, are also present. The same cells encountered or potentially present in loose connective tissue are also present or potentially so in this tissue. Normally, however, there are fewer cells in this tissue.

MORPHOLOGIC FEATURES:
1. A coarse network of collagenous fibers with some reticular and elastic fibers.
2. The reduced number of cells and increased

number of fibers when compared to loose connective tissue.

OCCURRENCE: Subepidermal connective tissue, capsules of organs (Plates I.3, IV.3).

Dense White Fibrous Connective Tissue—Regular. The significant feature of this connective tissue is the orderly, parallel orientation of collagenous fibers (Fig. 6.42). Although distinct bundles of fibers are present, they do not appear as such in routine preparations. Rather, the fibers (with H and E) form a relatively homogeneous pink-staining background. The fibrocytes seem to delimit the extent of individual bundles. The nuclei of these cells vary from oval to thin and elongated. They are dark-staining. Although present, it is rare that the thin processes of the cytoplasm will be distinct. The nuclei and fibers may appear wavy. Although other cell types may be present normally, they are extremely rare.

This connective tissue is the predominant type that forms *tendons* and *ligaments*. However, individual bundles of these highly organized fibers are held together by loose connective tissue. Also, the few blood vessels and nerves observed are surrounded by loose connective tissue. The ordered collagenous fiber arrangement resists the great amount of stress applied to tendons and ligaments.

DIAGNOSTIC FEATURES:
1. Very few cells, mostly fibrocytes.
2. Predominance of heavy collagenous fibers that appear as a relatively homogeneous background matrix between cells.
3. Longitudinal arrangement of fibrocytes.
4. Cells and fibers may appear wavy.
5. Collagen stains a light pink with H and E.

OCCURRENCE: Tendons (attachments of muscle to bone), ligaments (attachments of bone to bone), aponeuroses (thin, sheetlike tendons) (Plates IV. 5, IV. 6).

Elastic Connective Tissue. This type of connective tissue is a basic modification of the type previously discussed. The predominant fiber type is the elastic fiber, whereas the predominant cell type is the fibroblast (Fig. 6.43). The fibers are larger than collagenous fibers and branch and anastomose with each other. Individual elastic fibers are surrounded by areolar connective tissue. The elastic fibers are quite ordered as evidenced by the orderliness of the fibroblasts. Without careful examination, this tissue is easily confused with DWFCT. Upon careful examination, however, the presence of bright pink-staining fibers (with H and E) is a good distinguishing characteristic. With special staining, the elastic fibers are readily apparent (Fig. 6.44).

In cross-section, care must be taken to distinguish the extrafibrillar position of the nuclei (Fig. 6.45) of the fibroblasts. Otherwise, this tissue could be mistaken for others to be encountered later. Note also the large cross-sectional area of the fibers.

This tissue is of limited but important occurrence. It is extensively modified in the walls of arteries, wherein it forms a very resilient complex with smooth muscle.

DIAGNOSTIC FEATURES:
1. Predominance of elastic fibers in parallel and branched array.
2. Intense pink-staining of fibers with H and E.
3. Predominance of fibroblasts with few other cell types present.

OCCURRENCE: Nuchal ligament (ligamentum nuchae), some dorsal ligaments of spinal column, mural elements of arteries (Plate IV.4).

Special Connective Tissues

Reticular Connective Tissue. The predominant fiber in this tissue is the reticular fiber.

The fibrous network is complemented by a cellular reticulum (network) of reticular cells. Because this type of tissue is associated with *cytogenic organs* (*cell-producing*), careful examination is required to observe the cellular and fibrous reticulum through the mass of other cells normally present. Numerous cells (*stem cells, reticular cells, lymphocytes, agranulocytes, plasma cells, histiocytes*) may be present. In a section of spleen that has been flushed with physiologic saline, the reticulum is apparent. With special staining techniques for reticular fibers, the fibrous reticulum is easily observed (Fig. 6.9). Ordinary staining will not definitely demonstrate this tissue; however, the association with certain cell types is a good key to its identification.

Reticular fibers also constitute the finer interstitial connective tissue of some parenchymatous organs. In this instance, the defensive cells will be absent or of an occurrence similar to that expected in areolar connective tissue. In these areas the predominant cell is the fibroblast.

DIAGNOSTIC FEATURES:
1. A fine reticulum of fibers and cells; the fibers are argyrophilic.
2. Usually associated with cytogenic organs that produce defensive cells.

OCCURRENCE: Stroma (fibrous support) of lymphatic and hematopoietic organs; finer interstitial connective tissue of some organs.

Pigmented Connective Tissue. This tissue is areolar connective tissue in which pigment-containing cells occur (Fig. 6.34). It is of limited but significant occurrence.

DIAGNOSTIC FEATURE: occurrence of pigment-bearing cells.

OCCURRENCE: Iris and choroid coat; connective tissue associated with pigmented skin.

Adipose Tissue

The rationale for discussing adipose tissue apart from the proper connective tissues was discussed previously.

Form and Function. Adipose tissue is composed of a homogeneous population of cells, *adipocytes* or *fat cells*, that may occur as single cells, groups of cells or extensive masses of cells. Although this tissue consists of blood vessels, nerves and elements of loose and/or reticular connective tissue, the predominant feature is the adipocyte. The tissue, therefore, is very cellular. Although adipose tissue may occur in association with all of the loose connective tissue of the body, predilection sites do occur. Adipose tissue may form an extensive subcutaneous sheet, the panniculus adiposus; extensive quantities of this tissue often occur in association with the visceral, parietal and connecting mesothelial membranes of the celomic cavities. Additionally, adipose tissue occurs in regions otherwise devoid of other tissue components—the axillary region, inguinal region. The intimate and variable association of adipose tissue with the organs of the body is demonstrated best in the gross dissection laboratory. Most organs contain extensive quantities. Even the popular prime cuts of beef are a mixture of skeletal muscle, connective tissue and adipose tissue. The latter accounts for the characteristic marbling.

Adipose tissue subserves a variety of important functions. This tissue is a readily available source of energy. The stored fats of adipose tissue contain more energy per gram than corresponding quantities of proteins or sugars. (Fats supply 9 calories per gram whereas carbohydrates and proteins supply 4 calories per gram.) Adipose tissue is an important contributor to thermoregulation. Its placement throughout the body aids in the conservation of heat. Adipose

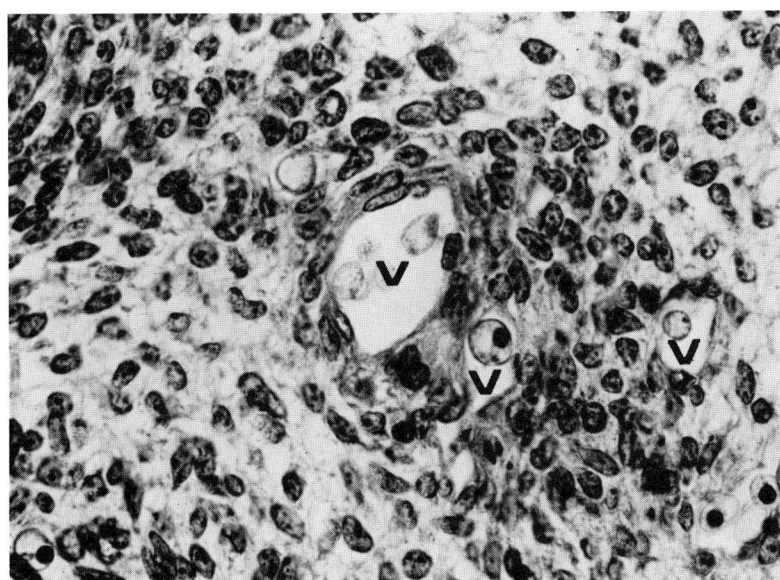

Fig. 6.35 Mesenchymal connective tissue from the limb bud of a hamster. Vessels (V) are scattered among the mesenchymal cells. The mesenchymal connective tissue will differentiate into other tissues derived from the mesoderm; it is a transitory tissue during development. ×160.

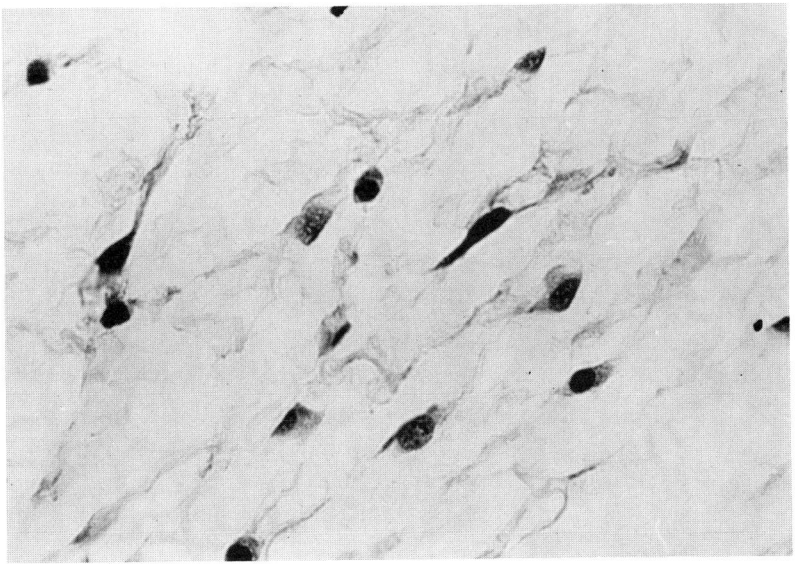

Fig. 6.36 Mucous connective tissue of the ovine umbilical cord. ×160.

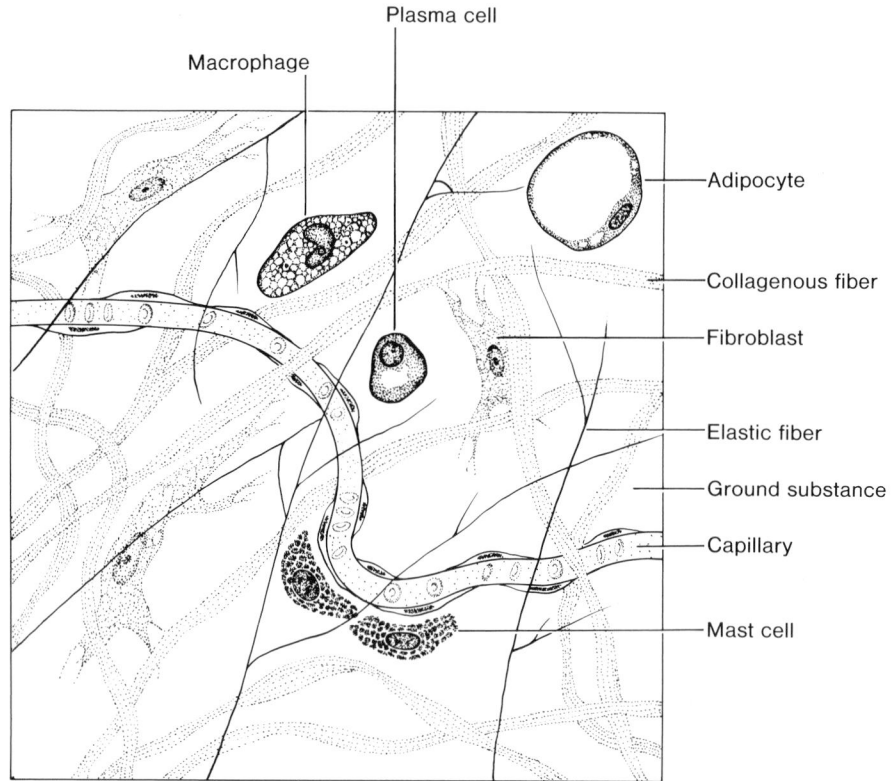

Fig. 6.37   Diagram of loose connective tissue. The major components of the tissue are labeled.

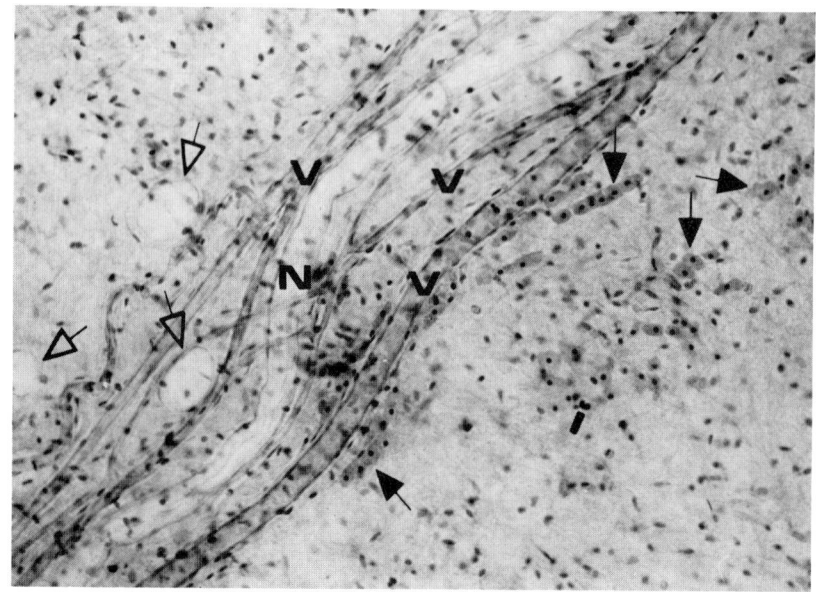

Fig. 6.38   Stretch preparation of loose connective tissue from the murine subcutis. Vessels (V) and a nerve (N) traverse the tissue. Mast cells (*solid arrows*), a macrophage (*bar*) and adipocytes (*open arrows*) are present. The remainder of the nuclei are those of fibroblasts. ×40.

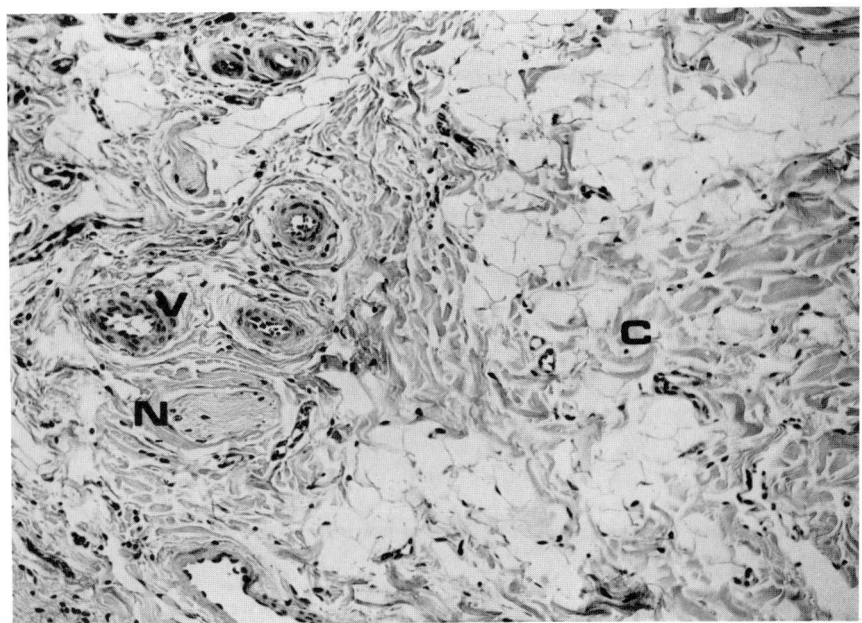

Fig. 6.39 A section of loose connective tissue. Collagenous fibers (C), nerves (N) and blood vessels (V) are scattered throughout the tissue. Fibroblasts and adipocytes are present also. ×40.

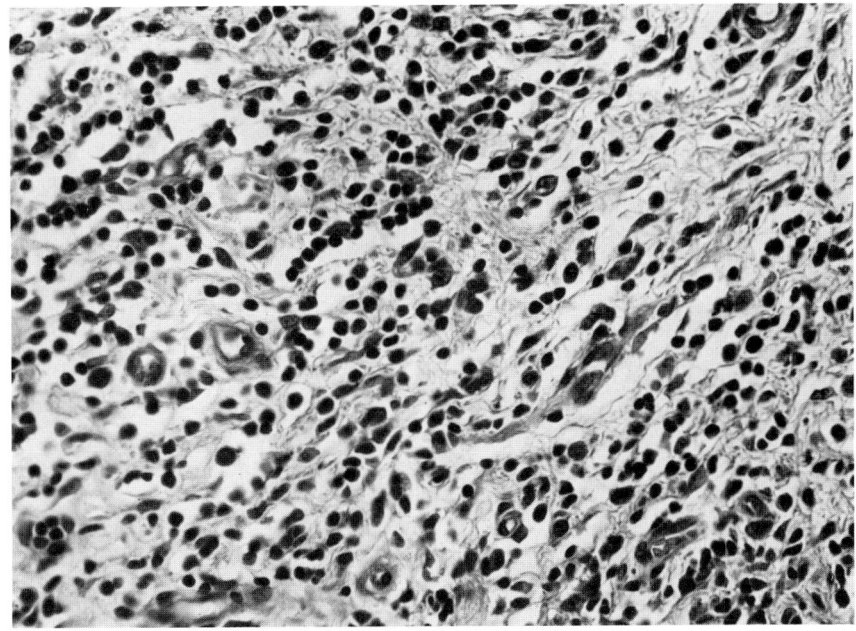

Fig. 6.40 A section of loose connective tissue from the upper digestive tract. The basic components are similar to those of Figure 6.38. The numerous dark nuclei are those of lymphocytes primarily. The mononucleated cells impart a hypercellular appearance to the tissue. This cellular population of loose connective tissue is typical of that which occurs in areas subjected continually to antigenic stimulation. ×100.

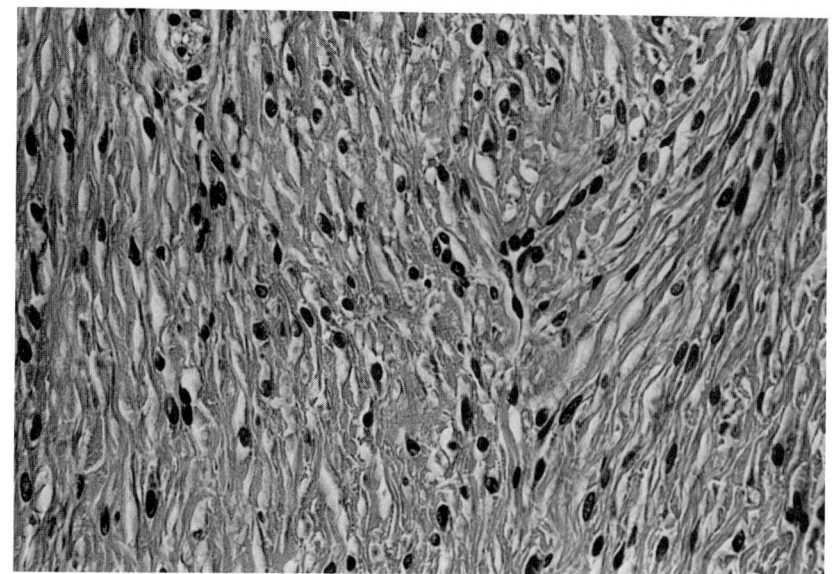

Fig. 6.41 A section of DWFCT, irregularly arranged, from the tunica albuginea of the canine testis. Collagenous fibers and fibroblasts are the predominant elements. ×100.

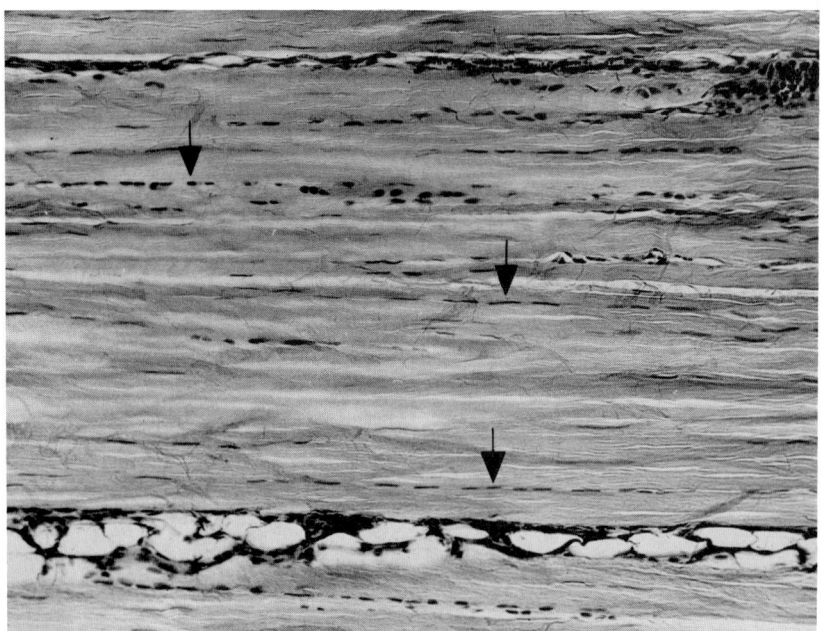

Fig. 6.42 A section of DWFCT, regularly arranged, from a tendon. The fibrocytes (*arrows*) are oriented parallel to the collagenous fibers. ×40.

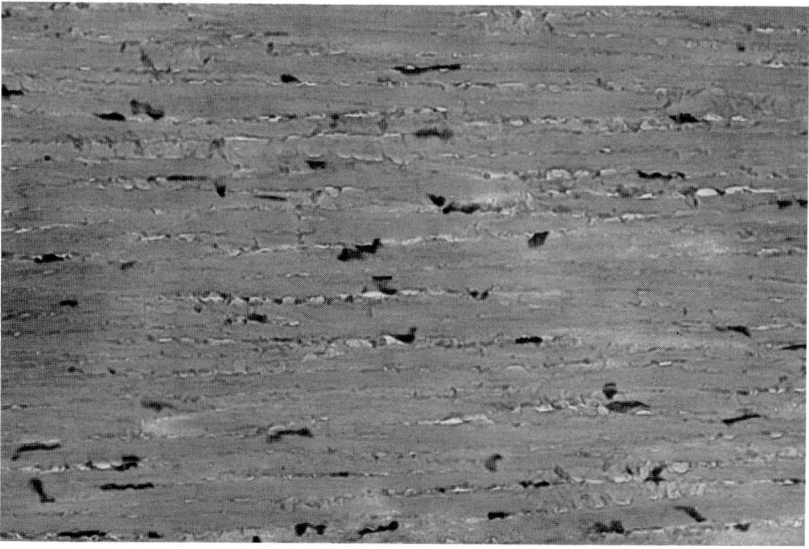

Fig. 6.43 A longitudinal section of the elastic connective tissue from a canine nuchal ligament. ×100.

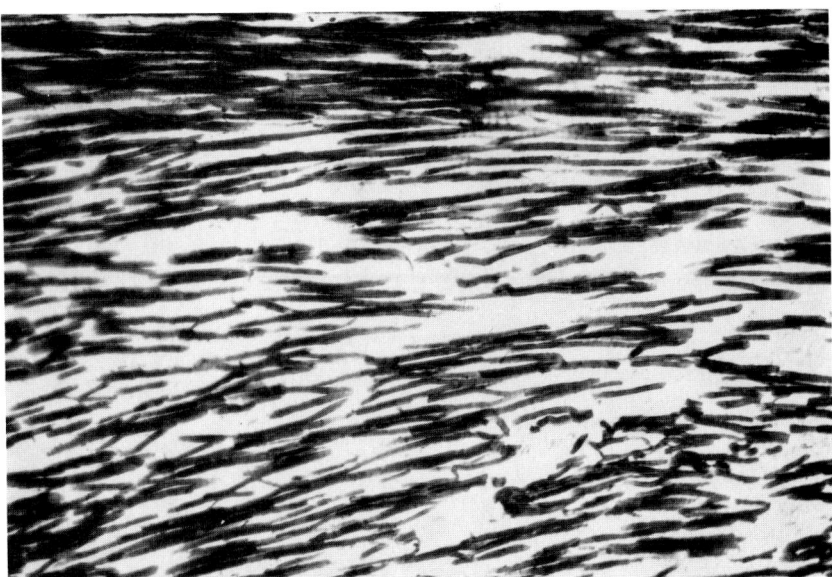

Fig. 6.44 A longitudinal section of the elastic fibers of a canine nuchal ligament. Only the elastic fibers are stained. ×40 (Verhoeff's stain).

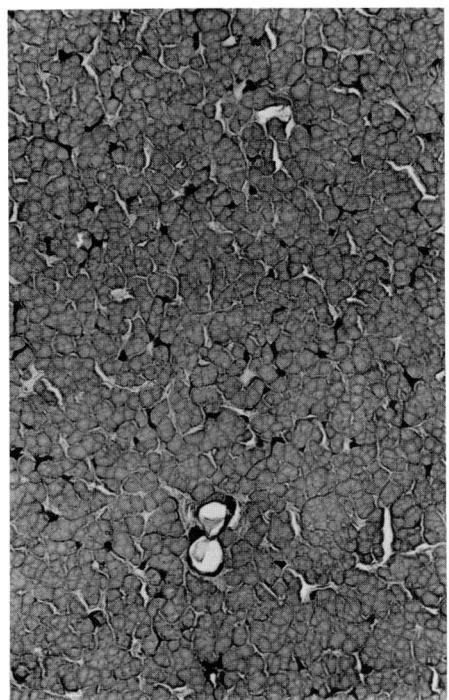

Fig. 6.45 Cross-section of the elastic connective tissue of a canine nuchal ligament. ×80.

tissue is also an important mechanical insulator. Its proper placement in association with the visceral organs and greater omentum helps to protect these organs from mechanical damage. The rich deposit of adipose tissue within the digital cushion of the equine foot is an important devise in the absoprtion of concussive forces associated with locomotion in this species. Also, adipose tissue associated with synovial membranes serves to absorb shock as well as afford some additional stability to diarthrodial joints.

Morphologically, two types of adipose tissue are identified—*white adipose tissue* and *brown adipose tissue.*

Origin of Adipose Tissue. The questions of the precise origin of fat cells and the relationship of white fat cells to brown fat cells have not been answered satisfactorily. An earlier popular view, one that still has proponents today, was fostered by Flemming in the late 19th century. He proposed that fat cells were formed by the simple accumulation of lipids by fibroblasts. Toldt, however, proposed that adipose tissue was a unique tissue, one that arose from lipoblasts that differentiated in specific parts of the animal body. Similarly, there are opposing views concerning the relationship of white and brown fat. Some believe that the populations are distinct, whereas others believe that brown fat represents a stage in the development of white fat. The evidence in the literature is exhausting and conflicting.

A reasonable consensus, however, seems to emerge. The special stem cell for adipocytes is probably the mesenchymal cell. This can account for specific predilection sites rather than adipocytes being spread ubiquitously throughout the body as a result of the fibroblastic accumulation of fat. Moreover, the presence of a basal lamina around individual adipocytes is difficult to explain if they are differentiated from fibroblasts. The occurrence of age and species differences relative to the propensity to accumulate fat, as well the anatomic sites in which the accumulation takes place support the idea of separate populations of fat cells.

White Adipose Tissue. This tissue is also called *white fat, unilocular fat* and *ordinary adipose tissue* (Plate V.11). The cells of white adipose tissue are very large, ranging to about 130 μm. They are spherical cells that may appear polyhedral. *Unilocular fat cells,* the predominant cell of this tissue,

have a signet-ring appearance (Fig. 6.46). The bulk of the cytoplasm is occupied by a single large fat droplet that is rimmed by a thin margin of cytoplasm. The nucleus, which is usually displaced to one side of the cell, accounts for the signet-ring configuration. In most planes of section, the nucleus will not be apparent (Fig. 6.47). In routine paraffin sections of fat cells, the space that was occupied by the lipids is all that remains; the solvents used in the process have leached out the fats. Special preparation techniques such as freezing and special stains (osmium tetroxide, Sudan stains) are required to demonstrate the lipids of fat cells (Fig. 6.48).

The lipids of these cells are triglycerides and certain fatty acids. They are mobilized through enzymatic hydrolysis (lipase) and free fatty acids enter the blood as an available source of energy. Although these substances turnover constantly, a continuous supply of glucose as an energy source precludes the release of these substances.

White adipose tissue may be subdivided into smaller units (lobules) by loose connective tissue septa. Reticular fibers extend from these septa and surround individual fat cells. The extensive vascular supply and nerves of this tissue gain access via these connective tissues.

Brown Adipose Tissue. This tissue consists of *multilocular fat cells* (Plate V.12). The predominant feature of these cells is the presence of numerous small fat droplets within the cytoplasm (Fig. 6.49). The rounded nucleus is not displaced to one side of the cell but may assume any position. Unless the special preparatory precautions mentioned previously are taken, the lipids are lost from these cells also. The resulting spaces from loss of lipids by routine preparation and scattered cytoplasmic components impart an acidophilic and foamy appearance to the cytoplasm of these cells (Fig. 6.49).

The brown color of this tissue results from numerous mitochondria and the corresponding high quantities of the cytochrome oxidase system. Brown fat cells contain more mitochondria than their white fat cell counterparts. Additionally, brown adipose tissue is more highly vascularized and innervated than white adipose tissue. Although connective tissue relationships in this tissue are similar to white adipose tissue, the lobular organization is sufficiently extensive to impart a glandular appearance.

The primary role of this tissue is the heating of the blood that passes through it. The metabolism of the stored lipids releases heat, warms the blood and raises body temperature. Brown adipose tissue has a limited but specific distribution. It develops during the prenatal period and is confined generally to the axilla, interscapular region, mediastinum, mesenteries and perirenal area. It may assist the young animal in resisting postnatal cold extremes. Hibernating rodents, similarly, have brown adipose

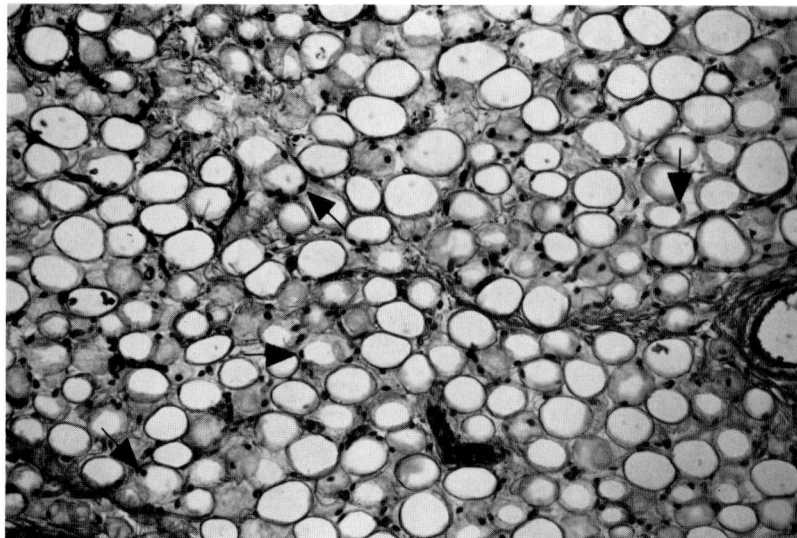

Fig. 6.46   A section of yellow adipose tissue. *Arrows*, nuclei of those cells in a typical signet-ring configuration. ×40.

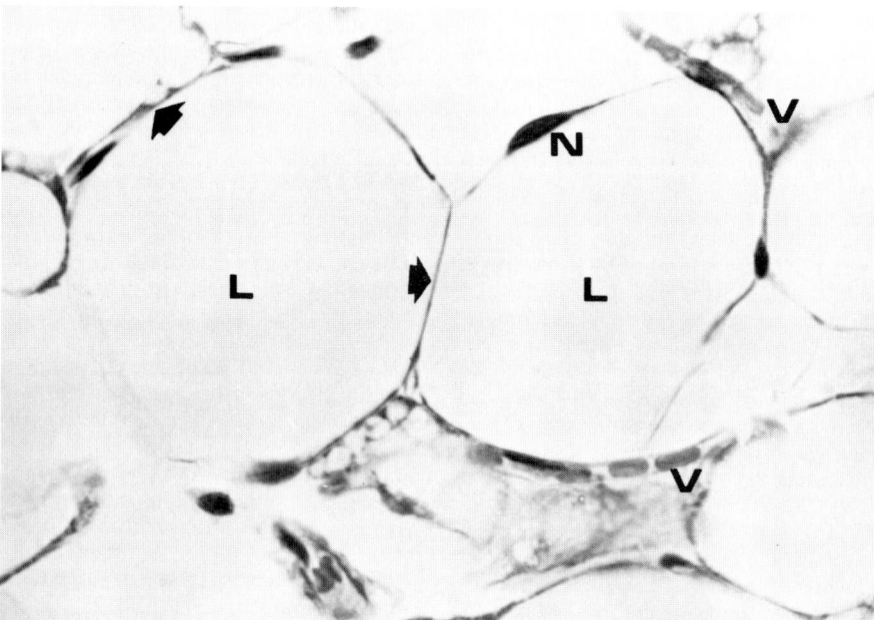

Fig. 6.47   A section of adipocytes from yellow adipose tissue. The signet-ring configuration is obvious. The nucleus (N) is displaced to one side of the cell. The cytoplasm is reduced to a thin margin at the periphery of the cell (*arrows*). The space that had been occupied by the lipid droplet (L) is the predominant cytoplasmic feature. Vessels (V) occur within the associated connective tissue. ×160.

gral parts of their tissue architecture and defense mechanisms. Unfortunately, it is easy to lose sight of their commonality of function—phagocytosis—because they are referred to by different names—microgliocytes, blood monocytes, Kupffer cells, alveolar macrophages, littoral cells of sinusoids (Fig. 6.50).

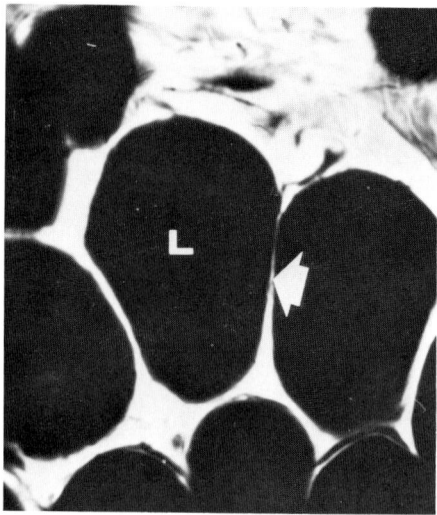

Fig. 6.48   A special stain for lipids. The large lipid droplet (L) remains as a dominant feature of the cytoplasm. The cellular margins, which have not been stained, are indicated by the *arrow*. ×125 (osmium tetroxide stain).

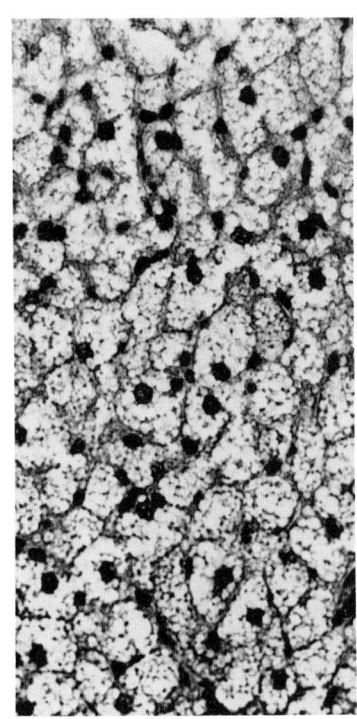

Fig. 6.49   A section of multilobular adipose tissue. Spaces which had been occupied by individual lobules of lipids are apparent within the cells. ×100.

tissue deposits in the areas specified previously. These depots assist with body temperature maintenance during hibernating periods.

The lipid droplets of both types of fat cells are not membrane-bound. Rather, they are rimmed by a condensation of cytoplasm that may contain some cytofilaments.

Two types of fat cell tumors occur in domestic animals, especially the dog. The benign lipoma is difficult to distinguish from typical white aidpose tissue histologically, whereas the malignant liposarcoma cells may look like multilocular fat cells histologically.

Reticuloendothelial System

Many cells of the body have the ability to ingest particulate matter (phagocytosis). Some cells, however, have an exceptional ability for phagocytosis. The *fixed and wandering macrophages* of the connective tissue compartment possess this ability and are important cellular defense components for the organism. The ability of macrophages to range "far and wide" within connective tissue affords a ready and mobile defense force that is associated with almost every tissue and organ of the body. Many organs of the body contain phagocytic cells that are inte-

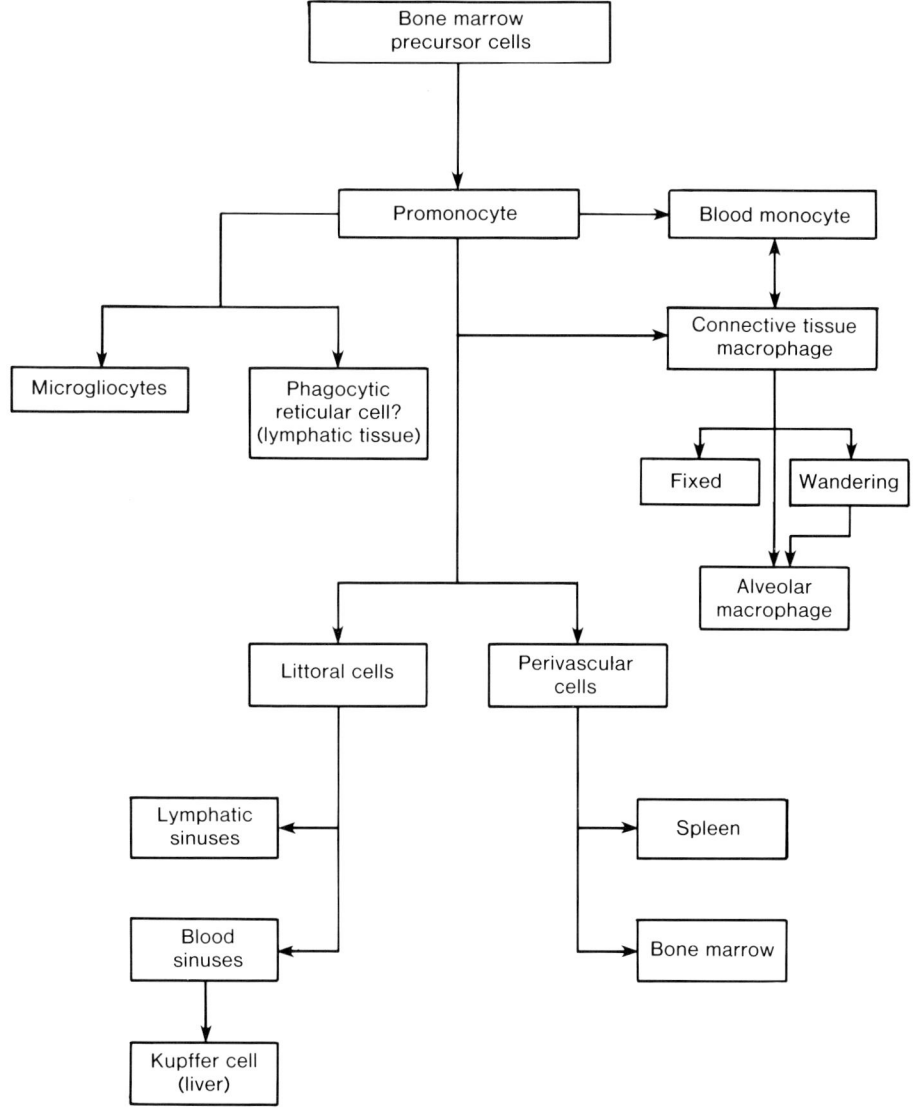

Fig. 6.50 Mononuclear Phagocyte System. The origin, distribution and relationships of the component cells are outlined. Littoral cells, not endothelial cells, of bone marrow and splenic sinuses may be phagocytic also. Conclusive evidence is lacking.

cesses within connective tissue. Connective tissue is not a static entity; cells and matrix components are in a constant state of flux. Old and/or damaged cells are removed and replaced by new fibroblasts. Similarly, matrix components that have been damaged or altered chemically are removed and replaced by new components. The macrophage is the key cell in this removal activity.

The ability of the fibroblast to mediate repair or regeneration is predicated upon a number of factors. This cell is capable of division. So, in times of need this cell is able to serve as its own "stem cell." Additionally, mesenchymal cells are scattered throughout connective tissue, especially in a pericapillary position. Mitotic activity and subsequent differentiation of some of these cells serves to replenish the fibroblastic population. The fibroblast is capable also of adding additional matrix components (collagen and glycosaminoglycans) to the connective tissue.

Fibrous connective tissue is not only capable of repairing itself, but it may be involved in the repair of other tissues. Following an acute myocardial infarction (heart attack), degenerative cardiac muscle is replaced by a scar of fibrous connective tissue. Skeletal muscle that has been injured severely is replaced similarly by a connective tissue scar. The result of chronic inflammation is the deposition of abnormal quantities of fibrous connective tissue, *fibrosis*. The formation of fibrous connective tissues in the repair process of other tissues may limit, reduce or obliterate the normal function of the repaired tissue.

Generally, the previous discussion relates to all proper connective tissues. The specific characteristic of repair of tendons and ligaments is discussed elsewhere.

This common function of phagocytosis was first recognized by Metchnikoff in the late nineteenth century. He looked upon these phagocytes as a diffuse cellular system of "big eaters" and coined the name *macrophage system*. Other cells, namely specialized endothelial lining cells and the cellular stroma (phagocytic reticular cell) of certain organs, were recognized to have well-developed phagocytic activity. This original system of phagocytes was expanded conceptually to include these reticular and endothelial cells. Thus, the name *reticuloendothelial system* was coined. It is still popular currently.

The bulk of evidence today controverts the reticular cell and endothelial cell contributions to the reticuloendothelial system. Reticular cells (fiber-forming cells) are not known to be phagocytic. Nor is the reverse true. Similarly, many endothelial cells, once considered to be phagocytic, are now considered to be specialized macrophages that

have established residence as littoral cells in many epithelial membranes. For these reasons, the name reticuloendothelial system has fallen into disfavor. A more descriptive name that is gaining acceptance is the *mononuclear phagocyte system* or *macrophage system*, the latter having been proposed by Metchnikoff almost 100 years ago.

This system includes numerous mononuclear cells of different organs that function through phagocytosis to protect the body from foreign materials and microorganisms. They also serve to rid the body of dead constituent cells and matrix materials. Importantly, they are involved in the processing of antigens as part of the cell-mediated immunity and humoral antibody responsiveness of the organism.

Regeneration and Repair

The fibroblast is the primary cell responsible for regenerative and reparative pro-

References

Extracellular Components

Bensley, S. H.: On the presence, properties and distribution of the intercellular ground substance of loose connective tissue. Anat. Rec. *60*:93, 1934.

Chain, E. and Duthie, E. S.: Identity of hyaluronidase and the spreading factor. Brit. J. Exp. Path. *21*:234, 1940.

Fahrenback, W. H., Sandberg, L. B., and Cleary, E. G.: Ultrastructural studies on early elastogenesis. Anat. Rec. *155*:563, 1966.

Greenlee, T. K., Jr., Ross, R. and Hartman, J. L.: The fine structure of elastic fibers. J. Cell. Biol. *30*:59, 1966.

Gross, J.: Collagen, Sci. Amer. *204*:120, 1961.

Hodge, A. J. and Petruska, J. A.: Recent studies with the electron microscope on ordered aggregates of the tropocollagen macromolecules. In *Aspects of Protein Structure*. Academic Press, New York, p. 239, 1964.

Lillie, R. D.: Histochemistry of connective tissues. Lab. Invest. *1*:30, 1952.

Mancini, R. E.: Connective tissue and serum proteins. Int. Rev. Cytol. *14*:193, 1963.

Petruska, J. A. and Hodge, A. J.: A subunit model for the tropocollagen macromolecule. Proc. Nat. Acad. Sci. USA *51*:871, 1964.

Schubert, M.: *A Primer on Connective Tissue Biochemistry*. Lea and Febiger, Philadelphia, 1968.

Spicer, S. S., Horn, R. G. and Leppi, T. J.: Histochemistry of connective tissue mucopolysaccharides. *In:* Wagner, B. M. and Smith, D. E. (editors). The Connective Tissue. pp 251–303. Williams & Wilkins, Baltimore, 1967.

Cellular Components

Carpenter, J. C., Perrelet, A. and Orci, L.: Morphological changes of the adipose cell membrane during lipolysis. J. Cell Biol. *72*:104, 1977.

Chapman, J. A., Gough, J. and Elves, M. W.: An electron microscopic study of the *in vitro* transformation of human leucocytes. II. Transformation to macrophages. J. Cell Sci. *2*:371, 1967.

Cohn, Z. A., Fedorko, M. E. and Hirsch, J. G.: The *in vivo* differentiation of mononuclear phagocytes. IV. The ultrastructure of macrophage differentiation in the peritoneal cavity and in culture. J. Exp. Med. *123*:747, 1966.

Cohn, Z. A., Fedorko, M. E. and Hirsch, J. G.: The *in vivo* differentiation of mononuclear phagocytes. V. The formation of macrophage lysosomes. J. Exp. Med. *123*:757, 1966.

Downey, H.: The development of histiocytes and macrophages from lymphocytes. J. Lab. Clin. Med. *45*:499, 1955.

Fawcett, D. W.: An experimental study of mast cell degranulation and regeneration. Anat. Rec. *121*:29, 1955.

Harrington, J. S.: Fibrogenesis. Environ. Health Persp. *9*:271, 1974.

Hayward, J. S., Lyman, C. P. and Taylor, C. R.: The possible role of brown fat as a source of heat during arousal from hibernation. Ann. N. Y. Acad. Sci. *131*:441, 1965.

Hunt, T. K. and Van Winkle, Jr., W.: *Fundamentals of Wound Management in Surgery—Wound Healing*: *Normal Repair*. Chirurgecom, Inc., South Plainfield, New Jersey, 1976.

Kolouch, F., Jr.: The lymphocyte in acute inflammation. Amer. J. Path. *15*:413, 1939.

Leibovich, S. J. and Ross, R.: The role of macrophages in wound repair. Am. J. Path. *78*:71, 1975.

Litt, M.: Eosinophils and antigen-antibody reaction. Ann. N. Y. Acad. Sci. *116*:964, 1964.

Maximow, A. A.: The morphology of the mesenchymal reactions. Arch. Pat. Lab. Med. *4*:557, 1927.

Movat, H. Z. and Fernando, N. V. P.: The fine structure of connective tissue. I. The fibroblast. Exp. Molec. Path. *1*:509, 1962.

Movat, H. Z. and Fernando, N. V. P.: The fine structure of connective tissue. II. The plasma cell. Exp. Molec. Path. *1*:535, 1962.

Padawer, J. (ed.): Mast cells and basophils. Ann. N. Y. Acad. Sci. *103*:1, 1963.

Sheldon, H., Hellenberg, C. H. and Winegard, A. I.: Observations on the morphology of adipose tissue. Diabetes *11*:378, 1962.

Smith, R. E. and Hock, R. J.: Brown fat: thermogenic effector of arousal in hibernation. Science *140*:199, 1963.

Taliaferro, W. H.: The cellular basis for immunity. Ann. Rev. Microbiol. *3*:159, 1949.

Weinstock, A. and Albright, J. T.: The fine structure of mast cells in normal human gingiva. J. Ultrastruct. Res. *17*:245, 1967.

West, G. B.: Function of mast cells. J. Pharm. Pharmacol. *14*:618, 1962.

7: Supportive Tissues—Cartilage

General Characteristics

Form and Function. Cartilage is a specialized connective tissue that consists of a few cells embedded within an amorphous, gel-like substance. In a manner similar to the activity of fibroblasts in other connective tissues, the cells of cartilage secrete various substances and become embedded in their own secretory products. However, these secretory products impart a firm but resilient quality to the matrix. These qualities suit cartilage to its functional role in *weight-bearing, movement* and *organ integrity.*

Cartilage does not have primitive mesenchymal cells scattered throughout it. Rather, the mesenchymal cells from which it arises, as well as those that allow growth, are located at the periphery of the cartilage in a membrane referred to as the *perichondrium.* These cells differentiate into *chondroblasts,* the cartilage-forming cells of the body. At a different stage in their life cycle, chondroblasts are referred to as *chondrocytes* (Fig. 7.1).

The chondroblastic line of differentiation is the means by which new cartilage is deposited upon pre-existing cartilage. This type of growth is called *appositional* growth. Once growth has occurred and the chondroblasts have become embedded in their own products, growth does not cease. Chondrocytes are capable of dividing within the confines of their *lacunae.* This mitotic activity from within causes expansion of the resilient matrix. This type of growth is *interstitial.* Most cartilage utilizes both mechanisms for growth.

Cartilage is an avascular tissue. Although large blood vessels pass through cartilage, there are no capillaries that directly supply the nutritional needs of this tissue. All metabolites must diffuse from the periphery to the cells in the depths of the tissue. The porosity of the matrix, therefore, is an important factor in maintaining the tissue. With age this task becomes more difficult. The natural fate of cartilage is to become mineralized. This increases the problem of percolation of metabolites through the matrix. The older cells die, the tissue is removed by phagocytic cells and bone is deposited in its place.

Also, cartilage proper is devoid of a nerve supply. Sensory innervation of this tissue is achieved by terminals of nerves scattered within the fibrous portion of the perichondrium.

Cartilage is the primary support tissue of the fetus. Support structures of cartilage develop in association with the upper and lower respiratory tract, the pinna and external auditory meatus, and pharyngotympanic tube. These cartilaginous structures continue to develop during adolescence and are maintained in the adult. Much of the cartilaginous mass of the fetus and neonatal organism is involved intimately with the developing musculoskeletal system. Certain structures, such as fibrocartilaginous intervertebral discs and fibrocartilaginous attachments of ligaments and tendons to bone, continue to develop and become integral parts of the supportive and locomotor structures of the musculoskeletal system. Much of the hyaline cartilage of the developing organism is involved in bone development. Most of the bones of the body are "preformed" in cartilage; a gradual but progressive reduction of the hyaline cartilage occurs until only the articular surfaces are composed of this tissue. The relatively small amounts of cartilage in the adult organism do not reflect its importance as a supportive tissue.

Origin of Cartilage. Cartilage, as one of the connective tissues, is derived from the mesenchymal cell. Sites within which cartilage is going to develop within the fetus are identifiable initially as sites of *mesenchymal cell condensation.* The mesenchymal cells withdraw their cellular processes, become round and form dense populations of cells. These presumptive sites of cartilage formation are called *chondrogenic centers.* The mesenchymal cells differentiate into chondroblasts. These cells enlarge and secrete their characteristic surrounding matrix. As the matrix or interstitial material increases, the cells become separated further from each other and each cell is bounded by its own secretory products. The space occupied by each cell is called a *lacuna.* Although these cells occupy *lacunae* (little lakes), their relationship to the embedding matrix is similar to that of the fibroblast and its surrounding matrix, which it also secretes.

Cells within lacunae, chondrocytes, are capable of mitosis. Division of these cells with a corresponding expansion of the matrix from within the mass of cartilage is termed *interstitial growth.* At the periphery of the developing cartilaginous mass, some of the mesenchymal cells condense to form

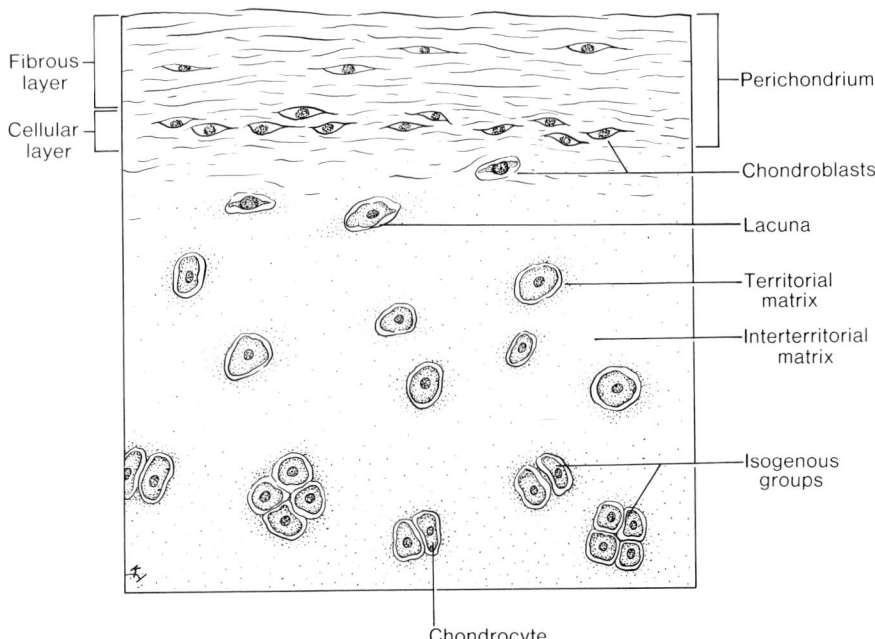

Fibrous layer
Cellular layer
Perichondrium
Chondroblasts
Lacuna
Territorial matrix
Interterritorial matrix
Isogenous groups
Chondrocyte

Fig. 7.1 Diagram of typical hyaline cartilage. Mitosis of cells within the perichondrium results in appositional growth. Mitotic activity within the matrix results in the formation of isogenous groups (cell nests) and interstitial growth. All light micrographs are labeled as the magnification with the microscope before photographic enlarging. All electron micrographs are labeled as total magnification, including photographic enlarging.

a covering layer of cells. This covering layer forms part of the perichondrium. Subsequent differentiation of the mesenchymal cells into cartilage cells accounts for the formation of cartilage on pre-existing cartilaginous surfaces, *appositional growth*. Interstitial and appositional growth mechanisms, as the name implies, are most active during development and growth. The potential for this type of activity is reduced in the adult.

Cells of Cartilage. Cartilage is composed of a homogeneous population of cells. Mesenchymal cells, either in a chondrogenic center of the embryo or in the perichondrium, differentiate into active cells that are capable of synthesizing and secreting large quantities of matrix components. These *chondroblasts* envelope themselves with their own secretions and eventually become isolated within lacunae. At this point, the cells are referred to as *chondrocytes*. They are the cells responsible for the maintenance and turnover of matrix materials. They perform the same functions as chondroblasts, but their level of activity is reduced when compared to the synthesis and secretion by chondroblasts. The chondroblast/chondrocyte relationship is probably best considered as the same cell in a different stage of its life cycle.

A third cell type may be observed in cartilage, especially during developmental stages. It is a multinucleated giant cell, the *chondroclast*. This cell is responsible for the removal of cartilage matrix and cells. Because of the morphologic and physiologic similarity of this cell to a cell of bone, the *osteoclast*, the chondroclast and the osteoclast are considered to be identical. Whether they are or not is yet to be determined. Even the origin of these cells is debated. Some argue that they are macrophages. Much evidence, however, supports their origin from chondrogenic cells. Chondroblastic cells probably fuse to form the multinucleated chondroclasts. As chondroclasts "eat" their way through cartilage, released chondrocytes are incorporated into the increasing mass of chondroclasts. (The same sequence of events is established for the giant cells in association with bone. If one assumes the chondroclast and osteoclast to be identical, then the sequence probably applies to cartilage. This assumption was made here.)

The chondroblastic and fibroblastic cell lines, as well as the osteoblastic cell line, are closely related populations of cells. All are derived originally from the mesenchymal cell. All secrete collagen and glycosaminoglycans. Yet, each is associated with a matrix that imparts distinctive characteristics to its respective tissues. Under varying circumstances, these tissues (fibrous connective tissues, cartilage and bone) occur in areas in which they are not expected. This abnormal transformation of an adult, fully differentiated tissue of one kind into another differentiated kind is called *metaplasia*. The mechanism or mechanisms responsible for this type of change are debated, but one fact is clear. These transformations do occur. Cartilage and bone can form de novo in fibrous connective tissue; bone and fibrous connective tissue can form in sites occupied by cartilage; and cartilage and fibrous connective tissue can form in sites occupied by bone. Experimental evidence has established clearly that the stem cell associated with these tissues is responsive to subtle but significant changes in its microenvironment. Under such circumstances, stem cells of a perichondrium, which under normal conditions would differentiate into cartilage cells, may produce one or both of the other fiber-producing cells. Similarly, stem cells of the covering of bone (periosteum) may differentiate into all three cell types. Although other mechanisms of metaplastic conversion are proposed, the presence and modulation of stem cells under varying environmental influences help to explain these observations.

Classification. Three types of cartilage are identified on the basis of the relative amounts of amorphous matrix and the amount and types of fibers embedded within the amorphous material. They are *hyaline cartilage*, *elastic cartilage* and *fibrocartilage*. Hyaline cartilage, the most common type, is most frequently encountered and is considered the type from which the other two are derived and modified.

Matrix Components

Fibers. The predominant fiber of cartilage is the fine collagenous fiber. In hyaline cartilage, these fibers are scattered in a random pattern throughout the matrix. In routine preparations they are observed rarely because their index of refraction is similar to that of the ground substance.

In fibrocartilage, however, the collagenous fibers are observed easily because they are the primary constituents of the cartilage. The amount of ground substance is reduced greatly.

The fibers of elastic cartilage include both collagenous and elastic fibers. Elastic fibers are visualized readily with normal preparatory techniques, as well as by special staining procedures.

Ground Substance. The principal constituents of the ground substance are the *glycosaminoglycans*. Minor differences in the quantities of specific glycosaminoglycans are related to age and location. Chondroitin-4-sulfate and chondroitin-6-sulfate are most abundant. Chondroitin-6-sulfate is more common in adult cartilage, whereas chondroitin-4-sulfate is more common in the cartilage of the young animal. Small quantities of hyaluronic acid may also be present in some cartilage. Keratan sulfate concentrations increase with age. These substances are chemically complexed with collagen, as well as with noncollagenous proteins, as proteoglycans. The presence of sulfate groups on these compounds imparts an acidic nature to the matrix. As such, the ground substance of cartilage is basophilic and stains appropriately with routine stains (H and E). The matrix of most cartilage, however, does not stain uniformly (Fig. 7.1). Young cartilage may be acidophilic while the matrix of the perilacunar margin (*capsular* or *territorial matrix*) of old cartilage stains intensely basophilic. The area of the matrix between individual cells or groups of cells, the *interterritorial matrix*, stains less intensely basophilic than the territorial matrix. The staining properties relate to the number of sulfate groups (basophilic components) and the acidophilic nature of the collagen. In young cartilage with fewer sulfate groups, the acidophilia of the collagen dominates. In the remainder of cartilage, the basophilic components dominate.

Although the sulfated glycosaminoglycans of cartilaginous matrix are PAS-negative, this matrix stains positively with PAS. The molecules responsible for this stain reactivity have not been determined.

The homogeneous nature of the intercellular material of hyaline cartilage appears differently when viewed with the electron microscope. Cellular/matrix relationships and the nature of the lacunar space also differ (Fig. 7.2). The chondrocytic lacunae are filled with fibrillar and granular materials. Some collagenous fibers may be ap-

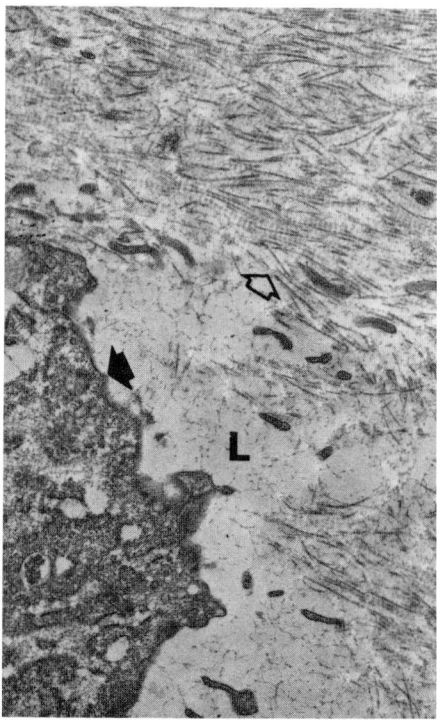

Fig. 7.2 An electron micrograph of growing cartilage. The cell margin (*solid arrow*) and lacunar margin (*open arrow*) are separated by the lacunar space (L). The lacunar space is filled with granular material (matrix granules), some sectioned collagen and cellular processes. X6800. (Courtesy of J. W. Newbrey)

parent also (Fig. 7.3). There is, then, a continuum of matrix materials from the cellular margin to the capsular or lacunar margin. The lacunar space is filled with *pericellular matrix* and is not the "empty space" seen with the light microscope. Enzyme digestion studies confirm that the granular materials, *matrix granules*, consist of complexes of glycosaminoglycans (chondroitin sulfates, keratan sulfate) and noncollagenous proteins. The fibrillar materials, *microfibrils*, are trypsin-labile, noncollagenous proteins. Collagen is obvious in the matrix proper. Matrix granules appear free in the matrix, in intimate association with microfibrils and juxtaposed to collagenous fibrils (Fig. 7.4). All of the matrix components are linked chemically to each other. Additionally, cytoplasmic processes project from the cells and extend into the matrix. An additional component is present in certain foci of hyaline cartilage. These are membrane-bound vesicles, *matrix vesicles*, that are pinched off from the cells or cellular processes and are located in the matrix. They occur in the mineralization zones of the hyaline cartilage of the growth plate. They are the sites utilized by the cartilage for the initiation of mineralization (Fig. 7.5).

Types of Cartilage

Hyaline Cartilage. Grossly, hyaline cartilage has a white, glassy appearance; thus the name (*hyalos* (Gr.), glass). In section this avascular tissue is separated from the surrounding tissue by the *perichondrium* (Fig. 7.6), which is analogous to the capsule of other organs. The perichondrium consists of a *fibrous* and a *cellular* portion. The fibrous portion is dense white fibrous connective tissue (DWFCT) that may blend insensibly with the surrounding connective tissue. Unless artifactual separation of the connective tissue occurs, the peripheral limits of the perichondrium are difficult to define. The cellular portion contains *mesenchymal cells* that give rise to fibroblasts of the fibrous perichondrium as well as to chondroblasts (Fig. 7.7). The cellular portion will be prominent in young growing cartilage only.

In young cartilage a definite gradation from *mesenchymal cells* to *chondroblasts* to *chondrocytes* is observed (Fig. 7.8). As mesenchymal cells differentiate into chondroblasts, these cells deposit matrix components and surround themselves in their own secretory products. As a result a small *lacuna* (lake) is formed. The cells reside within these spaces without any contact with other cells or the surface. Although the lacunae of cartilage may be devoid of cells in some sections, this is an artifact of sectioning. The lacunae, as well as the cells within them, are flattened with their long axis parallel to the surface. The matrix of this region is generally acidophilic.

Maturation of the chondroblasts into chondrocytes is accompanied by a cellular

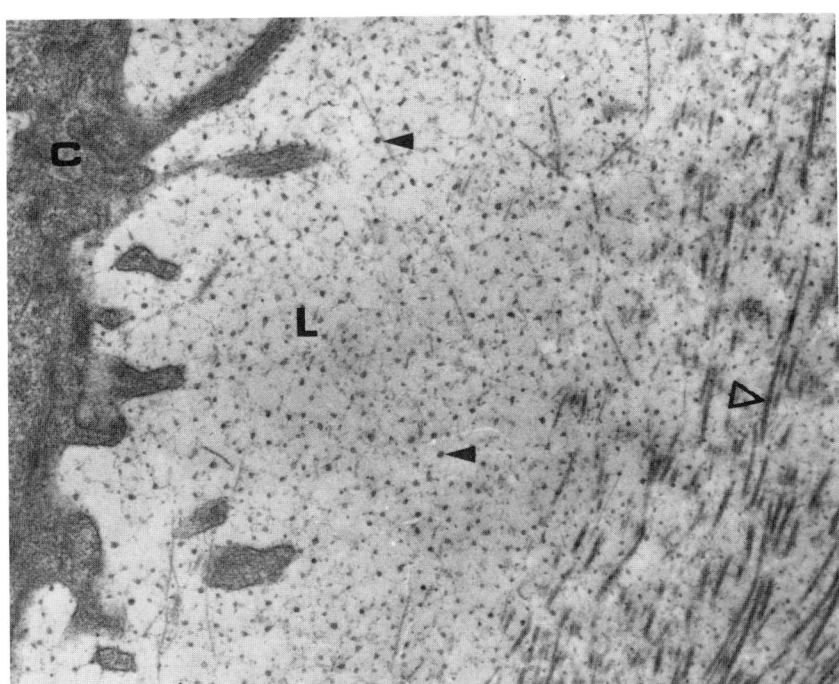

Fig. 7.3   An electron micrograph of growing cartilage. The chondroblast (C) has cellular processes that extend into and through the lacuna (L). The lacuna is filled with granular material or matrix granules (*solid arrows*). The small microfibrils within the lacuna are noncollagenous proteins. Collagenous fibers (*open arrow*) are apparent at the capsular margin of the lacuna. The preparation was stained with ruthenium red, an electron-dense stain for glycosaminoglycans. X15,000. (Courtesy of J. W. Newbrey)

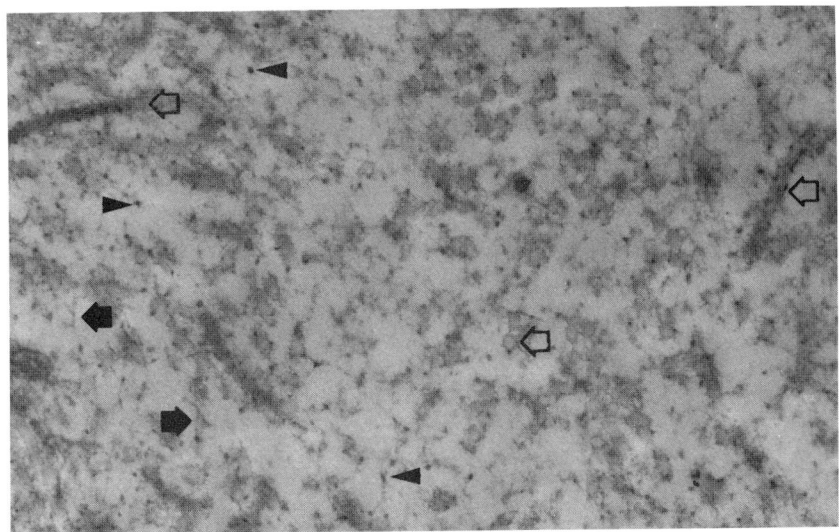

Fig. 7.4   An electron micrograph of the matrix of growing cartilage. The sample was stained with ruthenium red, a special stain for glycosaminoglycans. The intimate relationships of the biochemical matrix components is demonstrated. Matrix granules (*small solid arrows*) are juxtaposed intimately with microfibrils (*large solid arrows*) and collagenous fibers (*open arrows*). X36,000. (Courtesy of J. W. Newbrey)

hypertrophy, an enlargement of the lacunae and a change in lacunar shape to an ovoid or angular configuration (Fig. 7.9). Chondrocytes are also clustered as *isogenous groups* or *cell nests*. These cell nests represent the daughter cells of a single chondrocyte that underwent mitosis during the growth process. Further, these nests indicate that interstitial growth has been accomplished.

Interstitial growth is the means by which the growth plate contributes to the elongation of bones. The isogenous groups of cells in this structure assume a columnated relationship (Fig. 7.10). The significance of in-

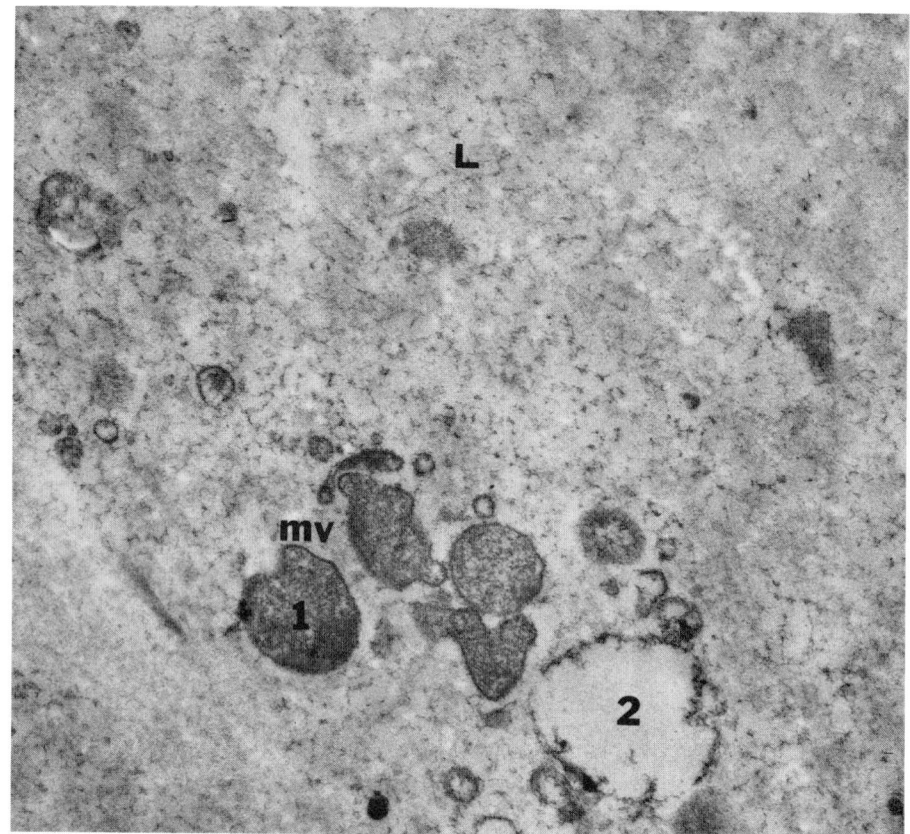

Fig. 7.5 An electron micrograph of mineralizing cartilage. Two types (1,2) of matrix vesicles (mv) are present in the matrix. The lacuna (L) is indicated. The matrix vesicles are foci of initial cartilage mineralization. X34,000. (Courtesy of J. W. Newbrey)

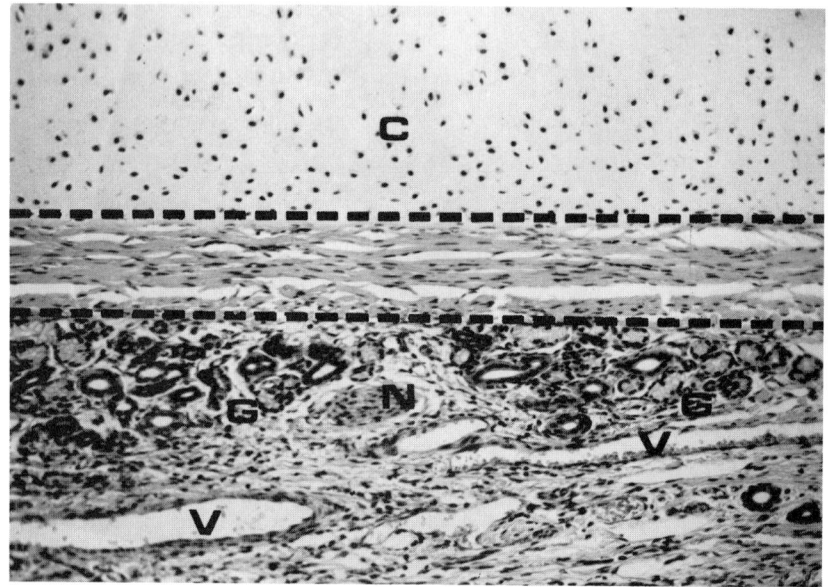

Fig. 7.6 Cartilage and associated tissue of an ovine turbinate. The cartilage (C) is surrounded by a perichondrium (*dashed lines*). The peripheral loose connective tissue (below perichondrium) contains nerves (N), glands (G) and blood vessels (V). X40.

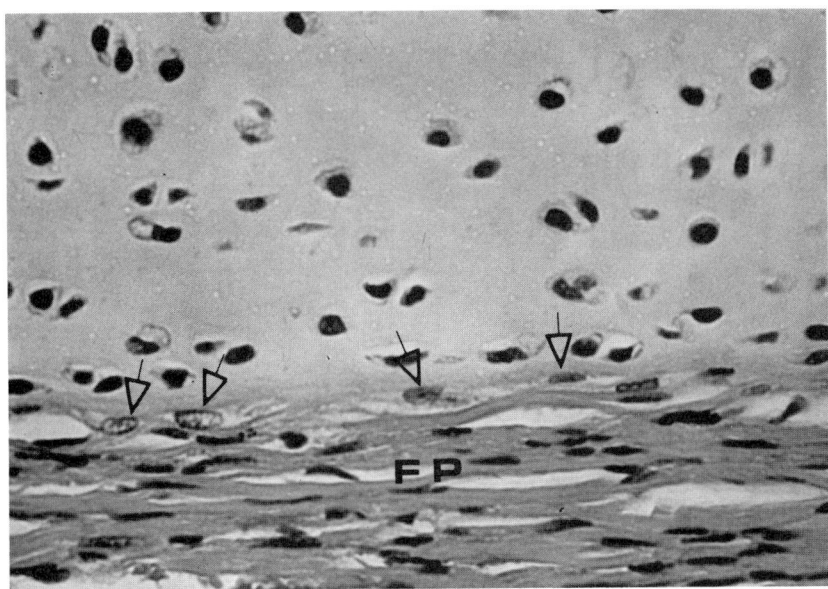

Fig. 7.7 Perichondrium of cartilage. The fibrous perichondrium (FP) consists of collagenous fibers and fibroblasts. The cellular perichondrium consists of mesenchymal cells (*arrows*). X160.

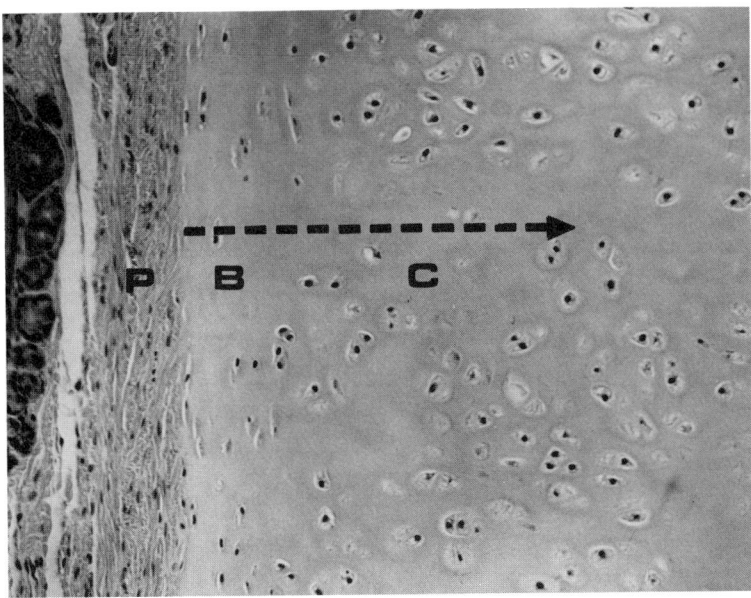

Fig. 7.8 Growing cartilage from the feline larynx. The perichondrium (P) is peripheral to the chondroblastic layer (B). Enlargement of chondroblasts and differentiation into chondrocytes (C) is apparent. *Dashed arrow*, progression of differentiation. X40.

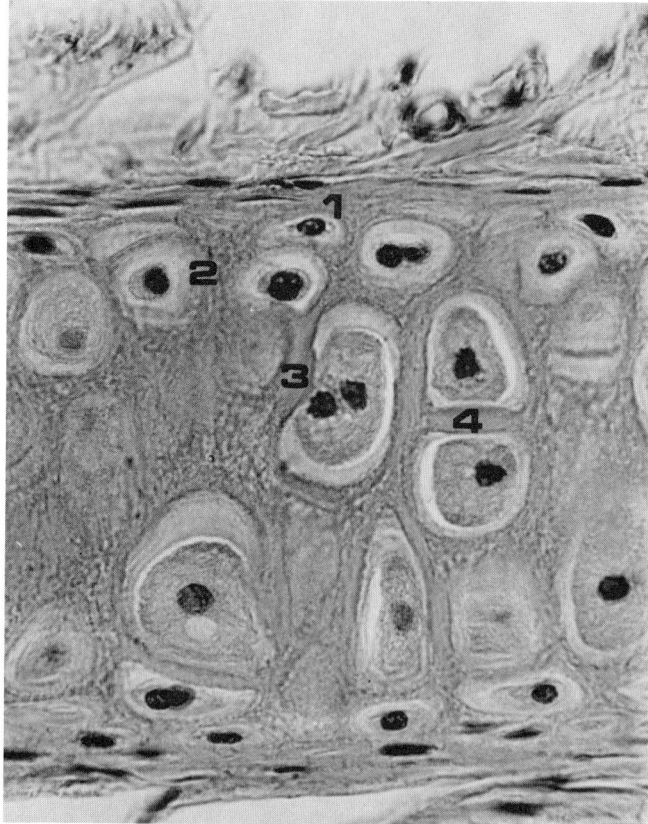

Fig. 7.9 Growing elastic cartilage of the porcine pinna. Chondroblasts (1) enlarge to become chondrocytes (2), chondrocytes may divide (3) to form isogenous groups (4). Interstitial growth consists of new cells and matrix added from within the mass of cartilage. X160.

Fibrous Cartilage. This tissue is also called *fibrocartilage* and is of limited occurrence in the body. Although of limited occurrence, it imparts additional strength to cartilage and DWFCT.

Fibrocartilage is an intermediate form between DWFCT and cartilage. Since visible collagenous fibers predominate, it may be considered a modified DWFCT.

Large collagenous *fascicles* (bundles) are oriented in an orderly array and are separated by isolated portions of cartilage (Fig. 7.16). The chondrocytes, located between the fascicles, secrete diminutive quantities of territorial matrix materials.

The classical appearance of this tissue is the *herringbone* configuration (Fig. 7.17) in which collagenous bundles are oriented to each other in the form of a V. Typically, however, the orientation of the fibers may not appear as orderly as that (Fig. 7.18).

Fibrocartilage is usually located at points of transition between DWFCT and cartilage and between DWFCT and bone. It imparts additional strength to these points of transition and/or attachment.

terstitial growth to the growth plate cartilage can not be overstated. This mechanism accounts for the achievement of the definitive height of individual animals. The amount of cartilage added to bones by this method is tremendous. Disruptions in the normal mechanism of elongation, such as occur in chondrodystrophic breeds of dogs can result in shortened limbs and/or brachycephaly.

Chondrocytes appear as smooth-surfaced cells that are withdrawn away from the lacunar margins (Fig 7.11). In fact, with the electron microscope the numerous processes of these cells are seen in intimate contact with the lacunar margins (Fig. 7.12).

The lacunar margin of individual chondrocytes or isogenous groups are more basophilic than other portions of the matrix. This marked basophilia delimits the *capsule* or *territorial matrix* of these cells, whereas the lighter area of basophilia marks the *interterritorial matrix*.

Although the perichondrium is generally a consistent feature of hyaline cartilage, the hyaline cartilage of the articular surfaces of bone secondarily loses its perichondrium (Fig. 7.13). This has significant implications upon the growth, repair and replacement potential of articular cartilage.

DIAGNOSTIC FEATURES:
1. Few cells embedded within a gel-like matrix which appears afibrillar.

2. Limits of the tissue are usually well marked by a perichondrium.
3. The matrix generally stains with basic dyes.

OCCURRENCE: Most bone-forming sites of the fetus and young animal; articular cartilages; airways of the respiratory tree; support structures of nose and larynx (Plates IV.8, IV.9).

Elastic Cartilage. Grossly, this tissue is yellow and is more resilient than hyaline cartilage due to the content of elastic fibers. Other than the presence of elastic fibers, this tissue is identical to hyaline cartilage. In some foci, more isogenous groups than those characteristic of hyaline cartilage may be apparent.

The elastic fibers are demonstrable with hematoxylin and eosin as pink-staining fibers scattered throughout the matrix (Fig. 7.14). They are more easily demonstrated with special staining techniques (Fig. 7.15).

DIAGNOSTIC FEATURES:

1. Identical to hyaline cartilage, except for the presence of elastic fibers.
2. Isogenous groups may be more frequently observed.

OCCURRENCE: External ear (pinna); external auditory canal; eustachian tube; parts of the laryngeal cartilages; epiglottic cartilage (Plate I.11, IV.10).

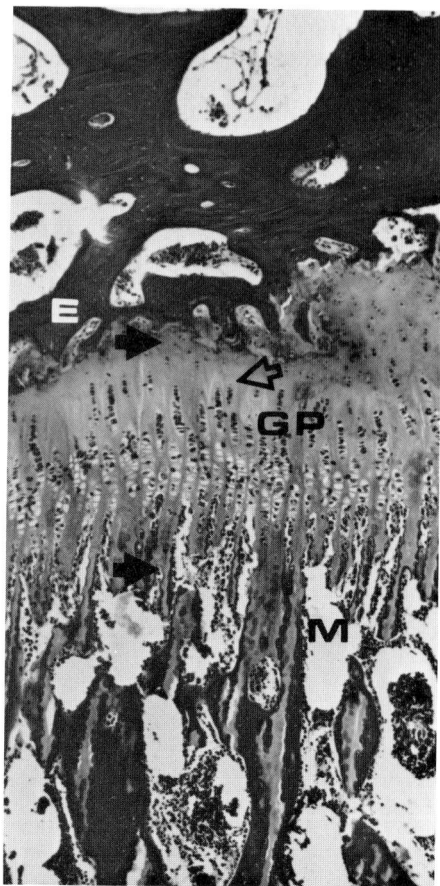

Fig. 7.10 Cartilage of the growth plate (GP). The growth plate is interdigitated between the epiphysis (E) and metaphysis (M). The approximate limits of the physis are indicated by *solid arrows*. Stacks of young chondrocytes (*open arrow*) divide and form ordered columns of maturing cells. The physis grows by interstitial mechanisms. X16.

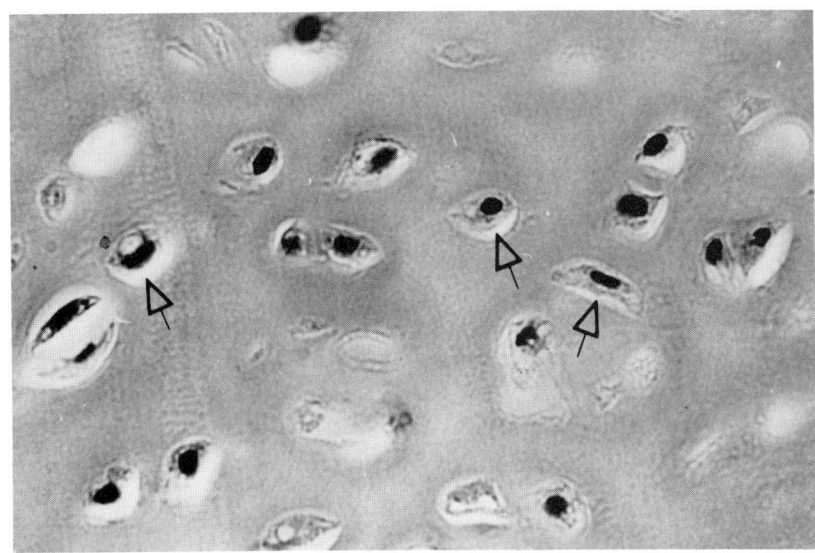

Fig. 7.11 Mature chondrocytes as single cells and components of cell nests. The cellular limits are withdrawn from the lacunar margins (*arrows*). X100.

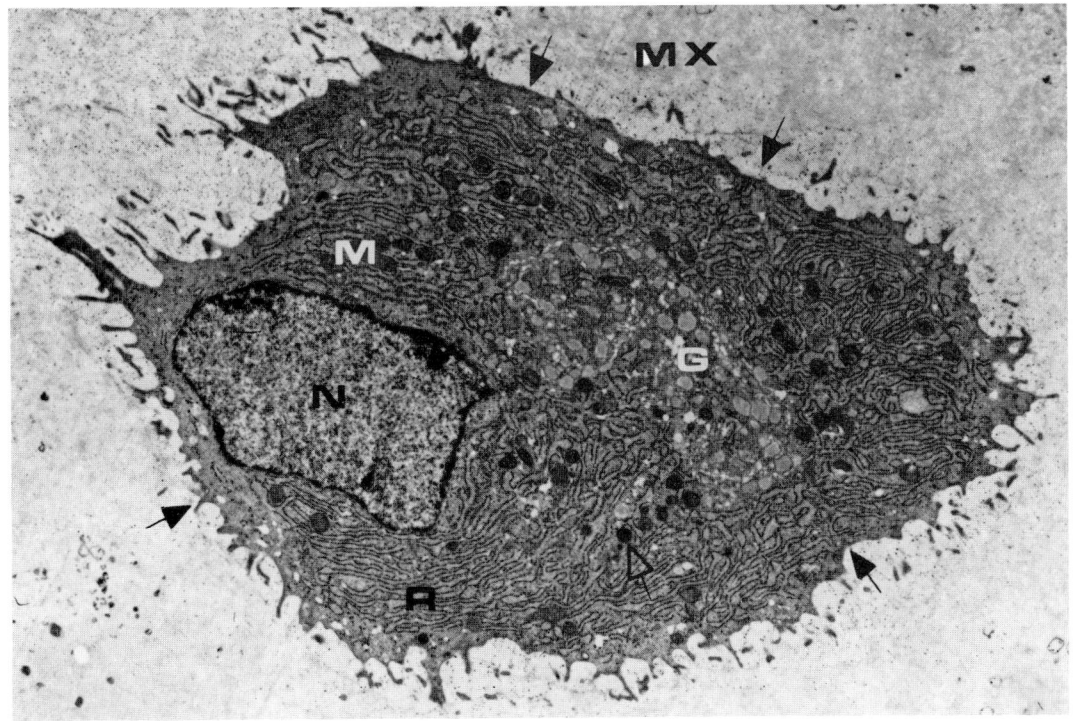

Fig. 7.12 An electron micrograph of a chondrocyte. The nucleus (N) is vesicular. The cytoplasm has an extensive Golgi apparatus (G) and rough endoplasmic reticulum (R). Mitochondria (M) and dense bodies (*open arrow*) are present also. The interface (*solid arrows*) between the cell and its matrix (MX) is intimate. Cellular processes extend into the matrix. The lacunar space of light microscopy is an artifact. X5,000.

This tissue does not have a perichondrium.

1. Predominance of coarse collagenous bundles in parallel and/or V-shaped orientation.

2. Presence of chondrocytes and limited amounts of matrix material between the bundles.

OCCURRENCE: Intervertebral disks; attachments of certain tendons and ligaments to bone; menisci (Plate IV.11).

Maintenance And Repair of Cartilage

Because cartilaginous tissues are avascular, they are dependent totally upon diffusion of metabolites from capillary beds within the perichondrium. Dependency upon diffusion is not unique to cartilage, but the distances through which metabolites must diffuse is a unique feature. Nutritional compromise of the chondrocytes leads to degenerative changes that are apparent especially in thick cartilaginous masses of aged animals. Mineralization of the matrix is a common sequel to the aging process of cartilage.

The hyaline cartilage of the growth plate normally undergoes mineralization. This "normal" process may be perceived as an acceleration of the aging process. As the cells are displaced further away from their blood supply, they may be compromised nutritionally and mineralization of the matrix results.

The actual maintenance of the cartilaginous matrix is the responsibility of the chondrocyte. These cells remove and replace fibrous and amorphous components. The intense basophilia of the capsular matrix reflects the ability of chondrocytes to add highly sulfated glycosaminoglycans to the matrix.

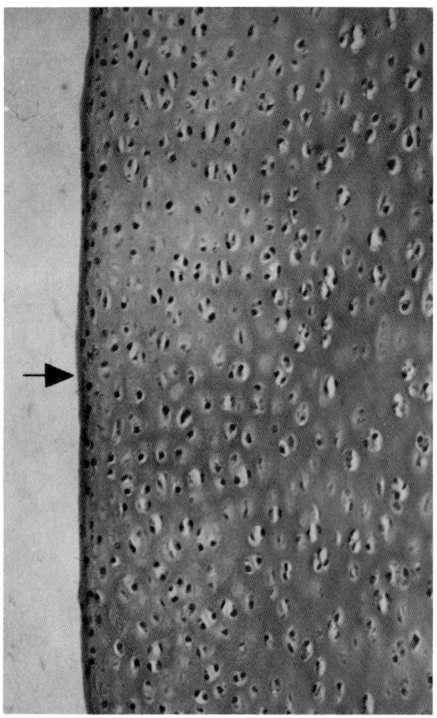

Fig. 7.13 Articular surface of the proximal head of a canine humerus. The hyaline cartilage of the articular surface (*arrow*) is devoid of a perichondrium. X38.

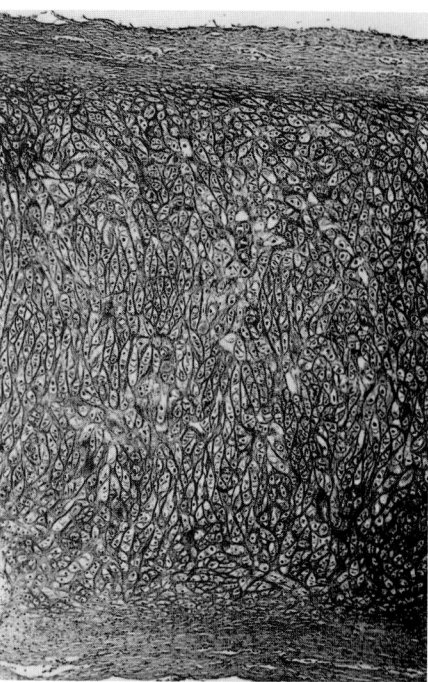

Fig. 7.15 Special staining of elastic cartilage. The elastic fibers are stained black. X13 (Verhoeff's stain).

Cartilage repair is not achieved to the same degree in all types of cartilage; nor, does the same type of cartilage achieve the same degree of repair in different locations. The age of the animals is a significant factor also.

The presence of a perichondrium insures an ample and readily available supply of mesenchymal cells. The continued proliferation and differentiation of mesenchymal cells of the perichondrium is a characteristic feature of young, growing animals. This is complemented by interstitial growth. Damage to hyaline or elastic cartilage during this period is repaired readily by the appositional growth of the perichondrium and by interstitial growth. In the adult, however, the perichondrium is not active and some of its regenerative ability is lost. Interstitial growth potential is lost also. Repair of adult cartilaginous tissues is mediated generally by a fibrous connective tissue that may be derived from the perichondrium or the dense white fibrous connective tissue of adjacent fascia. The newly added tissue, referred to as a granulation tissue by some authors, may be transformed gradually into cartilage. The new cartilage may retain a fibrocartilaginous character.

Fibrocartilage, however, reacts differently to injury. It is a dense tissue that is devoid of a perichondrium. The vascular supply to fibrocartilage is limited, especially in the menisci of the stifle joint and the intervertebral discs, to a few foci at its periphery. These vascular relationships coupled with a paucity of stem cells generally preclude

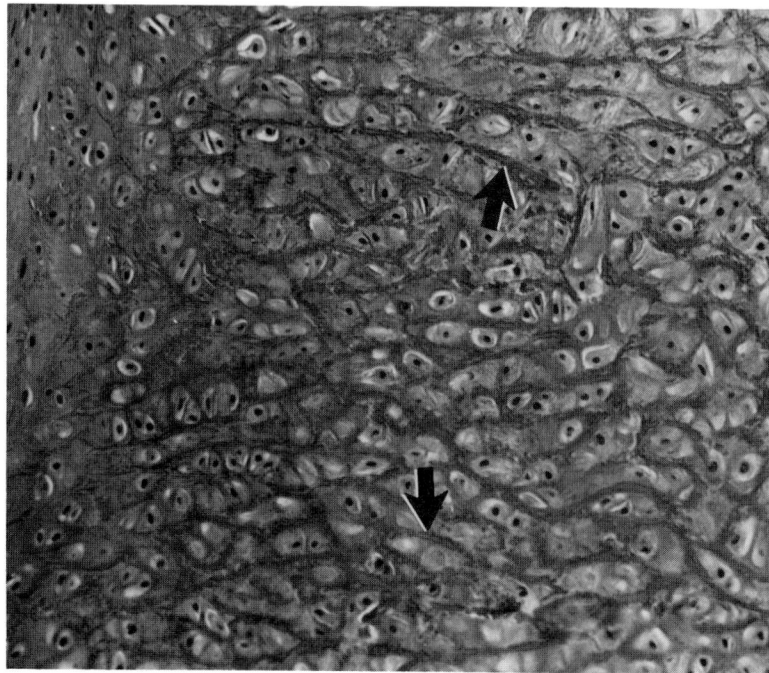

Fig. 7.14 Elastic cartilage from a bovine epiglottis. The elastic fibers (*arrows*) are predominant features of the matrix. X40.

good healing. Meniscal damage and intervertebral disc rupture usually compromise the vascular supply sufficiently to warrant the generalization that fibrocartilaginous repair potential is poor. This applies to the fibrocartilaginous interface at attachment points of ligaments and tendons to bone.

The hyaline cartilage of the articular surface is a unique focus that is devoid of a perichondrium. The interstitial mechanism is active until adulthood is achieved. Superficial damage to the articular surface may be repaired by this mechanism. Any minor blemish to the matrix of the articular surface, in the young or adult animal, may be repaired by an increased secretion of matrix components. In the adult, articular cartilage repair varies with the extent and location of the damage. On the weight-bearing surface, superficial damage can only be repaired by compensatory secretion by the chondrocytes. If the damage extends through the cartilage to the subchondral bone, then a number of possibilities exist. Stem cells associated with that region may differentiate into fibrous connective tissue, fibrocartilage

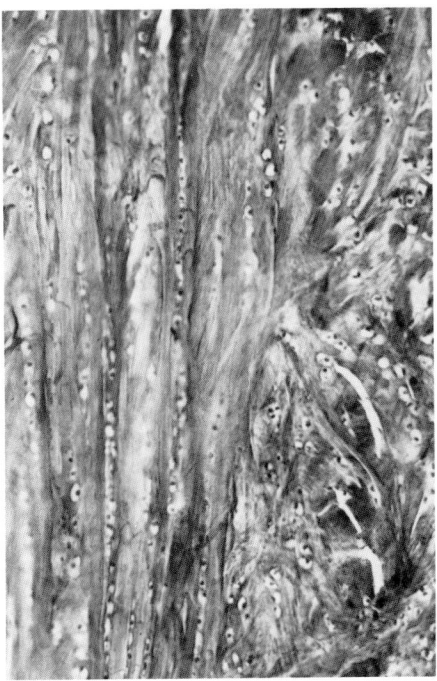

Fig. 7.18 Fibrocartilage from an intervertebral disc. The herringbone configuration is not as apparent as in Figure 7.17. X39 (Verhoeff's stain).

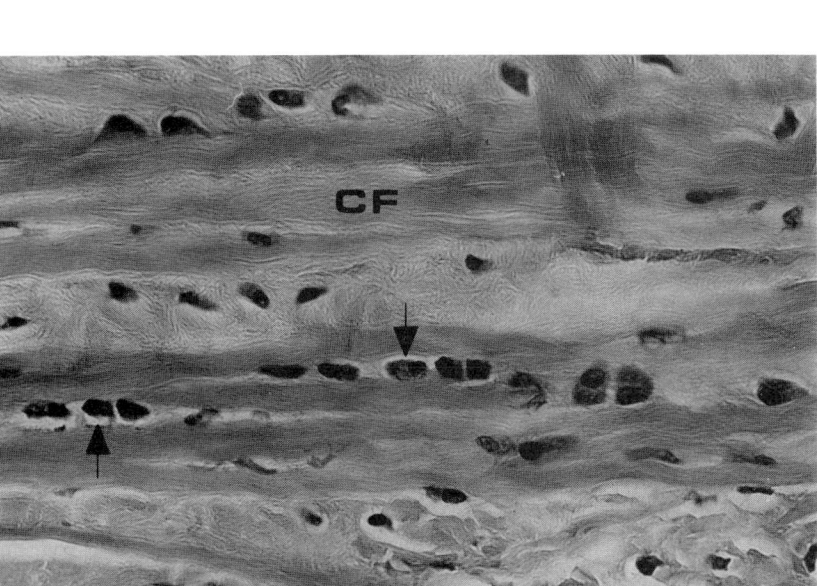

Fig. 7.16 Fibrocartilage. The collagenous fibers (CF) are predominant. Chondrocytes within their lacunae (*arrows*) are spaced in an orderly manner between the fibers. X100.

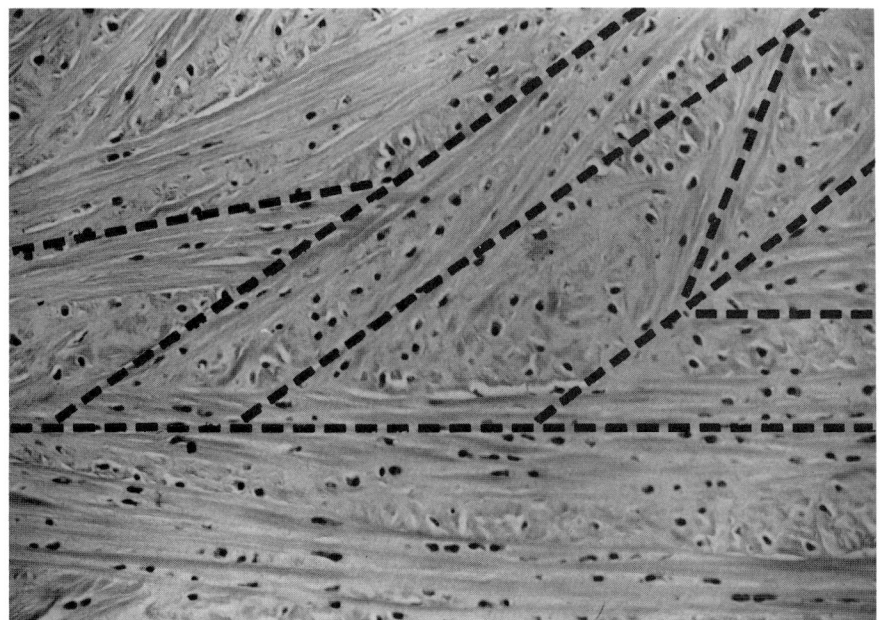

Fig. 7.17 Fibrocartilage from a meniscus of a canine stifle. The herringbone configuration (*dashed lines*) is apparent readily. X40.

or bone. Under carefully controlled experimental conditions these stem cells may give rise to hyaline cartilage. The replacement of the hyaline cartilage by bone represents a degenerative change called *osteoarthrosis*.

Along the nonweight-bearing surface at the periphery of the articular cartilage, damage generally results in replacement with fibrocartilage.

The most ideal repair would result in the replacement of a particular tissue with an identical type of tissue. The repair of cartilage, especially that of the articular surface of the adult, is less than ideal or satisfactory. The replacement tissues do not have the same properties; therefore, structure and function is usually compromised.

References

Amprino, R.: On the incorporation of radiosulfate in the cartilage. Experientia *11*:65, 1955.

Anderson, H. C.: Vesicles associated with calcification of the matrix of epiphyseal cartilage. J. Cell Biol. *41*: 59, 1969.

Cameron, D. A. and Robinson, R. A.: Electron microscopy of epiphyseal and articular cartilage matrix in the femur of the newborn infant. J. Bone Joint Surg. *40*:163, 1958.

Godman, G. C. and Lane, N.: On the site of sulfation in the chondrocyte. J. Cell Biol. *21*:353, 1964.

Godman, G. C. and Porter, K. R.: Chondrogenesis studies with the electron microscope. J. Biophys. Biochem. Cytol. *8*:719, 1960.

King, D.: The healing of semilunar cartilages. J. Bone Joint Surg. *18*:333, 1936.

Kuettner, K. E., Soble, L. W., Ray, R. D., Croxen, R. L., Passovoy, M. and Eisenstein, R.: Lysozyme in epiphyseal cartilage. II. The effect of egg white lysozyme on mouse embryonic femurs in organ cultures. J. Cell Biol. *44:*329, 1970.

Larsson, S. E. and Kuettner, K. E.: Microchemical studies of acid glycosaminoglycans from isolated chondrocytes in suspension. Calc. Tiss. Res. *14:*49, 1974.

Maroudas, A.: Distribution and diffusion of solutes in articular cartilage. Biophys. J. *10:*365, 1970.

Meachin, G.: The effect of scarification on articular cartilage in the rabbit. J. Bone Joint Surg. *45(B):* 150, 1963.

Nemeth-Csoka, M.: The influence of inorganic phosphate and citrate anions on the effect of glycosaminoglycans during collagen fibril formation. Exp. Pathol. *14:*40, 1977.

Palfrey, A. J. and Davies, D. V.: The fine structure of chondrocytes. J. Anat. *100:*213, 1966.

Pritchard, J. J.: A cytological and histochemical study of bone and cartilage formation in the rat. J. Anat. *86:* 259, 1952.

Sheldon, H. and Robinson, R. A.: Studies on cartilage. I. Electron Microscope observations on normal rabbit ear cartilage. J. Biophys. Biochem. Cytol. *4:*401, 1958.

Spycher, M. A., Moor H. and Ruettner, J. R.: Electron microscopic investigations on aging and osteoarthritic human articular cartilage. II. The fine structure of freeze-etched aging hip joint cartilage. Z. Zellforsch. *98:*512, 1969.

Svajger, A.: Chondrogenesis in the external ear of the rat. Z. Anat. Entwicklungsgesch. *131:*236, 1970.

Thyberg, J. and Friberg, U.: The lysosomal system in endochondral growth. Progr. Histochem. Cytochem. *10:*1, 1978.

8: Supportive Tissues—Bone

General Characteristics

Form and Function. Bone is a very specialized connective tissue that consists of a few cells embedded within a gel-like substance that becomes mineralized to varying degrees. The method of secretion and the manner in which the cells become embedded in the matrix are similar to those phenomena observed in cartilage. Although the fibrous and ground substance components of bone are similar to those of cartilage (collagen and acid mucopolysaccharides), the mineral phase of the matrix makes bone distinct from the other connective tissues. This mineral component consists of *amorphous calcium phosphate* and the *hydroxyapatite crystal.*

Three other characteristics significantly distinguish bone from cartilage. Whereas cartilage cells are embedded within a matrix without contact with each other or the surface, bone cells (*osteocytes*) are in contact with each other through cellular processes located in small canals (*canaliculi*) in the matrix. The cellular processes are not only a means through which coordinated activity may be mediated, but they and the canalicular space are significant in transport mechanisms through bone. Because materials diffuse less readily through mineralized matrices (as in mineralized cartilage), the significance of this canalicular system to bone viability cannot be overemphasized.

Whereas cartilage is avascular, bone is an extremely vascular tissue. Numerous blood vessels are scattered throughout bone. The cells of bone are rarely more than 2 mm from a supply of blood vessels.

Ossification, or the formation of bone, occurs in two distinct but related steps. The *osteoblasts* (bone-forming cells) secrete the *osteoid* (collagen and ground substance) which then undergoes *mineralization*. This mineralized matrix, unlike the normal cartilaginous matrix, is minimally expandable. Bone, therefore, is unable to grow by the interstitial mechanism. Appositional growth is the only mechanism by which bone can grow. This requires a copious supply of *stem cells* or *osteoprogenitor cells.*

The stem cells of bone are located in covering membranes called the *periosteum* and *endosteum*. The periosteum consists of a *fibrous* and *cellular layer* and is similar to the perichondrium. The endosteum is functionally similar to the periosteum but does not have a well-developed fibrous layer. A cellular layer is present, but the cells form a less definitive lining than the periosteum. Whereas the periosteum surrounds the outside or growing peripheral limits of bone, the endosteum lines the inside of bone and is intimately associated with the vessels that traverse the bone. Because of the periosteal and endosteal relationships to bone, all surfaces of bone (except some in old age) are covered by cells.

Besides its obvious function in the support and locomotion of the body, bone satisfies some very important metabolic requirements by virtue of its labile nature. Once formed, the mineral of bone is not irreversibly lost to the body. Rather, it may be removed by very distinct mechanisms. It functions, therefore, as an important dynamic store of calcium and phosphate. Calcium is significant in numerous metabolic activites (cardiac irritability, muscle contraction, enzyme activation and others), while phosphorous is the basis for a phosphate-based metabolism involving the production of energy-rich adenosine triphosphate.

Contrary to the perceptions that might be obtained from handling a dried portion of the skeleton in the gross anatomy laboratory, bone is not a dead tissue. Rather, it is metabolically active and in a constant state of change. The extensive vascular supply to bone gives some insights to its viability and metabolic activity. The cells of bone are responsive to numerous and varied stimuli. Calcium metabolism, which naturally must involve bone, is regulated by the activity of hormones (parathormone and calcitonin) that influence the manner in which bones and other organs handle available calcium. Numerous other hormones (estrogens, testosterone, thyroxine, glucocorticosteroids, growth hormone) act "in concert" upon bone, influencing directly its cellular activity and, indirectly, its intercellular substance. Also, bone is responsive to mechanical stimulation. Mechanical forces acting upon bone influence the amount of bone in the skeleton as well as its three-dimensional distribution.

To say that bone is not different than other tissues would be a definite overstatement. Nevertheless, all of the essential physiologic activities conducted by other tissues are conducted by bone. Cells must differentiate, die and be replaced. Cells must conduct the routine as well as the unique functions for which they are specialized. Cells must secrete, maintain and replace the secretory products that characterize them. All of these activities are characteristic of bone as a tissue. The significant difference is that bone must do all these things within the confines of an extensively mineralized matrix. This imposes some interesting features to bone.

One of the interesting features of bone as a tissue relates directly to its mineralized matrix. Whereas the turnover of matrix components in other connective tissues must be observed indirectly with various types of labels, the turnover of bone matrix may be observed directly. The amount, type, distribution and integrity of the matrix results from cellular activity. Observations of the matrix, therefore, afford useful insights into the tissue as a whole. The matrix of bone is to the histologist what the findings at an excavation site are to a paleontologist or archeologist. The matrix of bone is a telltale record of the events that had occurred previously.

Classification. Grossly, the bones of the skeleton are divided commonly into a number of classifications according to their shape and function. Bones, then, are either long, short, flat, irregular or sesamoid. Also, the pneumatic bones of birds are considered generally as a separate classification.

For the histologist, however, there are only two types of bone as a tissue. Bone is either *woven (immature, fibrous)* or *lamellar (mature)*. Both of these tissue types may be arranged in different manners so that they assume different *configurations*. These configurations are either *cancellous (spongy, trabecular) bone* or *compact (interstitial, osteonal, circumferential) bone* (Fig. 8.1). These configurations are visible grossly as well as microscopically.

It is important to remember that bone is both a tissue and an organ. Bone as a tissue can grow only by appositional growth. But, bone as an organ grows by appositional and interstitial growth. This is not a contradiction. Bone as an organ may contain a growth plate; the growth plate adds cartilage by the interstitial growth mechanism. One other example will clarify the necessity for careful usage of these terms. A long bone (as an organ) always develops by the replacement of cartilage by woven bone (as a tissue). Gradually, lamellar bone (as a tissue) is added to these trabeculae. The long bones of the adult continually add new bone (as a tissue) to the skeletal mass. This always results from the addition of lamellar bone

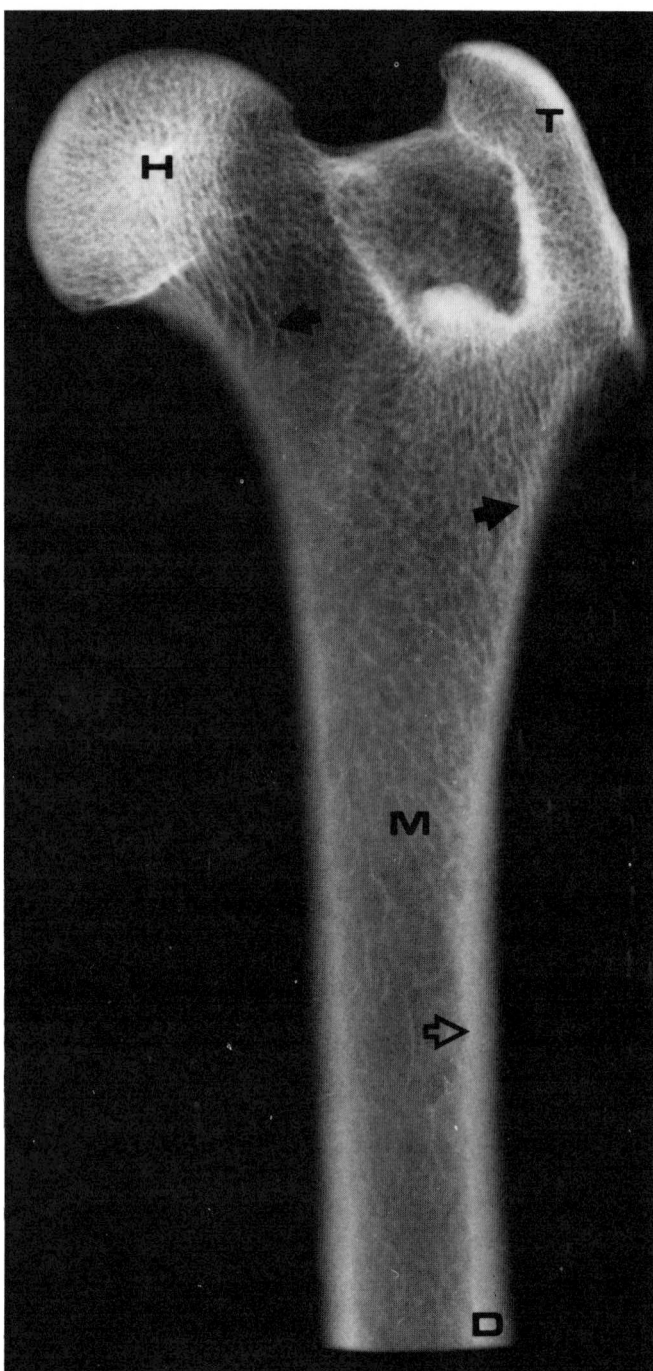

Fig. 8.1 A radiograph of the proximal portion of a longitudinally sectioned canine femur. Note the cancellous (*solid arrows*) and compact bone (*open arrow*). H, head; T, greater trochanter; M, marrow cavity; D, diaphysis XI. All light micrographs are labelled as the magnification with the microscope before photographic enlarging. All electron micrographs are labeled as total magnification, including photographic enlarging.

other in a helical pattern; each layer of a helix is oriented at a different angle to the previous layer (Fig. 8.2). The angle of collagenous fiber orientation between successive laminae may be acute, 90° or obtuse. The pattern of fiber orientation is responsible partially for the compressive and tensile properties of bone as a tissue and an organ. This pattern of collagen deposition imparts a lamellar appearance to mature bone (*lamellar bone*) that is especially apparent with polarizing microscopy (Fig. 3.7).

The collagenous fibers of *woven (immature) bone* are not as organized. Accordingly, the lamellar appearance, as well as the ordered appearance with polarizing microscopy, is lacking.

Ground Substance. The ground substance of bone is similar to that of cartilage. The acid mucopolysaccharide content of bone, however, is less than that of hyaline cartilage. The ground substance, therefore, usually is acidophilic. The mucopolysaccharides are conjugated to proteins. Numerous cross-linkages between the mucosubstances and collagen (glycoproteins) impart a rigidity to the ground substance.

Unmineralized ground substance is referred to as *osteoid*. Osteoid is the organic phase of bone matrix. It includes mucopolysaccharides, collagen and noncollagenous proteins.

Matrix. The amount of organic material in bone remains relatively constant throughout life. It usually comprises about 35% per unit volume. The remaining percentage, up to 65%, is occupied by the mineral phase of

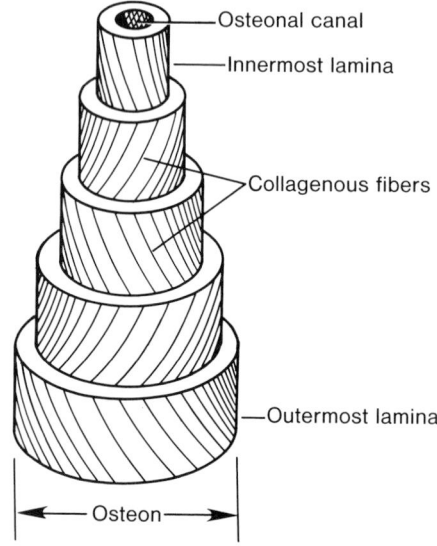

Fig. 8.2 A diagram of an osteon. The concentric laminae of bone have been removed partially to show the orientation of collagenous fibers within a lamina. In this example, collagenous fibers within laminae are oriented at approximately 90° to each other. The osteon is an elongated structure (cylinder) comprised of successive laminae of bone matrix. The relationship of the fibers to the apatite crystals is not indicated.

(as a tissue) to pre-existing lamellar bone (as a tissue). Therefore, the formation of a bone (as an organ) in the developing skeleton always involves woven and lamellar bone (as tissues). But the formation of bone (as a tissue) in adult bone (as an organ) always involves only the deposition of lamellar bone (as a tissue) under normal circumstances.

Matrix Components

Fibers. The fibrous component of bone is the typical fine collagenous fiber. Unlike most of the other connective tissues, the collagen of bone may be organized into highly ordered arrays. In *mature bone* this organization pattern is manifested as layers of collagenous fibers deposited upon each

bone. Bone mineral is not deposited maximally at the time osteoid is formed. Rather, there is a gradual deposition which begins with about 50% of the maximal mineral load. Gradually, 100% mineralization is achieved. The addition of mineral is at the expense of water in the matrix. Maximally mineralized bone contains less water than minimally mineralized bone. Although there are differences in the amount of mineral in bone, normal bone should contain about 65% mineral per unit volume. Any deviation from this value may be indicative of an abnormality.

The *hydroxyapatite crystal* is the predominant form of bone mineral. This is a complex lattice structure consisting of calcium, phosphorous and hydroxyl ions. The molecular formula for this crystalline structure is $Ca_{10}(PO_4)_6(OH)_2$. Although the formula $Ca_5(PO_4)_3OH$ is also correct, the spatial arrangement of the crystal cannot be satisfied with the latter. Numerous cations (Mg^{++}, Mn^{++}, Na^+ and others) and anions (lactate, citrate, carbonate, Cl^-, F^-) may be substituted into the crystalline structure, as well as being complexed to the surface of the molecule.

Amorphous calcium phosphate also occurs in variable quantities in bone mineral. This form of the bone salt may be a temporary deposition product during the formation of the hydroxyapatite crystal. Its precise role in the mineral phase of bone is currently the object of research.

Preparation of Bone Samples. The histologic study of bone may be approached by examination of either *demineralized* or *mineralized* (ground) sections. Demineralization is accomplished by two primary means, *chelation* or *acid hydrolysis*. Demineralization, sometimes referred to as *decalcification*, results in the removal of the mineral phase of bone. The organic material that remains after this type of treatment is called *osteoid*. Thin sections of bone may be obtained for study by this particular approach. Sections of bone prepared by this methodology retain near normal matrix relationships. Good cytologic detail is retained also. The use of mineralized samples complements the information available from demineralized bone sections. Mineralized samples must be cut with a diamond-tipped saw blade or ground on an abrasive material. With care, sample thickness of 50–100 μm can be obtained. Cytologic detail is not retained with this method; however, the nature of the matrix supplies valuable information about cellular activity. Special staining techniques can be applied to these sections and many inferences concerning the morphologic and physiologic states of the bone can be made. If bone-seeking labels (strontium, lead, tetracycline) are of interest, then this preparatory technique must be used. Demineralization removes the minerals as well as labels that may have been incorporated in vivo. Micrographs used in

this chapter are of bone samples that have been prepared by both of these techniques.

Envelopes of Bone

The cellular populations of bone are distributed throughout the tissue in two distinct loci. The osteocytic population is located within the intercellular substance. All of the other cells of bone are located on bone surfaces within distinct envelopes. These envelopes are the *periosteum* and the *endosteum*. The cells within these membranes may be considered subsets of the total cellular population that is responsible for various activities associated with bone. Mor-

phologically, the subsets of the total population of cells appear identical; however, they are not identical functionally. Numerous examples of different activities of the cellular components of the envelopes exist in health and disease. Also, these cellular populations appear to have different thresholds of response to the same stimuli.
Periosteum. The *periosteum* is the outer covering of a bone (Fig. 8.3). It covers the entire bone, except for the articular surfaces. It must be incised or removed before the underlying osseous tissue is visible directly. The periosteum consists of a fibrous and a cellular layer. The fibrous layer is dense white fibrous connective tissue and may be

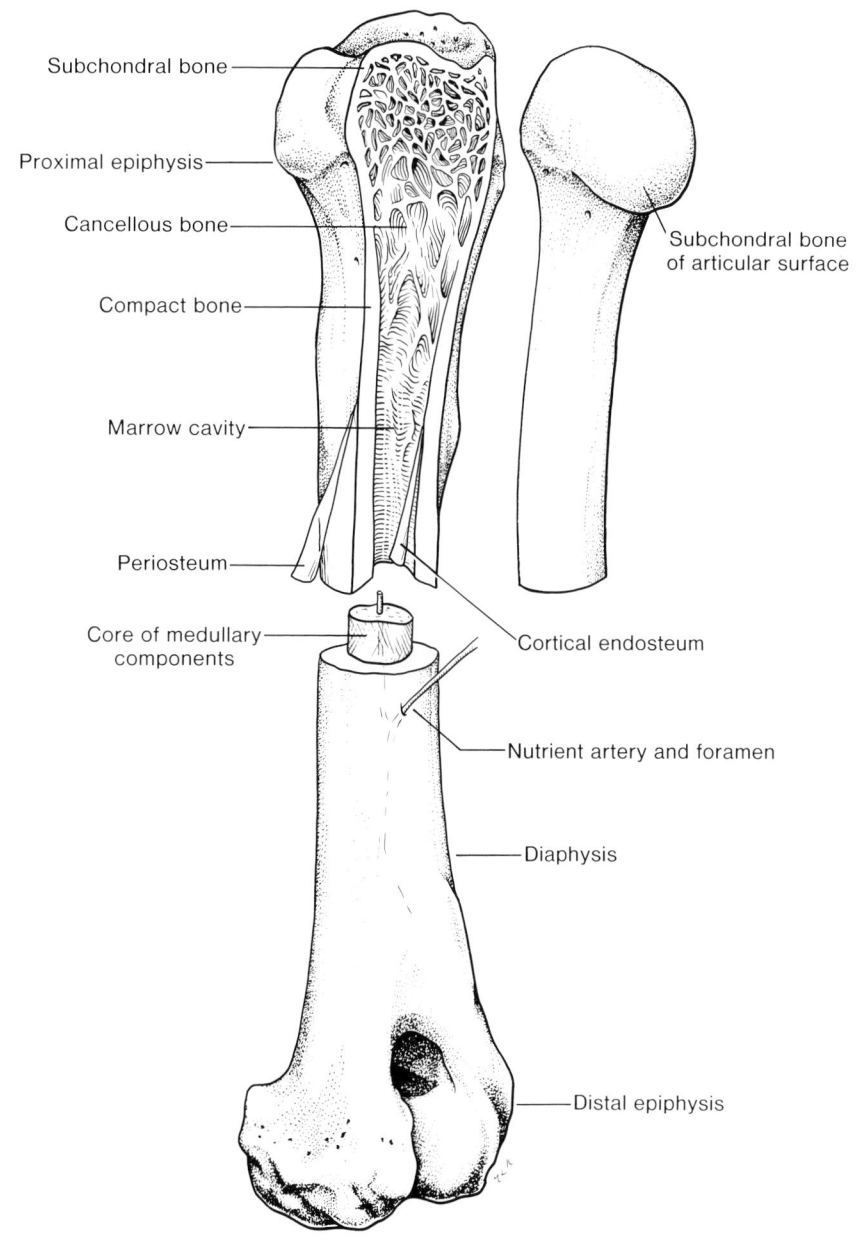

8.3 Drawing of canine humerus. Pertinent gross anatomic features are labeled. The preparation of the gross specimen resulted in the removal of the articular cartilage from the proximal and distal epiphyses. The periosteum covers all external bone surfaces except those of the articulations. The endosteum covers all internal bone surfaces. Compare with Figure 8.6.

considered the capsule of the organ (Fig. 8.4). Collagenous fibers of ligaments and tendons blend with and pass through this fibrous capsule before becoming anchored to the osseous tissue beneath it. The cellular layer of the periosteum consists of mesenchymal cells, osteoprogenitor cells, osteoblasts and osteoclasts. The mesenchymal cells differentiate into osteoprogenitor cells as well as the fibroblasts that are components of the fibrous layer. The periosteum is well-vascularized.

The cells of the periosteum are responsible for a number of important activities. During development, osteogenic cells of this envelope increase the diameter of the diaphysis. In the adult, the envelope is responsible for the maintenance of the associated bone surface. The proliferative activity of the periosteum is significant during fracture repair. Also, this envelope is responsive to various types of insults that result in *periosteal new bone* formation.

Endosteum. The *endosteum* is the inner covering of bone as an organ and tissue (Fig. 8.3). The compact bone adjacent to the marrow cavity, the trabecular bone of the marrow cavity and the osteonal canals within the substance of the compact bone are lined by elements of the endosteal envelope. Three subdivisions of the endosteum are named on the basis of their anatomic distribution within bones. More importantly, their identification as distinct envelopes is justified because of their differential activity under a variety of circumstances, despite their being continuous with each other. Although they consist of cells that are identical morphologically, they react differently to

what are perceived to be the same stimuli. The three subsets of the endosteum are the *cortical endosteum, trabecular endosteum* and the *osteonal endosteum*. The cortical endosteum is the envelope that covers the compact bone and defines the peripheral limit of the marrow cavity (Fig. 8.3). The trabecular endosteum is the envelope which covers trabeculae of bone that traverse the marrow cavity (Fig. 8.5). In most long bones, the trabeculae and their associated envelopes are confined generally to the proximal and distal epiphyses and metaphyses (Fig. 8.6). The osteonal endosteum lines the osteonal canals (Figs. 8.7, 8.8).

The cellular layer of the endosteum consists of cells identical to those which occur in the periosteum. The endosteum, however, does not have a heavy fibrous layer (Fig. 8.5). Rather, it is a loose connective tissue within which are located the typical cellular components of areolar connective tissue as well as the stem cells of bone.

Developmentally, the periosteum gives rise to and is continuous with all subdivisions of the endosteum. This continuity is apparent in the Volkmann's canals (Figs. 8.6, 8.7). Nevertheless, the classification of these functionally distinct envelopes is justified for the reasons discussed previously.

Cellular Components

Relationship of Cells. The fate of the mesenchymal cell in the connective and supportive tissues was discussed previously. Also, the close relationship between the fiber-forming cells—fibroblasts, chondroblasts and osteoblasts—was introduced in the pre-

vious chapter. Now, it is important to expand upon these relationships as they relate to the cellular populations associated with the envelopes of bone. Classically, the mesenchymal cell associated with bone has been described as differentiating into the specific cells of bone—osteoprogenitor cell, osteoblast, osteocyte and osteoclast. Moreover, these cell types have been described as being fixed post-mitotic cells, the products of mesenchymal cell differentiation. Current evidence shows that any one of these cells is capable of being transformed into any or all of the four cells which characterize bone. This temporary change in structure and function is termed *modulation*. The relationships of these cells and others are detailed in the accompanying diagram (Fig. 8.9).

Mesenchymal Cell. The morphology of this cell has been described elsewhere (Fig. 8.10). Some authors still describe the mesenchymal cell as the stem cell within the envelopes of bone. Although mesenchymal cells may be present in these loci, there is no evidence that the stem cell of bone is capable of differentiating into all of the typical mesenchymal cell derivatives. Rather, it has a limited potency to give rise to other cells. This cell is called the osteoprogenitor cell.

Osteoprogenitor Cell. The *osteoprogenitor cell* is also called an *osteogenic cell* by some authors. The former name seems more appropriate, because the activity of the cell is broader than just that associated with bone formative or osteogenic processes. These cells are similar morphologically to mesenchymal cells. They are identified on the basis of their location on bone surfaces or within the envelopes of bone, as well as their limited ability to be transformed into other cell types (Fig. 8.10). The osteoprogenitor cell is the only bone cell that actively divides, as evidenced by the active uptake of tritiated thymidine. This marker subsequently shows up in osteoblasts and osteoclasts, but this is interpreted to mean that the osteoprogenitor cells modulate into these more specialized cell types. Further, it is believed that the osteoblasts and osteoclasts are capable of modulating back to the less specialized osteoprogenitor cells.

The presence of mitotically active osteoprogenitor cells insures a plentiful supply of stem cells for this tissue. Notwithstanding the modulation of the osteoblasts and osteoclasts to this cell type, periods of growth and/or replacement require readily available supplies of osteoprogenitor cells.

Osteoblasts. These cells are the bone-forming cells of the body. They are responsible for the secretion of tropocollagen and acid glycosaminoglycans. Most importantly, they are also the storage cells of the mineral used in mineralization. This mineral is stored in these cells and is released upon some activation signal.

Osteoblasts or osteoprogenitor cells cover most bone surfaces. During periods of inactivity these cells assume a spindle shape

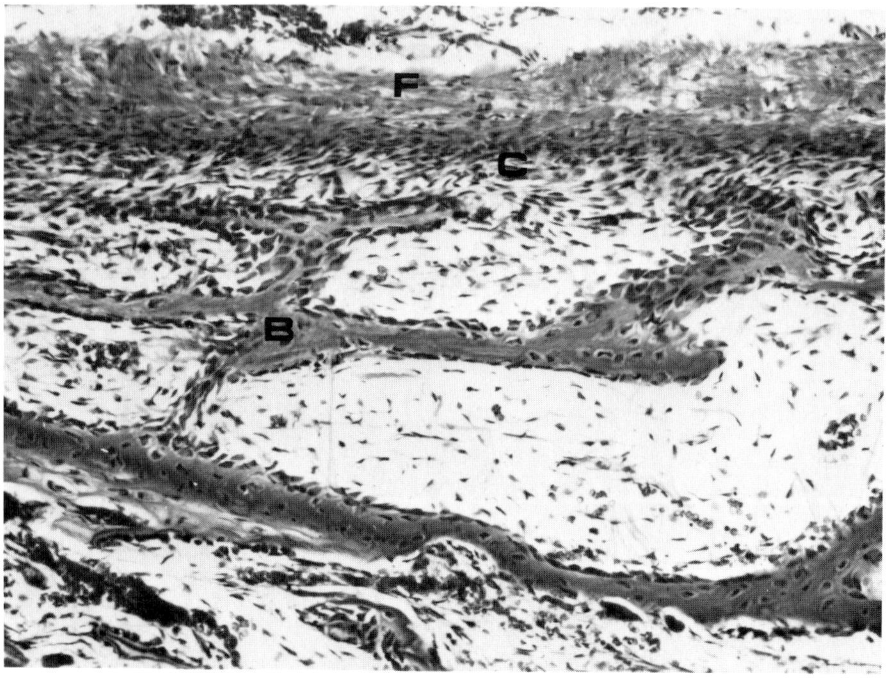

Fig. 8.4 Periosteum of a developing long bone. The fibrous (F) portion of the periosteum consists of DWFCT, whereas the cellular (C) portion consists of different types of bone cells. (B) bone. X40.

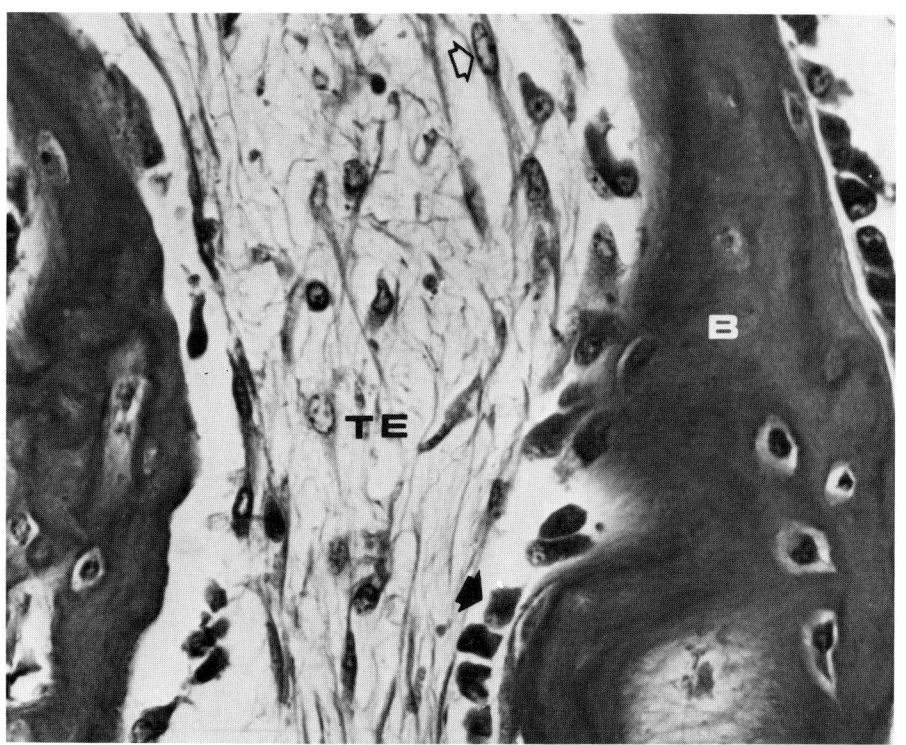

Fig. 8.5 Trabecular endosteum of bovine fetal jaw. The trabecular endosteum (TE) consists of loose connective tissue, stem cells (*open arrow*) and osteoblasts (*solid arrow*) or progenitor cells that cover the internal surfaces of bone. X100.

(Fig. 8.11). During inactive periods of their cycle they are called *inactive osteoblasts.* However, they may also be osteoprogenitor cells, because osteoblasts and/or osteoclasts may become apparent on these surfaces subsequently (Fig. 8.11). The cytoplasm is weakly basophilic and surrounds a single oval or round nucleus. During periods of activity the cells hypertrophy and become polarized (Fig. 8.12). They assume definite epithelioid characteristics. The single nucleus, with a prominent nucleolus, is displaced to the end of the cell away from the bone surface. The cytoplasm is moderately basophilic due to the high content of ribosomal ribonucleic acid. A well-developed Golgi apparatus and numerous mitochondria are characteristic (Plate II.5).

The activity of ostoblasts along a bone-forming surface is well-synchronized. The cells produce approximately 2 μm^3 of osteoid per day. This osteoid accumulates, layer upon layer, until a definitive *osteoid seam* is apparent that is approximately 10–15 μm thick. This osteoid seam, which has never been mineralized, is a lighter pink (H and E) than the osteoid that has been mineralized (Fig. 8.13). The osteoid seam is set apart from the remaining osteoid by a dark-staining *reversal band*, the region from which mineralization of the osteoid seam will progress. With mineralized sections and

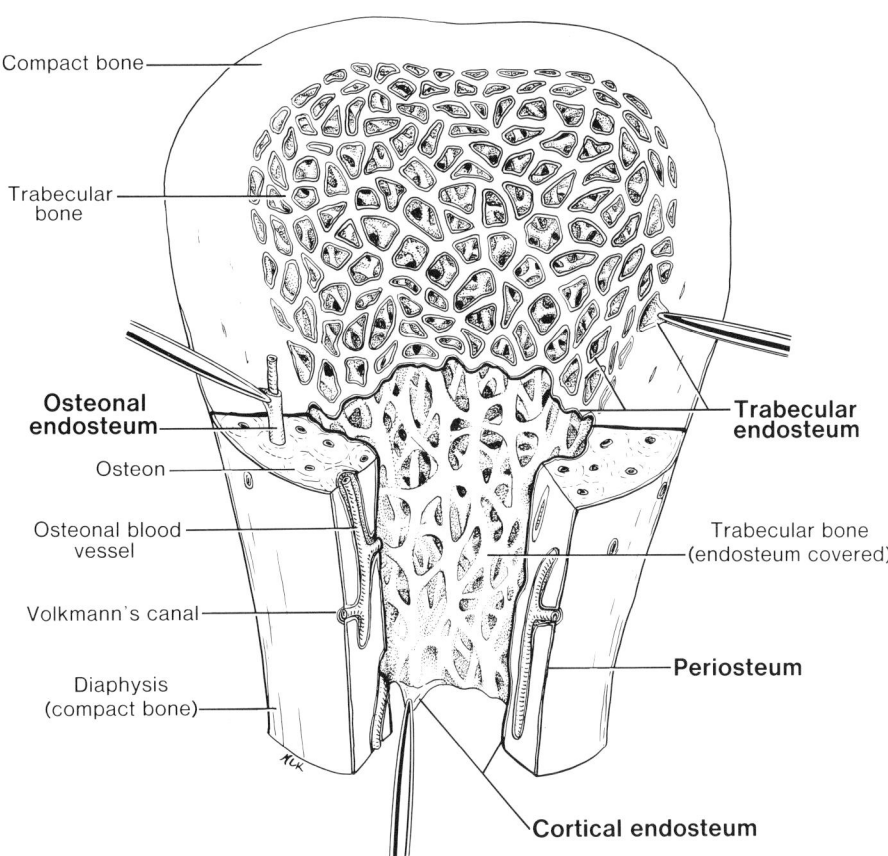

Fig. 8.6 Drawing of a sectioned long bone. The endosteum covers all internal bone surfaces.

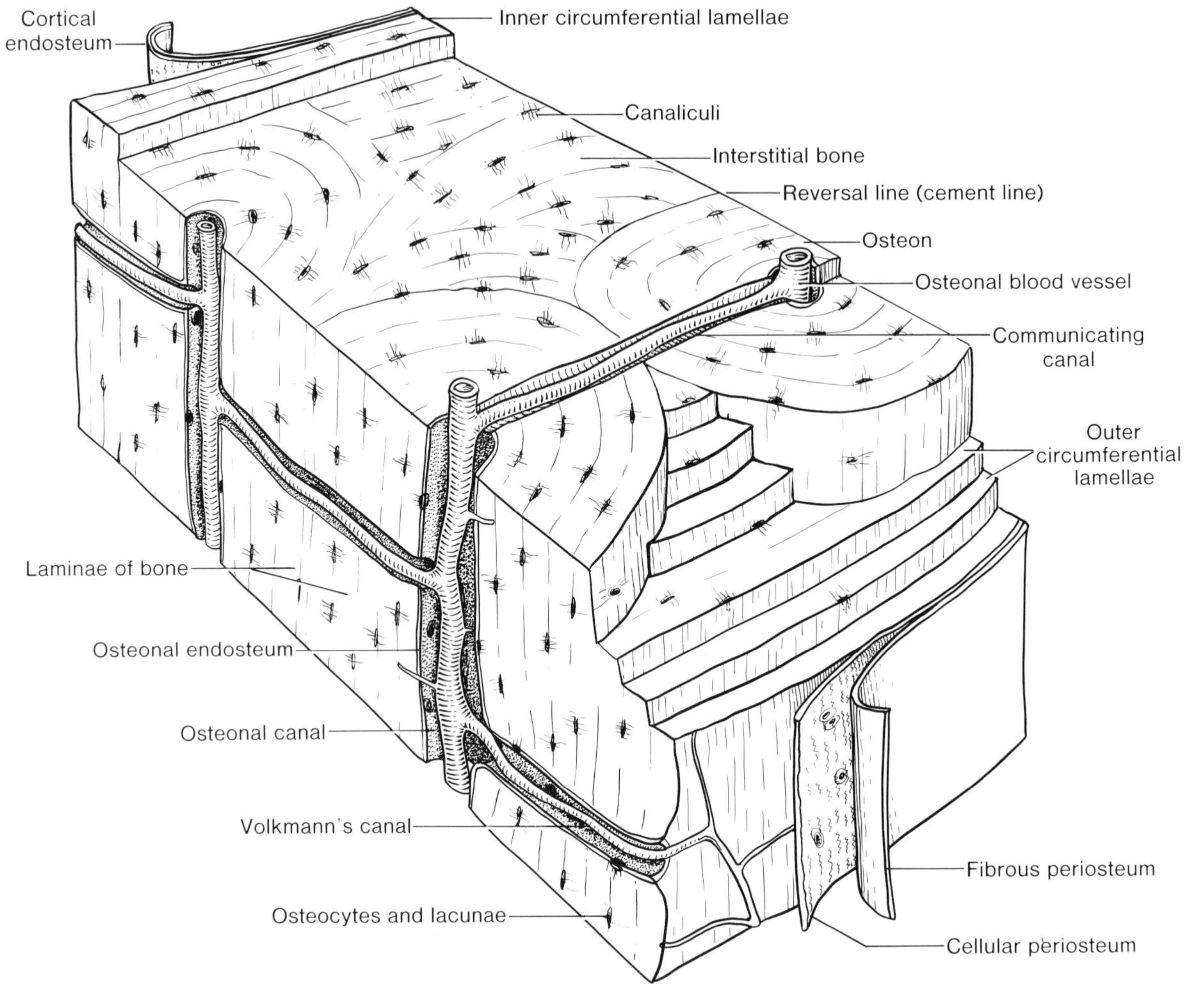

Cortical endosteum

Inner circumferential lamellae

Canaliculi

Interstitial bone

Reversal line (cement line)

Osteon

Osteonal blood vessel

Communicating canal

Outer circumferential lamellae

Laminae of bone

Osteonal endosteum

Osteonal canal

Volkmann's canal

Osteocytes and lacunae

Fibrous periosteum

Cellular periosteum

Fig. 8.7 Diagram of a section of compact bone of the diaphysis.

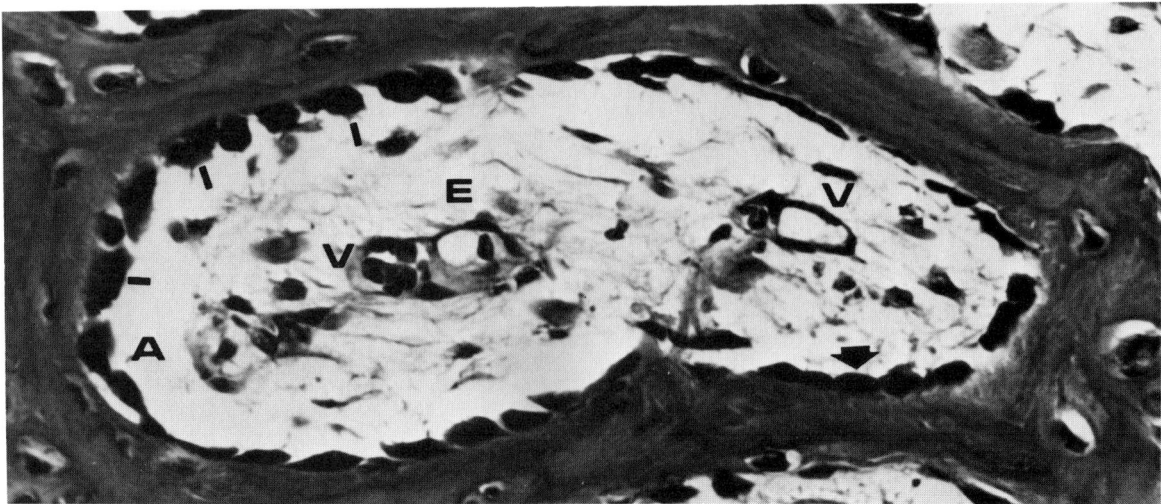

Fig. 8.8 Section of a developing osteon. The osteonal endosteum (E) is surrounded by bone which was formed by the cellular components of the endosteum. Loose connective tissue and blood vessels (V) are components of the envelope. Active osteoblasts (*bars*) and inactive osteoblasts (*arrow*) are present. The endosteum was separated from the bone (A) as a result of processing. Continuous centripetal deposition of bone along the peripheral margin of the endosteum will reduce the endosteal mass appreciably. Compare with Figure 8.32. X100.

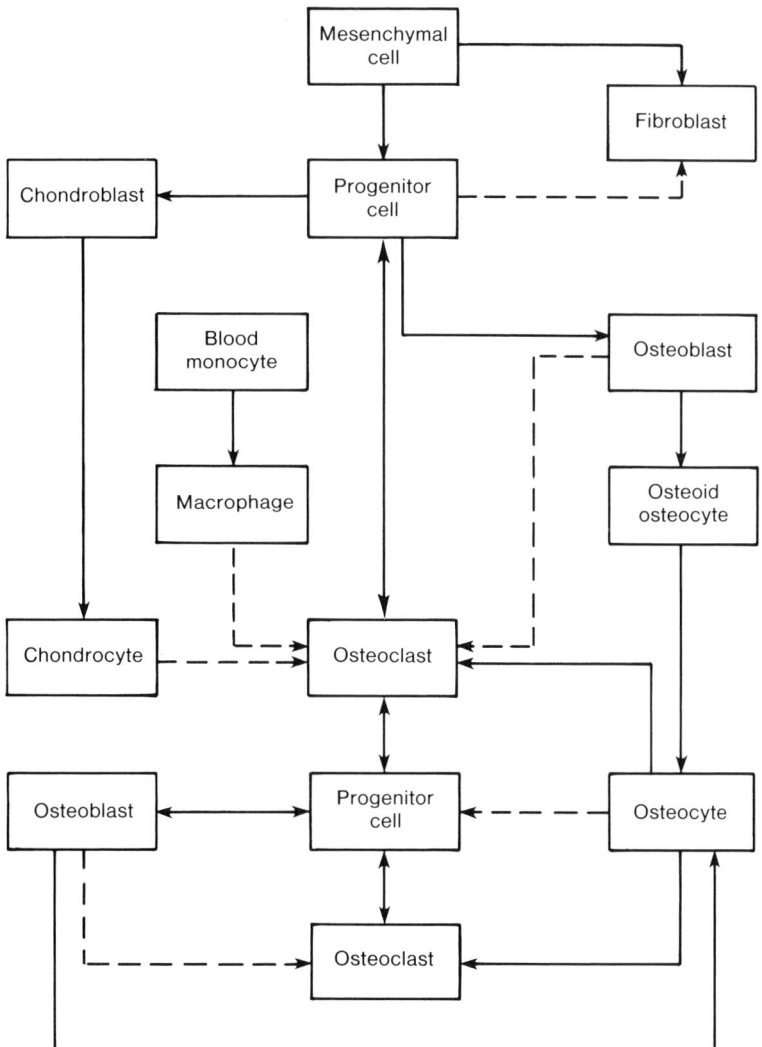

Fig. 8.9 Established and theoretical relationships among the cellular populations of bone. The *solid lines* indicate established relationships, whereas the *dashed lines* indicate theoretical relationships.

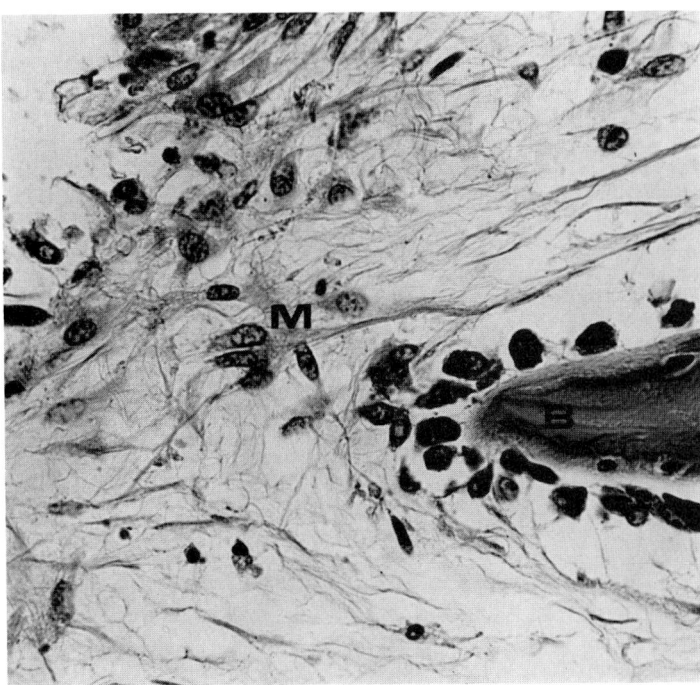

Fig. 8.10 Stem cells of bone located within an endosteal envelope. The stem cells (M) of bone have been considered to be the mesenchymal cells. The stem cells indicated may be mesenchymal cells or osteoprogenitor cells. A spicule of bone (B) is covered by osteoblasts. X100

special staining techniques, the osteoid seam is apparent; however, cellular detail is not preserved (Fig. 8.14 and Plate I.9).

The secretory activity of the osteoblast is biphasic. The first phase of activity involves the synthesis and secretion of organic materials. The tropocollagen polymerizes outside of the cell and becomes oriented in an orderly manner (Fig. 8.2). As with the fibroblast, the role of the osteoblast in this orientation process is not clear. Orientation of the collagenous fibers may result from osteoblastic influences, response to stress or a combination of both factors. The first phase culminates in the formation of the osteoid seam. The second phase of this activity is the mineralization of the osteoid. Calcium ions that had been stored in the osteoblast, especially in the mitochondria, are released from the cell and react with the

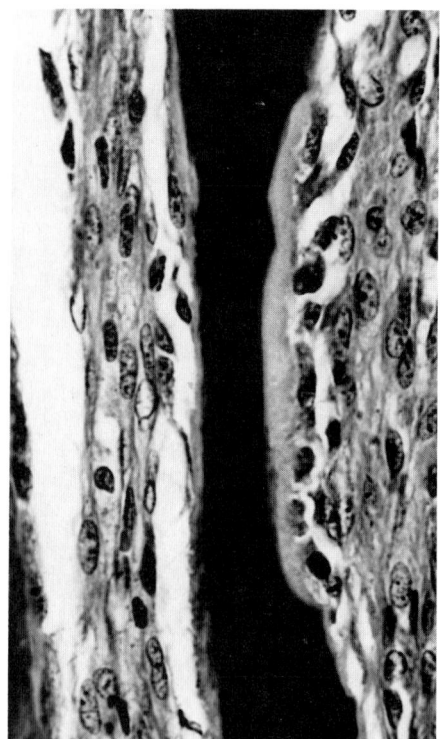

Fig. 8.13 Osteoid seam in a demineralized section of bone. The light-staining region adjacent to the black portion of the spicule is osteoid seam. X140.

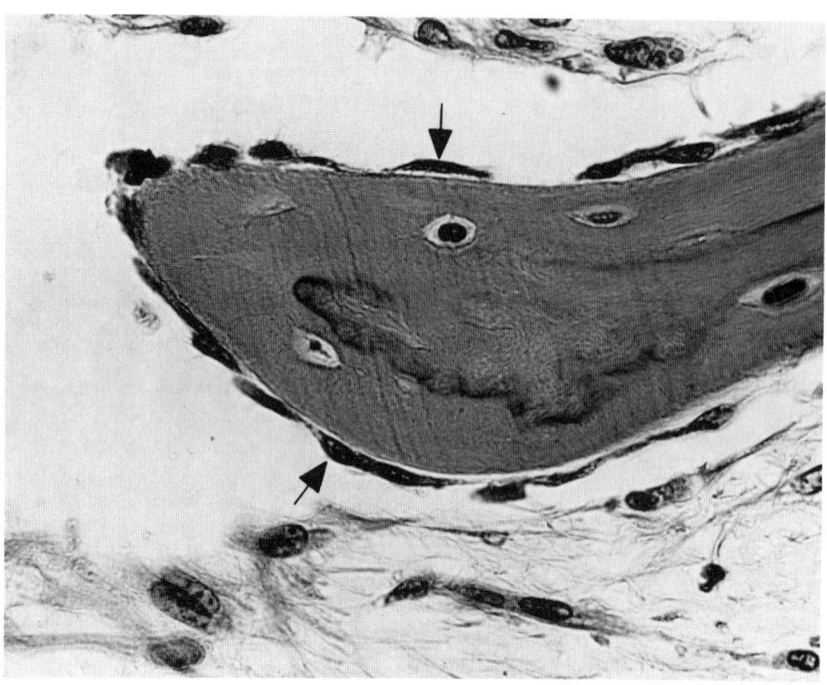

Fig. 8.11 Lining cells upon a spicule of bone. The lining cells (*arrows*) may be inactive osteoblasts or osteoprogenitor cells. X160.

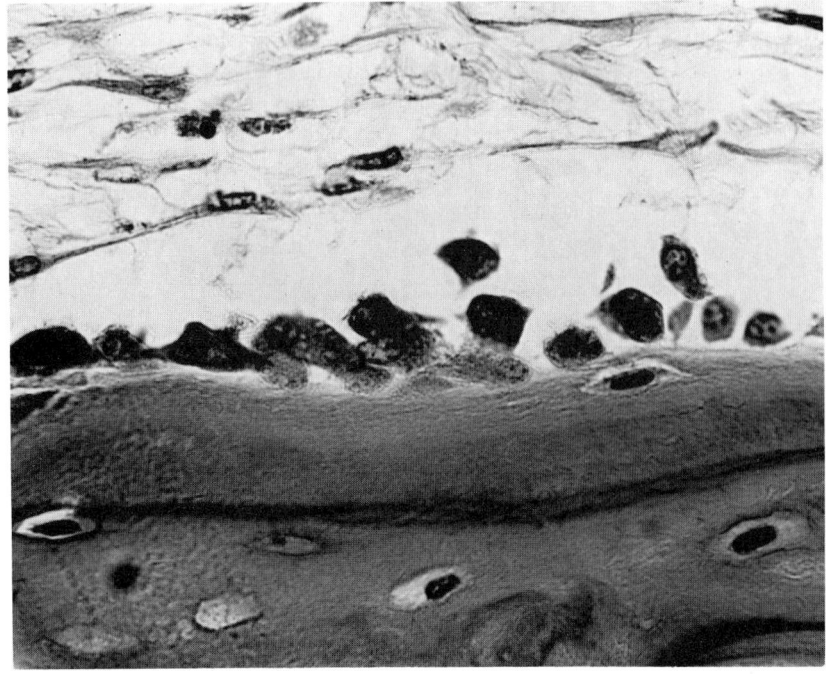

Fig. 8.12 Active lining cells upon a bone surface. The cuboidal cells are osteoblasts. X160.

collagen. Mineralization occurs first on the collagen with the formation of hydroxyapatite crystals adjacent to the fibers and subsequently within the collagenous fibers. The second phase is dependent upon the availability of the component minerals. The attachment of some glycosaminoglycans to collagen may serve to prevent mineralization of the osteoid seam during the first phase. Subsequent removal of some of these substances, then, may facilitate the mineralization of the matrix. Initial mineralization accounts for approximately one-half of the total holding capacity of the matrix. Gradual and progressive addition of mineral at the expense of water occurs over several months.

An understanding of this appositional and biphasic method of the formation of bone as a tissue explains a number of observations. The progressive formation and subsequent mineralization of osteoid seam accounts for the highly ordered and laminar characteristics of mature bone (Fig. 8.15). Disruptions and/or alterations in this orderly sequence can have significant effects upon the quantity and quality of bone that is formed. If the first phase does not occur, then the continual removal of bone by osteoclasts without the balanced formation by osteoblasts results in a quantitative reduction in bone—a *quantitative osteopenia*. If the second phase of the osteoblastic activity does not occur, then the organic matrix does

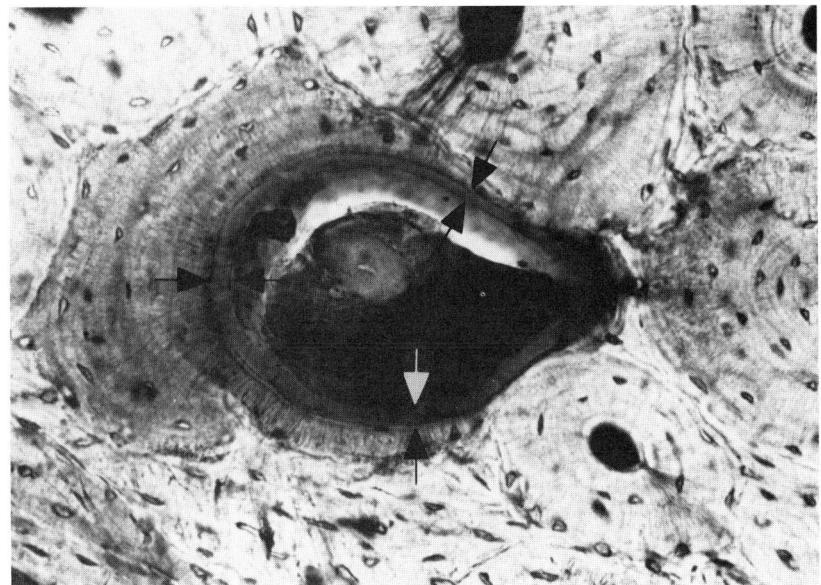

Fig. 8.14 Osteoid seam in a mineralized sample of bone. The arrows delimit the osteoid seam. The centripetal formation of bone in this filling osteon by the progressive deposition and mineralization of osteoid seams will reduce the diameter of the osteonal canal. A mature osteon will result (*lower right*). X25 (ground bone section).

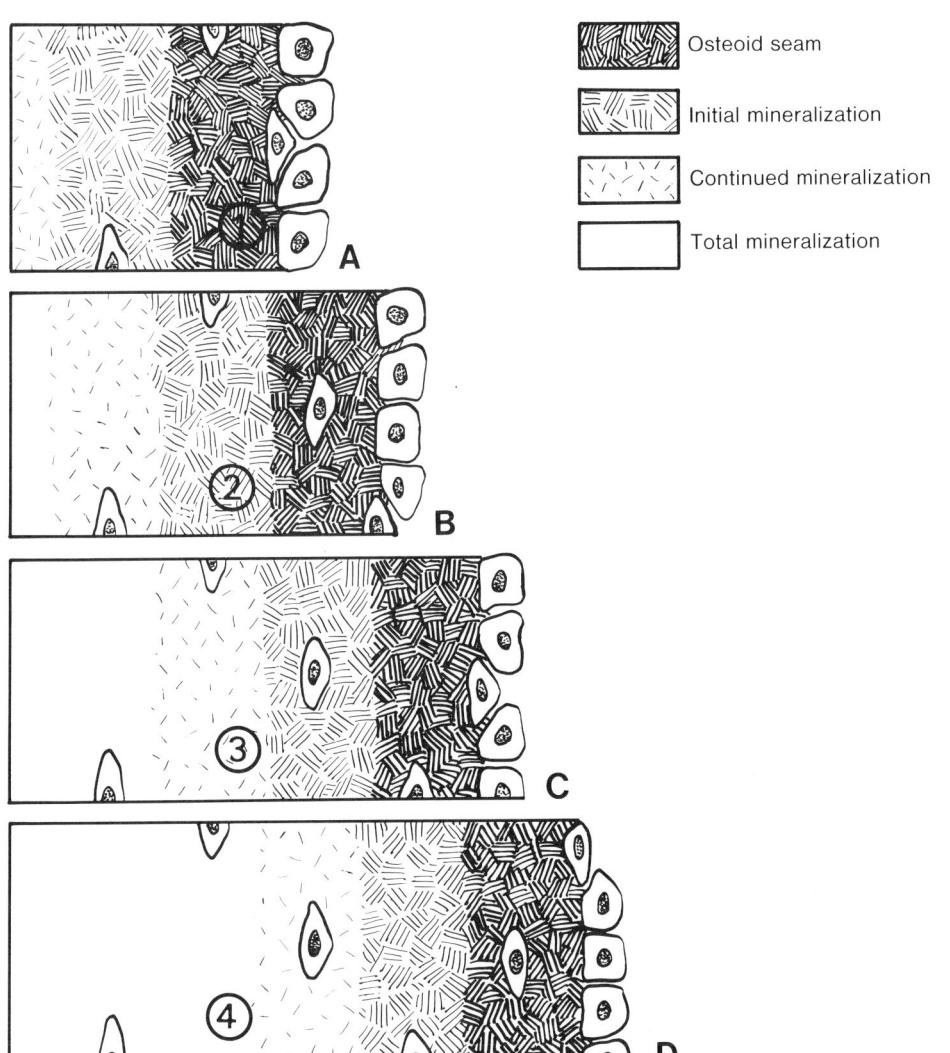

Fig. 8.15 Biphasic secretory activity of osteoblasts during bone formation. Bone formation in the adult occurs on preexisting bone surfaces. The initial stage of osteoblastic activity culminates with the formation of osteoid seam upon a pre-existing bone surface (A). Initial mineralization occurs within the most recent osteoid seam (B). New osteoid seam forms, while older osteoid seams become progressively more mineralized (C). This activity continues (D) until a specified amount of bone forms. Numbers 1–4 indicate the fate of the original osteoid seam formed.

not become mineralized. This results in a qualitative change in bone called a *qualitative osteopenia*.

A quantitative osteopenia is a reduction in bone mass. The bone that is present is normal; there just isn't enough of it. Cushing's syndrome, disuse osteoporosis and senile osteoporosis are diseases characterized by quantitative bone changes. The qualitative bone changes result from too little mineral in the matrix. There may be adequate to excessive amounts of matrix with insufficient amounts of mineral. Rickets, renal secondary hyperparathyroidism and nutritional secondary hyperparathyroidism are examples of diseases associated with qualitative bone changes.

As the osteoblasts secrete their products and retreat before the advancing front of osteoid, a few of the cells (about 1 of 10) become embedded in their own secretory products. At this point the osteoblasts are called osteocytes.

Osteocytes. *Osteocytes* are osteoblasts that have become embedded in their own secretory products. Osteocytes are sometimes observed shortly after they have become embedded in the osteoid seam. These cells are referred to as *osteoid osteocytes* (Fig. 8.16). Once the interstitial substance becomes mineralized, these cells are simply referred to as osteocytes.

The osteocytes appear similar to osteoblasts when examined with light micros-

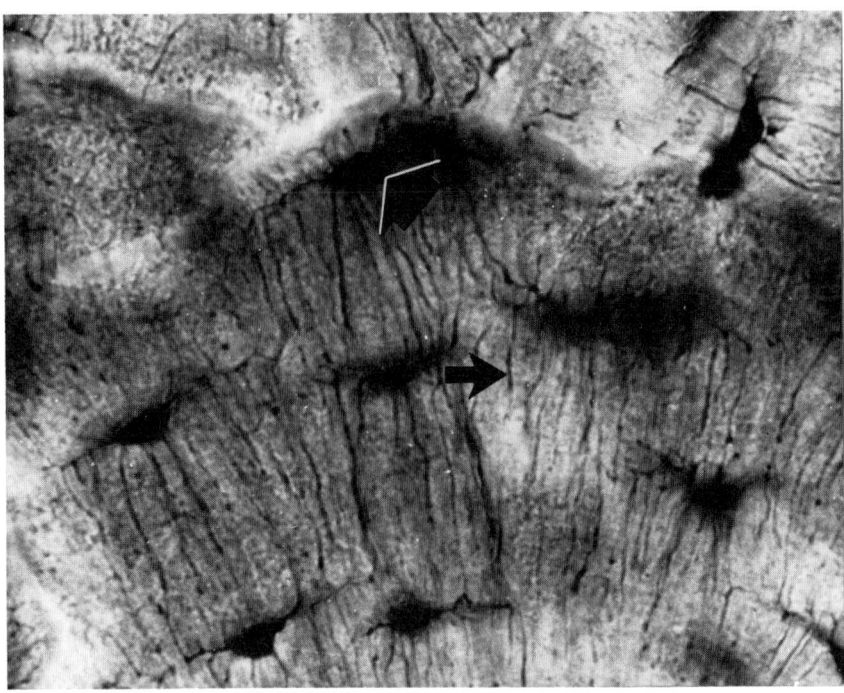

Fig. 8.17 The canalicular system of bone. Osteocytic lacunae (*large arrow*) are continuous with canaliculi (*small arrow*). X200 (ground bone section).

copy. However, osteocytic processes are prominent and the cytoplasm is either weakly basophilic or acidophilic. The osteocyte is a less active form of the osteoblast. The *lacunae*, and the cell as well, may vary from round to lenticular depending upon the type of bone in which they reside. As a result of fixation, osteocytes are retracted away from the lacunar surface. Occasionally, lacunae may appear empty; this is the artifactual result of sectioning. However, empty lacunae may also indicate pathologic changes in bone.

Although the cellular processes of osteocytes are not readily seen at the light microscopic level, the *canaliculi* are easily observed in mineralized sections (Fig. 8.17). Visualization of canaliculi in paraffin sections is enhanced by reducing the quality of the illumination. These canaliculi form an extensive communicative network between osteocytes and the cells on the bone surface (Fig. 8.18). Each canaliculus is occupied by a cellular process of an osteocyte (Fig. 8.19).

The osteocytes were once the "forgotten cells of bone." For years, these cells were considered to be circumstantial victims of the secretory activity of osteoblast. They occupied their position within the matrix and very little attention was directed to them. Today, their function is recognized as being significant. They are responsible for the maintenance of the matrix. They synthesize and secrete matrix materials; however, their activity level is less than that of osteoblasts. Also, they are capable of removing matrix substances. This process of removal of bone by osteocytes is termed *osteolysis*. The ability of these cells to add and

remove bone matrix is an important mechanism in the homeostatic maintenance of blood calcium levels.

The duplicity of function of osteocytes in the maintenance of bone matrix is compelling evidence that supports the concept of modulation of bone cells. They may act like osteoblasts as well as osteoclasts. Additionally, they contribute to the formation of osteoclasts by fusing with them as the osteoclasts move through bone. The subsequent fission of osteoclasts "releases" all of the contributing cells as a new population of osteoprogenitor cells.

Osteoclasts. *Osteoclasts* are multinucleated giant cells of the body that are responsible for the removal of bone. These cells possess the cellular mechanisms necessary for the dissolution of bone mineral as well as the digestion of the organic matrix. They release organic acids (citrate, lactate) which decrease the pH of the microenvironment. The acids dissolve the bone mineral and enhance the activity of lysosomal enzymes that are released—acid hydrolases actively hydrolyze the organic matrix. The process of bone removal mediated by osteoclasts is termed *osteoclasia*.

These cells have few to numerous nuclei contained within a foamy and acidophilic cytoplasm (Fig. 8.20). The cell is polarized; the nuclei are displaced to the cellular border away from the bone (Plate II.4). The cellular border adjacent to the bone is composed of numerous cellular processes—a *brush border* (Fig. 8.21). This brush or *ruffled border* terminates at a smooth zone peripheral to it. This smooth zone may serve as a tight seal between the cell and bone

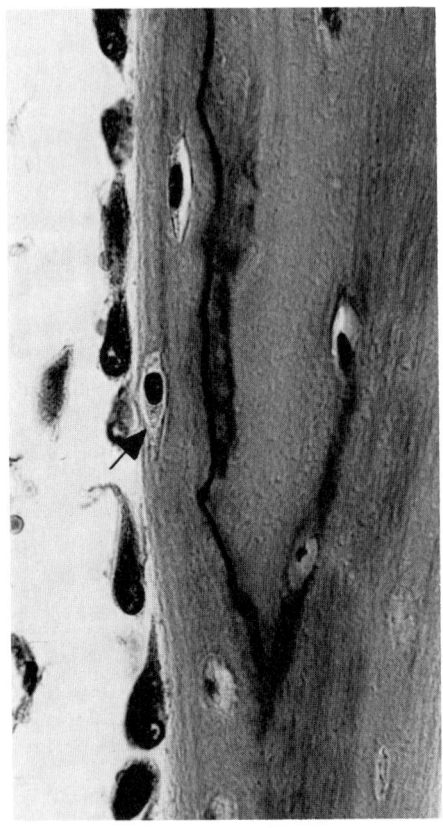

Fig. 8.16 Osteoblasts and osteocytes. An osteoblast was recently incorporated into bone as an osteoid osteocyte (*arrow*). X160.

surface to confine the microenvironmental change to the area subjacent to the active part of the ruffled border.

Osteoclasts reside on the surfaces of bones in concavities called *Howship's lacunae* (Fig. 8.22). They may be artifactually separated from the surface by sectioning. Osteoclasts may be observed along a bone surface in which bone deposition is occurring (Fig. 8.23), or an entire surface may be occupied by osteoclasts. Osteoclasts also develop within compact bone from the cells of the osteonal endosteum. In this instance, Howship's lacunae are continuous with each other as a *resorption space* (Fig. 8.24). The resorption space is the cross-sectional representation of a cylindrical portion of bone that is being removed by osteoclasia. The serrated edges of Howship's lacunae are sufficient evidence that bone resorption is occurring.

The origin and fate of osteoclasts was discussed previously (Fig. 8.9). Osteoprogenitor cells, osteoblasts and osteocytes contribute to the multinucleated giant cells. Some evidence suggests that they may be derived from the bone marrow. Because the osteoclast does not divide, the multinucleations are explained by the fusion with other cells. As these cells move through bone they incorporate other cells. The number of nuclei may correlate with the age and activity of osteoclasts. Upon completion of their resorptive activity, these cells may undergo fission and the cells that had been incorporated may be released as osteoprogenitor cells.

Types Of Bone

All of the bones of the animal body are composed of osseous tissues that are either woven or lamellar bone. These are the two types of bone as a tissue (Fig. 8.25).

Woven Bone. This type of bone is often referred to as *immature bone* or *coarsely bundled bone*, as well as *woven bone*. It is very cellular and the lacunae are very large and round (Fig. 8.26). The lacunae and their contained cells are dispersed randomly throughout the matrix. Bundles of collage-

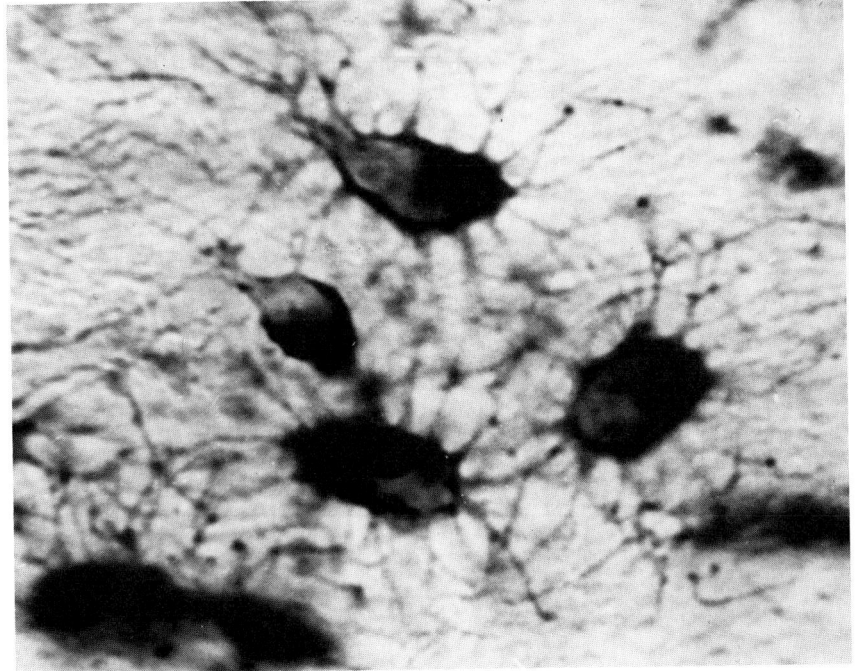

Fig. 8.18 Osteocytic processes and canaliculi. The extensive canalicular system contains osteocytic processes of adjacent cells. The canaliculi are in contact with each other. X320 (ground bone section).

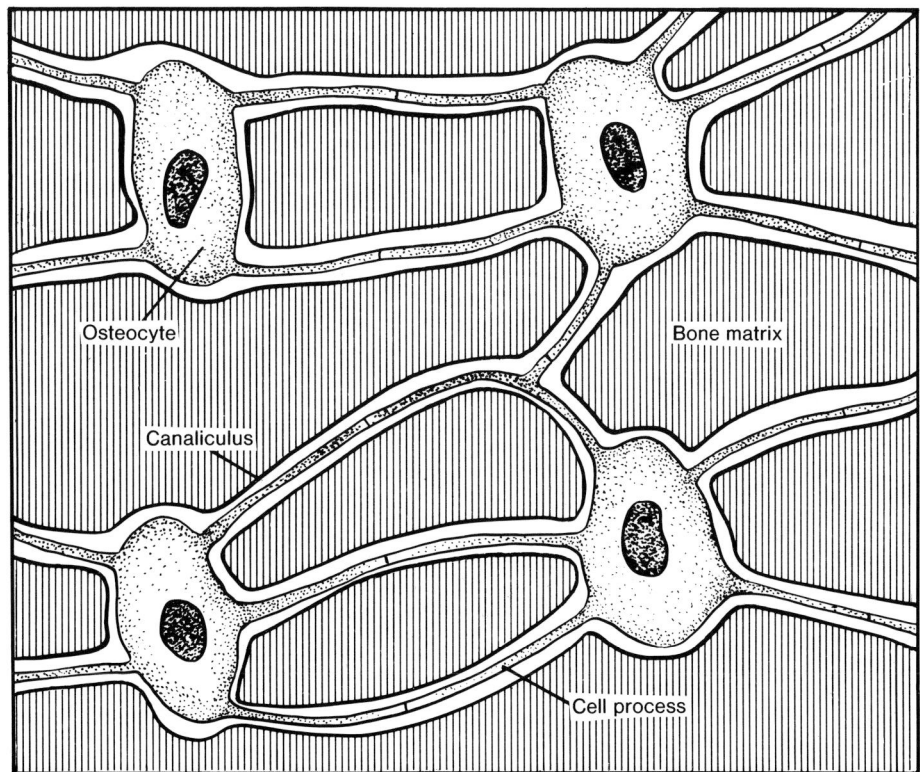

Fig. 8.19 A diagram of osteocytic relationships. Tight junctions occur at points of intercellular contact.

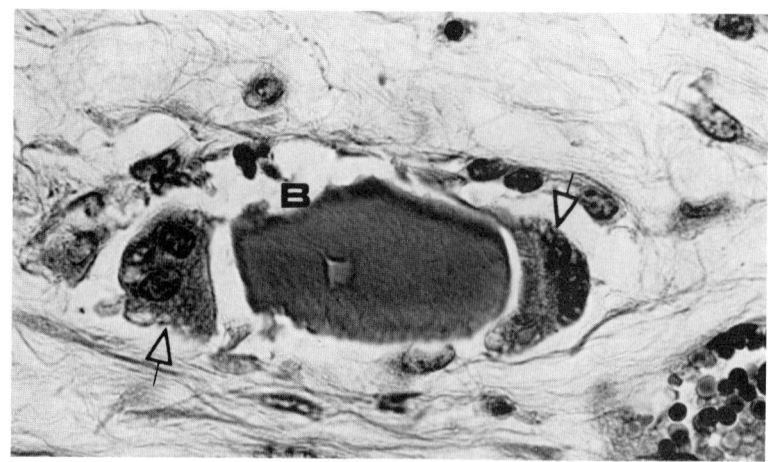

Fig. 8.20 A spicule of bone (B) is being removed by osteoclasia. Osteoclasts (*arrows*) are multinucleated giant cells. X160.

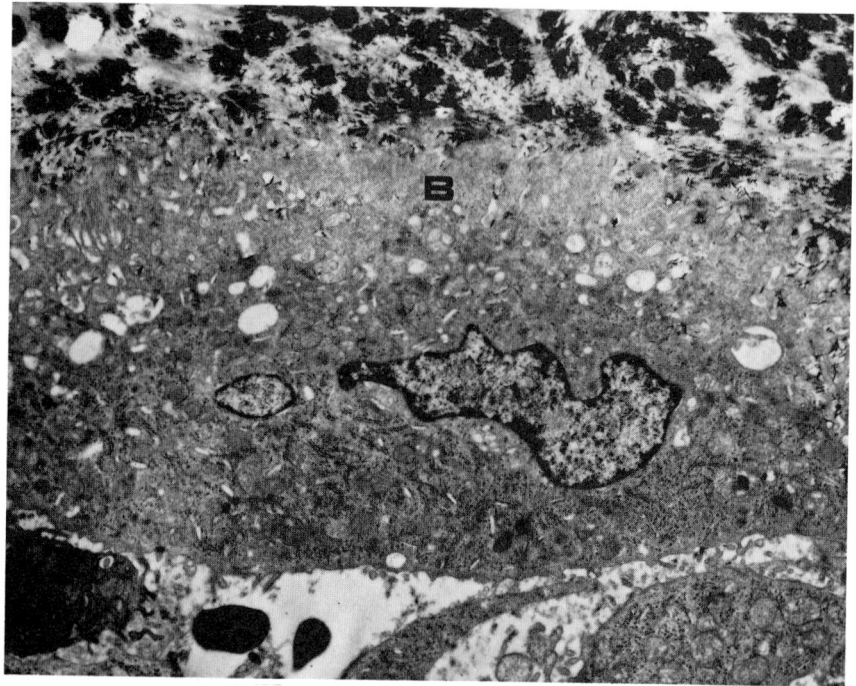

Fig. 8.21 An electron micrograph of an osteoclast. The cell is multinucleated and polarized. The brush border (B) is in contact with the bone surface. X5000.

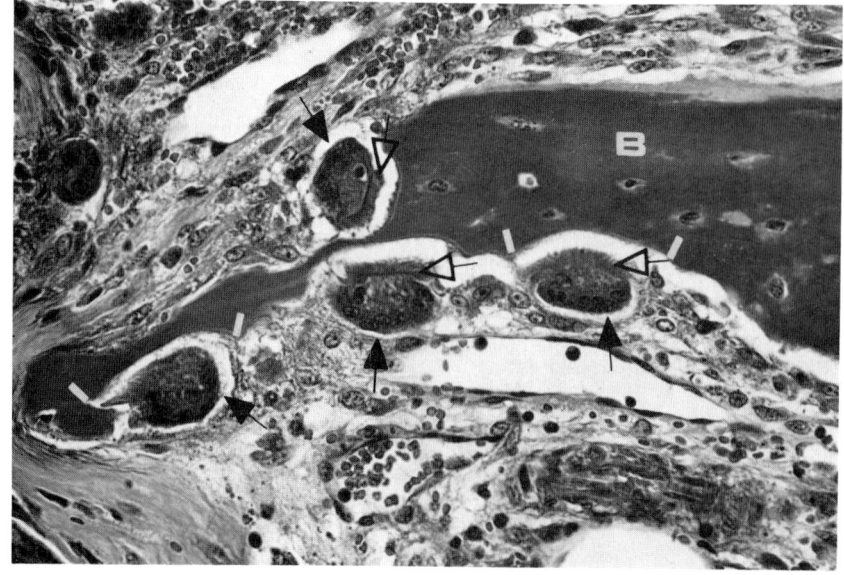

Fig. 8.22 A spicule of bone (B) is being removed and/or remodeled by numerous osteoclasts (*solid arrows*). The boundaries of Howship's lacunae are indicated by *white bars*. Note the brush borders (*open arrows*) and their relationship to the serrated margin of the bone. X100 (Masson's trichrome).

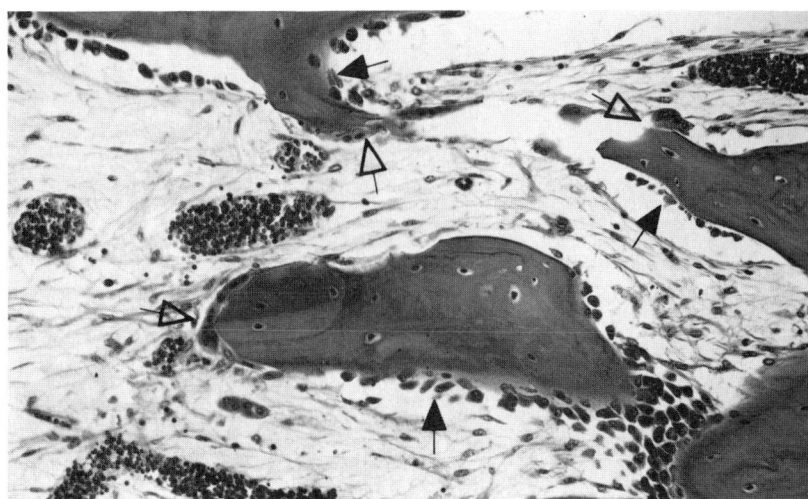

Fig. 8.23 Simultaneous deposition and removal of bone. Osteoblastic activity (*solid arrows*) and osteoclastic activity (*open arrows*) are occurring at the same time. X40.

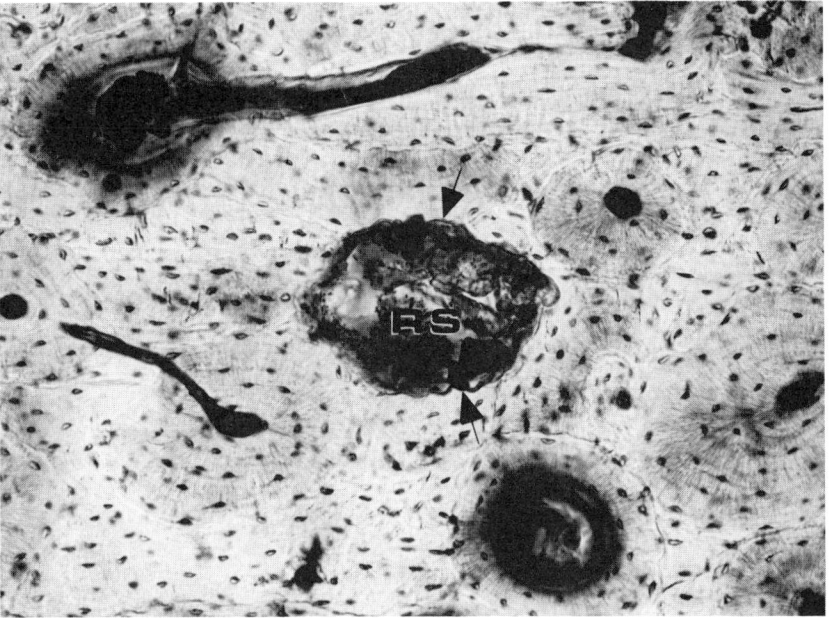

Fig. 8.24 A resorption space in bone. The resorption space (RS) has serrated edges (*arrows*) due to the confluence of Howship's lacunae. X40 (ground bone section).

nous fibers are arranged in a haphazard pattern; thus, there is no regular birefringent pattern with polarizing microscopy. The organic matrix is basophilic, stains unevenly and holds less mineral than mature bone.

Immature bone is the first bone that forms in ossification centers of the fetus and the primary spongiosa of developing adolescent bones. It is also the first bone that forms at the site of fracture repair. Certain types of bone tumors are characterized by this type of bone. Normally, it occurs in alveolar bone associated with teeth and at points of attachment of ligaments and tendons to bone.

Although this type of bone may vary in configuration from cancellous to compact, osteons are rarely composed of this tissue.

Under normal circumstances, this bone is always replaced by lamellar bone. It is a temporary tissue that affords support for the developing organism.

Lamellar Bone. This bone is also referred to as *mature bone*. It comprises the bulk of the adult skeleton. The lacunae, and thus the cells of this bone, are more lenticular than in immature bone (Fig. 8.27). Also, they are dispersed in an orderly fashion throughout the matrix in a pattern that reflects the ordered, lamellar arrangement of the collagen (Fig. 8.2). The collagenous fibers are deposited in helical array at varying angles in successive lamellae; thus, a very ordered pattern of birefringence is apparent with polarizing microscopy. The demineralized

organic matrix of mature bone stains lightly and evenly and is acidophilic.

Configurations Of Bone

Cancellous Bone. Cancellous bone is that bone that is arranged into *spicules* or *trabeculae*. These spicules may be either *woven bone* or *mature bone*. In the adult skeleton they are most probably composed of mature bone.

The diagnostic feature of cancellous bone is that there is more interosseous space than there is bone (Fig. 8.28). There are, however, numerous gradations of this type of configuration (Fig. 8.29).

Compact Bone. Compact bone represents the extreme in amount of bone formation. Characteristically, there is more bone than interosseous space (Fig. 8.30). In this configuration, there are gradations also. Compact bone may be organized into laminae (*lamellae*) or *osteons* (*Haversian systems*).

Organization Of Bone

Lamellae of Bone. This organizational pattern is typical of the bone-forming activity of the *periosteum* and portions of the *endosteum*. Successive *lamellae* or *laminae* of mature bone are deposited in extensive sheets of bone that are referred to as the *outer circumferential lamellae* or *periosteal lamellae* (Fig. 8.31). The cortical endosteum associated with the marrow cavity also gives rise to laminae or lamellae of bone. This bone constitutes the *inner circumferential lamellae* or *endosteal lamellae* (Fig. 8.32). These inner lamellae may be continued on trabeculae of bone comprising the cancellous bone of the marrow cavity.

Osteonal Bone. Osteonal bone is the lamellar bone that comprises *osteons* or *Haversian systems* (Figs. 8.33, 8.34). It is disposed in concentric laminae or sheets around an *osteonal canal* or *Haversian canal* (Fig. 8.35). The peripheral limits of the osteonal bone are marked by a *reversal line* or *cement line*. The osteonal canal contains blood vessels as well as cells of the osteonal endosteum.

Osteons are either primary or secondary. *Primary* osteons are formed on the periosteal surface. They are cylinders with small diameters that are composed of a few concentric laminae of bone. Their method of formation at the periosteal surface is depicted in Figure 8.36. They add strength to bone, smooth the surfaces at which they are formed and account for continuity of periosteal vessels with those of the compact bone. The formation of these structures not only demonstrates clearly the continuity of the envelopes of bone but demonstrates that the periosteum becomes the osteonal endosteum.

Secondary osteons are concentric laminae of bone that form within compact bone in response to various stimuli. The only prerequisite for their formation is the existence of a tunnel within the bone. The most ob-

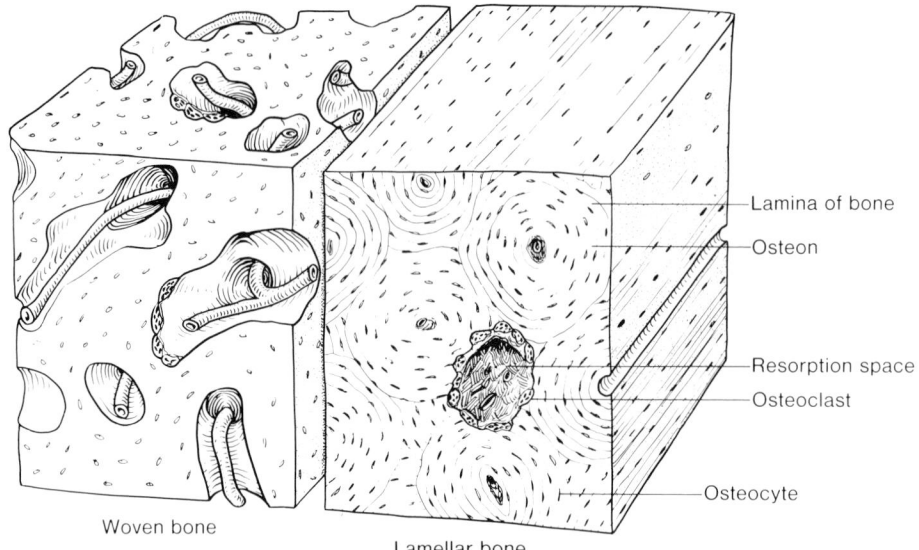

Lamina of bone

Osteon

Resorption space

Osteoclast

Osteocyte

Woven bone

Lamellar bone

Fig. 8.25 A diagram comparing the differences between woven and lamellar bone. The organizational differences are marked. Especially note the difference in the disposition of osteocytic lacunae. Lamellar bone comprises the bulk of the adult skeletal mass.

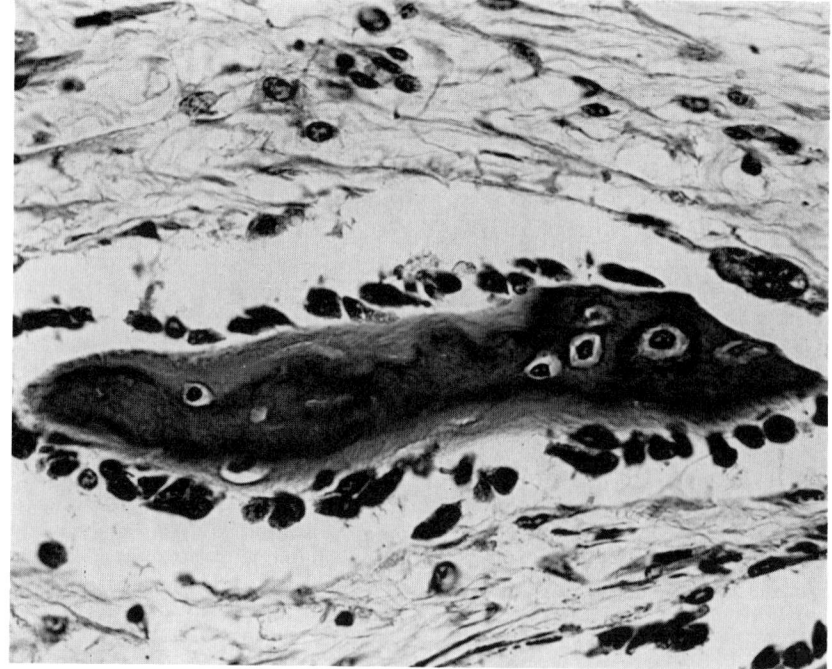

Fig. 8.26 Woven bone in the developing bovine mandible. Note the mottled appearance of the matrix, large osteocytes and random orientation of osteocytes. X100.

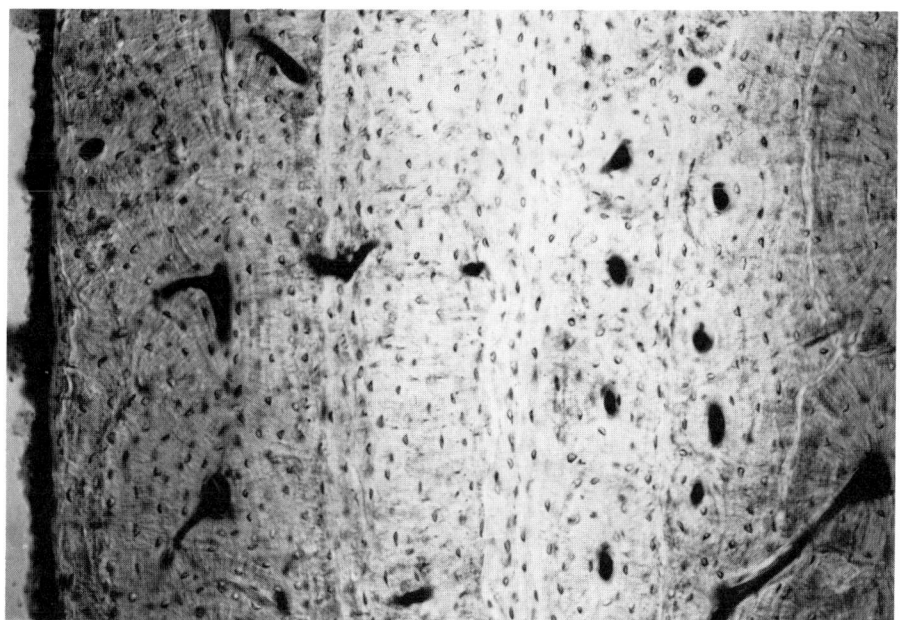

Fig. 8.27   Lamellar bone. The lamellar nature of the bone is indicated by the ordered disposition of osteocytic lacunae. X40 (ground bone section).

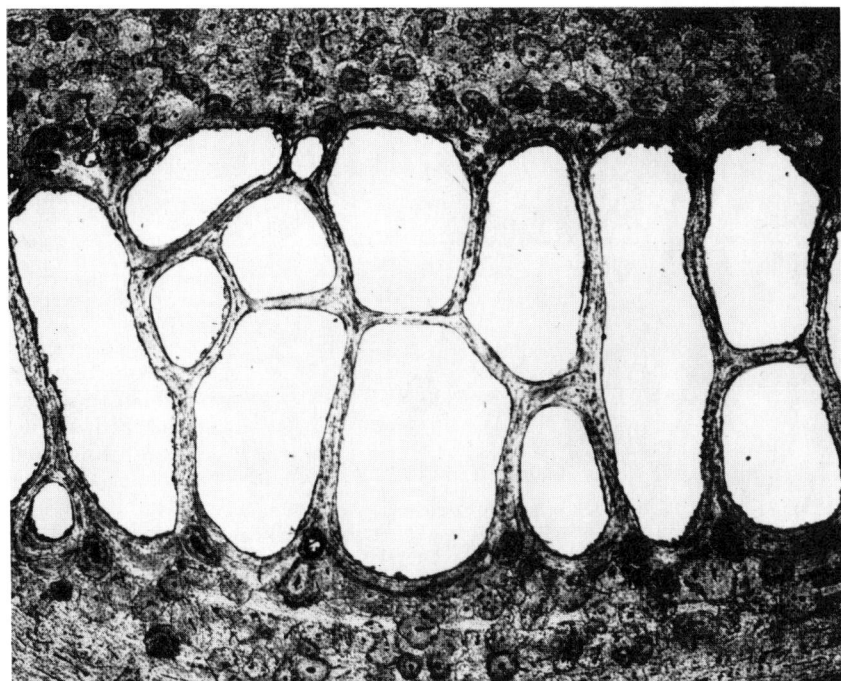

Fig. 8.28   Cancellous bone of the marrow cavity of a cervine rib. X10 (ground bone section).

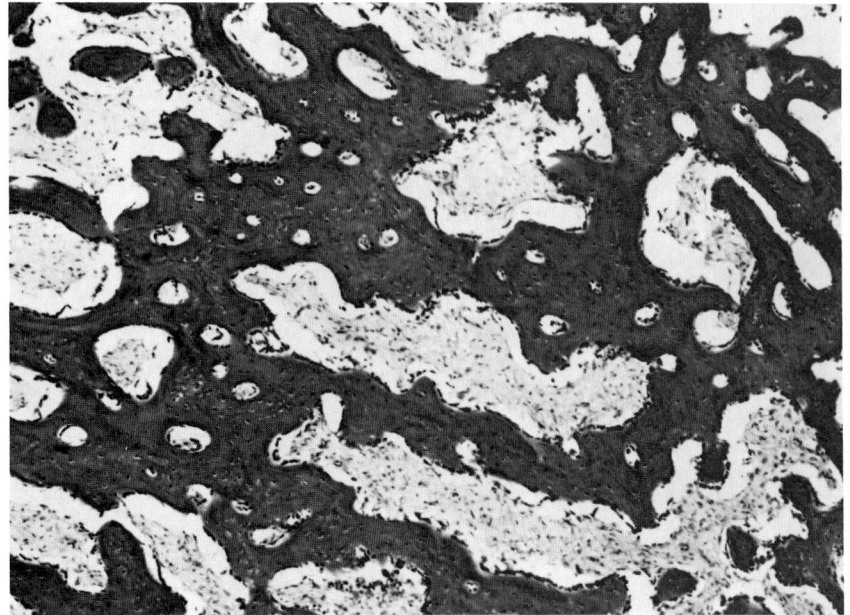

Fig. 8.29 Dense cancellous bone of a developing canine humerus. The interosseous space is reduced and the amount of bone is increased. Compare with Figure 8.27. X16.

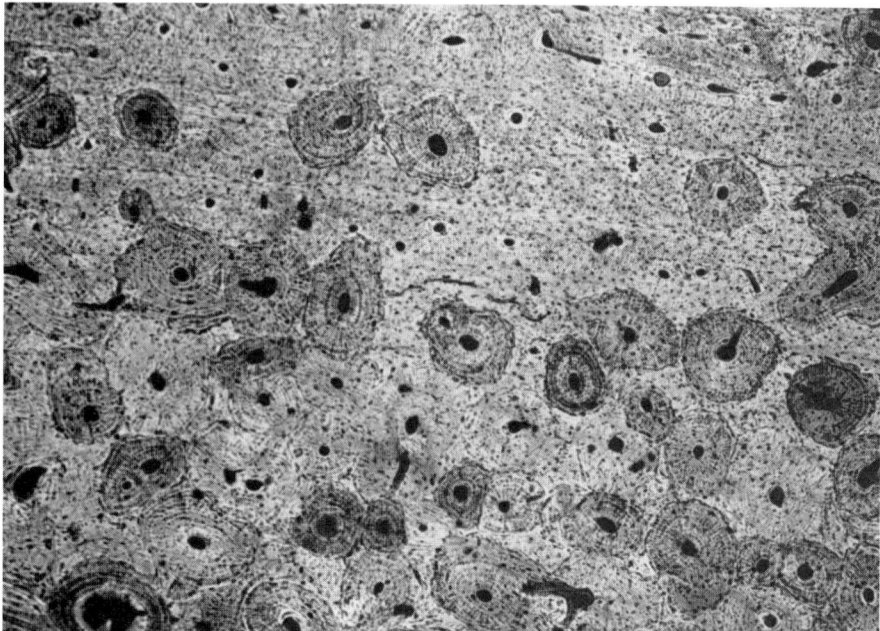

Fig. 8.30 Compact bone of an adult canine humerus. The interosseous space is reduced appreciably and is confined to the osteonal and communicating canals. This section of bone is comprised of portions of the outer circumferential lamellae, interstitial and osteonal bone. X16 (ground bone section).

tion of previously-formed osteons, the formation of new osteons and the formation of remnants of osteonal and circumferential bone. The remnants are called *interstitial bone* (Figs. 8.7, 8.34, 8.35 and 8.37). The secondary osteons may abut each other or may be separated by segments of interstitial bone. Also, secondary osteons may be isolated within circumferential bone.

Osteons are the *structural units of bone*. In their simplest form they are long cylinders with a hollow cavity, the osteonal canal, in their center. In actuality, they may be extensively branched. They are usually found in those areas where bone is subjected to great stress. Thus, they may be likened to bundles of reinforcing rods in concrete.

The blood vessels of bone, whether associated with circumferential lamellae or osteons, were entrapped during developmental stages. These vessels are connected with vessels at the periosteal or cortical endosteal surface through large *Volkmann's canals*. Osteonal vessels freely communicate with each other through *communicating canals* (Fig. 8.38). Thus, the internal vascular supply is extensively anastomotic and is in communication with cortical endosteal and/or periosteal vessels. The three-dimensional relationship of all these elements is important to keep in mind (Fig. 8.7).

Dynamics Of Bone

Internal Remodeling. Although the gross anatomic features of bones do not change appreciably throughout the life of the animal, constant changes occur within the substance of bone as a tissue. The process by which bones change their internal characteristics without altering gross morphology is termed *internal remodeling*. This special lifelong activity involves the removal of old lamellar bone and its replacement by new lamellar bone. Internal remodeling is the responsibility of the internal envelopes of bone (cortical, trabecular and osteonal endosteum). Although all three envelopes contribute to this activity, the most reliable data and greatest amount of information has been obtained for the internal remodeling activity that is osteonal envelope-associated. It is important to note, however, that trabecular bone is more labile than osteonal bone and trabecular endosteal remodeling activity may be as much as three times greater than osteonal activity. Again, the qualitative and quantitative study of compact bone turnover is easier to accomplish than the study of the turnover or internal remodeling of trabecular bone. The principles of compact bone turnover are applicable to that of trabecular bone turnover, but the stereological relationships are different. The subsequent discussion of this phenomenon is limited to the internal remodeling activity of the osteonal endosteum.

Numerous stimuli result in internal remodeling. Bones remodel throughout life in

vious tunnel is that of the primary osteon. The tunnel or osteonal canal of these structures contain the cells necessary for the formation of osteoclasts. Osteoclasts remove bone and expand the limits of the osteonal canal. The limit of this osteoclasia is defined by the *reversal line*. The reversal line, then, is the peripheral limit of bone removal and is the surface upon which new bone is deposited by osteoblasts. Thus, the term reversal line better describes the function of this osseous interface than the term *cement line*. The centripetal deposition of successive laminae of bone results in the formation of new osteons, secondary osteons (Figs. 8.34, 8.35, 8.37). This general term is applicable to all subsequent generations of osteons, whether they are secondary, tertiary or quarternary. This type of bone resorptive and formative activity results in the destruc-

response to all of the following: altered vascular relationships that require the repositioning of vessels within the compact bone to insure adequate nutrition for osteocytes; response to altered biomechanical stress upon bone that necessitates the repositioning and/or orientation of constituent osteons; response to stress that requires the replacement of primary osteons and circumferential bone by secondary osteons; the mobilization of bone mineral in response to dietary deficiencies and/or the malabsorption of adequate amounts of calcium; the immobilization and disuse generally associated with bones adjacent to a fracture site during the convalescent stages of fracture repair; the internal reorganization that actually results in the repair of a fracture; altered endocrine signals that can be associated with aging, endocrine diseases and/or imbalance, and prolonged use of certain chemotherapeutic agents. Importantly, internal remodeling is a normal process. It can be increased in response to any, all or a combination of the previously mentioned factors.

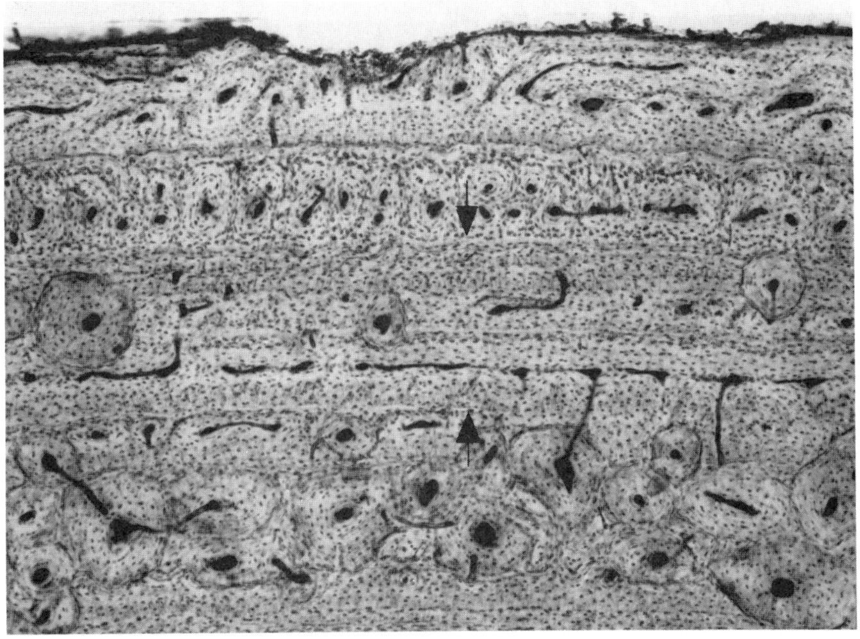

The evidence of internal remodeling, past or present, is recorded in the matrix. The histologist uses a number of keys to determine the extent of this process; primary and secondary osteons, interstitial bone, resorption spaces and the amount of bone present at a specific locus of compact bone. These morphologic features afford insights concerning the number and type of changes that have occurred in the matrix, as well as the balance of activity between formative and resorptive processes.

The homeostatic maintenance of skeletal volume is achieved through the balanced activity of osteoblasts and osteoclasts. These cells are the significant cells of an *osteonal remodeling unit*. (It is important to remember that these events of internal remodeling occur in all endosteal envelopes of bones, but they are best defined in terms of the osteonal endosteal envelope.) This unit includes these cells and the matrix features associated with their activity. In the normal, adult skeleton that is in perfect balance, the amount of bone formation must be equal to bone resorption. Moreover, the only possible way for internal remodeling to occur is to first remove bone from the compacta. This does occur in response to specific and varied stimuli. Subsequently, bone is replaced in the area from whence it was removed originally. The combined activity of the osteonal remodeling unit, internal remodeling, is described by the following relationships: IR = ARF; where IR is internal remodeling; A is activation; R is remodeling and F is formation. The activation signal stimulates osteoprogenitor cells and/or osteoblasts to modulate to osteoclasts. Bone is removed and is replaced subsequently. In the normal animal skeleton, R=F. Although there are numerous permutations for the relationship between R and F, the most significant is the quantitative reduction of bone (osteopenia) that results when R>F.

In any cross-section of bone, resorption spaces, mature osteons and filling osteons are apparent. The temporal and spatial relationships of these structures are more easily described when a longitudinal section is compared to cross sections (Figs. 8.39, 8.40, 8.41). Modulation of osteoprogenitor cells to osteoclasts occurs at a given point in an osteon in response to an activating stimulus. The osteoclasts proceed down the tunnel formed by the endosteal/bone interface and remove bone both longitudinally and centrifugally. This cavitation process expands the diameter of the osteonal canal, the peripheral limit of which becomes the reversal line. Although this osteoclastic activity progresses away from the point of activation via the *cutting cone*, osteoprogenitor cells modulate to osteoblasts at the same origination point. So, formation follows resorp-

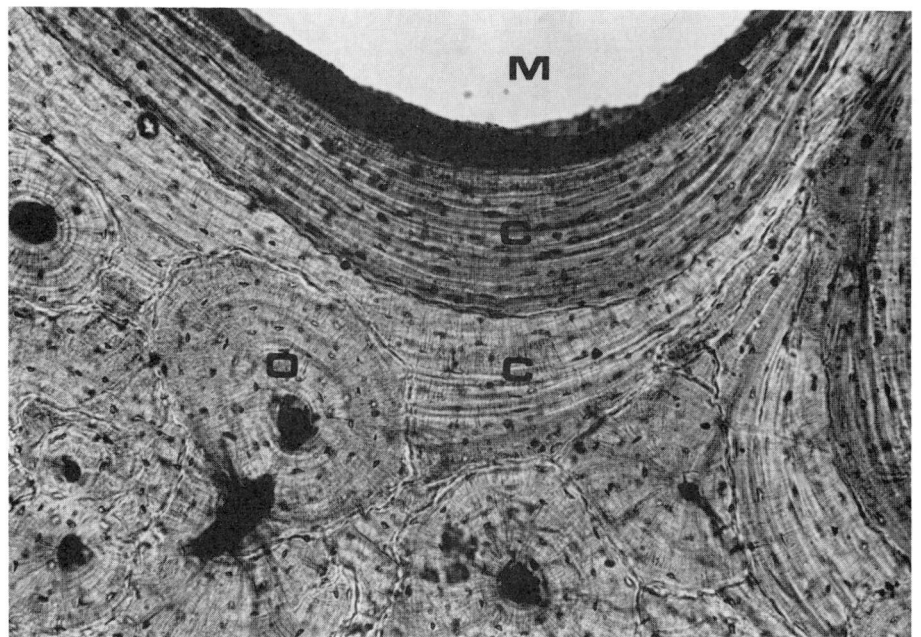

Fig. 8.31 Outer circumferential lamellae and primary osteons of a transverse section of juvenile bone. The circumferential lamellae occur between the *arrows*. The lamellae alternate with layers of primary osteons. X16 (ground bone section).

Fig. 8.32 Inner circumferential lamellae. The marrow cavity (M) is bordered by the inner circumferential bone (C). An osteon (O) has formed within part of the circumferential lamellae as a result of internal remodeling. X40 (ground bone section).

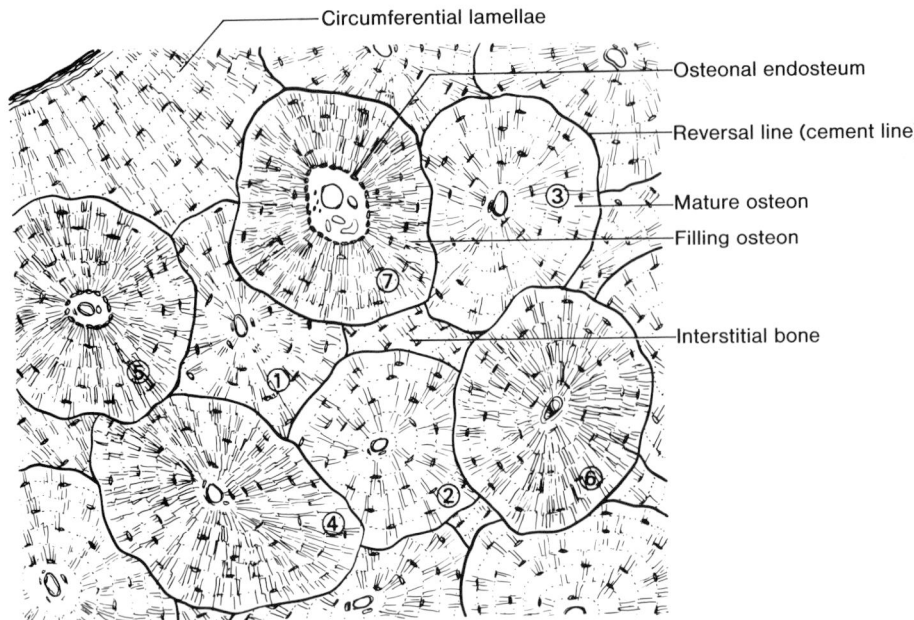

Fig. 8.33 A diagram of a cross-section of mature bone. All of the osteons are secondary; they formed as a result of internal remodeling. Interstitial remnants resulted from the formation of osteons 1, 2, and 3, the first generation of secondary osteons. Osteons 4, 6, and 7, *second generation osteons*, infringed upon osteons 1, 2 and 3 during their formation. Osteon 5, a third generation osteon, infringed upon the first and second generation osteons.

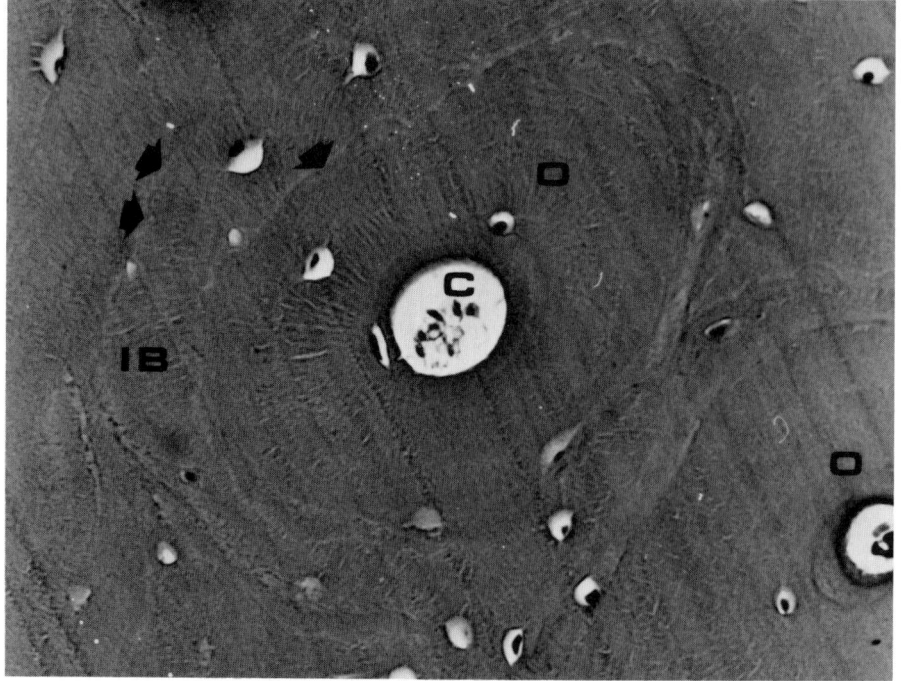

Fig. 8.34 Cross-section of compact bone. The limits of secondary osteons (O) are the reversal lines (*solid arrows*). A remnant of a previous generation osteon as interstitial bone (IB) is apparent. The reversal line of the old osteon is apparent (*double arrows*). The osteonal canal (C) contains endosteum. X100.

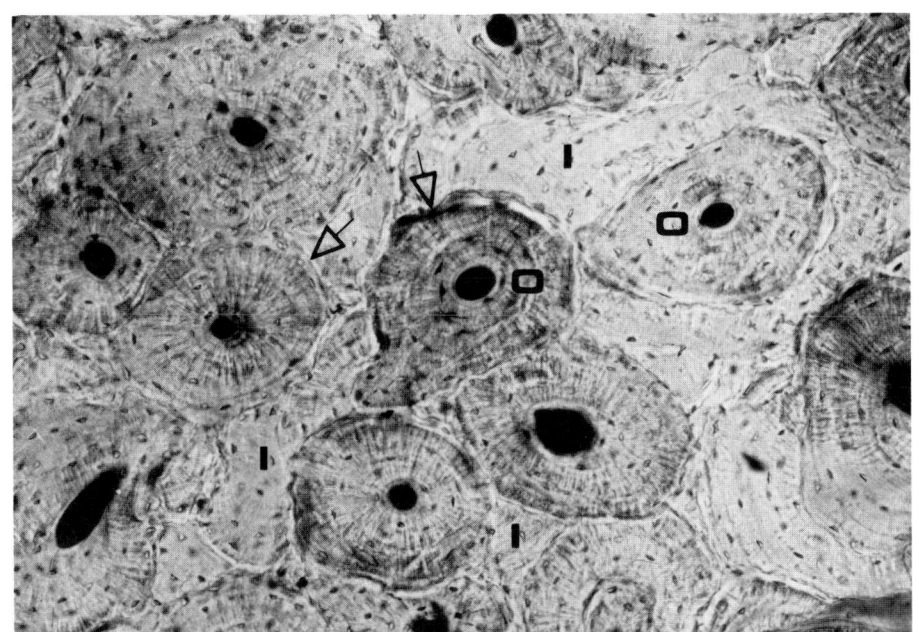

Fig. 8.35 Osteons, interstitial remnants and the compacta. I, interstitial; O, osteons. All of the osteons in this section are mature. The osteonal canals, dark areas within the osteon, are small. *Open arrows*, reversal lines. X40 (ground bone section).

tion. Eventually, osteoclastic activity ceases, whereas the osteoblasts continue to form new bone by apposition from the original reversal line. This centripetal process results in the formation of a new osteon. (Tetracycline labels may be given at timed intervals to determine bone apposition rates at a given locus (Fig. 2.5).

The resorption space is a cross-sectional representation of a sequence of events that resulted in the removal of an entire cylinder of bone (Fig. 8.40). The *filling osteons* represent various stages in the formation process that eventually culminates in the formation of *mature osteons* (Figs. 8.33, 8.35, 8.37, 8.38, 8.42). The timing of these events from osteoclastic activity to mature osteon is measured in months. When examining cross sections of bone it is important to remember that internal remodeling was responsible for the specific morphologic features of the compact bone. Further, the activity of the osteonal remodeling unit resulted in the distribution of its numerous components—secondary osteons, mature osteons, filling osteons, resorption spaces and interstitial bone. Successive and timed doses of tetracyclines aptly demonstrate the sequential centripetal growth of filling osteons (Fig. 8.43) (Plate I.10).

Hormones and Bone. Numerous hormones influence the structure of bone and are involved in the regulation, directly or indirectly, of calcium. One of the hormones exerting a regulatory effect upon bone is *parathormone (PTH)*. This hormone is released from the parathyroid glands by the direct influence of decreased blood calcium levels (hypocalcemia). Through its influence upon its target organs (bone, gut, kidney), it

favors the release of calcium into the blood. Thus, it is the *hypercalcemic factor*. PTH is released in periods of calcium need (*hypocalcemia*) and its most immediate effect upon bone is probably manifested upon the osteocyte. PTH stimulation results in osteolysis. Osteocytes and osteoblasts cooperate in the movement of bone mineral from the bone to the extracellular fluid space. Prolonged PTH stimulation results in the activation of osteonal remodeling units and the level of internal remodeling activity is increased. A delay or arrest in the formation stage of this process results in a net gain of released bone mineral. Because calcium and phosphate are released as a result of bone activity in response to PTH, the effect of this hormone upon the kidney is especially significant. Parathormone stimulates an increased absorption of calcium from the proximal convoluted tubule of the nephron. Under PTH stimulation, the resorption of phosphate by the proximal convoluted tubule is inhibited. This results in an increased loss of urinary phosphate. Because the product of the solubilities of calcium and phosphorus is equal to a constant, the increased phosphaturia aids the elevation of blood calcium levels. Also, PTH indirectly enhances the absorption of calcium and phosphate from the gut by stimulating the formation of an active metabolite of vitamin D.

Whereas PTH favors the elevation of blood calcium levels, *calcitonin* or *thyrocalcitonin (TCT)* favors the depression of blood calcium levels. It is released from the parafollicular cells of the thyroid gland in response to the direct stimulation of elevated blood calcium levels (*hypercalcemia*). Thus,

it is the *hypocalcemic factor*, because it favors the lowering of blood calcium levels. Although blood calcium is maintained at a homeostatic level (10 mg%), it constantly undulates slightly above and below this concentration. Both of these hormones, then, function synergistically to maintain 10 mg% (*normocalcemia*). PTH is released when calcium drops below normocalcemic levels and TCT is released when calcium goes above normocalcemic levels. The single target of TCT is bone. It favors the deposition of calcium in bone through the stimulation of osteoblastic and osteocytic formative activities. Calcium is deposited in bone in association with the collagen produced by these cells.

There are numerous species differences associated with the effects of the gonadal hormones upon the mature skeleton. The removal of the ovaries in a mature female leads to a loss of skeletal mass. A similar phenomenon occurs in the old (senile) female. *Estrogen* probably exerts an inhibitory effect upon osteoclasia. Removal of this inhibition results in an increased internal remodeling activity in which R>F. Although formation may be normal, resorption is increased. The effect of *testosterone* upon the mature skeleton seems to be similar to that of estrogen.

Glucocorticosteroids have an inhibitory effect upon the cellular components of the osteonal remodeling unit. However, the inhibition upon osteoblastic activity is greater than the inhibition upon osteoclasia. Thus, R>F and bone loss still results. This type of skeletal alteration can be a significant feature of Cushing's disease.

The *thyroid hormones* (T_3 and T_4) exert a direct stimulatory effect upon the metabolism of bone that favors an increased turnover of this tissue. In extreme cases of prolonged osseous stimulation, skeletal rarification can occur when resorption exceeds formation.

Although *somatotropin (growth hormone)* manifests its influence primarily upon the developing skeleton, this hormone is essential for normal repair processes of bone.

Vitamin D. The growth, maintenance and repair of the skeleton is dependent upon a number of nutritional factors. Calcium and phosphorus, in proper quantity and proper Ca/P ratio (1.4/1.0), are essential dietary constituents for a normal skeleton. Vitamin C is necessary in the diet for the synthesis of bone collagen; however, with the exception of primates and guinea pigs, domestic animals are able to synthesize vitamin C. Vitamin A is a dietary requirement for the development of a normal skeleton.

The significance of vitamin D in calcium metabolism has been recognized for years. Deficiencies of this substance in growing animals causes disruptions of the normal calcification mechanisms of cartilage and bone called *rickets*. In the adult, disruptions of bone mineralization from vitamin D de-

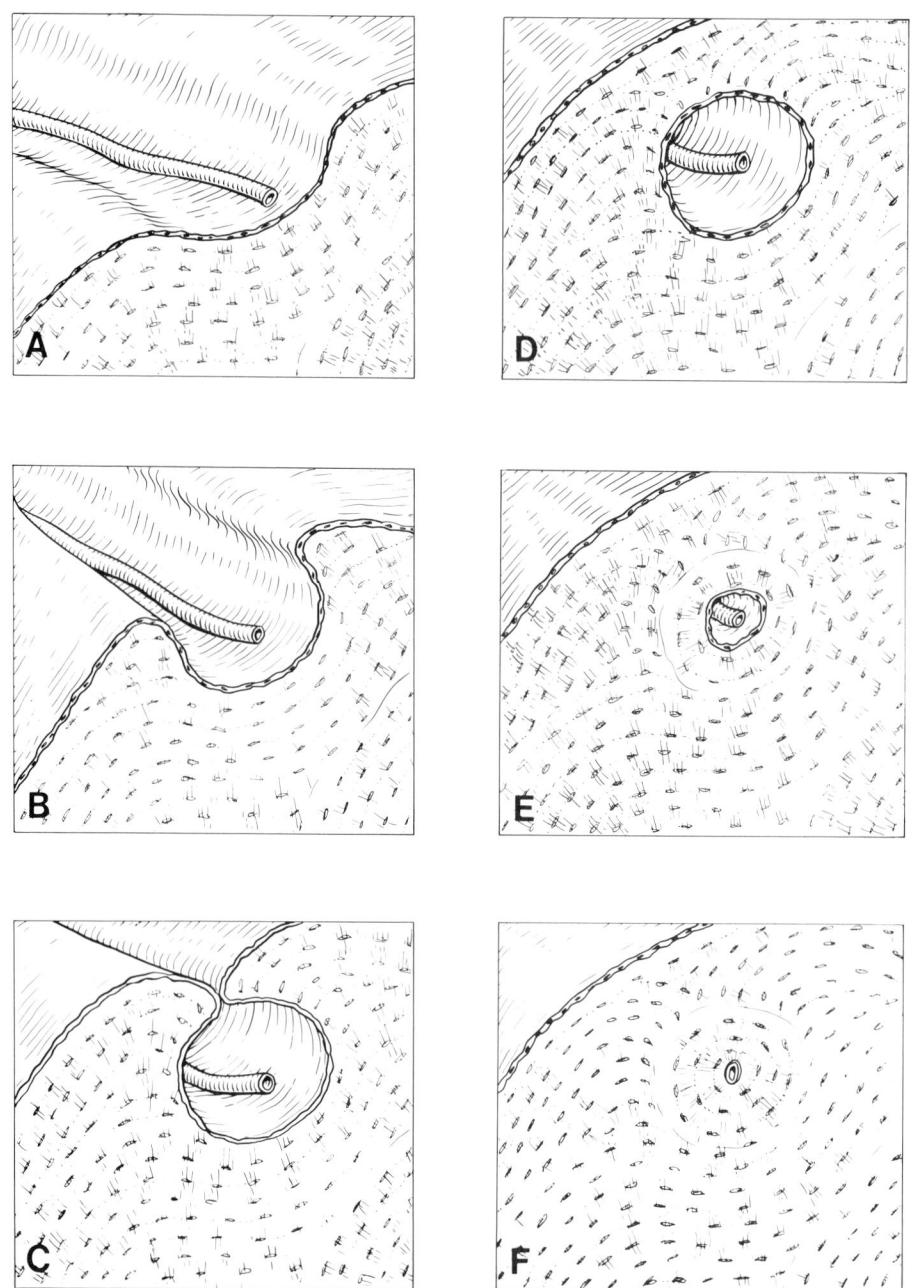

Fig. 8.36 A diagram of the development of primary osteons at the periosteal surface. Longitudinal depressions on the periosteal surface (A) become covered by bone (B and C) as a result of differential osteoblastic activity. Blood vessels and periosteal elements (D) become entrapped in the substance of the compact bone. The envelope is now called osteonal endosteum. Centripetal growth (E) results in the formation of a primary osteon (F). (Redrawn and modified from Ham, A. W.: Histology, 6th edition, J. B. Lippincott, Philadelphia, 1969).

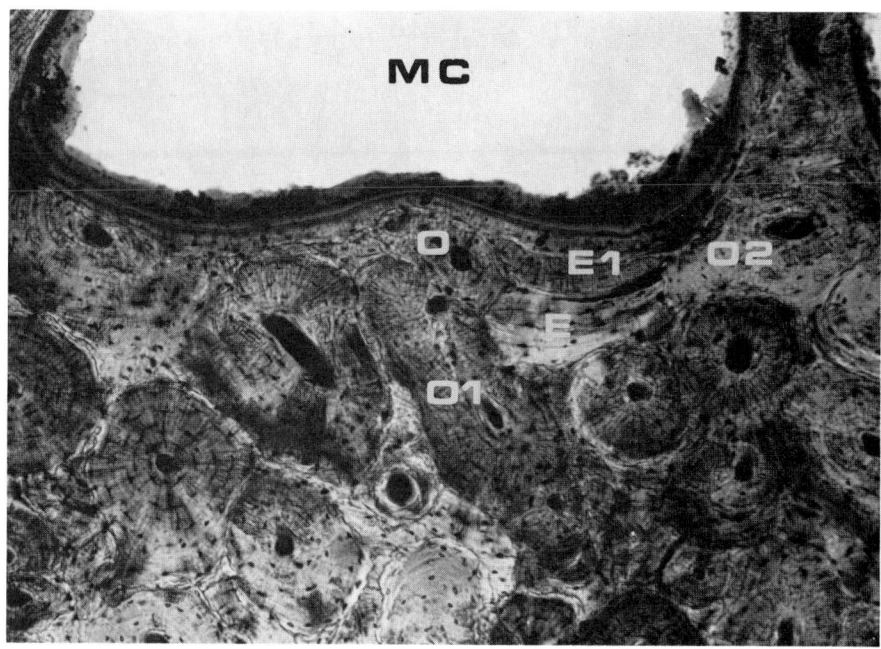

Fig. 8.37 Secondary osteons and interstitial bone. The marrow cavity (MC) is bordered by remnants of inner circumferential lamellae (E1) which are interrupted by an osteon (O). Osteons (O1, O2) also interrupt the endosteal bone (E). Compare with Figures 8.32, 8.33 and 8.35. X25 (ground bone section).

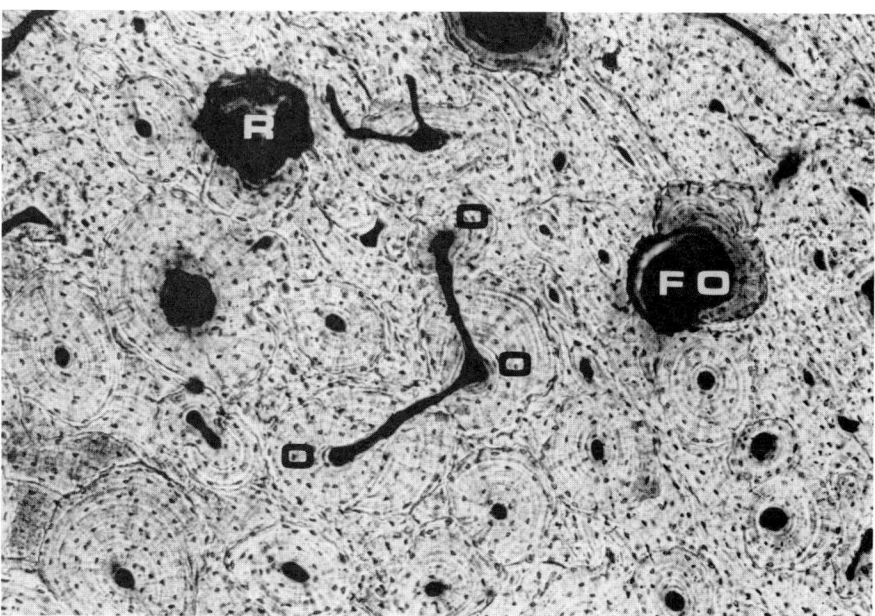

Fig. 8.38 Section of compact bone. Communicating canals connect with three osteonal canals (O). A resorption space (R) and a filling osteon (FO) are present. X25 (ground bone section).

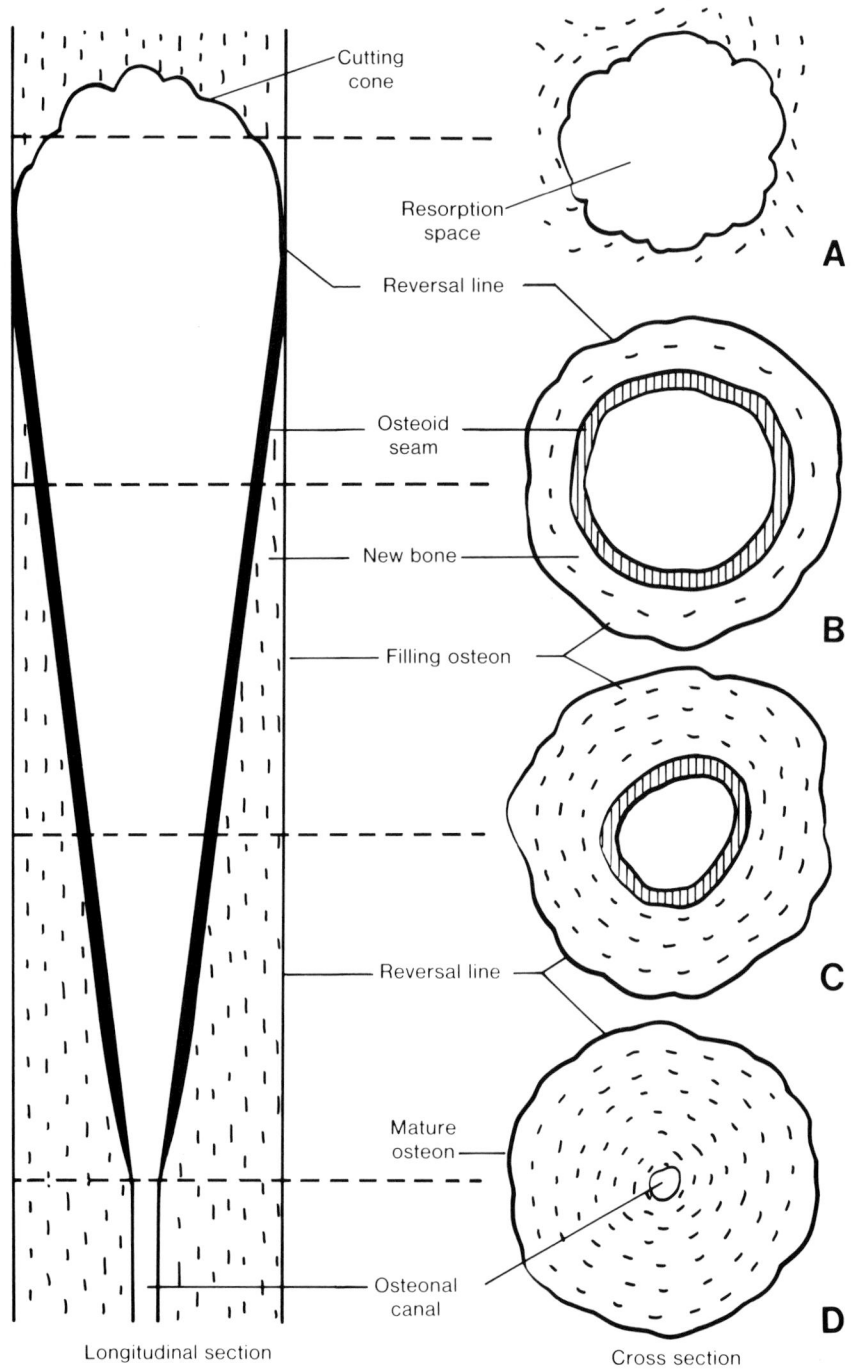

Longitudinal section

Cross section

Fig. 8.39 Diagram of longitudinal and cross sectional representations of an osteonal remodeling unit. The cutting cone, initiated at D, moved along the osteonal canal removing bone longitudinally and centrifugally. Point A represents the cutting cone. Gradual refilling with new bone (points B and C) resulted in the formation of a new osteon. Because the cavitation of the bone occurred initially at point D, the temporal relationship resulted in point D having more new bone—a mature osteon. Eventually, points B and C, filling osteons, would be converted to mature osteons. The reversal line truly represents a reversal of function and is the point at which osteoblastic activity replaces osteoclastic activity. It is evident from the diagram that the reversal line forms the peripheral limit of the osteon.

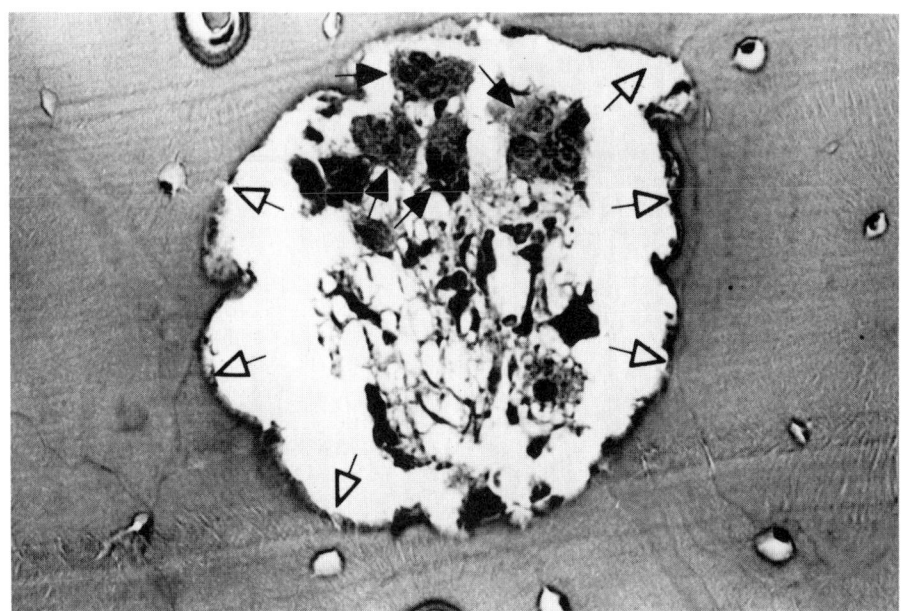

Fig. 8.40 Resorption space. The border of the resorption space is serrated because of the confluence of Howship's lacunae (*open arrows*). Osteoclasts (*solid arrows*) are displaced from the lacunae by the preparation techniques. X125. Compare with Figures 8.23 and 8.38.

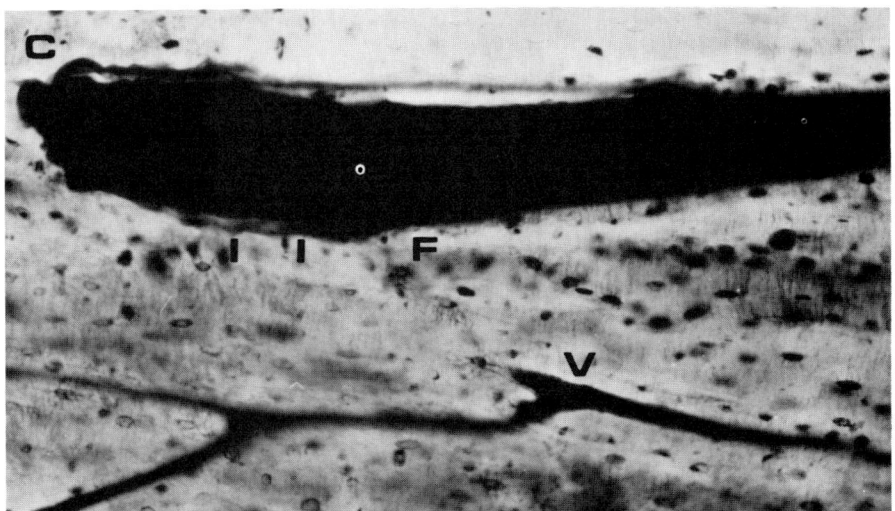

Fig. 8.41 A longitudinal section of compact bone. The cutting cone (C) is the front of osteoclasia. The reversal line (bars) is the peripheral limit of the newly forming osteon (F). The vessel (V) and osteonal endosteal elements comprise a narrow osteonal canal before and after cavitation of the bone. X40 (ground bone section).

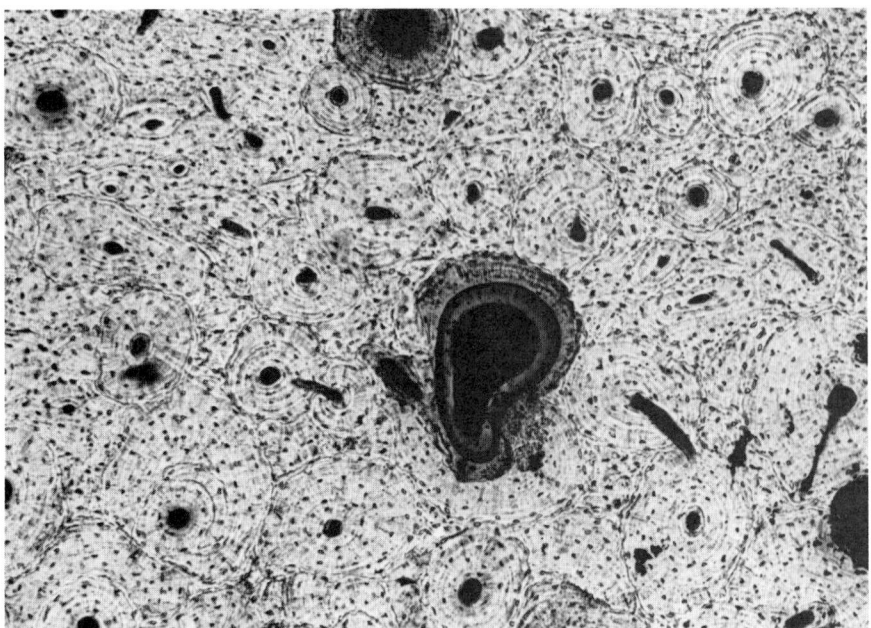

Fig. 8.42 Refilling osteon. The osteon in the center of the field is filling. Compare its morphology with the osteon in Figure 8.14. The osteon at the top of the micrograph is immature and inactive. Osteoid seam is not visible. The remaining osteons are mature. X25 (ground bone section).

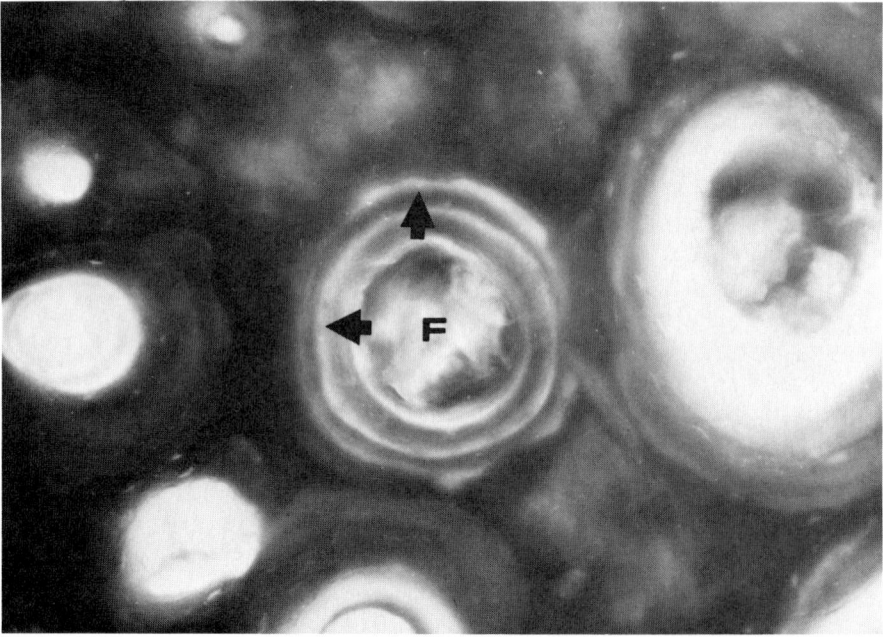

Fig. 8.43 A 50 μm section of the cortex of a canine bone. The successive layers of fluorescence (*arrows*) indicate the active deposition of bone in a filling osteon (F). (Courtesy R. W. Norrdin).

insures that only a relatively constant amount of 25-HCC is produced, whereas the remaining CC is stored in the liver for future use. Such a mechanism insures that the body is not subjected to the influence of high concentrations of vitamin D_3 and other less active metabolites. The 25-HCC form is not an active metabolite but is a necessary compound in the progress of conversion of CC to active metabolites.

The next step in the conversion process is the hydroxylation of 25-HCC in the 1 position to the compound *1,25-dihydroxycholecalciferol (1,25-DHCC)* within mitochondria of renal cells. Parathormone is necessary for this conversion to occur. Parathormone, then, exerts a significant effect upon the production of an active metabolite of vitamin D, 1,25-DHCC. This compound is the active metabolite responsible for the elevation of depressed blood calcium levels. Its sites of action are the gut, kidney, and bone.

Calcium is absorbed from the small intestine under the influence of 1,25-DHCC. Although the precise mechanism is not known, it is hypothesized that this is mediated through the synthesis of a Ca-binding protein, the formation of a Ca-stimulated ATPase in the striated border or the formation of an alkaline phosphatase in the lining cells. The first method is probably the most likely. This compound also functions synergistically with PTH in the conservation of urinary calcium by increasing proximal convoluted tubular reabsorption. Also, the PTH effects on bone are only manifested in the presence of 1,25-DHCC. This latter mechanism is probably the most significant means of quickly elevating blood calcium levels.

Whereas the formation of 25-HCC is a self-limiting conversion step, the conversion to 1,25-DHCC is influenced by several factors. PTH and hypophosphatemia influence the conversion of 25-HCC to 1,25-DHCC. Because calcium and phosphate are absorbed from the gut simultaneously under the influence of 1,25-DHCC, it is not surprising that hypophosphatemia will also stimulate this conversion to the active metabolite. Increased calcium demands upon the body during growth, lactation and gestation are associated with increased levels of 1,25-DHCC ostensibly stimulated by somatotropin, prolactin and placental lactogen, respectively.

Despite the careful regulation of 1,25-DHCC synthesis and its short life span, the fate of 25-HCC is regulated by a number of different factors. During periods of hypercalcemia, normophosphatemia, normocalcemia or when TCT and 1,25-DHCC are present, excess quantities of 25-HCC are hydroxylated in renal cells to *24,25-dihydroxycholecalciferol (24,25-DHCC)*. This compound may facilitate the deposition of calcium into bone. Its relationship to TCT has not been elucidated precisely.

The relationships of parathormone, cal-

ficiencies causes *adult rickets* or *osteomalacia* (a qualitative osteopenia). Recently, extensive research on this substance has broadened the understanding of the role of vitamin D and its metabolites in calcium metabolism.

Several different sterols belong to the vitamin D family. The most important of these is *vitamin D_3, cholecalciferol (CC)*. Vitamin D_3 is not the active form and other compounds are generated by its metabolism.

Its parent compound, *7-dehydrocholecalciferol*, is produced in the liver. It is converted to D_3 in the sebaceous glands of the skin by the action of ultraviolet light. The next step in the activation of CC is accomplished in the liver within the cytoplasm of hepatocytes (liver cells) wherein the 25-position of CC is hydroxylated. The compound *25-hydroxycholecalciferol (25-HCC)* is produced. The conversion of CC to 25-HCC is a self-limiting hydroxylation. This negative feedback

References

Amprino, R. and Engstrom, A.: Studies on x-ray absorption and diffraction of bone tissue. Acta Anat. *15:*1, 1952.

Ascenzi, R., Bonucci, E. and Bocciarelli, D. S.: An electron microscope study on primary periosteal bone. J. Ultrastruct. Res. *18:*605, 1967.

Belanger, L. F., Robichon, J., Migicovsky, B. B., Copp, D. H. and Vincent, J.: Resorption without osteoclasts (osteolysis). In *Mechanisms of Hard Tissue Destruction*, edited by R. F. Sognnaes. AAAS, Washington, D.C., 1963.

Bourne, G. H. (editor): *The Biochemistry and Physiology of Bone*. Volumes I–III, Academic Press, New York, 1972.

Cohen, J. and Harris, W. H.: The three dimensional anatomy of Haversian systems. J. Bone Joint Surg. *40A:*419, 1958.

Cooper, R. R., Milgram, J. W. and Robinson, R. A.: Morphology of the osteon: An electron microscopic study. J. Bone Joint Surg. *48A:*1239, 1966.

DeLuca, H. F.: The kidney as an endocrine organ for the production of 1,25-dihydroxyvitamin D₃, a calcium-mobilizing hormone. N. Engl. J. Med. *289:*359, 1973.

Frost, H. M.: *Bone Remodelling Dynamics*. C. C. Thomas, Springfield, 1963.

Frost, H. M.: *The Physiology of Cartilaginous, Fibrous, and Bony Tissue*. C. C. Thomas, Springfield, 1972.

Gonzales, F. and Karnovsky, M. J.: Electron microscopy of osteoclasts in healing fractures of rat bone. J. Biophys. Biochem. Cytol. *9:*299, 1961.

Hancox, N. M.: *Biology of Bone*. University Press, Cambridge, 1972.

Heller-Steinberg, M.: Ground substance, bone salts, and cellular activity in bone formation and destruction. Amer. J. Anat. *89:*347, 1951.

Hobdell, M. H. and Boyde, A.: Microradiography and scanning electron microscopy of bone sections. Z. Zellforsch. *94:*487, 1969.

Little, K.: *Bone Behavior*. Academic Press, New York, 1973.

Martin, J. H. and Matthew, J. L.: Mitochondrial granules in chondrocytes, osteoblasts and osteocytes. Clin. Orthop. *68:*273, 1970.

Nichols, Jr., G. and Wasserman, R. H. (editors): *Cellular Mechanisms for Calcium Transfer and Homeostasis*. Academic Press, New York, 1971.

Parfitt, A. M.: Mechanisms of calcium transfer between blood and bone and their cellular basis: Morphological and kinetic approaches to bone turnover. Metab. *25:*809, 1976.

Queener, S. F. and Bell, N. H.: Calcitonin: A general survey. Metab. *24:*555, 1975.

Rasmussen, H. and Goodman, D. B. P.: Relationships between calcium and cyclic nucleotide in cell activation. Physiol. Rev. *57:*421, 1977.

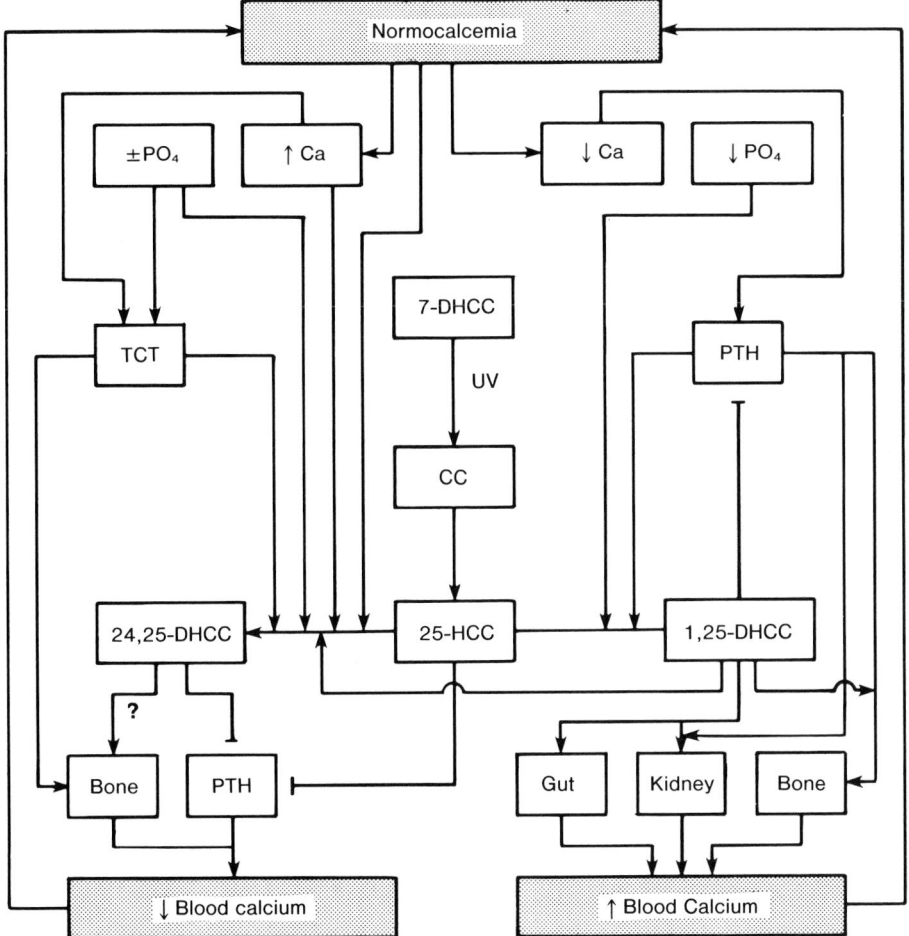

Fig. 8.44 Factors influencing the maintenance of normal blood calcium. Normocalcemia is maintained by a dual control mechanism involving parathormone (PTH) and calcitonin (TCT). The influence of vitamin D metabolites and target organs is outlined. *Arrows* indicate stimulation, whereas *bars* indicate blockage or suppression.

citonin and the active metabolites of vitamin D₃ to calcium metabolism are summarized in Fig. 8.44. Other metabolites of vitamin D₃ have been isolated also. Their precise roles in this regulation scheme await further insights from on-going and active research efforts. This dual control negative feedback loop is a finely tuned system for the maintenance of homeostatic levels of blood calcium (10 mg%).

9: Osteogenesis

Development of Bone

General Characteristics. Osteogenic processes, beginning in the embryo and continuing throughout the life of the animal, are mediated through the secretory activity of osteoblasts. These cells deposit a matrix that subsequently becomes mineralized. Although the actual cellular mechanism of bone deposition is the same in all osteogenic processes, the differentiation of mesenchymal cells into osteoprogenitor cells and subsequently into osteoblasts normally occurs in two different microenvironments. For this reason, two types of normal ossification processes are recognized, *intramembranous* and *endochondral*. The quality and appearance of the bone in both instances are identical; however, the primary association of osseous material with other tissues in the different environments greatly alters the appearance of the developing osseous organ.

In *intramembranous ossification*, the differentiation of osteoblasts occurs in an environment in which some mesenchymal cells have previously differentiated into fibroblasts. The presence of fibers and cells (mesenchymal and fibroblastic) imparts a fibrocellular or membranous quality to the microenvironment. The de novo formation of bone under these conditions, therefore, appears to occur in a minimally supported membranous environment.

In *endochondral ossification*, the differentiation of osteoblasts occurs in an environment in which cartilage has already been deposited. Foci of perivascular mesenchymal cells within certain areas of the cartilaginous tissue give rise to the osteoprogenitor cells. Bone deposition, as described previously, takes place. However, the cartilage is used as a temporary support or scaffold upon which bone is deposited. The cartilage is not transformed into bone but is eventually replaced by bone.

Occasionally, bone formation occurs in foci not normally occupied by osseous tissue. This *pathologic (metaplastic) ossification* may be observed in otherwise normal tissues of cicatrices, tracheal and laryngeal cartilage, lateral cartilages of the equine foot and other organs. Calcium salts may accumulate in tissues also. *Calcification* or *mineralization* of normal tissues, occurring in association with persistent hypercalcemia, is termed *metastatic calcification*. The calcification of degenerative or dead tissues is termed *dystrophic calcification*. Although some bone may be observed in metastatic and dystrophic calcification foci, the calcification process should not be confused with ossification processes.

Although the cellular mechanism of normal ossification is the same, it functions quite differently in the growing animal. Intramembranous ossification is responsible for the attainment of the definitive shape of those bones that are not preformed in cartilage. This includes longitudinal and latitudinal growth of a limited number of bones of the body. Endochondral ossification is responsible for the longitudinal growth of the bones of the body. Endochondral ossification, however, does not occur alone. The latitudinal or transverse growth of these bones is mediated through intramembranous ossification. Both of these ossification processes, prior to adulthood, are responsible for the *modeling* of bones or the attainment of the definitive, recognizable gross structure.

After the initial deposition of bone in a membranous or cartilaginous environment, subsequent bone formation occurs on preexisting bone surfaces by appositional growth. Continued deposition naturally leads to bone growth. The modeling of bones, however, is the combined result of osteoblastic and osteoclastic activity. The balance of these combined activities favors the deposition of bone during periods of growth.

Although osteogenic processes most noticeably occur during adolescence, they are not confined to this period. The deposition and removal of bone, without any significant alteration of the gross form of the structure, occur throughout life. This *internal remodeling* process complements the adolescent modeling of bones. Throughout the remainder of life, *internal remodeling* is maintained in a homeostatic balance. Any disruption to this balance during the pre- and/or postnatal period can result in serious metabolic bone disorders.

Intramembranous Ossification

Sequence of Development. This process begins in areas occupied by mesenchyme, the packing tissue of the embryo. The bones destined to form, either totally or partially in this manner, are the bones of the skull, mandible and clavicle, which are not weight-bearing structures.

Initially, the regions in which bone is to be formed are occupied by mesenchymal cells embedded within a homogeneous, fluid ground substance. The subsequent development of a *fibrocellular* tissue is brought about by the differentiation of some *fibroblasts* from mesenchymal cells (Fig. 9.1). The ability to distinguish one of these cells from the other is difficult. Generally, however, mesenchymal cells are larger and more pale-staining than their more differentiated counterparts, fibroblasts. *Collagenous fibers* are randomly scattered among the numerous *stellate cells*, which include fibroblasts and mesenchymal cells. Many of these cells are destined to become *osteoprogenitor cells*.

The next recognizable step in the differentiation process is the recognition of osteoblasts (Fig. 9.2). These cells stain quite darkly and are basophilic. During active secretion of their products they assume a cuboidal configuration. However, during periods of nonactivity they assume a spindle-shaped configuration. Although bone matrix is not always visible during early stages of differentiation, subsequent secretory activity by these cells will produce bone (Figs. 9.3, 9.4). Thus, these areas represent ossification centers in their early stages of development (Fig. 9.5).

Progressive development and differentiation produces recognizable spicules of bone (Fig. 9.6). A fibrocellular connective tissue with numerous blood vessels surrounds the developing bone. As osteoblasts deposit bone appositionally, some cells remain entrapped in their own secretory products (Fig. 9.7). Osteoblastic cells that become entrapped are then referred to as osteocytes. The bone being deposited in these ossification centers is the *woven* type. The large lacunae and the nonlamellar arrangement of the osteocytes are typical of this type of bone.

Woven bone serves as a temporary structure during development. A progressive reduction of the formation of woven bone occurs, while lamellar bone formation increases progressively. Osteoclasia accounts for the removal of woven bone as a temporary tissue until only lamellar bone remains (Fig. 9.8).

Osteoblastic and osteoclastic activities are integral components of bone formation (Fig. 9.9). The necessity for active osteoblasts is obvious. Besides the removal of woven bone, osteoclasts function to remove lamellar bone as well. The combined activity of the two cell types results in the movement of osseous spicules through space (Fig. 9.9). Osteoblastic activity on one side of a spicule and osteoclastic activity on the other side results in the movement of the spicule in the

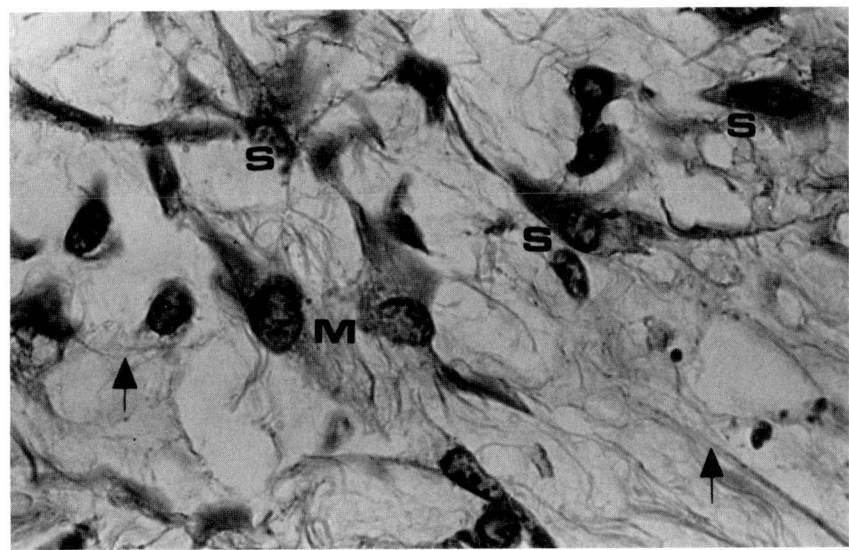

Fig. 9.1 Early cellular differentiation in intramembranous ossification (bovine fetal jaw). Many of the cells within a presumptive bone-forming site are spindle- or stellate-shaped cells (S). While some of them may be mesenchymal cells (M), others are osteoprogenitor cells. The morphologic distinction between the osteoprogenitor and mesenchymal cell is impossible. Some collagenous fibers are evident (*arrows*). X160. All light micrographs are labeled as the magnification with the microscope before photographic enlarging. All electron micrographs are labeled as total magnification, including photographic enlarging.

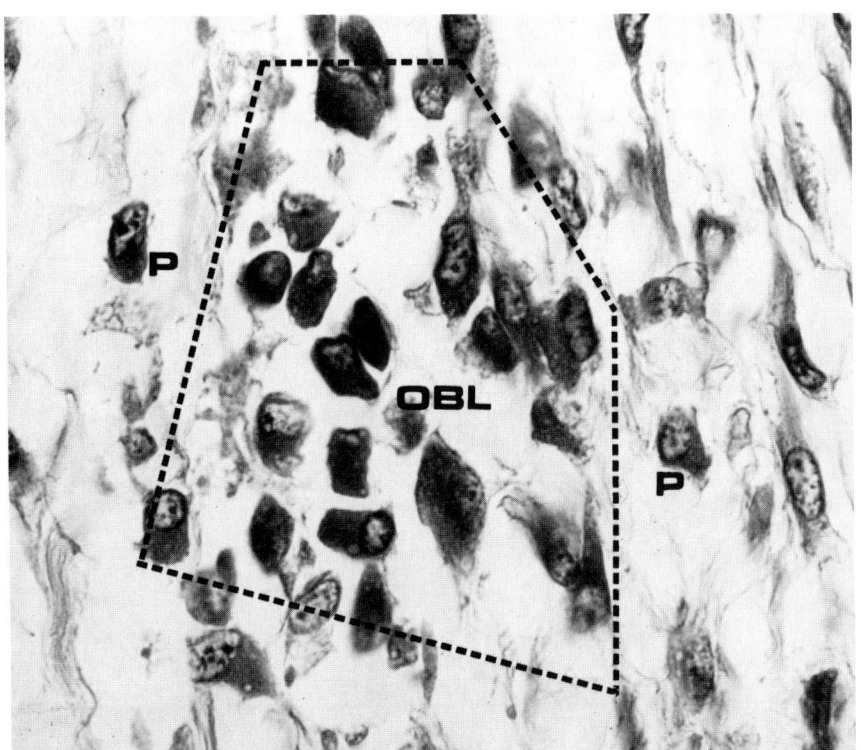

Fig. 9.2 Differentiation of osteoblasts within an intramembranous ossification center (bovine fetal jaw). The *outlined area* is an ossification center that contains osteoblasts (OBL). The light-staining cells at the periphery may be osteoprogenitor cells (P). The surrounding tissue is similar to that in Figure 9.1. X160.

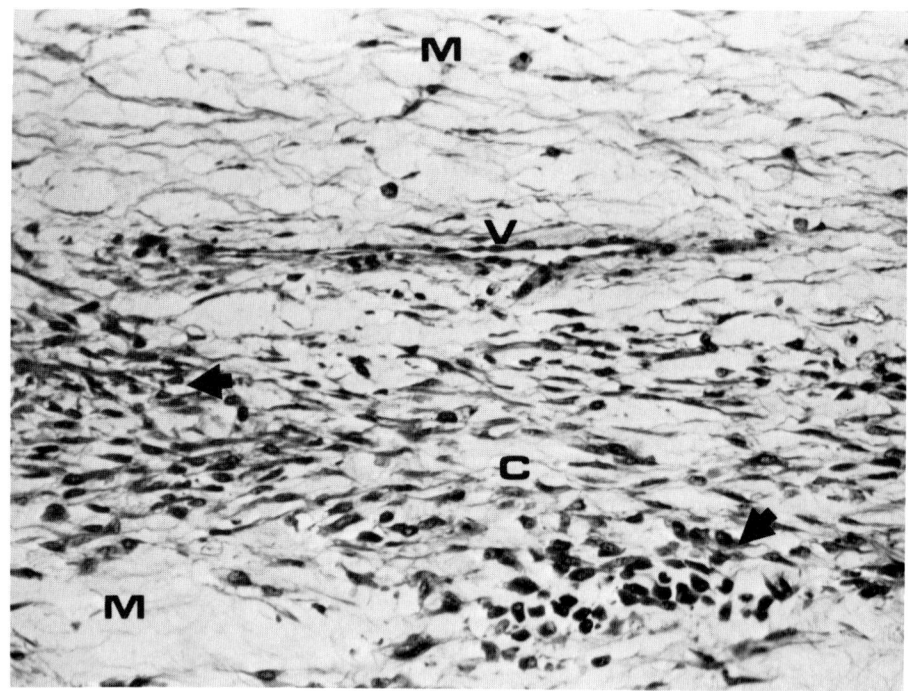

Fig. 9.3 Presumptive ossification center in the bovine fetal jaw. The mesenchyme (M) surrounds an area of mesenchymal condensation (C). Dark-staining cells (*arrows*) are osteoblasts. Bone matrix has not been formed at these sites yet. A blood vessel (V) has developed in association with the ossification center. X40.

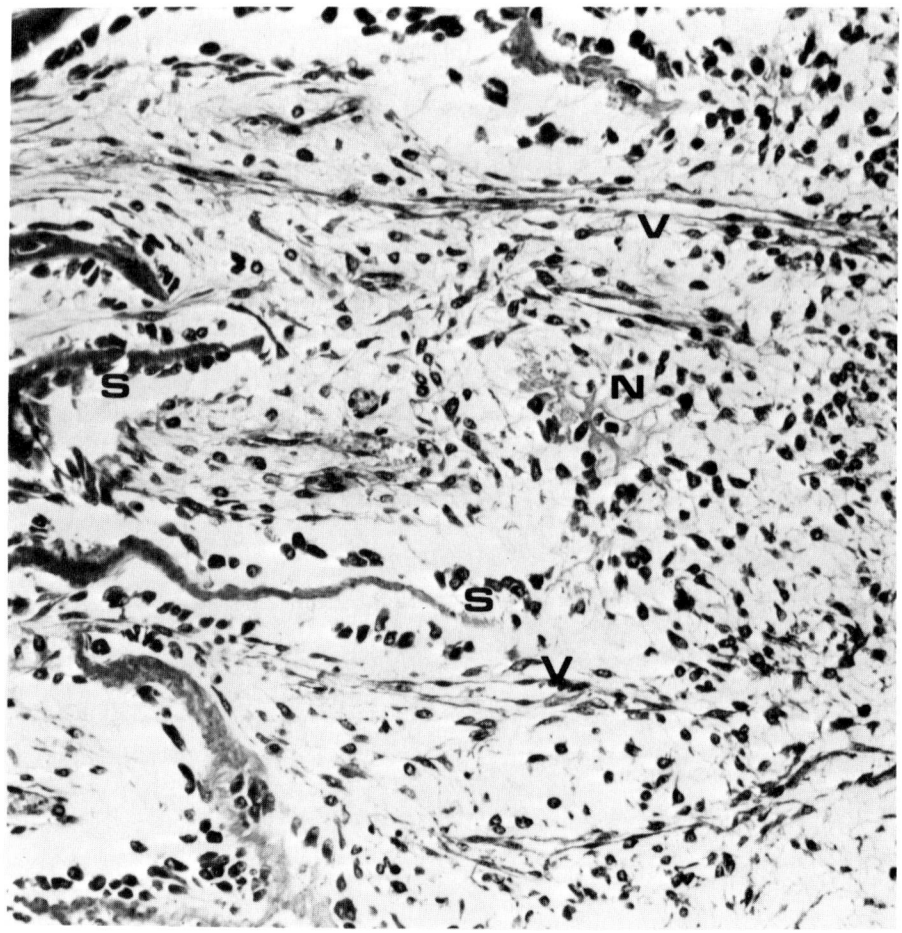

Fig. 9.4 Bone matrix formation within the ossification center (bovine fetal jaw). New matrix formation (N) is evident. Continued activity of osteoblasts forms progressively larger spicules (S) of bone. An extensive vascular bed (V) is developing also. X40.

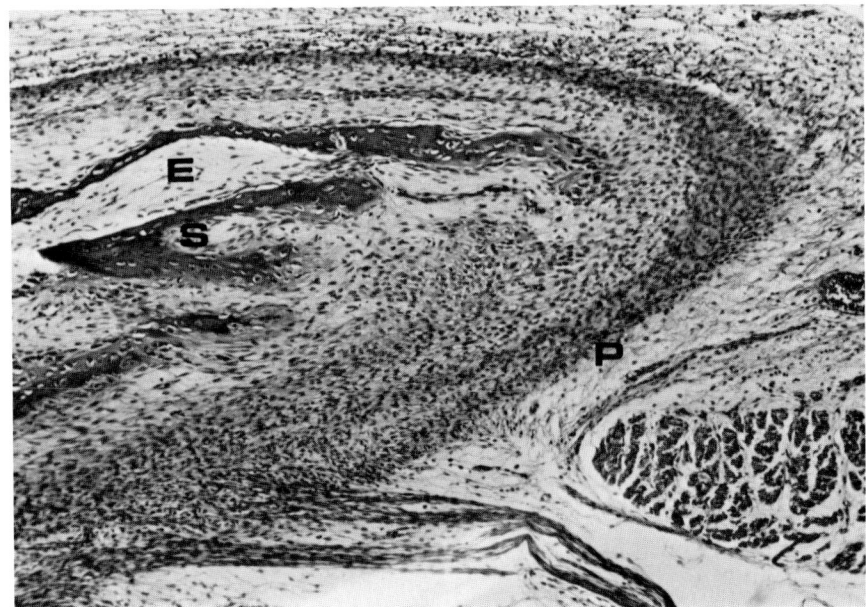

Fig. 9.5 Ossification center of the bovine fetal jaw. Bone spicules (S), endosteum (E) and periosteum (P) are evident. X20.

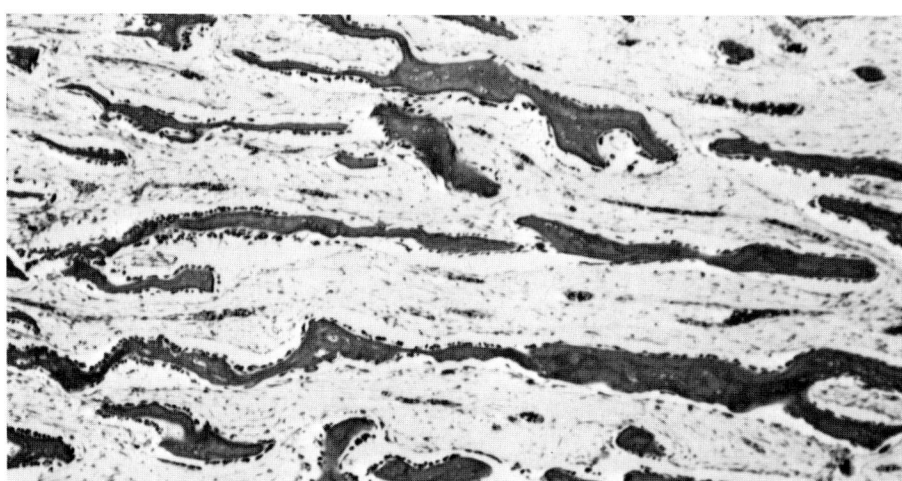

Fig. 9.6 Continued growth of the ossification center. Numerous bone spicules have developed and are separated by endosteum. X10.

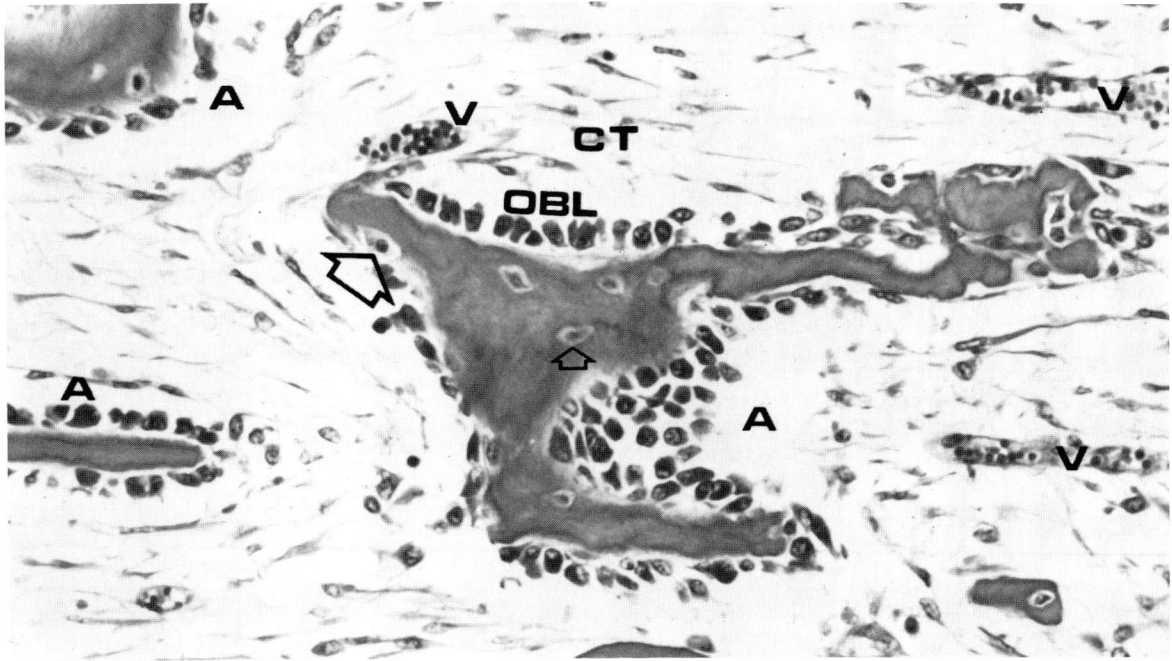

Fig. 9.7 Spicules of bone within an ossification center (bovine fetal jaw). Spicules of bone are surrounded by endosteum consisting of fibrocellular connective tissue (CT). Blood vessels are evident (V). The endosteum is artifactually separated from the bone (A). Osteoblasts (OBL) become entrapped in bone (*large arrow*) and are recognized eventually as typical osteocytes (*small arrow*). X63.

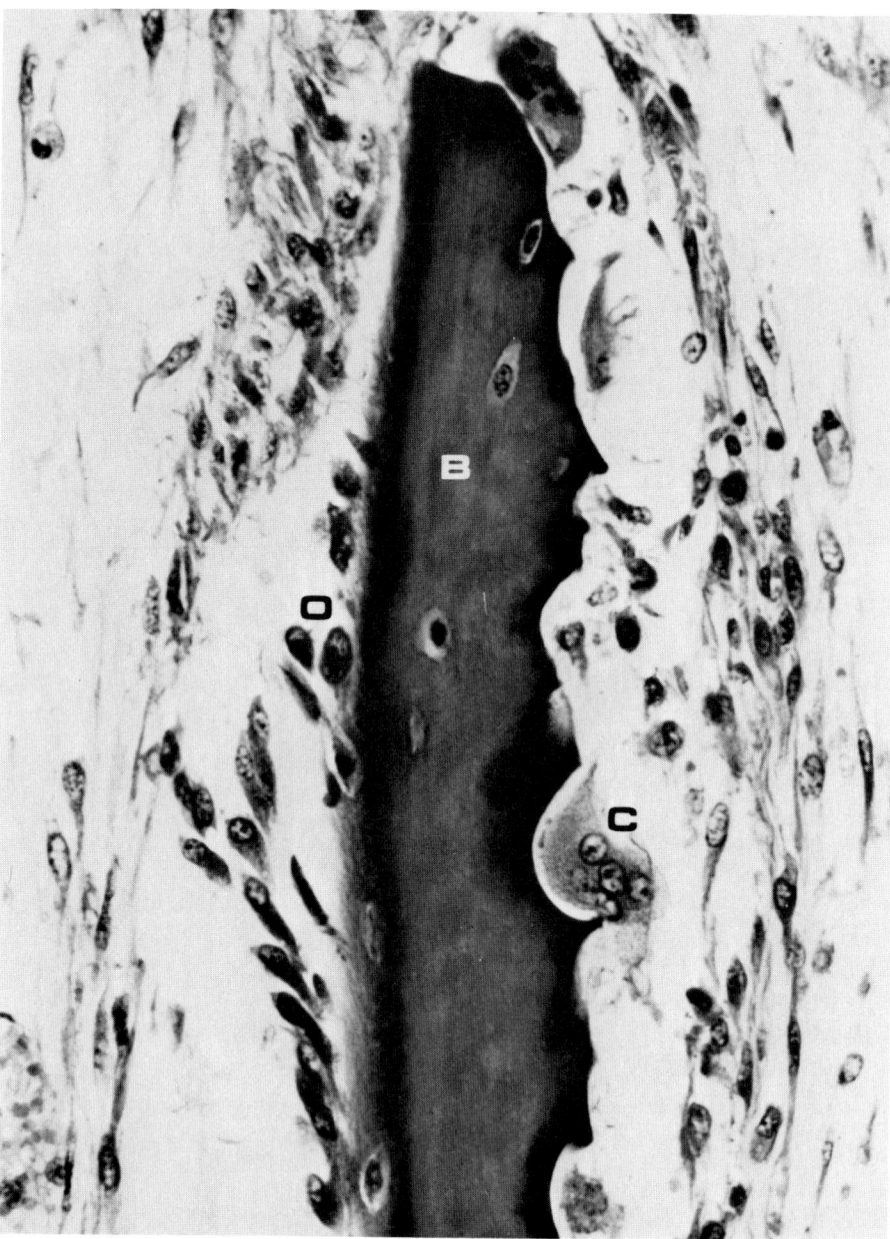

Fig. 9.8 Bone spicule (B) within an intramembranous ossification center. Osteocytes have been incorporated into the spicule. Osteoblastic (O) and osteoclastic (C) activity is evident. The spicule is composed of woven bone. X100.

The essence of this ossification mechanism is the de novo formation of bone in mesenchyme. Subsequent appositional bone growth on the recently formed spicules increases the mass of the ossification center (Fig. 9.11). Continual addition of bone results in the achievement of a definitive shape characterized by the appropriate distribution of cancellous and compact bone.

Endochondral Ossification

General Features. *Endochondral ossification* is also called *enchondral* or *intracartilaginous ossification.* These terms are descriptive, for the development of bone by this process occurs initially within a mass of cartilage. The essential feature of the endochondral ossification process is the preformation of future bones in hyaline cartilage models. The models are actually miniature versions of the future definitive bones (Fig. 9.12). The cartilage is removed gradually and is replaced continuously by bone. Endochondral ossification encompasses all of the activities responsible for the formation of the weight-bearing bones of the body. However, the formation of cartilage and its replacement by bone is the means by which the bones elongate. This elongation is achieved in such a way that the animal is able to bear weight while growth is being accomplished.

Alterations of the endochondral ossification process can have significant effects upon the skeletal mass. One of the most significant effects is the premature termination of endochondral ossification. In some species and breeds, the premature termination is considered an abnormality, although in certain breeds of dogs the early cessation of endochondral ossification results in shortened bones that are the normal standard for the breed. *Achondroplasia (chondrodystrophy, chondrodysplasia)* is the term that describes a premature termination of the endochondral ossification process. Achondroplasia is generalized in bulldogs and the Pekingese; localized to the head in Boxers and Boston Bull Terriers and is localized to the limbs of Dachshunds and Bassett Hounds.

Although the functions of endochondral ossification are few and seem relatively simple, they are vitally important to the animal. *Endochondral ossification provides for the elongation of most of the skeletal mass during growth.* This function is initiated prior to and during actual weight-bearing. The rate at which growth progresses, the duration of the process and the direction of the process in three-dimensional space is affected by numerous factors—genetic, nutritional, metabolic and mechanical. *Endochondral ossification contributes to the shape, size, spatial orientation and alignment of the articulations between bones.* Normal locomotor function is related directly to the modeling activity of this ossification process. *Endochondral ossification forms the majority of the cancellous bone of the body.* It effectively

direction of the osteoblasts. The ossification center is characterized by varied activities, all of which lead to the development of a definitive bone and its associated tissues. Spicules of bone form, move through space, coalesce and convert the ossification center into a recognizeable osseous structure. Areolar and dense connective tissue develop as integral components of periosteal and endosteal envelopes. Similarly, the characteristic vascular beds of bone develop within the mesenchyme of the ossification center.

Progressive expansion of the ossification center (increased size of the developing bone) is accompanied by an alteration of the configuration of the constituent osseous tissue. Isolated foci become more typically

cancellous bone (Fig. 9.10). Osteons also may form in the cancellous bone as some of it becomes compact bone. The cancellous nature of the bone within the forming marrow cavity is retained throughout adulthood. The periosteum, however, continually deposits laminae of bone in a compact configuration that serves to strengthen the bone and increase its diameter. The osteoclasts of the cortical endosteum continually remove bone. This effectively expands the marrow cavity while maintaining the essential thickness of the compact bone. During growth, then, the bone formed by the periosteum eventually will be removed by the cortical endosteum until the definitive diameter of the structure is achieved.

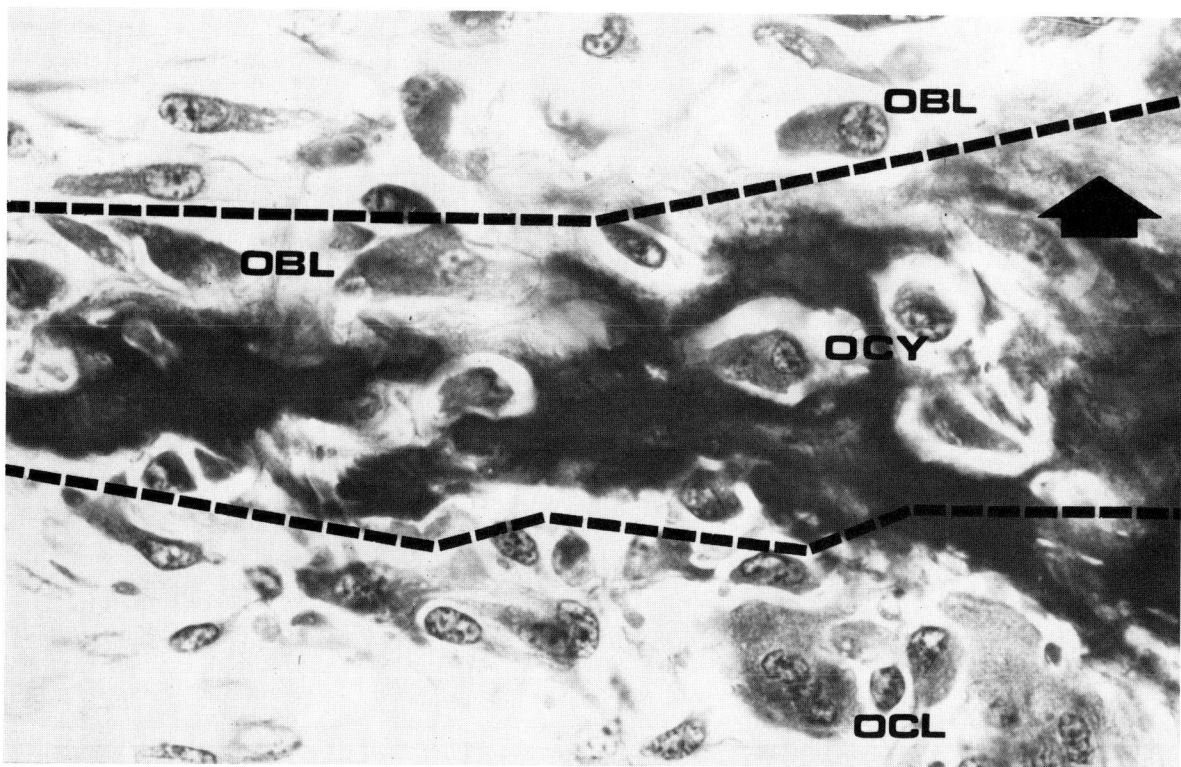

Fig. 9.9 Progressive development and activity of the ossification center (bovine fetal jaw). The osteoblasts (OBL) on the upper portion of the spicule are active; whereas, those on the lower portion of the spicule appear inactive. Osteoclasts (OCL) are present also. If the same relative cellular activity were to progress beyond the stage depicted, then the spicule would be altered as outlined. It would thicken in the left portion of the spicule and appear to move upward (*arrow*) in the right portion. Osteocytes (OCY) are oriented randomly in this immature bone. X160.

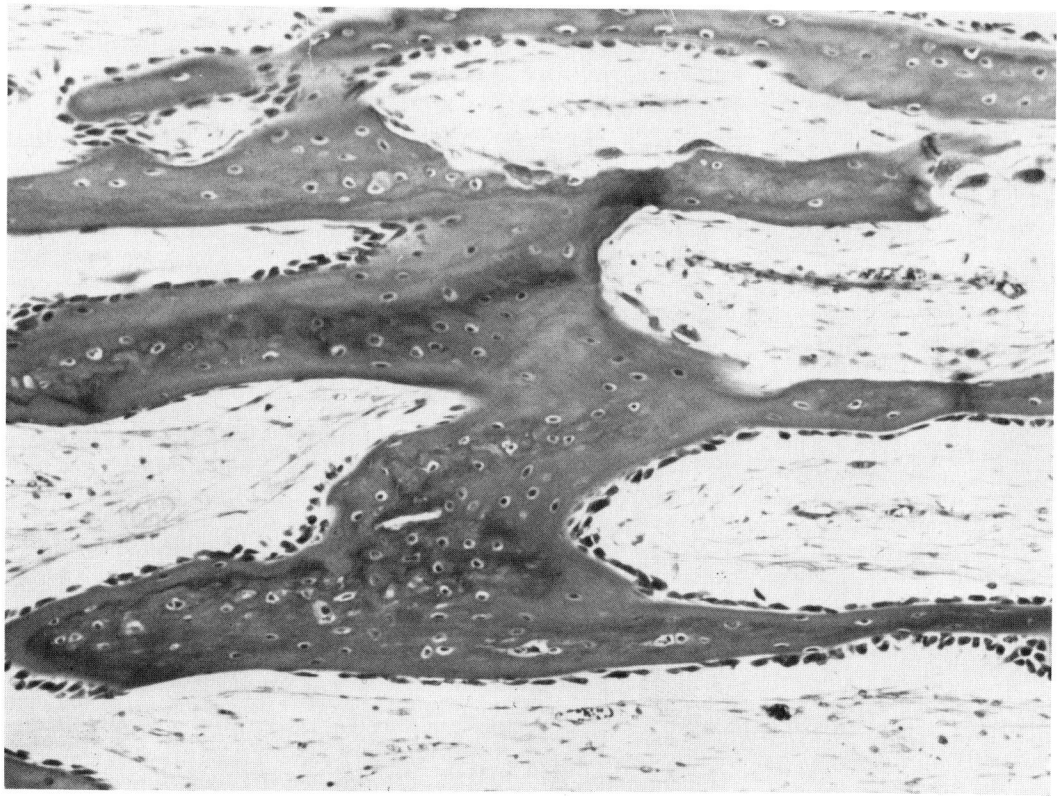

Fig. 9.10 Progressive growth of the ossification center (bovine fetal jaw). The union of spicules is occurring and the cancellous bone continues to develop. X63.

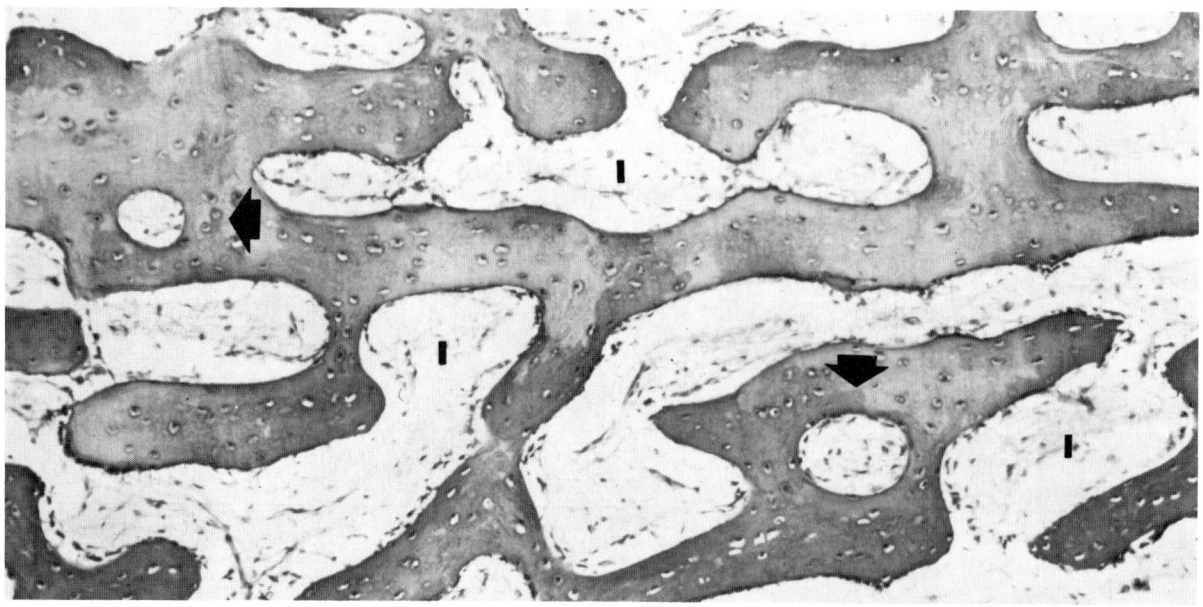

Fig. 9.11 Increased bone within the ossification center (bovine fetal jaw). The interosseous space (I) is being replaced by bone. Osteons may form at the sites indicated by the arrows. X63.

reduces the skeletal mass without compromising the ability to bear weight, because the trabeculae of cancellous bone, especially those of the epiphyses and metaphyses, are positioned for maximal mechanical advantage.

The general sequence of events of endochondral ossification is summarized diagrammatically in Figure 9.13. Continual reference to Figure 9.13 will be helpful.

Cartilaginous Model Formation. *Mesenchymal cell condensation* characterizes areas of the body in which bones will develop by endochondral ossification (Figs. 9.13A, 9.14). The condensation results from the mitotic activity of the cells and produces an area that is hypercellular. The relationships of future bones are apparent in the presumptive bone-forming sites (Fig. 9.15). The cells eventually differentiate into chondroblasts and form a chondrogenic center referred to as the *cartilaginous model* of the developing bone (Fig. 9.16). Commensurate with the differentiation of the cartilage, mesenchymal cells at the periphery of the model condense and form a *perichondrium* that encloses the entire model. Appositional growth activity of the perichondrium helps to lengthen and thicken the model. Interstitial growth of the model complements the appositional growth. As adjacent bone-forming sites lengthen, the perichondrium at the proximal and distal ends is lost. These sites eventually become the articular surfaces. Then, the model is dependent totally upon interstitial growth of cartilage for elongation.

The progressive lengthening and thickening of the model is associated with the maturation of the cartilage cells (Fig. 9.17). Those that differentiate first occupy the center of the model. They are older and more mature than those that follow. The young

cells, which are located proximally and distally, mature toward the center. Maturation is evidenced by a change in size. Young cells and their lacunae become progressively larger with maturation. Eventually, the lacunae of contiguous cells become sufficiently large to reduce the intervening matrix to a thin separating rim. Such older cells are hypertrophic (excessively enlarged). At the same time these maturation events are occurring, the perichondrium in the middle of the model (presumptive diaphysis) is invaded by blood vessels, and some of the cells in this envelope begin to modulate into osteoblasts and osteoclasts; thus, the *perichondrium* is converted to a *periosteum* (Fig. 9.13B). This envelope begins to form woven bone referred to as *collar* or *sleeve bone*. This bone, in fact, is the newly-forming diaphysis. At this point in development it is evident that bone has formed. The *diaphyseal ossification center* has been established (Fig. 9.13C).

Primary Ossification Center. The diaphyseal ossification center is also called the *primary ossification center*. The continued expansion and development of the primary ossification center is contingent upon the continued osteogenic activity of the periosteum and the fate of the mature chondrocytes that are surrounded by the sleeve bone (Fig. 9.13C). The matrix associated with hypertrophic chondrocytes in the center of the primary ossification center becomes calcified. (This was discussed in Chapter 7.) Classically, the stimulus responsible for this calcification process has been described as resulting from regressive and/or degenerative changes in the hypertrophic chondrocytes. The ultimate fate of the cells has been considered to be degeneration, death and dissolution. Again, the classical explanation has been the deprivation of a nutrient supply

as the diffusion distance to the cells increases with an increased size of the cartilage model of the primary ossification center. Current evidence indicates that the hypertrophic chondrocytes participate in the calcification process, and although some may die, others may eventually be released from their lacunae to give rise to other generations of cells.

There are three features of the primary ossification center at this point in development that are necessary to consider. The cartilaginous model is *avascular*. Blood vessels, located peripherally, are part of the periosteum but do not supply the cartilage. *No mesenchymal cells are within the cartilaginous model. Also, the bone that formed initially as sleeve bone is not the bone that forms as a consequence of endochondral ossification.* The sleeve bone is described classically as forming via intramembranous ossification. It is didactically useful to make a distinction between intramembranous ossification and the formation of this sleeve bone. The former involves the de novo formation of bone in a mesenchymal membrane free of any other supportive structures. Increased size is achieved subsequently by simple apposition of new bone on pre-existing bone. The first spicules of sleeve bone are formed *upon* the perimeter of the cartilaginous model. This model is the temporary supportive structure upon which the initial apposition of sleeve bone is manifested. It may be prudent to distinguish this initial spicule formation as *epichondral ossification*. Subsequent growth of periosteal bone is simple apposition of new bone to pre-existing bone.

After the calcification of the cartilage in the middle of the primary ossification center, cavities develop within this zone by dissolution of the cartilage matrix (Figs. 9.13D, 9.18). Blood vessels from the perios-

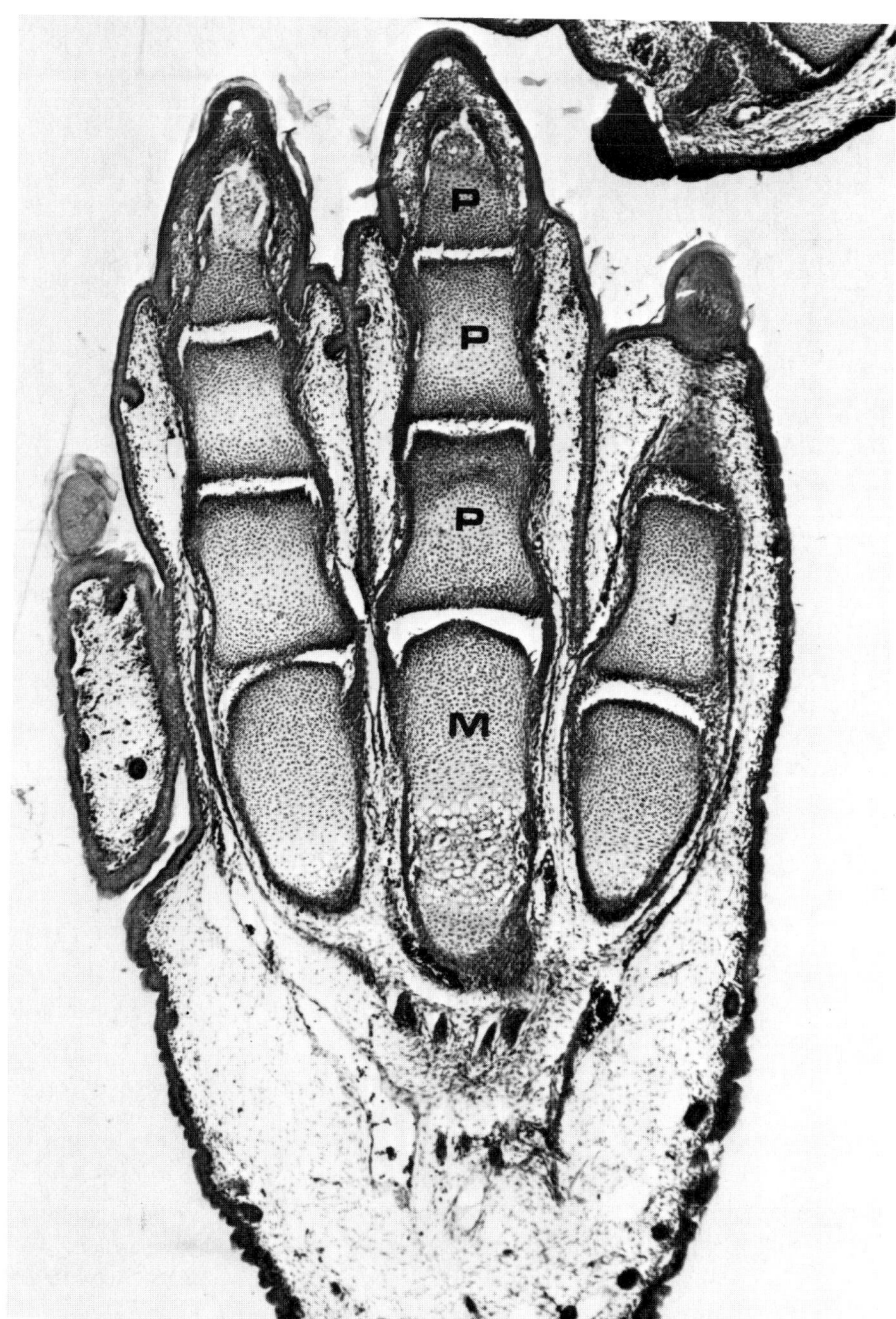

Fig. 9.12   Developing manus of a hamster. The bones of the manus (phalanges and metacarpals) are performed in cartilage. The metacarpal bones (M) and phalanges (P) are miniature versions of the adult structures. Note that the metacarpal-phalangeal joints and interphalangeal joints appear early in development. X10.

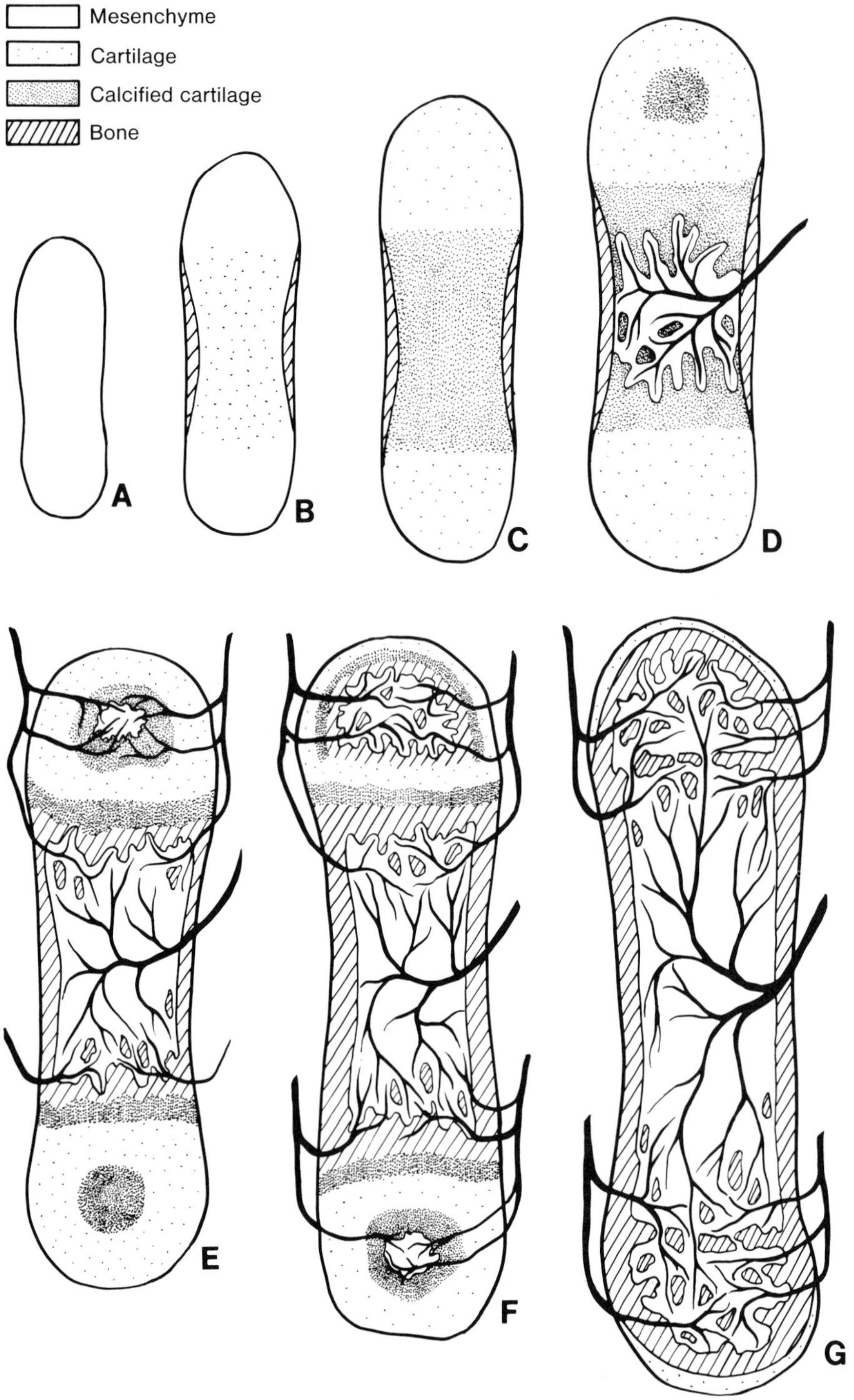

☐ Mesenchyme
▦ Cartilage
▨ Calcified cartilage
▨ Bone

Fig. 9.13 Diagram of the development of bones by endochondral ossification. Refer to the text for a complete description of the process.

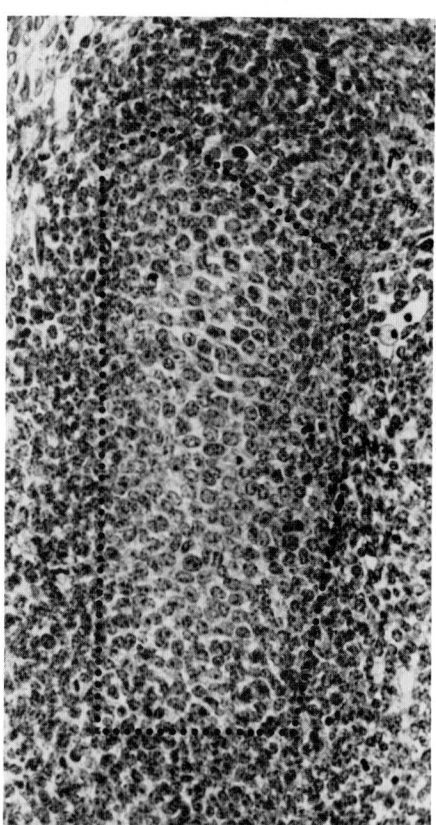

Fig. 9.14 Mesenchymal condensation in a presumptive bone-forming site (fetal hamster humerus). The mesenchymal cell condensation is outlined. A perichondrium will differentiate at the periphery of the condensation. X60 (PAS).

teum invade the newly-created mineralized cartilaginous matrix. A single, predominant vessel is responsible for the vascularization of this previously avascular cartilaginous model. This vessel and its associated mesenchymal cells which differentiate into *osteoprogenitor cells* is the *periosteal bud*. This vessel is destined to become the *nutrient artery* of the bone. Importantly, this vascular invasion seeds the primary ossification cen-

ter with bone cells. This is the event that establishes the periosteum giving rise to the endosteum. Osteoblasts develop and begin to form bone on remnants and spicules of the calcified cartilage. There is continuity between the woven bone deposited on the cartilaginous spicules and the woven bone from the periosteum.

Chondrocytes continue to divide at the proximal and distal ends of the model, ac-

counting for the continual increase in length (Fig. 9.18). Similarly, the periosteum continues to add new bone to the diaphysis to maintain the longitudinal relationship with the growing cartilage. Continued apposition of new bone also accounts for an increased bone diameter. The cells progress through the maturation stages described previously, and their matrix ultimately calcifies. Capillary loops from the periosteal bud, with their pericapillary populations of bone cells, advance into the calcified matrix removing cartilage by osteoclasia and creating new surfaces for bone formation (Fig. 9.19). The new surfaces are the contiguous chondrocytic lacunae. Removal of *transverse septa* between chondrocytes leaves the finger-like projections of the calcified *longitudinal septa* upon which woven bone is deposited. These events, interstitial growth of cartilage and metaphyseal osseous replacement, continue throughout the development of the bone. The removal of cartilage and the formation of bone on newly-created cartilaginous surfaces within the mass of the cartilaginous model are the essence of bone formation by endochondral ossification.

Some bones develop from a single ossification center. In these instances, the expanding osseous replacement reduces the growing cartilage to a zone that underlies

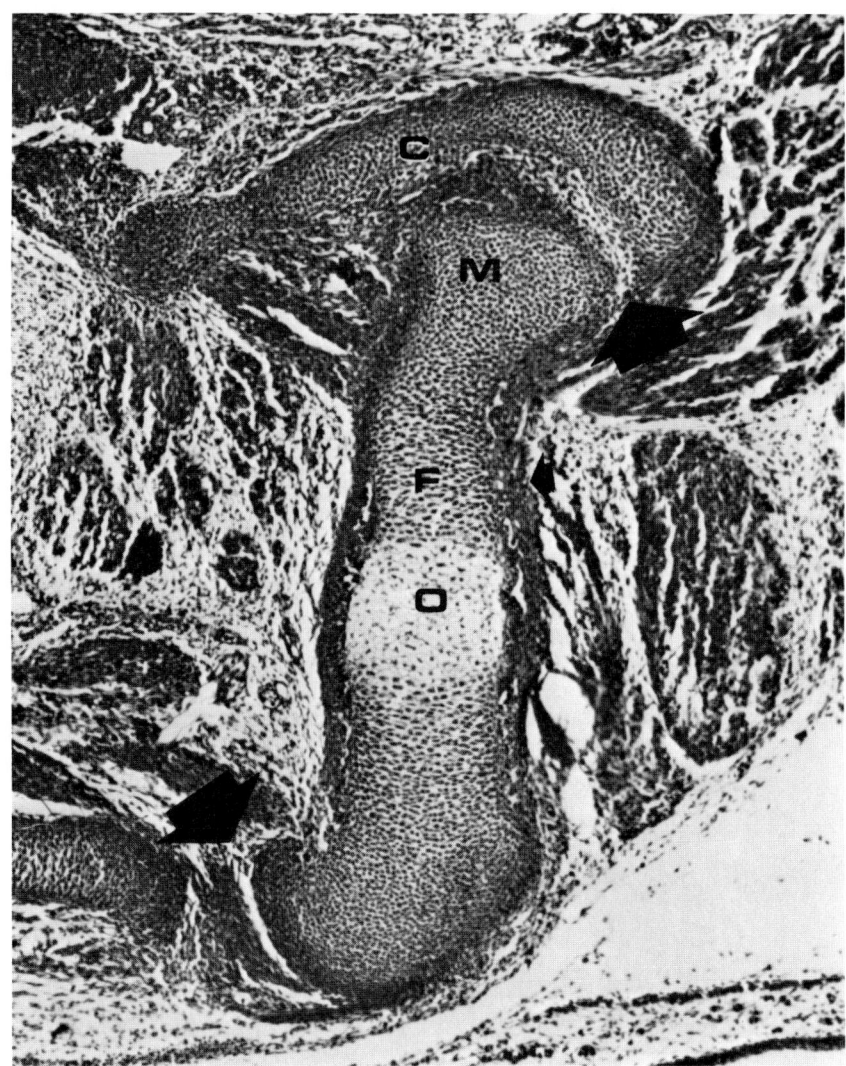

Fig. 9.15 Developing model of the os coxa and femur of a canine fetus. The general form of the femur (F) and os coxa (C) is apparent at this early stage of development. The majority of the model is composed of mesenchymal cells (M). The center of the model (O), composed of cartilage, is the early ossification center. The model is surrounded by a perichondrium (*small arrow*), while the cavitation of the acetabulum and stifle joint (*large arrows*) is apparent. X16.

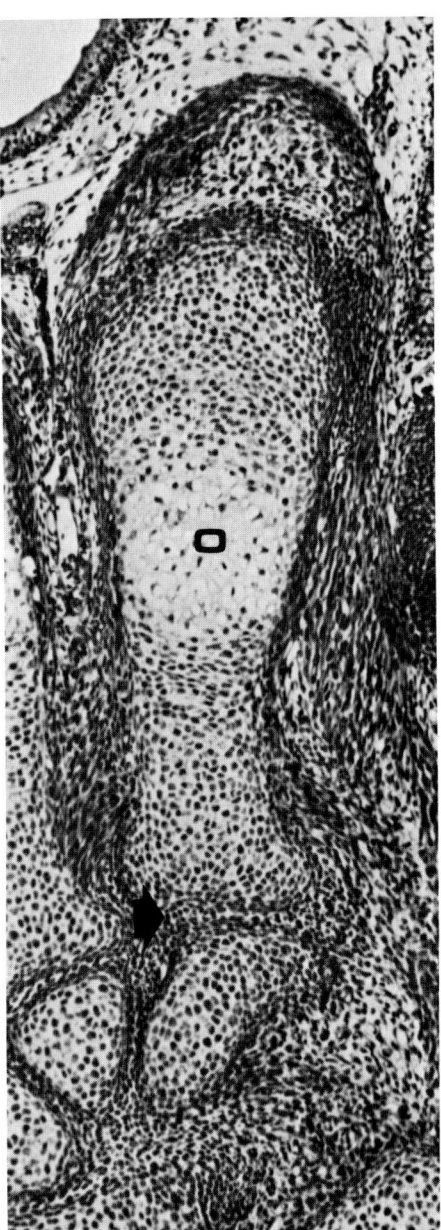

Fig. 9.16 Developing metacarpal and carpal bones of a fetal hamster. The models consist of cartilage. Mature cartilage occupies the metacarpal primary ossification center (O). A perichondrium surrounds the model, except at the point of formation of the carpal-metacarpal joint (*arrow*).

the articular cartilage. This zone of growth supplies new chondrocytes to the articular surface as well as to the maturation sequence that culminates in osseous replacement within the primary ossification center. Spicules of calcified cartilage and woven bone are used for the deposition of lamellar bone. The region of the ossification center that contains these three tissues (calcified cartilage, woven bone, lamellar bone) is called the *primary spongiosa* (Fig. 9.20). Gradually, calcified cartilage and woven bone (as well as some lamellar bone) are removed by osteoclasia and are replaced totally by lamellar bone. The *secondary spongiosa* is the region of the ossification center in which replacement by lamellar bone is accomplished completely.

In some bones, trabeculae of the primary spongiosa extend from proximal cartilage through the marrow cavity to the distal growth cartilage. In these bones, the secondary spongiosa, characterized by trabeculae of lamellar bone, expands longitudinally toward the growth cartilage. Upon cessation of growth, cancellous bone is continuous from both epiphyses through the marrow cavity. In other bones, the secondary spongiosa is a narrow zone of lamellar bone, because osteoclastic activity removes all trabeculae of bone from the marrow cavity. Upon cessation of growth the secondary spongiosa is confined to the proximal and distal epiphyses as trabecular bone, while the marrow cavity is hollow.

While these events occur within the ossification center and account for progressive elongation, the periosteum has been adding

bone continually and increasing the length and diameter of the organ. The increase in bone diameter is accompanied by an increase in marrow cavity diameter (Fig. 9.21). This means that the cortical endosteum removes bone, whereas the periosteum forms bone. Simultaneously, the trabecular endosteum forms bone at the point of metaphyseal osseous replacement and may remove bone if the marrow cavity is to be hollow.

These events lead to a definitive structure in those bones that develop from a single ossification center. Most bones of the body,

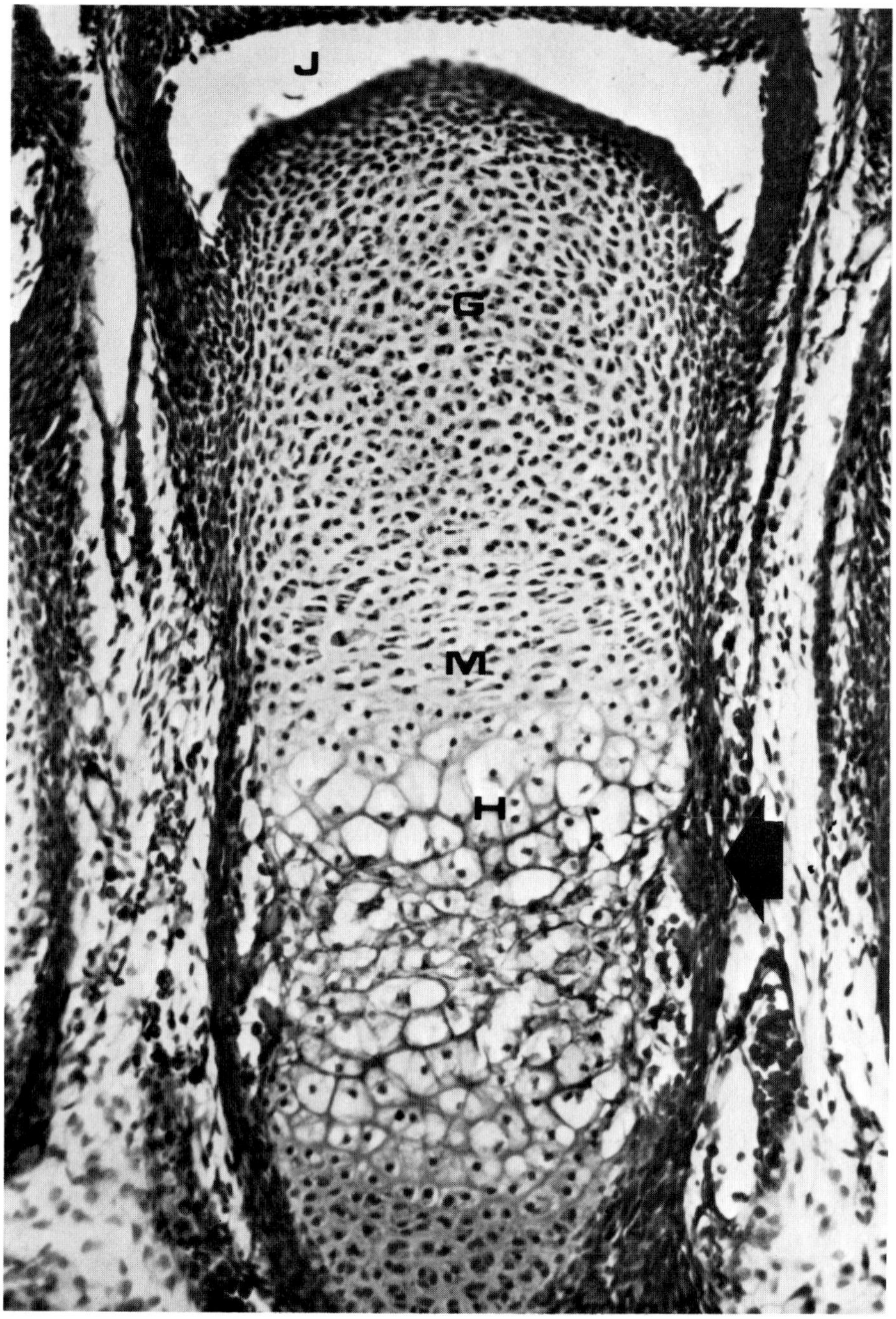

Fig. 9.17 Maturation of cartilage cells in the metacarpal ossification center of a fetal hamster. Chondrocytes are growing (G), maturing (M) and undergoing hypertrophy (H). The peripheral limits of the model are defined by a perichondrium (*arrow*). The metacarpal-phalangeal joint (J) has formed. X40.

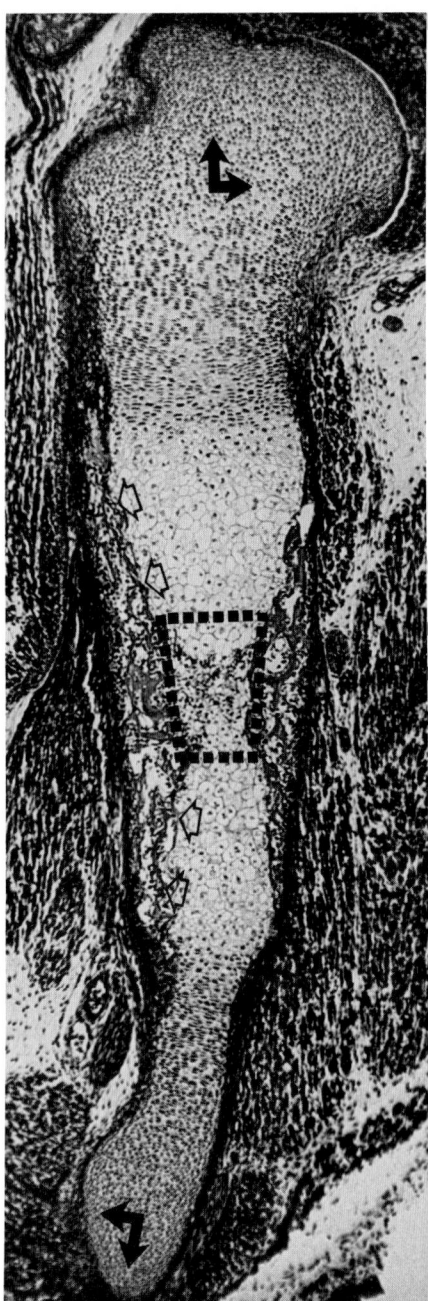

Fig. 9.18 Progressive development of the primary ossification center of a fetal hamster humerus. *Outlined area*, primary ossification center. Periosteal collar bone has developed (*open arrows*). The bone continues to grow in the directions indicated (*solid arrows*). X7.

however, develop from more than one ossification center.

Secondary Ossification Centers. Most of the long bones develop from at least three ossification centers. The primary ossification center accounts for the formation of the diaphysis, while *proximal* and *distal ossification centers* account for the formation of the proximal and distal epiphyses. These are referred to as *secondary ossification centers* (Figs. 9.13D, 9.13E). The number of ossification centers that characterize a developing

bone is a function of the degree of irregular shape of the specific bone (Fig. 9.22). All of these centers are called secondary ossification centers.

The sequence of events that lead to the formation of the secondary ossification centers and the events that occur within the secondary ossification center are essentially identical to those described for the primary ossification center (Figs. 9.13D, 9.13E, 9.13F). Cartilage cells mature in the center of the cartilage that comprises the ends of

the model. The central region of matrix subsequently calcifies. Dissolution of matrix and the formation of cavities within the calcified matrix are accompanied by vascular invasion similar to that which occurred in the primary ossification center. The epiphyseal arteries are responsible for this vascular invasion. Actually, *cartilage canals* are scattered throughout the presumptive secondary ossification centers. Cartilage canals,

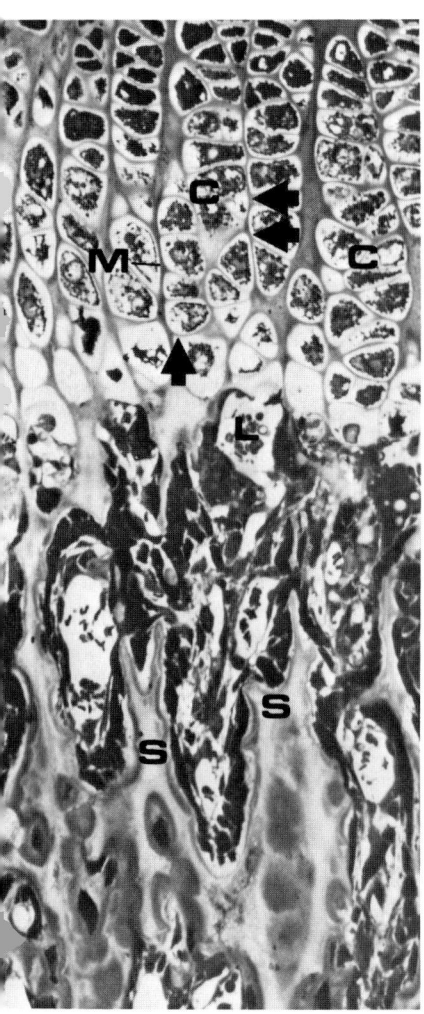

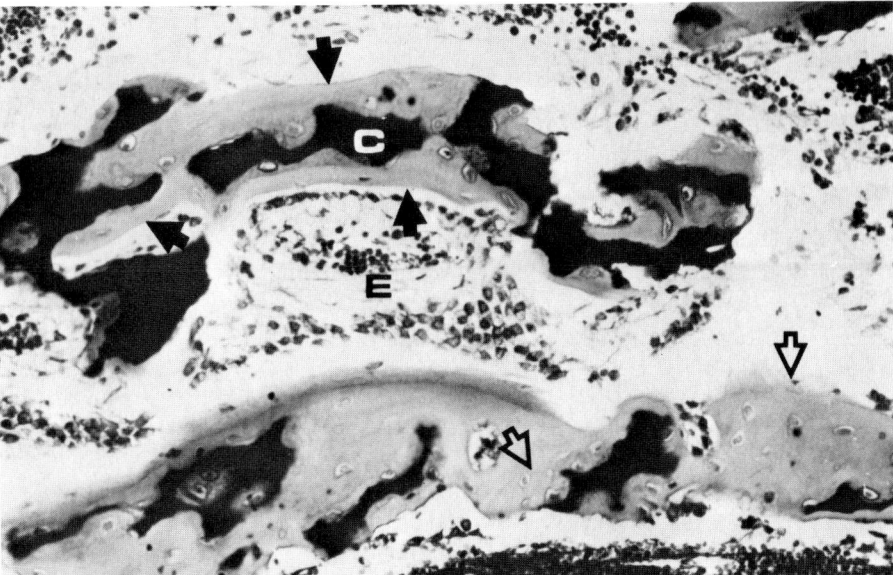

Fig. 9.20 Tissues of the primary spongiosa. Spicules of bone contain a core of calcified cartilage (C). Woven bone (*open arrows*) comprises the bulk of the osseous tissue. Lamellar bone formation is occurring upon the spicules (*solid arrows*). The interosseous tissues are endosteum (E) and myeloid elements. X40 (Aldehyde fuchsin).

ig. 9.19 Removal of calcified cartilage within he primary ossification center (mouse femur). he chondrocytes (C) within their lacunae are eparated from each other by thin rims of cartaginous matrix (M). Transverse septa (*arrow*) o not mineralize, whereas longitudinal septa *double arrows*) undergo mineralization. Capilary loops (L) are surrounded by numerous erivascular cells. Osteoclasts remove transerse septa and chondrocytes are released. he continuous lacunar surfaces and intervenng matrix become the surfaces (S) or longituinal septa upon which woven bone deposition ccurs. X160 (plastic-embedded, 1 μm secon).

resumably containing branches of the epihyseal arteries, are foci around which marix dissolution occurs (Fig. 9.23). Osseous eplacement occurs radially from the central egion in all directions. The amount of carilage is reduced progressively. Cartilage renains as an articular surface and cartilage emains as a disk or plate between the bone orming in the epiphyseal center and the one forming in the diaphyseal center (Fig. .24). This plate is called the *growth plate epiphyseal plate, epiphyseal disk, physis*). Cartilage is added continuously to the secndary ossification center by the interstitial

growth of the cells from the subarticular cartilage and the epiphyseal side of the growth plate. These zones of proliferative cells are continuous with each other at the peripheral margin of the cartilage of the epiphysis. The proliferative zone of the growth plate adds new cartilage cells to the diaphyseal and epiphyseal ossification centers simultaneously for a variable amount of time. Eventually epiphyseal osseous replacement adjacent to the growth plate overrides the proliferative capacity of the cartilage on this side of the growth plate. This results in the formation of an *endplate* of epiphyseal bone juxtaposed to the cartilage (Figs. 9.13F, 9.25). Two direct consequences occur as a result of endplate formation: 1) the growth and shaping of the epiphysis then is a function of the proliferative activity of the subarticular cartilage; 2) subsequent to endplate formation the growth plate only contributes cartilage to the diaphyseal ossification center.

Growth Plates. The formation of the growth plate occurs as a consequence of the development and expansion of a secondary ossification center (Figs. 9.13E, 9.13F, 9.24, 9.25, 9.26). The continued elongation of the diaphysis is a result of the interstitial growth of the cartilage within the growth plate. Mitotic activity within the reserve chondrocytic zone adds new cells constantly and moves the epiphysis further from the center of the diaphysis. This addition tends to thicken the growth plate; however, the growth plate maintains a relatively constant thickness throughout its functional existence. The constant thickness of the growth plate is maintained because the rate of proliferation of the reserve chondrocytic zone

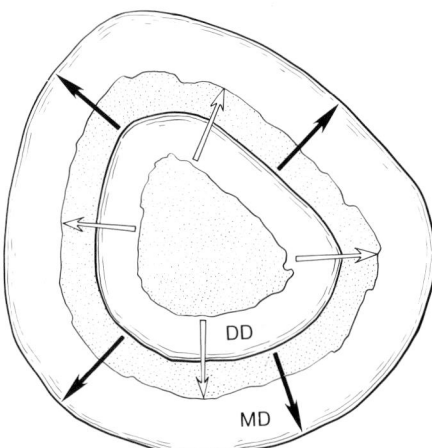

Fig. 9.21 Latitudinal movement of the diaphysis during growth. The developing diaphysis (DD) grows in width through the osteogenic activity of the periosteum (*solid arrows*). As periosteal bone is added, the cortical endosteum removes bone by osteoclastic activity (*open arrows*). The net result is a diaphysis with an increased diameter and an increased marrow cavity diameter (MD-mature diaphysis).

equals the rate of metaphyseal osseous replacement. Accordingly, the elongation of the diaphysis is coincident with the movement of the growth plate through space. Cessation of growth is achieved and the growth plate becomes progressively thinner and eventually closes when the rate of cartilage proliferation is exceeded by the rate of metaphyseal osseous replacement. Growth plates close at different times in different bones in different species. However, closure times for specific growth plates

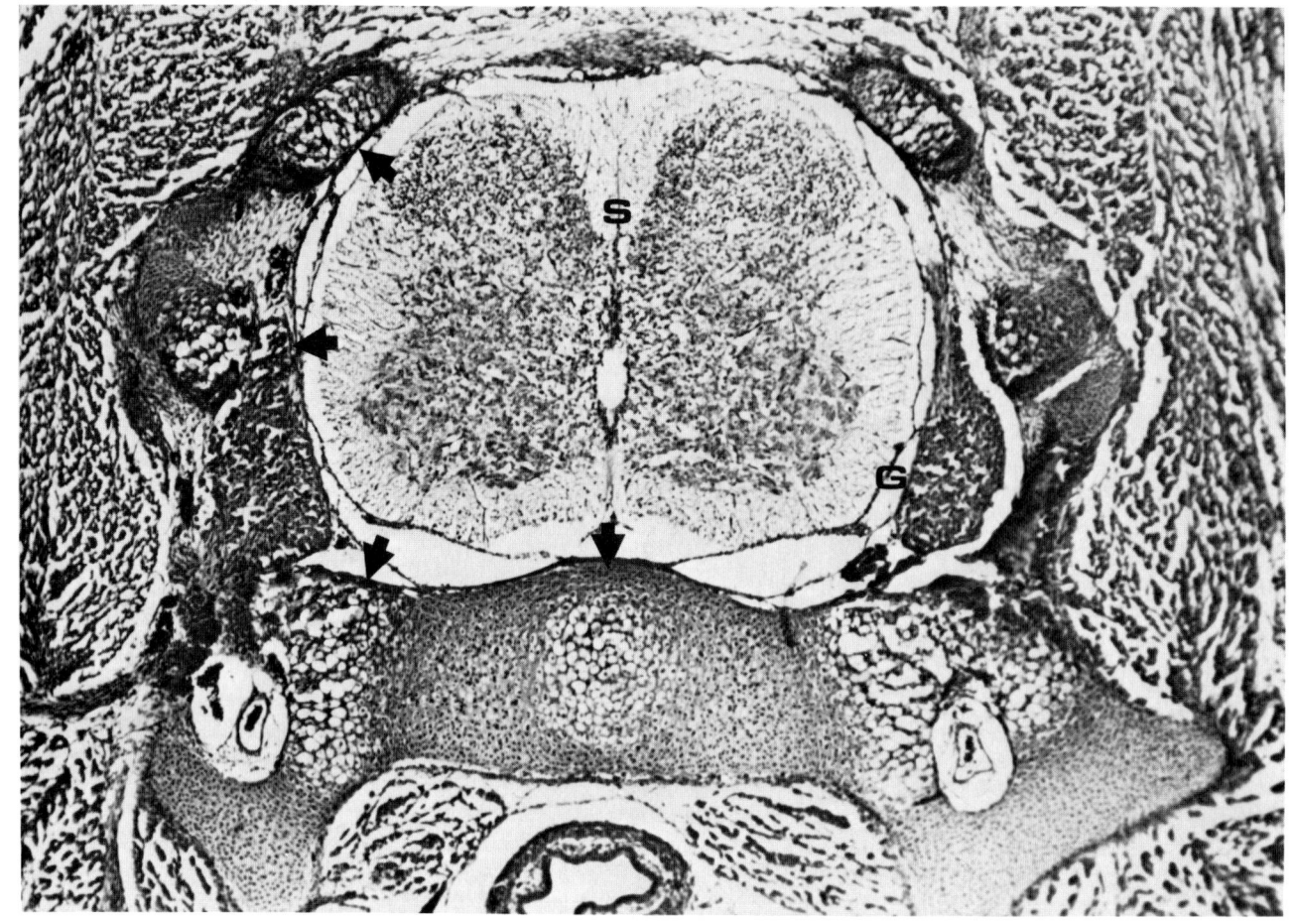

Fig. 9.22   Developing cervical vertebra of a fetal hamster. Numerous ossification centers (*arrows*) characterize the development of this irregular bone. The developing spinal cord and a dorsal root ganglion (G) occupy the spinal canal. X10.

in specific bones of a given species occur in a given time period. At closure, the trabecular bone of the metaphysis becomes continuous with the trabecular bone of the epiphysis (Figs. 9.13F, 9.13G).

The histologic organization of the growth plate is similar to that of the ossification center prior to plate formation. The events within the growth plate are identical to those described for the primary ossification center. This should not be surprising, since the growth plate is the proximal and/or distal limit of the expanding primary ossification center.

Five zones of cartilage cells are identifiable within the growth plate (Figs. 9.26, 9.27): 1) zone of resting chondrocytes, 2) zone of proliferative chondrocytes, 3) zone of maturing chondrocytes, 4) zone of hypertrophied chondrocytes and 5) the zone of calcified cartilage.

The *zone of resting chondrocytes* is juxtaposed to the epiphyseal endplate. These cells do not divide. Their primary function seems to be to weld the growth plate to the epiphysis.

The zone of *proliferative chondrocytes* is responsible for the elongation of the bone

as an organ. The zone is characterized by stacks of thin, wedge-shape cells that are actively mitotic. The stacks of cells represent isogenous groups or cell nests that are associated with interstitial growth. The activity of this zone is responsible for elongation as well as adding new cells to replace those lost to metaphyseal osseous replacement (Fig. 9.28).

The *zone of maturing chondrocytes* is the region in which various cellular characteristics may be observed. Cell and lacunar size increase progressively and lacunae become more rounded. The columnation of these cells is obvious. Mechanical influences upon the growth plate probably account for this columnation.

The *zone of hypertrophied chondrocytes* is a narrow zone adjacent to the maturation zone. Characteristically, the cells are large and the intercellular substance is reduced progressively. *Transverse septa* are especially thin. The *longitudinal septa*, the cartilage matrix between adjacent columns of cells, will eventually undergo calcification. This is the weakest zone of the growth plate. Fractures of growth plates (*epiphysiolysis*) generally occur through this zone.

The *zone of calcified cartilage* consists of cells, the matrix of which undergoes calcification. This calcification is associated with *matrix vesicles* (Chapter 7) and is confined generally to the longitudinal septa.

Perivascular cells of the capillary loops in this region of calcified cartilage remove the transverse septa (Figs. 9.28, 9.29). Chondrocytic lacunae become confluent and their contiguous surfaces are those upon which woven bone is deposited. These surfaces actually are the longitudinal septa. In longitudinal section they appear as finger-like projections into the metaphysis (Plate I.8). In actuality, they are tunnels the inner surfaces of which are used for bone deposition (Fig. 9.30).

The relationships of the *primary spongiosa* and *secondary spongiosa* in association with the growth plate are identical to those relationships described with the primary ossification center (Fig. 9.31).

Attainment of Definitive Morphology. Numerous events that are integral parts of the endochondral ossification process are responsible for the refinement of the structure that is characteristic of the definitive bone of the body.

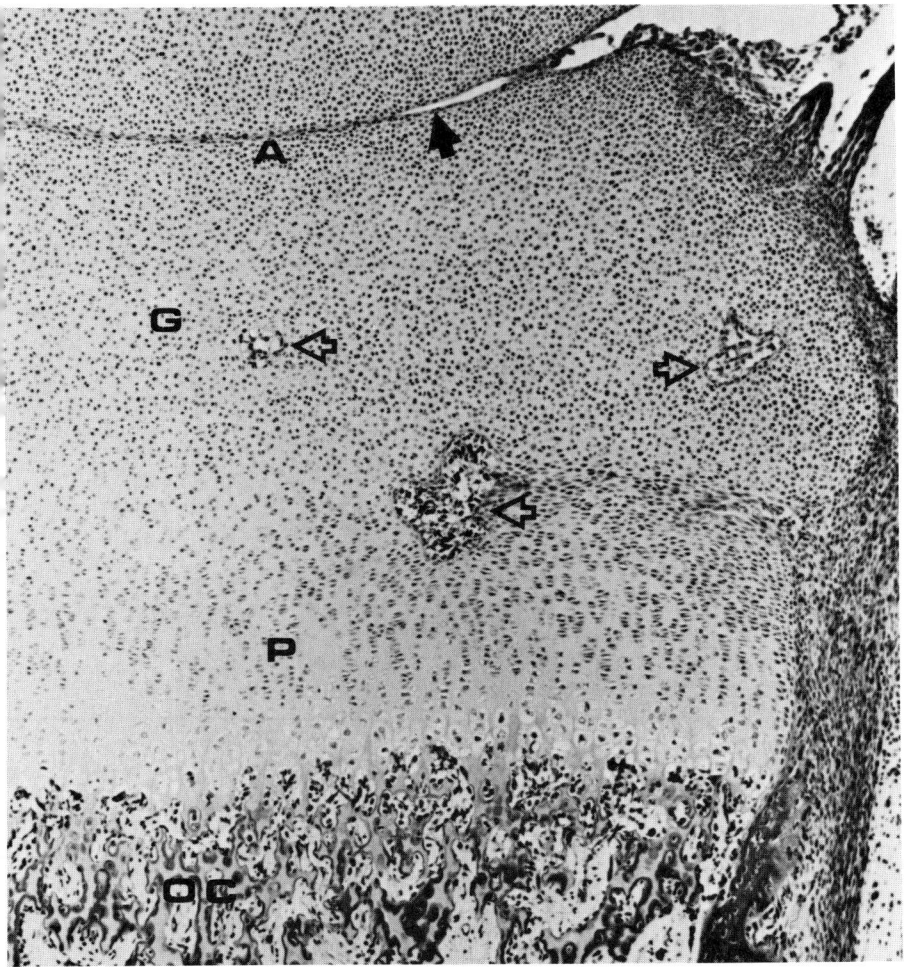

Fig. 9.23 Initiation of a secondary ossification center. The articular surface (*solid arrow*) is lined by chondrocytes (A) that are continuous through the growing cartilage (G) to the presumptive growth plate (P). The margin of the primary ossification center (OC) is beneath the presumptive physis. Cartilage canals (*open arrows*) are scattered throughout the presumptive secondary ossification center. X16.

the bones of the body. The activities that result in the three-dimensional morphology of a bone are called *modeling*. Modeling activities are complemented by internal remodeling; attendant internal changes accompany changes in gross morphology.

Hormonal Effects Upon Endochondral Ossification. Numerous and varied cellular activities are responsible for the integrated activities encompassed by endochondral ossification. Differentiation, modulation, mitosis, carbohydrate synthesis and secretion, protein synthesis and secretion, calcium metabolism and phagocytosis are integral functions of the cellular populations of the connective, cartilaginous, osseous and vascular tissues that are essential components of this developmental process. All of these events are regulated and influenced by numerous factors. The same factors that influence bone, as discussed in Chapter 8, have an effect upon developing bone as an organ and tissue.

The effects of *estrogens* upon endochondral ossification are diverse, complex and species-specific. Generally, the estrogens inhibit linear growth by favoring the closure of the growth plates. This involves an acceleration of metaphyseal osseous replacement and an inhibition upon the proliferative chondrocytes.

Testosterone exerts an effect similar to the estrogens. Skeletal maturation is dependent upon the presence of this hormone, because it favors bone formation. Its presence is important in the achievement of normal growth plate closure.

Excessive quantities of *glucocorticoids* inhibit skeletal growth and retard the development of secondary ossification centers. A decreased proliferation and hypertrophy of chondrocytes is a consistent developmental problem with excessive quantities of these substances. The phenomenon may be explained by the inhibitory effects of glucocorticosteroids upon protein synthesis. Osteoblastic activity within the primary and secondary spongiosa is reduced also. Similarly, they decrease the osteoblastic activity of the periosteum and endosteum of growing bones.

Growth hormone mediates its effect upon the growing skeleton by regulating the rate of mitosis of the proliferative chondrocytes. Excesses of growth hormone before growth plate closure result in *pituitary gigantism*. After growth plate closure, excesses result in a pronounced periosteal new bone formation called *acromegaly*.

Although the *thyroid hormones* (T_3 and T_4) affect the cellular metabolic activity of most cells, their effects upon the developing skeleton are manifested primarily in the cartilage. Thyroxine (T_4) is necessary for the proliferation and maturation of the chondrocytes. It also affects the proliferation and modulation of osteogenic cells of the primary and secondary spongiosa.

The attainment of definitive length is primarily the function of the growth plate. Although some length is achieved prior to the formation of a growth plate, the greatest amount of length results from the interstitial growth of the growth plate cartilage. Bone as an organ grows by the interstitial growth of the growth plate cartilage, but bone as a tissue can only grow by appositional growth.

The events responsible for the increased diameter of a bone were discussed previously. Importantly, periosteal bone deposition is balanced by the osteoclastic activity of the cortical endosteum. The majority of the compact bone of the diaphysis is derived from the periosteum. This includes primary osteons and outer circumferential lamellar bone. Secondary osteons represent osteonal endosteal modification of bone derived from periosteum.

The ends of long bones, generally are larger than the diaphysis (Fig. 9.32). The epiphyses and metaphyses are characterized by a distinct flair. After the formation of the epiphyseal endplate, the growth of the epiphysis occurs independently of the events of

the diaphyseal ossification center. The growing cartilage subjacent to the articular cartilage contributes to the expanded epiphysis. Naturally, the growing diaphysis must maintain a proper relationship with the enlarged epiphysis. This is achieved by selected modeling activities in the metaphyseal region. During growth, bone is resorbed on the periosteal side of the metaphysis, and bone is added to the trabeculae (tunnels) of the metaphysis as these join the endosteal side of the diaphysis. This facilitates a gradual flaring of the proximal and distal aspects of the bone.

The trabeculae of bone that are derived from the peripheral aspect of the growth plate are joined to the diaphysis (Fig. 9.33). The spatial orientation of the trabeculae is in the form of tunnels. The diaphyseal/metaphyseal union is strengthened by the progressive filling of these tunnels with bone. This is another way in which osteons may form during the conversion from cancellous to compact bone.

All of these activities combine to produce the definitive shapes that characterize all of

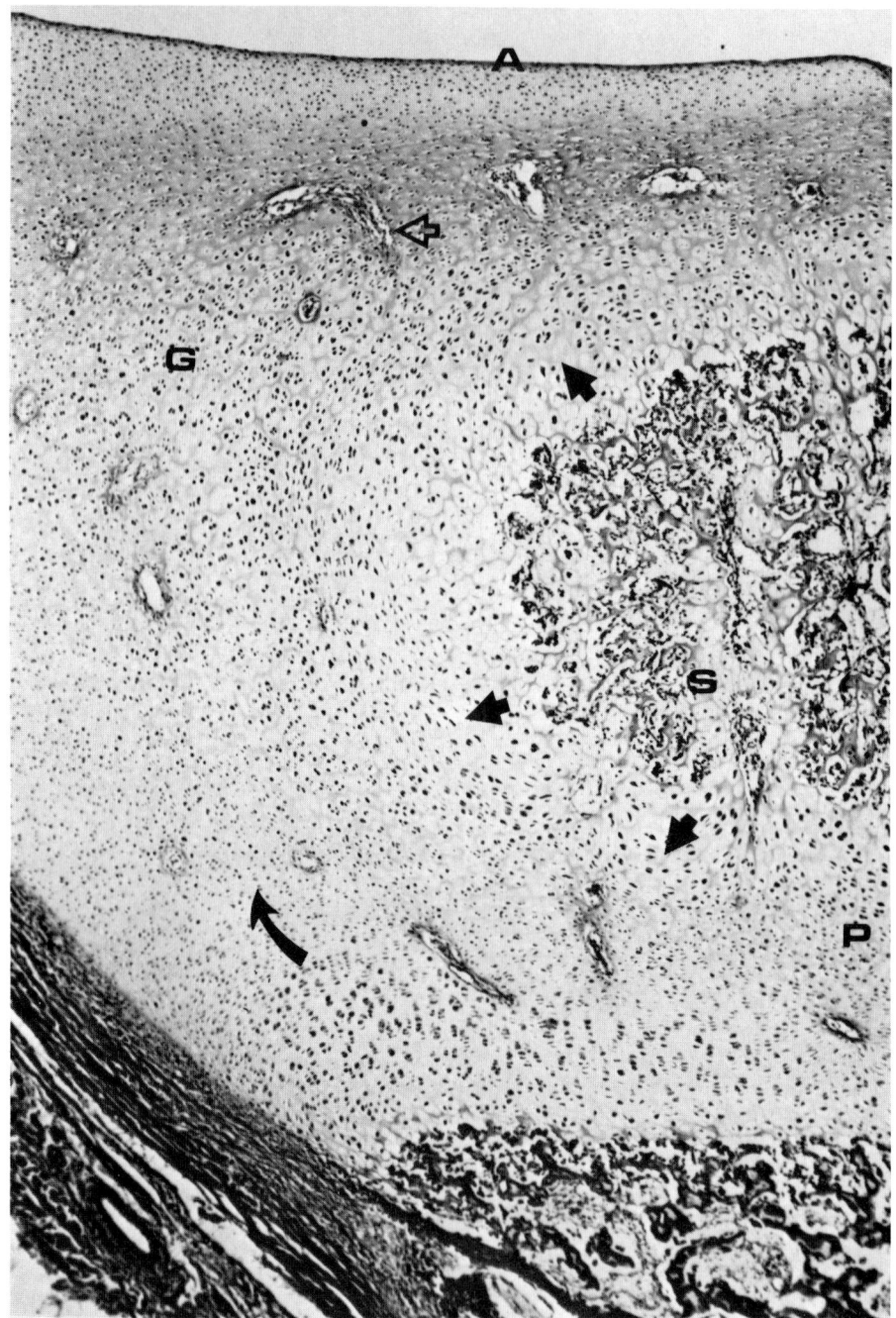

Fig. 9.24 A longitudinal section through a developing secondary ossification center. The cartilage of the epiphysis includes the articular cartilage (A), growing cartilage (G) and growth plate cartilage (P). The continuity of the growth plate cartilage (*curved arrow*) with the articular cartilage often is maintained throughout development. The secondary ossification center expands progressively (*solid arrows*) gradually reducing the epiphyseal and growth plate cartilage to narrow zones. X10.

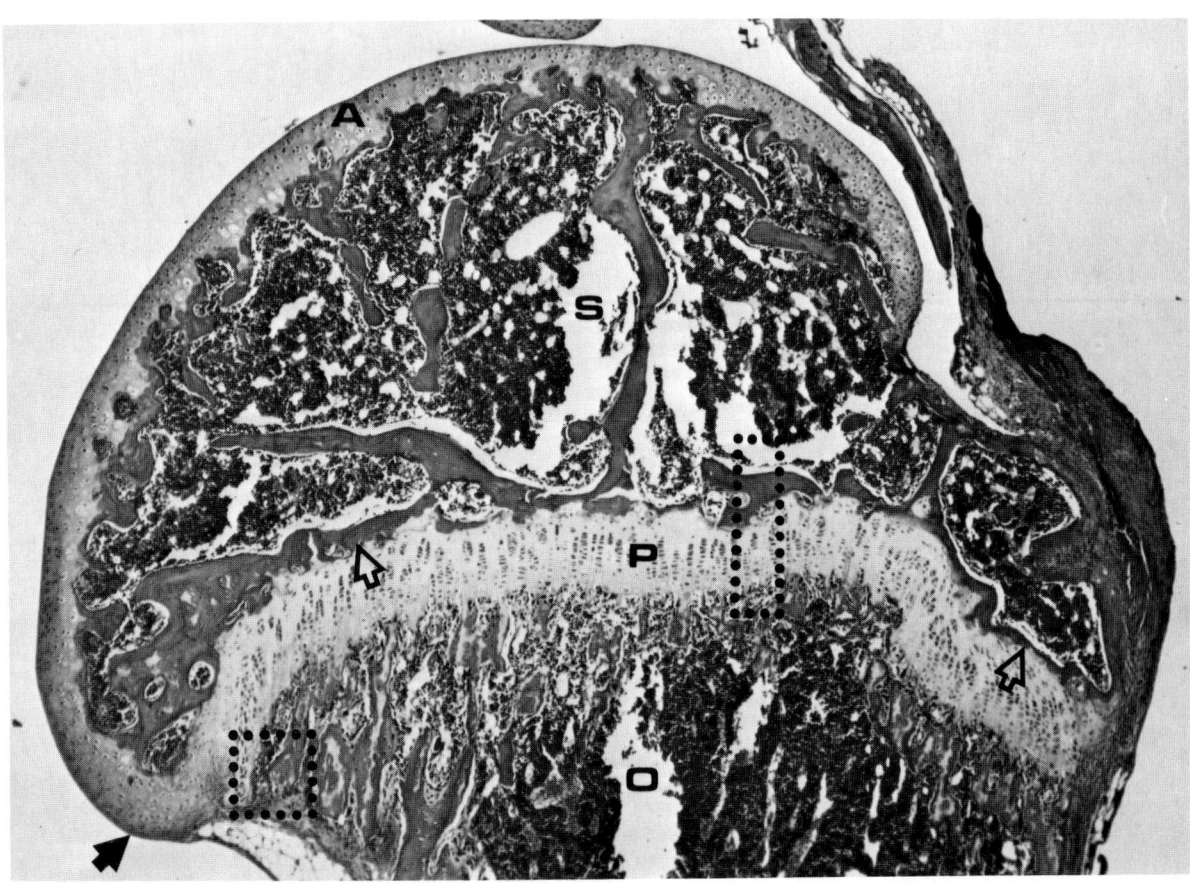

Fig. 9.25   The proximal humerus of a growing gerbil. The growth plate (P) separates the primary ossification center (O) from the secondary ossification center (S). The growth plate is continuous with the articular cartilage (*arrow*). Spicules of bone and calcified cartilage as well as myeloid tissue fill both ossification centers. The spaces are artifacts of preparation. The endplate (*open arrows*) resides upon the proximal margin of the physis. The *square area* is enlarged in Figure 9.33; the *rectangular area*, Figure 9.26. X10.

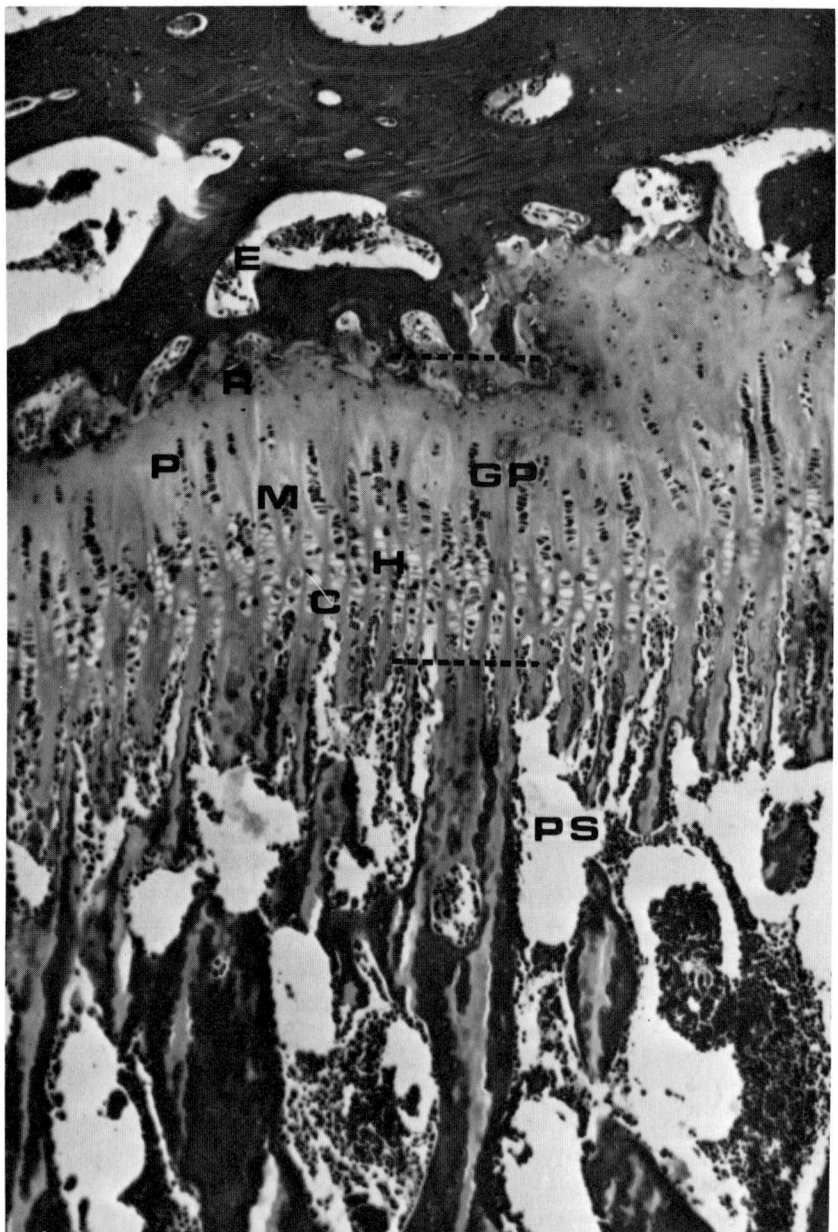

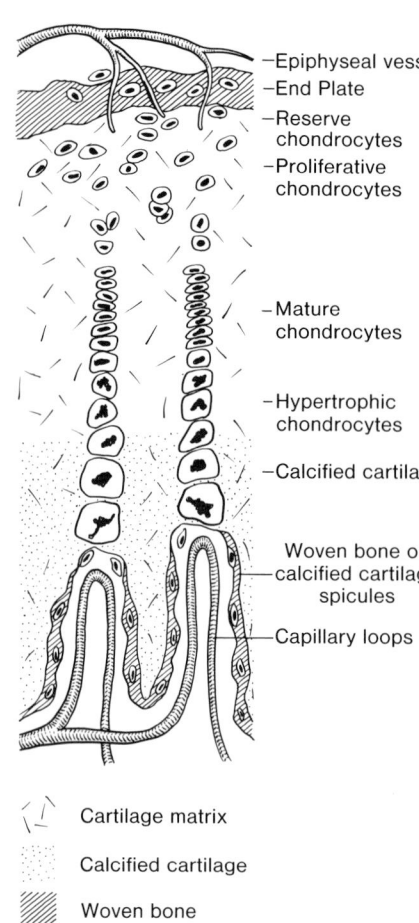

Epiphyseal vessels
End Plate
Reserve chondrocytes
Proliferative chondrocytes

Mature chondrocytes

Hypertrophic chondrocytes

Calcified cartilage

Woven bone on calcified cartilage spicules

Capillary loops

⟨ ⟩ Cartilage matrix

Calcified cartilage

Woven bone

Fig. 9.27 Diagram of a physis. Compare with Figure 9.26. The important components of the growth plate are labeled.

Fig. 9.26 Definitive growth plate. The endplate (E) has formed on the epiphyseal side of the growth plate. The approximate limits of the growth plate (GP) are indicated by *dashed lines*. The growth plate maintains a relatively constant thickness until closure occurs. The cells within the physis are columnated and are divisible into distinct yet related groups or zones. R-resting chondrocytes; P-proliferative chondrocytes; M-maturing chondrocytes; H-hypertrophied chondrocytes; C-zone of calcified cartilage. The primary spongiosa (PS) is just below the physis. X50.

Fracture Repair

General Features. Fractures may be defined simply as a loss of continuity or structural integrity in bones. Attendant changes may occur that may alter the normal function of the anatomic unit, may cause a loss of function of the anatomic unit or may affect changes elsewhere that may be symptomatic of the fracture. Fractures, however, may be accompanied by no apparent loss of normal function.

Various schemes are used to classify fractures: traumatic vs. pathologic, incomplete vs. complete, simple vs. compound, comminuted vs. noncomminuted. Also, many descriptors are used to describe the relationships of the broken fragments: tranverse, oblique, avulsive, overriding. Although various management procedures are utilized to facilitate the repair process, there are only a few ways that bone as an organ will respond to fracture, if normal repair is to be achieved. Bone will heal by *primary intention* or *secondary intention*. Before discussing the actual sequence of events that comprises these two mechanisms of repair, it is important to recognize that numerous factors can influence the course and outcome of the fracture repair process.

Nutritional and metabolic factors can exert a significant influence upon the repair of bone. A well-balanced *diet* is an essential component of good repair. The *age* of the animal is an important factor. Older animals tend toward a lower osteogenic activity than their younger counterparts. Similarly, the presence of intercurrent *disease* processes may alter significantly the outcome of the repair process. One of the most devastating influences upon fracture repair is the presence of *infection*, either naturally-induced during the fracture of the bone or introduced iatrogenically during the manipulation of the fracture.

Three other factors significantly affect the outcome of the fracture repair process; the *stability* and *immobilization* of the fracture site during the repair process, the maintenance of good *vascular integrity*, and the ability to return the fragments to their original relationship (*reduction*). These are factors over which the practitioner generally exercises some influence. Moreover, these factors generally influence whether fracture repair will proceed by primary or secondary intention healing.

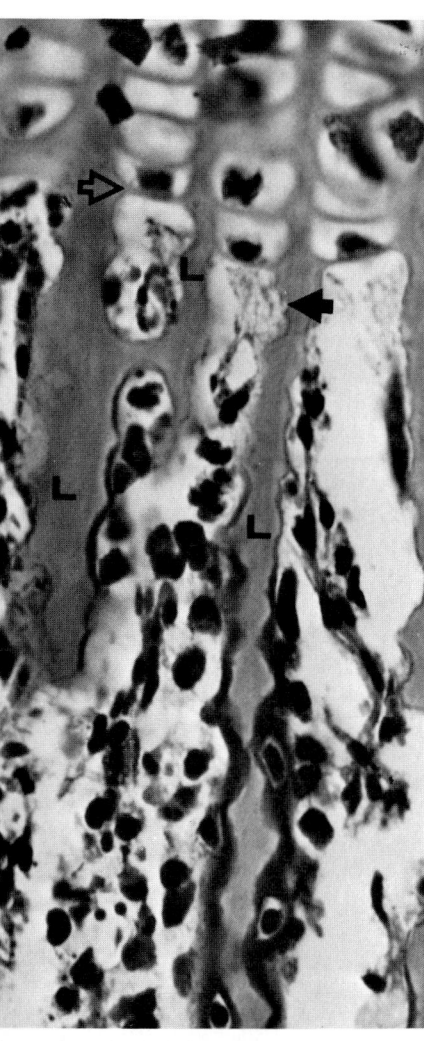

Fig. 9.28 Osseous replacement within the primary spongiosa. Chondrocytes are released from their lacunae (*solid arrow*) after disintegration of transverse septa (*open arrow*). These are the cells that are replaced by the proliferative zone of chondrocytes. Some chondrocytes have been displaced from their lacunae by the processing. The remaining longitudinal septa (L) have scalloped borders that correspond to confluent lateral margins of lacunae. The dark material deposited on the longitudinal septa is woven bone. Compare with Figure 9.19. X100.

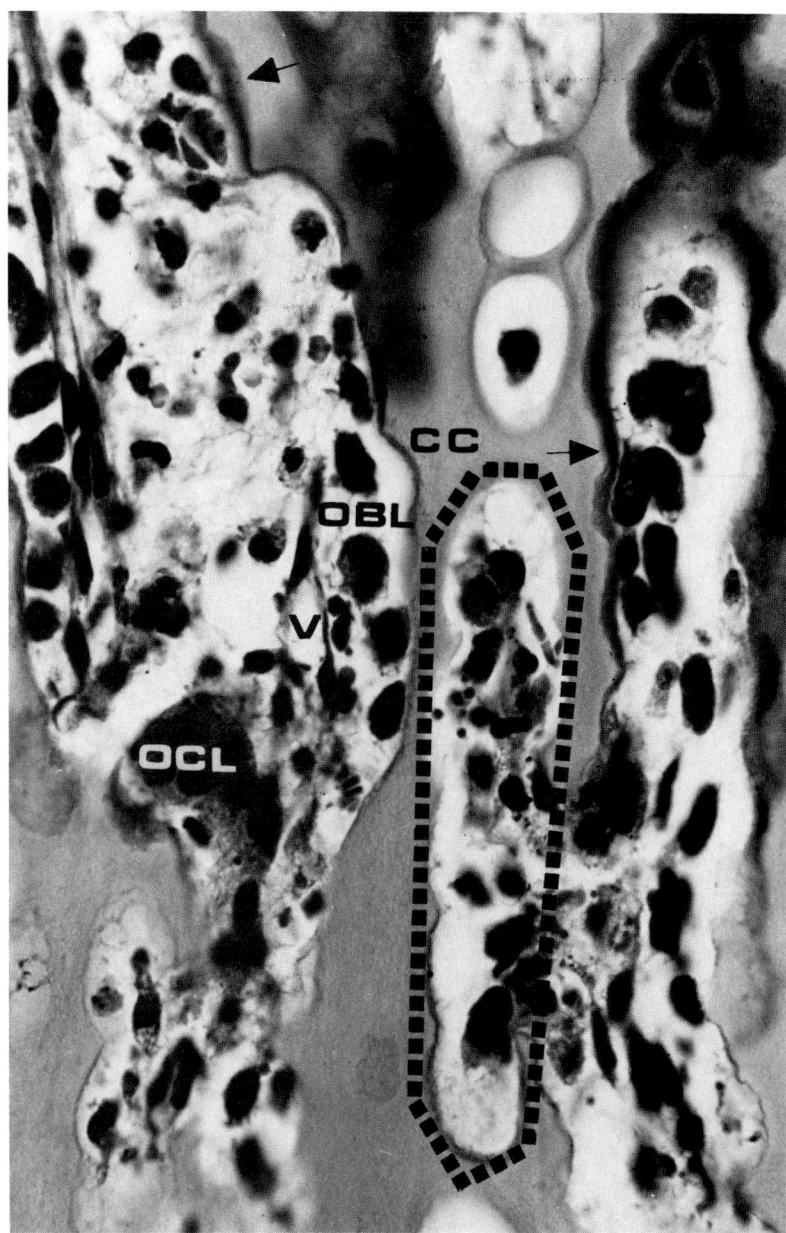

Fig. 9.29 Osteoblastic and osteoclastic activity adjacent to the growth plate. Confluent lacunae and their remaining longitudinal septa (*outlined area*) are the surfaces upon which osteoblasts (OBL) deposit woven bone (*arrows*). Osteoblasts and osteoclasts (OCL) comprise a major portion of the perivascular cell population associated with numerous vascular loops (V). X160.

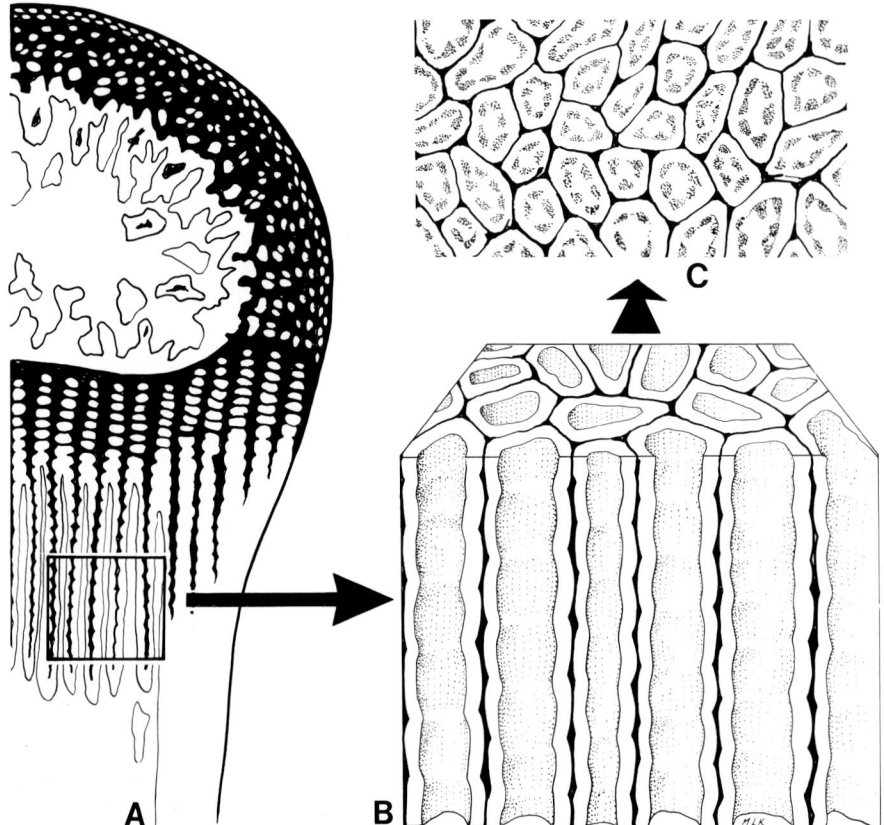

Fig. 9.30 Diagram of the morphologic relationships of components of the primary spongiosa. The retained longitudinal septa of calcified cartilage with woven bone deposited on the surface appear as spicules or finger-like projections in longitudinal section (A). The spicules are actually tunnels when viewed in three dimensions (B). The walls of the tunnels are formed of bone deposited upon a peripheral core of calcified cartilage. The tunnels become filled progressively with bone at their points of union with the diaphysis. Progressive centripetal deposition of bone within the tunnels (C) results in the formation of osteons within the metaphysis. (Redrawn and modified from Ham, A. W.: *Histology*, 7th edition, J. B. Lippincott, Philadelphia, 1974.)

vascular channels within the bone are disrupted. This results in the death of bone cells (osteoprogenitors, osteoblasts, osteocytes) and endothelial cells some distance back from the ends of the fractured fragments. This results in the fracture site being bordered by dead bone back to the level of the first viable anastomosis with functional vessels. Proliferation of osteoprogenitor cells and endothelial cells occurs within the viable bone adjacent to the dead bone bordering the fracture site. These cells grow toward the fracture site. Eventually, osteoclasts develop and begin to remove bone from the

Although the fracture repair process can be a complicated event, it is, in its simplest form, a reiteration of events studied previously. In primary intention healing, fracture repair is a variation of internal remodeling in which formation activity is greater than resorptive activity.

In secondary intention healing, fracture repair is essentially a reiteration of endochondral ossification.

The two examples used to describe the primary and secondary intention healing of bone must be considered stereotypical. Many variations of these basic themes exist. Nevertheless, an understanding of these basic themes is essential.

The process of fracture repair is a continuum of cellular events that progresses from the insult (impact) through the successful remodeling of the injured site. Although there is significant overlap in the type of activities that occur throughout the process, it is useful to divide the process into distinctive yet interrelated stages based upon the predominant activity apparent. The stages of fracture repair are: *Impact, Induction, Inflammatory, Reparative* and *Remodeling Stages*. Because these stages are more ob-

vious with second intention healing of bone, they will be described then.

Primary Intention Healing

General Characteristics. *Primary intention healing* of bone is characterized by the direct formation of bone without the formation of an intermediary cartilaginous supportive structure (*callus*). For the sake of clarification, this description of repair is predicated upon the following assumptions: vascular integrity is good, immobilization is excellent, reduction and alignment of the two fragments is excellent, and the ends of the fractured fragments are smooth. Rigid fixation, immobilization and reduction of the fracture site are achieved by the application of a metallic plate across the fracture site. These circumstances are rarely applicable to a naturally-induced fracture; however, they are conditions associated with experimental fractures. Nevertheless, the principles are applicable to naturally-occurring fractures.

Under the specified conditions, the following can be anticipated (Fig. 9.34): After the impact, soft tissue injury and inflammation will occur. As a result of the fracture,

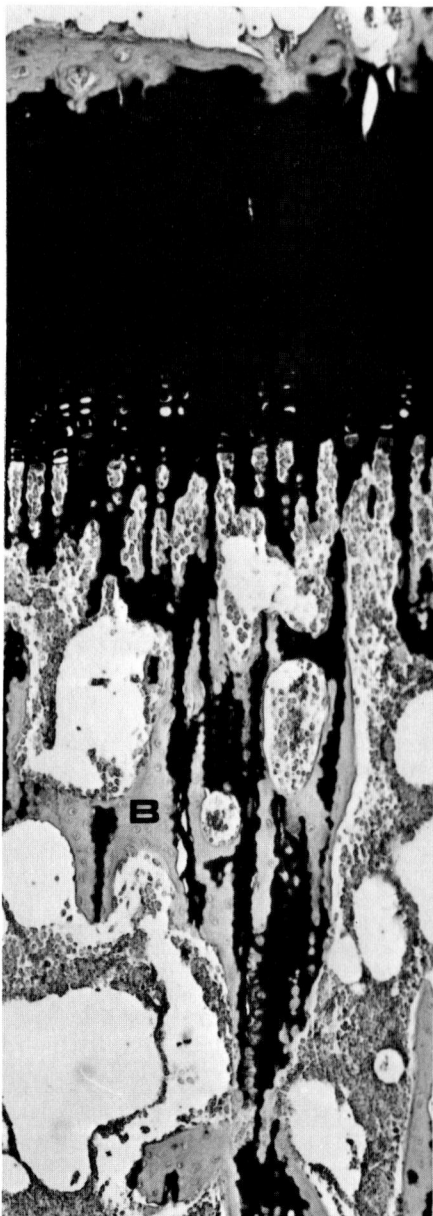

Fig. 9.31 Growth plate and primary spongiosa. Finger-like projections of dark-stained material, calcified cartilage, extend from the growth plate into the primary spongiosa. The progressive deposition of bone (B) is coupled to the continual removal of calcified cartilage. X16 (Aldehyde fuschin).

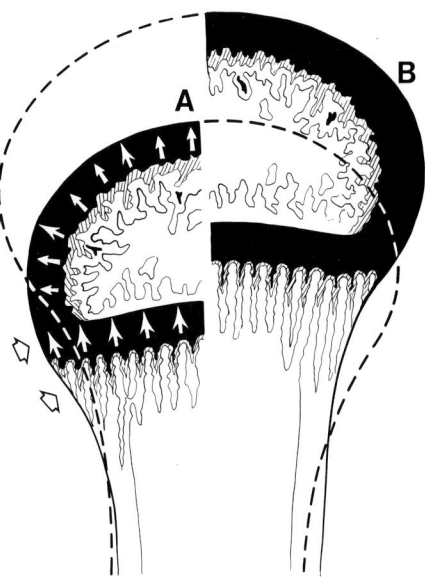

Fig. 9.32 A diagram of the activity associated with the modeling of epiphyses. The ends (epiphyses) of long bones are generally larger than the diaphyses. The growth plate and growth cartilage subjacent to the articular cartilage are responsible for the longitudinal movement of epiphyses through space. Interstitial growth of these components (*white arrows*) moves the epiphysis and articular surface from A to B. The epiphyseal flairing is accomplished by bone being resorbed by periosteal osteoclasts (*open arrows*) while deposition along the inner surface of the bone is accomplished via the trabecular endosteum associated with the tunnels of the primary spongiosa that are continuous with the diaphysis. (Redrawn and modified from Ham, A. W.: *Histology*, 7th edition, J. B. Lippincott, Philadelphia, 1974.)

osteonal canals in the same manner described with internal remodeling. The cutting cones cross the fracture site and establish the basis for the formation of new osteons.

Sometimes spaces may remain between the fractured fragments. This may occur when the fragments are irregularly fractured and perfect reduction is not achieved. Then, the space may be filled temporarily with woven bone that serves as a spot weld between the fragments. Canalization and new osteon formation still occurs as described. This process may be compared to the union of two pieces of wood with some glue (woven bone) and some dowels (new osteons).

Second Intention Healing

Second intention healing of bone involves the formation of an external supportive structure of cartilage, *callus*, during the fracture repair process. This type of healing can be anticipated when a rigid internal fixation device (metallic plate) is not used. It is generally the type of repair expected as a result of most management procedures involving the use of casts, pins and other devices. This

repair sequence occurs when vascular integrity may have been compromised, immobilization and stability of the fracture site are not perfect, and the reduction has not been achieved perfectly. For the sake of clarification, the following description assumes that the previously-described conditions relating to instability and reduction pertain to a simple, transverse, noncomminuted fracture in which the fractured fragments are smooth and fixation is achieved externally. The repair sequence is diagrammed in Figures 9.35–9.41.

Impact Stage. The energy absorbed upon impact of a bone is responsible for the type and extent of damage manifested. Because of their physical characteristics, bones fail (fracture) more readily with rapid loading than with slow loading. Also, they fail in tension. The impact not only accounts for the loss of osseous continuity, but it is responsible for the attendant soft tissue damage usually associated with such phenomena (Fig. 9.35). This results in the devitalization of previously normal tissues because of the disruption of vascular beds. The resultant hemostasis through clot formation exacerbates the vascular damage of the soft and

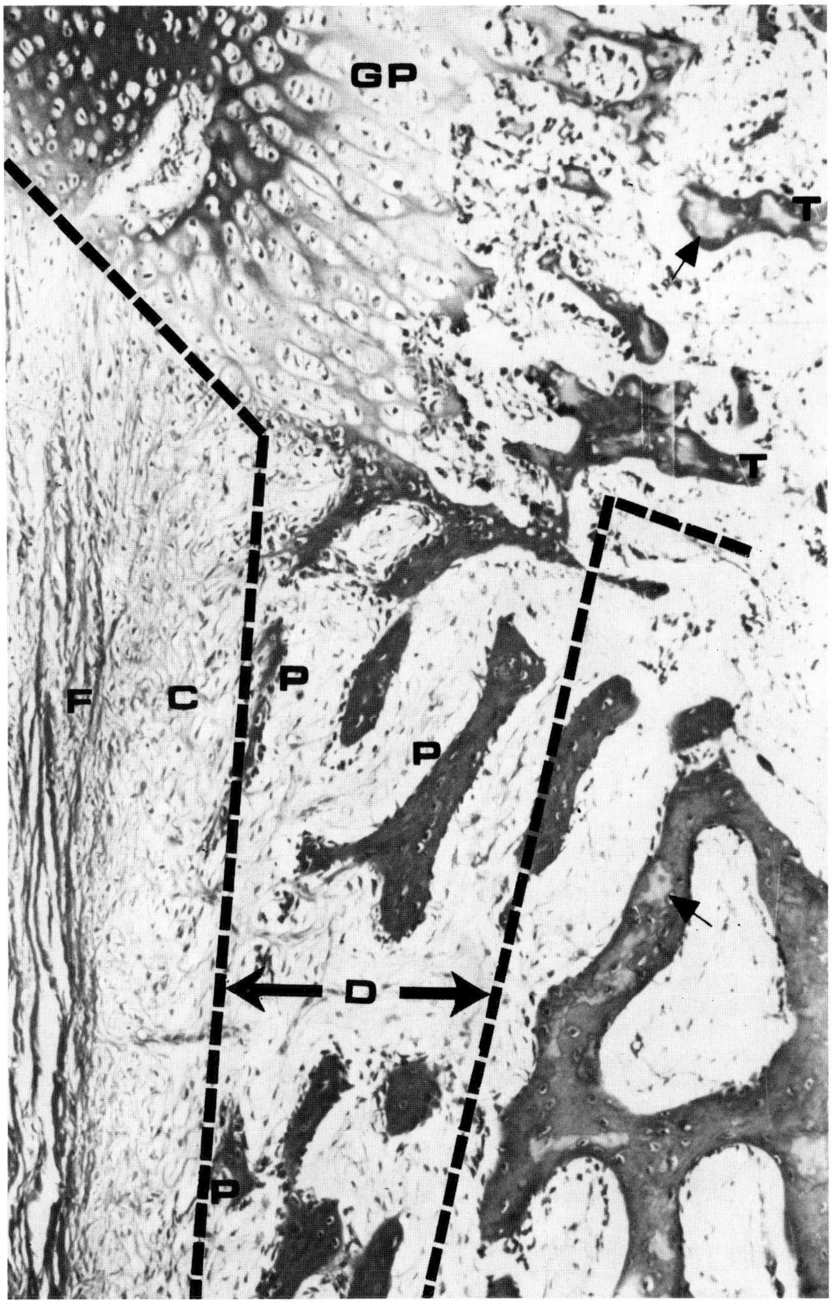

Fig. 9.33 Union of the growth plate to the diaphysis. The peripheral aspects of the growth plate (GP) are united to the diaphysis (D) by the tunnels (T) of calcified cartilage (*arrows*) and bone that comprise the primary spongiosa. The periosteum, fibrous (F) and cellular (C) components, covers the bone at this point of union (metaphysis). The periosteum may form bone (P) as well as remove it from this area. Removal results in the epiphyseal flairing characteristic of long bones. X25.

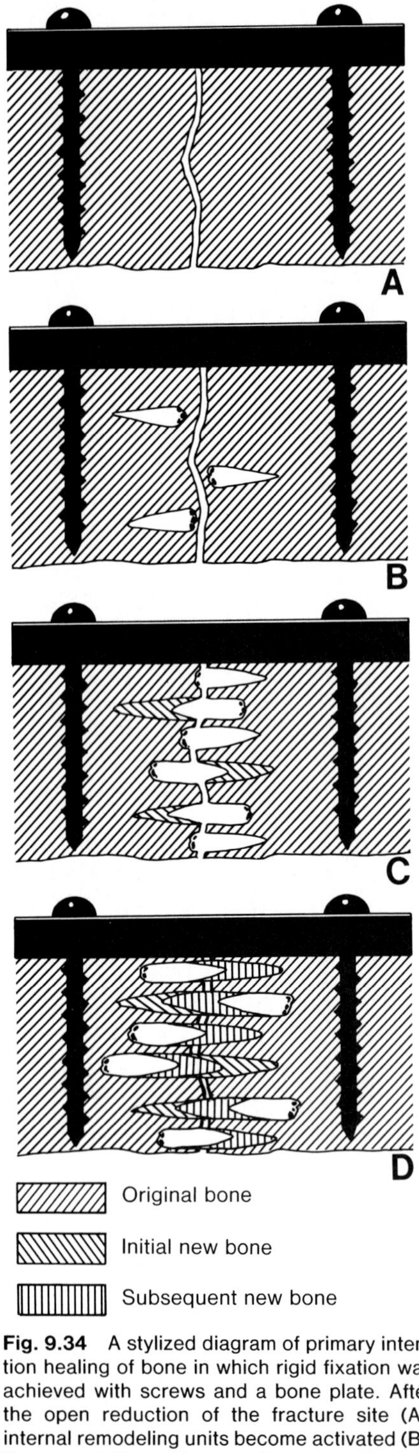

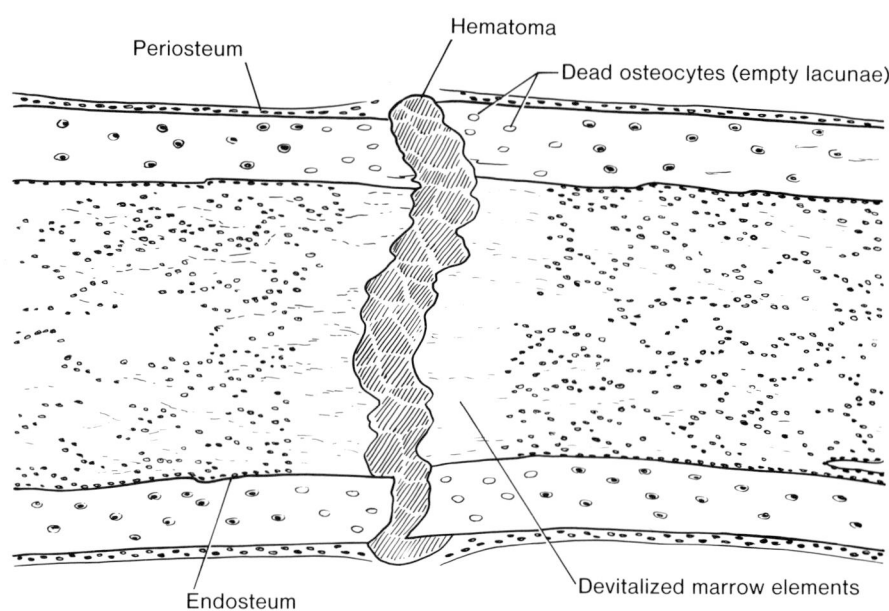

denced by the degeneration of osteocytes and empty osteocytic lacunae.

Induction Stage. The identification of this stage as a separate and distinct entity is probably quite artificial. Although it is initiated after the trauma, induction of new cells occurs throughout the fracture repair process. However, identifying it as a separate stage points to the significance of the events encompassed by it. Cells must be induced to proliferate, differentiate and modulate into new cellular populations to replace those that were damaged. Osteoblasts, osteoclasts, osteoprogenitor cells, chondroblasts, fibroblasts and endothelial cells comprise important replacement populations. The precise stimuli for the induction stage are unknown; however, local tissue hypoxia and related localized acidosis may be initial influential microenvironmen-

Fig. 9.35   Hematoma formation after fracture. Refer to the text for a complex description of the events involved in the fracture repair sequence as represented in Figures 9.35–9.41. (Figs. 9.35–9.41 were based upon, modified and expanded from the descriptions by Ham, A. W. and Harris, W. R.: Repair and transplantation of bone. *In:* Bourne, G. H. (editor), *The Biochemistry and Physiology of Bone*, Vol. III, pp. 337–399, Academic Press, New York, 1971.)

Original bone

Initial new bone

Subsequent new bone

Fig. 9.34   A stylized diagram of primary intention healing of bone in which rigid fixation was achieved with screws and a bone plate. After the open reduction of the fracture site (A), internal remodeling units become activated (B). The remodeling units cross the gap and establish a basis for osteonal bridging of the fracture site (C). The cutting cones form the cavity in which initial new bone formation occurs. The process continues (D) until new bone subsequently bridges the gap. Areas in the fracture gap between remodeling units may be "spot welded" with woven bone. The new osteons result in fracture repair having been achieved.

hard tissues. Periosteal and marrow elements, as well as endosteal components, and bone die back on either side of the fracture to a level coincident with the first functional vascular anastomosis. Bone death is evi-

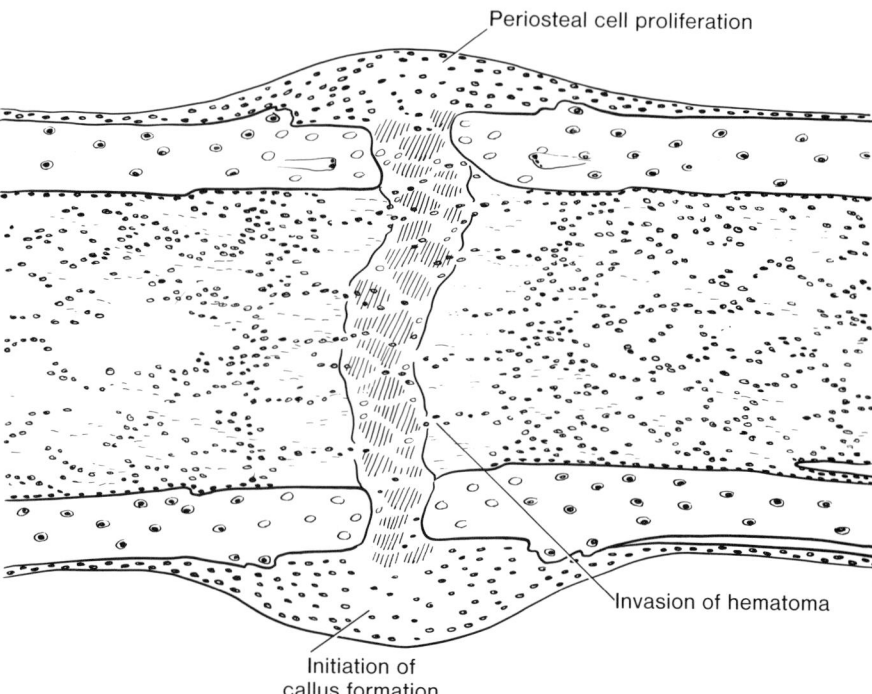

Fig. 9.36   Induction of cells from the marrow cavity, periosteum and endosteum. Invasion of the hematoma has occurred and callus formation is initiated.

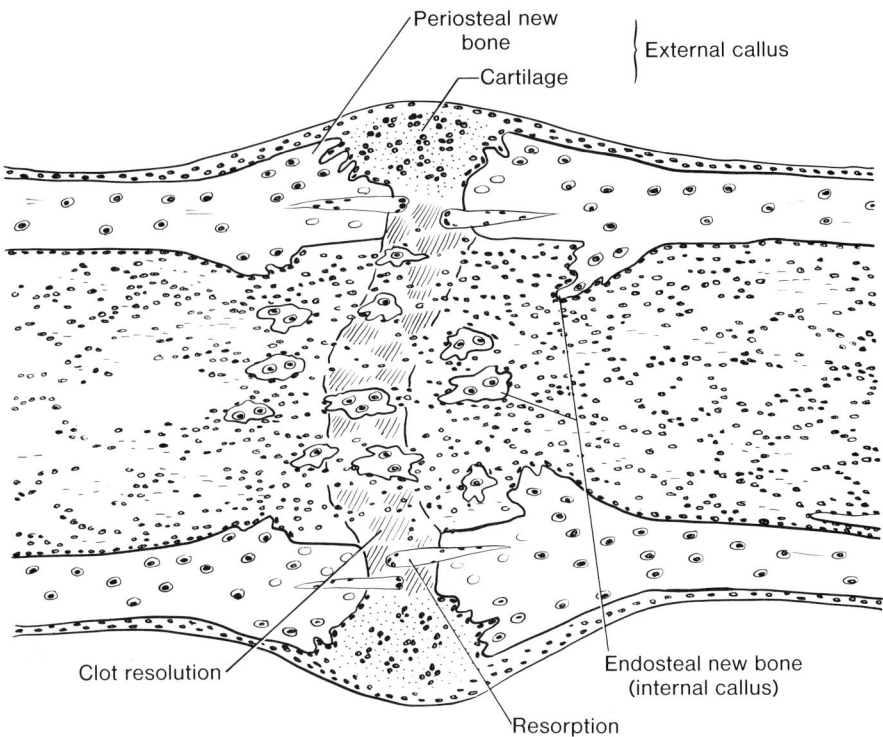

Fig. 9.37 Periosteal and endosteal bone formation at the fracture site. Bone formation in callus is initiated.

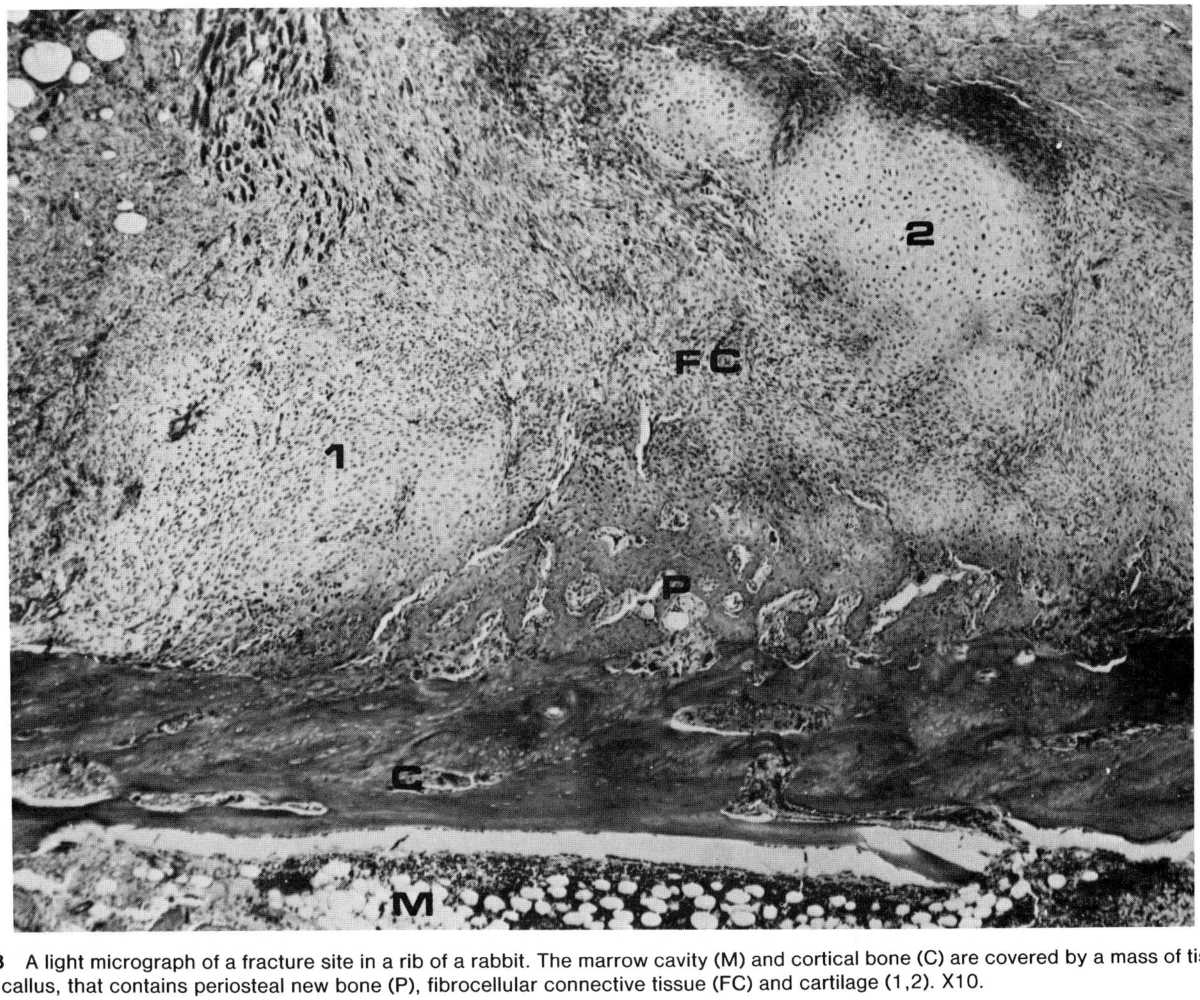

Fig. 9.38 A light micrograph of a fracture site in a rib of a rabbit. The marrow cavity (M) and cortical bone (C) are covered by a mass of tissue, the external callus, that contains periosteal new bone (P), fibrocellular connective tissue (FC) and cartilage (1,2). X10.

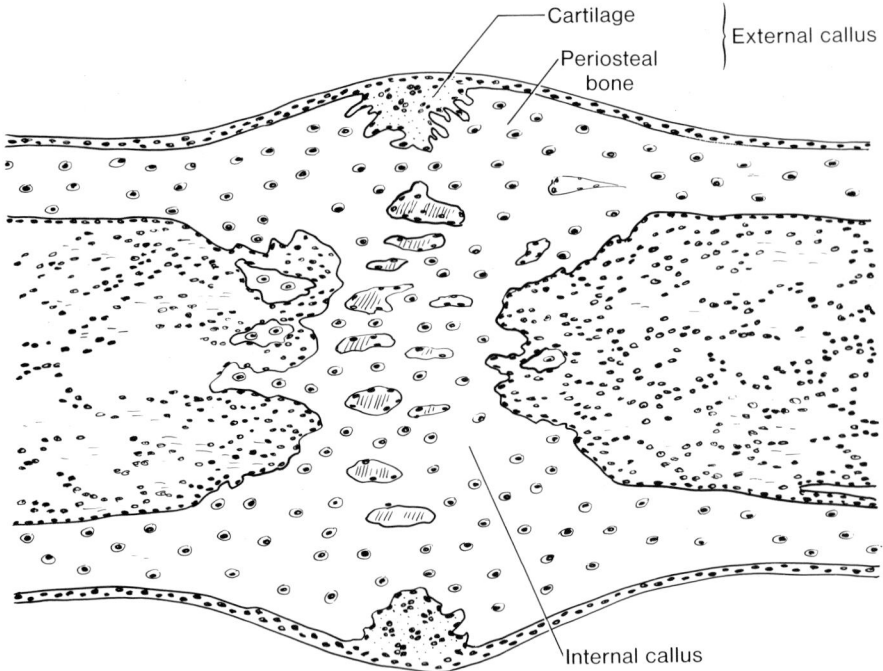

Fig. 9.39   Fracture site bridged with new bone. External and internal callus established.

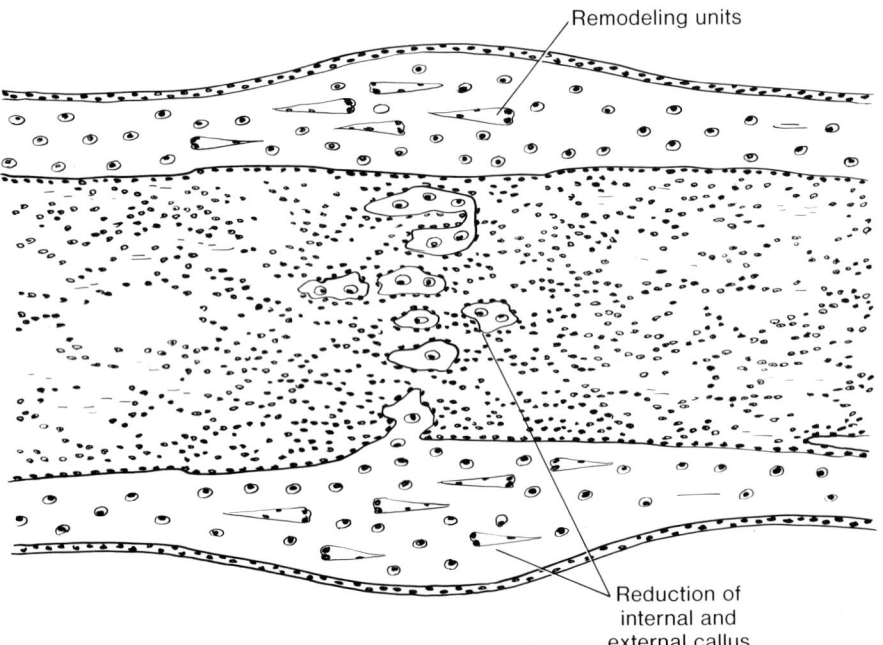

Fig. 9.40   Remodeling of internal and external callus. Bone mass is reduced and remodeled.

trabecular endosteum and osteonal endosteum are characterized by extensive mitotic activity of osteogenic and endothelial cells (Fig. 9.36). New cells and blood vessels from the endosteum migrate toward the fracture site, invade the hematoma and bridge the gap with a fibrocellular, hyperplastic tissue that eventually will form bone (Fig. 9.37). This tissue is the precursor of the bone that will form within the marrow cavity and within the gap between the fracture fragments. The new osseous tissue (woven bone) that is derived from the endosteum is called the *internal (endosteal) callus* (Fig. 9.37).

Concomitant with the endosteal events, the cells of the periosteum proliferate and produce a hypercellular mass that differentiates into bone and cartilage. These new cartilaginous and osseous tissues (woven bone) comprise the *external (periosteal) callus* (Fig. 9.37).

Callus Formation. *Callus* is that new tissue that forms around, between, within and adjacent to the fracture site. The formation of callus actually begins with the formation of the expansive, hyperplastic and fibrocellular tissue that forms from the endosteal and periosteal envelopes and ends with the deposition of bone across the fracture gap. Many terms are used to describe callus: *internal (endosteal) callus, external (periosteal) callus, bridging callus, permanent callus* and *provisional callus*. Despite the numerous names for this entity, only one callus forms in association with fracture repair. It changes character as the fibrocellular tissue from which it originates develops into bone, proliferates and is eventually remodeled. However, two important subdivisions of the callus exist that have different features and functions. These are the internal and external calluses.

External Callus. Proliferation of the osteogenic cells of the periosteum initially develops within an adequate vascular environment (Fig. 9.38). As a result, they produce new periosteal bone along the margin of the fracture some distance removed from the fracture gap. This osteogenic activity culminates in *periosteal new bone formation.* Eventually, this proliferating layer of cells bridges the gap of the fracture and forms a thickened cellular layer peripheral to the regressing hematoma. It is believed that the osteogenic cells in this region are proliferating faster than their associated periosteal vessels. Accordingly, they differentiate into chondroblasts. (Remember that the periosteum develops during endochondral ossification from the perichondrium.) Thus, the *external callus* consists of new bone peripherally and cartilage adjacent to the fracture gap. These tissues are covered peripherally by the periosteum (Fig. 9.39). As the cartilaginous mass continues to grow by appositional and interstitial mechanisms, this mass becomes further separated from its vascular supply. The chondrocytes along the cartilage/bone interface hypertrophy and their associated matrix becomes mineralized.

tal stimuli. The stimuli that sustain induction phenomena throughout repair of a fracture have not been identified.

Inflammatory Stage. This stage is initiated immediately after the insult. It results from the disrupted vascular supply, attendant hemorrhage and hematoma formation, and devitalization of tissue components. The resultant tissue necrosis is sufficient stimulation for the invasion by inflammatory cells (Fig. 9.36). During this stage devitalized tissue is removed and the hematoma is reorganized and removed. Inflammation is an

essential part of the repair process. The activities of this stage overlap with the reparative stage. Classically, this stage ends when the cardinal signs of inflammation (redness, pain, swelling and heat) are no longer apparent.

Reparative Stage. This stage involves numerous cellular activities that are initiated with induction, progress through inflammation and ultimately end with callus formation. As the hematoma is reorganized and invaded by phagocytic and fibroblastic cells, the periosteum, cortical endosteum,

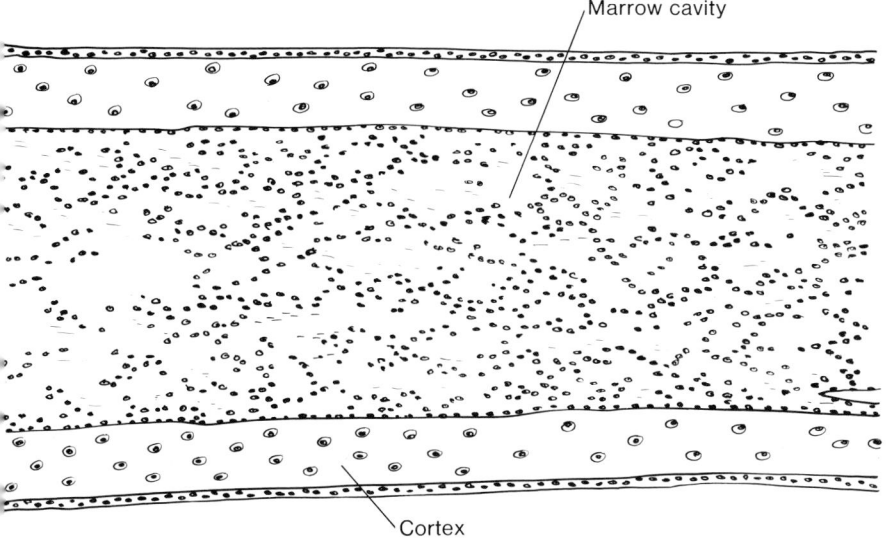

Marrow cavity

Cortex

Fig. 9.41   Return of bone to pre-fracture configuration.

from within outward from this interface there is a progression from calcified cartilage, hypertrophic chondrocytes, maturing chondrocytes and proliferating cells. Vascular invasion and osseous replacement are initiated at the cartilage/bone interface. These events continue until the cartilaginous mass is replaced by woven bone. This process, then, as it relates to the formation, maturation and alteration of the external callus is a reiteration of endochondral ossification.

The formation of an external callus under these circumstances of repair indicates that the repair process is progressing normally; in other circumstances the external callus is indicative of complications to repair that may lead to *delayed* or *nonunion*. The primary function of the external callus is the stabilization of the fracture site. The actual repair of the fracture site is achieved via the endosteal callus.

Internal Callus. The *internal (endosteal) callus* is that new tissue which develops from the endosteal envelopes and is responsible for the actual repair of the fracture (Figs. 9.37, 9.39). These events occur simultaneously with those events described for the periosteum. Proliferating cells from the trabecular and cortical endosteum invade the regressing hematoma and begin to form

bone that attaches to the inner surface of the bone on one side of the fracture, bridges the gap and is continuous with bone on the other side of the fracture. Eventually, woven bone is formed between the ends of the fracture fragments. There are two significant features of the internal callus. *Bone forms directly without a cartilaginous intermediary.* Also, *the internal callus is the tissue through which actual repair of the fracture is achieved.*
Remodeling Stage. The formation of the internal and external callus results in the deposition of cancellous woven bone. Progressive appositional growth converts this tissue configuration into dense cancellous and compact bone (Fig. 9.39). The new bone that is formed at or adjacent to the fracture site is bonded to dead and live bone. At this point in repair, the marrow cavity may be occluded with bone, the fracture gap is filled with bone and the fracture is surrounded by a sleeve of bone. Osteoclastic activity is responsible for removal of the live and dead bone that may fill the marrow cavity. Similarly, osteoclasia results in the progressive reduction of the external callus (Fig. 9.40). Simultaneously, internal remodeling activity, as described with primary intention healing, produces new osteons that traverse the fracture site. Eventually, only the cortical bone of the diaphysis remains (Fig. 9.41).

Fracture repair has been achieved successfully.

References

Bone Development

Anderson, C. E. and Parker, J.: Electron microscopy of the epiphyseal cartilage plate. Clin. Orthop. *58:*225, 1968.

Bassett, A. L.: Current concepts of bone formation. J. Bone Joint Surg. *44A:*1217, 1962.

Bonucci, E.: Fine structure of early cartilage calcification. J. Ultrastruct. Res. *20:*33, 1967.

Brookes, M.: Cortical vascularization and growth in foetal trabecular bones. J. Anat. *97:*597, 1963.

Clark, E. R. and Clark, E. L.: Microscopic observations on new formation of cartilage and bone in the living animal. Amer. J. Anat. *70:*167, 1942.

Frost, H. M.: Tetracycline-based histological analysis of bone remodelling. Calc. Tiss. Res. *3:*211, 1969.

Frost, H. M.: *Bone Modeling and Skeletal Modeling Errors.* C. C. Thomas, Springfield, 1973.

Kuettner, K. E., Sobel, L. W., Ray, R. D., Croxen, R. L., Passovoy, M. and Eisenstein, R.: Lysozyme in epiphyseal cartilage. J. Cell Biol. *44:*329, 1970.

Matthews, J. L., Martin, J. H., Lynn, J. A. and Collins, E. J.: Calcium incorporation in the developing cartilaginous epiphysis. Calc. Tiss. Res. *1:*330, 1968.

Odegaard, J.: Growth of the mandible studied with the aid of metallic implants. Am. J. Orthod. *57:*145, 1970.

Schenk, R. K., Spiro, D. and Wiener, J.: Cartilage resorption in the tibial epiphyseal plate of growing rats. *34:*275, 1964.

Schenk, R. K., Wiener, J. and Spiro, D.: Fine structural aspects of vascular invasion of the tibial epiphyseal plate of growing rats. Acta. Anat. *69:*1, 1968.

Scherft, J. P.: The ultrastructure of the organic matrix of calcified cartilage and bone in embryonic mouse radii. J. Ultrastruct. Res. *23:*333, 1968.

Weinmann, J. P. and Sicher, H.: *Bone and Bones,* C. V. Mosby, St. Louis, 1955.

Young, R. W.: Cell proliferation and specialization during endochondral osteogenesis in young rats. J. Cell Biol. *14:*357, 1962.

Fracture Repair

Ham, A. W. and Harris, W. R.: Repair and transplantation of bone. *In:* Bourne, G. H. (editor). *The Biochemistry and Physiology of Bone.* Vol. III. pp. 337–399. Academic Press, New York, 1971.

Heppenstall, R. B.: Fracture and cartilage repair. *In: Fundamentals of Wound Management in Surgery: Selected Tissues.* pp. 1–35, Chirurgecom, Inc., South Plainfield, New Jersey, 1977.

Jee, W. S. S.: The influence of reduced vascularity on the rate of internal reconstruction in adult long bone cortex. *In:* Frost, H. M. (editor). *Bone Biodynamics.* pp. 259–277. Little, Brown, Boston, 1964.

Peacock, Jr., E. E. and Van Winkle, Jr., W.: *Surgery and Biology of Wound Repair.* W. B. Saunders Co., Philadelphia, 1970.

Perrin, S.: Cortical bone healing. Acta Orthop. Scand. *Suppl. 125,* 1969.

10: Blood and Blood Cell Dynamics

Peripheral Blood

General Characteristics

Form and Function. Blood is considered a special type of connective tissue that consists of a large volume of fluid matrix and numerous formed elements. A fibrous component is also present during blood clotting when *fibrinogen* is converted to *fibrin*. Blood and its transudative components as tissue fluid are the most ubiquitous of the connective tissues.

The fluid phase of the blood is called *plasma*. All materials that pass to or from the cells through the connective tissue compartment occur as components of the liquid phase of the blood. This includes materials occurring normally as well as abnormally (bacteria, toxins, etc.). Also, the blood is often used as the carrier medium for many chemotherapeutic materials.

Upon removal of *fibrinogen* as *fibrin*, the remaining fluid is termed *serum*.

Suspended within the plasma are varied cells and/or fragments of cells. These formed elements serve numerous functions within the *intravascular space*, as well as within the *extravascular space*.

The functions of blood are numerous and varied. The *transport* of oxygen and carbon dioxide is an important complement to pulmonary and cellular respiration. Several important *buffer systems* occur in blood: carbonates, phosphates, hemoglobin and proteins. All food substances must pass through the blood; thus, *nutrition* is of considerable importance. An *excretory* function is obvious through the removal of metabolic waste products. The *maintenance of the water content* of the body is accomplished through a balance between the blood-vascular system, tissue fluid space, intracellular fluid space and lymphatics. Besides the necessity of fluids for the transport of various materials, the water content of the body is an important medium for *heat regulation*. Also, the transport of hormones gives the blood a *regulatory* function. These hormones may be transported free in the plasma and/or be attached to specific transport proteins. The blood is also an important *protective device* for the body through its cells and various suspended materials (antibodies, antitoxins, etc.)

Plasma. *Plasma* is the straw-colored and transparent fluid matrix of blood that is apparent when a blood sample to which an anticoagulant has been added has been centrifuged or the formed elements have been allowed to sediment to the bottom of a collection vial. The amount of plasma in the blood is species-dependent; generally, it comprises 35–50%. Numerous other factors (age, degree of hydration, disease, athletic conditioning) affect this percentage.

Plasma consists of approximately 90% water and 10% dissolved substances and solids. Dissolved inorganic ions (Na^+, K^+, Cl^-, HCO_3^-, Ca^{++} and others) constitute about 1% of the plasma. Plasma proteins (albumins, globulins, fibrinogen) comprise approximately 7% of the total plasma. Other organic substances (urea, uric acid, amino acids, fatty acids, glycerol and others) constitute 1%. Additionally, plasma normally contains various quantities of hormones, enzymes, pigments and vitamins and dissolved gases.

Many of the characteristics attributed to plasma are a function of its protein components. These substances are significant in the maintenance of intravascular osmotic pressure (colloid osmotic pressure), the transport of various plasma constituents (hormones, waste products), the clotting mechanism and the protection of the body by humoral antibodies (immunoglobulins). Electrophoretic separations are used commonly to characterize the protein constituents of plasma (or serum). Such characterizations demonstrate that plasma proteins consist of the following components: albumin, alpha globulins (alpha 1, alpha 2), beta globulins (beta 1, beta 2), gamma globulins and fibrinogen (Fig. 10.1). The globulin components vary with the species also.

Albumin is a small protein with a molecular weight of about 70,000. It accounts for approximately one-half of the total protein of the plasma and about 70% of the intravascular osmotic pressure. Albumin contributes significantly to the concentration gradient between blood and extracellular fluid; therefore, it helps to control the fluid balance between these compartments and to regulate total body fluids. Also, it binds and transports hormones (thyroxine), metabolites (bilirubin) and drugs (barbiturates).

The *alpha globulins* contribute to the osmotic pressure of the vascular bed as well as serving as carriers for various substances: copper by *ceruloplasmin*, hemoglobin by

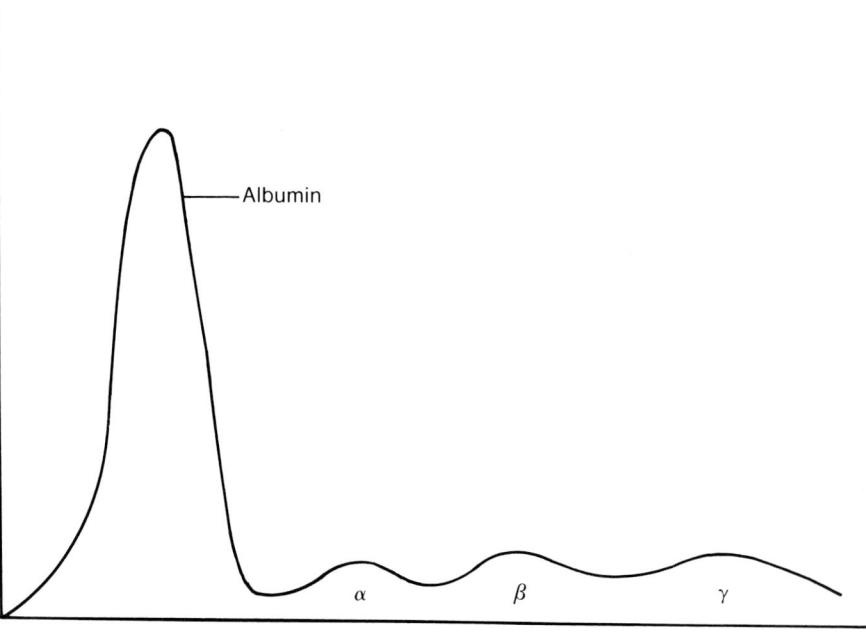

Fig. 10.1 An idealized electrophoretic pattern of a serum sample. Relative and absolute alterations in the components are valuable in diagnostic evaluations.

aptoglobin, thyroxine by *throxine binding globulin* (*TBG*), cortisol by *transcortin*. Lipoproteins of this fraction also transport triglycerides, fatty acids, vitamins and other substances. Additionally, this fraction contains cholinesterase, alkaline phosphatase, lactic dehydrogenase and factors involved in coagulation (factors V, IX and X).

The *beta globulins* contribute to oncotic pressure and serve as transport substances; iron is transported by *transferrin* and hemin by *hemopexin*. Lipoproteins, complement, fibrinogen and coagulation factors (VII, VIII) are present also.

The *gamma globulins* consist of the immunoglobulins, blood group globulins and the cryoglobulins. The immunoglobulins are discussed in Chapter 17.

Classification of Formed Elements. The formed elements of the blood include cells and/or fragments of cells that may be classified accordingly:

> Erythrocytes
> Leukocytes
>> Agranulocytes
>>> Lymphocytes
>>> Monocytes
>> Granulocytes
>>> Neutrophils (heterophils)
>>> Eosinophils
>>> Basophils
> Platelets and thrombocytes

Mammalian blood contains all of the previously mentioned elements except thrombocytes. Platelets are often referred to as thrombocytes, but in avian species the thrombocyte is a cell. In mammalian species the platelet is a cell fragment.

Of the cells that occur in the blood, there are numerous species differences concerning size, number and specific characteristics. Tables 10.1 and 10.2 represent normal values for the blood of various domestic and laboratory species.

The staining properties for the subsequent cells are described in terms of the use of Wright's or Giemsa stain.

Mammalian Blood Cells

Erythrocytes

Form and Function. The *erythrocytes* are also referred to as *red blood cells* (*RBC*), *red blood corpuscles* and *rubricytes*. The RBC is an anucleated, biconcave disk which is round in most mammalian species (Fig. 10.2). It is, however, oval in the members of the Camelidae (camel, dromedary, llama and alpaca). The diameter range is 3.5–7.5 μm in different species.

In smear preparations the biconcavity may be apparent because of the differential light transmission from the periphery to the central part of the corpuscle (Figs. 10.3, 10.4). However, if care is not taken with the preparation solutions, the RBC's may swell in hypotonic media or shrink in hypertonic media. All cells respond in this manner to

Table 10.1
Blood Parameters of Selected Domestic Species*

Parameter	Dog	Cat	Horse	Ox	Sheep	Goat	Pig	Rabbit	Rat	Guinea pig	Domestic Fowl
Packed cell volume (PCV, %)	45	37	42	35	38	35	42	48	45	40	36
Hemoglobin (gm %)	15	12	15	11	12	10	13	12	15	14.5	10.3
RBC's ($\times 10^6$/mm³)	6.8	7.5	9.5	7.0	12	13	6.5	5.6	8.5	5.6	2.8
RBC size (μm)	7.0	5.9	5.4	5.7	4.5	4.1	6.0	6.8	6.9	7.5	10.7×7.1
Total protein** (gm %)	6.0–7.5	6.0–7.5	6.0–8.0	6.0–8.0	6.0–7.5	6.0–7.5	6.0–7.0	6.0–7.2	6.1–7.1	5.1–6.3	4.0–5.2
Platelets ($\times 10^3$/mm³)	550	450	330	500	400	450	520	500	532	500	27.6
MCV ($\times 10^{-15}$L)	70	45	46	52	33	27	63	61	60	65	127
MCHC (gm/dl)	34	33	35	33	34	32	32	32	32	30	29
M/E ratio	1.2	1.6	1.6	0.7	1.1	0.7	1.8	1.0	1.6	1.5	—
WBC's ($\times 10^3$/mm³)	11.5	12.5	9.0	8.0	8.0	9.0	16.0	7.9	11.5	10.8	16.6

* These average parameters vary with age, sex, strain and breed of animal.
** Range of values.

varying tonicity, but it is most easily demonstrated in the RBC.

In sections stained by routine procedures, the RBC's will stain pink. Within the capillary beds, larger vessels and even as extravasated blood, RBC's may become stacked one upon the other in a typical *rouleaux* formation. Rouleaux formation, however, is species-specific. This formation is indicative

of the manner by which they move through the smallest blood vessels (capillaries). The occurrence of RBC's outside the vascular bed is usually an artifact of preparation techniques in normal tissues.

The RBC is uniquely modified to perform its primary function, carrying oxygen to the tissues in the form of *oxyhemoglobin* and carrying some carbon dioxide away from

the tissues in the form of *carboxyhemoglobin*. Most of the cellular organelles (nucleus, Golgi, mitochondria, etc.) are lost and the bulk of the cell is composed of *hemoglobin*. The structural modification as a biconcave disk also facilitates the movement of this entity through the capillary bed (Fig. 10.5).

Erythrocytic Variants. The previous description of erythrocytes applies to this particular corpuscle generally. Numerous variations occur in the morphology of the red blood cell. Some are attributable to improper processing of samples, whereas others are the result of disease processes. Some changes in morphology, however, cannot be explained. During the examination of peripheral blood smears from different species, many of the following changes will be observed. It is important to understand the significance of some of these morphologic variants.

Many erythrocytic variants are noted in the peripheral blood in a condition called *anemia*. Anemia is a condition in which there is a decreased number of circulating RBC's or a decrease in the amount of he-

Table 10.2
WBC Differential Counts of Selected Domestic Species*

Cells†	Dog	Cat	Horse	Ox	Sheep	Goat	Pig	Rabbit	Rat	Guinea pig	Domestic Fowl
Mature neutrophils	70	60	52	28	30	36	37	43	28	42	26
Immature neutrophils**	3	3	2	2	Rare	Rare	3	2	1	3	—
Lymphocytes	20	32	39	57	62	56	53	42	62	45	64
Monocytes	5.0	2.8	4.4	5.0	2.5	2.5	5.0	9.0	5.0	7.0	6.0
Eosinophils	4.0	5.2	4.1	8.8	5.0	5.0	3.5	2.0	2.0	5.0	2.0
Basophils	Rare	Rare	0.5	0.5	0.5	0.5	0.5	4.0	1.0	1.0	2.0

* These average parameters vary with age, sex, strain and breed of animal.
† Values are percentages of total WBC's.
** Values represent upper limits of normalcy.

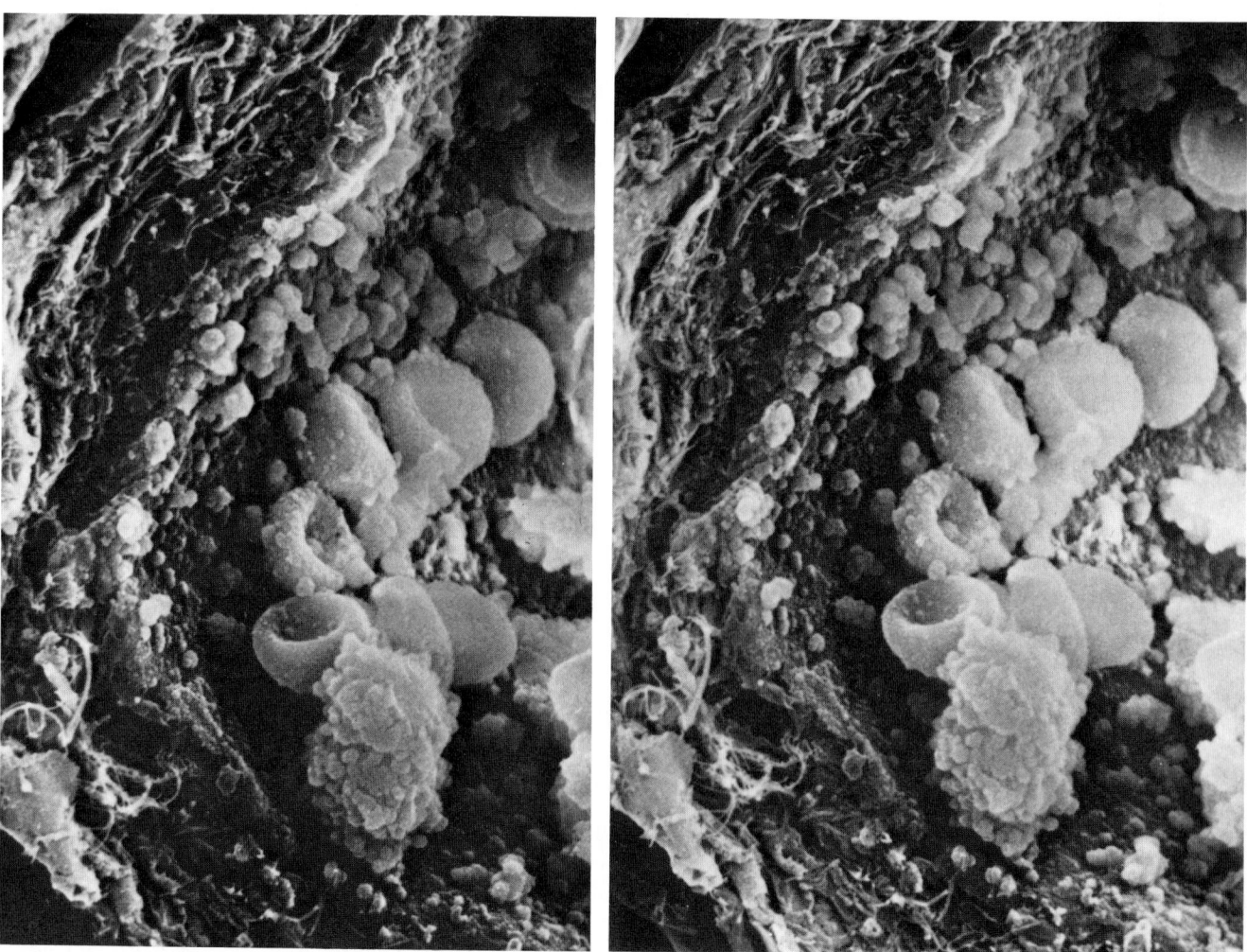

Fig. 10.2 A scanning electron micrograph of canine RBC's. The freeze-fractured sample is from the testis. The micrograph, a stereo pair, is comprised of one photograph with the specimen normal to the beam; the second photograph has a 6° tilt. The three-dimensional quality of the photographs will be apparent when viewed with stereo glasses. The large structure with numerous processes is a white blood cell. Note the central depression in the RBC's. Some of the RBC's are bowl-shaped. X4000. (Courtesy of C. J. Connell).

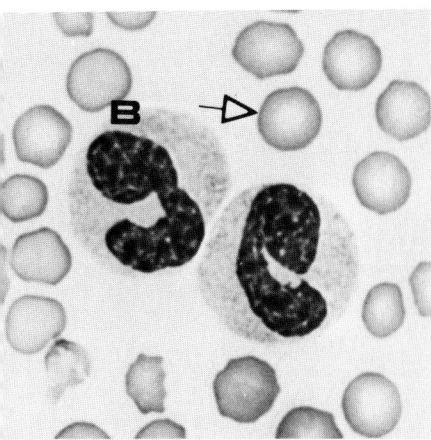

Fig. 10.3 Feline peripheral blood smear. The large cells in the center of the field are immature neutrophils—neutrophilic band cells (B). Central pallor is apparent in some corpuscles (arrow). The concavity is not developed equally in all species and is not apparent in all RBC's. X400. All light micrographs are labeled as the magnification with the microscope before photographic enlarging. All electron micrographs are labeled as total magnification, including photographic enlarging.

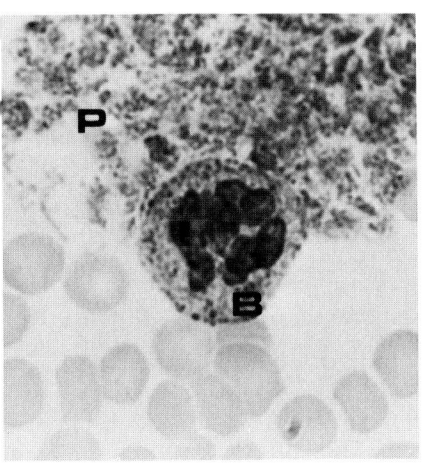

Fig. 10.4 Feline peripheral blood smear. A basophil (B) is surrounded by aggregated platelets (P) and RBC's. Variations in central pallor are obvious. X400.

noglobin. Although there are various ways of classifying anemias, one of the simplest and most useful is to classify them as *regenerative* or *nonregenerative*. A regenerative anemia is characterized by the bone marrow attempting to compensate by producing new RBC's. In nonregenerative anemia, the bone marrow is not responsive to the peripheral need for more RBC's.

Although the mature mammalian RBC is anucleated, it begins its life cycle as a typical nucleated cell. Sometimes, however, immature RBC's gain access to the peripheral circulation. One of these immature forms, *metarubricytes*, contain pyknotic nuclei (Fig. 10.6). Normally, the nuclei are extruded from the cells before their entry into the vascular bed. Metarubricytes in the periph-

eral circulation usually indicates regeneration.

Immature cells containing remnants of ribosomal material also gain access to the peripheral circulation. These corpuscles, characterized by a diffuse cytoplasmic basophila, are called *reticulocytes* (Fig. 10.7). Positive identification of these cells is predicated upon visualization of basophilic granules or a fibrillar network with supravital stains such as new methylene blue. *Polychromatophilic erythrocytes* are immature cells whose cytoplasm has a mixed affinity for the acid and basic dyes of Romanowsky stains. *Polychromasia* describes the condition of the blood when these entities are present (Plate. VII.4). The reticulocyte and the polychromatophilic erythrocyte are the

same cell stained differently. Polychromasia is indicative of regeneration and should not be confused with the *basophilic stippling* of erythrocytes that are stained with a Romanowsky stain (Fig. 10.8). The latter indicates regeneration in cats, cattle and sheep, but it can also indicate heavy metal poisoning that results in defective RBC formation. Moreover, basophilic stippling is not observed with new methylene blue.

Howell-Jolly (HJ) bodies are nonrefractile, nuclear remnants within RBC's which may be positioned eccentrically. Although HJ bodies indicate increased RBC production, they are observed routinely in 1% of the RBC's of feline and equine blood.

Erythrocyte refractile (ER) bodies are demonstrable in unstained wet mounts as

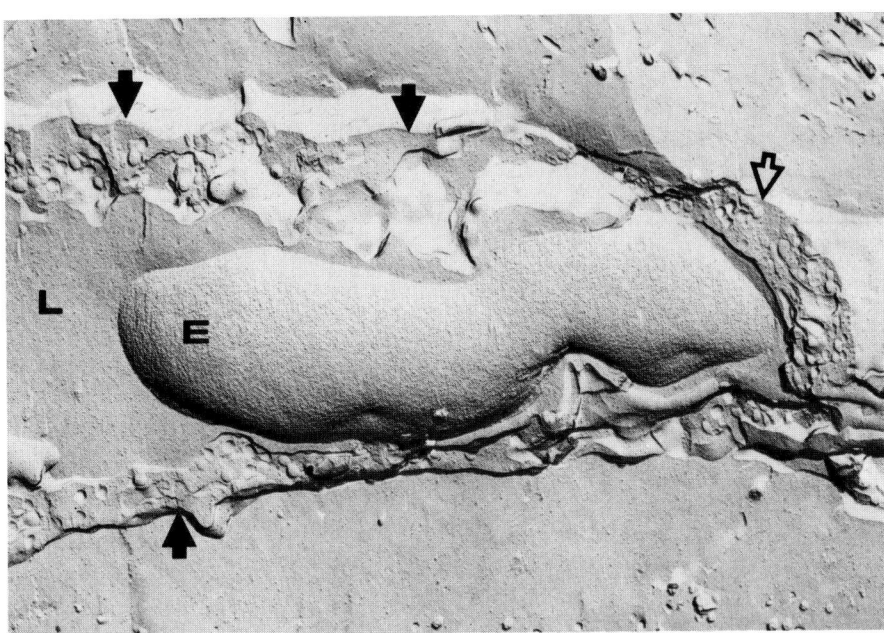

Fig. 10.5 An electron micrograph of a freeze-fractured capillary and RBC. The collapsed capillary is defined by the longitudinal (*solid arrows*) and cross (*open arrow*) sectioning of the endothelium. The capillary lumen (L) contains a single RBC (E) that conforms to the shape of the capillary. Red blood cells are capable of adjusting their shape to that of the capillary. Compare with Figure 2.13. X25,600 (Courtesy of J. E. Rash).

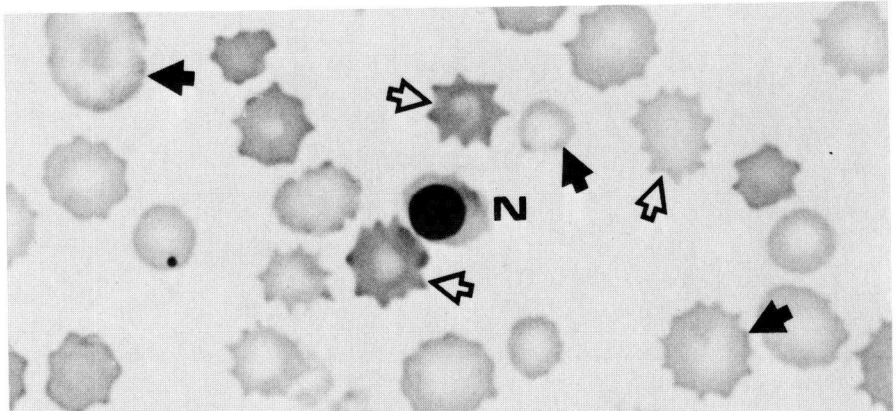

Fig. 10.6 Peripheral blood smear from a young piglet with a regenerative anemia. A nucleated RBC, metarubricyte, occupies the center of the field (N). Acanthocytes (*open arrows*) are present. Note the different sizes of the RBC's—anisocytosis (*solid arrows*). X400 (Giemsa stain).

highly refractile bodies near or protruding from the periphery of the RBC. The bodies appear as small circular pale areas at the periphery of the RBC with Wright's stain (Fig. 10.9). They may be observed in 10% of normal feline RBC's.

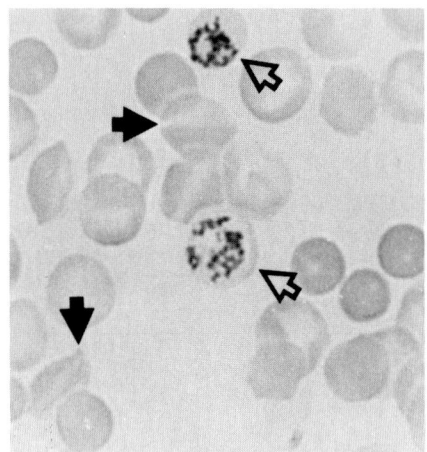

Fig. 10.7 Reticulocytes in a canine peripheral blood smear. The reticulocytes (*open arrows*) are surrounded by large RBC's (macrocytes) and small RBC's (microcytes). This condition is called anisocytosis. Note the leptocytes (*solid arrows*). X400 (new methylene blue stain).

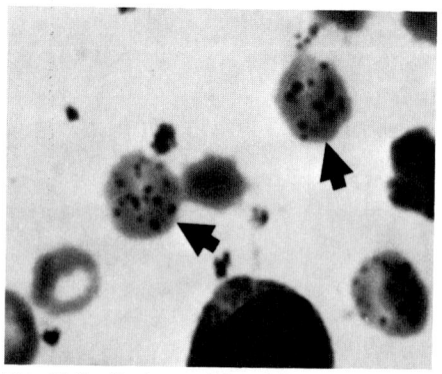

Fig. 10.8 Bovine peripheral blood smear. Basophilic stippling (*arrows*) is apparent. X400 (Giemsa stain).

Heinz bodies are peripherally-positioned intracytoplasmic masses of altered hemoglobin that appear as pale areas with Romanowsky stains and as refractile blue-black spheres with new methylene blue. The exact relationship between ER bodies and Heinz bodies, initially, was not clear. Heinz bodies were described originally as an erythrocytic response to certain toxic conditions, whereas ER bodies occurred under normal conditions in feline blood. Heinz bodies and ER bodies are the same structures which result from oxidation of hemoglobin by certain agents; feline hemoglobin is more susceptible to oxidation than other species.

The size, number, shape and staining properties of erythrocytes vary in different conditions of health and disease. These parameters are useful diagnostically.

Although the size of RBC's varies, it is constant for a given species. Red blood cells of normal size and hemoglobin content are referred to as *normocytic* (Figs. 10.3, 10.4). Any alteration to this normal size is referred to as *anisocytosis* (Fig. 10.10). Cells that are larger than normal are called *macrocytes*; cells that are smaller than normal, *microcytes*. Anemias in domestic animals are classified sometimes on the characteristic cell size as *normocytic anemia, macrocytic anemia* or *microcytic anemia*. *Normocytic anemia* is commonly a secondary disorder associated with various chronic diseases (infections, malignancies, nephritis). It is characterized by a suppression of the bone marrow in which the total RBC production is reduced, but the cells are normal in size and hemoglobin content. The most common cause of *macrocytic anemia* in domestic animals is the increased production and subsequent release of reticulocytes into the peripheral blood in response to blood loss or blood destruction crises. Because the anemia corrects itself once the crisis is met, this type is referred to as *transitory* or *pseudomacrocytic anemia*. True *macrocytic anemia* results from a maturation arrest in the bone marrow in which immature (large) cells gain access to the peripheral blood. A cobalt

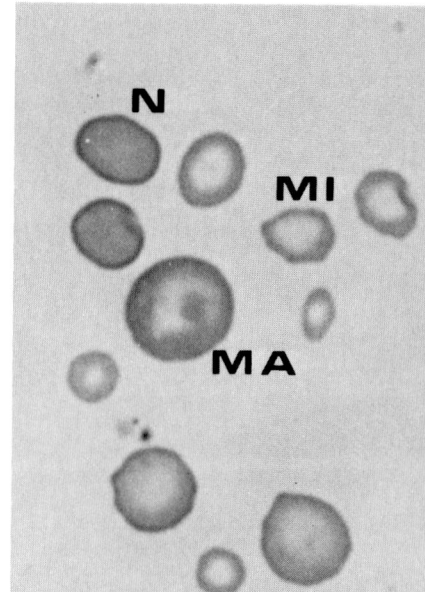

Fig. 10.10 Anisocytosis in a porcine peripheral blood smear. Macrocytes (MA), normocytes (N) and microcytes (MI) are evident. The microcytes are hypochromatic. X400 (Giemsa stain).

deficiency can cause this type of anemia in ruminants. A macrocytic anemia from vitamin B_{12} deficiency occurs in man due to a lack of *intrinsic factor*; however, domestic animals apparently do not need intrinsic factor for the absorption of vitamin B_{12}. A true macrocytic anemia occurs occasionally in felids with bone marrow proliferation disorders and has been reported in Miniature Poodles. The most common cause of a *microcytic anemia* is an iron-deficiency. Chronic blood loss is one of the most common causes of iron-deficiency. The mitotic activity and maturation of RBC precursors are linked to the iron (hemoglobin) content of the cells. An iron deficiency causes an additional division of the cells which results in smaller cells being produced.

The constant size of the RBC under normal conditions, as well as their presence in most tissue sections, affords the microscopist a "built-in micrometer." Although some shrinkage or swelling may result from tissue processing and alter the size of RBC's, they are generally about 5–6 μm in diameter. Species differences, however, must be noted.

The number of RBC's/mm^3 of peripheral blood is constant for a species and breed under normal conditions. The number of RBC's/mm^3 generally varies inversely with the size of the blood corpuscles. An increase in the numbers of RBC's/mm^3 is called *polycythemia*, whereas a decrease is called *oligocythemia*.

Any deviation from the normal shape of the RBC is termed *poikilocythemia*. There are numerous alterations to shape that are associated with many disease processes and/or faulty processing techniques. *Acanthocytes* have spine-like or blunt-processes pro-

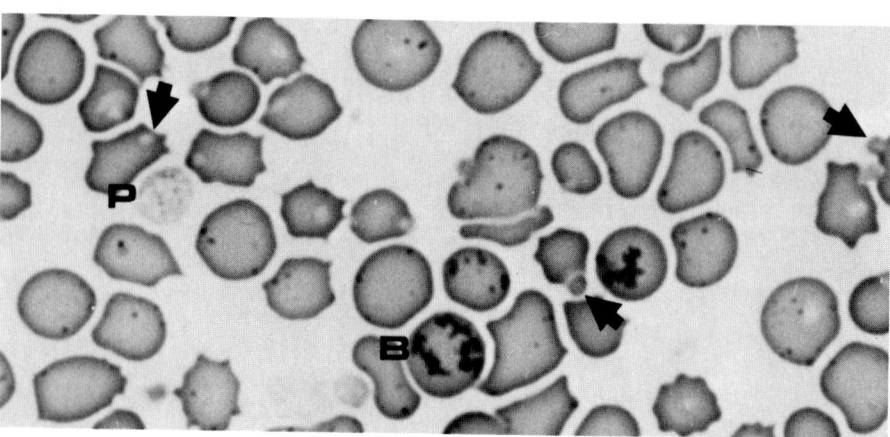

Fig. 10.9 Feline peripheral blood smear. Basophilic stippling (B) and Heinz bodies (*solid arrows*) are evident. P, platelet. X400 (Wright's stain).

ruding from their surfaces, and can result
rom various diseases (Fig. 10.6). Similar
morphologic changes can result during pro-
essing in which slow-drying fluids create a
ypertonic solution. Then the cells are
alled *crenated cells*. *Bowl or cup-shaped
RBC's* appear to have "punched-out" cen-
ers when observed in stained smears. RBC's
normally assume a parabolic shape as they
pass through capillaries (Fig. 2.13). Some
ype of cytoplasmic stromal defect does not
permit these cells to return to their normal
piconcave configuration. *Leptocytes* are
RBC's with a decreased volume and a normal to increased surface area (Fig. 10.11).
Leptocytes are either target cells or folded
cells. A *target cell* has a dense central zone
urrounded by a clear zone with another
dense zone at the periphery of the cell. These
ltered densities are generally attributed to
a heterogeneous distribution of hemoglobin.
Folded cells have a folded membrane across
he cell. *Ovalocytes* are eliptical erythrocytes
which may be encountered periodically.
They are normal in avian, piscine and ca-
meline blood. *Poikilocytes* are RBC's with
a variety of abnormal shapes. Most commonly they may have a "tear drop" shape.
They can indicate disease as well as slow
drying problems during processing. *Schis-
ocytes* are erythrocytic fragments with irregular shapes (Fig. 10.12). A spheroid cell with
a decreased volume compared to its diame-
er and without a central region of pallor is
called a *spherocyte*. Although it may be associated with other disease processes, it occurs commonly in autoimmune problems.
Stomatocytes have a linear region of central
pallor (Fig. 10.13). These cells are associated
with hereditary erythrocytic membrane defects.

The homogenous staining of RBC's, except for the area of central pallor, is a function of the amount and distribution of hemoglobin. The normal amount and distribution of hemoglobin is termed *normochromic*. A decrease in the hemoglobin content is *hypochromasia*. The release of reticulocytes from the bone marrow and iron

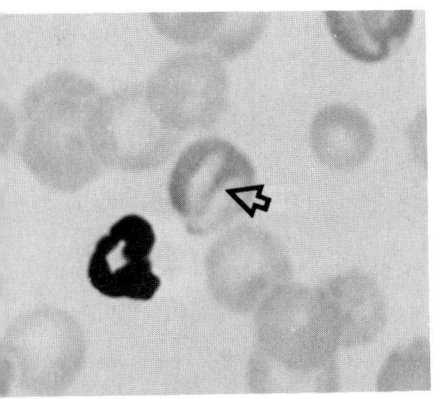
Fig. 10.11 A fold cell in a peripheral blood
smear of canine blood. A fold of membrane
(*arrow*) crosses the central area of pallor.
X400.

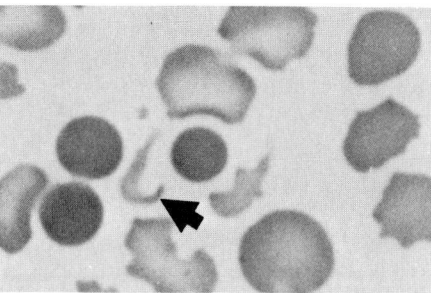
Fig. 10.12 Canine peripheral blood smear.
Arrow, schistocytes. X400 (Wright's stain).

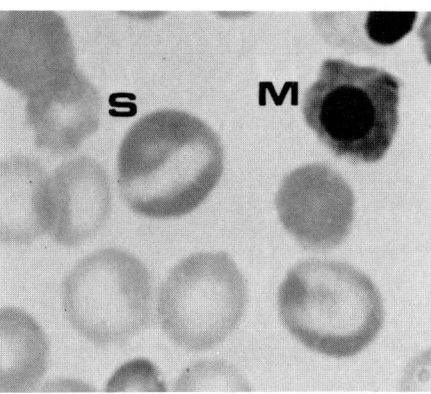
Fig. 10.13 Canine peripheral blood smear. S,
stomatocyte; M, metarubricyte. X400.

deficiency results in the appearance of hypochromasia. Reticulocytes contain hemoglobin, but the cells are larger than normal.
A *macrocytic hypochromic anemia* is characteristic of a regenerative anemia in all
domestic animals except the horse, which
does not release immature erythrocytes from
the bone marrow. A *microcytic hypochromic
anemia* results from an iron deficiency that
is commonly associated with chronic blood
loss (ectoparasites, endoparasites, gastric ul-
cers).

Of all the previous variations discussed
for the RBC, only the following are signs of
erythropoiesis in response to a peripheral
need (regenerative anemia): macrocytes, reticulocytes, nucleated RBC's polychromasia, HJ bodies and basophilic stippling (in
cats, cattle and sheep). The most reliable
sign of regeneration is polychromasia.

Granulocytes

Granulocytes are those *white blood cells*
or *leukocytes* of the blood that contain specific granules and have lobed or segmented
nuclei. They are important protective cells
that function within the vascular bed as well
as within the extravascular tissues. *Neutrophils*, *eosinophils* and *basophils* are granulocytes.
Neutrophilic Granulocytes. The *neutrophil,
heterophil* or *polymorphonuclear leukocyte*
(*PMN*) is the most frequently encountered
granulocyte (Plates VI, VII). The cell is
about twice the size of the RBC (9–12 μm)
and is characterized by a segmented nucleus

which may have from 3 to 5 lobes connected
by a fine strand of nucleoplasm (Figs. 10.14,
10.15, 10.16). The granules, usually described as neutrophilic, may vary from light
pink to purple depending upon the stain
used; thus, the term *heterophil*. In some species (rabbit, guinea pig) these particles stain
with acid dyes and the cells are usually
referred to as *pseudoeosinophils*. In some

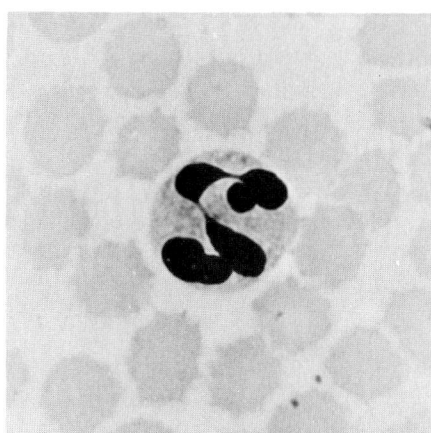
Fig. 10.14 A canine neutrophil in a peripheral
blood smear. X400.

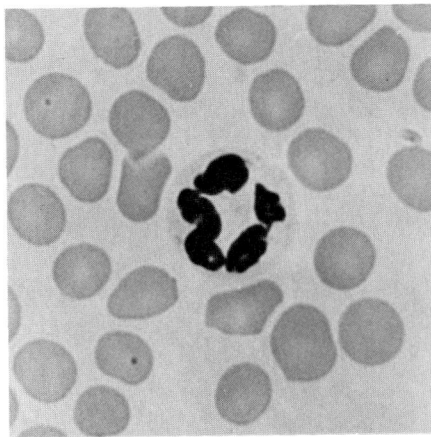
Fig. 10.15 A feline neutrophil in a peripheral
blood smear. Compare with Figure 10.3. X400.

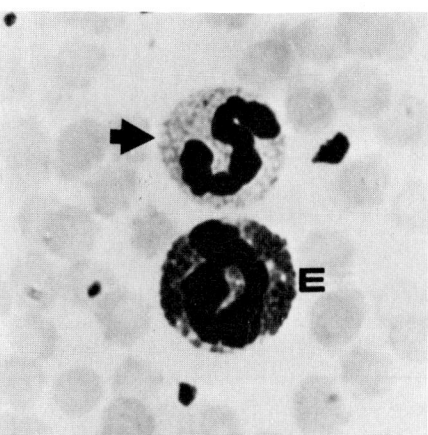
Fig. 10.16 An ovine peripheral blood smear.
An eosinophil (E) and an neutrophil (*arrow*) are
present. X400.

cases, due to preparatory techniques, the particles may not be apparent.

Electron microscopic examination and cytochemical studies have confirmed that these specific granules are lysosomes. Thus, the primary function of the neutrophil is phagocytosis of various particles, bacteria and other microorganisms. This activity is especially apparent in acute local inflammation during which time great numbers of these cells are present in the connective tissue.

Eosinophilic Granulocytes. The *eosinophil* or *acidophil* is the next most frequently encountered granulocyte (Plate VI). Its diameter is approximately 12–14 μm. Usually, the nucleus is bilobed, but it may be polymorphic (Fig. 10.17). Characteristically, the acidophilic granules are the distinguishing feature. They are uniform within a cell, but they do vary from species to species (Fig. 10.16). They are especially large in equids (Fig. 10.18). These granules also are lysosomes (Fig. 10.19).

The exact function of the eosinophil is not understood completely. They increase in numbers during allergic reactions (Type I Hypersensitivity) and during parasitic infections, and become especially numerous in

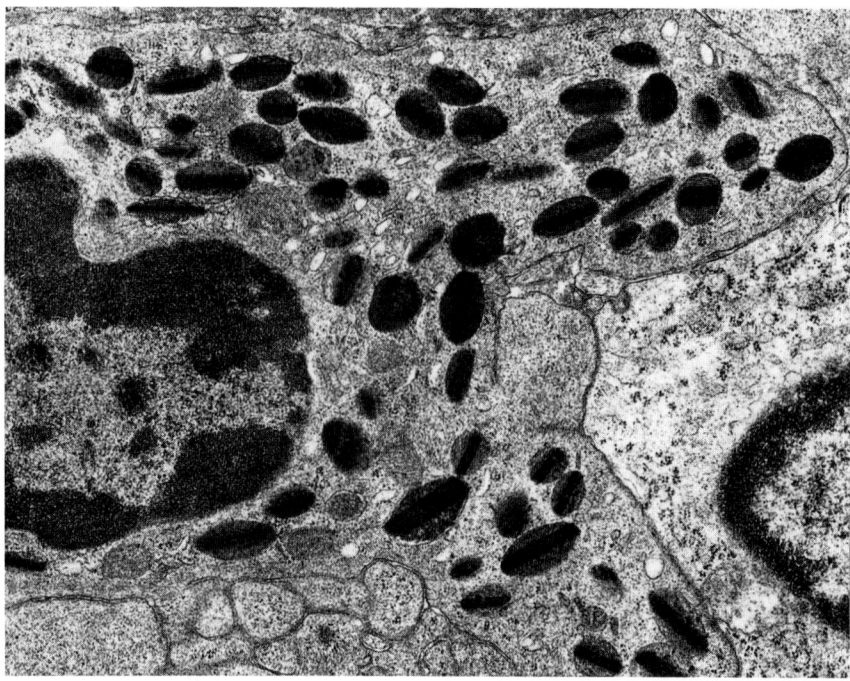

Fig. 10.19 An electron micrograph of an eosinophil. The dark bodies are the specific granules of the cell. X17,000 (Courtesy of A. M. Sheppard).

the extracellular space at sites of antibody/antigen reactions. They are phagocytic cells but to a lesser degree than the neutrophils. Their phagocytic activity may be limited to the antibody/antigen complexes with which they are associated. Their numbers are reduced by exogenous and endogenous corticosteroids. Their function in allergic reactions is discussed with immunity in Chapter 17.

Basophilic Granulocytes. The *basophil* or *basophilic leukocyte* is the least numerous of the granulocytes (Plate VI). It is about the same size as the neutrophil (9–12 μm). The nucleus is bilobed, although more lobes may be present. The granules are round, coarse and variable in size (Fig. 10.20). They usually stain much darker than the nucleus and may partially obscure it. These granules are basophilic and metachromatic (Figs. 10.20, 10.21).

The function of these cells is obscure. They rarely increase in number in pathologic conditions. They may increase in certain types of parasitism (canine heartworm disease). There is some evidence, however, that they are responsible for the elaboration of histamines and heparin in circulating blood.

Agranulocytes

The *agranulocytes* are white blood cells which do not contain specific granules; however, granules may be present. They are round cells with more or less rounded nuclei. *Lymphocytes* and *monocytes* are agranulocytes.

Lymphocytes. The *lymphocytes* are usually the most frequently encountered agranulocytes (Plate VI). They are characterized by a high nuclear/cytoplasmic ratio (Fig.

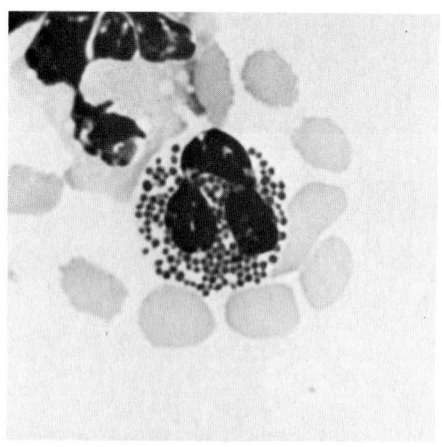

Fig. 10.17 An eosinophil in a bovine peripheral blood smear. X400.

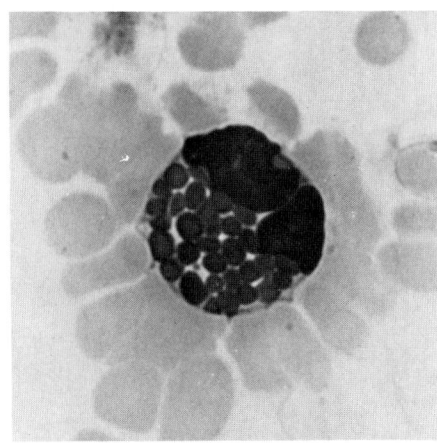

Fig. 10.18 An eosinophil in an equine peripheral blood smear. X400.

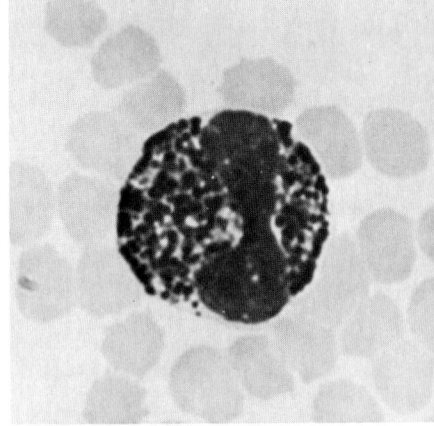

Fig. 10.20 A basophil in an equine peripheral blood smear. X400.

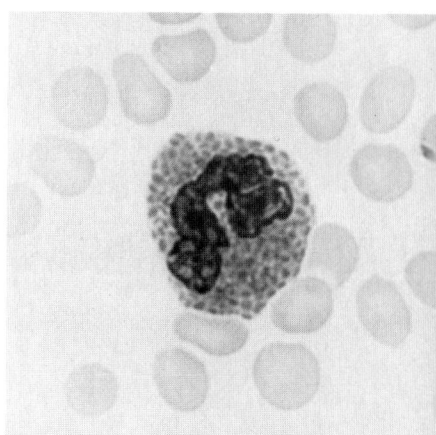

Fig. 10.21 A basophil in a feline peripheral blood smear. The specific granules are light-staining. X400.

.22). The nucleus is usually round and of
fficient density to obscure the nucleolus.
slight indentation of the nucleus may also
: seen (Fig. 10.23). The clear, basophilic
toplasm may contain some nonspecific,
urophilic granules (Fig. 10.24). Their oc-
rrence, however, is variable (Plate VII.2).
enerally, the nucleus is outlined by a pe-
pherally condensed heterochromatin that
adily diffracts light through the minimally
anulated cytoplasm. The predominant cy-
plasmic organelles are ribosomes, polyri-
osomes and rough endoplasmic reticulum.
he Golgi apparatus and mitochondria are
ant.

Lymphocytes vary appreciably in size.
mall lymphocytes have a diameter of 5–10
n and are the predominant lymphocytes
the circulating blood. *Medium-sized lym-
ocytes* range from 10–18 μm. The me-
um-sized lymphocytes are sometimes dif-
cult to distinguish from monocytes. *Large
mphocytes* typically occur in extravascular
ssues such as lymphatic tissue.

Whereas routine morphologic analyses
ly permit the distinction of lymphocyte
opulations based upon size, immunologic
chniques permit an evaluation of lympho-
ytes based upon function. Accordingly, two
istinct yet interrelated populations of lym-
hocytes have been identified. These popu-
tions are *B lymphocytes* and *T lymphocytes*.

B lymphocytes (B cells) are responsible for
e production of *antibodies (immunoglobu-
ns)* in response to antigenic stimulation.
hey are the basis for the blood-borne or
umoral antibody immunity of the organism.
heir cell surfaces are distinguished from T
lls by having specific receptors for antigen,
nmunoglobulin FC and C3b. They occur
the bone marrow, bursa of Fabricius (in
irds), germinal centers of lymphatic nod-
les and splenic follicles. Their origin is
iscussed with Agranulocytopoiesis in this
hapter. Their role in immunity is discussed
Chapter 17.

The *T lymphocytes (T cells)* represent a
ore functionally diverse population of

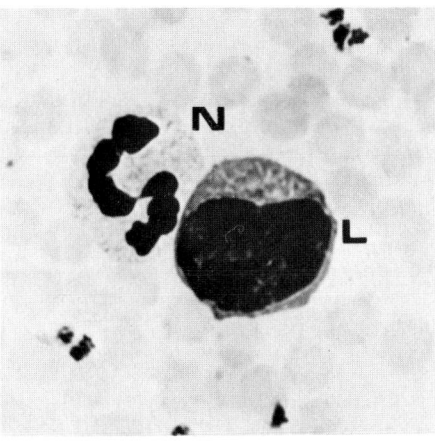

Fig. 10.23 An ovine peripheral blood smear. A lymphocyte (L) is adjacent to a neutrophil (N). X400.

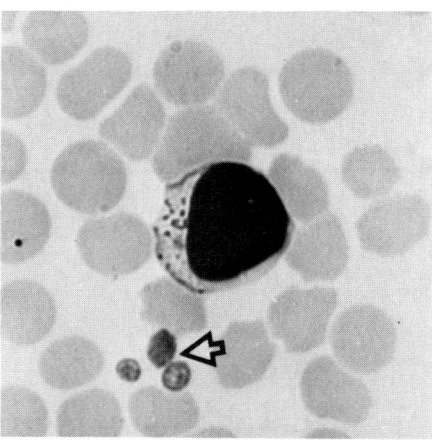

Fig. 10.24 A lymphocyte in an equine peripheral blood smear. Note the azurophilic granules within the cytoplasm. *Arrow*, platelets. X400.

cells than B cells. They are responsible for
cell-mediated immunity (CMI). In response
to antigenic stimulation, this population of
cells may become cytotoxic T cells (CMI),
T helper cells, T suppressor cells, memory
cells or may produce *lymphokines*. Lymphokines are low molecular weight proteins that
are produced primarily by T cell. However,
B cells can produce them in response to
certain stimuli. Some of the lymphokines
include: *MIF—Migration Inhibition Factor,
MAF—Macrophage Aggregating Factor,
MCF—Macrophage Chemotactic Factor,
MF—Mitogenic Factor* and *Interferon*. Migration Inhibition Factor prevents the migration of macrophages; MAF causes macrophages to aggregate; MF stimulates lymphocytes to divide; MCF attracts macrophages; Interferon prevents the replication
viruses. The surfaces of T cells generally
have a Thy-1 or theta antigen that distinguishes them from B cells. There are other
surface differences and stimulation responses that distinguish T cells from B cells.
T cells occur in the thymus, paracortical
zones of lymphatic nodules and the periarteriolar zone of splenic corpuscles. Their

origin and role in immunity is discussed
with the B cell in this Chapter and Chapter
17.

Most of the circulating lymphocytes in
most species are T cells. The life span of
lymphocytes may vary from hours to years.
The long-lived B and T lymphocytes are
believed to be the *memory cells*.

Monocytes. *Monocytes* are consistently the
largest of the blood vascular elements (Plate
VI). They range from 16–25 μm in diameter.
The nucleus is kidney-shaped or bean-
shaped, but it may be round as well as
trilobed (Fig. 10.25). The nuclear chromatin
is lighter and more reticular than the lymphocytic nuclear material (Fig. 10.26). With
appropriate staining, the cytoplasm is generally gray. The even distribution of clear
granules imparts a ground-glass appearance
to the cytoplasm. Scattered azurophilic
granules are contributory to this staining
quality. The nuclear configuration is an excellent and quite definitive diagnostic feature.

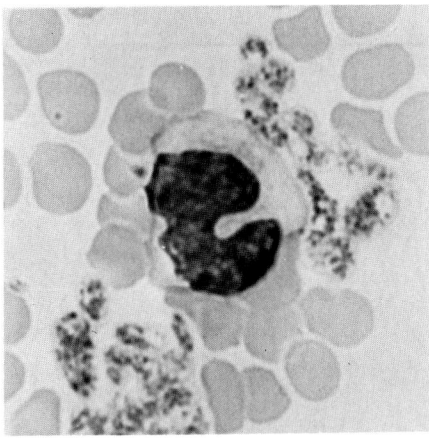

Fig. 10.25 A monocyte in a feline peripheral blood smear. The monocyte is surrounded by aggregated platelets. The nucleus of the monocyte is described as having a "spaghetti and meatball" appearance. X400.

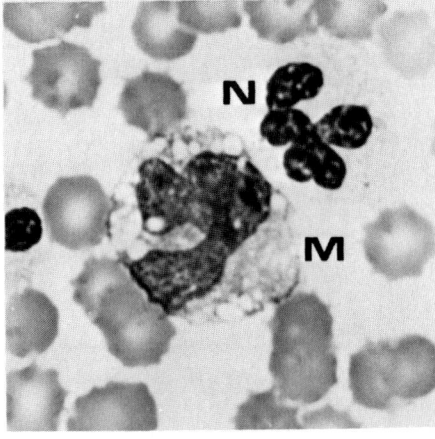

Fig. 10.26 A monocyte (M) and neutrophil (N) in a canine peripheral blood smear. X400.

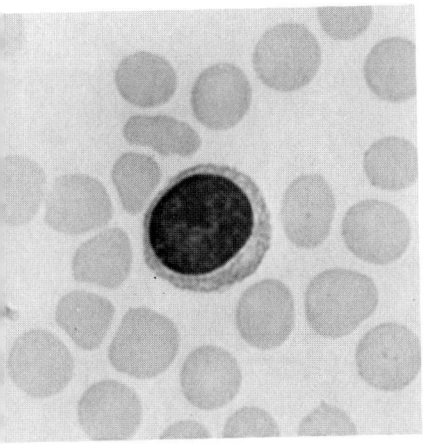

ig. 10.22 A lymphocyte in a feline peripheral lood smear. X400.

Monocytes are phagocytic cells that become macrophages once they have gained access to the extravascular space.

Plasma cells. The morphology and general function of *plasma cells* was discussed in Chapter 6. Their origin and relationship to B cells is discussed in this Chaper (*Agranulocytopoiesis*), whereas their immunologic function is discussed in Chapter 17.

Platelets

Blood platelets are small protoplasmic disks which are about 2–4 µm in diameter (Fig. 10.27). They are actually cytoplasmic fragments of a large cell, the *metamegakaryocyte*. The platelets are membrane-bound, round to oval fragments that contain a central, basophilic region (*chromomere*) and a pale, homogeneous peripheral zone (*hyalomere*). The chromomere contains mitochondria, endoplasmic reticular profiles and granules (Figs. 10.28, 10.29). The hyalomere may contain some glycogen, but it is usually

characterized by a homogeneous cytoplasmic matrix and microtubules. A nucleus is not present.

Platelets are functionally significant in hemostasis. (See Hemostasis.) Although their role in the cessation of bleeding may be their most prominent function, they subserve a variety of other functions. By virtue of their serotonin content, they are impo[rtant] tant mediators of vasoconstriction. By com[bining] bining with bacteria they aid phagocytos[is] by serving as opsonins. They may serve [a] similar function by combining with vir[us] particles.

Mammalian platelets are often referred [to] as thrombocytes.

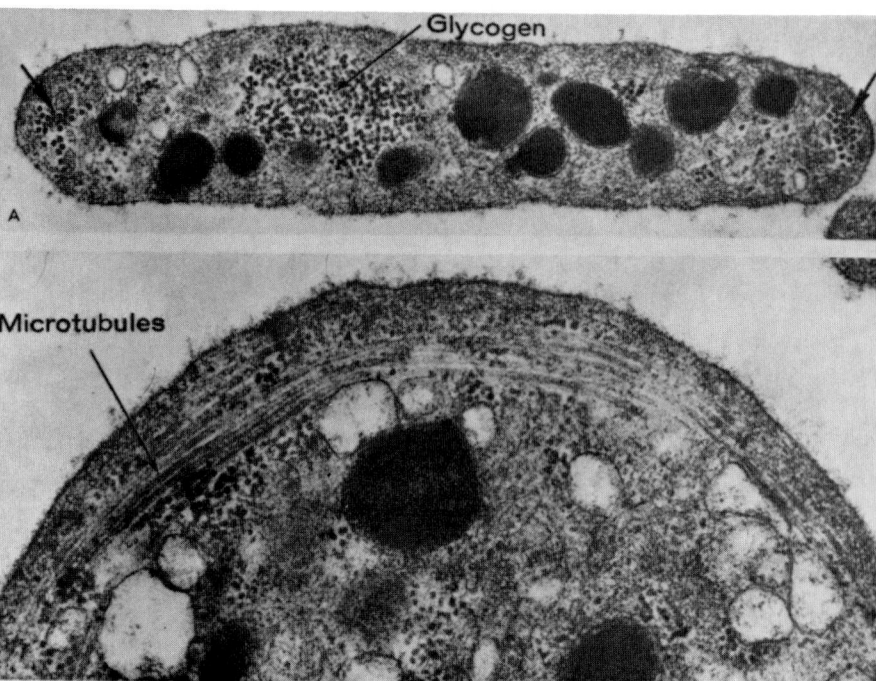

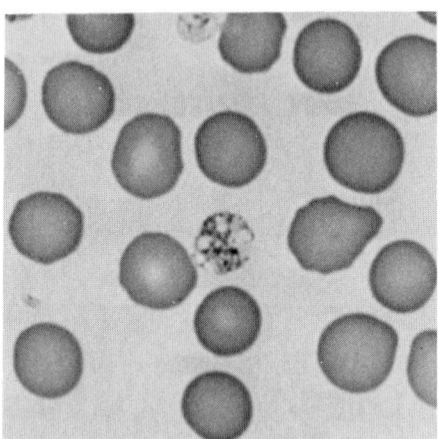

Fig. 10.27 A platelet in a canine peripheral blood smear. X400.

Fig. 10.29 Electron micrographs of platelets sectioned along the narrow surface (*upper*) an[d] parallel to the flat surface (*lower*). Glycogen granules are obvious within the granulomere, whi[le] microtubules (*arrows*) occur within the hyalomere. Upper, X31,000; Lower, X45,600. (Reprinte[d] with permission from Bloom, W. and Fawcett, D. W.: A Textbook of Histology. 10th edition, W. [B.] Saunders, Philadelphia, 1975.)

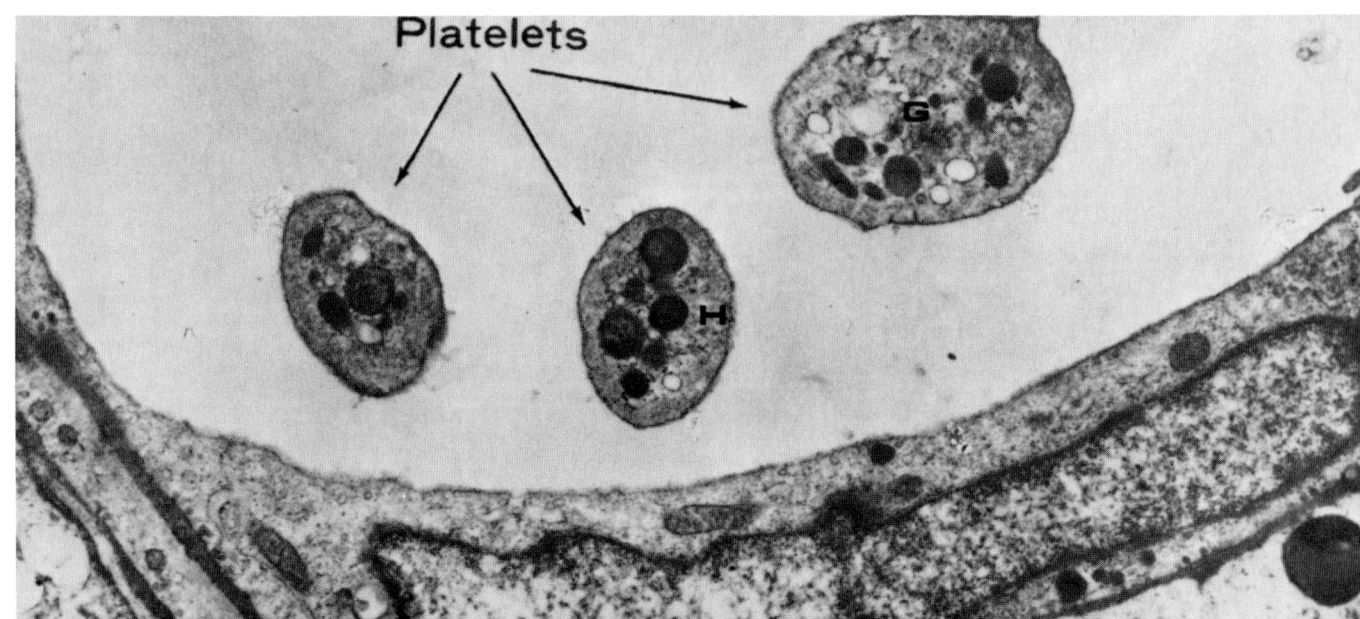

Fig. 10.28 An electron micrograph of platelets within a capillary. G, granulomere; H, hyalomere. (Reprinted with permission from Bloom, W. and Fawcett, D. W.: *A Textbook of Histology*, 10th edition, W. B. Saunders, Philadelphia, 1975).

Differences in Formed Elements— Selected Species

The blood cells of various domestic species are compared in color on Plates VI and VII.

Canine Blood Cells. The average size of the canine erythrocyte is 7.0 μm. These large cells usually have a well-defined central pallor. Occasionally, leptocytes are present. Although HJ bodies and nucleated erythrocytes are seen occasionally, they are not considered to be normal for the species. Reticulocytes normally should comprise less than 1% of the RBC's in an adult dog. Rouleaux formation occurs in canine erythrocytes.

The canine neutrophil contains an irregularly-lobed nucleus, the lobes of which are usually joined by a narrow strand rather than a true filament. The cytoplasm stains faintly a pink-gray color and contains fine, diffuse granules.

The eosinophil of canine blood consists of granules that vary in number and size. Also, these granules stain faintly with the acid dye (eosin). Usually, part or all of the nucleus is seen, since the granules are localized to a small part of the cytoplasm. The shape of this cell is variable.

The canine basophil contains granules that vary in size and number also. The intensity of the staining properties of the granules is variable. The number of granules is rarely sufficient to cover the nucleus or fill all of the cytoplasm. Because basophilic granules are water-soluble and easily removed during processing, this cell could be confused with a monocyte.

Although lymphocytes of the dog conform to the previous descriptions, the small lymphocyte is the predominant cell in the peripheral blood. Azurophilic granules occur rarely in these cells. Canine monocytes contain fine azurophilic granules and large nuclei. The nucleus is described typically as C-shaped with large blunt ends; however, the cell and nucleus are usually pleiomorphic.

Feline Blood Cells. The average size of feline RBC's is 5.9 μm. These corpuscles stain uniformly and the central pallor is not usually as prominent as in canine RBC's. Howell-Jolly bodies may occur in 1% of normal feline erythrocytes. Similarly, ER bodies may occur in 10% of the RBC's from normal cats. Nucleated erythrocytes may be encountered in the peripheral blood. Rouleaux formation is a prominent feature of feline RBC's.

The neutrophil of the cat contains a large nucleus that is usually coiled. Nuclear lobes may be connected by filaments or thin strands of nuclear materials. The fine pink granulations are contained within a gray cytoplasm.

The granules of the feline eosinphil are rod-shaped, refractile and numerous. They generally cover the nucleus.

Basophils are rarely encountered in the peripheral blood. They contain numerous, small, round light-staining lavender granules with occasional large dark granules.

The small lymphocyte is the predominant lymphocyte in the peripheral blood. Azurophilic granules are rare. The monocyte has a dull, blue cytoplasm that appears granular. Azurophilic granules are rare but cytoplasmic vacuoles may occur.

Equine Blood Cells. One of the most significant features of equine blood is the rapidity with which rouleaux formation occurs. Although single RBC's with a slight central pallor may be observed in blood smears, many cells will overlap in rouleaux formation. Howell-Jolly bodies may occur in normal erythrocytes. One of the most striking features of equine peripheral blood is the absence of immature erythrocytic forms. Reticulocytosis, even in anemia, is extremely rare.

The neutrophilic nucleus contains numerous foci of clumped heterochromatin. Interlobar filaments are rare. The gray cytoplasm contains fine, pink granules.

The eosinophil is the identifying feature of equine blood. The granules are large, round to oval, stain a bright red-orange and generally obscure most of the nucleus. The contour of the cell is defined by the granules.

The basophilic granulocyte contains purple granules that are scattered throughout the cytoplasm. Their shape and size are irregular; they may cover the nucleus.

Most of the peripheral lymphocytes are small. Large lymphocytes, however, may be as large as monocytes. Azurophilic granules are seen occasionally. The monocytic nucleus, most typically, is kidney-shaped. Small azurophilic granules may be scattered throughout the cytoplasm; small vacuoles may be present also.

Bovine Blood Cells. The small size of bovine RBC's and the absence of rouleaux formation is the reason bovine blood does not sediment readily. Anisocytosis is normal in this blood. The smallest RBC may be one-half of the diameter of the largest RBC. Normally, a central pallor is difficult to observe. Also, reticulocytes occur rarely in the peripheral blood of this animal.

The neutrophilic leukocyte has a lobed nucleus which generally has one lobe connected to the main part of the nucleus by a filament. Usually nuclear lobation is simply a partial constriction of the nucleus. The numerous, small granules may vary in staining properties from light pink to red. Neutrophils are the second most common white blood cell of bovine blood.

The eosinophil contains numerous, small, round, red granules which may fill the cytoplasm and cover the nucleus partially. Although the nucleus may be lobed, it is usually a C-shaped structure. The basophil, although rare, is typical.

The lymphocyte is the primary leukocyte of bovine blood. Small, medium and large lymphocytes occur in the peripheral blood. The large lymphocytes are confused easily with monocytes. Although the small and medium lymphocytes are typical, the large lymphocytes have a light-staining and eccentrically-positioned nucleus which is kidney-shaped, pale blue cytoplasm and numerous azurophilic granules. Cytoplasmic vacuolations may be apparent.

The morphology of monocytes is difficult to characterize; they vary in size and nuclear morphology is variable. A clover-leaf nucleus may be observed occasionally. The cell may be confused with large and medium lymphocytes; however, monocytic cytoplasm stains darker and is more granular than that of lymphocytes. The rare occurrence of azurophilic granules in the cytoplasm of monocytes is a useful distinguishing feature.

Ovine Blood Cells. The RBC's of sheep are smaller than those of bovids. A faint central pallor is observed, as well as a limited amount of rouleaux formation. All other characteristics of ovine RBC's are similar to those of the bovid.

The neutrophil is typically multilobed and these lobes are connected by fine filaments. The faintly-staining pink cytoplasm contains diffuse small granules. A few large granules occur also. As in bovine blood, these cells do not occur as frequently as in other nonruminant species.

The eosinophil contains red-orange granules which are equal in size, oval and refractile. These granules fill the cytoplasm and partially cover the nucleus. The basophil has granules that are dark with a red halo.

The lymphocytes vary from small to large but are difficult to categorize by size. All lymphocytes have nuclei with a smooth chromatin network that may stain with a red tint. Although the single nucleus is usually round, or oval and smooth, binucleated cells are encountered occasionally. The cytoplasm stains blue. Azurophilic granules may be observed also.

The monocytes have nuclei that may be oval, indented or even trilobed. Strands of intensely staining chromatin impart a lacy texture to the nucleus. The ground-glass-appearing cytoplasm stains more intensely than that of the large lymphocytes. Azurophilic granules are rare.

Caprine Blood Cells. The caprine RBC's are the smallest RBC's of domestic animals. They are round or triangular and devoid of a central pallor. Anisocytosis and rouleaux formation is not a common observation in adult blood. The blood of young goats, however, is characterized commonly by anisocytosis and poikilocytosis.

The neutrophil of the goat is similar to that of the sheep, except fewer lobes occur. The number of neutrophils is similar to other ruminants.

The eosinophil of the goat contains a nucleus which may vary from C-shaped to mono-, bi- or trilobed. The blue-stained cytoplasm contains numerous, small, round granules that stain an intense red. The basophil is typical; however, the purple granules have a red halo which imparts a red tint to the cytoplasm.

The caprine lymphocytes are small, medium and large. The nuclei are generally round to oval, but an occasional kidney-shaped nucleus is observed. The chromatin pattern in the nuclei of large lymphocytes is an important feature in differentiating these cells from monocytes. Large lymphocytes have coarsely clumped heterochromatin and nucleoli or nucleoli-like structures are present. Azurophilic granules of various sizes may be present.

The monocytes of the goat are similar to those of the sheep.

Porcine Blood Cells. Crenation and rouleaux formation occur, whereas the occurrence of central pallor is variable.

The neutrophil is characterized by an intensely stained nucleus that may be coiled. The lobes are connected by strictures; filaments are present rarely. The pale blue cytoplasm is filled with pale-staining small granules.

The eosinophil contains orange granules that fill the cytoplasm, obscure the cellular margin and partially obscure the nucleus.

The basophil is characterized by red-purple granules that assume coccoid or dumbell shapes.

The small lymphocytes of the pig are typical. The nucleus fills the cell and may be surrounded by a thin rim of pale blue cytoplasm. Large lymphocytes have a nucleus that is more vesicular than the smaller types. Azurophilic granules occur variably, tend to be rod-shaped and distributed along the cellular margin.

The monocyte is typical, but azurophilic granules are not a conspicous feature.

Avian Blood Cells

Erythrocytes

Morphology. The normal mature erythrocytes of avian blood are oval cells with oval nuclei (Fig. 10.30). These cells range from 10–13 μm long and from 6–7 μm wide. The elongated nucleus is about one-half of the dimensions of the cell. Nuclear heterochromatin may appear uniformly distributed in an oval nucleus. In a contracted nucleus, the heterochromatin may assume a more dense configuration. A nucleolus is not present. The cytoplasm may vary from orange-pink to red with routine blood stains. Numerous artifactual changes may alter the configuration and staining affinity of these cells. Erythrocytes of fishes and amphibians are morphologically similar to those of birds.

Granulocytes

The *granulocytes* of birds are the *heterophils, eosinophils* and *basophils.*

Heterophils. The *heterophil* of birds is the equivalent of the neutrophil in other species. The term heterophil is applied to these cells because of the great diversity of staining

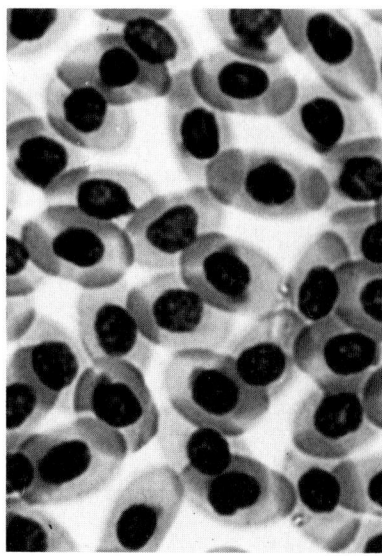

Fig. 10.30 Erythrocytes in an avian peripheral blood smear. X400.

reaction in various classes of vertebrates. Even in mammalian domestic species this could be appropriately applied.

The heterophil has a diameter of 6–9 μm. Despite its amoeboid properties, it is usually seen as a round cell in blood smears. The multilobed nucleus may have as many as 5 lobes and the heterochromatin is coarsely clumped. The distinguishing feature is the presence of brightly stained, eosinophilic rods with a fusiform configuration (Fig. 10.31). These specific inclusions are randomly scattered throughout the cell. They are easily dissolved in aqueous media and all that may remain is a red-stained *central body* or *vacuole*. As a result of this dissolution, the normally clear cytoplasm usually becomes acidophilic. Under these conditions the heterophils are easily confused with eosinophils.

Eosinophils. The avian *eosinophil* has a diameter between 5 and 9 μm. It has a multilobed nucleus with coarsely clumped heterochromatin. The cytoplasm, although usually obscured by tightly packed granules, stains a pale clear blue (Fig. 10.32). This characteristic is of diagnostic significance in distinguishing eosinophils from heterophils in which the rods have been partially dissolved. The granules of some eosinophils may appear as homogeneous bodies. In larger cells, the granules appear to be composed of three or four subunits which are combined in such a manner that a vacuity or clear space appears in the center of the complex. The eosinophilic granule is more refractive than that of the heterophil.

Basophils. The *basophil* of birds is similar to that of mammalian species. These cells are more numerous in avian blood.

Agranulocytes

The *agranulocytes* of avian blood are the *lymphocytes* and *monocytes.* Although the

relationship of the *thrombocyte* to the agranulocytic and erythrocytic series has not been clarified, the thrombocyte will be discussed with the agranulocytes.

Lymphocytes. The avian *lymphocyte* approximates the range of sizes reported for the comparable mammalian cell. Small, medium and large lymphocytes have been described. The cell is generally round with an even contour (Fig. 10.33). Cytoplasmic blebs, however, may be apparent. The nucleus is usually centrally located, but some cells may be polarized. Coarsely clumped heterochromatin is characteristic of this structure. Also, the nuclear/cytoplasmic ratio is high. A sharp indentation in the nucleus may also be apparent. Cytoplasmic characteristics are quite variable. The cytoplasm may stain faintly and be quite homogeneous, or it may stain intensely and be flocculated with basophilic material. The flocculation may be fine and slightly reti-

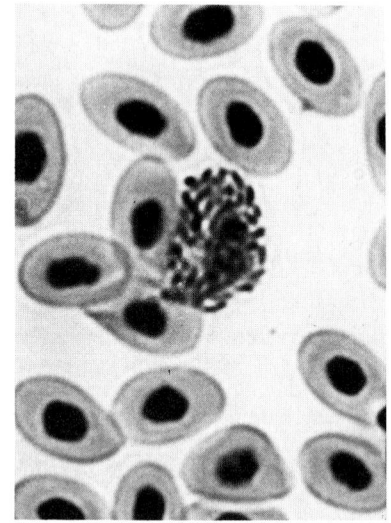

Fig. 10.31 Heterophil in an avian peripheral blood smear. X400.

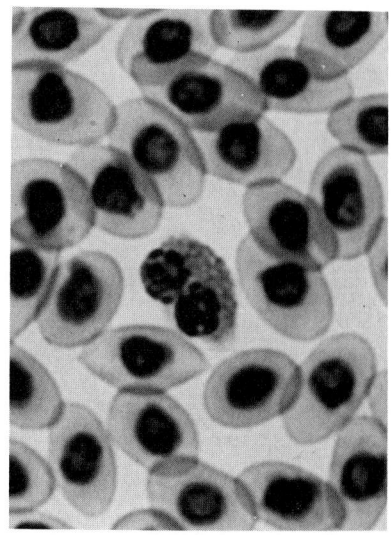

Fig. 10.32 An eosinophil in an avian peripheral blood smear. X400.

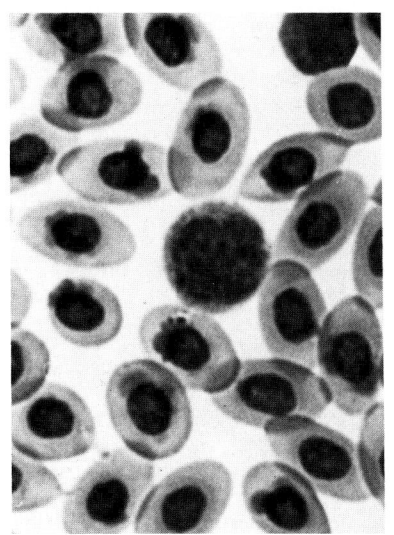

ig. 10.33   Lymphocyte in an avian peripheral
ood smear. X400.

ılated or heavy and coarsely reticulated.
ɔme magnenta-staining granules may be
·ident.

The discussion of the B cells and T cells
˙ the mammal is applicable to the bird.
˙he B cell was named on the basis of its
igin within the avian bursa of Fabricius.

Ionocytes. The avian *monocyte* is the larg-
·t cell of the mature elements of the agran-
locytic series. Usually, the average lym-
hocyte diameter approximates the diame-
r of the monocyte nucleus. Although the
ionocyte is usually round, numerous other
ɔnfigurations attest to its amoeboid char-
·teristics (Fig. 10.34). The nuclear/cyto-
lasmic ratio is smaller than that of the
mphocyte. The bean-shaped or kidney-
ıaped nucleus contains a fine reticulum of
·eterochromatin. The area of the cytoplasm
˙sociated with the nuclear indentation is
ıaracteristic for the monocytes. This jux-
.nuclear area contains orange granules or
˙ may be tinged orange. The ground-glass
ppearance of the cytoplasm, azurophilic
ˈranules and the juxtanuclear characteristics
·e diagnostic features for the monocyte.

ˈhrombocytes. The *thrombocytes* of birds
ıd other submammalian vertebrates are
ıcleated cells. These cells are somewhat
ıaller than erythrocytes and have average
imensions of 5 by 9 μm. The centrally
»cated, elongated nucleus is coarsely gran-
ˈar with heterochromatin (Fig. 10.35). The
ˈtoplasm is finely reticulated and baso-
ˈhilic and may contain a number of azuro-
ˈhilic, specific granules.

Besides functioning in hemostatis in a
ıanner similar to mammalian platelets, the
˙vian thrombocytes have been shown to be
·ephocytic and *phagocytic*.

Hemostasis

Hemostasis is a process in which a com-
ˈlex series of interactions culminate in the
·rmination of blood loss after vascular in-

jury. Because the maintenance of the integrity, volume and composition of blood is
essential to life, this process is a significant
part of homeostatic mechanisms. This
mechanism involves important contributions from the vasculature, platelets and coagulation factors.

Response of Vasculature. Vasoconstriction
immediately follows the rupture or cutting
of a normal vessel. This vasoconstriction
may be due to any one or a combination of
factors: 1) localized spasm (contraction) of
intramural smooth muscle; 2) reflex activity
involving vasomotor nerves of the sympathetic nervous system; and/or 3) the localized release of *vasoconstrictor substances*, especially *serotonin*. Vasoconstriction reduces
blood loss and facilitates the accumulation
of platelets at the site of injury. The denuded

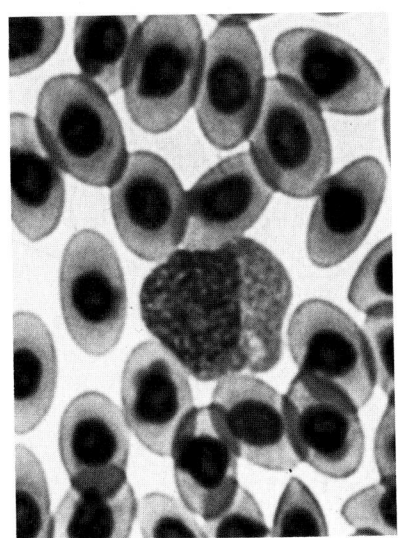

Fig. 10.34   Monocyte in an avian peripheral
blood smear. X400.

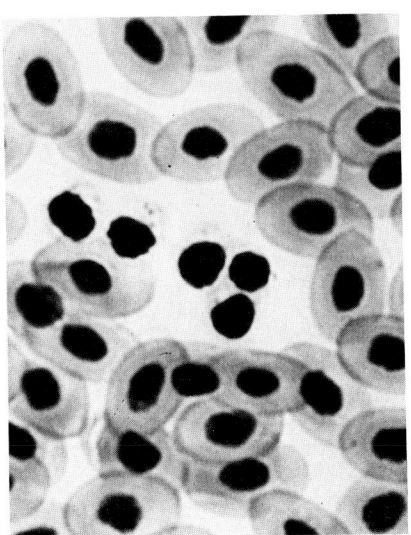

Fig. 10.35   Thrombocytes in an avian peripheral blood smear. X400.

or damaged endothelial surface of the vessel
exposes the subendothelial collagen, while
damaged cells release *adenosine diphosphate*.
These events facilitate platelet aggregation
by increasing the adhesiveness of their surfaces. The contact with the exposed collagen
activates intrinsic coagulative mechanisms,
while the release of tissue *thromboplastin*
(*Factor III*) activates extrinsic coagulative
mechanisms. *Plasminogen* is released at the
site of vascular injury also.

Platelet Function. Platelets which aggregate
at sites of injury are transformed into irregularly-shaped structures with pseudopodia.
These pseudopodia extend into the site of
injury and between the individual platelets
of the aggregate. The aggregation process
causes a *release reaction* in which the platelets secrete some of the products stored
within their granulomeres. These products
include ADP, serotonin, histamine and
platelet factor 3, a lipoprotein required for
coagulation. The lipoprotein catalyzes several reactions involved in the formation of
thrombin. This release reaction is called *degranulation*. Platelets, then, contribute to
continued aggregation of more platelets.
RBC's contain high concentrations of ADP.
Their entrapment and rupture within the
plug releases more ADP which enhances
more aggregation of platelets. The reversible
process of *platelet plug* formation stops the
blood loss from the site of injury. These
temporary plugs can be washed away from
the site of injury; rebleeding can occur as a
consequence. Additional mechanisms are
required to transform this temporary plug
into an irreversible aggregation of platelets.

Permanency is imparted to the platelet
plug through the interaction of *viscous metamorphosis* of platelets and *fibrin* generation.
Viscous metamorphosis is characterized by
irreversible morphologic changes of the
platelets within the plug. Filaments which
have contractile properties appear in the
platelets. This filamentous protein, *thrombosthenin*, occurs in the platelet as a monomer until activation converts it to a filamentous polymer that probably has the
same properties as the actin-myosin complexes of muscle. Fibrin attaches to the
platelet pseudopodia and the contraction of
thrombosthenin exerts tension on the fibri-
nous strands. This mechanism is believed to
account for *clot retraction*. Moreover, fibrin
deposition on the platelet aggregate is believed to be the activation mechanism for
viscous metamorphosis and the conversion
of the temporary platelet plug into an irreversible aggregate. Calcium is essential for
the contraction of thrombosthenin, whereas
cyclic AMP has been implicated as the regulator of viscous metamorphosis.

Coagulation. *Coagulation* is a complex series
of interactions in which the blood loses its
fluid characteristics and is converted to a
semisolid mass. The formation of the irreversible clot, resulting from the interaction
of damaged tissue, platelets and fibrin, is an
integral part of this process. The formation

of fibrin results from a complex process that involves tissue and/or blood factors.

The blood and tissue factors, except factor IV, are proteins, most of them are probably produced by the liver. The activation of the fibrin-producing mechanism which originates in the tissues is called the *extrinsic pathway*. That which originates in the blood is called the *intrinsic pathway*. These two pathways converge upon the *common pathway* that leads ultimately to fibrin formation. The numerous factors that comprise these pathways have many synonyms. Some of them are listed in Table 10.3. A coagulation scheme is outlined in Figure 10.36.

The sequence of events which leads to coagulation is considered to occur in three stages: (Stage I) the formation of a prothrombin-converting factor; (Stage II) the conversion of prothrombin to thrombin by the prothrombin-converting factor; (Stage III) the induction of fibrin formation from fibrinogen by thrombin. Stage I may be achieved by either the intrinsic or extrinsic pathways. Stages II and III are part of the common pathway.

Extrinsic Coagulation. The contact of blood with damaged tissue initiates the extrinsic pathway, which is dependent upon the release of the lipoprotein, *tissue thromboplastin* (factor III). The *kallikreins* are proteolytic enzymes that are released in response to localized damage. Although they are considered to be endogenous mediators of an increased vascular permeability, they may serve to initiate the conversion of *proconvertin* (factor VII) to its active form. Factor III, in the presence of calcium ions and phospholipids, acts on or with the activated factor VII to activate the *Stuart-Prower factor* (factor X). Activated factor X and activated *factor V* (*prothrombin accelerator*) may serve together to form the *prothrombin-*

converting factor. The remainder of the common pathway is detailed in Figure 10.36.

Intrinsic Coagulation. Blood which is separated from the body tissues retains its ability to coagulate. Because the ability to coagulate is inherent in the blood, this pathway is called the intrinsic mechanism. The surface contact activates the *Hageman factor* (*factor XII*), which in turn converts *prekallikrein* to *kallikrein*. Kallikrein then activates *factor XI* (*Plasma Thromboplastin Antecedent*). The latter activates *factor IX* (*Christmas factor*). Activated Christmas factor and the activated *antihemophilic factor* (*factor VIII*) then activate the *Stuart-Prower factor* (factor X). The remainder of the pathway is as described with extrinsic coagulation and is outlined in Figure 10.36.

Clot Formation and Fibrinolysis. The platelet is an essential component of clot formation and retraction. The necessity of fibrin in the formation of an irreversible platelet plug was discussed previously. Despite the so-called irreversibility of the platelet plug, blood clots are not permanent structures. The cascading effects of the clotting and coagulation mechanisms, once initiated, do not continue unregulated under normal circumstances. The devastating consequences of unchecked hemostatic mechanisms should be obvious. The fibrinolytic mechanism is outlined in Figure 10.37. Unfortunately, not all of the details of this mechanism are understood.

Proteolytic fragments of the *Hageman factor (factor XII)* and/or other tissue or plasma substances convert some activator from its inactive to its active form. This activator then converts *profibrinolysin* (*plasminogen*) to *fibrinolysin* (*plasmin*). Plasmin degrades the fibrin, *fibrin split products* are formed and the clot dissolves eventually.

A subtle balance exists between formation

and dissolution of a clot. Plasmin has a positive feedback effect upon the activated Hageman factor. As more plasmin is produced, it causes more proteolytic fragments to be formed from activated factor XII. This mechanism insures the eventual dissolution of a blood clot.

Blood Cell Dynamics— Hematopoiesis

General Characteristics

Form and Function. The replacement of all cells, as has been presented previously (Chapter 4), is predicted upon the occurrence of stem cells associated with the various tissues. Blood cell replacement is achieved through the activities of stem cells that are confined to specific areas. These areas of *hematopoiesis* differ in the prenatal, postnatal and adult animal. During early prenatal development, hematopoiesis begins in the blood islands associated with the yolk sac. It becomes widespread in the fetus and includes mesenchyme and blood vessels, liver, spleen, thymus, lymph nodes and bone marrow. Postnatal formation of erythrocytes, granulocytes and platelets is confined primarily to the red bone marrow. The spleen also is involved to a lesser degree in erythropoiesis. A progressive reduction in red bone marrow occurs throughout adolescence and hematopoietic activity is confined to the marrow cavities of the sternebrae, ribs, vertebrae and cranial bones. This reduction in hematopoiesis results from a conversion of *red bone marrow* to *yellow bone marrow*.

During early development, the thymus is the primary organ of lymphocytopoiesis. The spleen and remaining lymphoid tissues then become responsible for the production of agranulocytes throughout the life of the organism.

Hematopoiesis is one of the most controversial areas of histology. Although the progress of differentiation of specific cell types is easily described, the morphologic nature of the stem cell or cells has not been clarified satisfactorily. As a result there are three theories on the nature and fate of the stem cell or stem cells (Fig. 10.38). The *monophyletic* theory supports the premise that *all* blood cells arise from a single stem cell, the *hemocytoblast*. The *diphyletic* theory supports the premise that there is a separate stem cell, for the agranulocytes and a separate stem cell for the granulocytes and erythrocytes. The *polyphyletic* theory supports the idea that separate stem cells give rise to the erythrocytes and granulocytes, lymphocytes and monocytes.

The monophyletic theory seems to have the widest acceptance. However, the relationship of stem cells to specific cell lineages has not been clarified.

Trends in Development. The differentiation of mature red blood corpuscles and granulocytes is characterized by sequential

Table 10.3
Coagulation Factors of Hemostasis

International Committee Designation	Synonym
Factor I	Fibrinogen
Factor II	Prothrombin
Factor III	Tissue Thromboplastin*
Factor IV	Calcium Ion
Factor V	Labile Factor (Prothrombin Accelerator)
Factor VI	No Longer Applicable
Factor VII	Stabile Factor (Proconvertin)
Factor VIII	Antihemophilic Factor (Thromboplastinogen)
Factor IX	Christmas Factor (Plasma Thromboplastin Component)
Factor X	Stuart-Prower Factor
Factor XI	Plasma Thromboplastin Antecedent
Factor XII	Hageman Factor
Factor XIII	Fibrin-Stabilizing Factor
Platelet Factor	Platelet Factor 3†

* Occurs in tissues.
† Occurs in platelets.

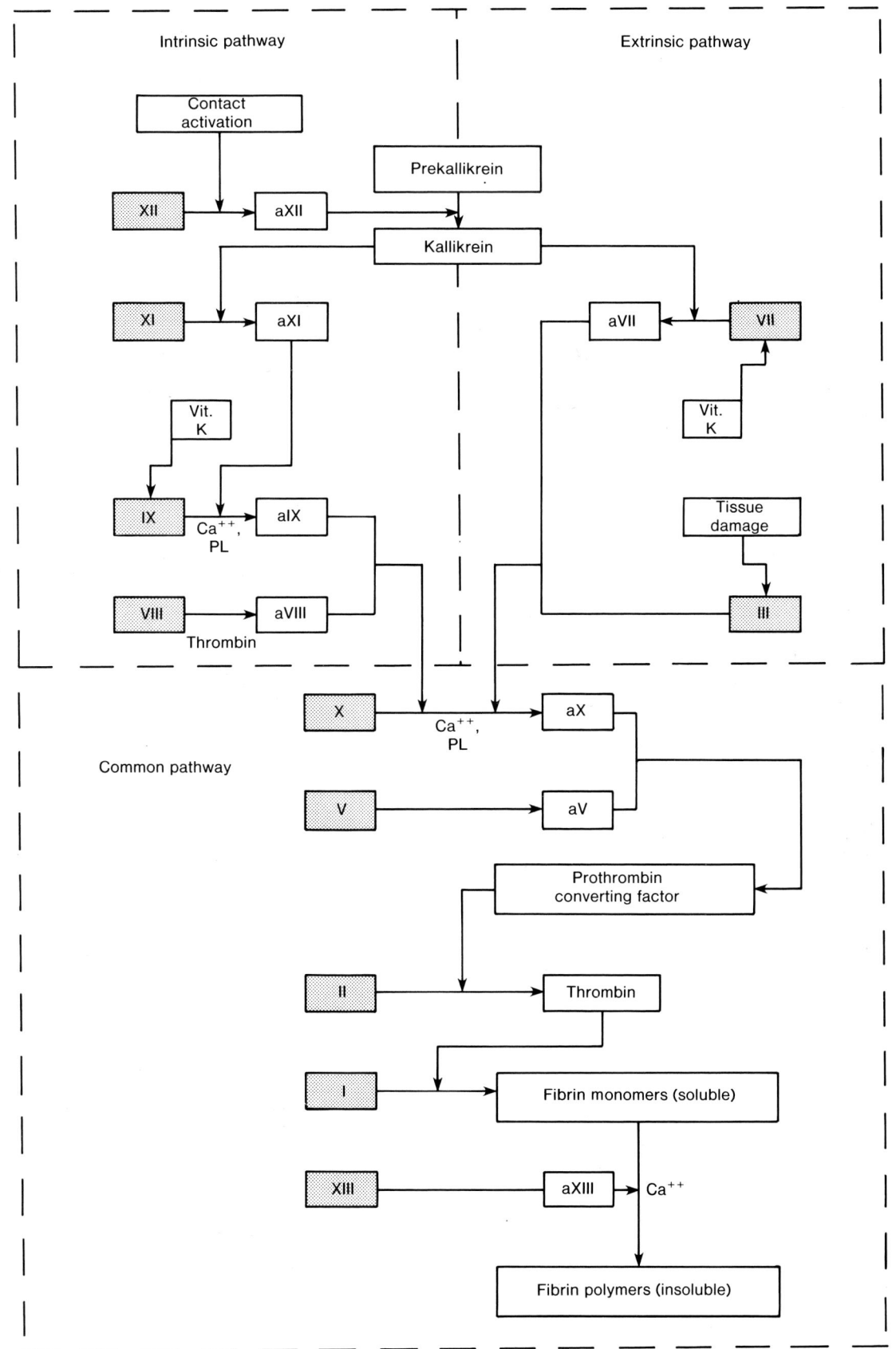

Fig. 10.36   A flow diagram of the coagulation scheme. a-activated; PL-phospholipid. Extrinsic and intrinsic pathways terminate with the activation of factor X, the first factor in the common pathway. Soluble fibrin monomers are converted to insoluble fibrin polymers in the common pathway.

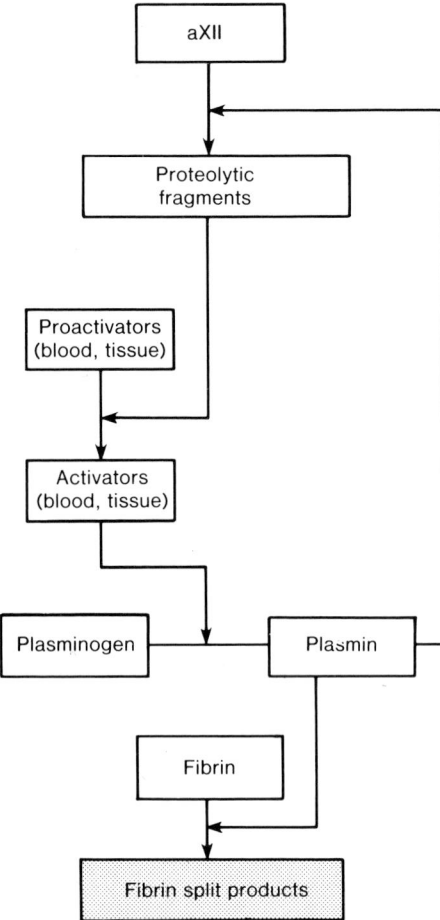

Fig. 10.37   A flow diagram of the fibrinolytic mechanism. Plasmin degrades fibrin into fibrin split products and exerts a positive feedback influence upon activated Hageman factor.

changes which typify the developmental process (Fig. 10.39).

The early cells in the sequence are large and become smaller with maturation. The nucleus, as well, is large and decreases with maturation. In the erythrocytic series, the nucleus is extruded from the cell.

The nucleus of early cells is light-staining and acidophilic. With maturation it becomes darker and basophilic. Similarly, the cytoplasm of early cells is basophilic and becomes progressively acidophilic with the maturation process.

The nuclei of stem cells are round and light-staining. The chromatin is disposed in a fine reticulated distribution. With maturation the nuclei become indented, lobed or segmented and the chromatin stains more darkly and is clumped.

Early cells are devoid of granules. In the granulocytic series, early granules are nonspecific and are replaced by the specific granulocytic inclusion granules.

Early cells have one or more nucleoli that are not apparent as development progresses toward the definitive cell type.

Also, mitotic activity is high in more primitive cells in normal development.

Similar trends are characteristic of the agranulocytic series also.

Bone Marrow

The marrow tissue is a hypercellular and highly vascularized form of connective tissue which is associated intimately with bone as an organ. It is contained within the *medullary cavity* (*marrow cavity*) as interosseous tissue in all bones of the soma. During development and growth, all of the marrow is *red bone marrow*. By adulthood, the red bone marrow is confined to a limited number of loci: sternebrae, ribs, vertebrae and cranial bones. The remaining loci will have been replaced with *yellow bone marrow*.

The marrow cavity first appears as an integral component of ossification processes and is involved in the development of bones. This involvement in bone is maintained throughout life, because the peripheral limits of the marrow contain elements of the cortical endosteum. Similarly, trabecular endosteum may be contained within the substance of the marrow tissues. The acquisition of blood-cell formative and blood-cell destructive functions, although acquired secondarily, is maintained throughout the life of the animal.

Red Bone Marrow. The red color of this type of bone marrow results from the accumulation of erythrocytes, erythrocytic precursors and their contained pigments. *Red bone marrow* is an hemopoietic tissue often called *myeloid tissue*. Erythrocytes, granulocytes and platelets are produced within this tissue. Agranulocytes also develop within this tissue as well as within the lymphatic organs.

The marrow consists of numerous vascular channels (arterial and venous), sinuses, a reticular fiber framework, free cells of the blood cell lineages, macrophages and some adipose tissue (Fig. 10.40). The marrow is divisible into two compartments: *vascular compartment* and *hematopoietic compartment*. The vascular compartment includes all of the vessels of the bone marrow. Classically, the sinuses of this tissue are described as being lined by phagocytic cells. The phagocytes are probably perivascular cells. The hematopoietic compartment comprises all of the irregular islands and columns of tissue between the vascular beds and includes a reticular fiber stroma, reticular cells, hemocytoblasts, phagocytic cells, intermediate and mature blood cell forms, adipose tissue and other typical connective tissue cells (plasma cells, mast cells). Primitive and phagocytic reticular cells are described classically as components of this tissue (Fig. 10.41). The nature, relationships and functional significance of these cells was discussed previously (Chapter 6). The primary function of the red bone marrow is blood cell production.

Yellow Bone Marrow. The amount of active bone marrow responsible for blood cell production is reduced appreciably by the time adulthood is achieved. Adipose tissue replaces most of the blood cell-producing elements of the hematopoietic compartment.

Under conditions of stress (including disease), the *yellow bone marrow* can revert to an active hematopoietic tissue.

Erythropoiesis

Cytology of Differentiation. The following cells comprise the erythrocytic series: *hemocytoblast, rubriblast, prorubricyte, rubricyte, metarubricyte, reticulocyte, mature red blood corpuscle* (Figs. 10.38, 10.39).

The *hemocytoblast* is approximately 15 μm in diameter and has a deeply basophilic cytoplasm and a large, round, pale-staining vesicular nucleus. It can undergo mitosis and may differentiate from more primitive stem cells.

The *rubriblast* (*proerythroblast, pronormoblast*) is an intermediate between the hemocytoblast and the prorubricyte which is described by some authors. The nucleus of this cell is primitive and somewhat smaller than that of the hemocytoblast. Also, the cytoplasm is more basophilic than that of the hemocytoblast. This cell is the first cell in the erythrocytic series.

The *prorubricyte* (*basophilic erythroblast, basophilic normoblast*) is smaller than the two previous forms and has a coarsely distributed chromatin in the nucleus and an intensely basophilic cytoplasm. The nucleoli are either poorly defined or absent. Mitotic activity is high.

The *rubricyte* (*polychromatophilic erythroblast, polychromatophilic normoblast*) is a small cell with a small, round and dense nucleus. Nucleoli are not apparent. The cytoplasm has a mottled basophilic and acidophilic appearance due to the presence of hemoglobin and ribonucleic protein (Plates VI.22, VII.5).

The *metarubricyte* (*orthochromatic erythroblast, normoblast*) is characterized by an acidophilic cytoplasm which is very similar to the mature red blood corpuscle (Plate VII.5). After extensive mitotic activity as a rubricyte, the nucleus becomes very condensed and eventually pyknotic. The nucleus is lost either by simple extrusion from the cell or by *karyolysis*.

The resulting enucleated cell is the *reticulocyte* (*polychromatophilic erythrocyte, diffusely basophilic erythrocyte*). The cytoplasm is diffusely basophilic, and with special staining techniques (supravital dyes such as cresyl blue or neutral red) a fine cytoplasmic reticulum is demonstrable. Although this reticulum is normally lost within the myeloid tissue during the transition to mature red blood corpuscles, some reticulocytes occur normally in the peripheral blood.

The increased cytoplasmic basophilia represents the accumulation of ribonucleoproteins for cellular synthesis. Hemoglobin, first synthesized by the rubricyte, results in a mottled cytoplasmic appearance. Increased synthesis of hemoglobin and a reduction of the appropriate cellular organelles characterizes the metarubricytic stage. A continuation of this process results in the

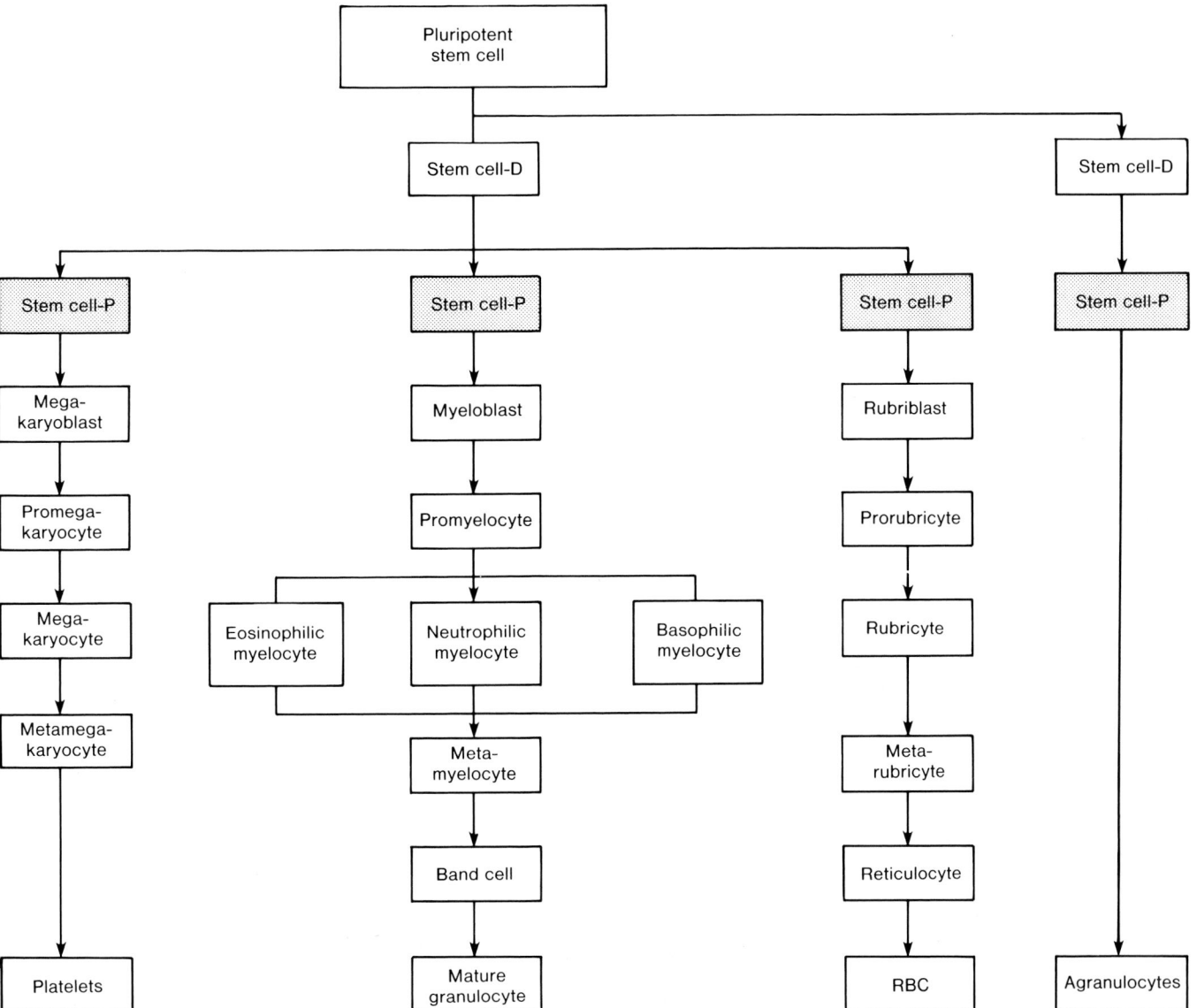

Fig. 10.38 A flow diagram of the origin and differentiation of blood cells. According to the monophyletic theory, a single pluripotent stem cell gives rise to all blood cells. The diphyletic theory states that separate stem cells (stem cells-D) give rise to lymphoid and myeloid elements, whereas the polyphyletic theory states that separate stem cells (stem cells-P) exist for each blood cell lineage.

mature RBC. Importantly, the circulating RBC's of the embryo are nucleated and probably represent metarubricytes.

Granulocytopoiesis

Cytology of Differentiation. The following cells comprise the granulocytic series: *hemocytoblast, myeloblast, promyelocyte, myelocyte, metamyelocyte, band cell, mature granulocyte* (Figs. 10.38, 10.39).

The *hemocytoblast* was described with the erythrocytic series.

The *myeloblast* has a diameter of 15–20 μm. The basophilic cytoplasm is unevenly stained and is darker at the periphery than in the perinuclear region. The nucleus is large, finely reticular and red-staining. Two or more nucleoli may be observed.

The *promyelocyte (progranulocyte)* is a large cell which may even be larger than the hemocytoblast. The nucleus is round with coarsely distributed chromatin. Nucleoli are not readily observed. The cytoplasm, although basophilic, contains acidophilic regions. Granules are present and vary from acidophilic to basophilic. There is a gradual decrease in *nonspecific granules* and a gradual increase in *specific granules*. A promyelocyte becomes a myelocyte when the specific granulocyte can be identified on the basis of the staining affinity, size and shape of the specific granules. Promyelocytic mitotic activity is high.

The *myelocyte (basophilic myelocyte, eosinophilic myelocyte, neutrophilic myelocyte)* is the first recognizable stage of the specific granulocytes. The nucleus is smaller and the chromatin is more coarse than the previous stages. Also, the nucleus is more oval than round and a slight indentation may be apparent. The decreased cytoplasmic basophilia is complemented by an increase in the number of specific granules. Mitotic activity of these cells is especially high.

The *metamyelocyte (basophilic metamyelocyte, eosinophilic metamyelocyte, neutrophilic metamyelocyte)* is characterized by a bean-shaped or horseshoe-shaped appearance. The cytoplasm is slightly acidophilic and filled with specific granules. Progressive indentation results in the lobed nuclear appearance of the mature granulocytes.

Neutrophilic granulocytes are the most predominate granulocytes of the myeloid tissue and peripheral blood. Immature forms of neutrophils are commonly encountered in the peripheral blood. A *neutrophilic metamyelocyte* is also referred to as a *juvenile*. The progressive indentation of the nucleus results in a neutrophil referred to as *neutrophilic band cell (neutrophilic stab cell, neutrophilic nonsegmented)* (Plates VI.23,

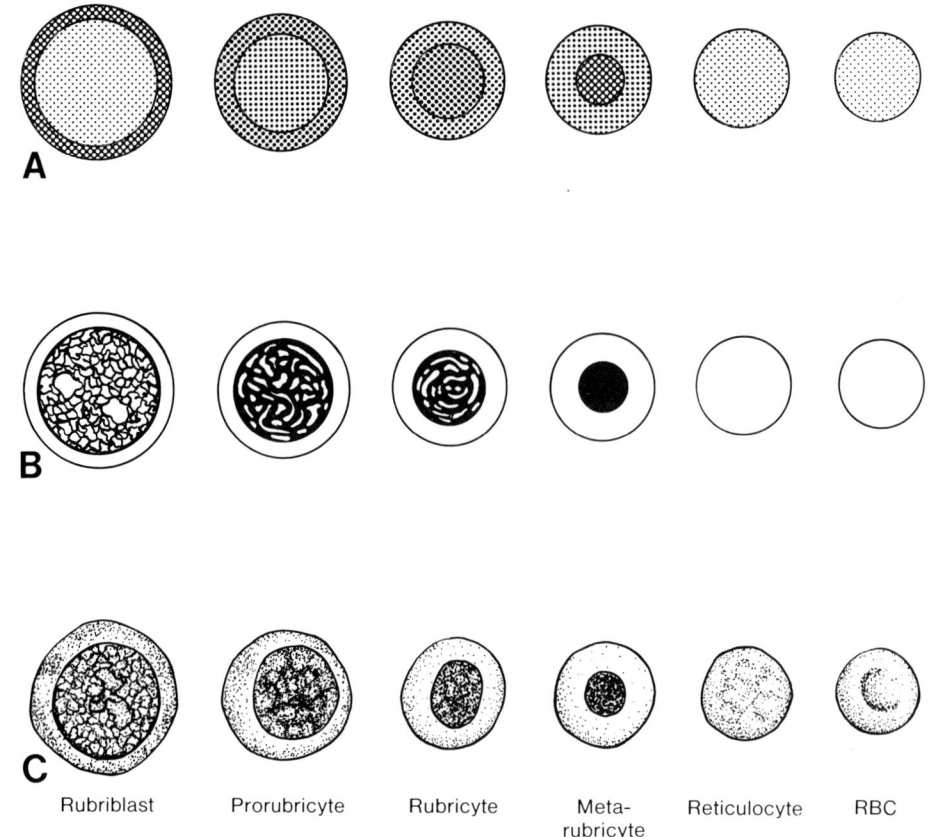

A

B

C

| Rubriblast | Prorubricyte | Rubricyte | Meta-rubricyte | Reticulocyte | RBC |

Fig. 10.39 A diagram depicting the cellular changes associated with the differentiation of blood cells. *A.* The large, pale-staining nucleus becomes progressively smaller with development. The nucleus is extruded in the erythrocytic series. The basophilic cytoplasm becomes progressively lighter as development progresses. *B.* Nuclear and cytoplasmic size is reduced during development, while more heterochromatin becomes obvious during the progress toward a mature cell. *C.* The stages of the development of erythrocytes may be compared with the generalities of *A* and *B*. (Modified and redrawn from Diggs, L. W., Sturm, D. and Bell, A.: *The Morphology of Blood Cells.* Abbott Laboratories, North Chicago, 1954.)

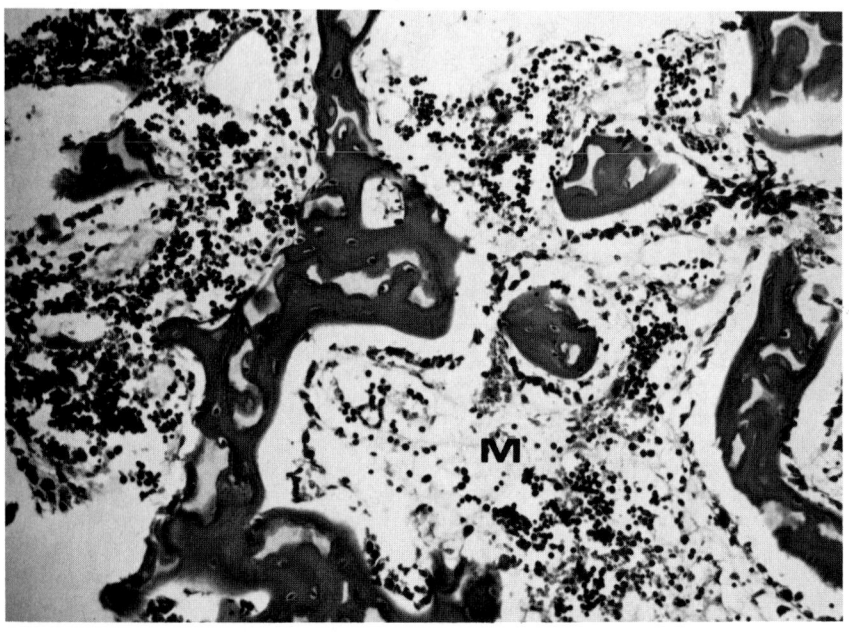

Fig. 10.40 Red bone marrow within the marrow cavity of a developing bone. The bone marrow (M) occupies the interosseous spaces between the developing bone and mineralized cartilaginous spicules of the primary spongiosa. X40.

VII.1, VII.3). The nucleus of this cell is characteristically horseshoe-shaped. The subsequent lobulation of the nucleus results in a mature cell referred to as a *neutrophilic segmenter* (*PMN, polymorphonuclear neutrophilic granulocyte, neutrophilic filamented, neutrophilic polymorphonuclear or, simply, neutrophil*).

Thrombocytopoiesis

Cytology of Differentiation. The cells that comprise the platelet formation series are *hemocytoblast, megakaryoblast, promegakaryocyte, megakaryocyte, metamegakaryocyte* and *platelets* (Fig. 10.38).

The *hemocytoblast* was described with the erythrocytic series.

The *megakaryoblast* has a lightly basophilic cytoplasm and a nucleus that stains red and is finely granular. The peripheral cytoplasm has pseudopods and a foamy appearance.

The *promegakaryocyte* is larger than the previous cell type and two nuclei may be present. The cytoplasm is slightly basophilic and contains numerous basophilic granules. Cytoplasmic blebs with a foamy appearance may be apparent at the periphery of the cell

The *megakaryocyte* is larger than the previous cell type. Karyokinesis occurs and as
many as 16 nuclei may form. These, however, subsequently fuse to form the characteristic bulged and lobed nucleus of this cell.
The cytoplasmic volume is large and acidophilic. Vacuoles and pale-staining areas
are scattered among the evenly distributed,
lightly basophilic granules.

The *metamegakaryocyte* is the largest cell
in the series. Except for the aggregation of
cytoplasmic granules and the appearance of
platelets at the cellular periphery, it is similar to the megakaryocyte.

This series of cellular changes is characterized by an increase in size and number of
nuclei per cell—the reverse in the general
trend in the aforementioned series. Mitoses
occur in which nuclear separation (*karyokinesis*) is not accompanied by a cytoplasmic
separation (*cytokinesis*). Platelets form from
metamegakaryocytes by an exocytotic process in which they pinch off from the cell
surface.

Agranulocytopoiesis

General Characteristics. The developmental sequence for the agranulocytes (lymphocytes, monocytes, macrophages and plasma
cells) occurs in the lymphoid organs as well
as in the bone marrow. For this reason,
some authors refer to these organs as *lymphomyeloid organs*. The developmental sequences leading to the mature forms of these
cells are not as clearly defined as they are in
the previously described sequences. Moreover, the location and nature of all stem
cells, specific areas in which development
occurs and the relationships of these mononucleated cells to each other needs further
clarification. Figure 10.42 represents a summary of the known relationships among
these cells.

Lymphocytopoiesis and Plasma Cells. The
lymphatic organs were thought for years to
be the only sites of lymphocytopoiesis. Current evidence has established that this process occurs in the myeloid tissue also. The
precise nature of the stem cell for this sequence has eluded research efforts. The
primitive reticular cell, classically, has been
considered the cell which gave rise to the
hemocytoblast. The uncertainty of the functional significance of the primitive reticular
cell was discussed in Chapter 6 (Reticular
Cells).

The stem cell, *hemocytoblast*, was described with the section on erythropoiesis. It
is assumed that this cell is capable of differentiating into all of the agranulocytes.

The *lymphoblasts* are the largest cells of
this series. They have large, round vesicular
nuclei with one or more prominent nucleoli,
and have a basophilic cytoplasm. (These
cells are sometimes called *large lymphocytes*.) Progressive differentiation and mitosis results in a smaller cell with a nucleus
that contains more coarsely clumped heter-

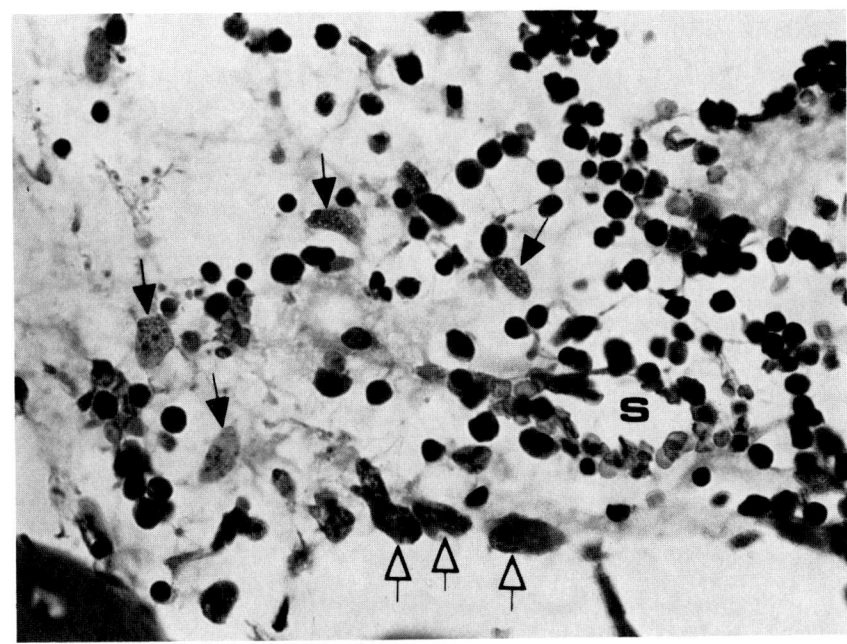

Fig. 10.41   Elements of red bone marrow. Reticular cells (*solid arrows*) comprise a cellular
reticulum. Numerous free blood cells are in various stages of development. A sinusoid (S) and
artifactually displaced osteoblasts (*open arrows*) are present. X160.

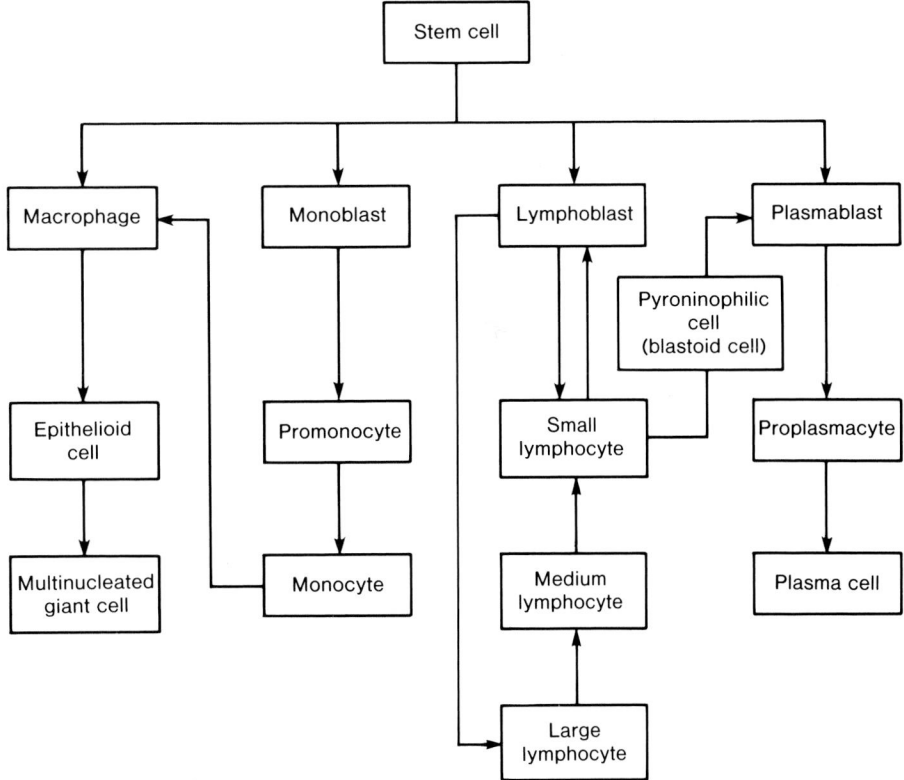

Fig. 10.42   A flow diagram of the established relationships among agranulocytes.

ochromatin. These are *large lymphocytes*
that may be called *prolymphocytes* or *medium lymphocytes* by some authors. The subsequent division of these intermediate forms
results in *small lymphocytes*. Although the
progression appears to be from lymphoblast
to small lymphocyte, any of these cells can
enter the peripheral circulation.

Small lymphocytes are not fixed postmi-
totic cells. Under appropriate stimulation

they can dedifferentiate into lymphoblasts
which then can give rise to more small
lymphocytes. Also, with appropriate antigenic stimulation, the small lymphocyte is
converted to a *pyroninophilic cell*. These cells
contain large quantities of RNA, which is
stainable with pyronin, and are sometimes
called *immunoblasts*. The cells are characterized by a *blastoid transformation* which
permits them to become *plasmablasts*. *Plas-*

mablasts and *proplasmacytes* are not distinct and identifiable cytologic intermediates in the differentiation of *plasma cells.*

Origin of Lymphocytes. During embryonic life, stem cells are produced sequentially in the yolk sac, liver, and spleen (Fig. 10.43). Lymphocytes differentiate in the liver and spleen. Stem cells then populate the bone marrow. The bone marrow functions as the major source for two distinct yet interrelated populations of lymphocytes.

One population of stem cells leaves the bone marrow and populates the thymus. These cells proliferate and differentiate within this organ and eventually *peripheralization* occurs. Lymphocytes from the thymus, *T lymphocytes,* populate specific areas of the *secondary lymphatic organs—paracortical zone of lymphatic nodules* and *periarteriolar zone of splenic corpuscles.* These cells are responsible for cell-mediated immunity and interact with B lymphocytes in an undetermined way to induce antibody formation (Fig. 10.43).

The organs involved in the development of *B lymphocytes* in the mammal have not been characterized completely. Stem cells leave the bone marrow and populate the bursal equivalent. In birds, these cells infiltrate the bursa of Fabricius and subsequently populate secondary lymphatic organs. Because mammals do not have a bursa of Fabricius, extensive research has been directed to defining a bursal equivalent. It

tissue (GALT) was the bursal equivalent. Now, it is conjectured that the bone marrow may assume the role of the bursa of Fabricius. Additional research is required to clarify these relationships. After the population of the bursal equivalent, these cells populate the secondary lymphatic organs—*germinal centers of lymphatic nodules.* The B cells produced in these areas synthesize antibodies (humoral antibody response) and are capable of transformation into plasma cells (Fig. 10.43).

The B cells and T cells cooperate in the immunologic responsiveness of the organism (Chapter 17).

Monocytopoiesis. The origin, distribution and relationships of the mononucleated phagocytic cells of the body were discussed in Chapter 6 (Reticuloendothelial System). Although the precise nature and morphology of the stem cell for monocytes has not been clarified, it is clear that monocytes originate in the bone marrow. Immature monocytes in the bone marrow are larger than but similar to their mature counterparts. The large oval or round nucleus has numerous nucleoli. These *promonocytes* are difficult to distinguish from granulocytic precursors.

Blood Cell Dynamics—Circulation, Regulation, Destruction

The finite existence of the formed elements of the blood requires that old and/or damaged cells be removed from the circulation and new elements be added by the lymphomyeloid tissues. The rate at which these two processes occur normally accounts for the usual populations of cells that comprise the peripheral blood. Any alteration to the formative and/or removal processes can result in abnormal parameters. The dynamics of this balanced activity are referred to as *blood kinetics.* Many organs contribute to the formation and/or destruction of blood cells, directly or indirectly. The bone marrow and thymus are important lymphomyeloid organs involved in hematopoiesis. The spleen, lymph nodes and lymph nodules are important contributors to hematopoiesis. The bone marrow, spleen and other organs with RES potential are involved also in the destruction of cells. The liver contributes significantly to iron metabolism and retains its fetal potential for hematopoiesis. Additionally, it produces most of the plasma proteins. Portions of the gastrointestinal system contribute to erythrogenesis by their absorption of iron and production of *intrinsic factor.* Intrinsic factor exists in man but may not occur in domestic animals. Besides contributing to the degradation and excretion of hemoglobin metabolites, the kidney is important in the regulation of erythropoiesis through its involvement in the generation of *erythropoietin.* The balance between production and turnover is affected readily by disruptions to the normal contribution by these numerous organs.

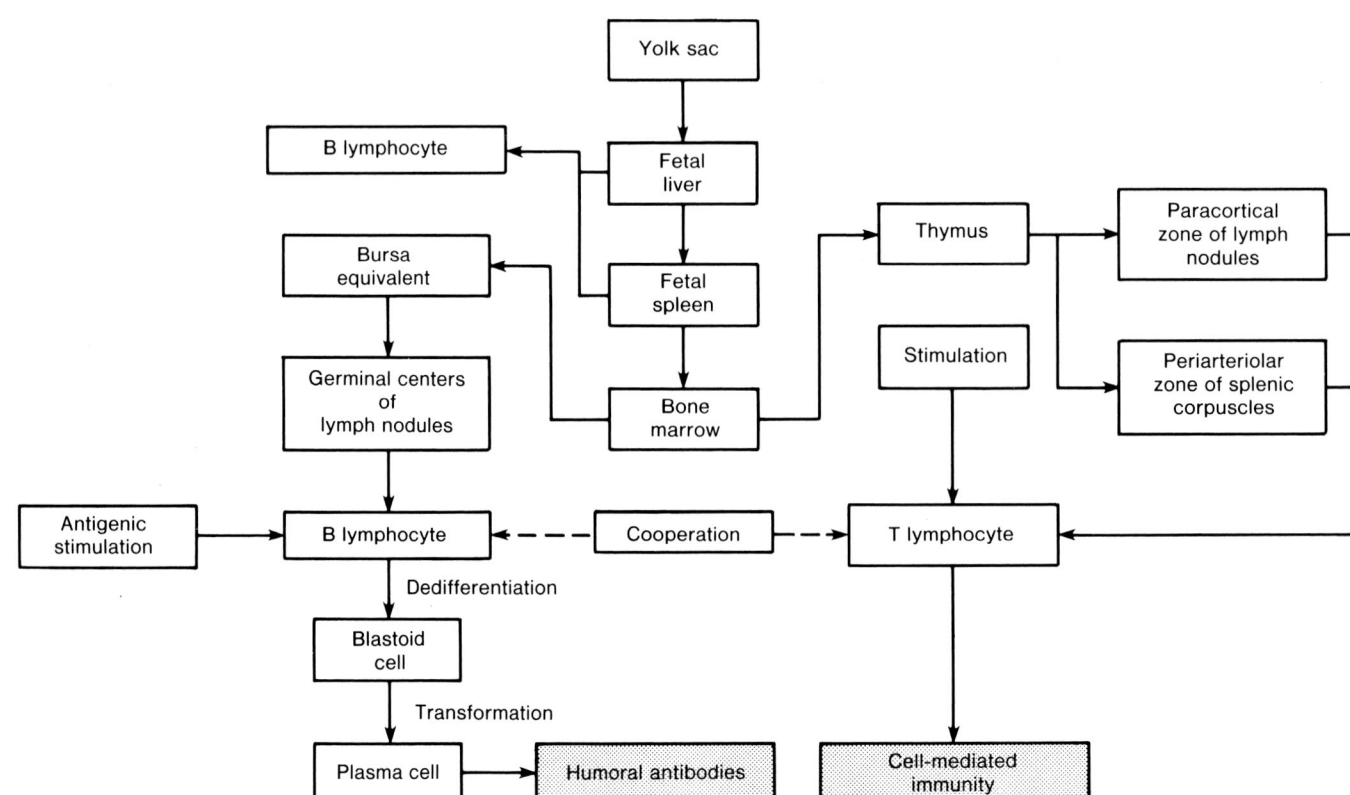

Fig. 10.43 A flow diagram of the origin, fate and function of B and T lymphocytes.

Erythrokinetics

Life Cycle of Erythrocytes. Beginning as a nucleated cell, the erthrocyte undergoes a differentiation process that suits it ideally for its basic function of carrying oxygen to the tissues. The extrusion of its nucleus, the synthesis of hemoglobin and its biconcave shape insure that it has a maximum oxygen carrying capacity and a good volume to surface ratio. Although numerous conditions are associated with an increased production of RBC's, the ultimate stimulation for erythropoiesis is related to its basic function. Thus, a reduced amount of oxygen in the tissues (*tissue hypoxia*) is the ultimate stimulus. The relationship of tissue hypoxia and blood cell production is outlined in Figure 10.44.

The kidney and other organs respond to hypoxia by releasing *renal erythropoietic factor (REF)*, *erythrogenin*. Nephrectomized dogs, however, do not produce REF. This factor reacts with a plasma globulin produced in the liver, *erythropoietinogen*, to produce *erythropoietin (EP)*. Then, erythropoietin stimulates uncommitted stem cells,

erythropoietin-sensitive cells (*EPS cells*) to differentiate into rubriblasts. Erythropoietin stimulation also increases the amount of the enzyme *aminolevulinic acid synthetase*, an enzyme necessary for the synthesis of heme.

Although such stimulation is immediate, increased numbers of red blood cells are not noted in the peripheral circulation for about 3 days. The normal proliferation and differentiation cycle within the bone marrow takes about 3–5 days. Deleted mitoses and the early release of immature forms can occur, but the number of RBC's is not increased.

An erythropoietin-sensitive cell and its descendants will undergo four mitotic divisions in a span of 5 days to produce 16 erythrocytes. Not all of the cells of the rubricytic series, however, have the same potential for mitotic activity. Mitotic activity ceases in the late rubricytic stage.

The life span of the erythrocytes of domestic animals is variable. Average life spans are listed in Table 10.4. Reticulocytes occur rarely in normal blood of animals with an average RBC life span that is greater than 100 days. As erythrocytes age, they are

Table 10.4
Average Life Span of Erythrocytes

Species	X life span-days
Canid	120
Felid	73
Equid	145
Bovid	159
Ovid	110
Caprid	125
Porcid	67

removed from the circulation by the cells of the RES, especially those of the spleen. Although there are no morphologic alterations visible with normal erythrocytic aging, metabolic pathways are altered and the cells are removed from the circulation. Because the number of erythrocytes is a homeostatic parameter of the blood, *erythropoiesis must equal erythroclasia*. A medium-sized dog will produce and destroy approximately 5×10^7 erythrocytes/minute.

Hemoglobin Synthesis, Destruction and Reutilization. *Hemoglobin* is a *chromoprotein* (conjugated protein) that consists of a *heme* and *globin*. Heme is a protoporphyrin plus ferrous iron that is synthesized in the mitochondria, whereas globin is a protein. Hemoglobin constitutes approximately 95% of the dry weight of the mature RBC. Variations in the amino acid sequence of the globin account for different types of hemoglobin (embryonic, fetal and adult) that occur in many species.

Old erythrocytes are removed from the circulation by the phagocytic cells of the RES. Although the spleen is the primary organ for erythroclasia, it does occur in other organs (bone marrow, liver). Subtle membrane alterations and increased RBC fragility probably account for the phagocytic process. All components of the hemoglobin molecule are reutilized by the body. The extravascular metabolism and reutilization of components are detailed in Figure 10.45. This figure describes the events that occur when hemoglobin is removed and metabolized outside of the vascular system. A different sequence of events and different plasma components are utilized for intravascular hemolysis.

Hemoglobin is split into its two components, *heme* and *globin*. The globin is hydrolyzed to its component amino acids which become part of the body's circulating amino acid pool. Iron is removed from the heme, leaving the protoporphyrin. Iron is bound to plasma transferrin and then transported to the bone marrow for reutilization. Ferritin and hemosiderin are the storage forms of the iron in the reticuloendothelial cells of the bone marrow and spleen. The protoporphyrin is converted to *biliverdin* and then *bilirubin*. Bilirubin is transported in the plasma bound to plasma proteins. Although it is bound, this is the *unconjugated* form of bilirubin. Bilirubin enters the hepatocytes and is conjugated to a glucuronide by the activity of the enzyme *glucuronyl transferase*.

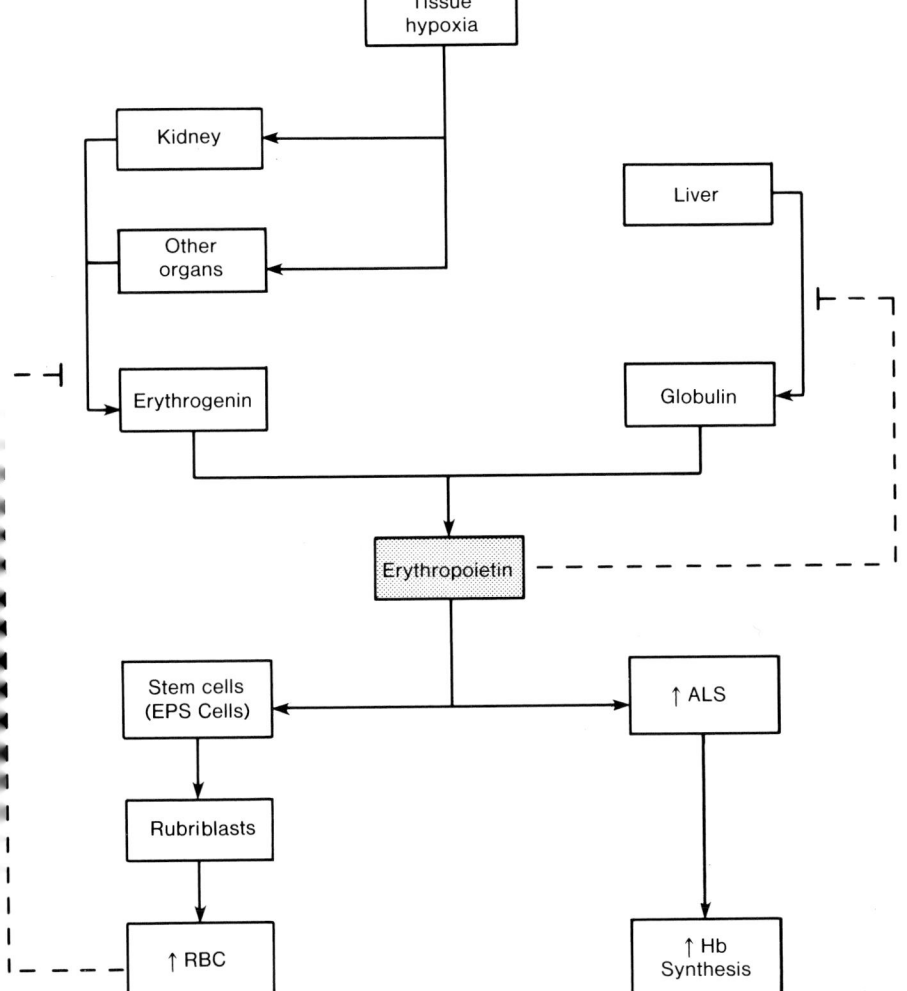

Fig. 10.44 A flow diagram demonstrating the factors involved in the regulation of erythropoiesis. *Arrows* represent direction of flow and/or stimulation. *Bars* represent inhibition. EPS cells, erythropoietin—sensitive cells; ALS, amino-levulinic acid synthetase; Hb, hemoglobin.

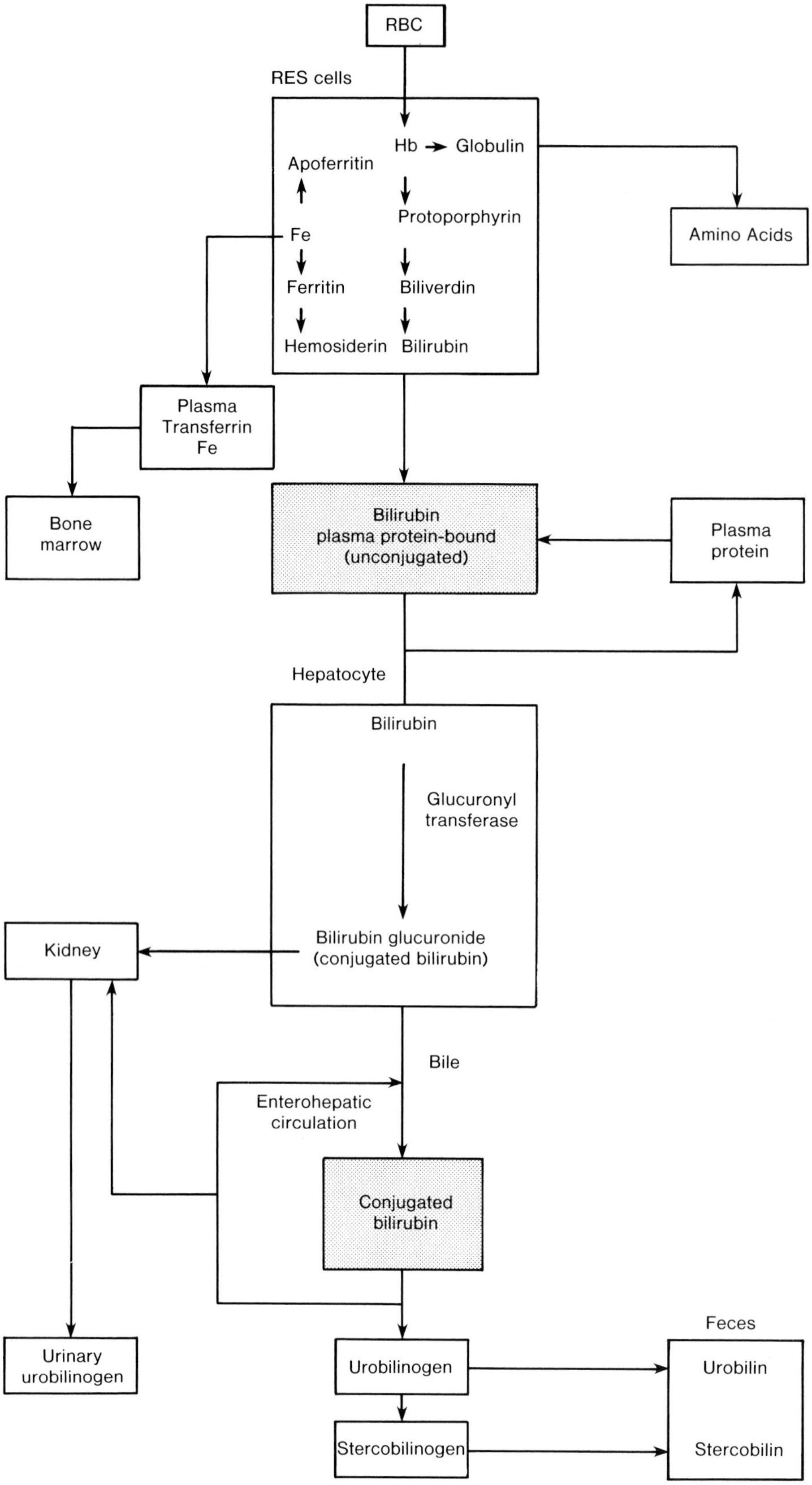

RBC

RES cells

Hb → Globulin

Apoferritin

Fe

Protoporphyrin

Ferritin

Biliverdin

Hemosiderin

Bilirubin

Amino Acids

Plasma
Transferrin
Fe

Bone
marrow

Bilirubin
plasma protein-bound
(unconjugated)

Plasma
protein

Hepatocyte

Bilirubin

Glucuronyl
transferase

Bilirubin glucuronide
(conjugated bilirubin)

Kidney

Bile

Enterohepatic
circulation

Conjugated
bilirubin

Urinary
urobilinogen

Feces

Urobilinogen

Urobilin

Stercobilinogen

Stercobilin

Fig. 10.45 A flow diagram demonstrating the extravascular metabolism of hemoglobin. Refer to the text for a complete description of the process.

This conversion (*conjugation*) to *bilirubin glucuronide* is a detoxification (biotransformation) process which makes bilirubin water-soluble. A small amount of this compound reenters the circulation and is ex-

creted by the kidney as *urobilinogen*. Most of the conjugated bilirubin is secreted by the hepatocytes as the major bile pigment in the bile. Bilirubin absorbed by the small intestine recirculates back into the liver by the

enterohepatic circulation. Further alteratio of bilirubin occurs in the intestines and th resultant compounds, *urobilin* and *stercoh ilin*, are eliminated in the feces. These pi ments impart the characteristic color to fec material.

An excessive amount of bilirubin impar a yellow color to the tissues. This conditio *jaundice* (*icterus*), can occur under vario circumstances. An evaluation of blood fc conjugated and/or unconjugated bilirubi is an important diagnostic aid. Excessive re blood cell destruction (*hemolytic jaur dice*) is characterized by increased quantitic of unconjugated bilirubin. Bile duct obstruc tions are characterized by increased quar tities of conjugated bilirubin.

Granulokinetics

Neutrophils. Neutrophilic granulocytes prc liferate and mature within the bone marro (Fig. 10.46). They are released to the vas culature wherein they comprise a *circulatin* and *marginal pool*. They leave the vascula compartment and enter the *tissue pool*. The do not return from the tissues to the circu lating pool.

Five mitoses are characteristic of the de velopmental sequence of this cell. Myelc

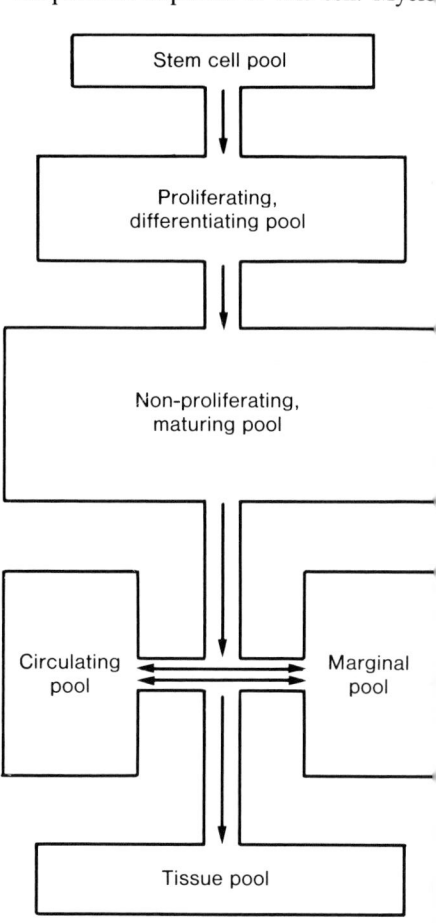

Fig. 10.46 A diagram of the flow and distri bution of neutrophils within various pools withir the body. The proliferating, differentiating poc consists of myeloblasts, progranulocytes, and myelocytes, whereas the non-proliferating, ma turing pool consists of metamyelocytes, band cells, and mature cells.

blasts and progranulocytes each divide once, while myelocytes divide three times. Five days are required for myelocytes to become mature, fully differentiated neutrophils. A 3–5 day lag period occurs before an increased or decreased response from the bone marrow will be noted in the peripheral blood. However, an increase in circulating neutrophils can occur rapidly by mobilizing the neutrophils that comprise the marginal pool. The marginal pool consists of neutrophils which marginate along the walls of small vessels. This pool may equal the circulating pool (dog) or may be 2–3 times the circulating pool (cat).

The half-life of neutrophils within the circulating pool is approximately 6 hours. The circulating pool of neutrophils is replaced approximately every 10–12 hours. The replacement occurs directly from the maturation pool. Under normal conditions of peripheral neutrophil utilization, the reserve pool in the canine bone marrow contains about a 5-day supply of cells. Mature cells are the first neutrophils that are mobilized from the maturation pool. As the demand for neutrophils increases, progressively younger cells are released from the bone marrow. Even neutrophilic myelocytes may occur in the circulation during periods of extreme demand and excessive depletion of the maturation pool.

The regulation of granulocytopoiesis is not understood completely. Serum inducing factors and releasing factors have been implicated in the regulation of production and release. A humoral substance, *chalone*, that has a specific tissue inhibitory effect on mitosis and an *antichalone* have been implicated in the regulation process also.

Neutrophilia, an increased number of circulating neutrophils, can occur in response to various physiologic and disease conditions. *Neutropenia*, a decreased number of circulating neutrophils, can occur from excessive utilization and/or a decreased production. A neutrophilia with a slight to moderate increase in the number of immature neutrophils (>3%) is called a *regenerative left shift*. A *degenerative left shift* is characterized by a low to slightly elevated neutrophil count in which the number of immature forms is greater than the number of mature neutrophils. A *right shift* is characterized by an increased number of older cells in which nuclear hypersegmentation is obvious. Various types of shifts characterize the response of the body to different disease processes.

Eosinophils. The maturation pattern, production time, life span and circulation of the eosinophil is similar to the pattern described for the neutrophil. The production time for the eosinophil is about 3–6 days. Although circulating numbers of eosinophils are low, approximately 300 cells to every circulating eosinophil comprise the maturation pool, whereas about 100 cells for every circulating cell comprises the proliferating pool.

Although the eosinophil is associated with allergic reactions, the ultimate stimulation for an increased number of eosinophils is the release of histamine from degranulated mast cells. Although the local release of histamine serves as an eosinophilic chemotactic factor, this is not always associated with an *eosinophilic leukocytosis (eosinophilia)*. Circulating histamine probably accounts for eosinophilia.

Basophils. The small numbers of these cells within the body complicates kinetic studies of them. Their life span is approximately 10–12 days. The functions of these cells are similar to the mast cell.

Kinetics of Agranulocytes

Lymphocytes. T lymphocytes are more numerous in the peripheral blood than B lymphocytes. T cells are long-lived cells that may remain in the body for months or years. Thymocytes, however, are short-lived (3–4 days) and most of them degenerate within the thymus. B cells that are responsible for the *primary immune response* are short-lived, whereas those responsible for the *secondary immune response* are long-lived. Accurate data concerning the life span of lymphocytes are difficult to obtain because of the recirculation of lymphocytes.

Large and medium lymphocytes of the bone marrow, spleen and lymph nodes seem to generate in about 8 hours, whereas small lymphocytes within these organs may require at least 4 days. In the dog, a sufficient number of lymphocytes enters the vasculature from the thoracic duct to indicate that all lymphocytes may be replaced every 12 hours.

Except for thymocytes, the common stimulator for lymphopoiesis is the presence of antigen.

Circulating lymphocytes can gain access to lymph nodes by leaving the circulation through venules in the paracortical zones of lymph nodes. These venules, redundantly referred to as *postcapillary venules*, afford immunologic advantages to the organism. Once inside the parenchyma of the lymph node, these lymphocytes may return to the vascular bed via the postcapillary venules. The lymphocytes may enter the lymph node within the circulation and exit the vasculature at the postcapillary venules, enter the efferent lymphatics and eventually be returned to the circulation through the thoracic duct. The *recirculation* phenomenon insures that immunocompetent cells are distributed widely throughout the body and that numerous lymphocytes are exposed to a local antigen. The phenomenon facilitates a generalized immunologic response to localized antigens. Evaluation of lymphatic outflow from lymph nodes indicates that 95% of these lymphocytes may be of blood origin, whereas 5% are of nodal origin. T cells appear to recirculate as much as 5 times faster than B cells.

Lymphocytosis is an increase in the number of lymphocytes, whereas *lymphopenia* is a decrease in the number of lymphocytes. Certain types of disease processes cause a lymphocytosis (bacterial infection); others (viral) cause a lymphopenia.

Monocytes. The origin, distribution and relationships of these cells was discussed previously (Chapter 6). Monocytes marginate in the vascular bed; this marginal pool may be five times as large as the circulating pool. Because young monocytes leave the bone marrow rapidly, the maturation pool is considered to be small. Once these cells gain access to the vascular compartment they enter the tissues randomly. The tissue pool of histocytes may be 400 times greater than the circulating pool of monocytes. Whereas the circulating half-life of human monocytes is about 8 days, the life span of histocytes probably exceeds 100 days.

Evaluation of Blood and Bone Marrow

The morphology of formed elements in the blood and bone marrow is an important criterion when conducting an evaluation of these tissues. Subjective impressions are usually complemented by less subjective, quantitative data. The previous portions of this chapter emphasized the importance of structural features and relationships; the following is intended to acquaint the student with the quantitative aspects of *hematology*.

Whole blood evaluations invariably involve the use of substances that will inhibit coagulation. Such substances, *anticoagulants*, include *EDTA (ethylenediamine tetraacetic acid)*, *heparin, sodium citrate* and various salts of oxalic acid (*sodium oxalate, potassium oxalate*). Heparin interferes with the generation of fibrin by functioning as an antithrombin and antithromboplastin. The other compounds arrest coagulation by forming insoluble salts with calcium. Often, hematologic evaluation will require the use of a blood sample with an anticoagulant added, a clotted blood sample for serum evaluations and a blood smear for qualitative and quantitative evaluations.

Peripheral Blood Parameters. Counting of RBC's and WBC's is an important part of the evaluation. *Erythrocyte and white blood cell counts* can be accomplished with automated systems, but the use of a *hemocytometer* is a quick, easy and inexpensive counting method. Red blood cells and total white blood cells are reported as the number of cells/mm^3 of blood. Often, the erythrocyte count is not accomplished but is replaced by the *packed cell volume (PCV)*. The PCV is a valuable parameter that is related to RBC numbers and size. Moreover, this parameter is useful in the determination of other valuable RBC parameters.

The *differential count* of white blood cells is accomplished on a stained blood smear. The count is predicated upon identifying the frequency of occurrence of different white blood cells when 100 or 200 white blood cells are counted. Identification of mature and immature forms is an important part of this subjective evaluation. It is customary to note also other distinguishing characteristics of the cells (anisocytosis, polychromasia, toxicity), as well as the presence of nucleated RBC's and any other notable features. A differential leukocyte count generates *relative values* for WBC's. The percentages are converted to *absolute values* by multiplying the total white cell count by the percentage of occurrence of each cell type, mature and immature. This evaluative technique is necessary for insights concerning normalcy, regenerative left shifts and similar phenomena.

The *mean corpuscular volume (MCV)* is an important parameter that is useful in determining the size of RBC's. Because anemias may be normocytic, microcytic or macrocytic, this is a diagnostic parameter of anemia. The MCV is determined by multiplying the PCV by 10 and dividing by the RBC count. The MCV is expressed in femtoliters (1×10^{-15} liters).

Hemoglobin concentration is determined routinely with a *hemoglobinometer*. This simple technique is the determination of *oxyhemoglobin* by its light absorption. Although the values obtained by this method are less accurate (+10%) than wet chemical methods for *cyanomethemoglobin*, they are useful for clinical evaluations. The *mean corpuscular hemoglobin concentration (MCHC)* is a useful parameter for distinguishing anemias as normochromic or hypochromic. The MCHC in g/dl is determined by dividing the hemoglobin concentration (g/dl) by the PCV and multiplying by 100.

The *erythrocyte sedimentation rate* is determined by using a tube of blood to which an anticoagulant has been added and noting the amount of erythrocyte settling that occurs in a given time period.

Total protein determinations can be made on serum or plasma proteins by refractometry. This is a simple and quick determination. *Electrophoresis* can be accomplished on the sample also. The *albumin/globulin ratio (A/G ratio)*, normally 0.7–1.0, is a valuable diagnostic parameter that is determined by electrophoresis.

Bone Marrow Evaluation. Bone marrow evaluations are important diagnostic procedures that can be used to offer more insights concerning peripheral blood observations. Bone marrow biopsies are surgical procedures which require aseptic techniques. Different biopsy sites are used in different domestic animals: cat—trochanteric fossa; dog—iliac crest, trochanteric fossa; cattle, sheep—rib, sternum; horse—tuber coxae, sterum, rib.

A bone marrow evaluation requires complete familiarity with the cytology of differentiation. Many subjective evaluations are made on the stained smear of bone marrow. A differential count of 500 cells is a valuable parameter. The *myeloid/erythroid ratio (ME ratio)* is determined by dividing the total number of granulocytic cells by the total number of nucleated erythrocytic cells of the differential count.

References

Erythrocytes

Baker, R. F.: Ultrastructure of red blood cells. Fed. Proc. *26:*1785, 1967.

Fisher, J. W. and Gordon, A. S.: Conference: erythropoietin. Ann New York Acad. Sci. *149*, 1968.

Hevesy, G. and Ottesen, J.: Life-cycle of the red corpuscle of the hen. Nature *156:*534, 1945.

Koehler, J. K.: Freeze-etching observations on nucleated erythrocytes with special reference to the nuclear and plasma membranes. Z. Zellforsch. *85:*1, 1968.

Marks, P. and Rifkind, R. A.: Protein synthesis: its control in erythropoiesis. Sci. *175:*955, 1972.

Schalm, O. W.: Hematologic characteristics of autoimmune hemolytic anemia in the dog. Calif. Vet. *23:*19, 1969.

Granulocytes

Archer, G. T. and Hirsch, J. C.: Motion picture studies of degranulation of horse eosinophils during phagocytosis. J. Exp. Med. *118:*287, 1963.

Dolowy, W. C., Cornet, J. and Henson, D.: Particles in leukocytes of normal human beings after negative staining in electron microscopy. Nature *209:*1358, 1966.

Franklin, D. A.: Electron microscopic study of human basophils. *29:*878, 1967.

Hamre, C. J.: Origin and differentiation of heterophil, eosinophil and basophil leucocytes of chickens. Anat. Rec. *112:*339, 1952.

Hersch, I. G. and Cohn, Z. A.: Degranulation of polymorphonuclear leucocytes following phagocytosis of microorganisms. J. Exp. Med. *112:*1005, 1960.

Miller, F., DeHarven, E. and Palade, G. E. The structure of eosinophil leukocyte granules in rodents and in man. J. Cell Biol. *31:*349, 1966.

Natt, M. P. and Herrick, C. A.: Variation in the shape of the rodlike granule of the chicken heterophil leucocyte and its possible significance. Poult. Sci. *33:*828, 1954.

Agranulocytes

Elves, M. W.: *The Lymphocytes.* Lloyd Luke Ltd., London, 1966.

Fiore-Donati, L. and Hanna, M. G., Jr.: *Lymphatic Tissue and Germinal Centers in Immune Response.* Plenum, New York, 1969.

Gowans, J. L.: The life history of lymphocytes. Brit. Med. Bull. *15:*50, 1959.

Gowans, J. L.: The immunological activities of lymphocytes. Progr. Allerg. *9:*1, 1965.

Greaves, M. F., Owen, J. J. T. and Raff, M. C.: *T and B Lymphocytes: Origins, Properties and Roles in Immune Responses.* North-Holland Publishers, New York, 1975.

Hoshino, T., Takeda, M., Abe, K and Ito, T.: Early development of thymic lymphocytes in mice, studied by light and electron microscopy. Anat. Rec. *164:*47, 1969.

Mackay, L. J., Jarrett, W. F. H. and Coombs, R. R. A.: Two populations of lymphocytes in a cat. Vet. Rec. *96:*41, 1975.

Movat, H. Z. and Fernando, N. V. P.: The fine structure of the lymphoid tissue during antibody formation. Exp. Molec. Path. *4:*155, 1965.

Tizard, I. R.: *An Introduction to Veterinary Immunology.* W. B. Saunders, Philadelphia, 1977.

Tompkins, E. H.: The monocyte. Ann. N. Y. Acad. Sci. *59:*732, 1955.

Platelets and Thrombocytes

Behnke, O.: Electron microscopic observations on the membrane systems of the rat blood platelet. Anat. Rec. *158:*121, 1967.

Carlson, H. C., Sweeney, P. R. and Tokaryk, J. M.: Demonstration of phagocytic and trephocytic activities of chicken thrombocytes by microscopy and vital staining techniques. Avian Dis. *12:*700, 1968.

Clarke, J. A., Hawkey, C. and Salisbury, A. J.: Surface ultrastructure of platelets and thrombocytes. Nature *223:*401, 1969.

Rodman, N. F. and Mason, R. G.: Platelet-platelet interaction: Relationship to hemostasis and thrombosis. Fed. Proc. *26:*95, 1967.

Simpson, C. F.: Ultrastructural features of the turkey thrombocyte and lymphocyte. Poult. Sci. *47:*848, 1968.

Comparative Hematology

Afonsky, D.: Blood picture in normal dogs. Amer. J Physiol. *180:*456, 1955.

Archer, R. K.: *Haematological Techniques for Use in Animals.* Blackwell Scientific, Oxford, 1965.

Benjamin, M. M.: *Outline of Veterinary Clinical Pathology.* 3rd edition. Iowa State University Press, Ames 1978.

Calhoun, M. L. and Brown, E. M.: Hematology and Hematopoietic Organs. *In* Dunne, H. W. (editor) *Swine Diseases* pp. 33–75. Iowa State University Press, Ames, 1975.

Diggs, L. W., Sturm, D. and Bell, A.: *The Morphology of Human Blood Cells,* Abbott Laboratories, North Chicago, 1970.

Ferguson, L. C., Irwin, M. R. and Beach, B. A.: On variation in the blood cells of healthy cattle. J Infect. Dis. *76:*24, 1945.

Holman, H. H.: A negative correlation between size and number of the erythrocytes of cows, sheep, goats and horses. J. Path. Bact. *64:*379, 1952.

Lucas, A. M.: A discussion of synonymy in avian and mammalian hematological nomenclature. Amer. J Vet. Res. *20:*887, 1959.

Rich, L. J.: *The Morphology of Canine and Feline Blood Cells with Equine References,* Ralston Purina, St Louis, 1974.

Schalm, O. W., Jain, N. C. and Carroll, E. J.: *Veterinary Hematology.* 3rd edition, Lea and Febiger, Philadelphia, 1975.

Wintrobe, M. M.: *Clinical Hematology.* 7th edition. Lea and Febiger, Philadelphia, 1974.

Wintrobe, M. M., Shumacker, H. B., Jr. and Schmidt W. J.: Values for number, size and hemoglobin content of erythrocytes in normal dogs, rabbits and rats. Amer. J. Physiol. *114:*502, 1936.

Hemostasis

Bennett, B. and Douglas, A. S.: Blood coagulation mechanism. Clin. Haematol. *2:*3, 1973.

Day, H. J.: Role of platelets in hemostasis and thrombosis. Ser. Haematol. *8:*23, 1974.

Dodds, W. J.: The diagnosis, management and treatment of bleeding disorders. I and II. Mod. Vet. Prac. *58:*680, *58:*756, 1977.

Hall, D. E.: *Blood Coagulation and Its Disorders in the Dog.* Bailliere, Tindall, London, 1972.

Kirk, R. W. (editor): *Current Veterinary Therapy VI. Small Animal Practice.* pp. 421–492, 1977.

Hematopoiesis

Ackerman, G. A.: Ultrastructure and cytochemistry of the developing neutrophil. Lab. Invest. *19:*290, 1968.

Behnke, O.: An electron microscope study of the megakaryocyte of the rat bone marrow. I. The development of the demarcation membrane system and the platelet surface coat. J. Ultrastruct. Res. *24:*412, 1968.

Calhoun, L. M.: Bone marrow of horses and cattle. Science *104:*423, 1946.

Calhoun, L. M.: A cytological study of costal marrow. I. The adult horse. Amer. J. Vet. Res. *15:*181, 1954; II. The adult cow. Amer. J. Vet. Res. *15:*395, 1954.

Campbell, F. R.: Nuclear elimination from the normoblast of fetal guinea pig liver as studied with electron microscopy and serial sectioning techniques. Anat. Rec. *160:*539, 1968.

Fedorko, M.: Formation of cytoplasmic granules in human eosinophilic myelocytes: An electron microscopic autoradiographic study. Blood *31:*188, 1968.

Johnson, F. R. and Roberts, D. B.: The growth and division of human small lymphocytes in tissue culture: An electron microscopic study. J. Anat. *98:*303, 1964.

Kaihotsu, N.: Electron microscopic studies on the maturation process of neutrophilic leucocytes. Kobe J. Med. Sci. *13:*47, 1967.

Kato, K.: Monophyletic scheme of blood cell formation for clinical and laboratory reference. J. Lab. Clin. Med. 20:1243, 1935.

Loutit, J. F.: Transplantation of haemopoietic tissue. Brit. Med. Bull. 21:118, 1965.

Osoba, D.: Precursors of thymic lymphocytes. Ser. Haematol. 7:427, 1974.

Pease, D. C.: An electron microscopic study of red bone marrow. J. Hemat. 11:501, 1956.

Scott, R. E. and Horn, R. G.: Fine structural features of eosinophil granulocyte development in human bone marrow. J. Ultrastruct. Res. 33:16, 1970.

Stanley, E. R., Hanson, G., Woodcock, J. and Metcalf, D.: Colony stimulating factor and the regulation of granulopoiesis and macrophage production. Fed. Proc. 34:2272, 1975.

Wetzel, B. K., Horn, R. G. and Spicer, S. S.: Fine structural studies on the development of heterophil, eosinophil and basophil granulocytes in rabbits.

Lab. Invest. 16:349, 1967.

Wu, A. M., Till, J. E., Siminovitch, L. and McCulloch, E. A.: A cytological study of the capacity for differentiation of normal hemopoietic colony-forming cells. J. Cell Physiol. 69:177, 1967.

Yamada, E.: The fine structure of the megakaryocyte in the mouse spleen. Acta Anat. 29:267, 1957.

Kinetics

Everett, N. B., Caffrey, R. W. and Rieke, W. D.: Recirculation of lymphocytes. Ann. New York Acad. Sci. 113:887, 1964.

Finch, C. A.: Some quantitative aspects of erythropoiesis. Ann. New York Acad. Sci. 77:410, 1959.

Firth, J. L.: Life-span, recirculation and transformation of lymphocytes. Int. Rev. Exp. Pathol. 5:1, 1966.

Giblett, E. R.: The plasma transferrins. Prog. Med. Genet. 2:34, 1962.

Greenwalt, T. J. and Jamieson, G. A.: *Formation and*

Destruction of Blood Cells. J. B. Lippincott, Philadelphia, 1970.

Lajtha, L. G., Pozzi, L. V., Schofield, R. and Fox, M. Kinetic properties of hemopoietic stem cells. Cell Tiss. Kinet. 2:39, 1969.

Leblond, C. P. and Walker, B. E.: Renewal of cell populations. Physiol. Rev. 36:255, 1956.

Morley, A. A.: A neutrophil cycle in healthy individuals. Lancet 2:1220, 1966.

Perutz, M. F.: The hemoglobin molecule. Proc. R. Soc. (London) (Biol.) Ser. B. 173:1113, 1969.

Schalm, O. W.: Interpretation of leukocyte responses in the dog. J. Am. Vet. Med. Assoc. 142:147, 1963.

Schalm, O. W., Hughes, J. and Hardy, D.: Dynamics of the neutrophilic leukocyte and a unique response in acute indigestion in the cow. Calif. Vet. 21:20, 1967.

Weed, R. I.: The importance of erythrocyte deformability. Am. J. Med. 49:147, 1970

11: Muscle Tissue

General Characteristics

Form and Function. The structural element of muscular tissue is the *muscle cell* or *muscle fiber*. Unlike the connective tissue fiber that is noncellular and the nerve fiber that is a cellular process, the term *fiber*, in this context, refers to an entire cell. Although all cells possess the ability to contract to one degree or another, *contractility* in muscle fibers is an especially well-developed characteristic.

Muscle comprises the majority of the "flesh" (*sarcos*, Gr., flesh) or "meat" of an organism. It is also a primary mural (wall) element of tubular organs.

Muscle fibers are elongated cells that may be uninucleated or multinucleated. They are enclosed by a *sarcolemma* (the combined *plasmalemma* and *basal lamina*) and *fine reticular fibers*. The *sarcoplasm*, or cytoplasm, contains typical organelles as well as contractile elements. These *contractile elements* are myofilaments composed of the proteins, *actin* and *myosin*. The *myofilaments* are grouped as *myofibrils*. The organization of the contractile elements is different in the various types of muscular tissue.

The characteristic property of muscle, contractility, is translated into the development of tension upon stimulation. This tension is the means by which work is accomplished. The work may be locomotion, expression of secretions from glands, movement of blood through the cardiovascular system, movement of materials through the digestive system and a host of related functions.

Functionally, muscle may be *voluntary* or *involuntary*. Structurally, it may be *smooth* (*nonstriated*) or *striated*. Through the combination of these characteristics, the following classification is derived:

1. Smooth muscle: nonstriated, involuntary.
2. Skeletal muscle: striated, voluntary.
3. Cardiac muscle: striated, involuntary.

Smooth Muscle

Histologic Structure. Smooth muscle fibers are elongated, spindle-shaped cells with finely tapered ends. The central region in which the nucleus is located is the widest part of the cell. These cells may be as short as 20 μm as mural elements of a small tubule or as long as 0.5 mm in the wall of a gravid uterus. Although the fibers are as described,

this appearance is not always apparent in a single section. Often the cytoplasmic portions of the cells are tightly packed and appear to blend as a homogeneous mass (Fig. 11.1). The elongated, cylindrical nucleus is rounded at the ends and contains a fine chromatin network. Clumped heterochromatin may be apparent along the inner nuclear membrane. Two to several nucleoli may be apparent. The nuclei may be twisted and wrinkled or assume a helical configuration. This may be indicative of active contraction at the time of fixation or a passive distortion due to agonal changes. The nucleus, together with a bright, homogeneous, acidophilic cytoplasm is the key to identification (Plates V.1, V.2).

The appearance of these cells varies with the plane of section. In longitudinal section, they appear as described previously. Because of their shape, however, not all nuclei will be included in any given section. Only those cells that have been sectioned through their thickest profiles will have nuclei apparent. These cells are staggered; the thickest portion of one is adjacent to the tapered portion of another. The appearance of nuclei reflects this staggering.

In cross-section, the cells are round to oval (Fig. 11.2). The nuclei are round and centrally located or slightly eccentric in position. Again, the nuclei are not seen in all cells sectioned as a result of the staggered relationship.

Smooth muscle fibers are intimately associated with fine reticular fibers (Fig. 11.3). These fibers, although they wrap around the cells, are not in contact with the muscle fibers. Each muscle fiber is surrounded by a polysaccharide-rich basal lamina in which reticular fibers may be embedded. Bundles of muscle fibers may be intimately associated with connective tissue as in the corium. In other areas, the muscle cells are arranged in extensive sheets, a few to many layers thick. In these instances, the finer reticular fibers are eventually continuous with the connective tissue surrounding the entire sheet. These sheets are often arranged so that the muscle fibers of one sheet are at right angles to the muscle fibers of another. In cross-section through a tubular organ, such as the gut, one sheet (circularly oriented and inner) is longitudinally sectioned. The adjacent sheet (longitudinal and outer), at 90° to the other, is cross-sectioned (Fig.

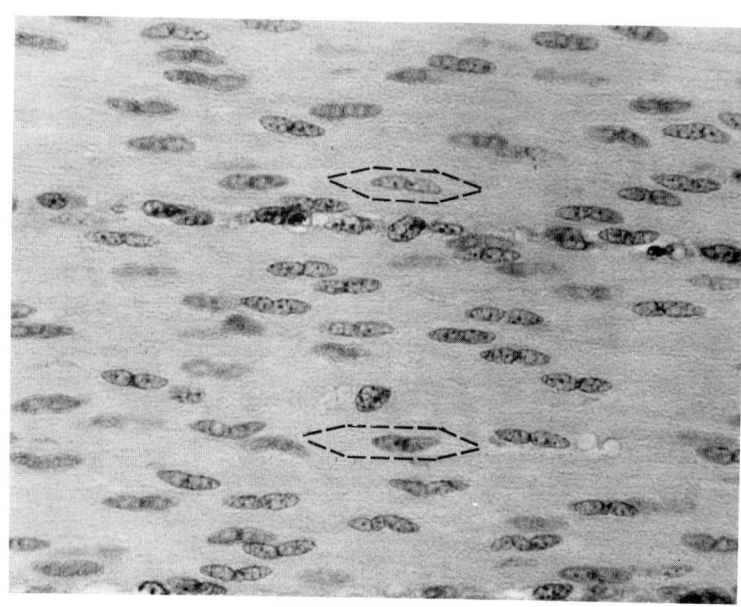

Fig. 11.1 Longitudinal section of smooth muscle. *Dashed lines*, approximate cellular limits. The elongated nuclei are oriented parallel to the long axis of the muscle fiber. Cellular limits are difficult to discern in longitudinal sections of sheets of smooth muscle. Some of the torpedo-shaped nuclei appear to be twisted. This an indication that the cells are contracted. X160. All light micrographs are labeled as the magnification with the microscope before photographic enlarging. All electron micrographs are labeled as total magnification, including photographic enlarging.

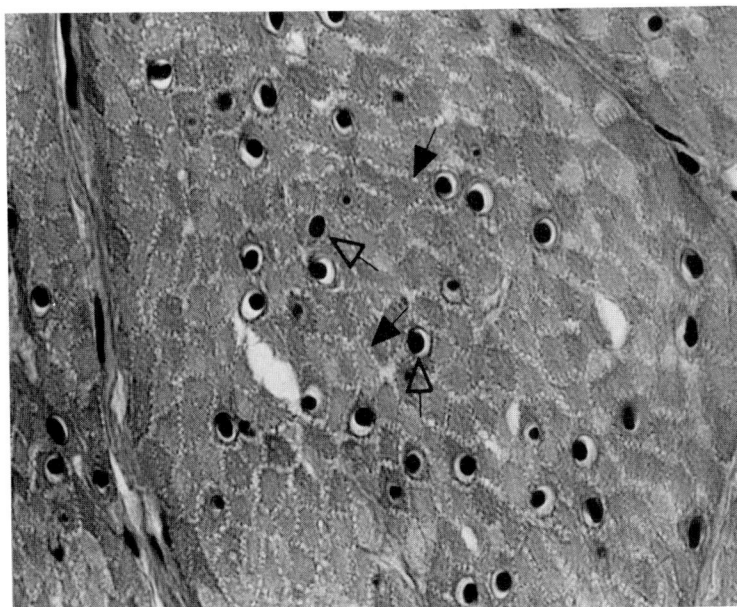

Fig. 11.2 Cross-section of smooth muscle. The nuclei (*open arrows*) and cellular limits (*solid arrows*) are apparent. Most of the nuclei are out of the plane of section. X160.

11.4). Naturally, in longitudinal section of an organ the reverse occurs.

Re-examine sections of regular DWFCT in longitudinal and cross-sections and note the differences between it and smooth muscle.

MORPHOLOGICAL FEATURES OF SMOOTH MUSCLE:

1. A homogeneous, brightly acidophilic cytoplasm.
2. Elongated nuclei with a fine chromatin network.
3. Nuclei may be smooth-surfaced, wrinkled, twisted or helical.
4. Cells are tightly packed and cellular boundaries are indistinct.

Ultrastructure. At the electron microscopic level, the smooth muscle cell reflects its light microscopic appearance (Fig. 11.5). The nucleus is elongated and finely granular with peripherally clumped heterochromatin. The organelles are confined to the perinuclear regions of the cell, especially at the poles of the nucleus. Mitochondria, rough endoplasmic reticulum, free ribosomes and a small Golgi apparatus are present. Parallel, discontinuous, spirally-oriented bundles of myofilaments occur within the cytoplasm. These bundles vary in thickness and are oriented generally along the long axis of the cell. Dense, amorphous, round bodies are scattered throughout the cell and appear to be points of attachment for the myofilaments within the cytoplasm and at the cell surface (Fig. 11.5). These dense bodies are considered to be analogous to Z lines in skeletal muscle. The myofilaments consist of *actin* and *myosin*.

The *plasma membrane* of smooth muscle cells is typical; however, it contains numerous caveolae, and many pinocytotic vesicles are juxtaposed to it (Fig. 11.6). The basal lamina covers the entire cell, except at points of cell-to-cell contact, *nexi* (Fig. 11.5). A *nexus* or gap junction is an intimate contact point between adjacent cells which functions to facilitate the spread of excitation from one cell to another. These are regions of low electrical resistance.

Functional Correlates. Smooth muscle is slow to contract; it is characterized by a sustained contraction that is resistant to fatigue. Although the contraction mechanism is not understood fully, it is probably based upon the sliding filament mechanism which is described for skeletal muscle. This mechanism involves the myofilaments, actin and myosin.

Upon contraction, the spindle-shaped, elongated, smooth-surfaced cell is converted to a shortened cell with numerous dimples on the surface. The dimples result from the bulging of cytoplasm between points of contact between the anchoring plaques and the plasma membrane. This imparts the characteristic thickening and twisting of the cell during contraction. The twisting and the absence of an orderly sarcomeric arrangement permits the smooth muscle cell to shorten more in proportion to its length than skeletal muscle.

Calcium is an essential ion for activating and sustaining smooth muscle contraction. Varying levels of cytoplasmic calcium are involved in this contraction mechanism. Most likely the influx and outward movement of calcium is associated with the sarcoplasmic reticulum and caveolae.

Although neuronal stimulation can initiate smooth muscle contraction, not all smooth muscle cells are innervated. The spread of excitation can occur by nexi through which adjacent cell contractile mechanisms are activated. The morphologic distortion of cells can be transmitted to ad-

jacent cells by the generation of forces through the connective tissue fibrous coverings. Also, smooth muscle is responsive to humoral agents. One of the most important stimuli to contraction of smooth muscle is its responsiveness to stretch. This local stimulus is important in the normal function of the hollow visceral organs.

Although smooth muscle may be considered a single morphologic entity, additional distinctions among this tissue type are possible on the basis of physiologic and pharmacologic properties. *Vascular smooth muscle* or *multiunit smooth muscle* has a high density of nerves which innervate the fibers. Functionally, this smooth muscle type acts like skeletal muscle because of its dependency upon nervous stimulation. However, not all of the cells are innervated. There is no evidence for *ephaptic conduction*; i.e., nexi are not observed between adjacent cells. The release of neurotransmitters from nerve endings probably accounts for the stimulation of adjacent cells which are not innervated. *Visceral smooth muscle* or *single unit smooth muscle* has a lower density of innervation than the multiunit type of smooth muscle. Visceral smooth muscle cells act as single units and the spread of excitation is dependent upon ephaptic conduction mechanisms. This smooth muscle type is characterized further by different kinds of contraction—*rhythmic contraction* and *tonic contraction*. Rhythmic contraction is initiated by the spontaneous and periodic activation of "pacemaker cells" within the muscle mass. The *tonic contraction* accounts for the characteristic partial contraction or *tone* of smooth muscle. It may be attributed to the responsiveness of smooth muscle to stretch. An *intermediate type* of smooth muscle exists in which there is an innervation density greater than that observed in unitary smooth muscle in addition to nexi.

Smooth muscle is also influenced by hormones secreted by the gastrointestinal tract. Hormones may inhibit or excite visceral smooth muscle of the stomach and intestines. Uterine smooth muscle is responsive to the hormones associated with estrus, pregnancy and parturition. Epinephrine has a significant influence on smooth muscle also.

Smooth muscle is an integral component of the walls of hollow visceral organs. This intramural mass of muscle contributes to the size of the lumen, the tone of the walls and the movement of materials through the organs. Smooth muscle is not confined to the hollow viscera; it occurs also in the eye and orbit (iris, ciliary body, eyelid, 3rd eyelid, periorbita and splenic capsule). In the vascular system the smooth muscle of the vessel wall actively contributes to peripheral resistance which assists in the maintenance of blood pressure.

Skeletal Muscle

Histologic Structure. The skeletal muscle fiber is an elongated cell that is slightly

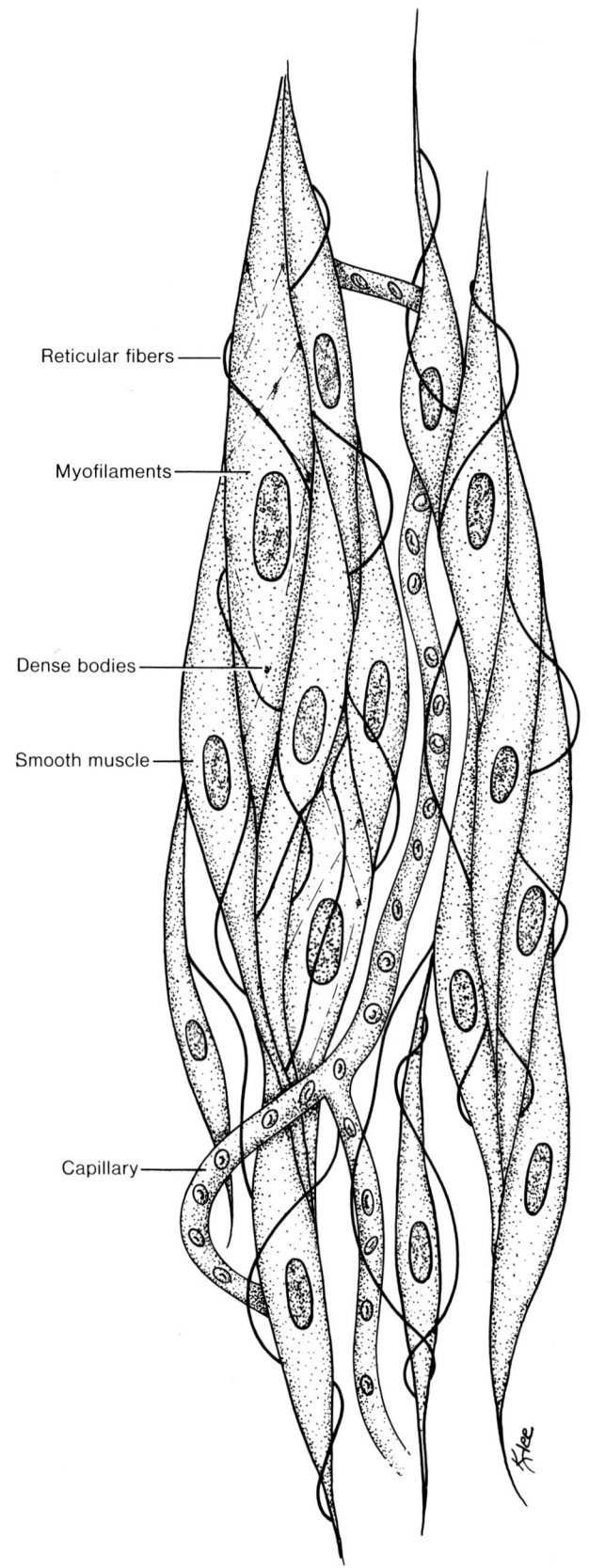

Reticular fibers —

Myofilaments —

Dense bodies —

Smooth muscle —

Capillary —

Fig. 11.3 Diagram of the three-dimensional relationships between smooth muscle cells and associated tissue. Myofilaments are scattered throughout the cytoplasm and are attached to the surface and within the cytoplasm by dense bodies.

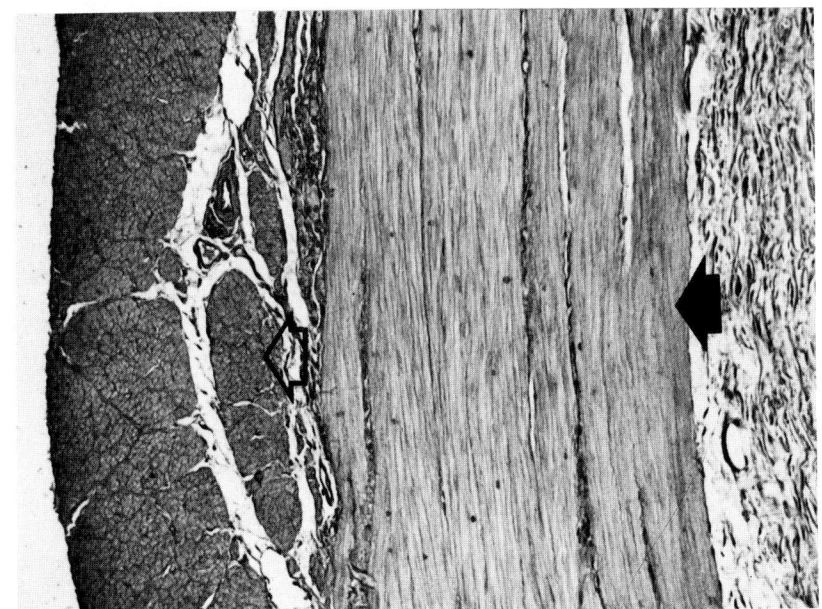

Fig. 11.4 Tunica muscularis of the wall of the gastrointestinal tract. The inner circular muscle (*solid arrow*) is sectioned longitudinally; the outer longitudinal muscle (*open arrow*) is cross-sectioned. X40.

apered or blunt at the ends. Although there s great variability in length, most muscle ibers are between 1 and 40 mm. They vary from 10–100 μm in diameter. Two conspicuous features are immediately apparent. These cells are multinucleated and striated Fig. 11.7). The oval nuclei have moderately abundant quantities of peripherally lumped heterochromatin. The nuclei are ocated at the periphery of the cells. Some nuclei will appear to be centrally located. This, however, is usually an artifact of sectioning; i.e., the section may be close to the sarcolemma above or below the observation plane.

The cross-striations, or dark and light bands, are oriented perpendicular to the ong axis of the muscle fiber (Plate V.3). Upon higher magnification the regularity of he banding is resolved (Fig. 11.8). The ighter *I bands* separate the darker *A bands*. Contained within the I bands are dense ines, the *Z lines* (Plate II.12). A *sarcomere*, he *unit of muscular contraction*, includes the nyofilaments contained between two adjacent Z lines.

Individual muscle fibers are oriented in an unbranched, parallel array and are separated from one another by loose connective issue that contains blood vessels and nerves. Naturally, a basal lamina separates the connective tissue compartment from the associated muscle fibers.

In cross-section, the peripheral relationship of the nuclei to the muscle fibers is observed more readily (Fig. 11.9). Also, the myofibrils are seen as clumps (*Cohnheim's fields*) of acidophilic dots (Plate V.4).

Ultrastructure. The detailed morphology of a sarcomere has been clarified with the electron microscope (Fig. 11.10). One sarcomere

extends between two adjacent Z lines in a myofibril and includes one-half of the I bands on either side of the A band (Fig. 11.11). The only myofilaments contained within the I bands are the thin actin filaments. The A band, however, contains both the thin actin filaments and the thick myosin filaments. The actin filaments do not extend uninterruptedly from the Z line through the A band. Rather, there are two separate actin filaments extending from each Z line through the A band. The gap between their ends within the A band is the H band. Upon contraction, the I band is shortened, the H band is obliterated and a dense M line is formed in the space previously occupied by the H band.

A small and inactive Golgi apparatus is juxtaposed to many of the nuclei. Mitochondria are numerous and scattered throughout the cell. They occur at nuclear poles, beneath the sarcolemma and interdigitated among the myofibrils. The intimate relationship between the mitochondria and the myofibrils is significant in the contractile mechanism.

The *sarcoplasmic reticulum* is comprised of an extensive network of cisterns and tubules (*sarcotubules*) which occur among and on the myofibrillar units (Fig. 11.12). This canalicular network corresponds to the smooth endoplasmic reticulum. Most of these tubular profiles are oriented longitudinally to the myofibrils. At specific loci within the cell these tubules become confluent and form *terminal cisterns* that are oriented perpendicular to the long axis of the cell. At these specific loci two terminal cisterns are separated from each other by a transversely-oriented, slender *transverse tubule*. Transverse tubules are invaginations

of the plasmalemma which comprise the *transverse sarcotubular system* (*T tubular system*). Two terminal cisterns and a transverse tubule comprise a *triad* (Figs. 11.12 and 11.13). In the skeletal muscle of amphibians, the triads are located at Z lines. In mammalian skeletal muscle, triads are located at A-I junctions of a sarcomere, resulting in two triads per sarcomere.

The transverse tubules are not part of the sarcoplasm and are not part of the sarcoplasmic reticulum. There is no patent communication among the components of the triad. Substances within the transverse tubules are actually outside of the cell, because these tubules are slender invaginations of the cell membrane. The relationships of the sarcoplasmic reticulum and transverse tubules to the cell and sarcomeres are depicted in Figure 11.14.

Myofibrillar Organization. The myofibrils that comprise a sarcomere are composed of two different kinds of myofilaments, *actin* and *myosin* (Fig. 11.15). The disposition and registration of the myofilaments within and between sarcomeres account for the typical striated pattern of skeletal muscle.

Myosin is a thick filament that is approximately 10 nm in diameter by 1.5 μm long. It is the principal component of the A band wherein these parallel filaments are separated by a distance of 45 nm. Thick filaments have a smooth and thick central portion that tapers toward each end. The slender portion of these filaments have radial projections. The isolation and dissociation of thick filaments yields *myosin*. Myosin is a cone-shaped molecule approximately 150 nm long with a globular portion or head at one end. The thick filaments of the A band are formed by the association of myosin molecules such that the elongated, rod-shaped part of the molecules projects toward the thicker central portion of the filament. The globular heads project in the opposite direction and account for the radial projections associated with the slender portions of the thick filaments of myosin. Digestion of myosin with trypsin yields two major fragments, *light meromyosin* (*LMM*) and *heavy meromyosin* (*HMM*). The LMM fragment comprises the rod-shaped portion of the molecule, while the HMM fragment comprises the radially-projecting globular heads.

The thin *actin* filaments are approximately 5 nm in diameter and 1 μm long. They originate from the Z line, comprise the I band exclusively and extend into the A band between the thick myosin filaments. Each thin filament of actin consists of two strands of *fibrous actin* (*F actin*) disposed in a double helix. F actin is a polymer of about 200 *G actin* (*globular actin*) monomers. A fibrous protein, *tropomyosin*, occupies the space between the F actin, while *troponin*, a globular protein, occupies a specific locus at each half-turn in the helix. Tropomyosin and troponin are regulatory proteins in the contractile mechanism.

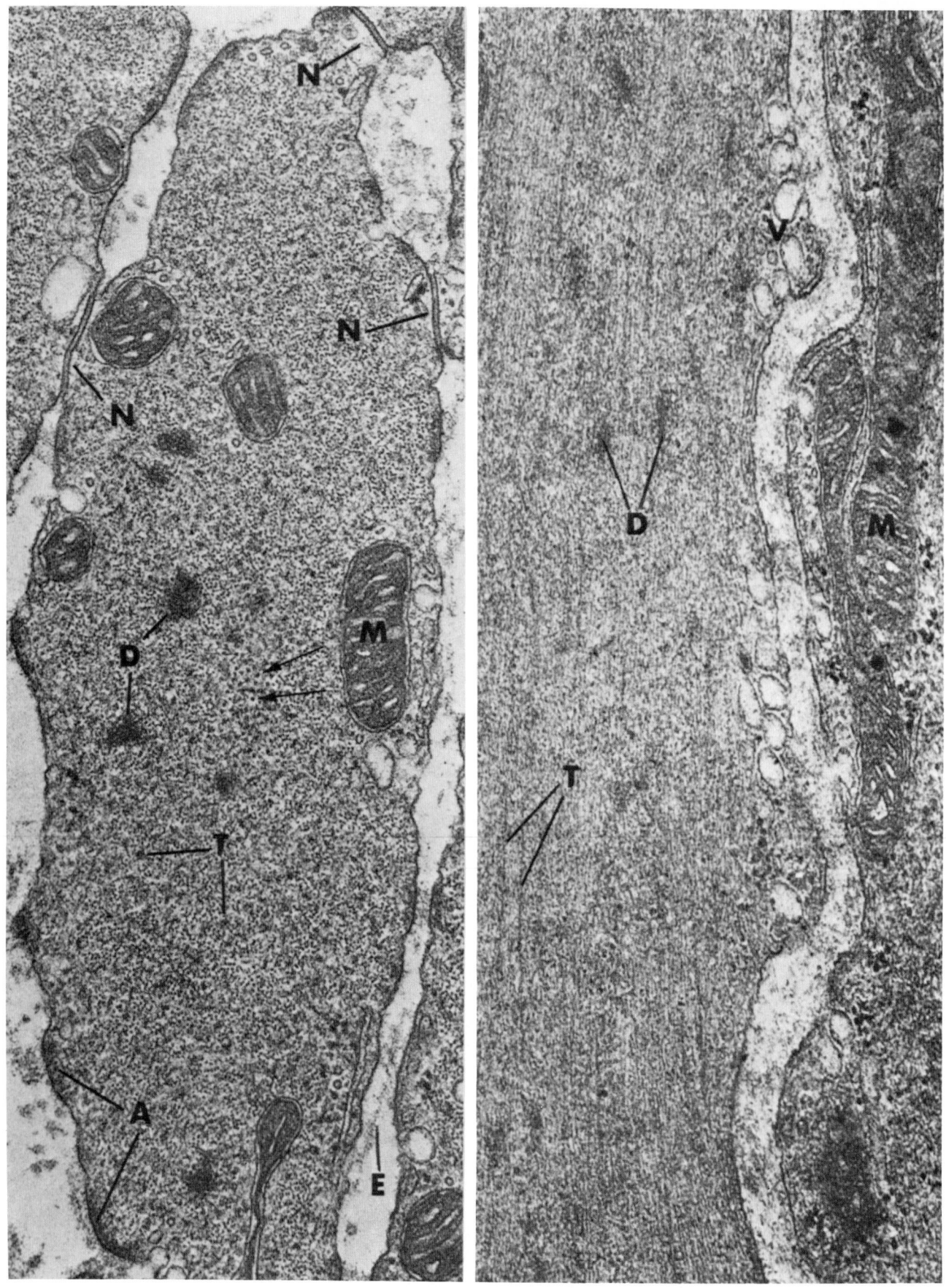

Fig. 11.5 An electron micrograph of smooth muscle cells from a rat small intestine. The cells on the *left* are cut transversely. Thick filaments (T), probably myosin, are scattered among numerous thin actin filaments. A third type of filament (arrows) are non-contractile intermediate size filaments. Attachment plaques (A) anchor the myofilaments to the cell membrane and dense bodies (D) anchor the filaments within the cytoplasm. Nexi (N) between adjacent cells are apparent. Mitochondria (M) are present. The cells on the *right* are sectioned longitudinally. Pinocytotic vesicles (V) are evident along the cell membrane. E, basal lamina. X89,600. (Reprinted with permission from: Copenhaver, W. M., Kelly, D. E. and Wood, R. L.: *Bailey's Textbook of Histology*, 17th edition, Williams & Wilkins, Baltimore, 1978.)

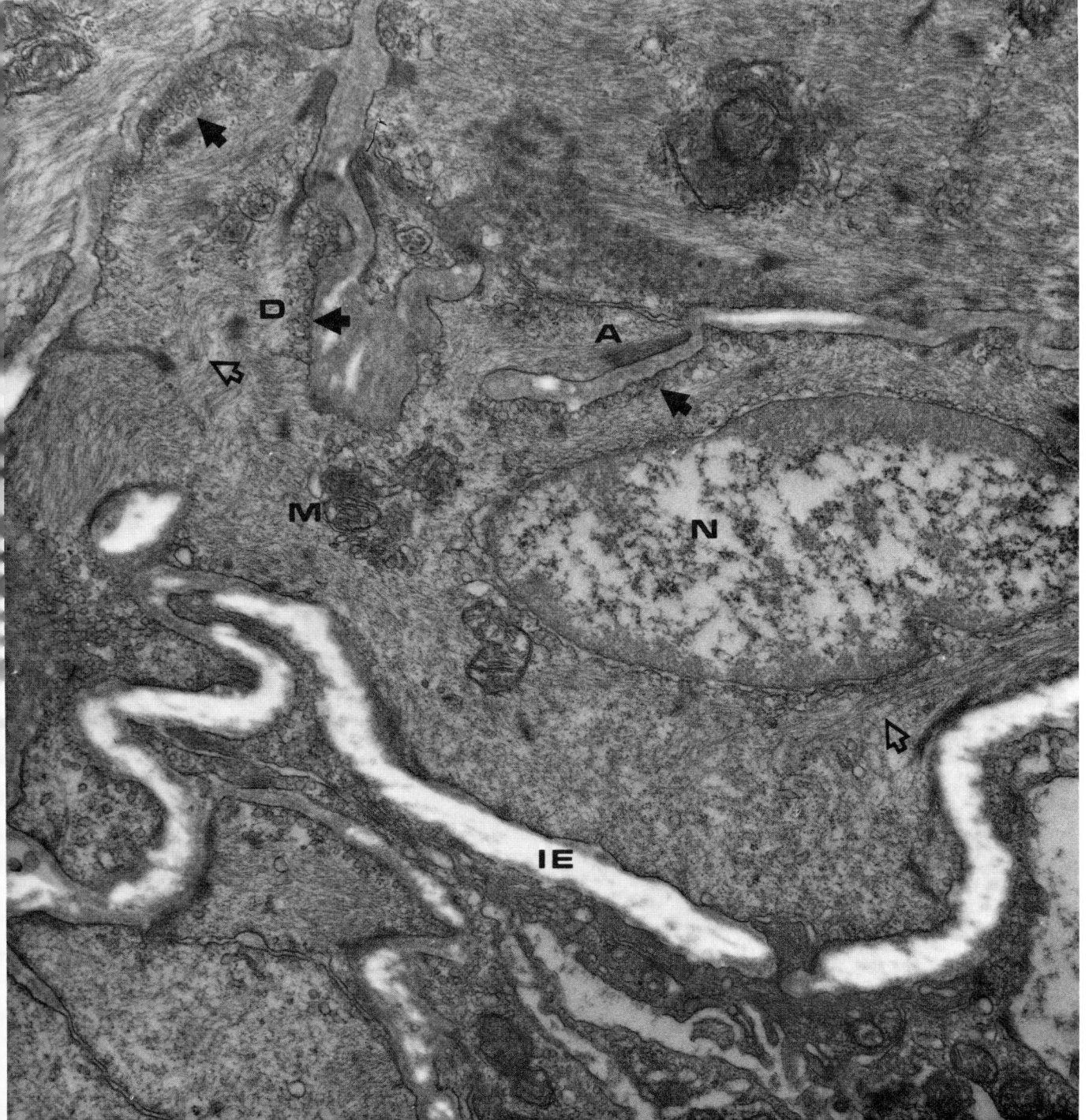

Fig. 11.6 Longitudinal section of smooth muscle of an arteriole. Mitochondria (M) are confined to the pole of the nucleus (N). Numerous filaments (*open arrows*) are scattered throughout the cytoplasm. The plasma membrane is studded with numerous caveolae (*solid arrows*), a characteristic feature of smooth muscle cells. Anchoring points (A) on the cell membrane and dense bodies (D) are evident within the cytoplasm. The basal lamina surrounds the cell and is apparent as dense material on either side of the internal elastic membrane (1E). X27,000.

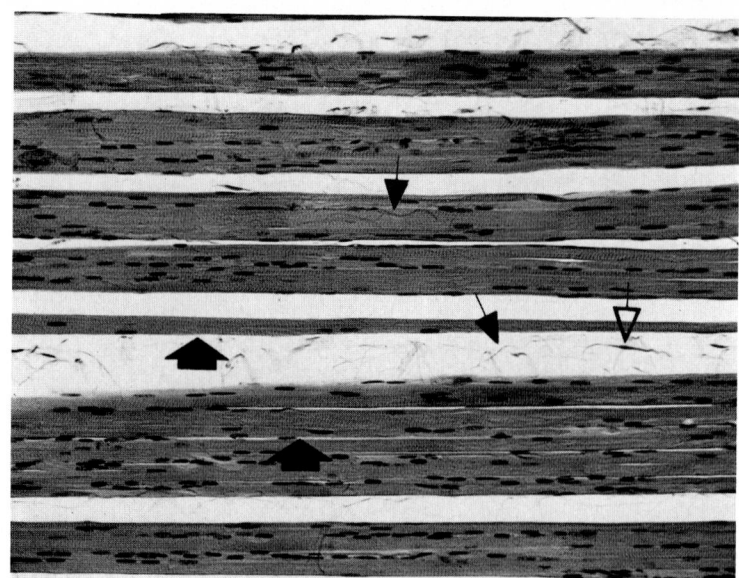

Fig. 11.7 Longitudinal section of skeletal muscle. Individual muscle fibers (*large arrows*) are striated and multinucleated. Compare the muscle fiber size with the connective tissue cell (*open arrow*). Endomyseal connective tissue (*solid arrows*) surrounds the muscle fibers. X40.

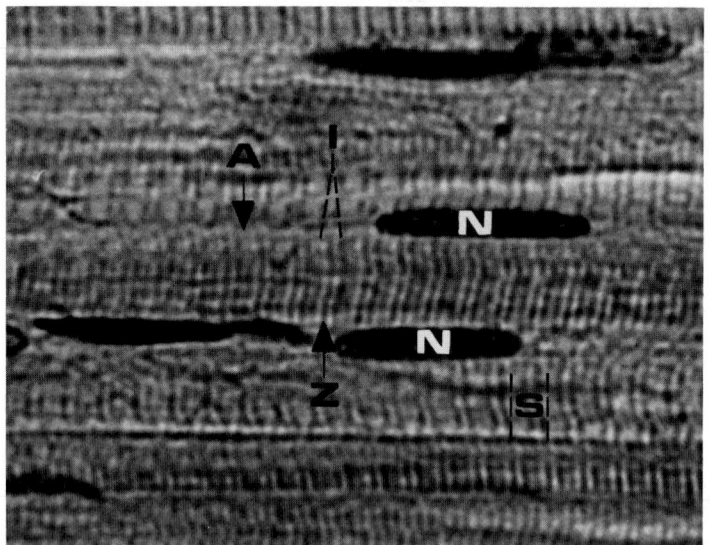

Fig. 11.8 Striations of skeletal muscle. The nuclei (N), A band (A), I band (I) and Z lines (Z) are indicated. The sarcomeres are in register. The sarcomere (S) below the S is outlined with *dashed lines*. The sarcomere extends from Z line to Z line. X400.

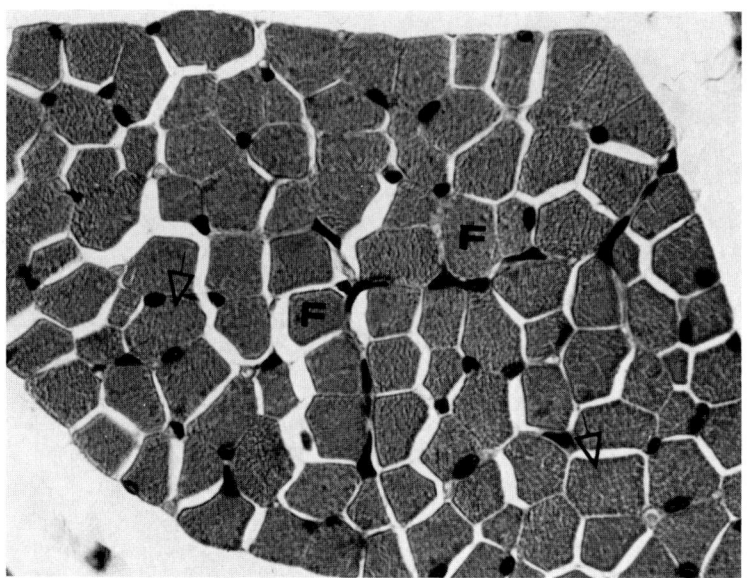

Fig. 11.9 Cross-section of skeletal muscle. The fibers (F) are grouped in bundles or fascicles. The grouping of myofibrils as Cohnheim's areas (*arrows*) is apparent. The nuclei are positioned peripherally. X160.

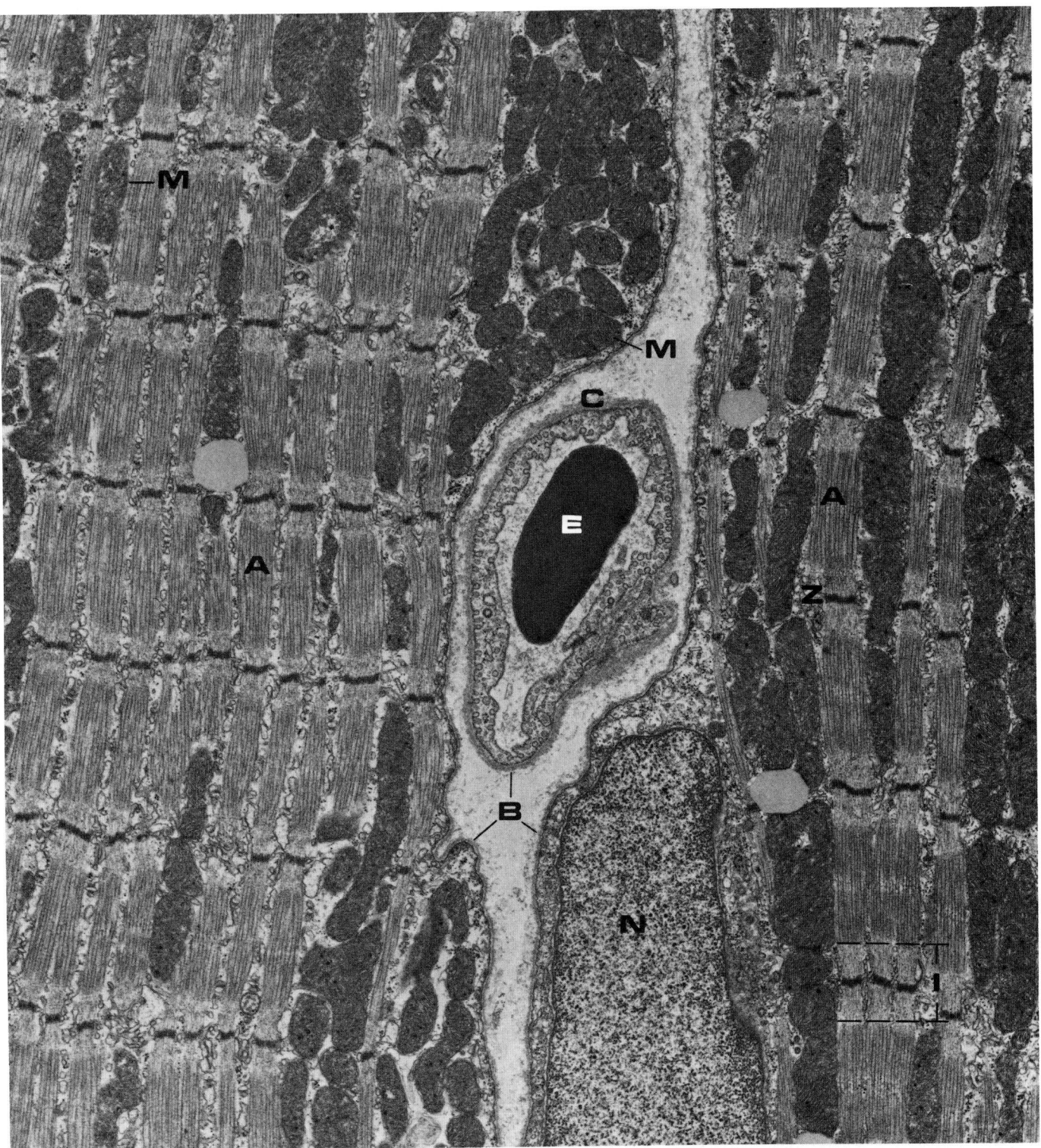

Fig. 11.10 An electron micrograph of longitudinally sectioned skeletal muscle from the extrinsic eye muscles of a slow loris. Two muscle fibers are separated by the endomyseal connective tissue space which is bounded by a basal lamina (B). The connective tissue space contains a capillary (C) with an erythrocyte (E). Caveolae and pinocytotic vesicles are contained within the endothelial cell of the capillary. The A bands (A) or anisotropic bands are darker than the I bands (I) or isotropic bands. Z lines (Z) occur in the middle of the I bands. Mitochondria (M) occur between the myofibrils and beneath the sarcolemma (subsarcolemmal). A nucleus (N) of one muscle fiber is included in the section. X14,600. (Micrograph courtesy of D. E. Kelly and included with permission from Copenhaver, W. M., Kelly, D. E. and Wood, R. L.: *Bailey's Textbook of Histology*, Williams & Wilkins, Baltimore, 1978.)

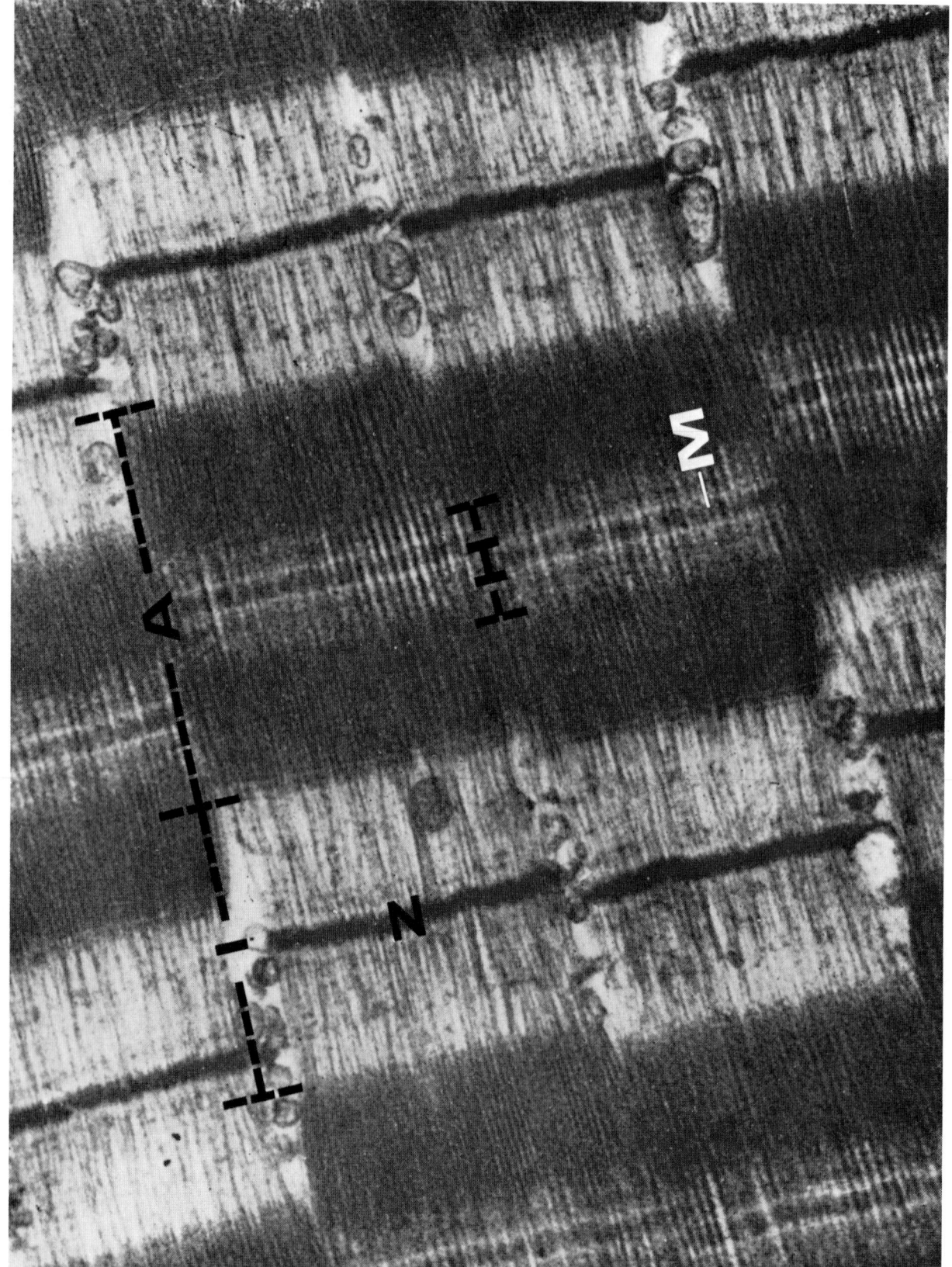

Fig. 11.11 An electron micrograph of myofibrils from the psoas muscle of a rabbit. The dark A bands (A) contain a lighter H band (H). An M line (M) bisects the H band. The light I bands (I) contain a dark Z line (Z). X52,000. (Reprinted with permission from: Copenhaver, W. M., Kelly, D. E. and Wood, R. L.: *Bailey's Textbook of Histology*, Williams & Wilkins, Baltimore, 1978.)

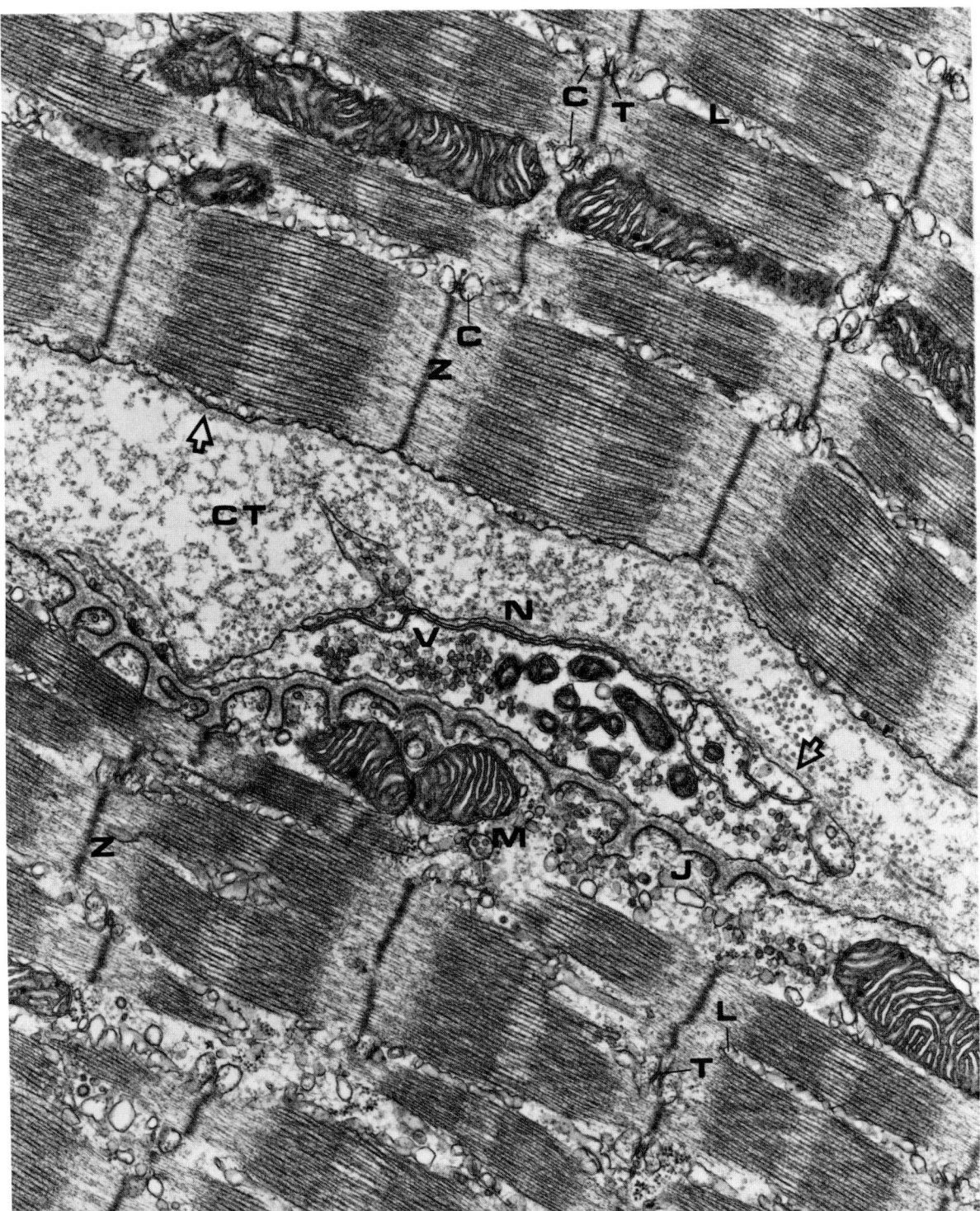

Fig. 11.12 An electron micrograph of longitudinal sections through two fibers of amphibian skeletal muscle. The longitudinally oriented (L) and terminal cisterns (C) of the sarcoplasmic reticulum extend between the myofibrils. The terminal cisterns (C) and transverse tubules (T) form triads at the level of the Z line (Z). Mitochondria (M) occur in subsarcolemmal and interfibrillar positions. A nerve ending (N) forms a neuromuscular complex with the muscle cell. Note the clear (ACH-containing) presynaptic vesicles (V) within the nerve ending and the junctional folds (J) of the sarcolemma. The plasmalemma of the muscle cells and nerve ending are covered by a basal or external lamina (*open arrows*). The connective tissue (CT) between the muscle fibers contains collagen in longitudinal and cross-section. X26,000. (Micrograph courtesy of D. E. Kelly and included with permission from: Copenhaver, W. M., Kelly, D. E. and Wood, R. L.: *Bailey's Textbook of Histology*, Williams & Wilkins, Baltimore, 1978.)

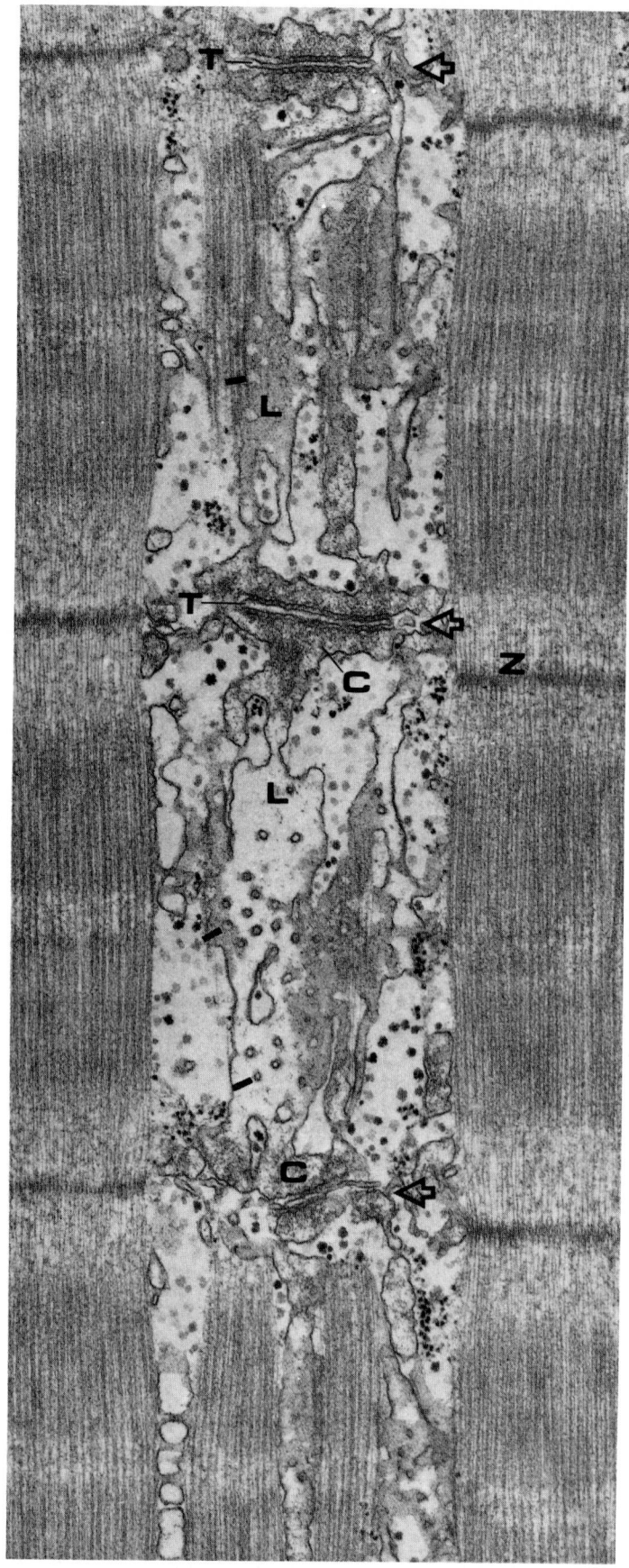

Fig. 11.13 An electron micrograph of a longitudinal section of amphibian skeletal muscle. The triads (*open arrows*) occur at the level of Z lines (Z). The membranes of the longitudinal components (L) of the sarcoplasmic reticulum contain numerous perforations (*bars*). Longitudinal components terminate as dilated cisterns (C) in association with transverse tubules (T). Two cisterns and a transverse tubule comprise a triad. Three triads are evident in this section. Glycogen as dark-staining granules is scattered throughout the cytoplasm. X34,000. (Micrograph courtesy of D. E. Kelly and included with permission from: Copenhaver, W. M., Kelly, D. E. and Wood, R. L.: *Bailey's Textbook of Histology*, Williams & Wilkins, Baltimore, 1978.)

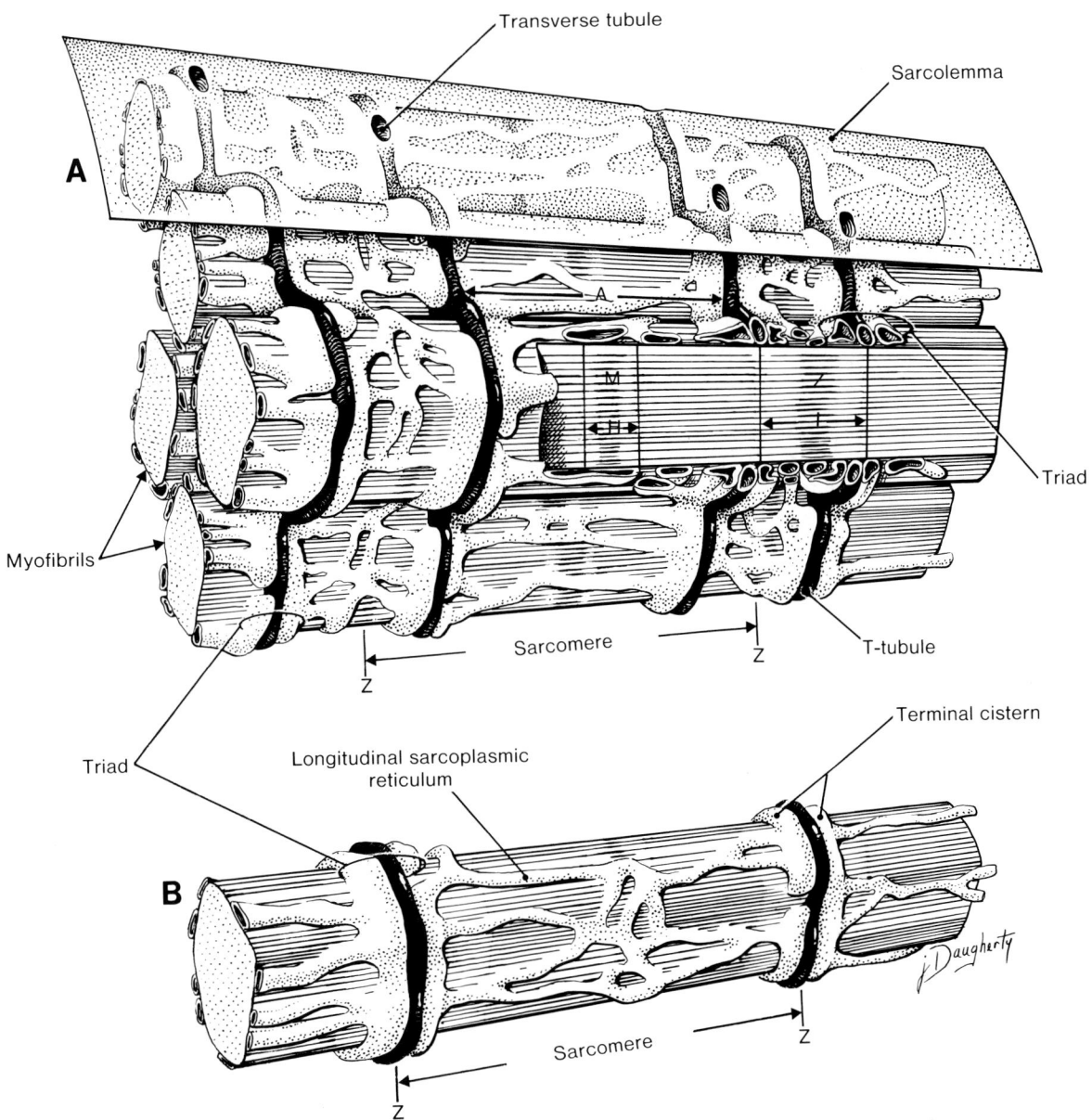

Fig. 11.14 A diagrammatic three-dimensional drawing to demonstrate the relationships of myofibrils, sarcoplasmic reticulum and T tubules in mammalian skeletal and cardiac muscle. A, skeletal muscle; B, cardiac muscle. The triads of mammalian skeletal muscle occur at the AI junctions; thus, two triads characterize each sarcomere. The triads of cardiac muscle and amphibian skeletal muscle occur at the Z lines (Z). The T tubules are invaginations of the sarcolemma that surround the myofibrils at specific locations in association with the terminal cisterns of the sarcoplasmic reticulum. (Redrawn and modified from Peachey.)

Contractile Mechanism. The contraction of skeletal muscle is initiated at the motor endplate (Fig. 11.12). The action potential reaches the presynaptic area and *acetycholine*, a cholinergic neurotransmitter, is released. The activation of cholinergic receptors culminates in the generation of an endplate potential that results in an action potential which spreads from this site along the cell membrane of the muscle fiber and into the depths of the cell via the transverse sarcotubular system. This inward movement of the wave of depolarization causes the release of calcium from the sarcoplasmic reticulum and initiates contraction (Fig. 11.16). These events comprise *excitation-contraction coupling*. The thick and thin filaments and adenosine triphosphate (ATP) are essential components in the contraction coupling.

The release of calcium into the sarcoplasm probably evokes a conformational change in troponin which detects the altered calcium levels and causes the movement of tropomyosin. Tropomyosin, which normally blocks the active sites of actin and myosin during relaxation, is displaced sufficiently to remove this inhibition and permit the interaction between the globular heads (HMM) of the myosin with the G actin monomers of actin. This interaction occurs as a result of the outward movement of the globular heads and is dependent upon the conversion of ATP→ADP with the release of energy. This occurs with each make and break event. ATPase, which is present in the globular heads, is responsible for this conversion and release of energy. The outward movement is facilitated by the flexibility of the neck region which connects LMM with globular heads (Fig. 11.17).

The thick and thin filaments may be visualized as two interacting worm gears. Contraction is envisioned as the sequential connections, disconnections, and reconnections between the globular heads of myosin with G actin. Each reconnection at an adjacent G actin monomer site results in the incremental shortening of the sarcomere. The number of reconnections, each equivalent to the approximate 56Å diameter of G actin,

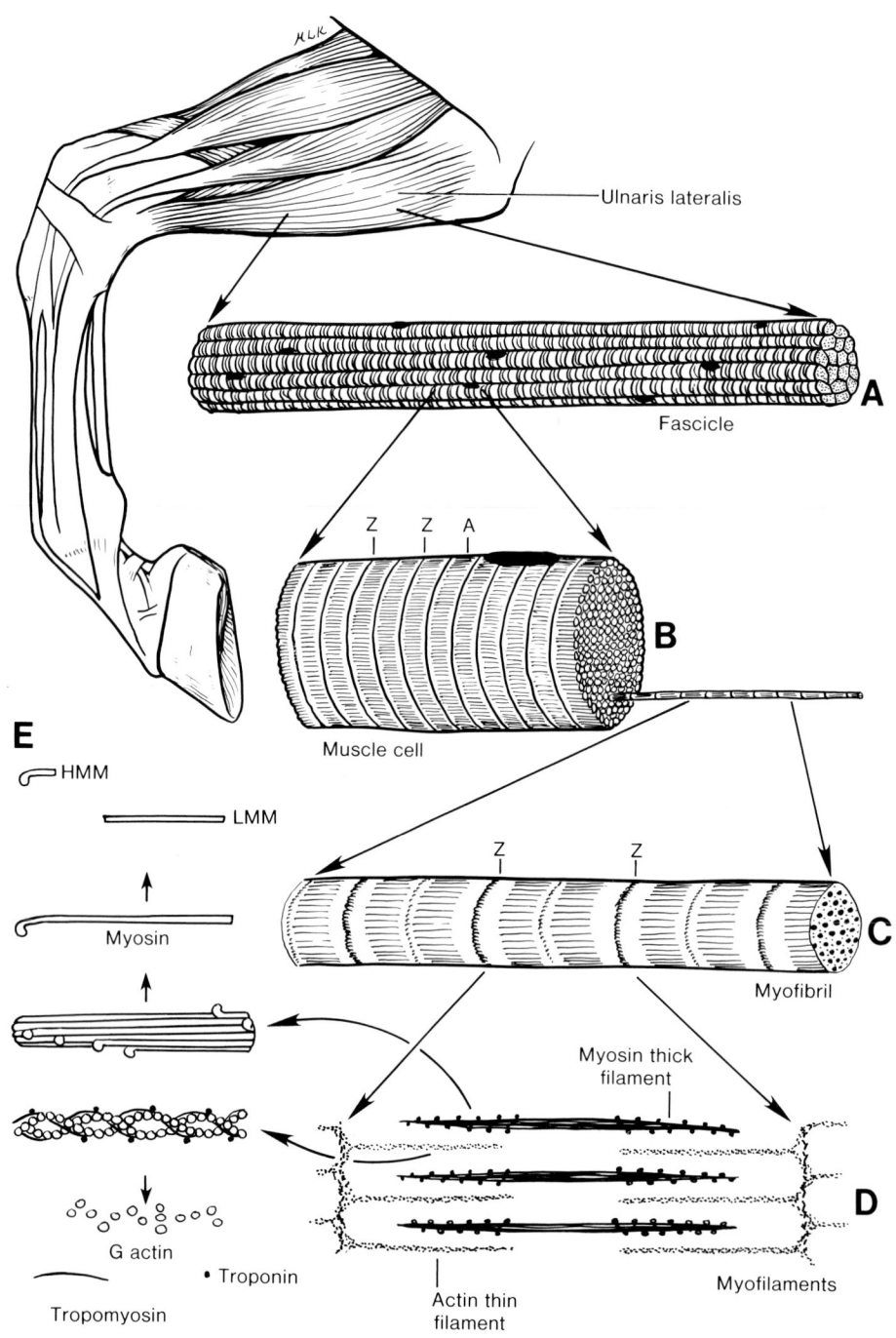

Ulnaris lateralis

Fascicle **A**

Z Z A

B

Muscle cell

E

⌐ HMM

LMM

Myosin

C

Myofibril

Myosin thick
filament

G actin

• Troponin

Tropomyosin

Actin thin
filament

Myofilaments

D

Fig. 11.15 A diagram demonstrating the gross, histologic, ultrastructural and biochemical relationships of skeletal muscle. The equine thoracic limb demonstrates the gross relationships. Low magnification examination of a muscle fascicle with a light microscope reveals elongated striated cells (A). High magnification light microscopy (B) demonstrates Z lines, A bands and I bands. The examination of myofibrils with the electron microscope (C and D) reveals the intimate relationships between myofilaments of the sarcomere. Biochemical analyses (E) have been used to characterize the thin and thick myofilaments. (Redrawn and modified from Bloom, W. and Fawcett, D. W.: *A Textbook of Histology*, 9th edition, W. B. Saunders, Philadelphia, 1968.)

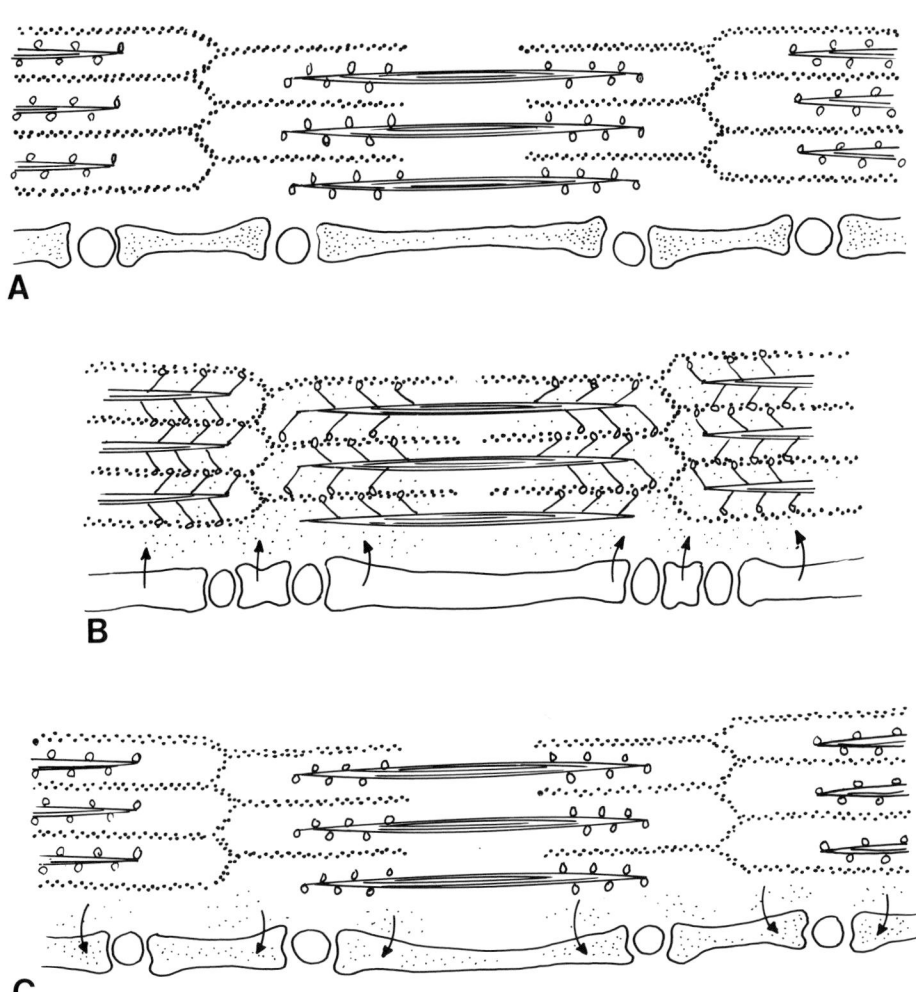

A

B

C

Fig. 11.16 Calcium and the contractile mechanism. During relaxation (A), calcium is stored in the sarcoplasmic reticulum. The wave of depolarization moves along the sarcolemma and probably alters the membrane potential of the transverse tubules. The altered membrane potential presumably induces a change in the sarcoplasmic reticulum that permits the movement of calcium into the cytoplasm (B). The inhibition is removed and the globular heads of myosin contact the G actin monomers. The return to the resting state (C) is achieved upon return of calcium to the sarcoplasmic reticular profiles.

cycles, an M line may appear as actin filaments slide past the myosin filaments and overlap or interact in the center of the A band. During extremes in contraction, a *contraction zone* may appear adjacent to the Z line. This may represent an overlap of myosin thick filaments at the Z line.

When muscle is stretched, the length of the A band remains constant, while the I band and H band length is increased.

The sliding filament hypothesis is a reasonable explanation of the morphologic changes associated with relaxation and contraction. The physiologic events explained previously are consistent with the morphologic alterations and support this hypothesis.

Types of Muscle Fibers. Skeletal muscle fibers do not comprise a homogeneous group of contractile fibers. Classically, *red, white* and *intermediate fibers* have been identified. Grossly, a muscle mass is described in a similar manner.

Red muscle fibers are small muscle cells that have numerous mitochondria and an abundance of the pigment *myoglobin.* The respiratory pigments (cytochrome system) of the mitochondria and the myoglobin impart the red color. The extensive mitochondria with their numerous cristae occupy interfibrillar and subsarcolemmal positions. Sarcoplasmic reticular profiles, especially in the region of the H band, are more complex than described previously. Also, Z lines are thick. An extensive capillary bed surrounds these muscle fibers. The transport of oxygen from the capillary bed to the cytochrome system of the mitochondria is facilitated by myoglobin, which has a high affinity for oxygen. Generally, red fibers respire by oxidative mechanisms and are characterized by slow contraction cycles. Prolongation of contraction and relaxation times means that these types of fibers are not fatigued easily. Storage of oxygen by myoglobin may help preclude fatigue.

White muscle fibers are large muscle cells that have very small amounts of myoglobin and a minimal number of mitochondria. Sarcoplasmic reticular profiles are simple and Z lines are thin. The scant amount of myoglobin requires that oxygen is transferred directly from the capillary bed to the few mitochondria. Because mitochondria are scant, metabolism is primarily anaerobic. The contraction cycle of white muscle fibers is shorter than their red counterparts. Accordingly, the white fibers are easily fatigued; lactic acid accumulates readily.

Intermediate muscle fibers, as their name implies, have characteristics of both the other fiber types.

Functional Correlates. The contractile mechanism is dependent upon ATP as a source of energy. The hydrolysis of ATP results in the formation of ADP and inorganic phosphate with the release of energy for this process. Unfortunately, there is an insufficient supply of ATP in a muscle cell to sustain contraction for a long period of

is summed as the total shortening of the sarcomere and the contraction of the muscle fiber.

ATP also supplies the energy for the active transport or pumping of calcium from the sarcoplasm to the sarcoplasmic reticulum where it is stored in the terminal cisterns. This event causes relaxation. The ADP is phosphorylated to ATP, troponin and tropomyosin assume their precontraction relationships, the globular heads of myosin swing back to their relaxed configuration and the muscle fiber is ready for the next contraction.

Relaxation/Contraction Morphology. The previously-described events comprise the *sliding filament hypothesis* of muscle contraction. These events coincide with the morphology of the sarcomere as observed with the light and electron microscope. The ultrastructure of the sarcomere is schematically presented in Figure 11.18. At rest, the sarcomere appears as described with the

ultrastructure of the cell. The I band, consisting of actin thin filaments, is the light-staining region of the sarcomere. It is divided in half by the Z line. The A band, consisting of myosin thick filaments and actin thin filaments, is the dark-staining region of the sarcomere. Because the actin thin filaments do not extend through the entire width of the A band, a light-staining H band is apparent in the middle of the A band. A sarcomere includes a Z line, 1/2 I band, A band, 1/2 I band and a Z line.

The morphology of the contracted state depends upon the degree of contraction. As muscles contract they become shorter and wider than their resting length and width. Commensurate changes are noted in the sarcomere. The I bands decrease in length and are eventually obliterated when 50% contraction is achieved. The H band changes proportionally with the I band alterations. Although the A band does not change length during normal contraction

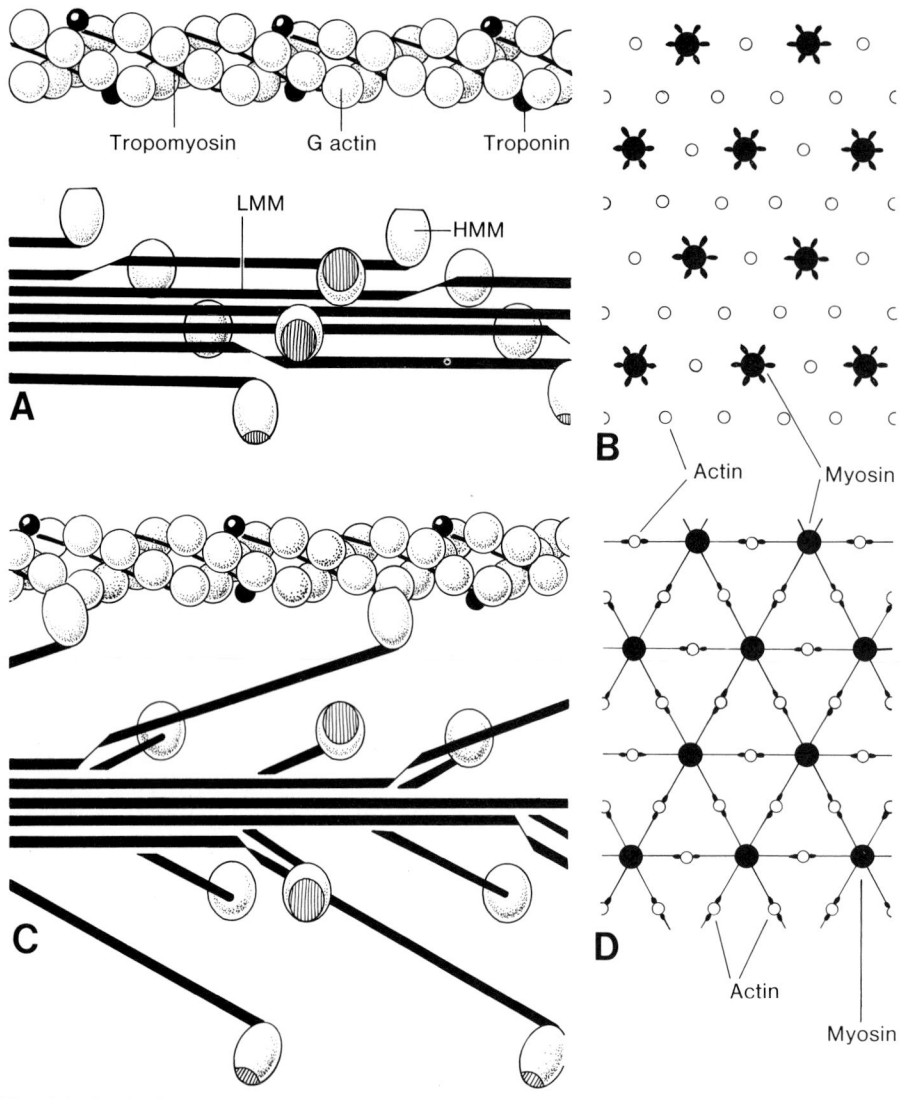

Fig. 11.17 A diagram of the relationships between actin and myosin during relaxation and contraction. The globular heads radiate around the myosin thick filament in close association with the actin thin filaments (A). Cross-sections (B) through myofilaments reveals that six actin thin filaments surround each myosin, but actin thin filaments are shared by adjacent myosin thick filaments. Upon contraction (C), the globular heads swing laterally and contact G actin monomers. Each actin thin filament is contacted by two globular heads (D). The scales between the longitudinal (A, C) and cross-sectional (B, D) representations are not equal. (Redrawn and modified from Ham, A. W.: *Histology*, 7th edition, J. B. Lippincott, Philadelphia, 1974.)

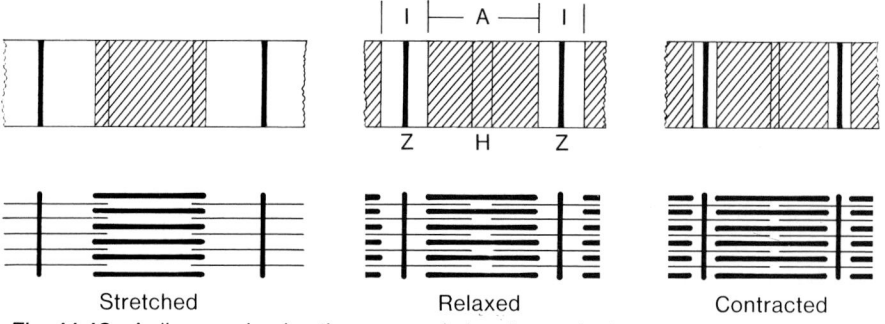

Fig. 11.18 A diagram showing the sarcomeric banding and relationships of the myofilaments during three different physiologic conditions. Refer to the text for a complete description of these relationships.

time. Most muscle cells have a storage of ATP that would last less than 1 second. Active and continual contraction requires that ATP be replenished rapidly. This occurs through glycolysis and the tricarboxylic acid (TCA) cycle. Additionally, muscle fibers have developed a backup and storage system that replenishes ATP rapidly. This system utilizes a *phosphagen, creatine phosphate* (*CP, phosphocreatine*) that functions to store phosphate bond energy (Fig. 11.19).

During periods of low demand, ATP reacts with *creatine* to form CP. The ratio of CP:ATP is approximately 30:1. The ATP for the production of CP is derived from the metabolism of glucose through glycolytic and tricarboxylic acid pathways. The TCA cycle is 19 times more efficient in the production of ATP than is glycolysis.

During periods of exercise, ATP is being degraded constantly to ADP, whereas CP constantly rephosphorylates ADP and makes more ATP available for contraction. This phosphorylation is catalyzed by the enzyme *creatine phosphokinase* (*CPK*). As long as an adequate oxygen supply is maintained to muscle during exercise, the high ATP yield from aerobic metabolism and the TCA cycle continuously charges the creatine and forms CP. The CP is the most readily available reserve source of ATP.

During strenuous exercise, the oxygen supply is inadequate to drive the TCA cycle. Muscle metabolism then switches to anaerobic respiratory mechanisms. Pyruvic acid is converted to lactic acid instead of being metabolized to carbon dioxide and acetyl-coenzyme A as it is under aerobic conditions. This results in a diminished supply of ATP, an inadequate charging of the creatine and the accumulation of lactic acid. The accumulation of lactate involves an *oxygen debt* that must be satisfied during its metabolism back to pyruvate. Lactate leaks from the cell and causes a localized vasoconstriction that exacerbates the problems. Lactate is carried in the blood to the liver where it is metabolized. The local accumulation of lactate accounts partially for the muscular soreness associated with strenuous exercise. Lactate is converted back to pyruvate within the muscle as the oxygen supply relative to contractile activity is increased.

The energy for muscular contraction is generated by the degradation and metabolism of glycogen stores in the muscle cells. Aerobic respiration is the most efficient energy-generation process and is the source of energy for protracted muscular activity. Such events are dependent upon good glycogen stores and an increased ability for oxygen consumption. The lactic acid system, anaerobic respiration, is the source of energy for short, demanding periods of muscular activity. Because the CP-ATP system is depleted rapidly, these other sources of energy are essential for the types of activities described.

Besides serving as the source of energy for contraction, ATP is required for the movement of calcium from the sarcoplasm into the sarcoplasmic reticulum. Depletion of ATP results in the accumulation of calcium and the inability of the myosin globular heads to release from the G actin. This contraction after the cessation of stimulation may account for *muscle cramps* as well as *rigor mortis*.

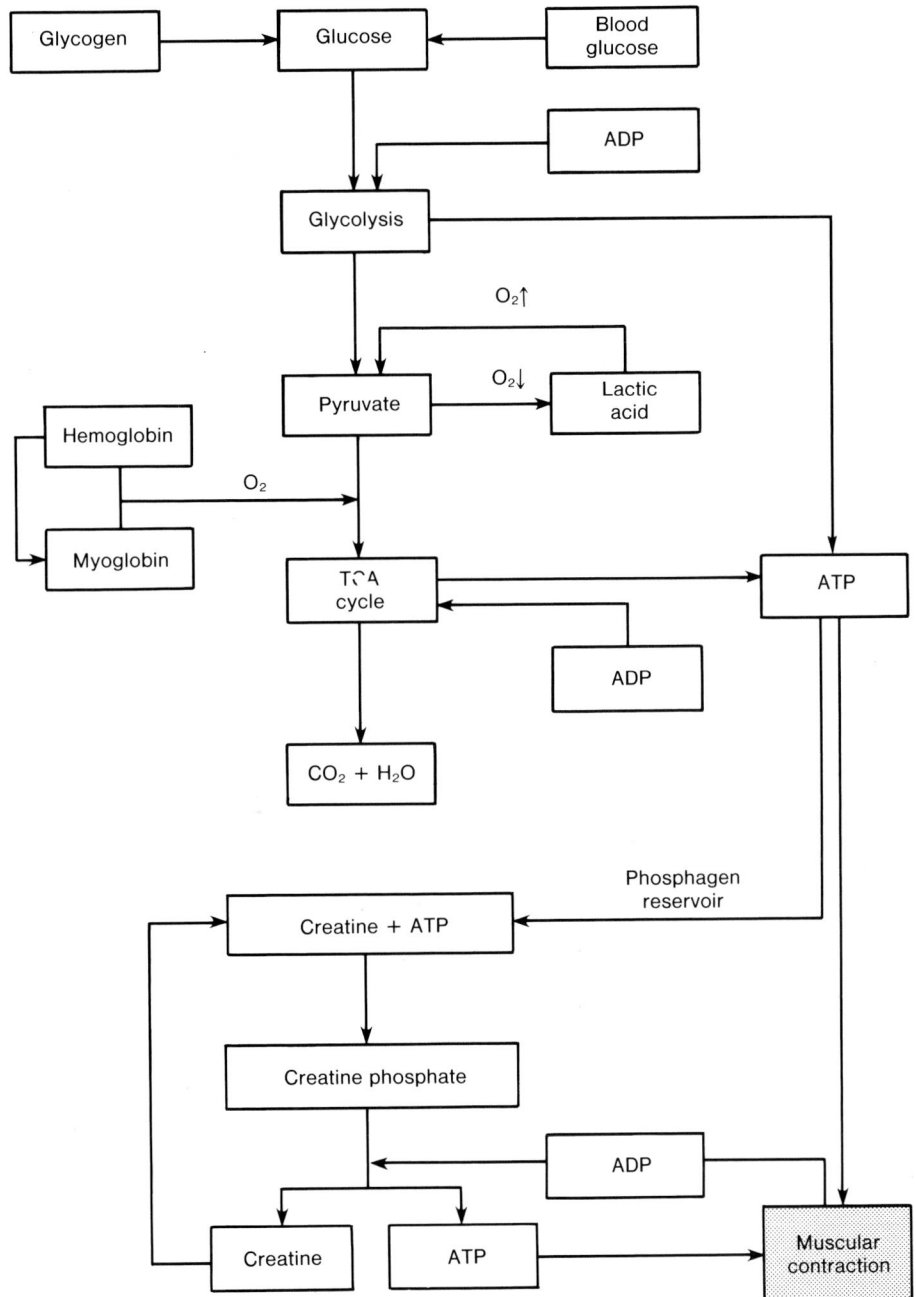

Fig. 11.19 Energy sources and muscle contraction. Muscle metabolism is discussed in the text.

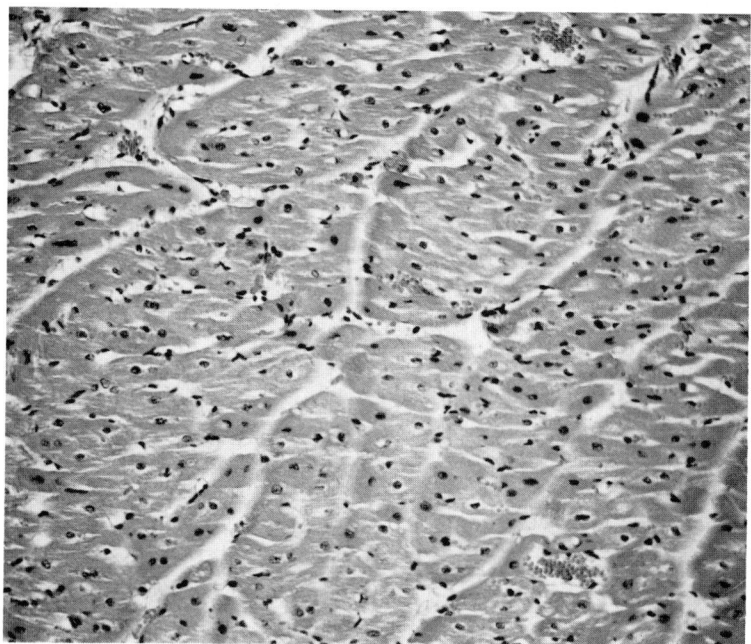

Fig. 11.20 Section of cardiac muscle. The branched fibers contain nuclei located in the center of the sarcoplasm. X40.

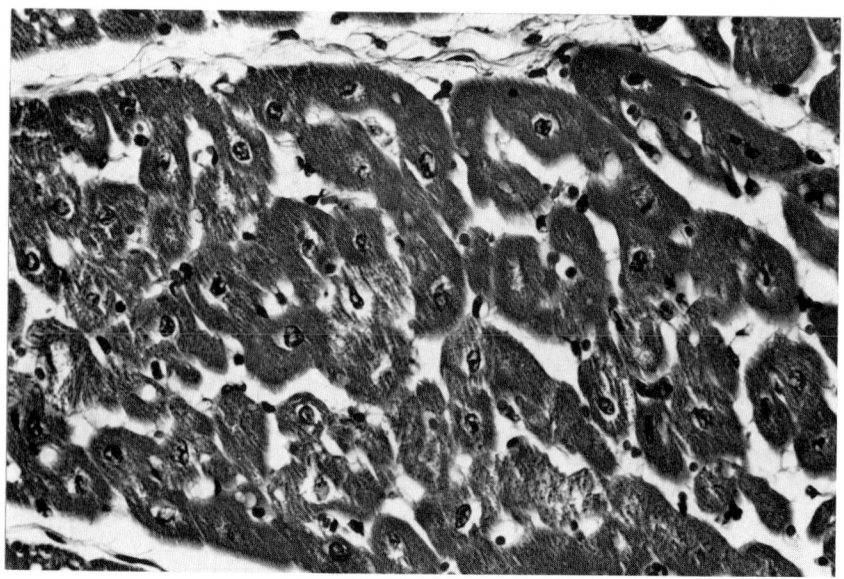

Fig. 11.21 Section of cardiac muscle. The central location of the nuclei and perinuclear halos are prominent features of the branched muscle fibers. X100.

Although intracellular calcium is essential for the contractile mechanism, extracellular calcium is required to maintain proper membrane permeabilities and the excitability of nerve cells and muscle cells. A reduction of blood calcium is associated classically with a *hypocalcemic tetany.* Despite the depletion of extracellular calcium, muscle cells do not readily lose their intracellular calcium. Hypocalcemia results in a hyperexcitability of motor nerve fibers and muscle cells that results in the tetanic stimulation and response of the muscle fibers. A sufficient amount of extracellular calcium must

be present to permit the release of the neurotransmitter *acetycholine.* Hypocalcemic tetany usually occurs as a sequel to acute calcium loss. Canine *eclampsia,* hypocalcemic tetany in the postpartum lactating female, is a classic example. However, tetany is not always a sequel to acute calcium loss. *Bovine milk fever, post-parturient paresis,* is a hypocalcemic condition characterized by a flaccid paralysis rather than tetany. This apparent paradoxical situation is explained in a number of ways. The most compelling explanation seems to be that neurotransmitter release is disrupted at

higher calcium levels than those that would cause the eventual hyperexcitability of the nerve cell.

Skeletal muscle fibers are adaptive morphologically to the functional demands made upon them. Increased use results in an increased gross muscle size. The increased muscle mass results from the *hypertrophy* of individual muscle fibers. Cytoplasm and the amount of contractile proteins increase. Ribosomes are responsible for the synthesis of these contractile proteins. The addition of new actin and myosin is accomplished by the addition of new myofibrillar units, be-

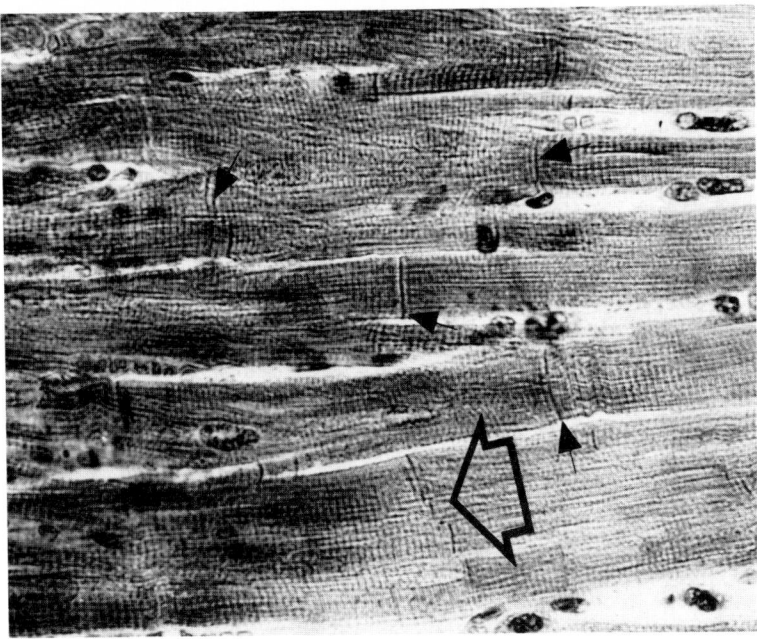

Fig. 11.22 Intercalated disks of cardiac muscle. The disks, *solid arrows*, delimit the end-to-end boundaries of adjacent muscle cells. The intercalated disks may appear as straight boundaries or have a stepwise appearance (*large arrow*). X160.

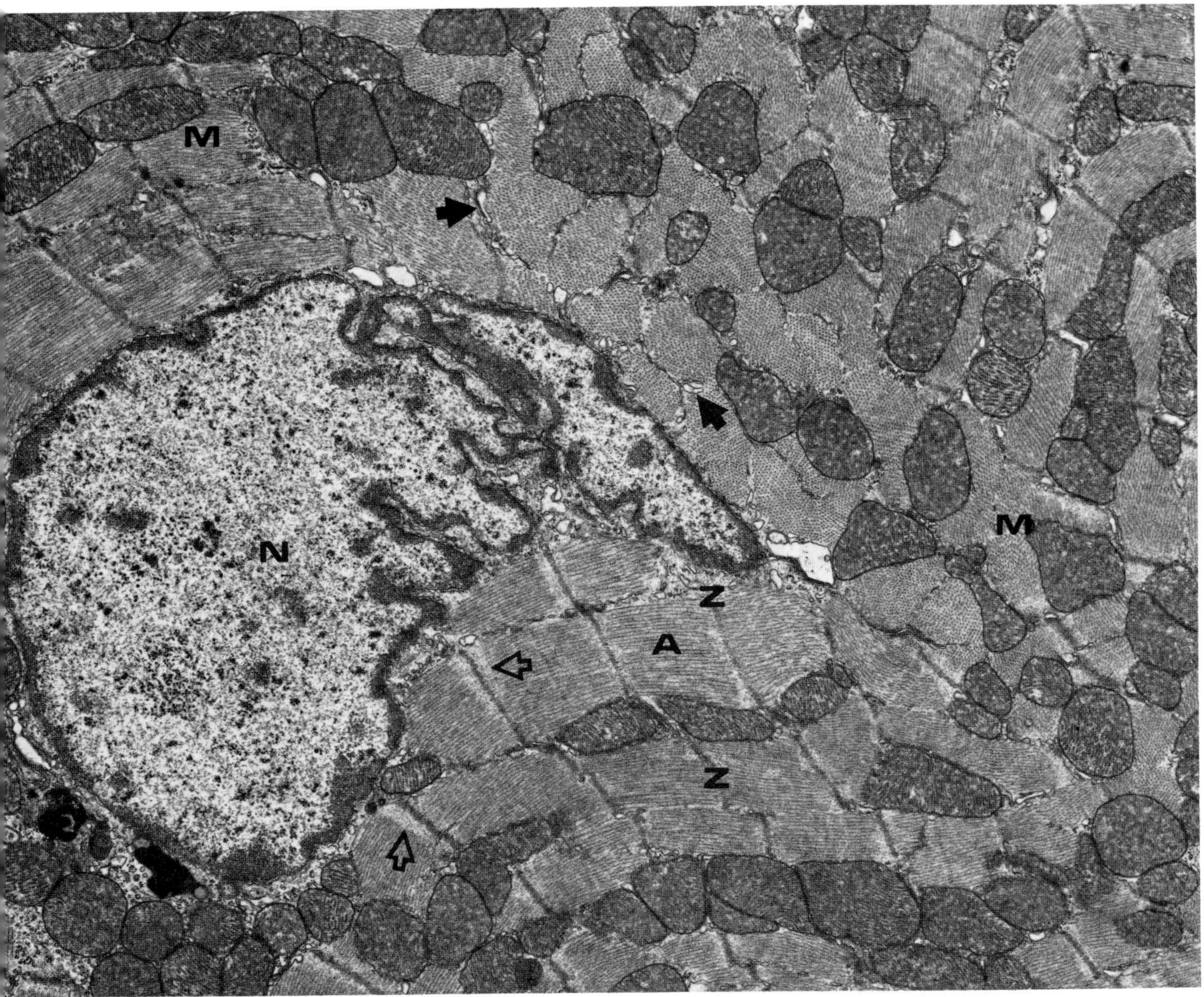

Fig. 11.23 An electron micrograph of a cardiac muscle cell. The nucleus (N) is surrounded by bundles of myofilaments that are longitudinally and cross-sectioned. Z lines are not in register (Z) and I bands (*open arrows*) are almost obliterated. A bands (A) are adjacent to Z lines. Numerous mitochondria (M) surround the nucleus and are scattered among the myofibrils. Profiles (*solid arrows*) of the sarcoplasmic reticulum surround the myofibrils. X11,400.

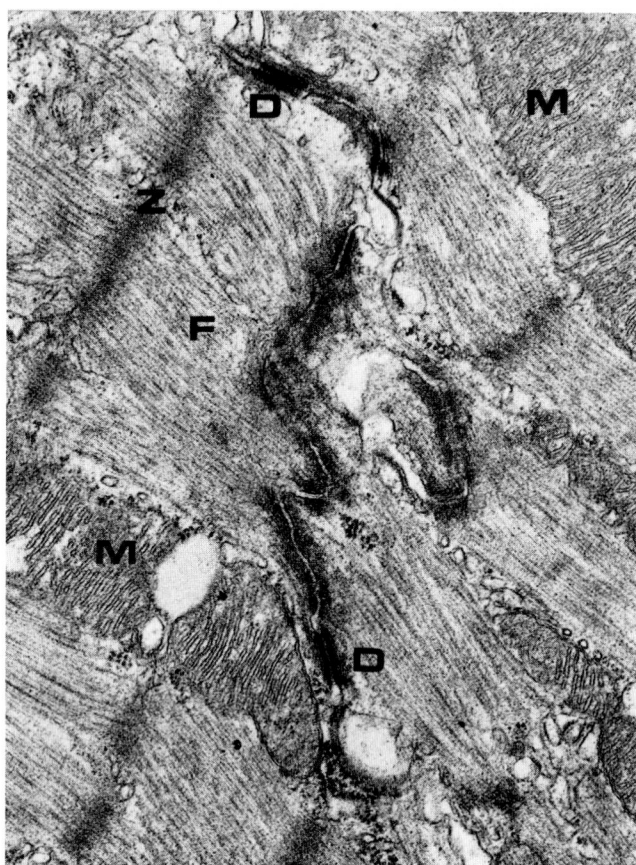

Fig. 11.24 An electron micrograph of an intercalated disk. The tortuous path of the disk is apparent. Desmosomes (D) are components of the disk. Myofilaments (F) extend from Z lines (Z) and terminate at the disk. Mitochondria (M) are indicated. X26,000.

cause hypertrophy results in an increased number of myofibrils, not an increase in myofibrillar thickness. A thickness limit probably exists beyond which functional efficiency is lost. Myofibrils are known to split during the growth process.

Disuse of a muscle or group of muscles results in *atrophy*. Atrophy is a decreased size of individual fibers and a loss of contractile protein. The atrophy of disuse may result from confinement, immobilization associated with fracture repair and loss of innervation. Because muscular contraction is essential to maintain the integrity of skeletal elements with which they are associated, the muscular atrophy resulting from fracture immobilization also results in a loss of skeletal mass in the local area. Muscular atrophy is also an important clinical sign of neurologic diseases involving the *final common pathway* (*lower motor neuron*, *α-motor neuron*). Nervous stimulation and exercise are essential for the maintenance of muscular mass.

Cardiac Muscle

Histologic Structure. This tissue is very similar to skeletal muscle. Both are striated; however, cardiac muscle is involuntary. Only those features characteristic of cardiac muscle will be presented here. If a specific characteristic is omitted, the student is to assume that it is similar to skeletal muscle.

There are six morphologic features of cardiac muscle that are quite distinct and are aids in identification. The cardiac muscle fibers are branched (Plates V.5, V.6). In any given section, longitudinally, transversely and obliquely sectioned fibers may be present (Fig. 11.20). The connective tissue surrounding each muscle fiber is more prominent here than in skeletal muscle.

The nucleus of a cardiac muscle cell is centrally located and surrounded by a pale-staining cytoplasmic region—a *perinuclear halo* (Fig. 11.21). The sarcoplasm contains myofilaments that are arranged in a manner previously described. Bundles of myofilaments, however, reflect the branching of the muscle fibers. Moreover, the striations that are readily apparent in skeletal muscle are not as prominent in cardiac muscle. Distinct, transversely-oriented, dark-staining bands are scattered throughout the cardiac muscle. These *intercalated disks* are points of end-to-end contact between contiguous muscle fibers. They appear as stepwise striations in the muscle mass (Fig. 11.22).

Ultrastructural Features. The ultrastructural features of cardiac muscle cells are similar to those described for skeletal muscle (Fig. 11.23). Only the significant differences are discussed herein.

The intercalated disks, as points of contact and adhesion between adjacent cardiac muscle cells, are composed of various types of junctional complexes between terminal Z lines (Fig. 11.24). These complexes include *desmosomes*, *gap junctions* and *fasciae adherentes* (Fig. 11.25). Focal areas of dense filamentous materials represent the attachment points of actin filaments to the sarcolemma. These regions are the fasciae adherentes (singular, fascia adherens) which are similar to the zonula adherens of epithelial tissues, except that the former are irregular and discontinuous regions rather than distinct belt-like zones. The desmosomes are typical and serve as points of adhesion between cells. The laterally-oriented cellular interfaces consist of gap junctions or nexi. Nexi are points of low electrical resistance that couple the cells together electrically. The fasciae adherentes couple the cells together mechanically.

The *sarcoplasmic reticulum* consists of longitudinally-oriented and highly anastomotic profiles. Although terminal cisterns are absent, sarcoplasmic reticular profiles make intimate contact with *transverse tubules* (*T tubules*) as diadic structures. These *diads* generally occur at the level of Z lines. T tubules are larger than their counterparts in skeletal muscle and contain basal lamina material. Mitochondria occur in greater numbers than in skeletal muscle. Cardiac muscle fibers of the atria contain dense, membrane-bound granules the function of which is yet to be determined. *Atrial granules* do not occur in ventricular muscle cells.

Functional Correlates. The contractile mechanism of cardiac muscle is the same as described for skeletal muscle. The spontaneous and rhythmic contraction of this tissue is a unique functional characteristic, whereas the spread of excitation from one fiber to another is similar to visceral or single unit smooth muscle. The presence of *pacemaker cells* establishes a beat that may be modified by the nerve fibers of the autonomic nervous system. Sympathetic nerve fibers have a positive chronotropic effect (increase heart rate) or induce a *tachycardia*, whereas parasympathetic nerve fibers have a negative chronotropic effect (decreased heart rate) or induce a *bradycardia*.

Although the metabolism of cardiac muscle is similar to skeletal muscle, significant differences do occur. Cardiac muscle cells have an extensive vascular supply, abundant mitochondria and large quantities of myoglobin. Hypoxic conditions that lead to anaerobic metabolism can not support cardiac muscle contraction because of inadequate energy production.

The cardiac muscle cell is capable of hypertrophy, which accounts for its increased size during growth and is one of the mechanisms by which the heart responds to an increased work load.

Purkinje Fibers. *Purkinje fibers* are specialized cardiac muscle cells that are modified as impulse-conducting cells (Fig. 11.26). These fibers conduct impulses from the A-

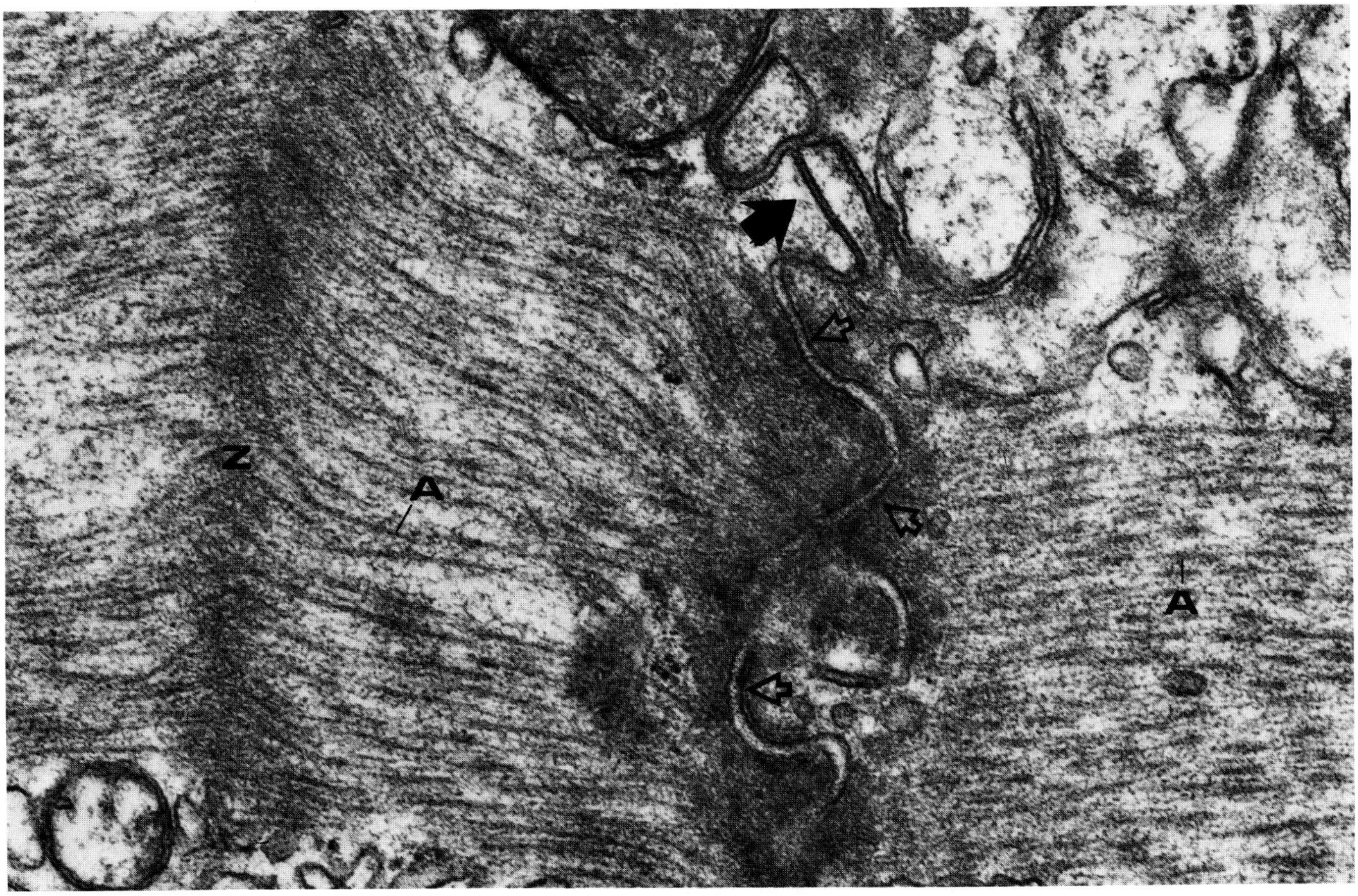

Fig. 11.25   An electron micrograph of an intercalated disk. Actin filaments (A) extend from Z lines (Z) and are embedded in the dense material associated with fasciae adherentes (*open arrows*). Gap junctions (*solid arrow*) are apparent also. X62,000.

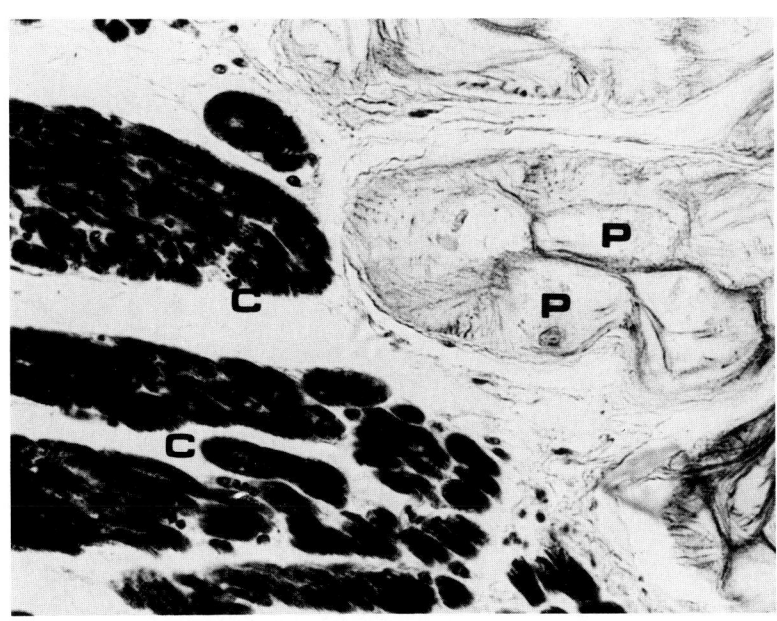

Fig. 11.26   Cardiac muscle cells and Purkinje fibers. The Purkinje fibers (P) are larger than the cardiac muscle cells (C). X100 (phosphotungstic acid-hematoxylin (PTAH)).

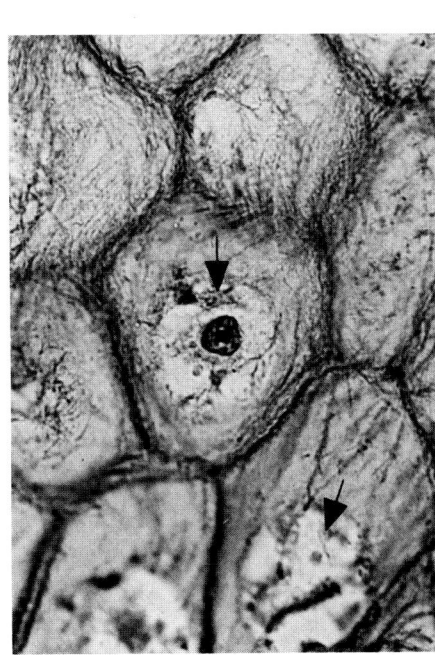

Fig. 11.27   Cross-section of Purkinje fibers. Note the perinuclear halos (*arrows*) and paucity of myofibrils. X160 (PTAH).

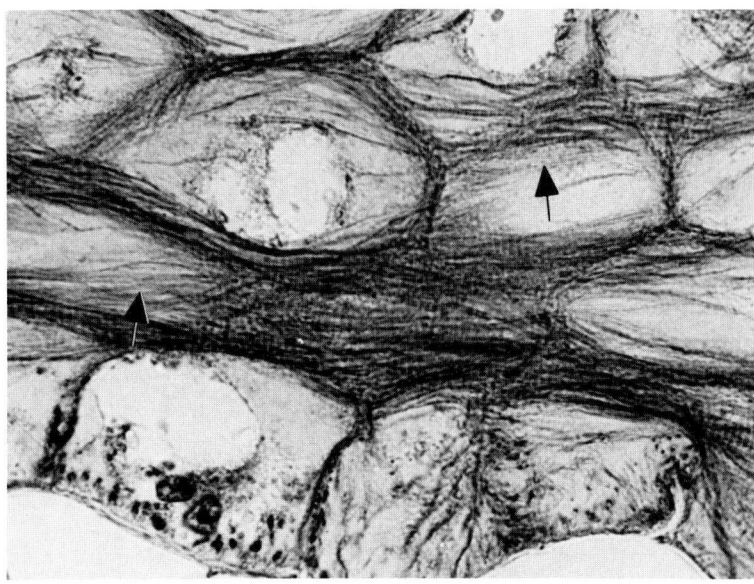

Fig. 11.28 Longitudinal and oblique sections of Purkinje fibers. The myofibrils (*arrows*) are apparent in the periphery of the fibers. X160 (PTAH).

V node through the interventricular septum to the ventricles.

In cross-section the Purkinje fibers are much larger than typical cardiac muscle cells (Fig. 11.27). Also, the Purkinje fibers have an abundant pale-staining, acidophilic sarcoplasm that is rich in glycogen. Myofibrils are few and, when present, are usually located peripherally. Nuclei are centrally located.

In longitudinal section these fibers appear as swollen cardiac muscle cells with scattered myofibrils. These fibers are joined to cardiac muscle cells by intercalated disks (Fig. 11.28).

Repair and Regeneration

Smooth Muscle. Mitotic activity has been noted in smooth muscle cells. This activity appears to be limited and may not be a major factor in repair and regeneration of damaged cells. New smooth muscle cells may be derived from pericapillary mesen-chymal cells also. The regenerative powers of smooth muscle are limited; healing occurs primarily through the formation of a connective tissue scar.

Skeletal Muscle. The regeneration of damaged skeletal muscle fibers is limited. Healing occurs primarily by scar tissue formation. There are instances, however, during which new skeletal muscle fibers are derived from *myoblasts. Satellite cells* may be myoblasts which have persisted from fetal into adult life. These cells proliferate, fuse and form typical skeletal muscle cells. The simultaneous formation of scar tissue rarely permits the return to 100% function.

Cardiac Muscle. Cardiac muscle cells do not regenerate. Repair is achieved by the formation of scar tissue.

References

Smooth Muscle
Ashton, F. T., Somlyo, A. V. and Somlyo, A. P.: The contractile apparatus of vascular smooth muscle: Intermediate high voltage stereo electron microscopy. J. Mol. Biol. *98:*17, 1975.

Kelly, R. E. and Rice, R. V.: Ultrastructural studies on the contractile mechanism of smooth muscle. J. Cell Biol. *42:*683, 1969.
Garamvolgyi, N., Vizi, E. S. and Knoll, J.: The regular occurrence of thick filaments in stretched mammalian smooth muscle. J. Ultrastruct. Res. *34:*135, 1971.
Lane, B. P.: Alterations in cytological detail of intestinal smooth muscle cells in various stages of contraction. J. Cell Biol. *27:*199, 1965.
McNutt, N. S. and Weinstein, R. S.: The ultrastructure of the nexus. J. Cell Biol. *47:*666, 1970.
Osvaldo-Decima, L.: Smooth muscle in the ovary of the rat and monkey. J. Ultrastruct. Res. *29:*218, 1970.

Skeletal Muscle
Close, R. I.: Dynamic properties of skeletal muscle. Physiol. Rev. *52:*129, 1972.
Franzini-Armstrong, C. and Porter, K. R.: The Z disc of skeletal muscle. Z. Zellforsch. *61:*661, 1964.
Hanson, J. and Huxley, H. E.: Structural basis of the cross-striations in muscle. Nature *172:*530, 1953.
Huxley, A. F.: Muscular contraction. J. Physiol. (London). *243:*1, 1974.
Huxley, H. E.: The contraction of muscle. Sci. Amer. *199:*67, 1958.
Jones, J. K., Cohen, C., Szent-Gyorgyi, A. G. and Longley, W.: Paramyosin: Molecular length and assembly. Science *163:*1196, 1969.
Knappeis, G. G. and Carlsen, F.: The ultrastructure of the M line in skeletal muscle. J. Cell Biol. *38:*202, 1968.
Peachey, L. D.: The sarcoplasmic reticulum and transverse tubules of the frog's sartorius. J. Cell Biol. *25:*209, 1965.
Shafiq, S. A., Gorycki, M., Goldstone, L. and Milhorat, A. T.: The fine structure of fiber types in normal human muscle. Anat. Rec. *156:*283, 1966.
Squire, J. M.: Muscle filament structure and muscle contraction. Ann. Rev. Biophys. Bioeng. *4:*137, 1975.

Cardiac Muscle
Johnson, E. A. and Sommer, J. R.: A strand of cardiac muscle. Its ultrastructure and the electrophysiological implication of its geometry. J. Cell Biol. *33:*103, 1967.
Katz, A. M.: Contractile proteins of the heart. Physiol. Rev. *50:*63, 1970.
Legato, M. J.: Sarcomergenesis in the human myocardium. J. Mole. Cell Cardiol. *1:*425, 1970.
Rhodin, J. A., Missier, P. and Reid, L. C.: The structure of the specialized impulse-conducting system of the steer-heart. Circulation *24:*349, 1961.
Simpson, F. O. and Oertelis, S. J.: Relationship of the sarcoplasmic reticulum to the sarcolemma in sheep cardiac muscle. Nature *189:*758, 1961.
Sommer, J. R. and Waugh, R. A.: The ultrastructure of the mammalian cardiac muscle—with special emphasis on the tubular membrane systems. Am. J. Pathol. *82:*191, 1976.
Spiro, D.: The ultrastructure of heart muscle. Trans. N. Y. Acad. Sci. *24:*879, 1962.

12: Nervous Tissue

General Characteristics

Form and Function. Classically, the study of nervous tissue is integrated with a study of the various organs that comprise the nervous system. This chapter, however, presents the basic histologic components of nervous tissue upon which a study of organology is predicated. The organs of the nervous system are presented separately (Chapter 15).

Nervous tissue is distributed throughout the soma and is intimately associated with most of the tissues and organs of the body. The anatomic unit of nervous tissue is the neuron. Although there are numerous types of neurons, their primary function is to receive stimuli from the internal (*interoception*) and external (*exteroception*) environment. The subsequent transmission of signals throughout the body or the specific transmission of information to effector organs of the body are also integral parts of their functional significance.

The well-developed cytoplasmic characteristics of *irritability* and *conductivity* uniquely suit them to their task. Moreover, their well-developed cellular processes ensure contact with most parts of the body. These processes are the anatomic bases for the transmission of information throughout the soma. Intimate contact between neurons and cellular processes is achieved through junctional regions called *synapses.*

Neurons are intimately associated with other cell types called *neuroglia.* These cells are responsible for the protection, nutrition and structural integrity of nervous tissue. Neurons also may be intimately associated with other cells of the basic tissues.

Although the elements of nervous tissue are few, numerous modifications to neurons and the structural relationships among them allow for a great diversity in the organization of the nervous system.

Neuronal Organization

Neurons. Neurons are the genetic, morphologic, functional and trophic units of the nervous system. This statement, the *Neuron Doctrine,* recognizes that: 1) each neuron is derived from an embryonic stem cell, a *neuroblast,* and contains all the necessary coded information to fulfill its functions; 2) each neuron is a separate and distinct structural unit that makes contact with other units but have structural continuity; 3) chains of these cells comprise the conduction mechanism for the nervous system; 4) each neuron is

responsible for the nutrition, metabolism and maintenance of its component parts.

Neurons assume various shapes and sizes. Although no single description encompasses all neurons, they do have characteristics in common despite the diversity of three-dimensional morphology. A neuron or *nerve cell* consists of *cell body* (*cyton, soma*) and a

variable number of cellular processes. The cellular processes are the *dendrites* and *axon* (Fig. 12.1). The *perikaryon* is that portion of the cell body surrounding the nucleus.

Classification of Neurons. The morphologic diversity of neurons is manifested in numerous ways. Neurons vary in size, shape, number of processes and length of processes

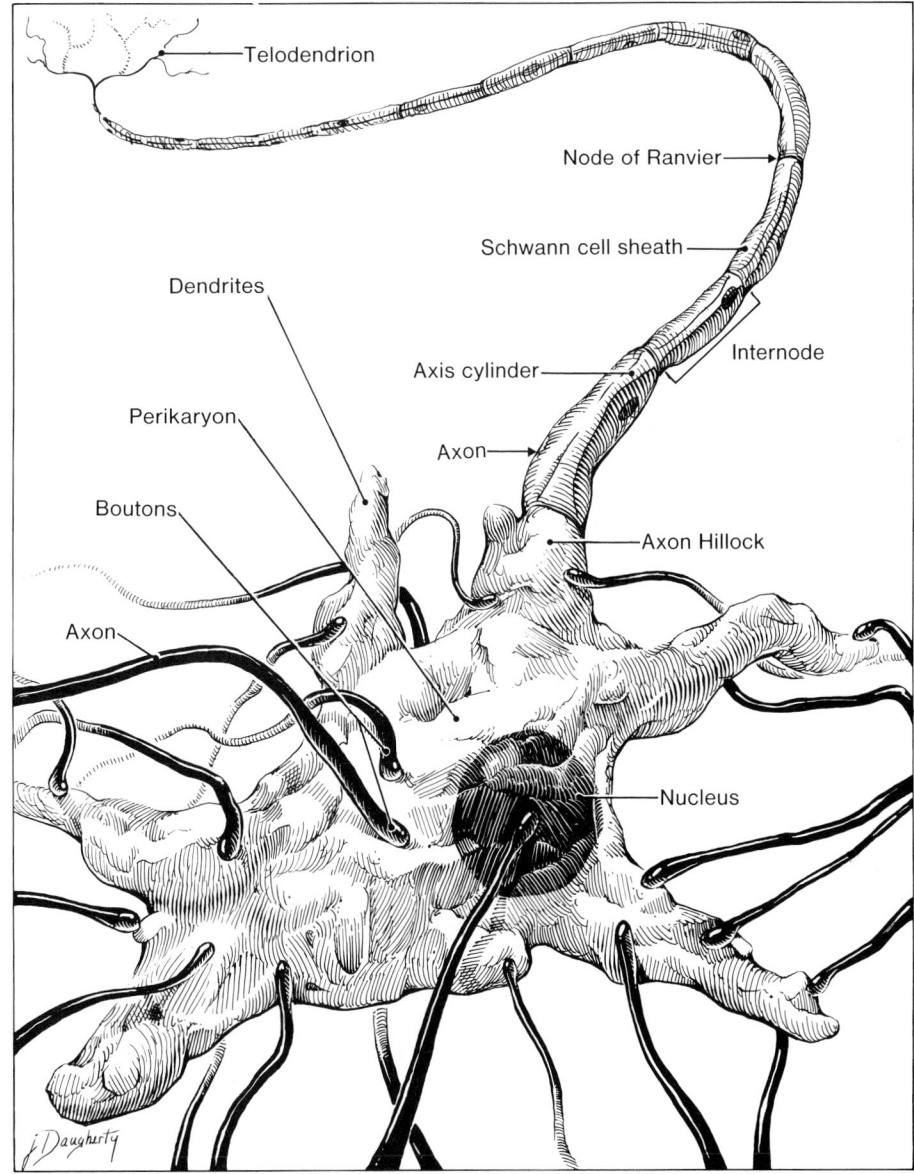

Fig. 12.1 Stylized drawing of a neuron. All light micrographs are labeled as the magnification with the microscope before photographic enlarging. All electron micrographs are labeled as total magnification, including photographic enlarging.

(Fig. 12.2). These different morphologic features represent adaptations to the numerous and diverse functional demands made upon these cells.

Although attempts at classification schemes are worthwhile, such schemes are rarely all-inclusive. Neurons may be divided into two general groups—transmission neurons and neurosecretory neurons (Fig. 12.3). *Transmission (conducting)* neurons comprise the majority of the neuronal types. These cells have dendrites, a cell body and an axon. Various morphological features are used to classify conducting neurons. *Golgi type I* neurons have numerous dendrites and a very long axon. The ventral horn cells of the gray column of the spinal cord (α-motor neurons), the sympathetic and parasympathetic preganglionic neurons, the sympathetic postganglionic neurons and other motor neurons of the nervous system are examples of Golgi type I neurons. *Golgi type II* neurons have numerous dendrites and a short axon. Interneurons and cells of the cerebral and cerebellar cortex are examples. Golgi type I and II neurons are commonly called *multipolar* neurons in recognition of their numerous dendritic processes. *Bipolar* neurons have one main dendrite and an axon that are located at opposite poles of the cell body. These cells are confined to areas of special visceral and somatic sensation. *True unipolar* neurons have only an axon and are confined generally in distribution to the developing nervous system. *Pseudounipolar* neurons have an axon and a dendrite that are fused close to the cell body, but separate some distance from the cell body. Both processes appear morphologically as axons. These are typical neurons of the cranial and spinal ganglia. Some neurons, such as the amacrine cells of the retina, do not have axons and are referred to as *anaxonic* neurons. Some of these neuronal types are diagrammed in Figure 12.4.

Neurosecretory neurons are specialized cells that synthesize, transport along their axons as Herring bodies and release various hormones into the blood. The relationship of these cells to blood vessels is referred to as *neurohemal organs* (Fig. 12.3) Some neurosecretory cells of the hypothalamus elaborate *oxytocin* and *antidiuretic hormone* into the capillaries of the neurohypophysis of the pituitary gland. Other neurosecretory cells of the hypothalamus elaborate *releasing factors (releasing hormones)* or *inhibiting factors (inhibiting hormones)* which regulate the secretory activity of the cells of the adenohypophysis of the pituitary gland. (These are discussed in detail in Chapter 22).

Classic morphologic considerations of neurons always include detailed descriptions of the dendrites, cell body and axon. Furthermore, classic discussions of the functional relationships of these three components invariably included the following: 1) the dendrites became stimulated and carried information to the cell body (*afferent*); 2)

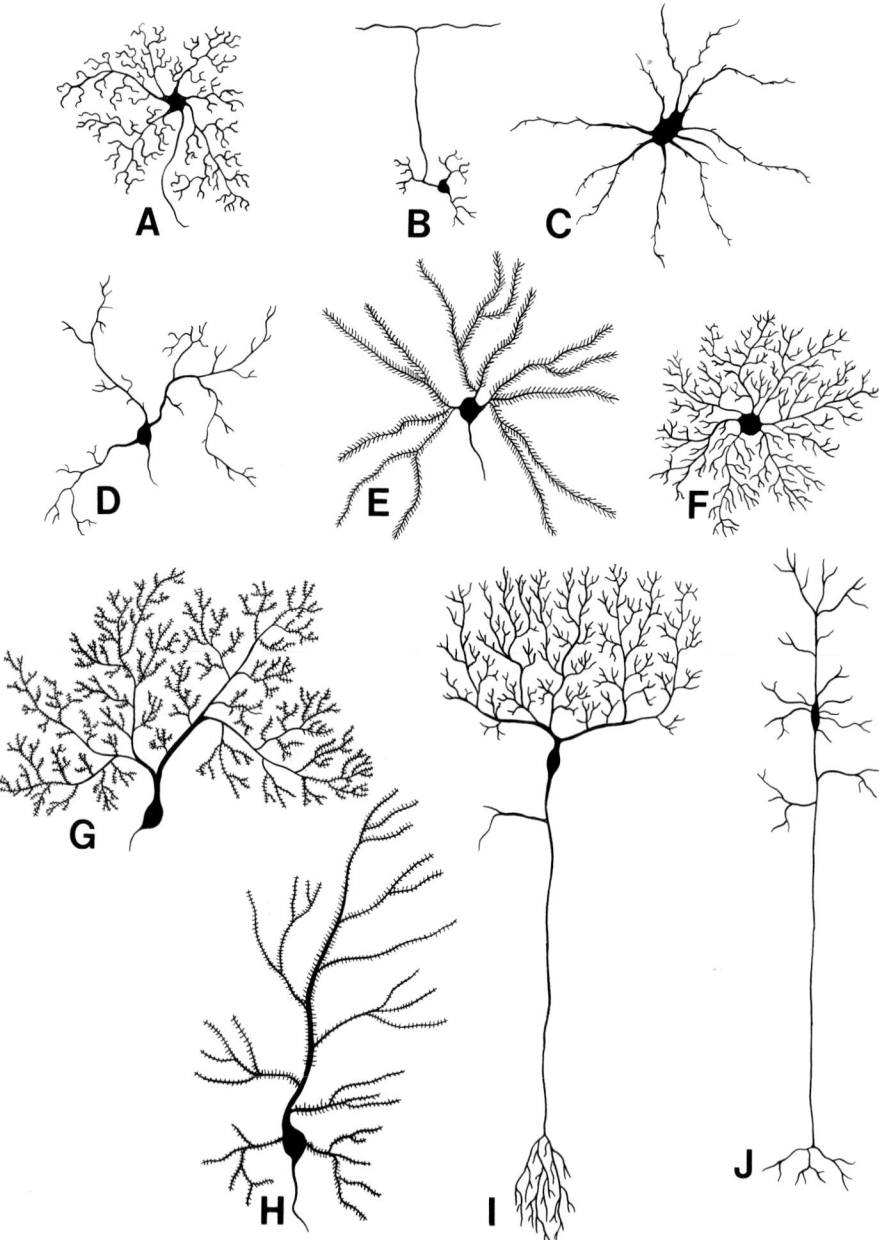

Fig. 12.2   A diagram of examples of different neurons that are components of the central nervous system. A, neuron of olivary nucleus; B, granule cell of cerebellar cortex; C, neuron from reticular formation; D, large neuron of spinal nucleus of the trigeminal nerve; E, neuron of basal ganglia; F, neuron of thalamic nuclei; G, Purkinje cell of cerebellar cortex; H, pyramidal cell of cerebral cortex; I, Purkinje cell and its long axon; J, Pyraminal cell and its long axon. The cells are not drawn to scale. (Redrawn and modified from: Truex, R. C. and Carpenter, M. B.: *Human Neuroanatomy*, 5th edition, Williams & Wilkins, Baltimore, 1966.

the axon then carried information away from the cell body (*efferent*); 3) this information eventually was transferred to the next element in the series, another neuron or effector organ. The relationship of the cell body to these afferent and efferent components is variable; however, the location of the cell body for specified types of neurons is constant. The specific location of the cell body in relation to the geometric organization is not important when the excitation, conduction and information transfer functions are considered. According to the *Bodian classification*, the three functionally significant zones are dendritic zone, axonic zone and telodendritic zone (Fig. 12.5). The *dendritic zone* is the area of the neuron that is subject to excitatory and inhibitory stimulation. It includes the dendrites, cell body and initial segment of the axon. Impulses impinging upon these surfaces may or may not result in the propagation of an action potential. The response is graded. The *axonic zone* includes the initial segment of the

xon, axis cylinder and part of the arborizing nerve terminal. It is the all-or-none conducting portion of the neuron. The *telodendritic zone* includes those terminal modifications that permit the transfer of information, electrically or chemically, to the next element in the pathway, neuron or effector organ. Activity in these elements resulting from the electrical or chemical activity of the telodendria results in a graded response.
Neuronal Cell Bodies. Although the cell body of a neuron is usually large, it may vary from 4–135 μm in diameter. A prominent, round, large vesicular nucleus is usually centrally located. A prominent nucleolus is present also (Fig. 12.6).

The cytoplasm is granular and basophilic. The abundant, granular basophilic inclusions are the *Nissl bodies* (*Nissl substance, tigroid granules*). They are scattered throughout the perikaryon and the cytoplasm of the dendrites (Fig. 12.7) but are not present in the axon. A clear area, the *axon hillock*, delimits the origin of the axon in the perikaryon (Fig. 12.8). Nissl substance varies in shape, size and distribution within the neuron; however, these basophilic aggregates of granules assume characteristic patterns in different types of neurons. The granules are actually clusters of rough endoplasmic reticulum, free ribosomes and free polysomes (Fig. 12.9). Because most neurons do not synthesize proteins for extracellular transport, the occurrence of Nissl substance is somewhat enigmatic. Neurons may renew as much as one-third of their proteins per day; these organelles may be involved in the maintenance and renewal process. Nissl substance is quite labile and may dissolve (*chromatolysis*) when the cell body and/or its processes are injured. The process of

chromatolysis has been considered for years to be strictly a degenerative change in neurons. Because the dissolution of Nissl substance is accompanied by an increase in smooth endoplasmic reticular profiles, an increase in the amount of free ribosomes and polysomes and an increase in the total cellular RNA content, chromatolysis is now considered to be a restorative process. However, chromatolysis may still indicate degeneration in some neurons. The restorative aspects of this change are dependent upon the neurons involved, the severity of the injury and the location of the injury to the cell.

Although a Golgi apparatus is present in the perikaryon, its function, too, is enigmatic. Its function may relate to the formation of lysosomes, the condensation and segregation of cellular products and/or the replenishment of the plasmalemma. Mitochondria occur in large numbers within the cell body and the nerve cell processes (Fig. 12.9). *Lipofuscin*, a yellow-brown pigment, was described in Chapter 4. Its occurrence in nerve cells may be linked to the high rate of metabolism and organelle turnover that characterize these cells. The lipofuscin pigment is thought to be contained within residual bodies from autophagocytic phenomena. Its presence within these cells is associated with cellular dysfunction. *Neurofilaments* and *neurotubules* (*microtubules*) are present in the cell body and the cellular processes (Fig. 12.9). Although the plasmalemma is typical morphologically and conforms to the fluid mosaic model, it is not structurally and functionally uniform.
Dendrites. The *dendrites* are the cellular processes of the cell body which increase the surface area of the neuron. They are like the

branches of a tree (Gr.; *dendron*, tree). The dendritic processes are usually shorter than the axon, branch continuously and gradually taper at the ends (Fig. 12.1). The surface of these processes, as well as that of the cell body, are covered with numerous *spines* or *gemmules* which represent the synaptic connections with *axon terminals* of other nerve cells. The cytoplasmic content of these processes is similar to the cell body. Nissl substance is confined to the proximal portions of the processes, although neurotubules, neurofilaments and mitochondria are present also. Classically, the dendrites are considered to carry information toward the cell body.
Axon. The *axon* or *axis cylinder* arises generally from the *axon hillock* region of the perikaryon (Figs. 12.1 and 12.8). This single process has a smooth surface and a uniform diameter. It branches extensively as the *telodendrion* before its termination on an effector. (Effectors can be muscles, glands or other neurons.) The plasma membrane of the axon is termed the *axolemma*. Although the cell membrane of the axon is typical, it has functional and morphologic alterations at various points along its course. The *initial segment* of the axon as it emerges from the cell body is the point at which myelination begins. Also, the initial segment has a lower threshold of excitation than the dendrites and cell body. Nodes of Ranvier occur along myelinated axons and are foci of discontinuity in the myelin sheath at which points the axons are covered by cytoplasmic processes of the glial cells. The axon may be thicker at nodes of Ranvier. Functionally, the nodes account for *saltatory conduction* of impulses; i.e., the jumping of the wave of depolarization from node to node. Axon terminals are modified in various ways to facilitate information transfer.

The cytoplasm of the axon is termed the *axoplasm*. Mitochondria, neurotubules, neurofilaments and smooth endoplasmic reticular profiles are the conspicuous organelles. Nissl substance does not occur in the axon hillock and axon. The spatial orientation and length of the nerve cell processes creates special transport problems for the neuron, since most of the synthesis of molecules occurs in the cell body. Transport problems are especially manifest in the axon. Materials move constantly away from (*somatofugal*) and to (*somatopetal*) the cell body. Somatofugal movement has been characterized by experimental techniques as *slow axoplasmic flow* and *fast axoplasmic flow*. Most of the materials within the axoplasm move slowly at rates of 0.5–5.0 mm/day and are believed to involve large molecules utilized in the maintenance, turnover and repair of the axon. Some materials, however, move very rapidly at rates of 10–200 mm/day. The materials involved in fast axoplasmic flow utilize neurotubules for their transport. These materials are believed to be those involved with the synaptic func-

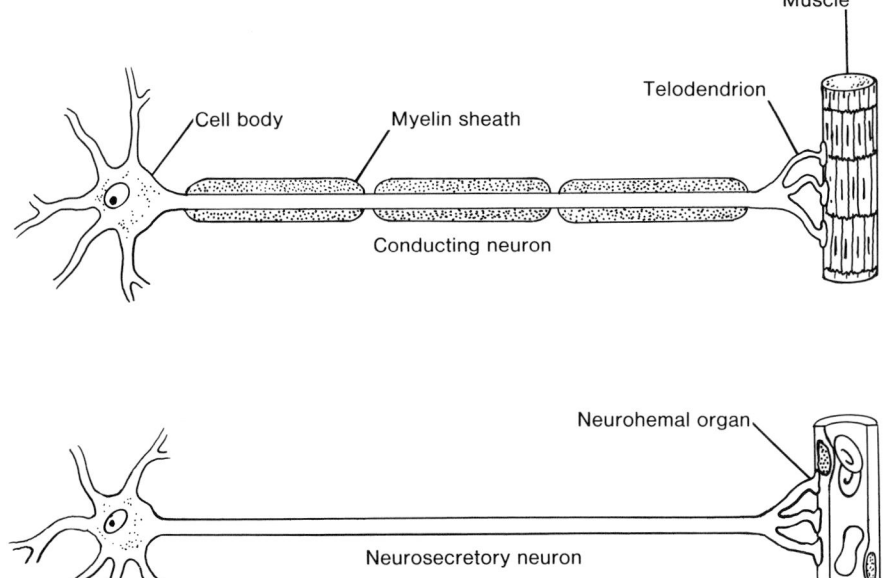

Fig. 12.3 A diagram of conducting and neurosecretory neurons.

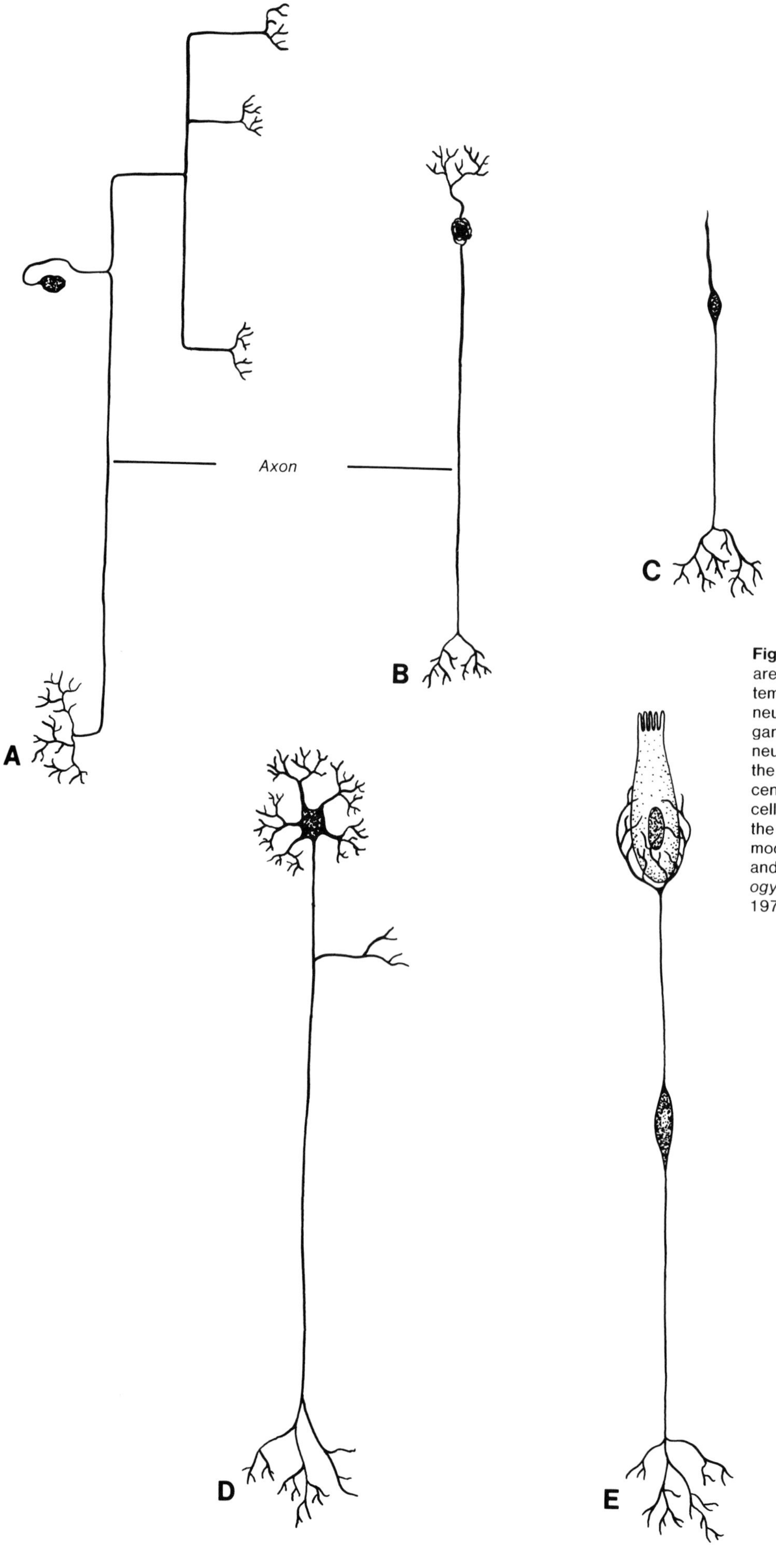

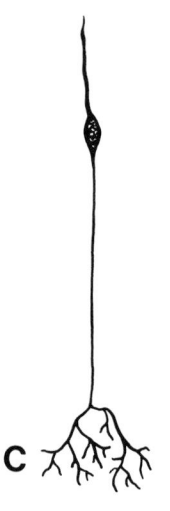

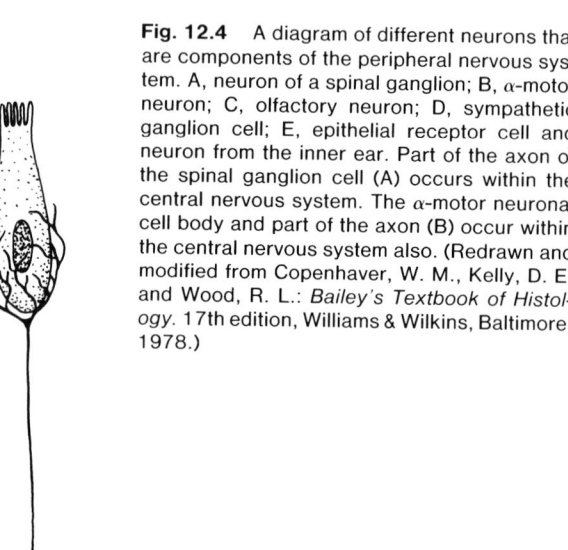

Axon

A

B

C

D

E

Fig. 12.4 A diagram of different neurons that are components of the peripheral nervous system. A, neuron of a spinal ganglion; B, α-motor neuron; C, olfactory neuron; D, sympathetic ganglion cell; E, epithelial receptor cell and neuron from the inner ear. Part of the axon of the spinal ganglion cell (A) occurs within the central nervous system. The α-motor neuronal cell body and part of the axon (B) occur within the central nervous system also. (Redrawn and modified from Copenhaver, W. M., Kelly, D. E. and Wood, R. L.: *Bailey's Textbook of Histology.* 17th edition, Williams & Wilkins, Baltimore, 1978.)

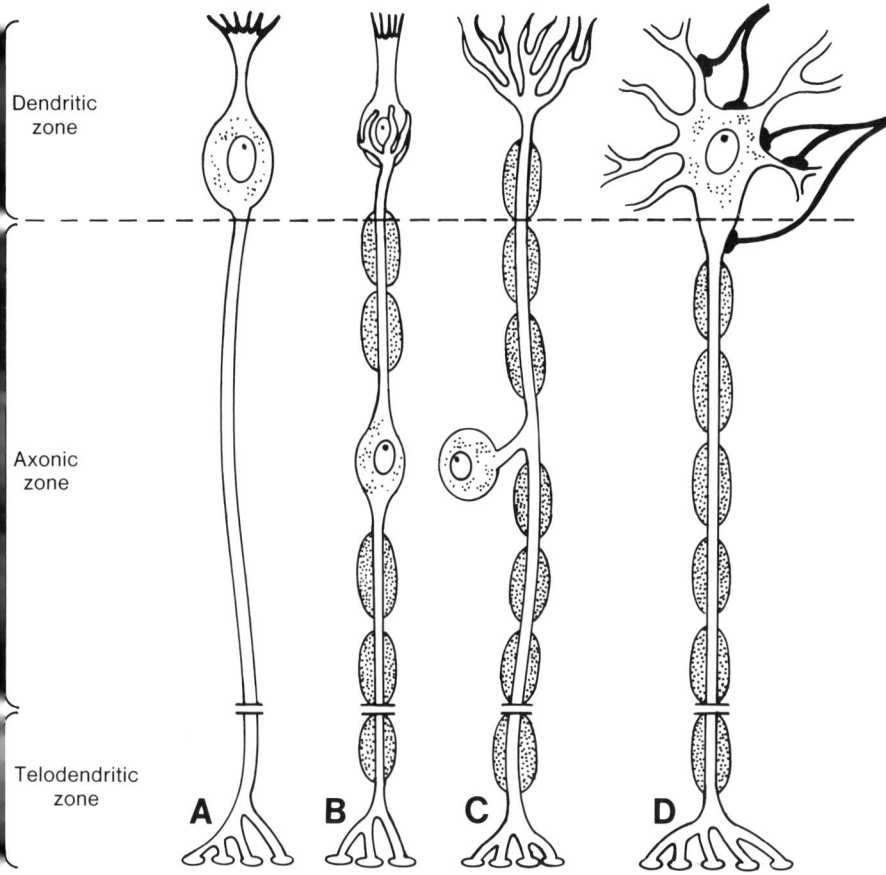

Fig. 12.5 The Bodian classification of neuronal components. The position of the cell body may vary, but three distinct yet related zones occur. A, olfactory neuron, B, epithelial cell and neuron of inner ear; C, dorsal root ganglion cell; D, α-motor neuron.

The left portion of the figure is labeled:
- Dendritic zone
- Axonic zone
- Telodendritic zone

A, B, C, D

tions of the axon. Because the cell body is responsive to alterations in its axon, *retrograde* (somatopetal) *flow* occurs also.

Information Transfer

Neurons are modified uniquely for generating and conducting information throughout the body in the form of electrical messages. Equally important to these functions is the ability to transfer information to effector organs and/or other neurons. The transfer of information occurs by two different mechanisms–*electrotonic* and *electrochemical transmission.*

Electrotonic Transmission. *Electrotonic transmission* in nervous tissue occurs at specific sites called *ephapses, electrotonic junctions* or *electrical synapses.* In tissues discussed previously, these sites of electrical transmission between cells (Figs. 11.5, 11.25) were called *gap junctions (nexi).* The essence of this relationship is the ionic coupling of intimately apposed cellular membranes with minimal intercellular space (Fig. 12.10). Electrical stimulation of cells related in this manner allows the unpolarized spread of excitation by ionic current flow between junctional components. Since the relationships are intimate, the contributing cell membranes function as a single unit and transmission is achieved rapidly.

Synapses. *Synapses* are *electrochemical transmission* sites that occur more commonly than ephapses. The electrical activity of the *presynaptic* nerve cell membrane causes the release of a neurotransmitter substance which traverses the intercellular space and joins to a *receptor site* on the adjacent *postsynaptic* cell membrane. The union of the neurotransmitter substance with the receptor site results in subsequent events in the adjacent cell which may be excitatory or inhibitory. The events associated with the release, diffusion and union of the neurotransmitter substance at the receptor site results in an increased transmission time referred to as *synaptic delay.*

Despite numerous variations, the following description is applicable to most synapses. Ultrastructural studies have clarified these relationships. Axonal terminations comprise the *presynaptic* membranous elements, while the adjacent cell or effector organ comprise the *postsynaptic* membranous elements. The pre- and postsynaptic membranes are separated by an intercellular space (*synaptic cleft*) which varies in width from 6–20 nm (Fig. 12.11) and contains electron-dense materials and fine filaments. Filamentous densities associated with the postsynaptic membrane comprise the *subsynaptic web.* The presynaptic terminal consists of mitochondria, neurofilaments, neurotubules and *synaptic vesicles.* Cytoplasmic densities may be associated with both the pre- and postsynaptic membranes (*symmetrical synapse*) or either membrane (*asymmetrical synapses*). However, intermediate forms exist also. Unlike electrotonic junc-

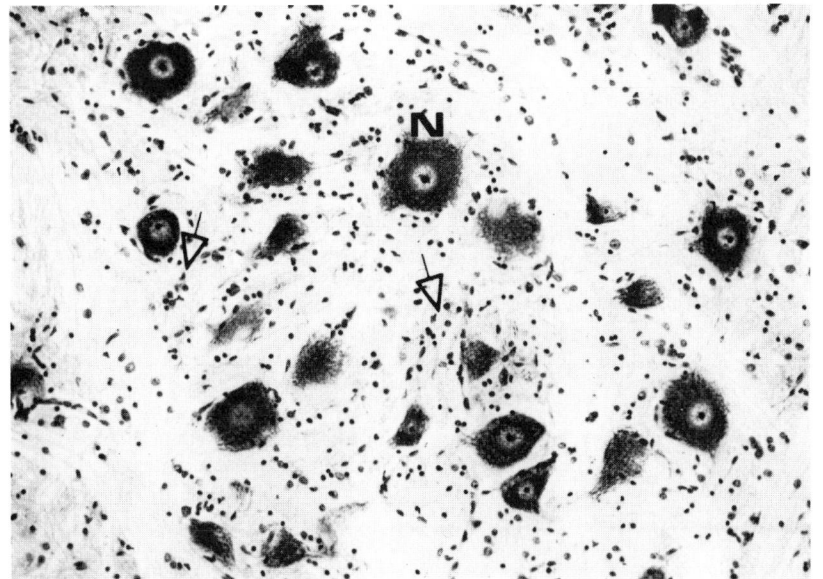

Fig. 12.6 Nervous tissue from the brain stem of a pig. The neurons (N) are distributed among numerous neuroglial cells (*open arrows*). The cell body at N is stained darkly. The round, pale-staining nucleus, with a prominent nucleolus, is located centrally. X40.

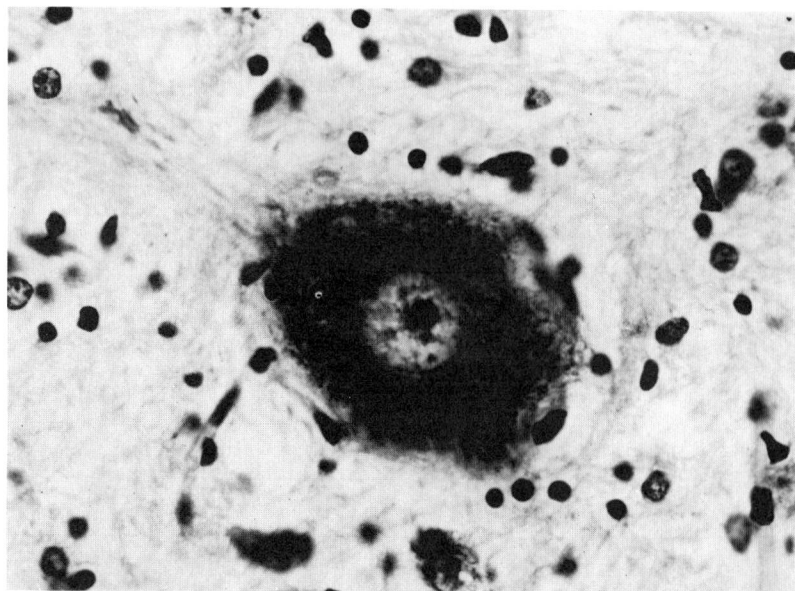

Fig. 12.7 Nissl substance of a neuron. The Nissl substance is the dark material in the cytoplasm. The nuclei of cells surrounding the neuron are those of neuroglial cells. Note the size difference. X160.

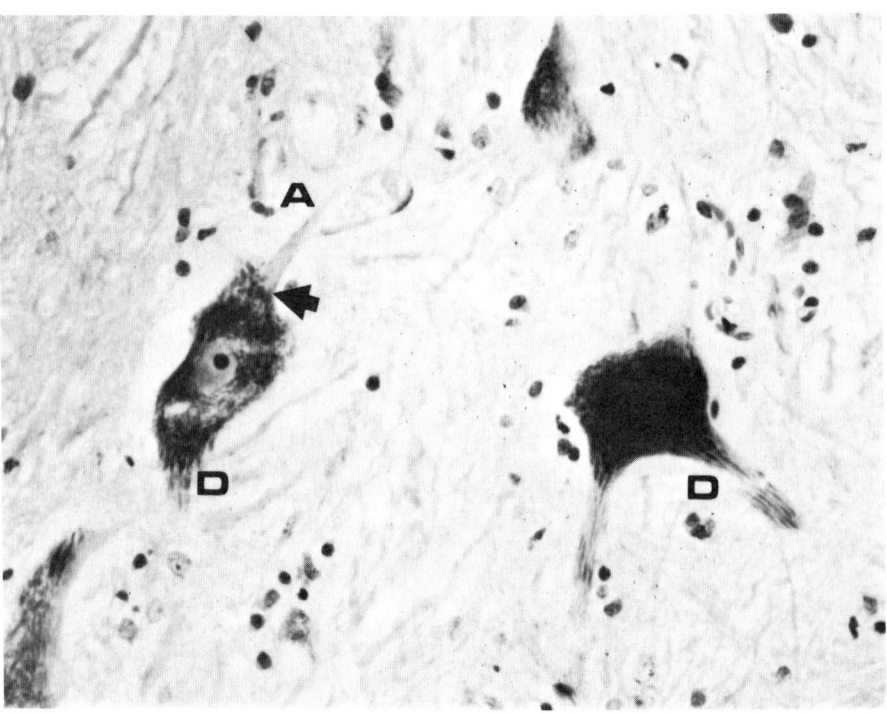

Fig. 12.8 Neurons from the brain stem of a dog. The axon hillock (*arrow*), devoid of Nissl substance, delimits clearly the origin of the axon within the cell body. X100. (Nocht's stain). A, axon; D, dendrites

synapses. *Axo-somatic synapses* involve the axon of one neuron and the cell body of another. In reverberating circuits the axon may stimulate its perikaryon of origin through an interneuron. *Axo-dendritic synapses* are variable but involve the axon of one neuron and the primary or secondary dendrites or dendritic spines of another neuron. *Axo-axonic synapses* involve two axons. Axon terminals are not the only structures that can comprise the presynaptic element of a synapse. *Dendro-dendritic*, *somato-dendritic* and *somato-somatic* synapses have been identified.

The *neuromuscular junction* is a special type of synaptic relationship between neurons and striated muscle. (See Chapter 14.)

Neurotransmitters and Receptors. *Neurotransmitters* are special chemical compounds that functionally link the presynaptic neuron to the postsynaptic neuron or effector organ. Although many compounds have been implicated as being neurotransmitter substances, only a few qualify on the basis of supportive experimental evidence. These include *acetycholine, norepinephrine, gamma-aminobutyric acid*, and *serotonin*. *Glycine, dopamine* and *glutamic acid* have been suggested also.

The presynaptic enlargement contains numerous *synaptic vesicles*. Presumably neurotransmitter substances are contained within or are bound to these vesicles. Upon appropriate presynaptic electrical stimulation, exocytosis occurs. These vesicles fuse with the presynaptic membrane and release their contents into the synaptic cleft. Subsequent binding to the receptor site accounts for the electrical activity of the postsynaptic membrane.

Two distinct populations of synaptic vesicles are identifiable. *Clear vesicles* occur in those neuronal terminals in which *acetylcholine* is the neurotransmitter. *Dense core or granular vesicles* occur in association with neurons that release *norepinephrine* or other catecholamines. *Cholinergic nerves* release acetycholine as the neurotransmitter, while *adrenergic nerves* utilize norepinephrine as the neurotransmitter substance. Cholinergic and adrenergic synapses have the ability to synthesize, secrete, degrade and reutilize all or portions of the neurotransmitters.

Acetylcholine is synthesized from choline and *acetyl-coenzyme A* (Fig. 12.14). This reaction is catalyzed by *choline acetylase*. The enzyme is active in the nerve terminals and is a specific marker for cholinergic nerves. Acetylcholine is stored in clear synaptic vesicles in synaptic terminals of these neurons and is released into the synaptic cleft upon nervous stimulation. *Acetyl-cholinesterase* (*true cholinesterase, specific cholinesterase*) occurs in the postsynaptic cell membranes and is responsible for the hydrolysis and subsequent inactivation of this neurotransmitter at cholinergic receptor sites.

The synthesis of norepinephrine (and epinephrine) occurs according to the scheme in

tions, chemical synapses have a distinct morphologic presynaptic to postsynaptic polarity that is manifested functionally as a polarized or unidirectional flow of information from the presynaptic membrane to the postsynaptic membrane.

The presynaptic portion of the axis cylinder expands into bulb-like processes called *end bulbs, end feet* or *boutons* (Fig. 12.12). These expansions at the ends of the axons are called *boutons terminaux*, whereas such enlargements along the course of the axis cylinder are called *boutons en passage*. Boutons en passage occur along the axons of unmyelinated nerves or at nodes of Ranvier of myelinated nerves.

The axonal terminals can form synapses with various parts of other neurons (Fig. 12.13). Accordingly, they are designated axo-somatic, axo-dendritic and axo-axonal

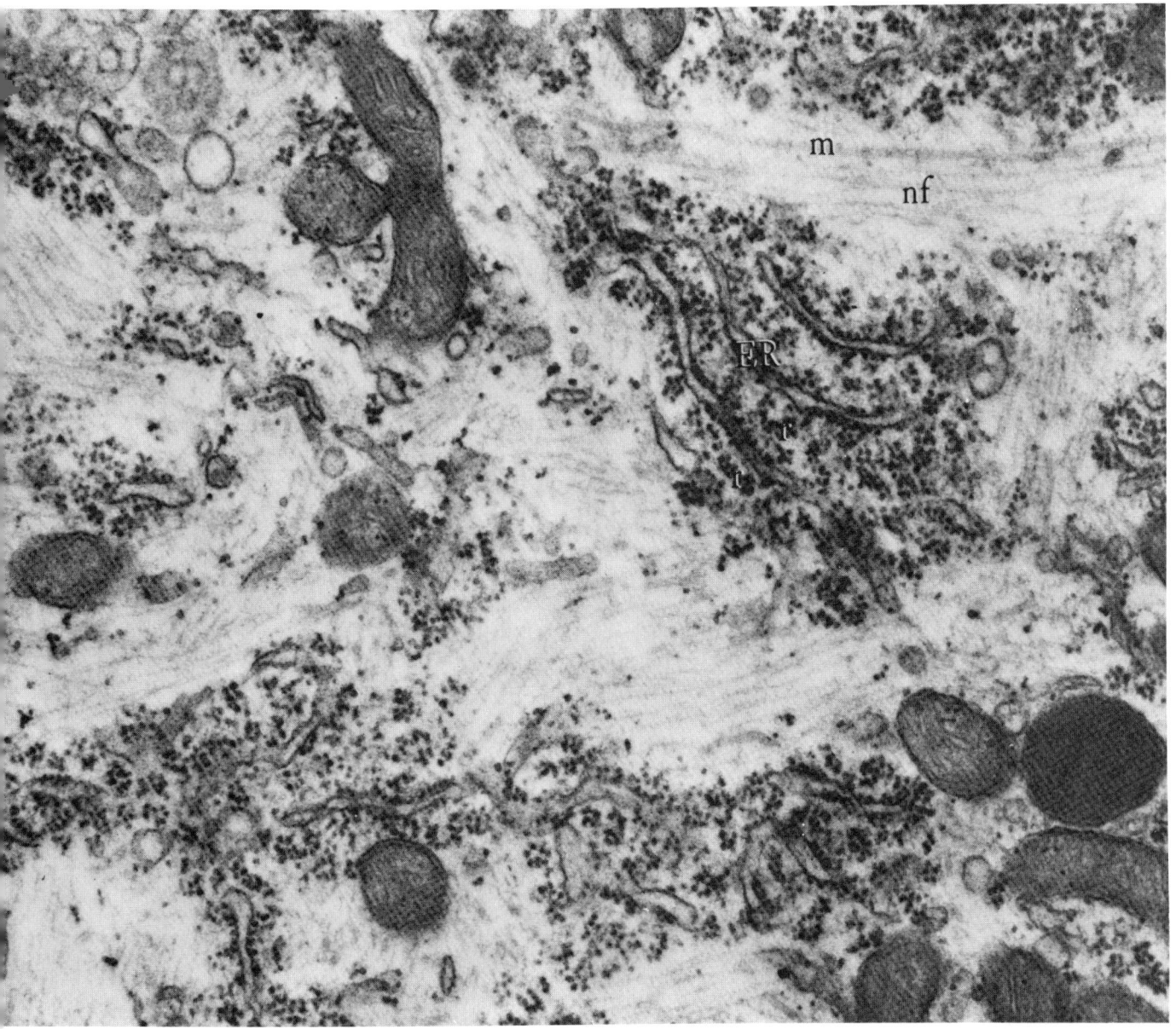

ig. 12.9   An electron micrograph of the cytoplasm of a murine dorsal root ganglion cell. The cytoplasm contains discrete Nissl substance omposed of rough endoplasmic reticulum (ER) and free ribosomes (r) and polysomes. Numerous neurofilaments (*nf*) and microtubules (m) are cattered throughout the cytoplasm. X49,000. (Reprinted with permission from Peters, A., Palay, S. L. and Webster, H. F.: *The Fine Structure of the ervous System: The Neurons and Supporting Cells.* W. B. Saunders, Philadelphia, 1976).

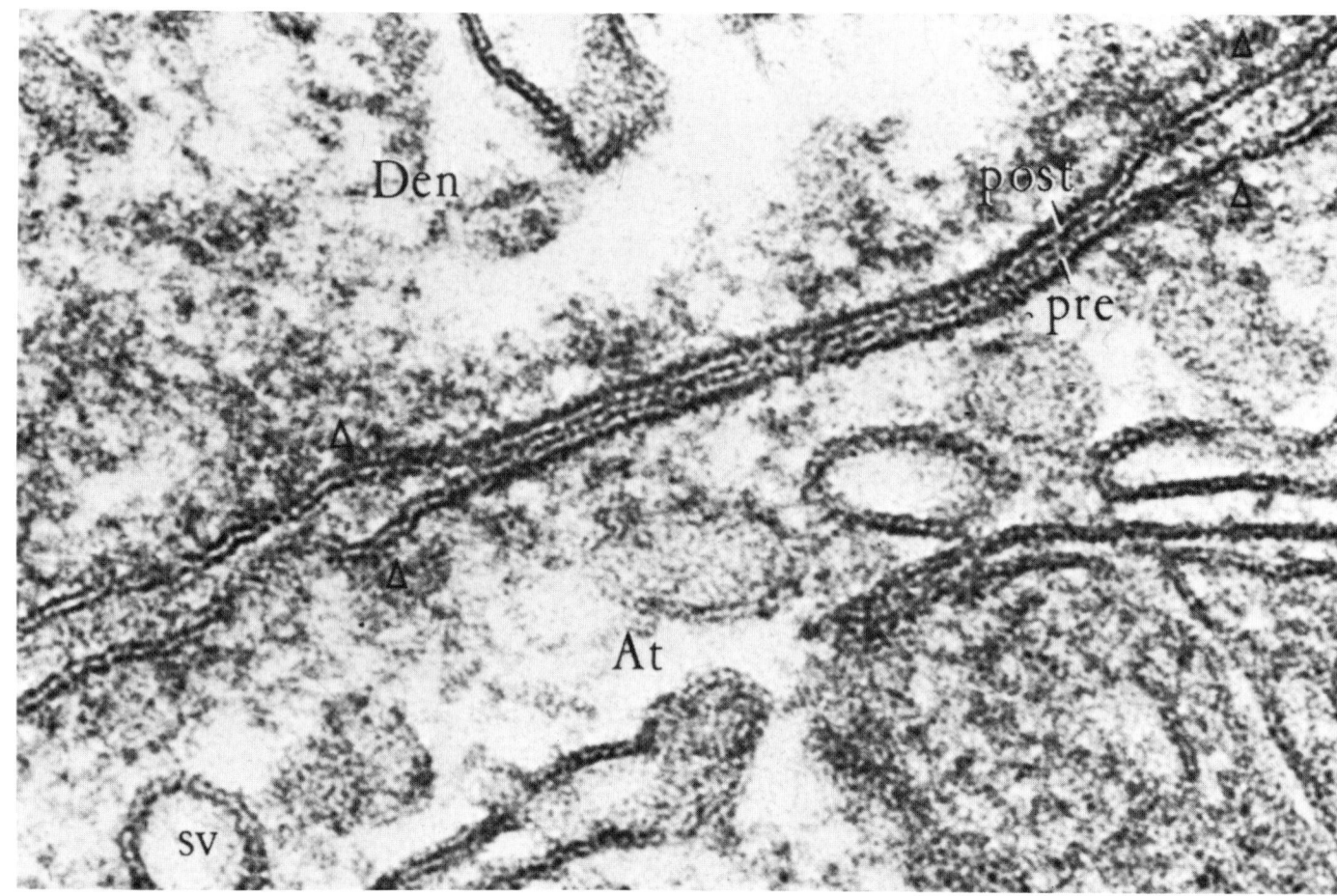

Fig. 12.10   An electrical synapse between a mossy fiber (*At*) and a granule cell dendrite (*Den*) within the cerebellum of a viper. Note the intimate juxtaposition of the pre- and postsynaptic membranes which diverge at the margins (△) of the gap junction to form punctate junctions. Synaptic vesicles (*SV*) are present within the mossy fiber also. X305,000. (Reprinted with permission from Peters, A., Palay, S. L. and Webster, H. F.: *The Fine Structure of the Nervous System: The Neurons and Supporting Cells.* W. B. Saunders, Philadelphia, 1976).

Figure 12.15. Most of the synthesis occurs within the dense-cored vesicles of adrenergic neurons. The degradation of norepinephrine (and epinephrine) is complex and is detailed in Fig. 12.16. The most important process in terminating the activity of norepinephrine (and epinephrine) is their reentry into the adrenergic neuronal terminals wherein they are oxidized by a mitochondrial enzyme, *monoamine oxidase* (*MAO*). The deaminated metabolites gain access to the blood and are excreted in the urine. The kidney and liver may deactivate norepinephrine (and epinephrine) also. *Catechol-o-methyl transferase* (*COMT*) of the kidney, liver and postsynaptic membrane may assist in the deactivation process by the methylation of these substances. The inactivated metabolites resulting from COMT and MAO activity may be conjugated with glucuronides via the activity of the hepatic enzyme *glucuronyl transferase*. Such conjugates are subject to excretion in the bile and recirculation via the enterohepatic pathway.

A *receptor* on or within the postsynaptic membrane is conceived as a molecular structure with which a single neurotransmitter substance reacts. The site may be an enzyme and/or a structural protein component of the membrane. Conformational changes of the receptor protein after its fusion with the neurotransmitter may account for membrane permeability alterations that follow this interaction. The stimulation of a receptor site results in two important postsynaptic events—excitation or inhibition. *Excitation* as a result of receptor stimulation is associated with a decreased polarity (*hypopolarization*) of the postsynaptic membrane. The alteration in polarity can be measured electrically as an *excitatory postsynaptic potential* (*EPSP*). Inhibition as a result of receptor stimulation is associated with an increased polarity (*hyperpolarization*) of the postsynaptic membrane. This altered polarity is measurable as an *inhibitory postsynaptic potential* (*IPSP*). The receptor site probably functions as a chemical gate in which stimulation results in a flow of ions that, in one case, increases the negative potential (hyperpolarization) beyond the normal resting potential of −70 mv. In the other case, the flow of ions decreases the negative potential (hypopolarization) to some value less than −70 mv. The potential for excitation or inhibition of the postsynaptic membrane resides with the receptor site, because a given neurotransmitter may elicit excitatory and inhibitory postsynaptic events.

The generation of an EPSP means that the postsynaptic membrane permeability status is more likely to lead to an action potential, while the generation of an IPSP means that the permeability status and increased potential is less likely to lead to an action potential. The *spatial* and *temporal summation* of EPSP's and IPSP's generally determine the ultimate response of the postsynaptic element (neurons or effector organs).

The receptor sites for cholinergic nerves may result in excitatory or inhibitory events. The fusion of acetylcholine with the receptor sites at a neuromuscular junction of skeletal muscle results in the influx of sodium ions, the depolarization of the cell membrane above the threshold for action potential generation and the activation or firing of the cell. In the heart, the fusion of acetylcholine with the cardiac muscle receptor sites results in an increased potassium

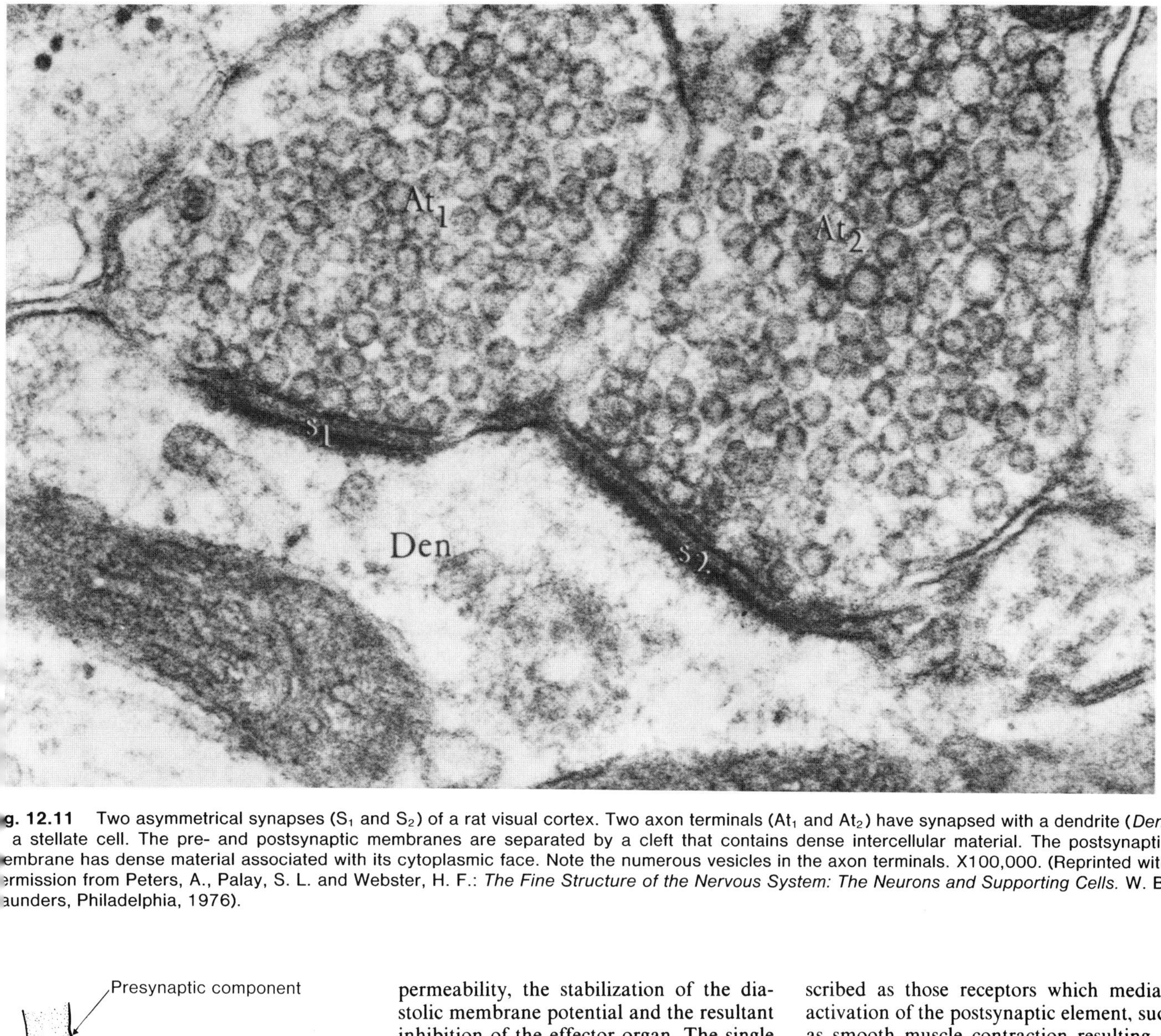

ig. 12.11 Two asymmetrical synapses (S₁ and S₂) of a rat visual cortex. Two axon terminals (At₁ and At₂) have synapsed with a dendrite (*Den*) a stellate cell. The pre- and postsynaptic membranes are separated by a cleft that contains dense intercellular material. The postsynaptic embrane has dense material associated with its cytoplasmic face. Note the numerous vesicles in the axon terminals. X100,000. (Reprinted with ermission from Peters, A., Palay, S. L. and Webster, H. F.: *The Fine Structure of the Nervous System: The Neurons and Supporting Cells.* W. B. aunders, Philadelphia, 1976).

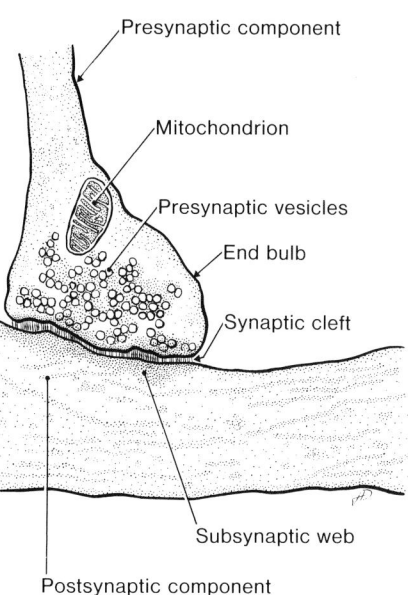

ig. 12.12 Diagram of a synapse. The pri-
nary constituents of the synapse are labeled.
synaptic morphology varies.

permeability, the stabilization of the diastolic membrane potential and the resultant inhibition of the effector organ. The single neurotransmitter, acetycholine, results in two different physiologic effects that are clearly the result of different acetylcholine receptors.

Adrenergic receptor sites are responsive to norepinephrine, the neurotransmitter substance of adrenergic fibers. Also, these adrenergic sites are responsive to the secretion of the adrenal medulla—*epinephrine*. Importantly, although norepinephrine manifests local effects, the effects of epinephrine are manifested throughout the body. These two substances are classified as *catecholamines*.

On the basis of the differential effects of epinephrine and norepinephrine (and other drugs) upon adrenergic receptor sites, two different receptors are defined. These are α and β receptors. Alpha receptors are stimulated by epinephrine and norepinephrine, whereas β receptors are affected by epinephrine and to a lesser extent by norepinephrine. Classically, the α receptors are de-

scribed as those receptors which mediate activation of the postsynaptic element, such as smooth muscle contraction resulting in vasoconstriction. However, there is one exception—α receptors are inhibitory to the smooth muscle of the intestines. Beta receptors are now divided into two types: β_1 and β_2 receptors. *Beta₁* receptors are stimulatory to the myocardium and inhibit smooth muscle of the intestines. The β_1 receptor stimulation of the heart results in an increased cardiac rate (*positive chronotropy*) and an increased strength of contraction (*positive inotropy*). *Beta₂* receptor activation is manifested as inhibition of smooth muscle contraction in the bronchioles, vascular beds and uterus.

The large body of evidence that permits the classification of adrenoceptors has created the illusion that these entities are morphologic realities and well-defined static membrane components. More than likely, they are dynamic structures with considerable molecular plasticity. The previous definitions of α, β_1 and β_2 receptors are the classical ones; i.e., organs would be supplied

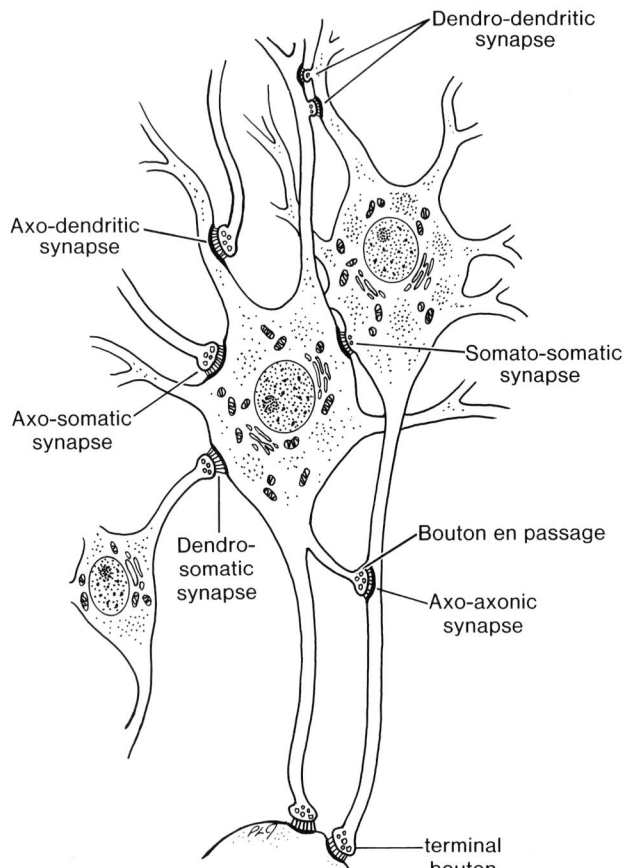

Fig. 12.13 A diagram showing different types of synaptic patterns. Although all of the synapses are drawn as the asymmetrical type, other patterns exist.

with unchanging α and β receptors or a combination of both. The equilibrium between the two (including β₁ and β₂ receptors) would dictate the type of response expected upon adrenergic stimulation.

Current evidence indicates that α and β receptors may represent different conformations of a metabolically controlled single molecular entity. Such modulation of receptor structures with its concommitant functional manifestations would permit the organism to respond to varying physiologic and/or pathologic conditions. Evidence in support of this includes the deviation from the expected response of adrenergic stimulation associated with temperature alterations, neurectomies, varying hormone levels (thyroid hormone, steroids) and specific adrenergic blockade. Further, such induced conformational changes may contribute to or result from various disease processes. Additionally, these conformational changes and the factors that may govern them may account for intraspecific and interspecific differences noted upon adrenergic stimulation in domestic animals. The diversity of response to these substances is vested in the uniqueness of the adrenergic receptors. Adrenergic receptors and the physiologic activities associated with them are discussed in detail in Chapter 15.

Neuroglia

General Considerations. The connective tissues of the body form an essential framework for most of the organs of the body. This framework serves not only a supportive role but is the means by which vascular components spread throughout the parenchyma. The intimate pattern of association and dependency is part of the structural aspects of the peripheral nervous system. These intimate relationships are not apparent in the central nervous system. The cells of the central nervous system, as well as some of its peripheral cellular components, are derivatives of the ectoderm. These cells are actually uniquely modified epithelial cells. Epithelia are dependent upon the connective tissues but are separated from them. The development of the central nervous system is characterized by the proliferation of closely juxtaposed cells and the differentiation of these cells into two distinct populations. One population, the neurons, develop complex geometrical patterns. The other population of cells develop between the neurons. By virtue of the intimate relationships of these cells to neurons, the second population of cells develop complex geometrical patterns. The second population of cells, the *neuroglia*, serves as the supportive network

or stroma of the central nervous system. The neuroglia constitute the "neural glue" that binds the neurons together. Besides a supportive function, they also protect, nourish and perform other functions vital to the integrity of the neurons. The peripheral nervous system also has neuroglial cells associated with it.

The neuroglial cells may be subdivided on the basis of their size. The *macroglia* include oligodendrogliocytes, astrocytes, ependyma, amphicytes, Schwann cells and Müller cells. The *microglia* are the microgliocytes. The neuroglia may be subdivided also on the basis of their association with the central or peripheral nervous systems. The *central glia* includes oligodendrogliocytes, astrocytes, ependyma, Müller cells and microgliocytes. The *peripheral glia* includes the amphicytes and Schwann cells.

Routine staining techniques are not useful for the demonstration of the cell bodies and cytoplasmic processes of most neuroglial cells. The routine identification of the central glial elements is predicated upon nuclear morphology. Special staining techniques, however, demonstrate their morphology well (Fig. 12.17). Peripheral glial elements are usually identified easily on the basis of their relationships to elements of the peripheral nervous system.

Neuropil is a term used to describe the complex, felt-like network in which the nerve cell bodies of the central nervous system are embedded. The neuropil consists of nerve cell processes (axonal and dendritic) and neuroglial elements of the gray matter. **Oligodendrogliocytes.** The *oligodendrogliocytes* of the central glia are the most numerous of the neuroglial elements (Fig. 12.18). These cells are characterized by a small, oval or round nucleus that contains a fair amount of heterochromatin. The nucleus,

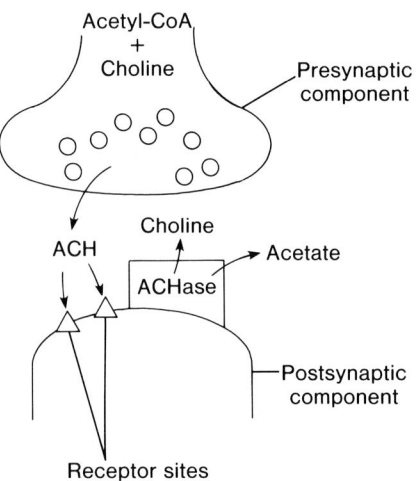

Fig. 12.14 A diagram of a cholinergic synapse. After attachment at the receptor sites ACH is degraded to acetate and choline by ACHase. Acetate diffuses into the surrounding tissues, whereas choline is returned to the presynaptic terminal.

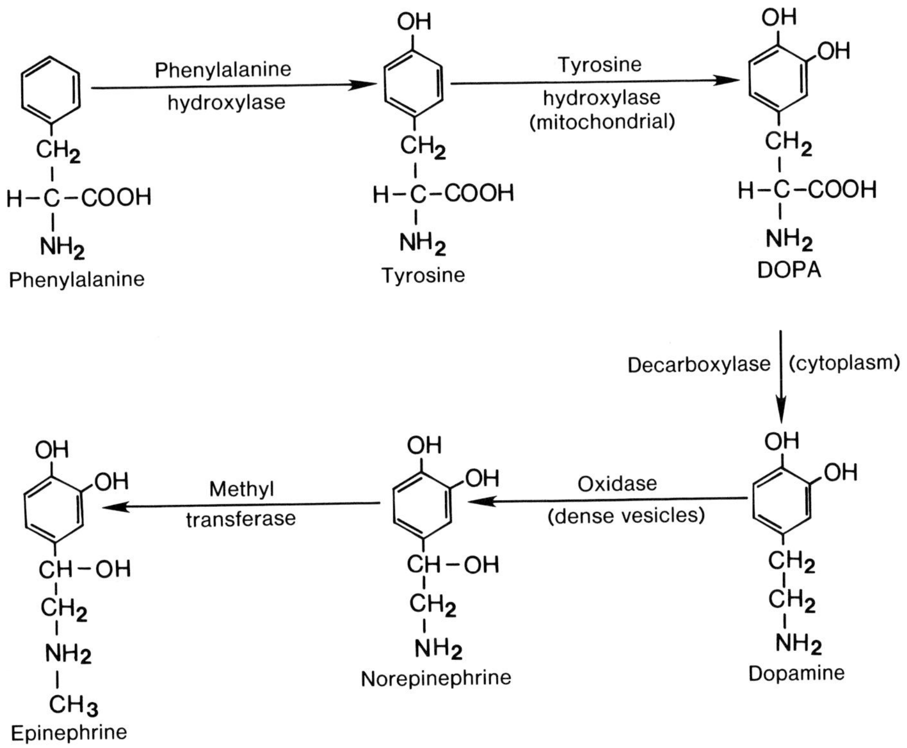

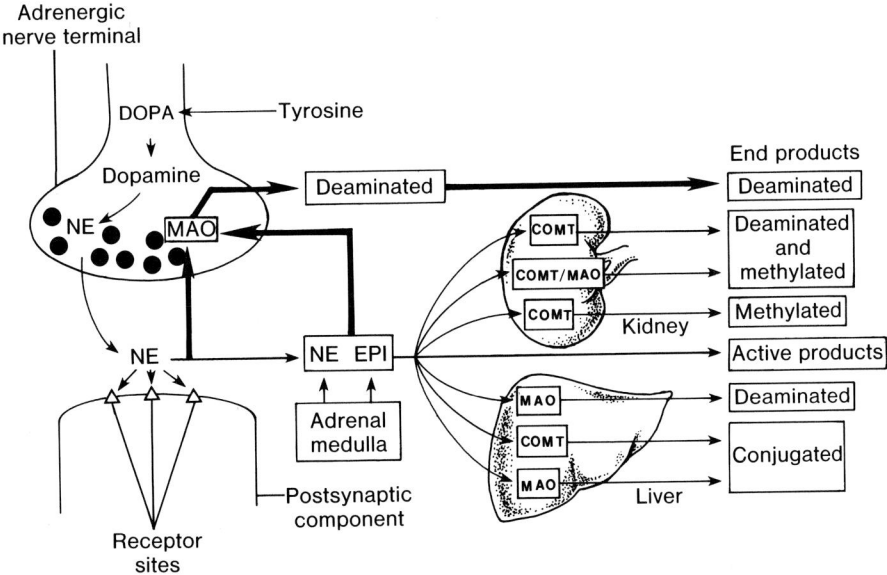

Fig. 12.15 The biosynthesis of catecholamines.

Fig. 12.16 The secretion and degradation of norepinephrine (NE) and epinephrine (EPI). Deaminated, methylated and conjugated products of epinephrine and norepinephrine are removed from the body by excretion and elimination. The most important inactivation process involves the deamination of the active products by the adrenergic nerve terminals.

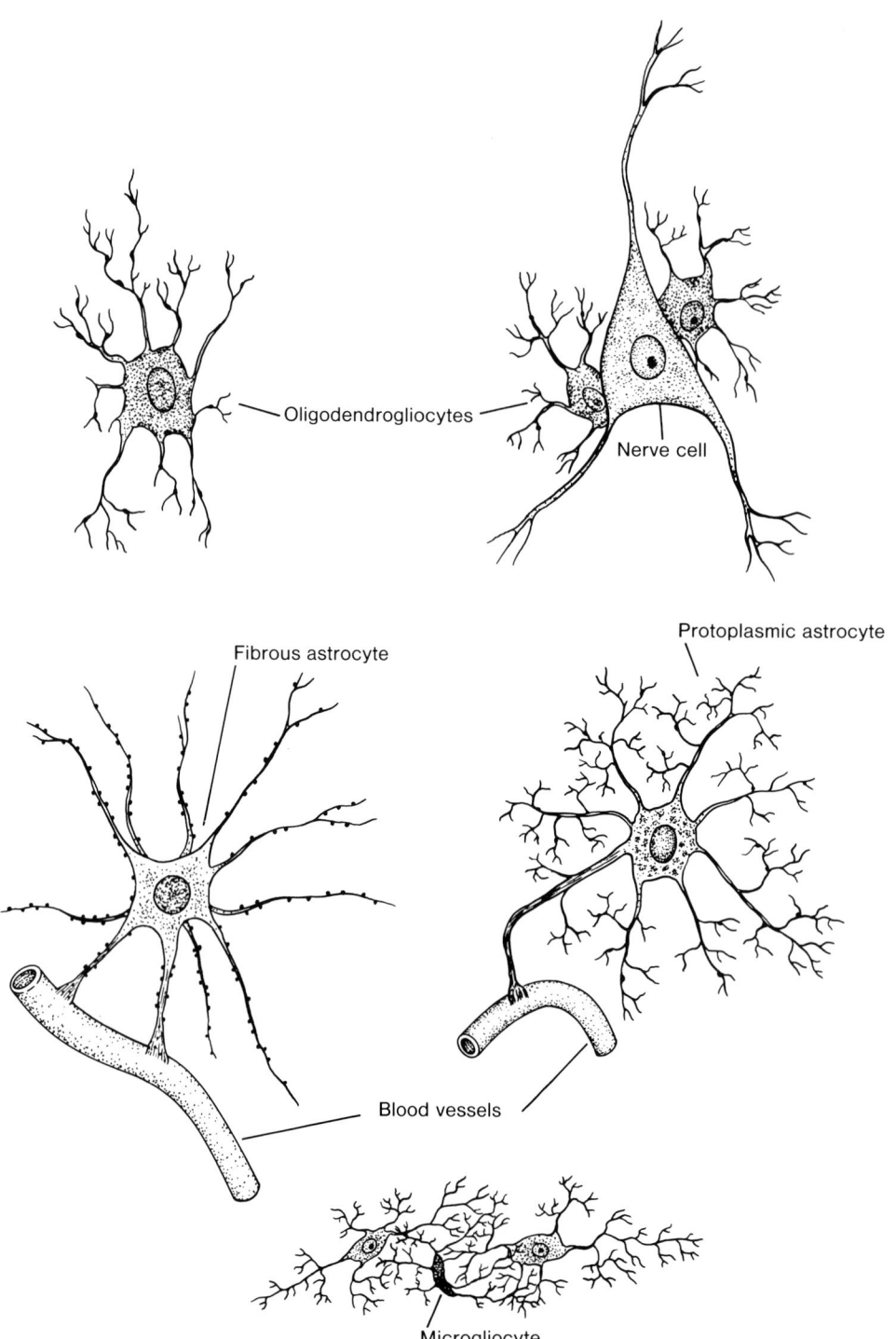

Fig. 12.17   A diagram of the morphology of central neuroglial cells as visualized with silver staining techniques. (Redrawn and modified from Copenhaver, W. M., Kelly, D. E. and Wood, R. L.: *Bailey's Textbook of Histology*, 17th edition, Williams & Wilkins, Baltimore, 1978.)

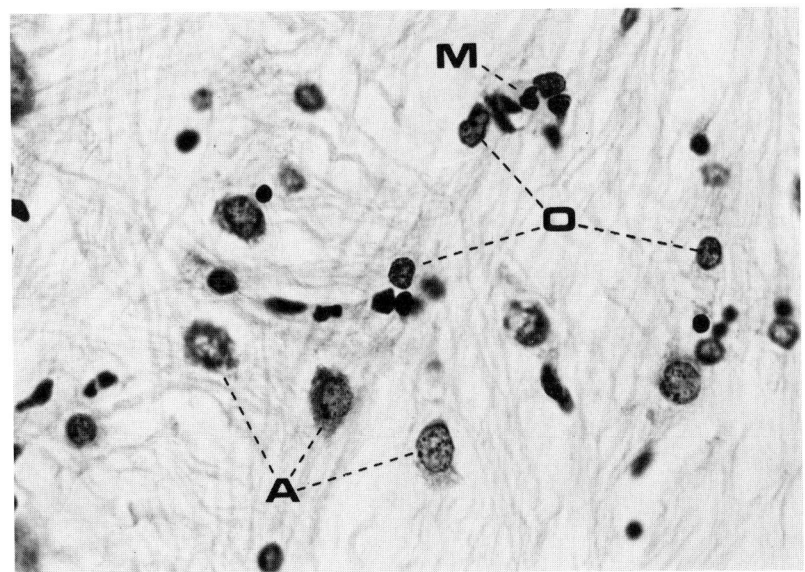

Fig. 12.18 Neurogliocytes from the brain stem of a pig. The oligodendrogliocytes (O), astrocytes (A) and microgliocytes (M) are indicated. X160.

however, may vary from large and pale to small and dark. Generally, this nucleus is smaller and more round than that of the astrocyte. The oligodendrogliocyte contains scant amounts of cytoplasm and few cellular processes. These cells are interdigitated between nerve cell processes and nerve cell bodies. Also, they are intimately associated with the capillaries of the vascular bed. Oligodendrogliocytes, therefore, may be perineuronal, perivascular or interfascicular. Perineuronal oligodendrogliocytes may perform some type of nutritional function. In some regions of the feline brain as much as 90% of the surface area of the cell body may be covered by these cells.

Oligodendrogliocytes are responsible for myelination of nerve cell processes within the central nervous system. This function influences the speed of conduction along nerve cell processes.

Astrocytes. The *astrocytes* are the next most frequently encountered neuroglial cells of the central nervous system (Fig. 12.18). Astrocytes or spider cells are divided into two different types, *fibrous* and *protoplasmic*. The major difference between these cell types is that one has more cytoplasm than the other. The fibrous type is abundant in the white matter and the protoplasmic type is common in the gray matter. Both have a large, round or oval nucleus which is usually quite pale. Chromatin granules are fine but may be clumped next to the inner nuclear membrane.

Astrocytes are important cells in the structural support of the brain and spinal cord. The fibrous processes, especially, impart a weave-like texture and supportive framework around the neuronal processes. Astrocytes form the *outer glial limitans*. These cells are responsible for the repair of nervous tissue defects and the formation of central

nervous system scars. Astrocytes can become hypertrophic, hyperplastic and phagocytic. Astrocytes serve to isolate neuronal receptor surfaces by serving an insulating function. Clasically, these cells contribute to the *blood-brain boundary* or *barrier*.

Microgliocytes. The *microgliocytes* are scattered throughout the central nervous system and are characterized by a scant cytoplasm which contains a small, dark nucleus (Fig. 12.18). The nucleus may be round, indented or irregularly-shaped. The cell body has numerous short processes. These cells are considered generally to be members of the macrophage system which are derived from promonocytes from the bone marrow (Fig. 6.49). However, this view is not shared by all investigators. Microgliocytes seem capable of phagocytosis in response to minor injury. Subsequent to extensive injury, phagocytic cells migrate from the blood vessels and accomplish functions ascribed to microgliocytes.

Müller Cells. *Müller cells* are neuroglial elements that are associated with the neurons that comprise the retina. These cells are discussed with the eye in Chapter 25.

Ependyma. *Ependymal cells* are neuroglial elements that line the neural canal (Fig. 12.19). Because of the nature of the embryologic origin of the nervous tissue, a tube is formed which is lined with epithelium that may vary from squamous to columnar. The epithelial lining is retained in the adult and is observed as the lining of the central canal of the spinal cord and the four ventricles of the brain. This lining is especially prominent and modified in areas where the *choroid plexuses* are formed. Embryonic ependyma are ciliated cells of a low cuboidal or low columnar configuration. The latter is retained in the adult; islands of cilia may be observed projecting from the brushlike lu-

minal border. These cells have large, pale nuclei with one or more nucleoli. The basal borders, in the adult, reside on a basement membrane and are separated from the nervous tissue. In younger animals, however, the basal modifications are quite complex and cellular processes may extend through the mantle layer of the developing nervous tissue.

The functions of the ependymal cells are varied. Ependymal cells contribute significantly to the formation of cerebrospinal fluid. This formative process is not confined to areas in which the ependyma is juxtaposed to the choroid plexuses but occurs at scattered sites throughout the ventricular system of the central nervous system. The ciliated ependymal cells are responsible for the movement of cerebrospinal fluid within the ventricular system. Nerve endings within the ependymal lining impart a sensory function to this layer of cells. The cerebrospinal fluid and thus the ependymal cells which help form this modified transudate may be involved in the transport of hormones. *Tanycytes* are specific cells of the ependymal lining which occur principally in

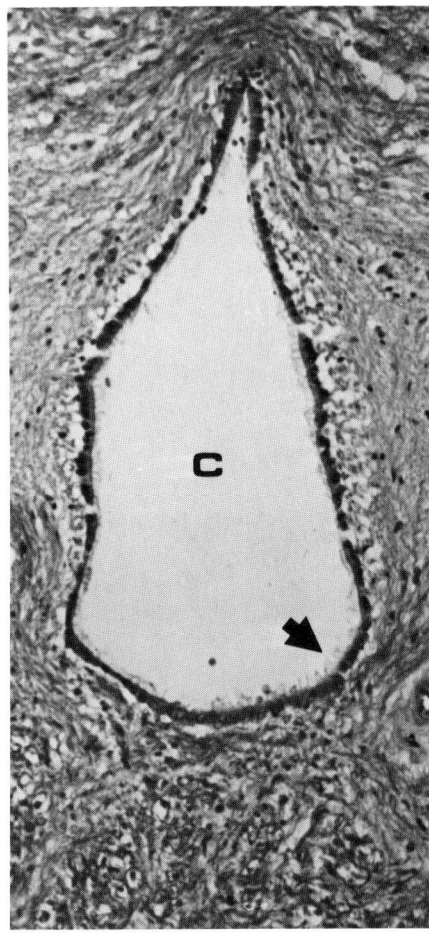

Fig. 12.19 Ependymal cells lining the neural canal of a canine spinal cord. The canal (C) is lined by columnar cells that are ciliated (*arrow*). X40.

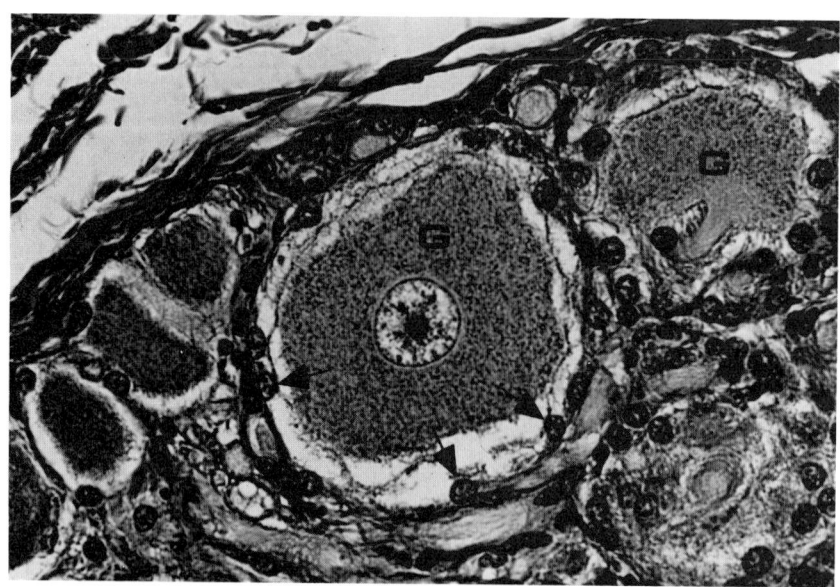

Fig. 12.20 Amphicytes and ganglion cells of a dorsal root ganglion of a dog. The amphicytes (*arrows*) surround the ganglion cells (G). The amphicytes have been separated from the ganglion cells artifactually by processing. X125.

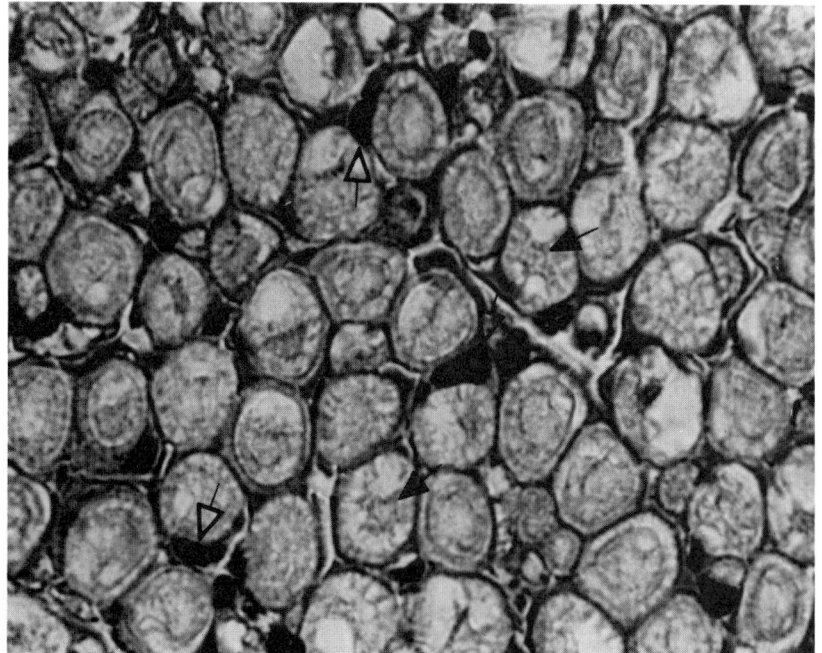

Fig. 12.21 A cross-section of peripheral nerve fibers. The Schwann cells (*open arrows*) surround the nerve cell processes. The axoplasm (*solid arrows*) is surrounded by the myelin sheath. X160.

the walls of the third ventricle. These cells have long, unbranched basal processes which extend into the subependymal area. The processes are juxtaposed to subependymal capillaries. Although they seem to serve a structural function, as evidenced by their morphologic configuration, they may be involved in transport and/or secretory activities. A clarification of their functional significance awaits further research.

The *subependymal organ* or region may be responsible for the replacement of neuroglial cells throughout the life of the organism.

Amphicytes. The *amphicytes (satellite cells, capsule cells)* of the peripheral glia are those neuroglial cells that surround the neurons of ganglia (Fig. 12.20). Although the capsule that they form is confined to the perikaryon, it is probably continuous with the sheath of Schwann. Amphicytes are probably closely related to oligodendrogliocytes.

Schwann Cells. *Schwann cells* of the peripheral glia are associated with nerve cell fibers (Fig. 12.21). They surround these fibers and are responsible for the formation of myelin. These cells, also, are probably closely related to oligodendrogliocytes.

Cellular Investments of Neurons

By virtue of their integrated development, the neurons of the central nervous system are associated intimately with the central neuroglial cells. These neuroglial elements comprise the cellular investments of cells of the central nervous system. Oligodendrogliocytes establish unique relationships with neurons by virtue of myelin sheath formation on nerve cell processes within the central nervous system. Nerve cell processes and certain neurons (ganglion cells) occur in the peripheral nervous system and are invested by neuroglial elements that assume relationships to the nerve cell bodies and processes similar to those described for the central nervous system.

The relationship of these cellular sheaths may assume various forms. The amphicytes of ganglion cells comprise a simple cellular covering over the cells. Unmyelinated nerves are contained within plasmalemmal invaginations of Schwann cells. Myelinated nerves also occur within invaginations of Schwann cells but are invested with wrappings of the plasma membrane which comprise the myelin sheath.

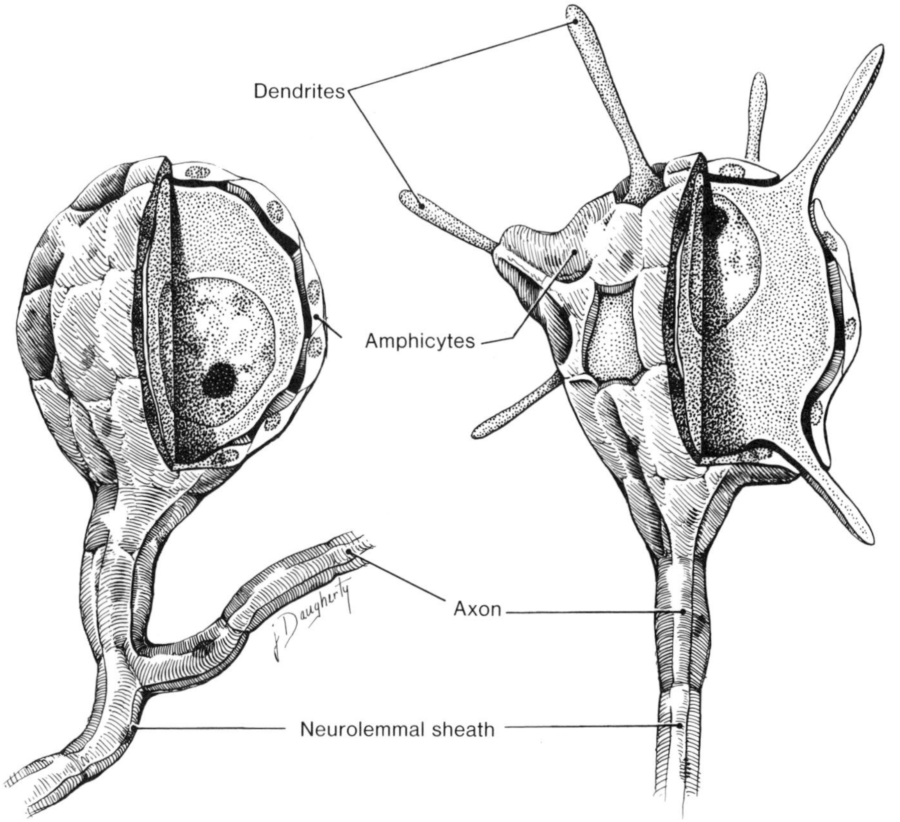

Ganglion Cell Sheaths. *Ganglion cells* are nerve cells that occur as part of the peripheral nervous system. Accumulations of their nerve cell bodies are called *ganglia*. The nerve cell bodies are covered by a layer of cells called *amphicytes* (Fig. 12.22). Although amphicytes usually form a continuous covering over the ganglion cells as in the dorsal root ganglia, the covering may be incomplete in autonomic ganglia. The investment is not confined to the cell body but may cover part of the dendrites as well as the initial segment of the axon. Amphicytes terminate at points of Schwann cell initiation. The distinction between amphicytes and Schwann cells may be artificial.

Unmyelinated Nerve Fibers. The Schwann cell forms the cellular investment for nerve cell processes. *Unmyelinated fibers*, or the *fibers of Remak*, are small fibers that are either unmyelinated or are invested only by a trace of myelin. Such fibers are contained within elongated invaginations in the Schwann cell (Fig. 12.23). The fibers, however, are not within the Schwann cell cytoplasm but are covered by the plasmalemma of the investing cell. Such investments are called *sheaths of Schwann* or *neurolemmal sheaths*. Similarly, Schwann cells are also called *neurolemmal cells*. The juxtaposed plasmalemmal components of the Schwann cell that encircle the axis cylinder are called *mesaxons*. A single Schwann cell can invest many nerve cell fibers.

Because a single Schwann cell only invests a nerve process over a limited distance, the neurolemmal sheath is composed of numerous juxtaposed Schwann cells. A basal lamina, located peripheral to the neurolemmal sheath, covers the Schwann cell and separates it from the surrounding connective tissue space (Fig. 12.23).

The exact function of the Schwann cell in this type of relationship is not clear; however, these cells are important in the repair process. Unmyelinated nerve fibers are small processes with relatively slow impulse conducting speeds.

Myelinated Nerve Fibers. These nerve fibers are the largest and most rapidly conducting fibers in the body. The myelin functions in a manner similar to the insulator on an electrical conductor. The oligodendrogliocytes and the Schwann cells are responsible for the formation of myelin. Although their methods and end products are slightly different, the result is that the nerve fiber is invested with a sheath of myelin.

The *axis cylinder* or nerve cell process contains axoplasm and is limited by a cell membrane, the *axolemma* (Fig. 12.21). The space adjacent to the axis cylinder is occupied by the myelin sheath. In routine preparations, however, the removal of lipids seriously alters the appearance of these membranous whorls. All that remains is the nonlipid component of the myelin sheath, *neurokeratin* (Fig. 12.24). Finger-like projec-

Dendrites

Amphicytes

Axon

Neurolemmal sheath

Dorsal root ganglion cell   Autonomic ganglion cell

Fig. 12.22 A diagram of the relationship of amphicytes to ganglion cells. The amphicytes form a complete covering around the ganglion cells of the dorsal root ganglion. The covering may be incomplete in autonomic ganglia.

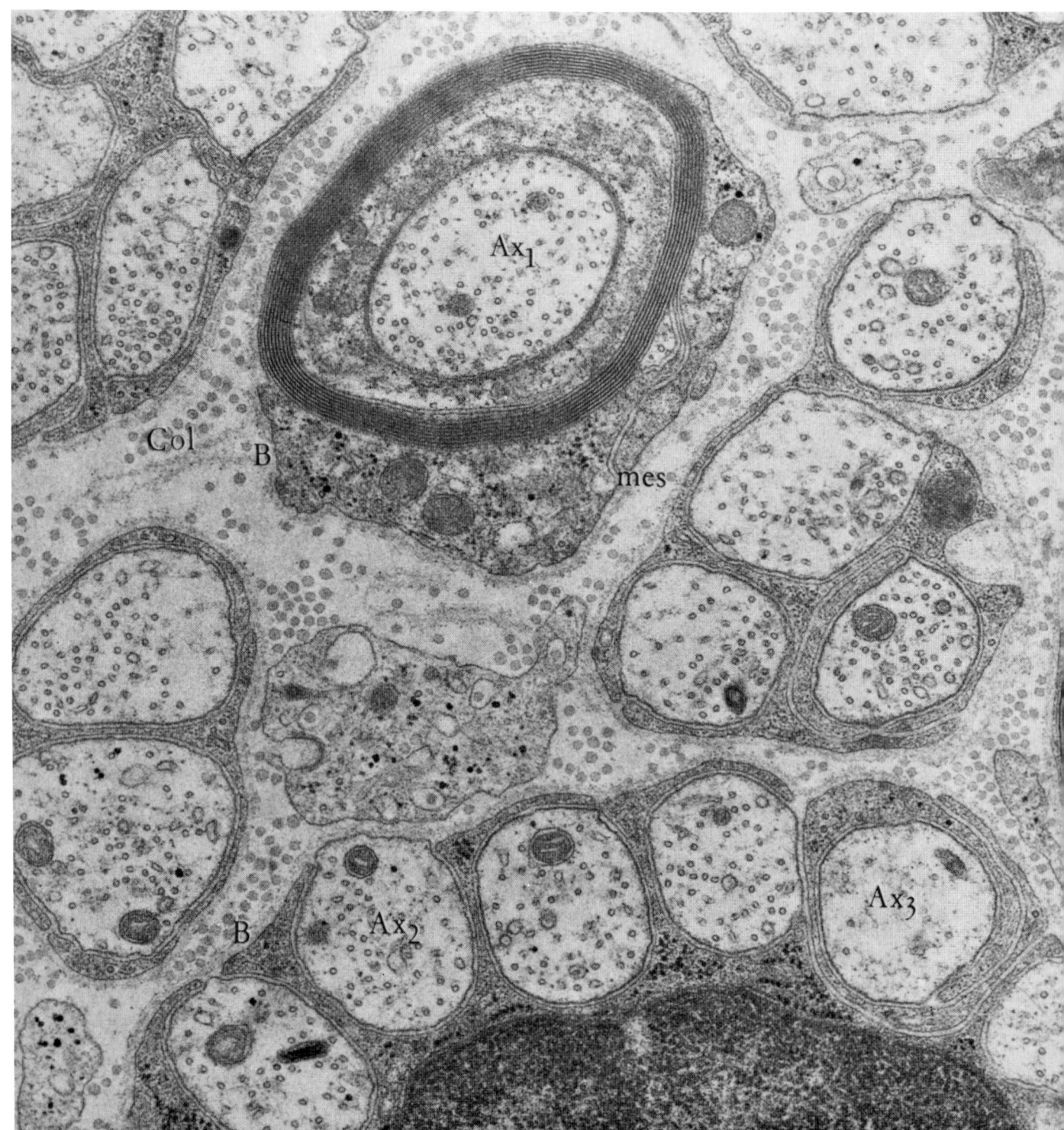

Fig. 12.23   A cross-section of the ischiatic nerve of an adult rat. A myelinated nerve fiber (top) is surrounded by a basal lamina (B) and collagenous fibers (Col). The axon (Ax$_1$) is juxtaposed to the Schwann cell cytoplasm. Note the outer mesaxon (mes) and its continuity with the myelin. Other axons are unmyelinated. Note the Schwann cell relationship to Ax$_2$, which is covered incompletely. A finger-like process of the Schwann cell surrounds Ax$_3$. The collagen is part of the endoneurium. X48,000. (Reprinted with permission from Peters, A., Palay, S. L. and Webster, H. F.: *The Fine Structure of the Nervous System: The Neurons and Supporting Cells.* W. B. Saunders, Philadelphia, 1976).

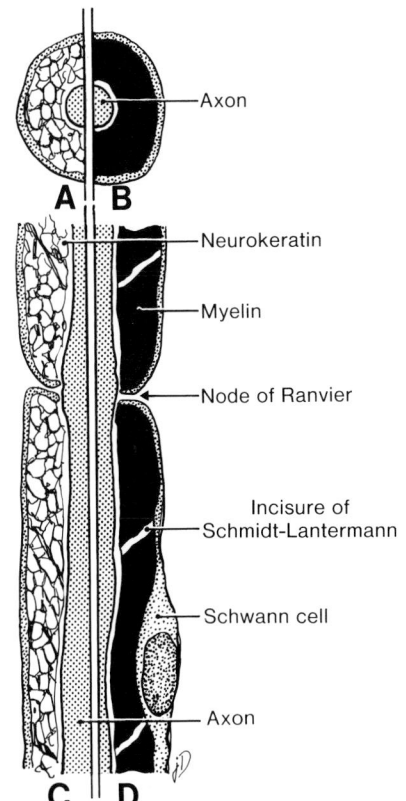

Fig. 12.24 A diagram of a cross-sectioned (A,B) and a longitudinally sectioned (C,D) peripheral nerve fiber. The routine preparation of nerve fibers by the paraffin technique alters the appearance of myelin (A,C). The protein remnants are called neurokeratin. Preservation of lipids and staining with osmium (B,D) presents the nerve fiber differently. Compare A and C with Figures 12.21 and 12.25. Compare B and D with Figures 12.26 and 12.27. (Redrawn and modified from Bloom, W. and Fawcett, D. W.: *A Textbook of Histology.* 10th edition, W. B. Saunders, Philadelphia, 1975.)

tions of neurokeratin appear as the spokes of a wheel. Peripheral to the remnants of the myelin sheath are the cells responsible for its formation, Schwann cells. These cells have a large, vesicular nucleus in which chromatin is clumped peripherally. The cytoplasmic, circumscribing remnants of Schwann cells are referred to as the *neurolemma* or the *sheath of Schwann.*

A single Schwann cell does not invest a nerve cell process along its entire length. Rather, the cell and associated meylin sheath extend a certain distance at which point another Schwann cell and associated myelin sheath are encountered. These breaks in continuity are referred to as *nodes of Ranvier* (Fig. 12.25). One Schwann cell covers the nerve cell process between two nodes. The nodes appear as constrictions along the nerve fiber at which point the myelin configuration stops, but the processes of the Schwann cell continue to contact the axolemma (Figs. 12.26, 12.27). Although the meylin sheath stops at the node, the axis cylinder continues through the nodal region uninterruptedly (Fig. 12.28).

Ultrastructural studies have clarified the relationships of the myelin sheath to the axis cylinder and neuroglial element (Figs. 12.23 and 12.28). The myelin sheath consists of continuous whorls formed by cytoplasmic processes of the neuroglial cell (Fig. 12.29). An *inner mesaxon* is formed by juxtaposed cellular processes of the Schwann cell adjacent to the nerve cell processes. An *outer mesaxon* represents the same relationship at the periphery of the myelin. The outer portion of the myelin sheath is covered by the cytoplasm of the neuroglial cell responsible for the myelination. A basal lamina covers the Schwann cell of peripheral nerve cell processes and separates it from the surrounding connective tissue.

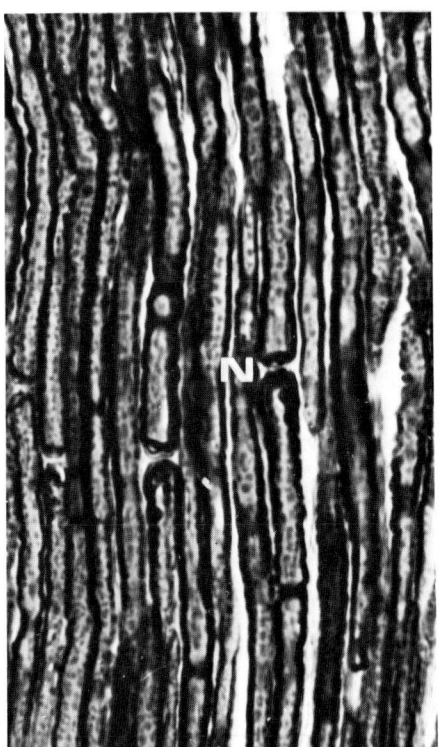

Fig. 12.26 A longitudinal section of the ischiatic nerve stained with osmium tetroxide. N, Node of Ranvier, Compare with Figure 12.24. X100.

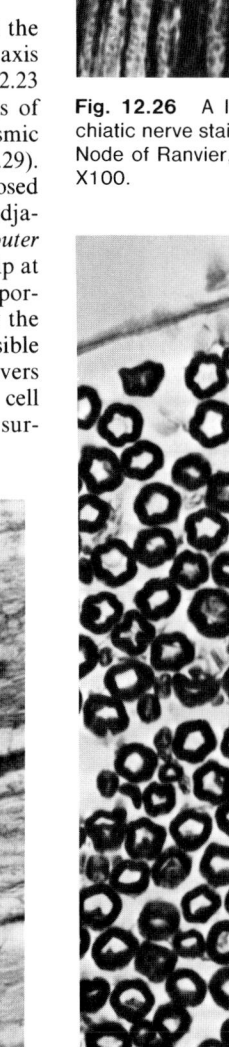

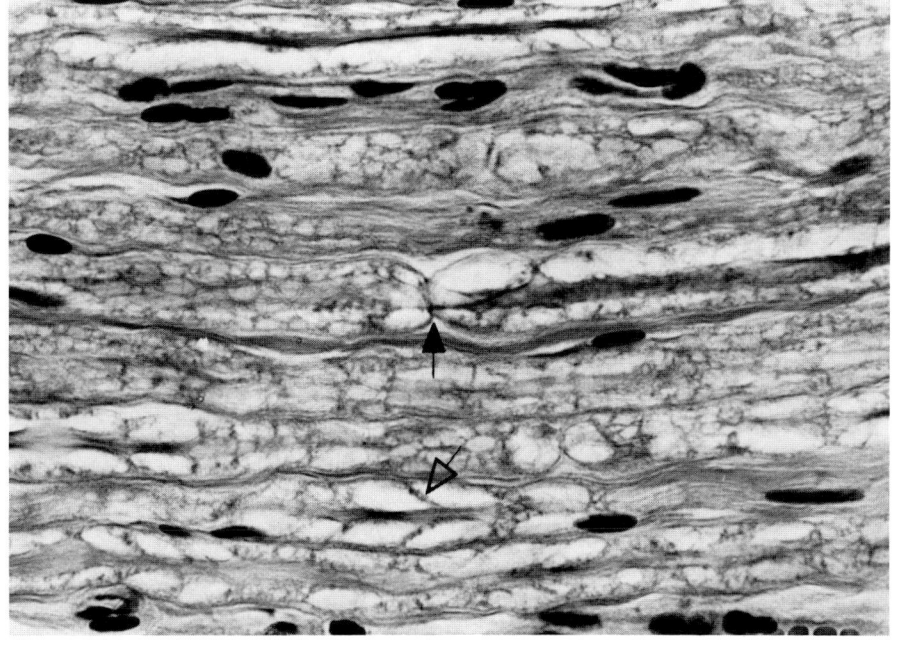

Fig. 12.25 A longitudinal section of nerve fibers. A node of Ranvier (*solid arrow*) and a cleft of Schmidt-Lanterman (*open arrow*) are visible. X160.

Fig. 12.27 A cross section of the ischiatic nerve stained with osmium tetroxide. The axis cylinders are unstained. Compare with Figure 12.24. X100.

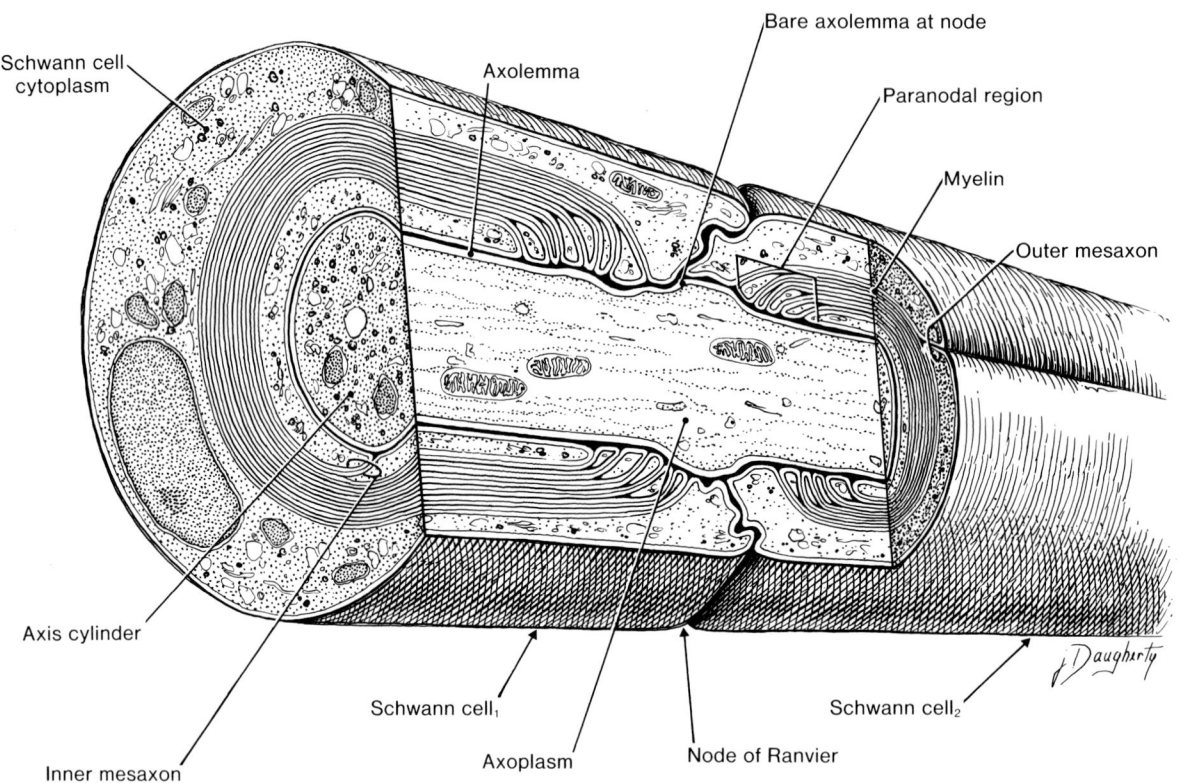

Fig. 12.28   A diagrammatic representation of the components of a myelinated nerve cell process. (Redrawn and modified from Bloom, W. an Fawcett, D. W.: *A Textbook of Histology*, W. B. Saunders, 10th edition, Philadelphia, 1975.)

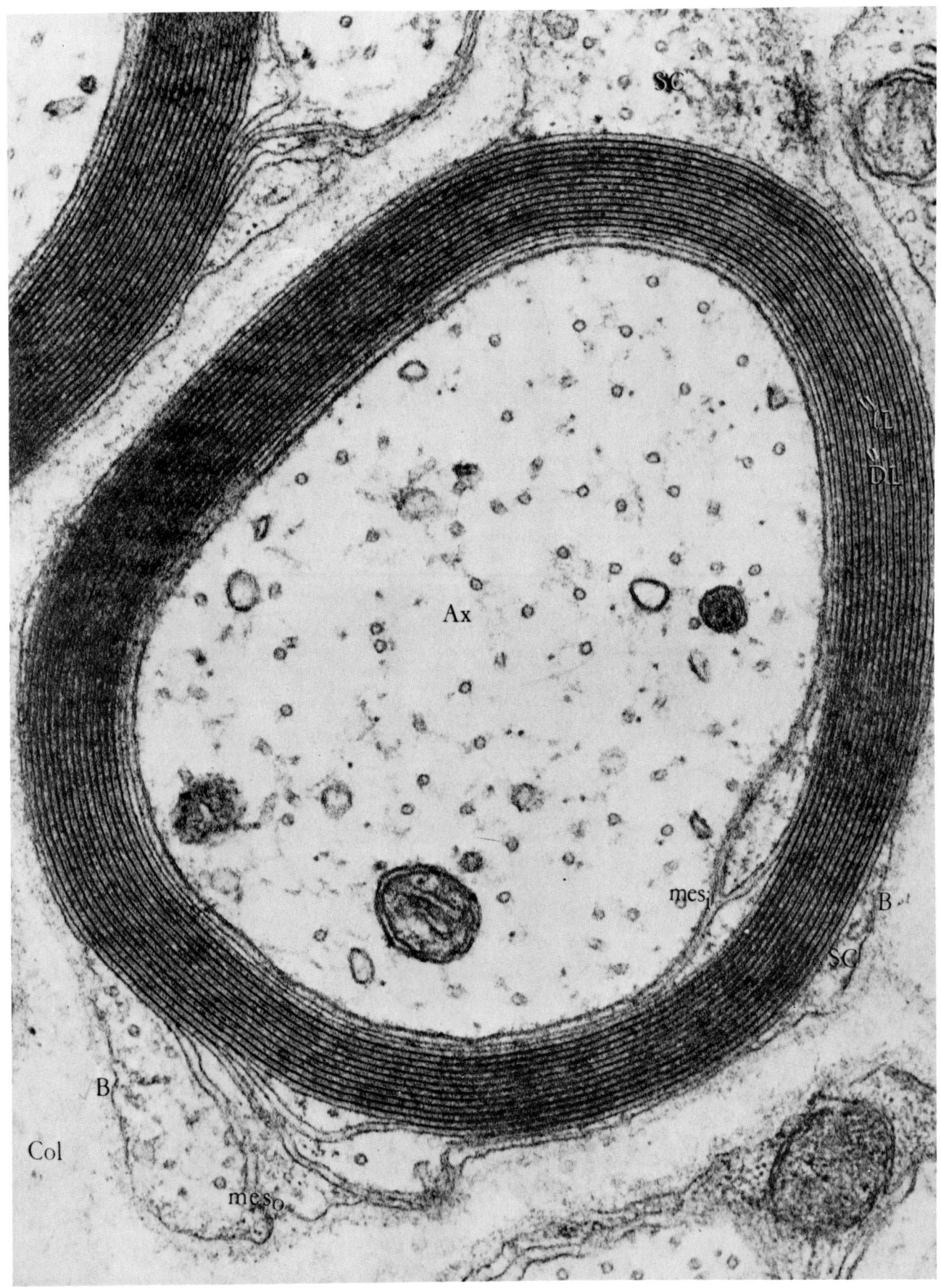

Fig. 12.29 A cross-section of a myelinated nerve fiber from the ischiatic nerve of an adult rat. The axis cylinder (*Ax*) is surrounded by a myelin sheath composed of spiralled sheets of the Schwann cell plasma membrane. Note the inner mesaxon (mes$_i$) and outer mesaxon (mes$_o$). SC, Schwann cell; B, basal lamina; Col, collagenous fibers. Major dense period lines (DL) and intraperiod lines (IL) are apparent. X100,000. (Reprinted with permission from Peters, A., Palay, S. L. and Webster, H. F.: *The Fine Structure of the Nervous System: The Neurons and Supporting Cells.* W. B. Saunders, Philadelphia, 1976).

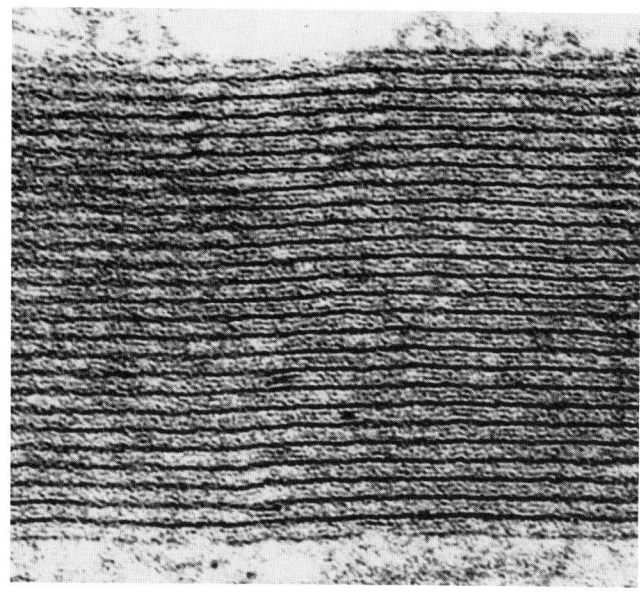

Fig. 12.30 An electron micrograph of myelin. The dark, major period lines and light, interperiod lines are visible. X154,000.

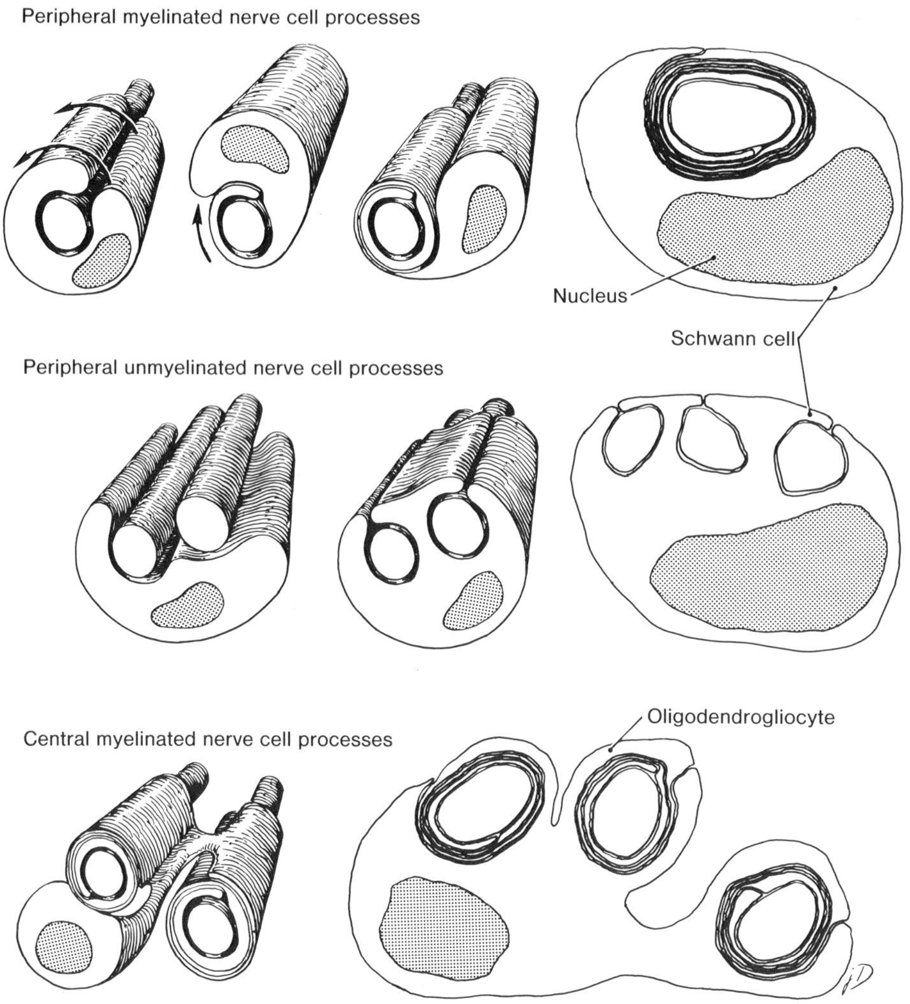

Peripheral myelinated nerve cell processes

Peripheral unmyelinated nerve cell processes

Nucleus

Schwann cell

Oligodendrogliocyte

Central myelinated nerve cell processes

Fig. 12.31 A diagrammatic representation of myelination in the central and peripheral nervous systems and the relationship of unmyelinated fibers to Schwann cells. See text for complete description.

The juxtaposition of successive layers of plasma membrane accounts for myelination. The outer leaflets of contiguous membranes fuse to form *intraperiod lines*, while the inner leaflets of adjacent plasma membranes fuse to form the *major dense lines* as the cytoplasm is extruded from the encircling process (Fig. 12.30).

Myelination. The *myelination* of a nerve cell process in the peripheral nervous system results from the intimate relationship established between these processes and Schwann cells. Similar relationships between nerve cell processes and oligodendrogliocytes result in central myelination. The relationships between unmyelineated fibers and neurolemmal cells, myelinated fibers and Schwann cells and myelinated fibers and oligodendrogliocytes are detailed in Figure 12.31.

Numerous unmyelinated fibers are associated intimately with a single Schwann cell (Figs. 12.23, 12.31). During *peripheral myelination*, a single nerve cell process occupies an invagination along a Schwann cell. A tongue-like projection of the Schwann cell winds around the axis cylinder (Fig. 12.31). As the cytoplasm within this process is lost, the plasma membranes become juxtaposed and fusion of membrane components occurs as described previously. The degree of myelination, or thickness of the myelin sheath, is proportional to the number of whorls that occurs during this process (Figs. 12.23, 12.29). A single Schwann cell is responsible for the internodal myelination of one nerve cell process and one internodal region. Moreover, the Schwann cell is associated intimately with the invested nerve fiber.

Although the process of *central myelination* by oligodendrogliocytes is similar to that which occurs peripherally, a few differences exist (Fig. 12.31). Connective tissue elements are not associated intimately with central nervous tissue; adjacent myelinated nerve fibers are not separated by a basal lamina. The repetitive unit of intraperiod and major dense lines is narrower in central myelin than in peripheral myelin. Centrally-myelinated nerve fibers do not have much oligodendrogliocytic cytoplasm associated with the myelin sheath. The cell body of the oligodendrogliocytes is not juxtaposed to the myelin sheaths but is connected to them by cellular processes. Also, one oligodendrogliocyte may myelinate more than one nerve fiber as well as more than one internodal region along the same fiber.

The neuroglial cells are important for the maintained integrity of the myelin sheath as well as being responsible for the re-myelination after demyelination that accompanies some diseases and injuries (Chapter 15).

References

Cellular Components
Bodian, D: The generalized vertebrate neuron. Science *137*:323, 1962.
Bondareff, W. and Hyden, H.: Submicroscopic structure

of single neurons isolated from rabbit lateral vestibular nucleus. J. Ultrastruct. Res. 26:399, 1964.

Eccles, J. C.: *The Physiology of Nerve Cells*. Johns Hopkins Press, Baltimore, 1957.

Fogelson, M. H., Gonates, N. K., Rorke, L. B. and Spiro, A.: Oligodendroglial lamellar inclusions. Arch. Neurol. 19:150, 1968.

Glees, P.: *Neuroglia; Morphology and Function*. C. C. Thomas, Springfield, 1955.

Hamberger, A., Hansson, H. and Sjostrand, F.: Surface structure of isolated neurons. J. Cell Biol. 47:319, 1970.

Luse, S. A.: Ultrastructure of reactive and neoplastic astrocytes. Lab. Invest. 7:401, 1958.

Palay, S. L. and Palade, G. E.: The fine structure of neurons, J. Biophys. Biochem. Cytol. 1:69, 1955.

Peters, A., Palay, S. and Webster, H. F.: *The Fine Structure of the Nervous System: The Neurons and Supporting Cells*. W. B. Saunders, Philadelphia, 1976.

Quarton, G. C., Melnechuk, T. and Schmitt, F. O.: *The Neurosciences*. Rockefeller University Press, New York, 1967.

Sandborn, E. B.: Electron microscopy of the neuron membrane systems and filaments. Canad. J. Physiol. Pharmacol. 44:329, 1966.

Vaughn, J. E.: An electron microscopic analysis of gliogenesis in rat optic nerve. Z. Zellforsch. 94:293, 1969.

Nerve Cell Processes

Bischoff, A. and Moor, H.: Ultrastructural differences between the myelin sheaths of peripheral nerve fibers and CNS white matter. Z. Zellforsch. 81:303, 1967.

Cravioto, H.: The role of Schwann cells in the development of human peripheral nerves. J. Ultrastruct. Res. 12:634, 1965.

Douglas, W. W. and Ritchie, J. M.: Mammalian nonmyelinated nerve fibers. Physiol. Rev. 42:297, 1962.

Hursh, J. B.: Conduction velocity and diameter of nerve fibers. Am. J. Physiol. 127:131, 1939.

Napolitano, L. M. and Scallen, T. J.: Observations on the fine structure of peripheral nerve myelin. Anat. Rec. 163:1, 1969.

Peters, A.: Observations on the connections between myelin sheaths and glial cells in the optic nerves of young rats. J. Anat. 98:125, 1964.

Uzman, B. G. and Nogueira-Graf, G.: Electron microscope studies of the formation of nodes of Ranvier in mouse sciatic nerves. J. Biophys. Biochem. Cytol. 3:589, 1957.

Transmission

Akert, K. and Waser, P. G. (editors): Mechanisms of Synaptic Transmission. Progr. Brain Res. 31, 1969.

DeRobertis, E. D. P.: *Histophysiology of Synapses and Neurosecretion*. The Macmillan Company, New York, 1964.

DeRobertis, E. D. P.: Ultrastructure and cytochemistry of the synaptic region. Science 156:907, 1967.

Dewey, M. M. and Barr, L.: Intercellular connection between smooth muscle cells: The nexus. Sci. 137:670, 1962.

Grundfest, H.: Synaptic and ephaptic transmission. In Quarton, G. C. et al. (editors). *The Neurosciences*. pp. 353–372, Rockefeller University Press, New York, 1967.

Gobel, S. and Dubner, R.: Axo-axonic synapses in the main sensory trigeminal nucleus. Experientia 24:1250, 1968.

Jones, D. G.: The morphology of the contact region of vertebrate synaptosomes. Z. Zellforsch. 95:263, 1969.

Katz, B.: *Nerve, Muscle and Synapse*. McGraw-Hill, New York, 1966.

Katz, B.: *The Release of Neural Transmitter Substances*. C. C. Thomas, Springfield, 1969.

Priedkalns, J. and Oksche, A.: Ultrastructure of synaptic terminals in nucleus infundibularis and nucleus supraopticus of *Passer domesticus*. Z. Zellforsch. 98:135, 1969.

Takeno, K., Nishio, A. and Yanagiya, I.: Bound acetylcholine in the nerve ending particles. J. Neurochem. 16:47, 1969.

COLOR PLATES

Plate I: Various Stains of Selected Tissues and Organs

Fig. I.1   A section of haired skin. The stratified squamous epithelium stains purple, whereas the dense connective tissue of the dermis is blue. The hairs are yellow, whereas the associated sebaceous glands are pale red. X40 (Masson's trichrome).

Fig. I.2   Bovine haired skin. The hair follicle in the center of the field is surrounded by yellow-staining dense connective tissue. A sebaceous gland is in the upper left. X40 (hematoxylin-phloxine-safran).

Fig. I.3   Dense white fibrous connective tissue (irregularly arranged). Collagenous fibers are pink. Sections of arterioles, a venule and nerve fibers are apparent in the upper part of the micrograph. X40 (Hematoxylin and eosin. This is one of the most popular stains used in histology.)

Fig. I.4   A section of porcine cerebellum. Large Purkinje cells occupy the interface between the granular (*right*) and molecular (*left*) layers. X40 (Hematoxylin and eosin).

Fig. I.5   A section of porcine cerebellum similar to that of Figure I.4. The dark-staining cells are Purkinje cells. X40 (silver impregnation).

Fig. I.6   A section of a feline ovary. Two vesicular follicles occupy the center of the field. The pink band around the oocyte is the zona pellucida. Primordial follicles are apparent along the right margin. X40 (Hematoxylin and eosin).

Fig. I.7   A section of a feline ovary similar to that of Figure I.6. The vesicular follicle is more mature and larger than those in the previous figure. X40 (Lendrum's phloxine tartrazine).

Fig. I.8   A section of a canine proximal femoral growth plate. The cartilage of the growth plate and primary spongiosa stains dark blue. Bone is pale blue. The bone marrow imparts a high cellularity to the primary spongiosa. X40 (alcian blue).

Fig. I.9   A ground section (50 μm) of lamellar bone. Pale-staining areas are old bone. Orange represents newer bone. Red is the newest bone. The green band internal and adjacent to the newest bone (*red*) is the osteoid seam. A resorption space is apparent (*upper left*). X40 (tetrachrome stain of Villenueva and Frost).

Fig. I.10   A tetracycline-labeled, ground section (50 μm) of bone from the fracture repair site of an equine third carpal bone. The fluorescent bands indicate bone deposition at the times of injection of tetracycline. X40 (fluorescence microscopy).

Fig. I.11   A section of elastic cartilage. A perichondrium (*yellow*) surrounds the mass of cartilage (Pentachrome stain).

Fig. I.12   Equine intestinal mucosa. Goblet cells are stained purple. X40 (Periodic acid-Schiff).

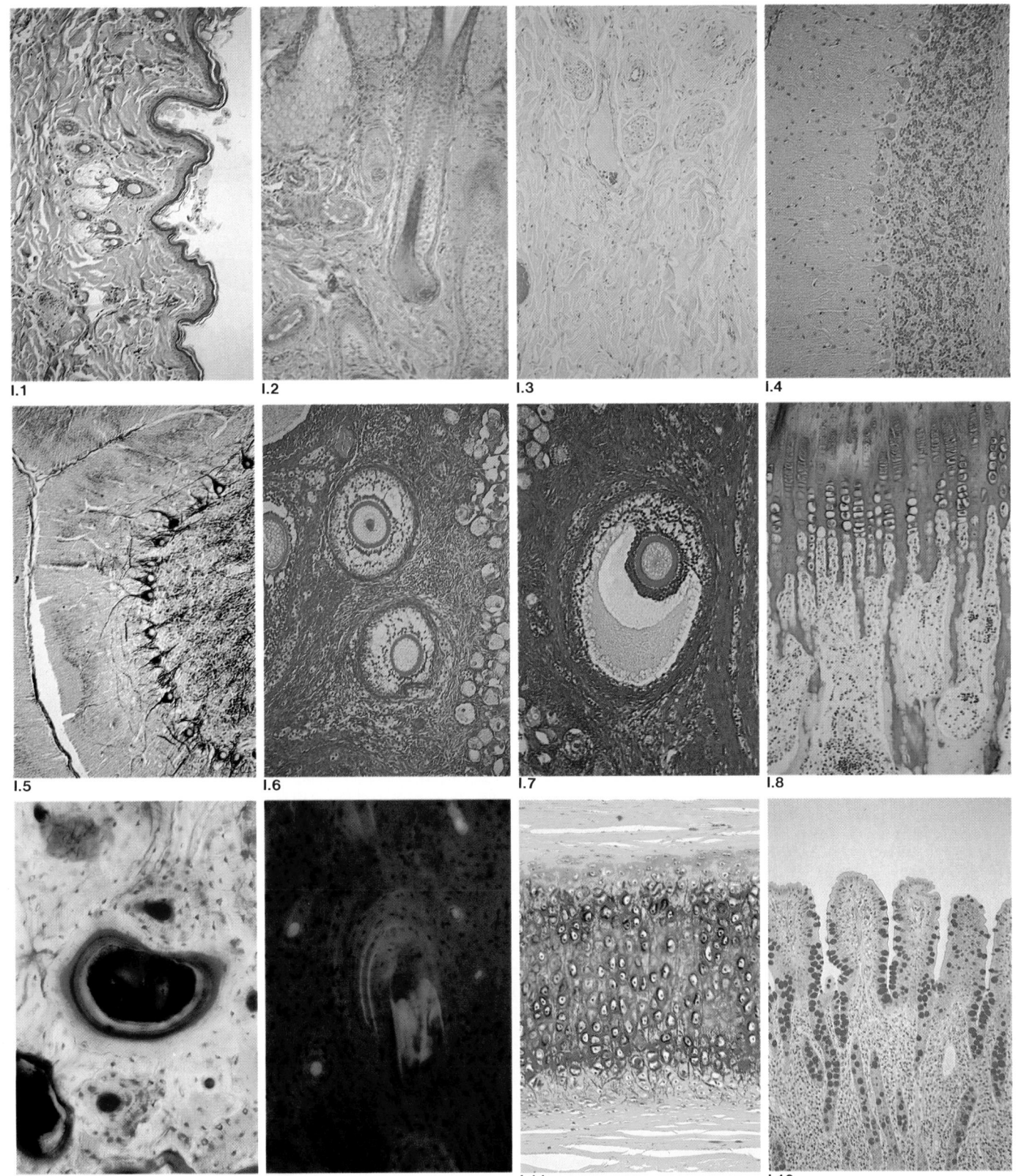

I.1   I.2   I.3   I.4

I.5   I.6   I.7   I.8

I.9   I.10   I.11   I.12

PLATE I

Plate II: Characteristics of Selected Cells

Fig. II.1   Leydig cells of a porcine testis. These steroid-producing cells have an acidophilic cytoplasm that may appear foamy. X400 (Hematoxylin and eosin).

Fig. II.2   A seminiferous tubule of a porcine testis. A Sertoli cell (*lower center*) has a large triangular nucleus that is positioned along the basal border of the cell. The cytoplasm is difficult to discern. Identification of the cell is predicated upon nuclear morphology. Spermatocytes (*round nuclei*) and spermatazoa (*elongated nuclei*) are evident also. X400 (Hematoxylin and eosin).

Fig. II.3   Steroid-producing cells of the zona fasciculata of an equine adrenal cortex. The cells have a vesicular nucleus and an acidophilic, foamy cytoplasm. X400 (Hematoxylin and eosin).

Fig. II.4   An osteoclast from bone. The large cell is multinucleated. The acidophilic and finely granulated cytoplasm contains numerous vacuoles. The brush border is evident along the bone-cell interface. X400 (Hematoxylin and eosin).

Fig. II.5   Osteoblasts from developing bone. The osteoblasts line the surface of a spicule of bone (*center*). The active cells have a vesicular nucleus and a basophilic cytoplasm. The cytoplasmic basophilia is from the extensive quantities of rough endoplasmic reticulum. Note the negative-staining Golgi zone in one of the cells (*left center*). X400 (Hematoxylin and eosin).

Fig. II.6   Mesenchymal cells from loose connective tissue. The large vesicular nucleus is the prominent cellular feature. The slightly basophilic cytoplasm is barely evident among the acidophilic collagenous fibers. X400 (Hematoxylin and eosin).

Fig. II.7   Cells of the bovine abomasum. The round to oval cells with bright pink cytoplasm are parietal cells. The cytoplasmic granularity results from numerous mitochondria. The cells secrete hydrochloric acid. The foamy cells in the center of the field are mucous-secreting cells. X400 (Hematoxylin and eosin).

Fig. II.8   Serous cells associated with the olfactory mucosa. The cuboidal cells have a centrally positioned nucleus surrounded by a finely granulated acidophilic cytoplasm. X400 (Hematoxylin and eosin).

Fig. II.9   Mucous cells from the glands associated with an equine ureter. The low columnar cells have a foamy cytoplasm and a basally positioned and flattened nucleus. X400 (Hematoxylin and eosin).

Fig. II.10   A cross-section through a pancreatic acinus (*arrow*). The pancreatic acinar cells have an apical acidophilia and a basal basophilia. The basophilia results from the accumulation of ribosomes and rough endoplasmic reticulum in the basal part of the cell, while the apical acidophilia is from zymogen granules. X400 (Gomori's chrome alum-hematoxylin). (Courtesy of R. A. Kainer.)

Fig. II.11   Nerve cell and satellite cells of a dorsal root ganglion. The ganglion cell has a large vesicular nucleus with a prominent nucleolus. Nissl substance is barely evident as a focal cytoplasmic basophilia. A nerve fiber is sectioned longitudinally (*right*). X400 (Hematoxylin and eosin).

Fig. II.12   A longitudinal section of skeletal muscle. The striations result from the registration of myofibrils. A dark A band is separated by a light I band. The I band contains a Z line. The *arrow* indicates connective tissue elements of the endomysium. X400 (Hematoxylin and eosin). (Courtesy of R. A. Kainer.)

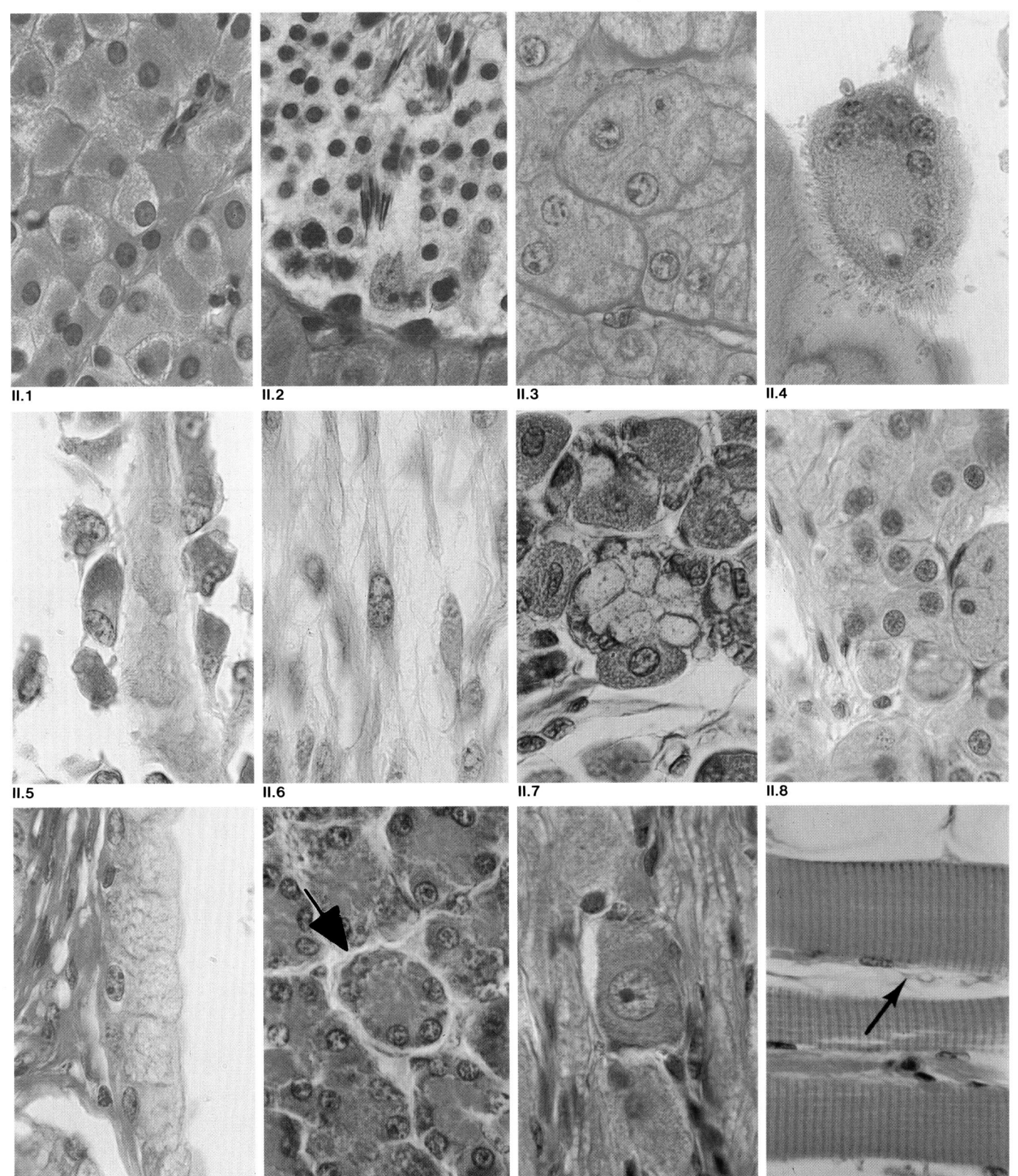

II.1

II.2

II.3

II.4

II.5

II.6

II.7

II.8

II.9

II.10

II.11

II.12

PLATE II

Plate III: Surface and Glandular Epithelia

Fig. III.1 Simple cuboidal epithelium of a salivary gland duct. X100 (Hemotoxylin-phloxine-satran).

Fig. III.2 Simple columnar epithelium of a canine stomach. The apcial borders of the cells are clear. X100. (Hematoxylin and eosin).

Fig. III.3 Simple columnar epithelium and goblet cells of the feline jejunum. The pale blue cells are goblet cells. X100. (Mallory's azan).

Fig. III.4 Simple columnar epithelium and goblet cells of the equine intestinal mucosa. The goblet cells and striated border are stained purple. X100. (Periodic acid-Schiff).

Fig. III.5 Keratinized stratified squamous epithelium of the canine muzzle. The pale-staining material (*top*) is keratin. Note the epidermal pegs and dermal papillae. X100. (Hematoxylin and eosin).

Fig. III.6 Nonkeratinized stratified squamous epithelium of the canine esophagus. X100. (Hematoxylin-phloxine-safran).

Fig. III.7 Pseudostratified ciliated columnar epithelium with goblet cells from a murine trachea. Bundles of smooth muscle fibers are present in the lamina propria mucosae. X100. (Hematoxylin and eosin).

Fig. III.8 Adenomere of an apocrine tubular gland surrounded by dense white fibrous connective tissue. X100. (Masson's trichrome).

Fig. III.9 Sebaceous glands. The alveolar glands are associated with a hair follicle. X100. (Masson's trichrome).

Fig. III.10 Equine pyloric glands. Note the typical mucous cell characteristics. X100. (Hematoxylin and eosin).

Fig. III.11 Mucous and serous cells within adenomeres of glands associated with respiratory mucosa. X100. (Hematoxylin and eosin).

Fig. III.12 Hepatocytes of the procine liver. The epithelial cells are arranged in cords. X100. (Hematoxylin and eosin).

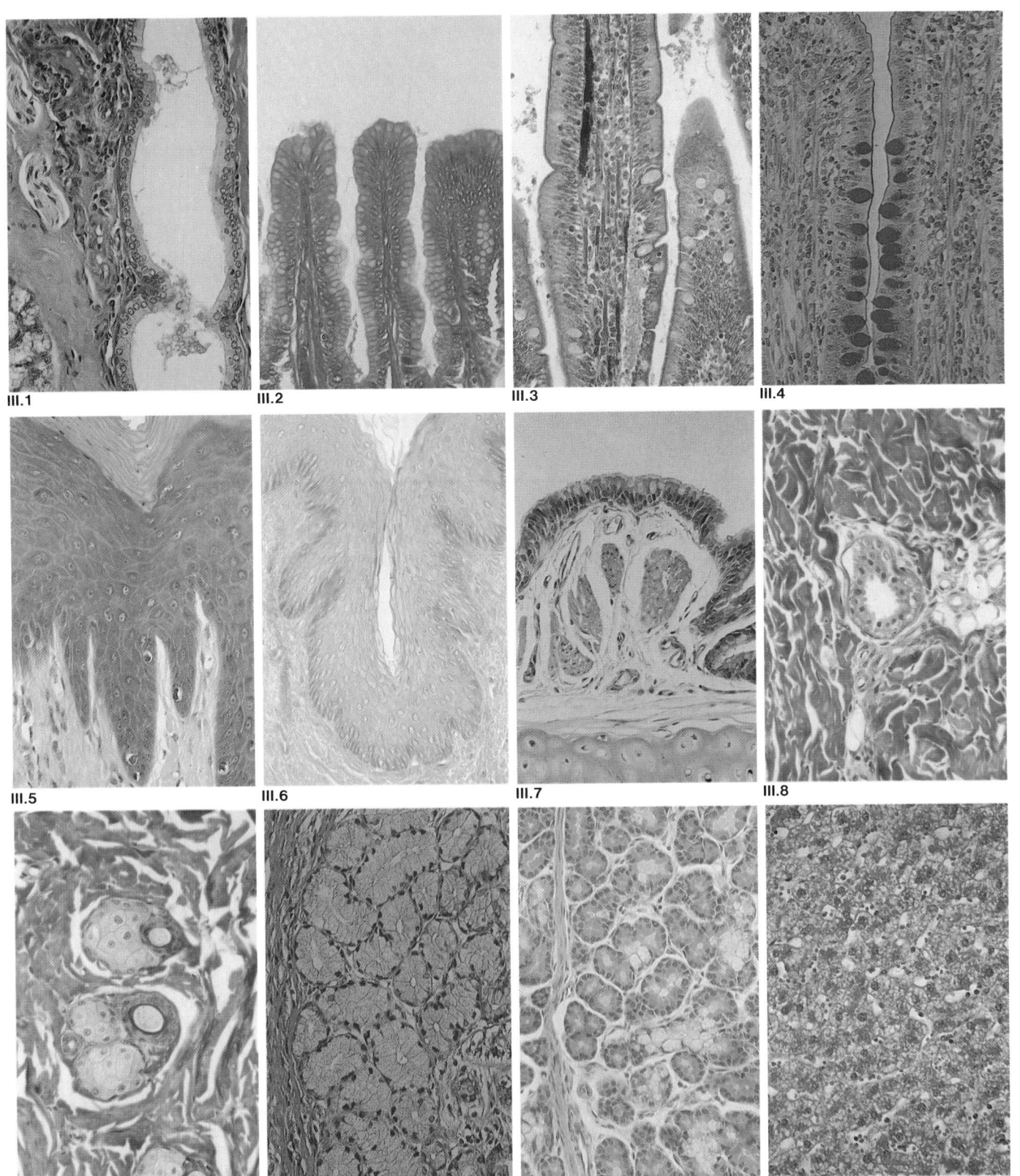

III.1

III.2

III.3

III.4

III.5

III.6

III.7

III.8

III.9

III.10

III.11

III.12

PLATE III

Plate IV: Connective Tissue

Fig. IV.1   Loose connective tissue. The connective tissue is comprised of a loose array of collagenous fibers and typical cells. A venule (*top left*), arteriole (*top right*) and a nerve fiber (*lower left*) are evident. X100. (Hematoxylin and eosin).

Fig. IV.2   Hypercellular loose connective tissue of the pharyngeal mucosa. Numerous mononuclear cells comprise part of the cell population. X100. (Hematoxylin-phloxine-safran).

Fig. IV.3   Dense white fibrous connective tissue (*irregularly arranged*) with pink-staining elastic fibers. X100. (Hematoxylin-phloxine-safran).

Fig. IV.4   A longitudinal section of the nuchal ligament of a lamb. X100. (Hematoxylin and eosin).

Fig. IV.5   A longitudinal section of a tendon. X100. (Hematoxylin and eosin).

Fig. IV.6   A longitudinal section of a tendon. X100. (van Gieson).

Fig. IV.7   Section of hyaline cartilage. The capsular margin stains a dark purple. The interterritorial matrix is light purple. X100. (Hematoxylin and eosin).

Fig. IV.8   Hyaline cartilage. The cells are contained within lacunae. X100. (Hematoxylin and eosin).

Fig. IV.9   Hyaline cartilage of the articular surface (*top*) and growth plate (*lower right*). The epiphyseal and metaphyseal bone (*pink*) contain cores of calcified cartilage. X100. (Hematoxylin-phloxine-safran).

Fig. IV.10   Elastic cartilage. The elastic fibers are red and are especially obvious in the young cartilage adjacent to the perichondrium (*bottom*). X100. (Pentachrome stain).

Fig. IV.11   Fibrocartilage from a canine meniscus. Note the columns of chondrocytes between the collagenous fibers. X100. (Hematoxylin and eosin).

Fig. IV.12   Osteons within lamellar bone. X100. (Mallory's).

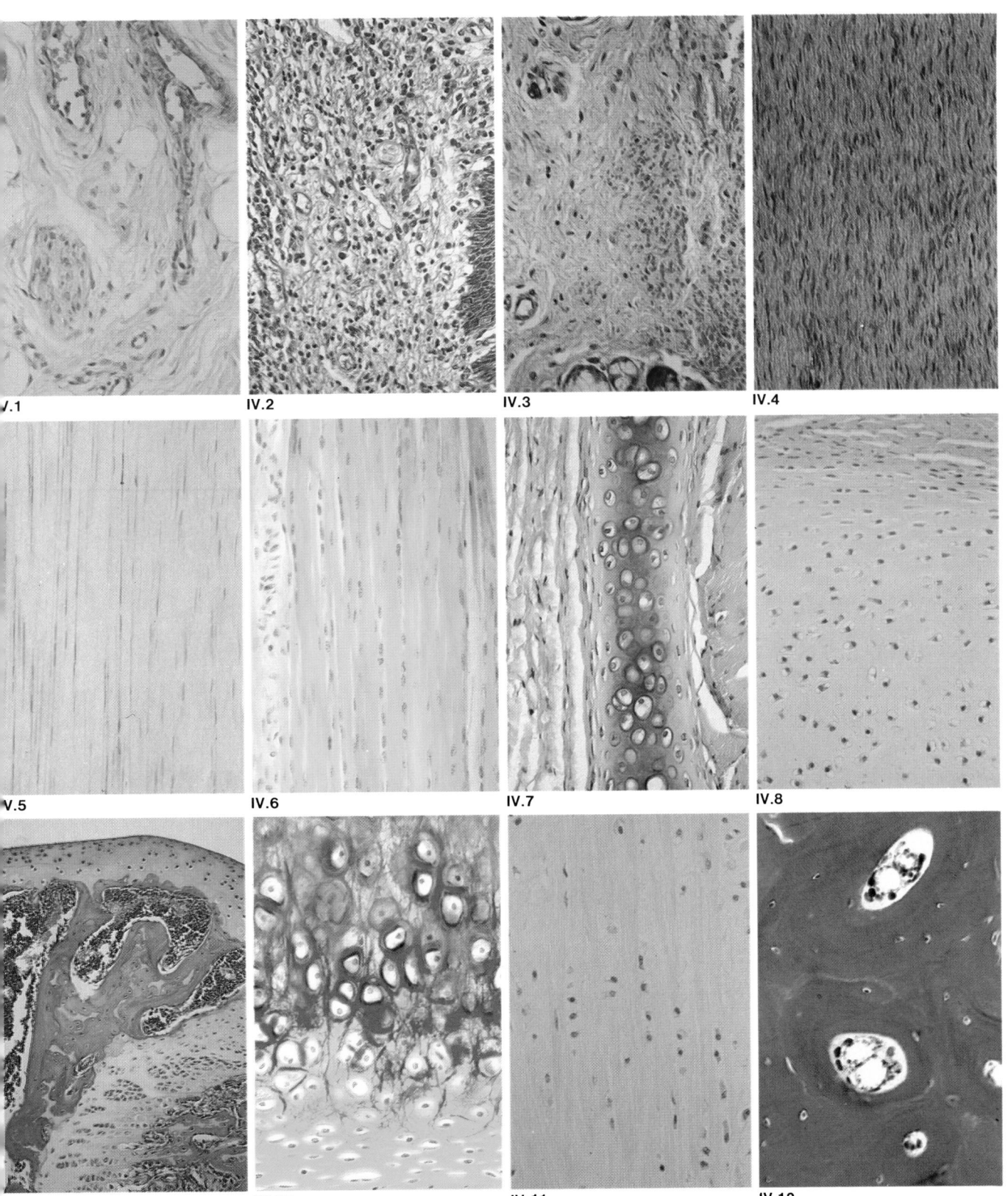

IV.1 IV.2 IV.3 IV.4

IV.5 IV.6 IV.7 IV.8

IV.9 IV.10 IV.11 IV.12

PLATE IV

Plate V: Muscular, Nervous and Adipose Tissue

Fig. V.1   A longitudinal section of a sheet of smooth muscle from the tunica muscularis of the intestine. X100. (Hematoxylin and eosin).

Fig. V.2   A cross-section of bundles of smooth muscle. X100. (Hematoxylin and eosin). (Courtesy of R. A. Kainer).

Fig. V.3   A longitudinal section of skeletal muscle. X100. (Hematoxylin and eosin). (Courtesy of R. A. Kainer).

Fig. V.4   A cross-section of skeletal muscle. Note the groups of contractile elements within individual fibers. X100. (Masson's trichrome).

Fig. V.5   Longitudinal section of cardiac muscle. Striations are not always evident. X100. (Hematoxylin and eosin).

Fig. V.6   A cross-section of cardiac muscle. X100. (Hematoxylin and eosin).

Fig. V.7   A longitudinal section of a peripheral myelinated nerve. X100. (Hematoxylin and eosin).

Fig. V.8   A longitudinal section of a peripheral myelinated nerve. X100. (Osmium tetroxide).

Fig. V.9   A cross-section of a fascicle of a peripheral myelinated nerve. X100. (Hematoxylin and eosin).

Fig. V.10   A section of the brain stem of a pig. A neuron occupies the center of the field. The cytoplasmic blue-staining material is Nissl substance. The small nuclei are those of the neuroglial cells. X100. (Nocht's stain).

Fig. V.11   Yellow adipose tissue. X100. (Hematoxylin and eosin).

Fig. V.12   Brown adipose tissue. X100. (Hematoxylin and eosin).

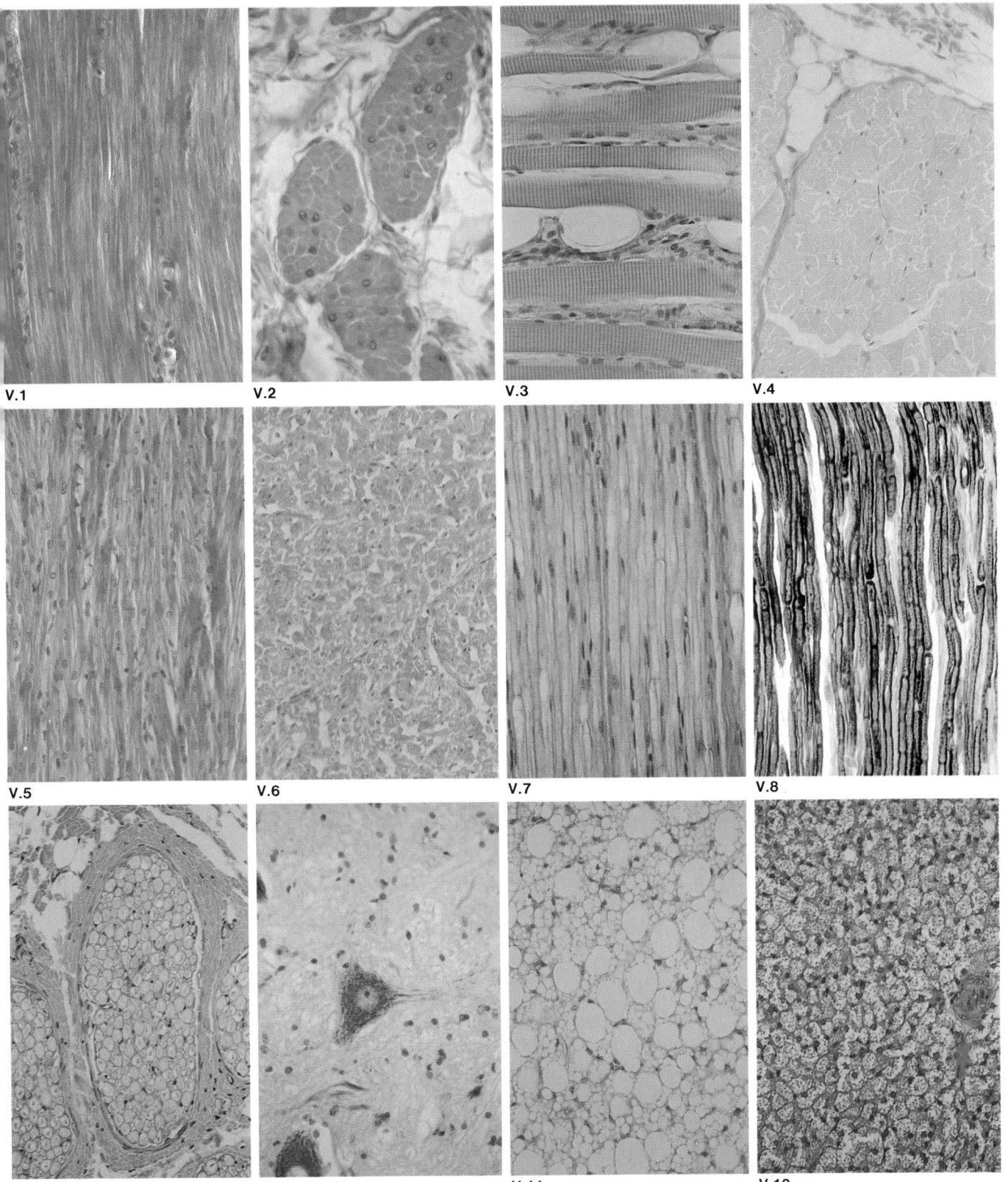

V.1

V.2

V.3

V.4

V.5

V.6

V.7

V.8

V.9

V.10

V.11

V.12

PLATE V

Plate VI: Peripheral Blood
All of the blood smears were stained with a Romanowsky stain and photographed at 400X.

Fig. VI.1   Canine neutrophil.
Fig. VI.2   Feline neutrophil.
Fig. VI.3   Equine neutrophil.
Fig. VI.4   Bovine neutrophil.
Fig. VI.5   Canine lymphocyte.
Fig. VI.6   Feline lymphocyte.
Fig. VI.7   Equine lymphocyte.
Fig. VI.8   Bovine lymphocyte.
Fig. VI.9   Canine monocyte.
Fig. VI.10   Feline monocyte.
Fig. VI.11   Equine monocyte.
Fig. VI.12   Bovine monocyte.
Fig. VI.13   Canine eosinophil. (Courtesy M. A. Thrall).
Fig. VI.14   Feline eosinophil. (Courtesy M. A. Thrall).
Fig. VI.15   Equine eosinophil. (Courtesy R. A. Kainer).
Fig. VI.16   Bovine eosinophil. (Courtesy M. A. Thrall).
Fig. VI.17   Canine basophil.
Fig. VI.18   Feline basophil.
Fig. VI.19   Equine basophil.
Fig. VI.20   Bovine basophil.
Fig. VI.21   Canine lymphocyte. Note the indented nucleus.
Fig. VI.22   A canine rubicyte in a peripheral blood smear.
Fig. VI.23   Toxic neutrophilic bands in a feline peripheral blood smear. Note the Barr body.
Fig. VI.24   Erythrophagocytosis by a blood monocyte.

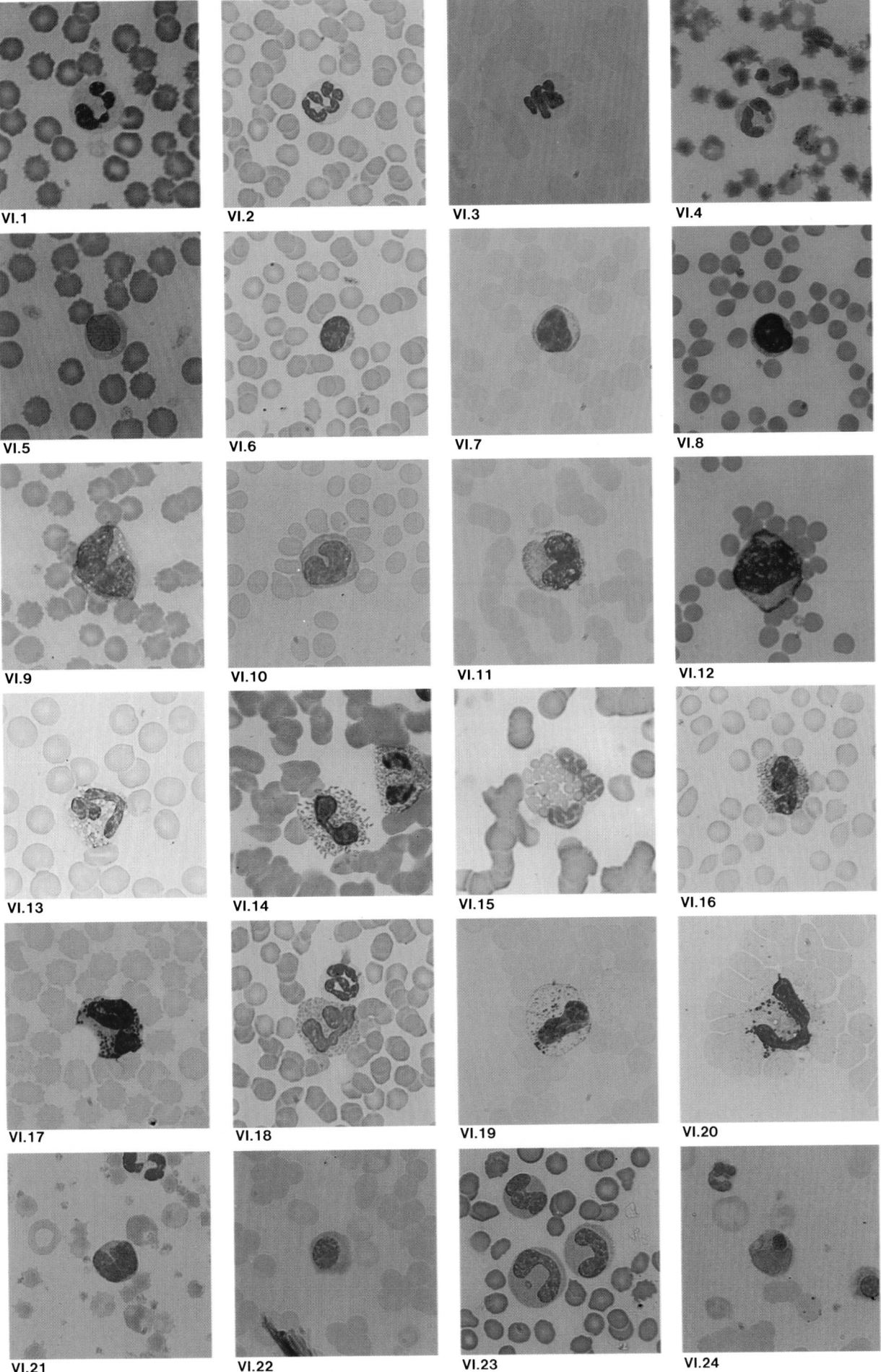

VI.1 VI.2 VI.3 VI.4
VI.5 VI.6 VI.7 VI.8
VI.9 VI.10 VI.11 VI.12
VI.13 VI.14 VI.15 VI.16
VI.17 VI.18 VI.19 VI.20
VI.21 VI.22 VI.23 VI.24

PLATE VI

Plate VII: Peripheral Blood and Exfoliative Cytology

All of the specimens were stained with a Romanowsky stain and photographed at 400X.

Fig. VII.1 Feline neutrophilic band with toxic granulation.

Fig. VII.2 Bovine lymphocyte with azurophilic granules.

Fig. VII.3 Canine monocyte (*top*), neutrophilic band (*middle*) and neutrophil (*bottom*).

Fig. VII.4 Polychromasia in a canine peripheral blood smear.

Fig. VII.5 Canine peripheral blood smear. *Top to bottom*—platelet, monocyte, rubricyte, metarubricyte.

Fig. VII.6 Macrophage with hemosiderin in cerebrospinal fluid from a dog with head trauma.

Fig. VII.7 A reactive canine lymph node with a large lymphoblast (*upper left*), mature lymphocytes, plasma cells (*center*) and a Mott cell (*lower right*). A lymphoglandular body is in the *center* of the field.

Fig. VII.8 A canine popliteal lymph node with metastatic mast cell tumor cells (*upper left*), plasmablast (*upper center*), and a plasma cell (*upper right*). Mast cell granules from ruptured cells are scattered throughout the sample.

Fig. VII.9 Transitional epithelial cells from an impression smear of the urinary bladder of a normal dog.

Fig. VII.10 Ciliated columnar cells from a tracheal wash of a normal dog.

Fig. VII.11 A tracheal wash from a dog with chronic bronchitis. Vacuolated macrophages, neutrophils and a reactive lymphocyte are present.

Fig. VII.12 Thyroid follicular cells from a normal dog.

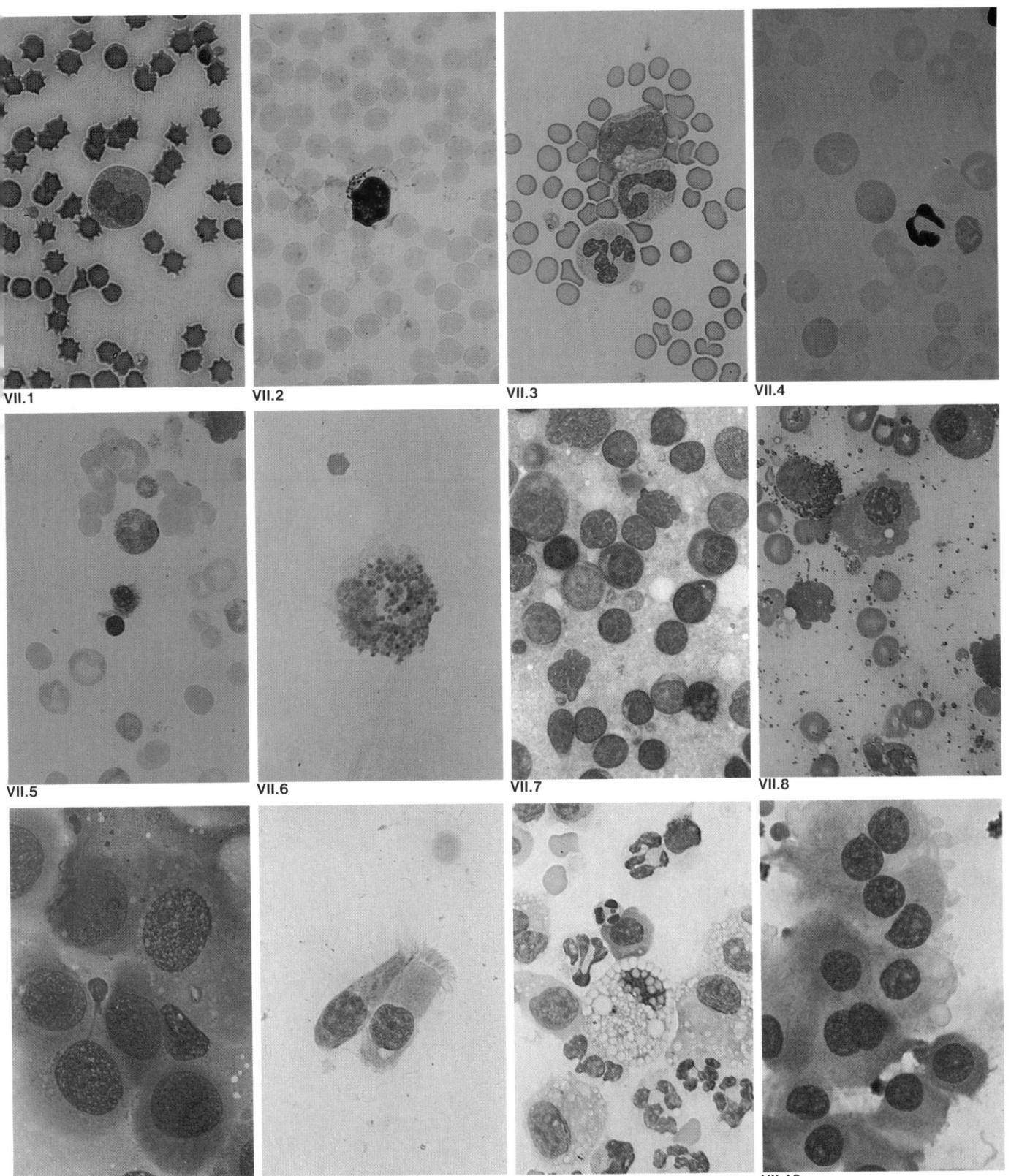

VII.1

VII.2

VII.3

VII.4

VII.5

VII.6

VII.7

VII.8

VII.9

VII.10

VII.11

VII.12

PLATE VII

Plate VIII: Exfoliative Cytology

All of the specimens were stained with a Romanowsky stain and were photographed at 400X.

Fig. VIII.1   Thyroid follicular cells with dark blue cytoplasmic granules from a normal dog.

Fig. VIII.2   Secretory cells from an aspirate of a canine salivary gland. Compare with Figure VII.11.

Fig. VIII.3   Normal prostatic epithelial cells from a canine prostate gland.

Fig. VIII.4   Aspirate of a canine hyperplastic prostate gland. The cells are more columnar than normal.

Fig. VIII.5   Aspirate of a canine prostate gland with adenocarcinoma. The large binucleated cell has prominent nucleoli.

Fig. VIII.6   Aspirate of a canine prostate gland with squamous cell metaplasia. The cells have pyknotic nuclei and abundant cytoplasm.

Fig. VIII.7   Canine vaginal smear in early estrus. Cornified epithelial cells have numerous bacteria on their surfaces. Some RBC's are present.

Fig. VIII.8   Vaginal smear from a dog in diestrus. Intermediate epithelial cells contain neutrophils.

Fig. VIII.9   A smear of abdominal fluid from a normal horse. Clusters of mesothelial cells, neutrophils and macrophages are evident.

Fig. VIII.10   A smear of abdominal fluid from a normal horse. Neutrophils, macrophages, RBC's and a neutrophil with a pyknotic nucleus (*center*) are present.

Fig. VIII.11   Epithelial cells from a conjunctival scraping from a normal dog.

Fig. VIII.12   Goblet cells from a conjunctival scraping from a dog with keratoconjunctivitis sicca.

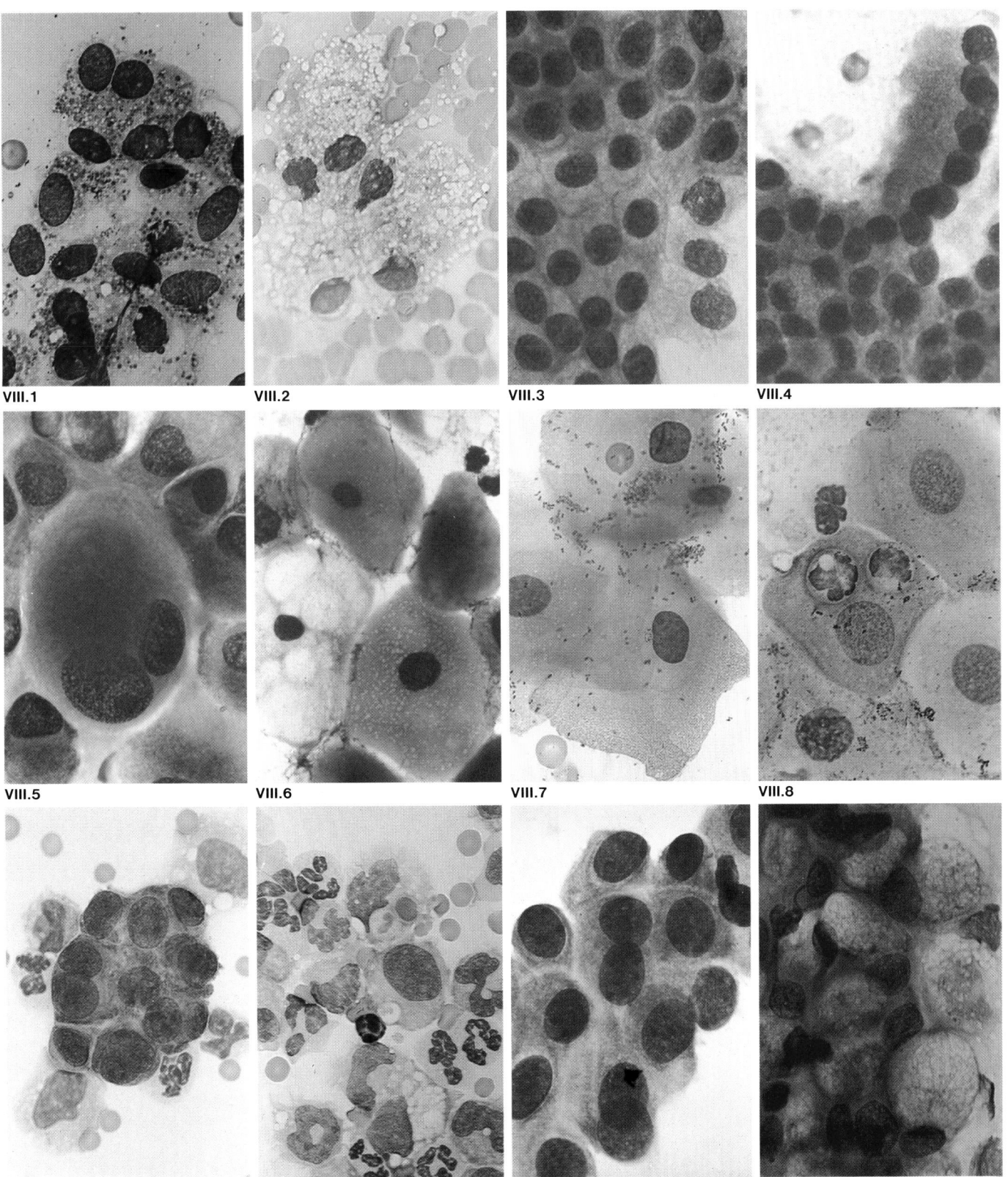

VIII.1

VIII.2

VIII.3

VIII.4

VIII.5

VIII.6

VIII.7

VIII.8

VIII.9

VIII.10

VIII.11

VIII.12

PLATE VIII

SECTION IV:

COMPARATIVE ORGANOLOGY

13: Organization of Organs

Organization of Tubular Organs

Form and Function. All of the organs of the body are formed by a combination of one or more of the basic tissues. Besides the specific cellular differences that may characterize an organ, the amount, types and distribution of various tissues are diagnostic features.

Most tubular organs consists of four concentric layers which are called *tunics* Fig. 13.1). These are, from the luminal surface to the periphery: the *tunica mucosa, tunica submucosa, tunica muscularis* and the *tunica adventitia* or *tunica serosa*. All of the tunics may be present, one or more may be reduced or eliminated, or one or more may be modified to meet specific local needs. These variations, in conjunction with other factors, permit identification of an organ.

The tunica mucosa is the innermost or luminal coat and consists of three layers: *lamina epithelialis mucosae, lamina propria mucosae* and the *lamina muscularis mucosae* (Fig. 13.2).

The *lamina epithelialis* is the epithelial layer of an organ. It may consist of one or more types of epithelial cells as per the specific function of an organ or portion of an organ. It is a consistent lamina of this tunic. A basement membrane is a constant feature between epithelial cells (and other nonconnective tissues) and the subjacent connective tissue. Some authors include the basement membrane as a layer of the tunica mucosa and call it the *lamina membrana propria mucosae*.

The *lamina propria mucosae* is the connective tissue which underlies the epithelial layer. It is usually areolar and/or reticular connective tissue. Small vessels, nerves and infoldings of the lamina epithelialis mucosae occupy this space. The connective tissue of this space may contain large numbers of protective cells either free or as lymph nodules. Besides a defensive function, this layer is the means by which the epithelium is nourished and controlled.

The *lamina muscularis mucosae* is one or more layers of smooth muscle cells. An inner circular and an outer longitudinal layer may be present.

This lamina is of variable occurrence. When present it serves as a means by which local mobility of organs is achieved. Also, it serves to express secretory products from the glands which may invaginate into the lamina propria mucosae (Fig. 13.3). When present, it serves as a sharp line of demarcation between the connective tissue of the lamina propria mucosae and the tunica submucosa. When absent, these two connective tissue spaces blend together insensibly.

The *tunica submucosa* consists of areolar connective tissue which is more coarsely arranged than the connective tissue of the lamina propria muscosae (Fig. 13.4). Large blood vessels, nerves, nerve plexi and autonomic ganglia are present. In some organs,

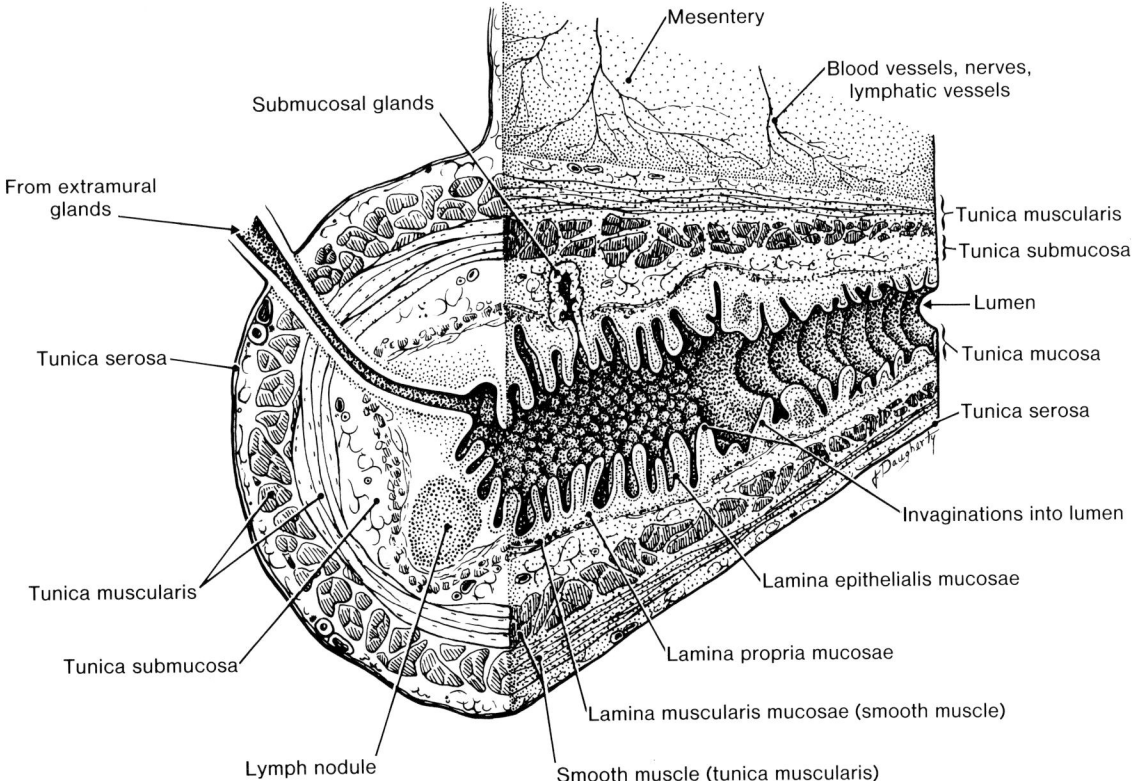

Fig. 13.1 A stylized drawing of a typical tubular visceral organ. Refer to text for a complete description of components. All light micrographs are labeled as the magnification with the microscope before photographic enlarging. All electron micrographs are labeled as total magnification, including photographic enlarging.

glands may be present also. This tunic permits motility of the tunica mucosa. In the absence of a lamina muscularis mucosae, the lamina propria mucosae and the tunica submucosa are usually referred to simply as the lamina propria mucosae, *lamina propria-submucosa* or simply tunica submucosa.

The *tunica muscularis* is usually well-developed and consists of two layers of muscle (Fig. 13.5). In some organs, however, it may be absent. Although these layers usually consist of smooth muscle, in some instances they may be comprised of skeletal muscle. The most common arrangement of this tunic is a division into inner circular and outer longitudinal layers. Although described as circular and longitudinal, the inner layer is disposed in a tighter helical pattern than the outer, more loosely oriented helix. Vascular and neural plexi and autonomic ganglia usually separate the two layers. This tunic is responsible for the tone of the organ, size of the lumen and the movement of materials through the hollow organ.

The *tunica adventitia* is a collection of loose connective tissue over the periphery of an organ. Blood vessels, nerves, ganglia and adipose tissue may occur within this tunic. Organs that are intimately associated with the coelomic cavities are surrounded by a layer of mesothelium. In these cases, the most peripheral tunic is referred to as the *tunica serosa* (Fig. 13.6). It is composed, therefore, of mesothelium and connective tissue. It is through the tunica adventitia and/or tunica serosa that the vascular, lymphatic and nerve supplies gain access to an organ. Further, these tunics are responsible for the suspension of organs either through the union of the tunica adventitia with surrounding connective tissue or by the reflection of mesothelium and associated connective tissue as mesenteries.

Although there are numerous variations of this scheme, this organization is basic to tubular organs.

Surface and Glandular Modifications. Invariably, the tubular organs of the body are associated with the transport, secretion, absorption and diffusion of various types of materials (ingesta, fluids, blood, gas). Many methods are utilized by these organs to increase their surface areas. Some of these modifications, especially as they relate to the digestive system, are detailed in Figure 13.7. The cellular elements of a flattened tunica mucosa may evaginate into the lumen of the organ and form villous projections (Figs. 13.7B, 13.8), rugae (Fig. 13.7F) and

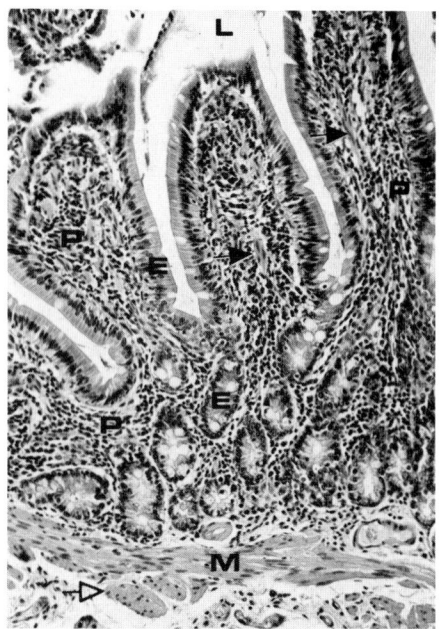

Fig. 13.2 Tunica mucosa of the equine duodenum. The lamina epithelialis mucosae (E) is adjacent to the lumen (L) and invaginates into the lamina propria mucosae (P). The lamina propria mucosae is very cellular. The lamina muscularis mucosae (M) consists of an inner circular and outer longitudinal layer (*open arrow*) of smooth muscle. Extensions of the lamina muscularis mucosae (*solid arrows*) are apparent within the lamina propria mucosae. X29.

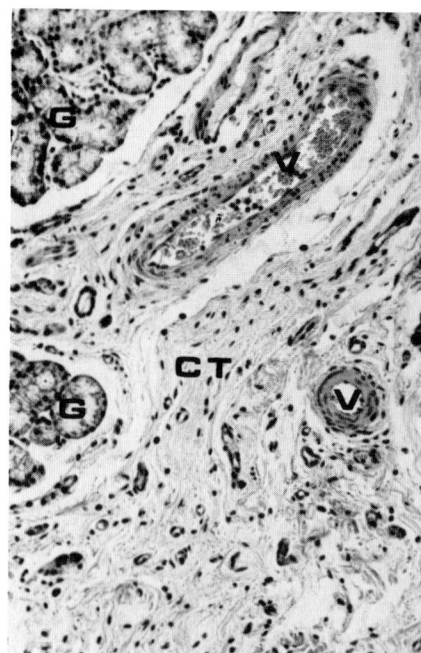

Fig. 13.4 Tunica submucosa of the equine duodenum. The areolar connective tissue (CT) surrounds vessels (V) and glands (G) within the tunica submucosa. Nerves and lymphatic vessels are present also. X34.

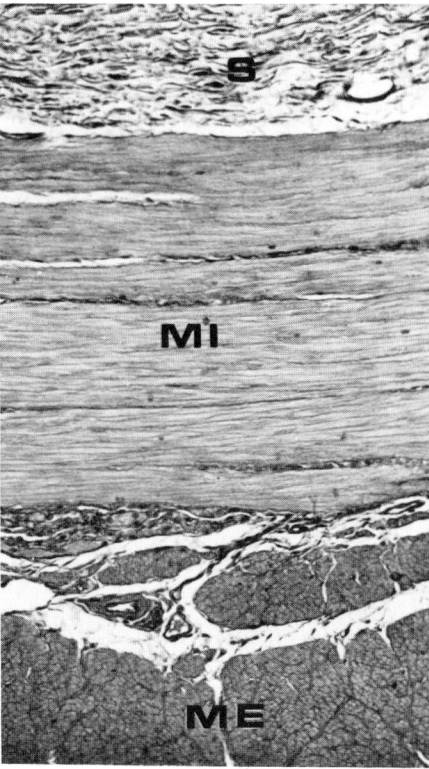

Fig. 13.5 Tunica muscularis of the feline stomach. The tunica muscularis is peripheral to the tunica submucosa (S). The tunica muscularis consists of inner (MI) and outer (ME) layers of smooth muscle. Compare with Figure 11.4. X40.

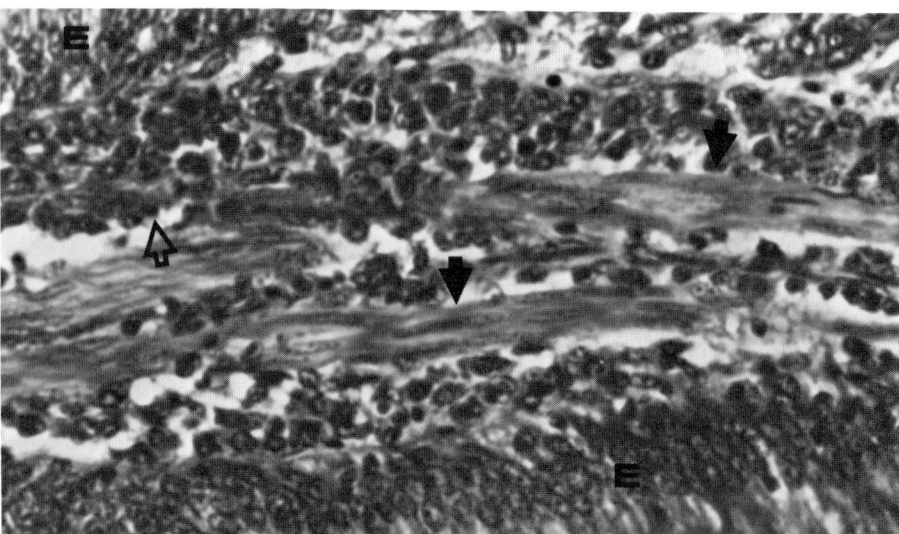

Fig. 13.3 Lamina propria mucosae of the equine duodenum. The villus is covered by the lamina epithelialis mucosae (E) and contains a very cellular connective tissue core (*open arrow*). Smooth muscle (*solid arrows*) from the lamina muscularis mucosae extends into the lamina propria mucosae. X125.

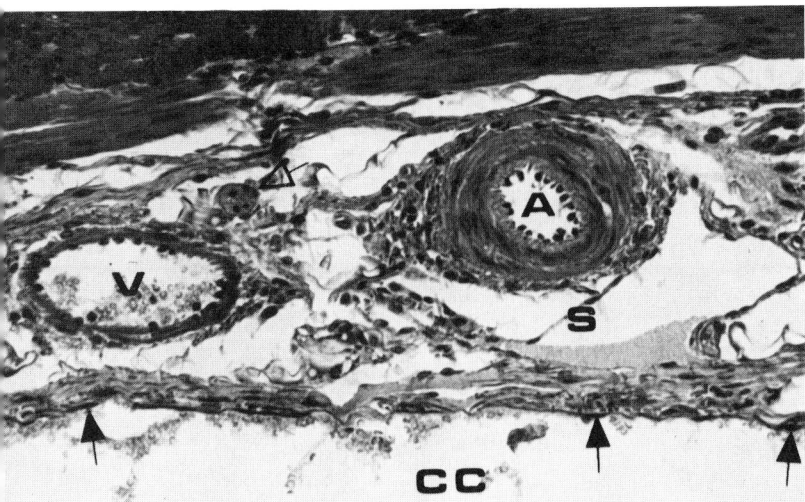

Fig. 13.6 Tunica serosa of the feline stomach. The tunica serosa, visceral peritoneum, is the outer covering of the organ. The celomic cavity (CC) is bounded by the mesothelial cells (*solid arrows*) that comprise serosal membranes, visceral and parietal. Subserosal connective tissue (S) is areolar. Arteries (A), veins (V) and nerves (*open arrow*) are present. The spaces within the connective tissue are artifacts of sectioning. X63.

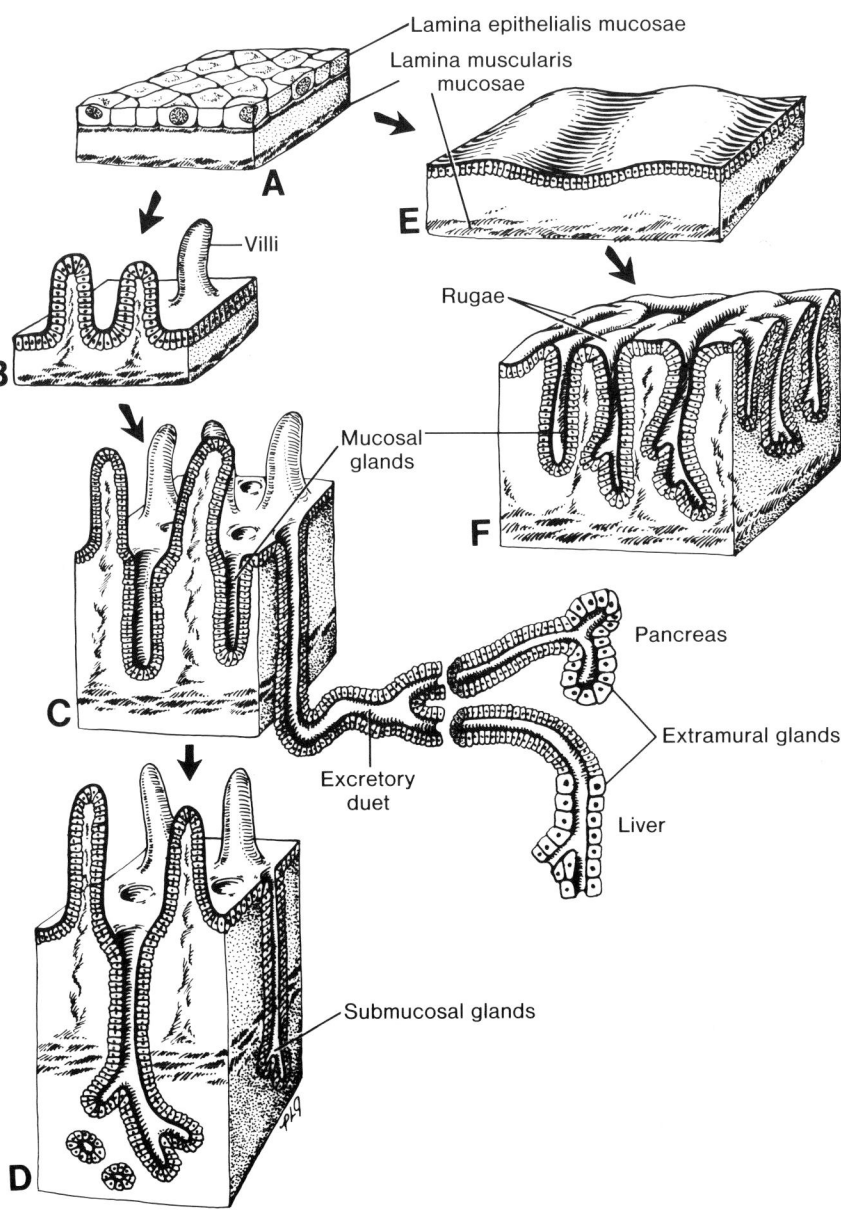

Fig. 13.7 A diagram of the development of surface modifications and glands associated with the mural elements of tubular visceral organs. A flat epithelial surface (A) may undergo differential growth (E) and form mucosal glands (F) by invaginations of the lamina epithelialis mucosae into the lamina propria mucosae. Surface alterations resulting from differential growth form villous projections into the lumen (B). Differential growth also may form invaginations between the villi as mucosal glands (C). Continued growth of the epithelium forms the ducts and/or adenomeres of extramural glands (C). The growth of the lamina epithelialis mucosae through the lamina propria mucosae into the tunica submucosa establishes submucosal glands (D).

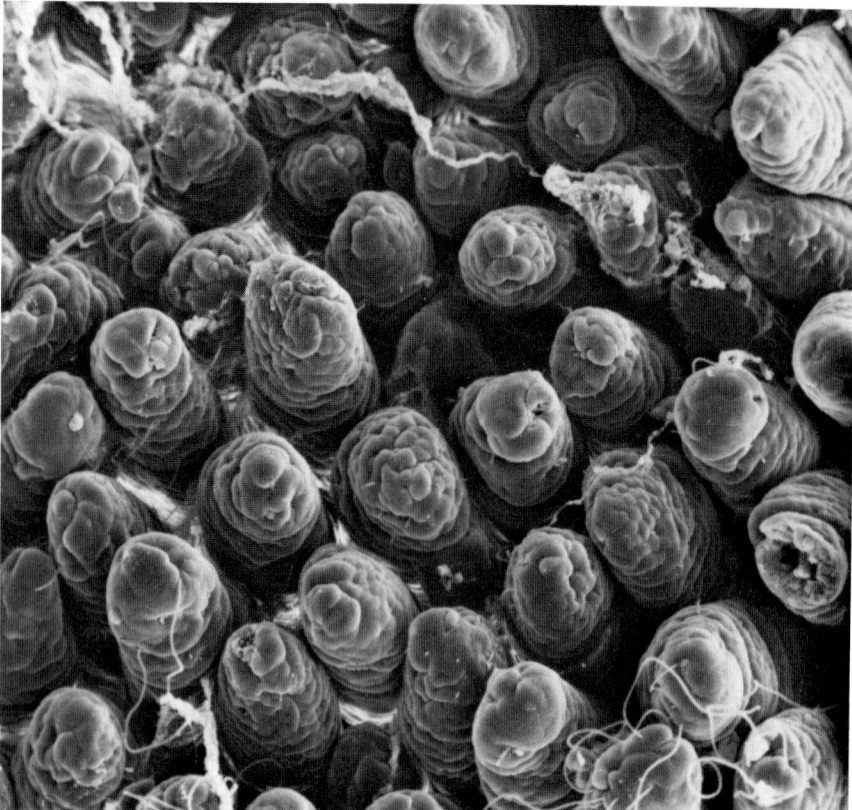

Fig. 13.8 A scanning electron micrograph of villi from the jejunum of a mouse. The villi project from the mucosal surface into the lumen of the organ. (Micrograph courtesy of D. L. Eisenbrandt).

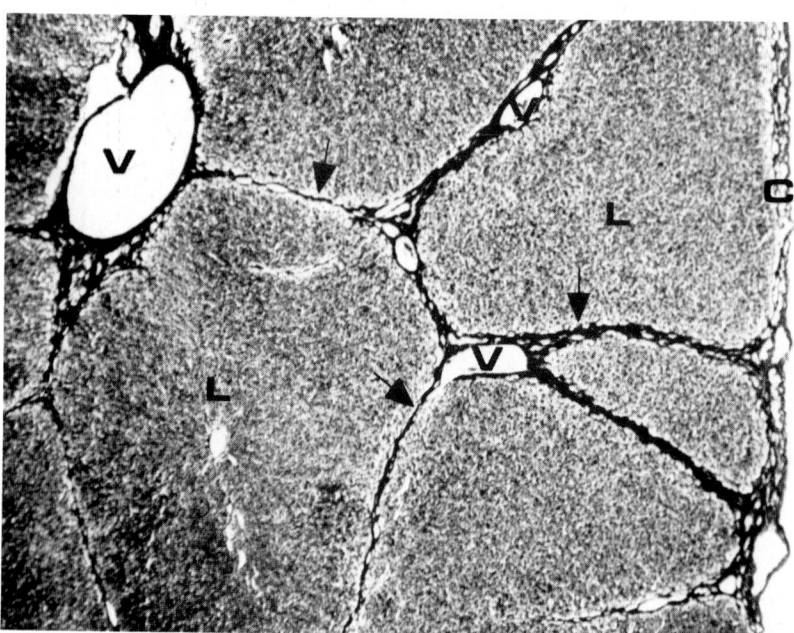

Fig. 13.9 The organization of a solid organ (porcine liver). The connective tissue capsule (C) is continuous with large trabeculae (*arrows*) that subdivide the organ. Fine reticular fibers extend a short distance into the lobules (L). Large vessels (V) are located within trabeculae. X10 (Snook's reticulum stain).

called *mucosal glands* (Fig. 13.7C,D,F). Invaginations of the lamina epithelialis mucosae may perforate the lamina muscularis mucosae and the adenomeres may occupy the tunica submucosa. Such glandular structures are called *submucosal glands* (Fig. 13.7D). In specialized cases, the lamina epithelialis mucosae is continuous with glandular structures positioned remotely from the lumen of the organ (Fig. 13.7C). This type of organization typifies the relationship of the liver and pancreas to the gut lumen.

Organization of Parenchymatous Organs

Form and Function. The solid or parenchymatous organs of the body are also composed of a combination of one or more of the basic tissues. Their organizational pattern is somewhat different from that described for tubular or hollow organs.

The components of solid organs may be divided into two definitive subgroups. The *parenchyma* is the specific functional component of a specific organ, whereas the *stroma* includes those tissues (connective tissue, vasculature, nerves, lymphatics) that

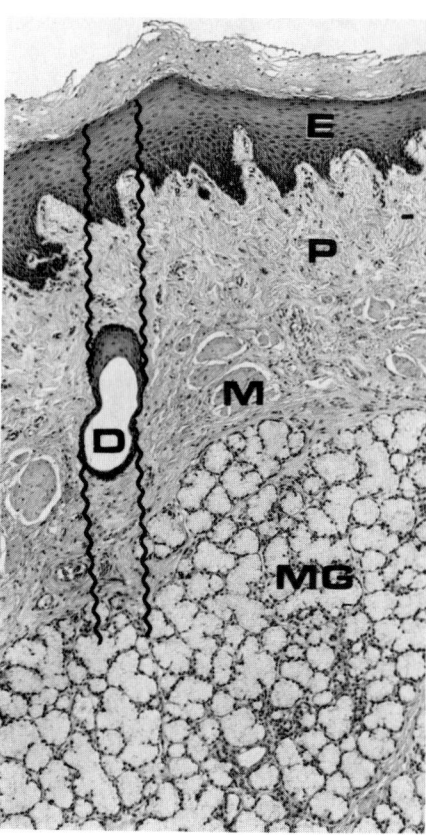

Fig. 13.10 A mucous membrane lined by stratified squamous epithelium (porcine esophagus). The lamina epithelialis mucosae (E) is covered by a mucoid secretory product and underlaid by the lamina propria mucosae (P). The lamina muscularis mucosae (M) is discontinuous. Mucosal glands (MG) are responsible for the moistened surface. Their secretory products reach the surface (*wavy lines*) through the excretory duct (D) and its continuations. X16.

other effacable and noneffacable folds. The cellular elements of the tunica mucosa may invaginate into the lamina propria mucosae independent of surface projections (Fig. 13.7F) or in association with surface projections (Fig. 13.7C). This usually results in the thickening of the lamina propria mucosae,

and elements of the lamina muscularis mucosae may interdigitate between these invaginations of the lamina epithelialis mucosae (Figs. 13.7C,D,F) and extend into the evaginations of the tunica mucosa (Figs. 13.7B,C,D,F). Glandular structures that remain within the lamina propria mucosae are

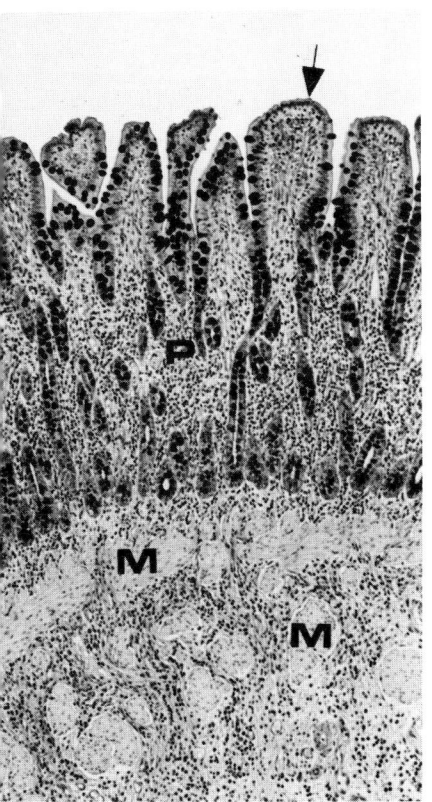

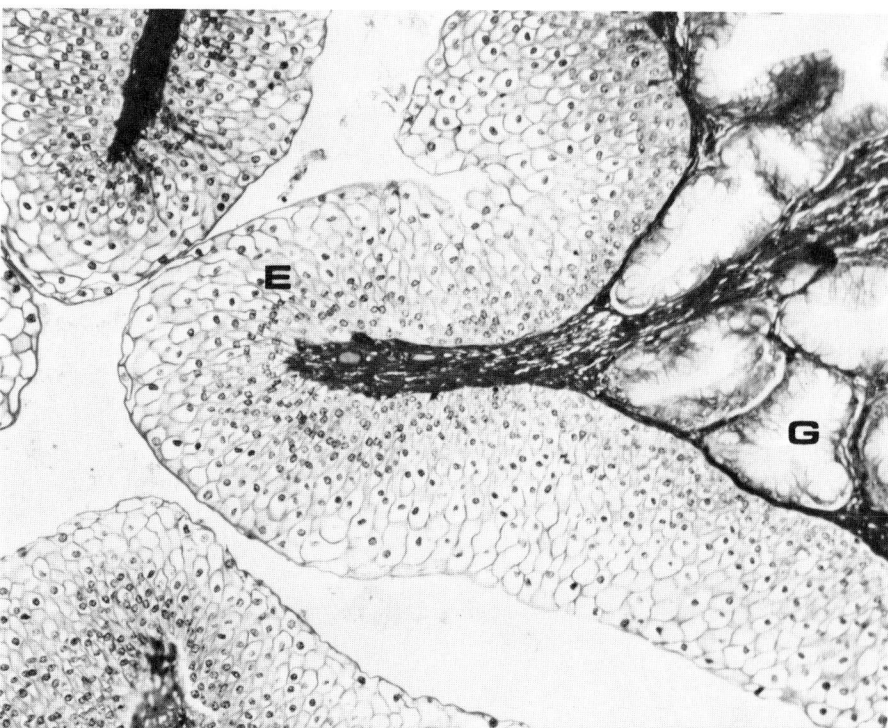

Fig. 13.12   A transitional mucous membrane from an equine ureter. Mucous glands (G) moisten the surface of the transitional epithelium (E). X40.

Fig. 13.11   A mucous membrane lined by simple columnar epithelium (canine jejunum). The epithelium (*arrow*) invaginates into the lamina propria mucosae (P). The lamina muscularis mucosae (M) consists of longitudinal and circular muscle. The dark-staining cells of the lamina epithelialis mucosae are goblet cells and other mucus-secreting cells. X16 (Alcian blue and PAS).

metabolically and/or structurally support as well as control the parenchyma.

In its greatest simplicity, the following scheme is applicable to these organs whether they are muscle, nerve trunks or glands (Fig. 13.9). Small groups of parenchyma are surrounded by a fine meshwork of areolar or reticular connective tissue in which vessels and nerves are located. Small groups of parenchyma may be grouped as a unit and surrounded by a more coarse areolar connective tissue, or the connective tissue of these small groups may be continuous with coarse areolar connective tissue *trabeculae*. In either case, the connective tissue is progressively more dense and is continuous with the dense white fibrous connective tissue of the capsule. This type of connective tissue continuity affords structural support and facilitates the entry and/or exit of vessels and nerves. This scheme or minor variation thereof typify the organization of solid organs.

Mucous and Serous Membranes

Membranes as Simple Organs. *Mucous membranes* include some or all of the components of the tunica mucosa. These membranes are kept moist by secretions from cells within the lamina epithelialis and/or

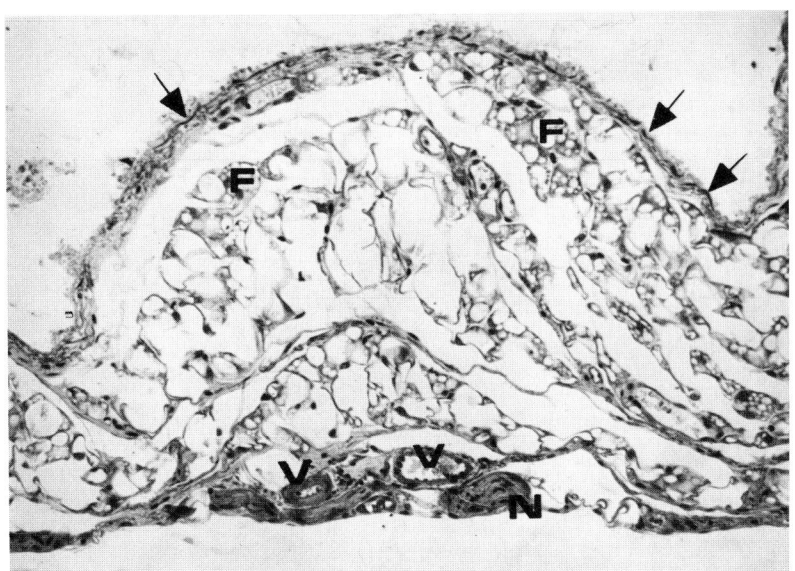

Fig. 13.13   A serous membrane (tunica serosa). The mesothelium (*solid arrows*) and its associated connective tissue are underlaid by a subserosal connective tissue (areolar) that contains adipocytes (F), vessels (V) and nerves (N). Compare with Figure 13.6. X40.

from glands located within the lamina propria mucosae and/or tunica submucosa. The lamina epithelialis mucosae may consist of stratified squamous, cuboidal, columnar or pseudostratified columnar epithelium.

A mucous membrane consisting of stratified squamous epithelium typically occurs in the digestive and reproductive systems (Fig. 13.10). Mucous membranes lined by columnar, cuboidal or pseudostratified columnar epithelium occur typically in the digestive, respiratory and reproductive systems (Fig. 13.11). Those lined by transitional epithelium occur in the urinary system (Fig. 13.12).

Serous membranes consist of a layer of mesothelium and associated connective tissue (Fig. 13.13). They line the coelomic spaces and are moistened by the fluids contained within these spaces.

These membranes are simple organs.

References

Specific references for the subject material of this chapter are included in subsequent chapters that cover specific organs.

14: Musculoskeletal System

General Characteristics

Form and Function. The form of this system is as varied as the form of the muscles and bones of which it is comprised. Some representatives of all of the basic tissues contribute to the formation of this system. The structural component of the system, bone, gives support to the body as well as serving as points of attachment against which the muscles can operate. The contractile portion, skeletal muscle, is the means by which the contractility of the fibers is converted into the work involved in support and locomotion. Dense white fibrous connective tissue in ligaments and tendons constitutes the mechanism for attachment of bone to bone and muscle to bone. Cartilage facilitates growth as well as serving as the substrate for bone to bone contact (articular surfaces). The proper connective tissues bind various parts of the system together and allow for the free passage of blood vessels, lymphatics and nerves. As an integrated system with numerous component parts, the primary functions are the support and movement of the body.

Bone as an Organ

Physical Properties of Bone

The matrix components of bone impart some unique and important physical properties that influence its characteristics and behavior in biologic systems. The hardness, strength and rigidity of the skeleton are a function of its physical properties.

Density and Composition. One of the most important physical properties of bone is its *density*, because many of its mechanical properties relate directly to this property. Although density may be determined a number of ways for bone, density data are usually reported as the mass/unit volume of fully-hydrated, defatted bone. The density of compact bone normally is in the range 1.9–2.1. Trabecular bone is approximately 15% less dense than compact bone. These figures actually represent the density of the osseous tissue. The methods used compensate for any discontinuities (osteonal canals, communicating canals, interosseous space) in the bone.

The mineral content of bone contributes significantly to bone density. Although the mineral content is usually reported maximally as 65% of the defatted dry weight, variations occur that depend upon the de-

gree of mineralization of the bone. Newly formed bone which is incompletely mineralized is *low density bone*, whereas older bone that may approach complete mineralization is *high density bone*. Although the organic content is constant at about 35% of the defatted dry weight, the additional mineral is added at the expense of water.

The ash content of a bone represents the inorganic residue following the incineration of a bone sample. *Ash/unit volume* is generally 65% of the defatted dry weight. A straight line relationship exists between density and ash/unit volume. The principal constituents of the ash are calcium and

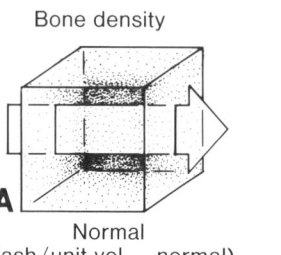

Bone density

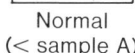

Radiographic Density

Normal

A

Normal
(ash/unit vol.—normal)

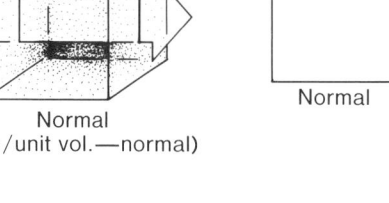

Normal
(ash/unit vol.—normal)

Normal
(< sample A)

B

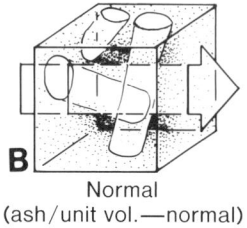

< Normal
(ash/unit vol. < normal)

< Normal

C

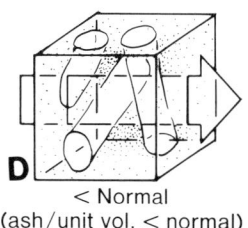

< Normal
(ash/unit vol. < normal)

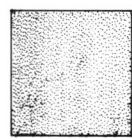

≪ Normal

D

phosphorus. These occur in a 2:1 weight/weight ratio. Calcium is 25% and phosphorus is 12% of the defatted dry weight. Carbonate, sodium, magnesium, chloride and trace elements are present also.

Density and ash/unit volume are important parameters useful in characterizing bone. A reduction in bone mass without a change in ash content represents a *quantitative* change in bone. A reduction in ash content with or without a decrease in bone mass indicates a *qualitative* change in bone. Bone density, as discussed herein, is not equivalent to radiographic density. Figure 14.1 compares bone density, ash/unit volume and radiographic density.

Piezoelectricity. In 1870, Wolff observed that "every change in the form and function of bones or their function alone is followed by certain definite changes in their configuration in accordance with mathematical laws." Today, this statement is known as *Wolff's Law*. This law identifies some important characteristics of bone: 1) the morphology of bone is capable of changing; 2) the morphology changes in a predictable

Fig. 14.1 A diagram comparing bone density, ash/unit volume and radiographic density. A. A cube of dense cortical bone has a normal density that translates radiographically as a specified amount of radiolucency. The ash/unit volume is normal. B. A cube of bone, despite numerous vacuities and cavities (osteonal canals, resorption spaces, Volkmann's canals), has a normal density and a normal ash/unit volume (quantitative change). The same cube of bone could be a sample of trabecular bone in which the cavities represent the interosseous space associated with cancellous bone. The radiographic density of the sample would be normal; however, the radiographic density would be less than the radiographic density of sample A. C. A cube of bone similar to sample A may not contain the proper amount of mineral (qualitative bone change). The density and ash/unit volume would be less than normal. These parameters might be indistinguishable from the parameters for sample B. The radiographic density of sample C would be similar to and indistinguishable from sample B. D. A cube of bone with decreased mineral (qualitative change) and increased cavities and/or increased interosseous spaces (quantitative changes) would have a low bone density and low ash/unit volume. The decreased density results from the qualitative change, not the quantitative change. The radiographic density of sample D would be much less than normal. Based upon radiographic density only, it is impossible to distinguish between samples B, C and D.

manner; 3) morphology and function are linked intimately; 4) bone may perceive stimuli and respond to them. Today, additional insights expand the basic concepts of Wolff's law and broaden the basis for meaningful application of this information.

Bone has the ability to react to mechanical energy by first converting (transducing) the energy into a useable signal (stimulus). The transducer property of bone is a function of the highly ordered, crystalline nature of hydroxyapatite and the ordered arrangement of collagen. The transduced information is in the form of electrical energy which affects the cells' electrical environment and controls their behavior. Presumably, the generation of an electrical potential results from a separation of charge through the movement of ions. This generation of electrical potential in response to mechanical stimulation is termed *piezolectricity*. It explains the responsiveness of bone as predicted by Wolff's Law (Fig. 14.2).

Biomechanical Properties of Bone

Stress and Strain. Bones are subjected continually to various forces acting upon them. The magnitude, direction, duration and rate at which a force (*stress*) is applied influences the responsiveness of the organ. The stress may be sufficient to fracture the structure or may alter its three-dimensional relationship to the rest of the skeletal mass. When a stress is applied to a bone, the bone responds by the development of a *strain* within it. The strain is a measurement of the amount of deformation that occurs in the structure. If the strain results in an elongation of the structure, then the strain is *tensile*. If the strain results in a shortening of the structure, then it is *compressive*. Tension and compression are two of the most significant types of strain which influence the integrity and spatial orientation of bones. Flexure, shearing and torque are influential also.

The collagenous fibers of bone impart the tensile strength, whereas the hydroxyapatite crystals impart the compressive strength. Together they provide bone with good tensile and compressive properties. The collagenous fibers may be compared to the reinforcing rods in concrete, while the components of the concrete are comparable to the mineral portion of the matrix. The compressive properties of bone are greater than the tensile properties. Accordingly, bone failure (fracture) generally occurs in tension.

Flexure-Drift Relationships. The application of a flexural stress of sufficient magnitude to bone may cause the structure to bend (Fig. 14.3). When this occurs, compressive strain is developed along the concave surface, whereas a tensile strain is developed upon the convex surface. If this flexural force were repeated and/or maintained for a protracted period of time, then the bone would drift through space toward the concave surface (Fig. 14.4). This movement is predicated upon a separation of

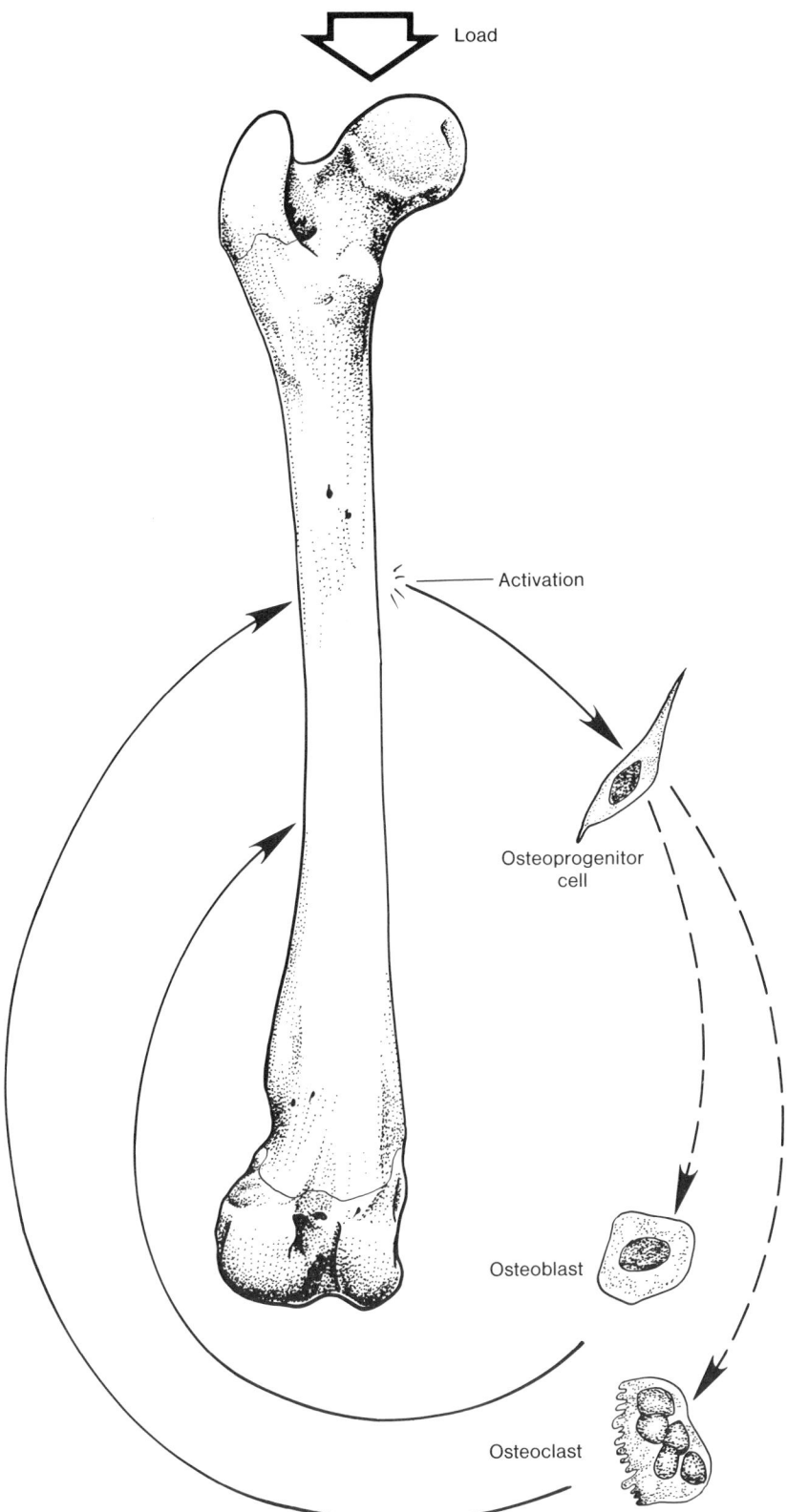

Fig. 14.2 A diagram indicating the responsiveness of bone to mechanical stimuli. The loading of a bone, especially manifested if the loading is abnormal, activates osteoprogenitor cells within the osseous envelopes. The modulation of the osteoprogenitor cells into osteoblasts and/or osteoclasts determines the type of response—formation or resorption—manifested by the organ.

charge resulting from piezoelectricity. Osteoblastic activity occurs on the compressive or concave surface in association with a negative potential. Osteoclastic activity occurs on the tensile or convex surface in association with a positive potential.

This type of osseous spatial adjustment does occur under various circumstances. The autocorrection or realignment of misaligned fracture fragments is an application

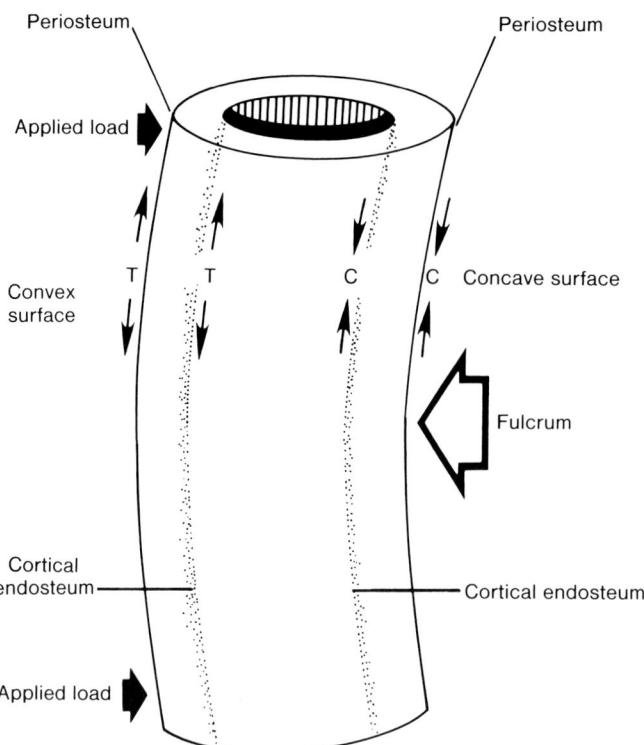

Fig. 14.3 A diagram demonstrating the type of strain developed within a loaded, living bone. The loading of the bone as indicated induces compressive strain along the concave surface and tensile strain along the convex surface. The tension and compression are greatest along the periosteal surfaces.

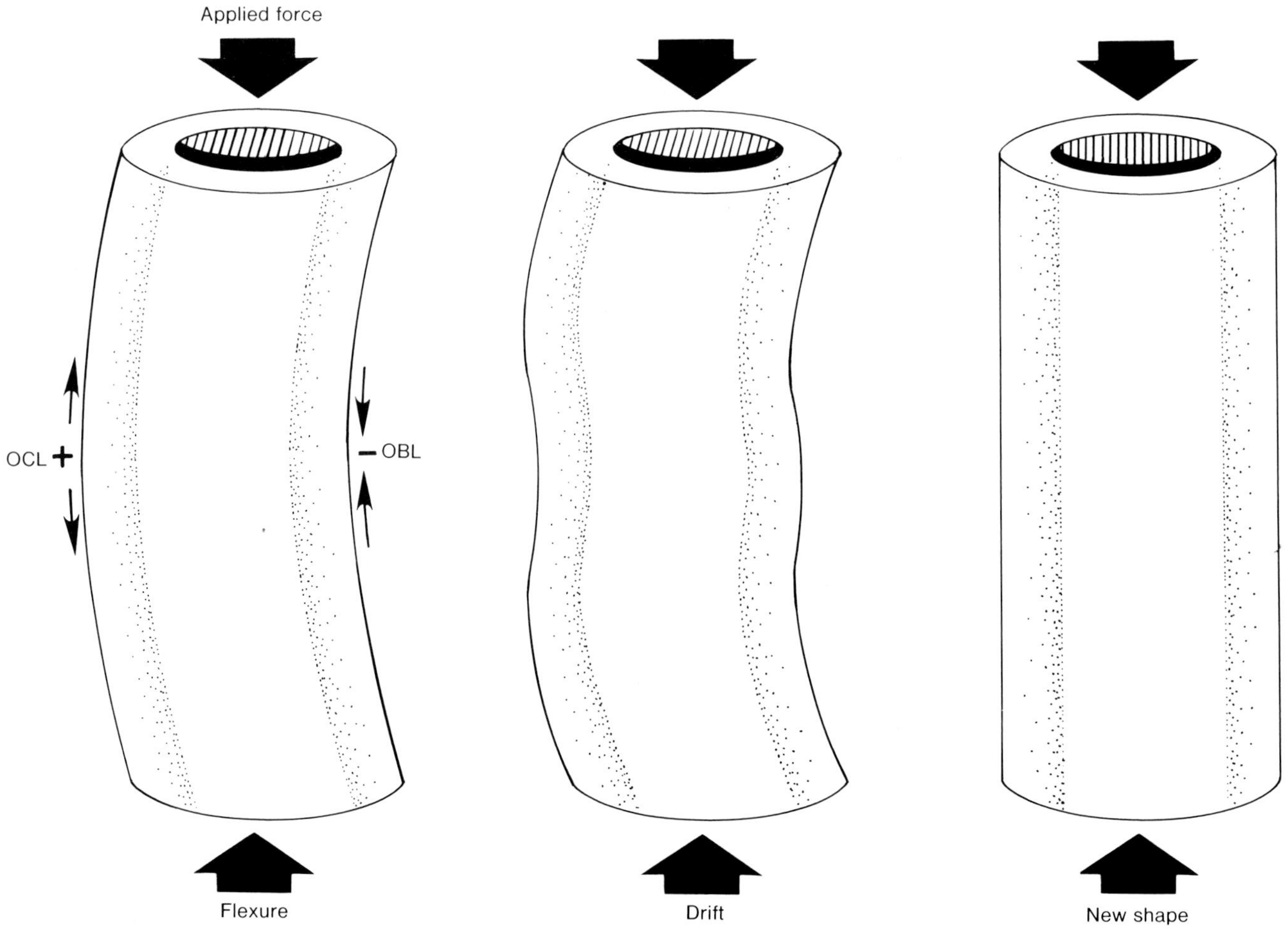

Fig. 14.4 Flexure-drift relationships in bone. The sustained applied force induces a flexure in the bone associated with a separation of charge (biopotential). The concave surface, associated with compression, drifts as a result of osteoblastic (OBL) activity. The surface under tension, the convex surface, drifts as a result of osteoclastic (OCL) activity. The new shape of the bone results from the predictable activity of bone cells under the specified loading conditions. Bones will drift toward the concave surface.

f this principle. Similarly, the osseous remodeling associated with the sub-luxation
and luxation (dislocation) of joints, or any
other alteration in normal weight-bearing,
results from this mechanism. This does not
imply that bones with natural curvatures
will eventually assume a straightened configuration. The normal curvatures and positions of bones are designed to neutralize
the effects of flexural stress that results from
loading (weight-bearing) with those opposite forces generated by the pull of muscles.
Cartilage and Bone Modeling. The role of
cartilage in the formation of the long bones
was discussed previously (Chapter 9). The
columnation of the cells of the growth plate
may represent a response to the orientation
of mechanical forces applied to this structure. The growth plate itself is generally
oriented perpendicular to applied forces.
The presence of collagen in the growth plate
probably permits the generation of piezoe-
lectric alteration of biologic electrical potentials. Thus, stress influences growth plate
orientation, columnation of cells within the
plate and the responsiveness of the growth
plate to altered stress patterns.

Two types of growth plates or growth
cartilage configurations exist in developing
bones (Fig. 14.5). One is a *pressure growth
plate* (*compression growth plate, pressure epiphysis*) that is subject generally to compressive forces. The capital femoral growth plate
and epiphysis are good examples. The other
is a *tension growth plate* (*tension epiphysis,
traction epiphysis*) that is subject generally to
tensile forces. The greater trochanter of the
femur is a good example of a traction epiphysis. This discussion will be confined to
pressure growth plates.

The application of normal, even and sustained compression upon pressure growth
plates results in the even growth of the plate
and the proper spatial orientation of the
bone. However, these plates are differentially responsive to compression. Increased
compression within the normal range accelerates growth of the plate, whereas an increased compression in the abnormal range
retards growth of the plate. An uneven and
sustained loading of a bone surface can
result in an altered spatial orientation of the
growth plate and associated articular surface
(Fig. 14.6).

The principles can be used to correct angular limb deformities (Fig. 14.7). Some
animals are born with angular limb deformities of the carpus in which the distal portion
of the limb projects laterad (carpus valgus).
If the problem is attributable to the distal
radial growth plate, then the principles of
growth plate response to compression are
applicable. A nonexpandable fixation device is bridged across the medial aspect of
the distal radial physis and is anchored in
the adjacent metaphysis and epiphysis. As
the plate continues to grow, it is assumed
that nonphysiologic compressive forces retard the growth of the plate on that side.
The lateral aspect of the plate continues to

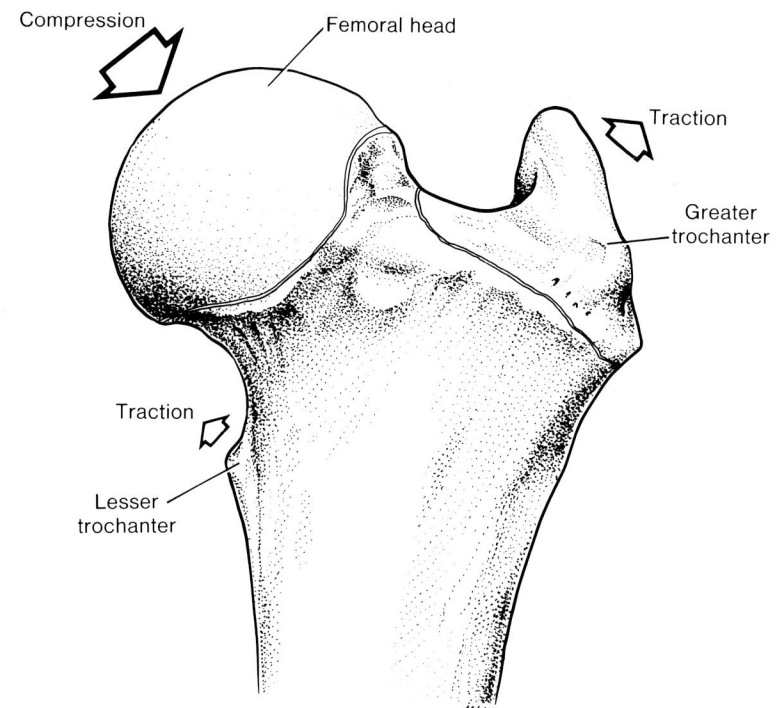

Fig. 14.5 A diagram depicting pressure and traction epiphyses of the proximal femur.

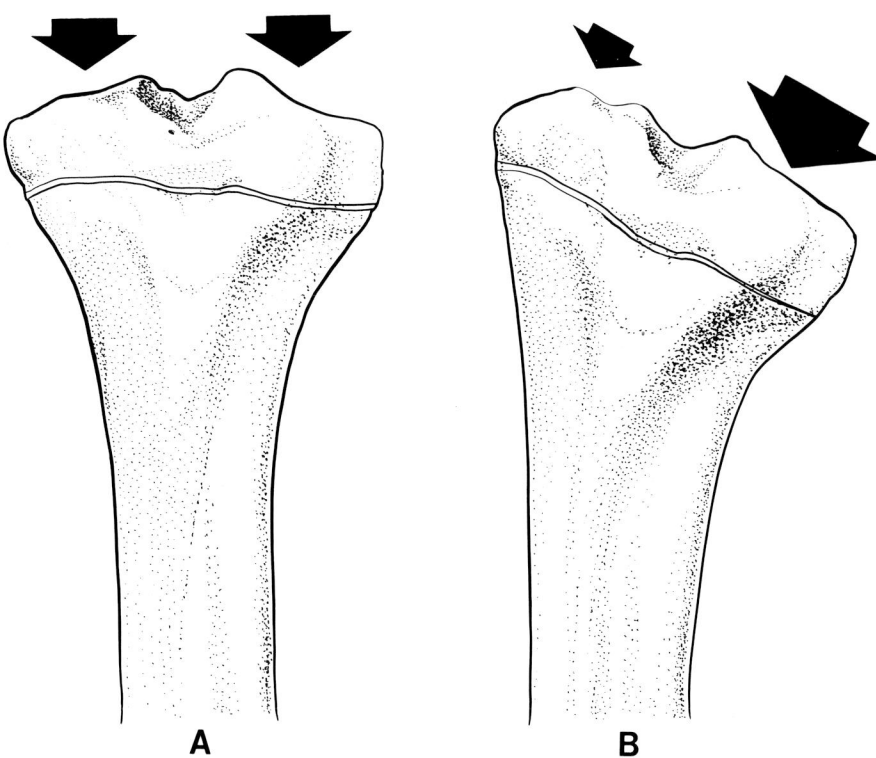

A   **B**

Fig. 14.6 A diagram depicting the result of uneven loading of the proximal tibial growth plate. A, even distribution of a normal load. B, an uneven distribution of an abnormal load. The growth of the physis has been retarded (B) under the excessive load, causing the tibial plateau to change spatial orientation.

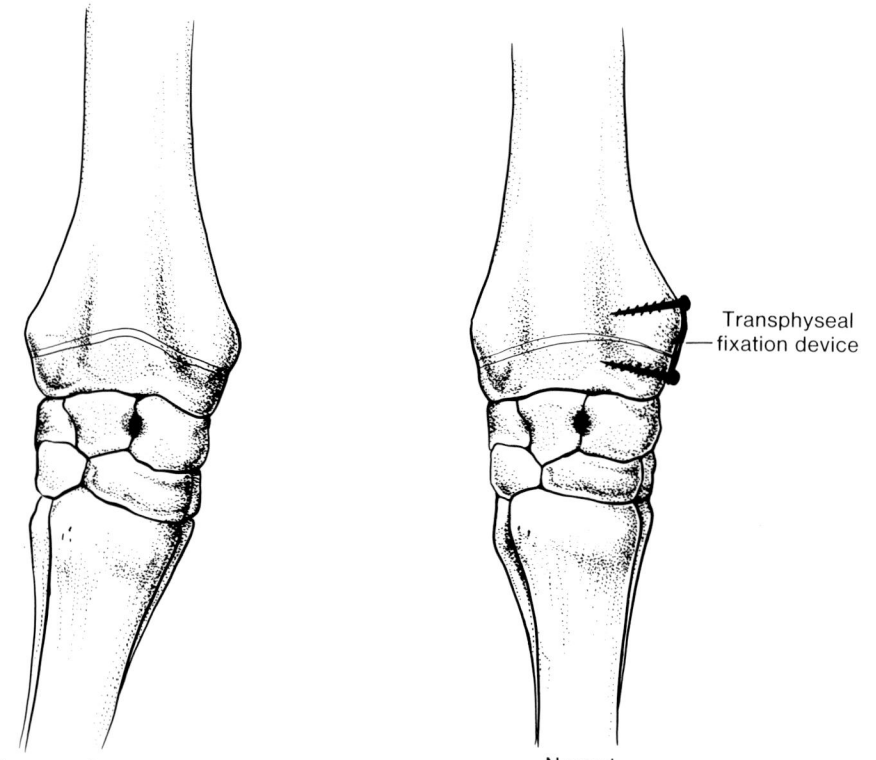

Carpus valgus Normal

Fig. 14.7 A diagram depicting the use of a trans-physeal fixation device to correct an angular limb deformity in a foal attributable to an altered growth rate in the distal radial physis. Nonphysiologic compression retards the physis after the application of the devise. The lateral side, growing normally, straightens the limb. If the device were not removed after straightening, then a medial deviation would result.

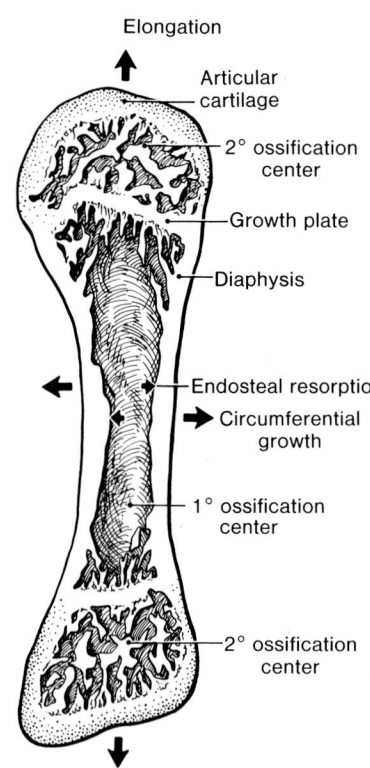

Fig. 14.8 The growth of a long bone. The growth plate is responsible for elongation. The periosteum adds new bone, whereas the cortical endosteum removes bone. These combined activities result in circumferential growth of the diaphysis and enlargement of the marrow cavity.

grow normally and eventually the lateral growth compensates with a resultant correction of the limb. The fixation device is then removed.

Biologic Properties of Bone

Dynamic Properties. The dynamic properties of bone are: endochondral ossification, internal remodeling, modeling, repair and calcium metabolism. These processes establish clearly that bone is a viable, and dynamic tissue.

As a tissue, bone consists of those elements discussed previously (Chapter 8). As an organ, however, the interaction of various tissues results in complex relationships which permit a different perspective of form and function. Developing osseous systems are a good example of the complexity of this integrated activity (Chapter 9).

As the long bones of the body grow, they move through space in three dimensions (Fig. 14.8). This growth phenomenon is, of course, the result of integrated cellular and tissue activity. The growth plate is responsible for elongation. The final three-dimensional configuration of the distal and proximal heads results from the activities of the secondary ossification centers. The periosteum is responsible for the thickening or centrifugal growth of the diaphysis, whereas the endosteum is responsible for the thinning of the diaphysis. Of no little significance is the realization that these two en-

velopes result in *osseous drift*, the three-dimensional movement of the diaphysis through space. Numerous factors influence the activity at the growth plate and diaphysis. *Modeling* is the response of these activities to varied influencing factors and results in the definitive form of a bone (Fig. 14.9).

The growth plate is an example of a joint between two bones, those of the epiphysis and diaphysis. This type of joint is a *synchondrosis* (Fig. 14.10). With age the cartilage of the growth plate is totally replaced by bone. This *synchondrosis* then becomes a *synostosis*. Naturally, this transition represents the completion of bone elongation. Of no little significance, also, is the recognition of what the closure of the growth plate represents. During growth the definitive thickness of the plate was maintained because of the balanced activity of the proliferative cartilage zone and the region of osseous replacement. At closure, the balance of these activities favored the total replacement of the cartilage.

The completion of growth and the achievement of the definitive adult form does not mark the completion of bone changes. *Internal remodeling* still occurs (Chapter 8).

Vascular, Neural and Lymphatic Components of Bone. The active metabolism and dynamic nature of bone is reflected in its vascular supply. Bones are well-vascularized organs. The blood supply permits access to

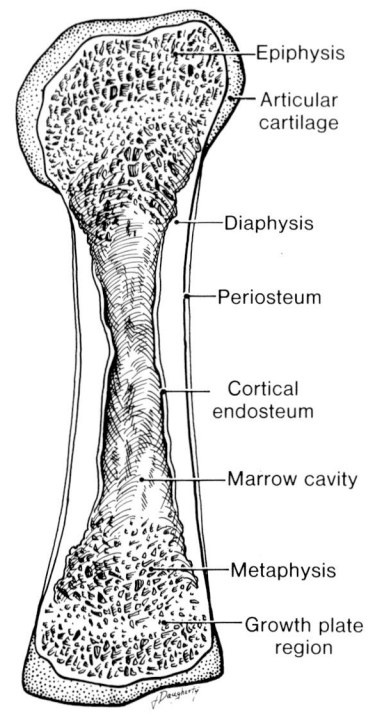

Fig. 14.9 The definitive form of a long bone results from the modeling activities during development. The growth plate becomes a synostosis upon closure.

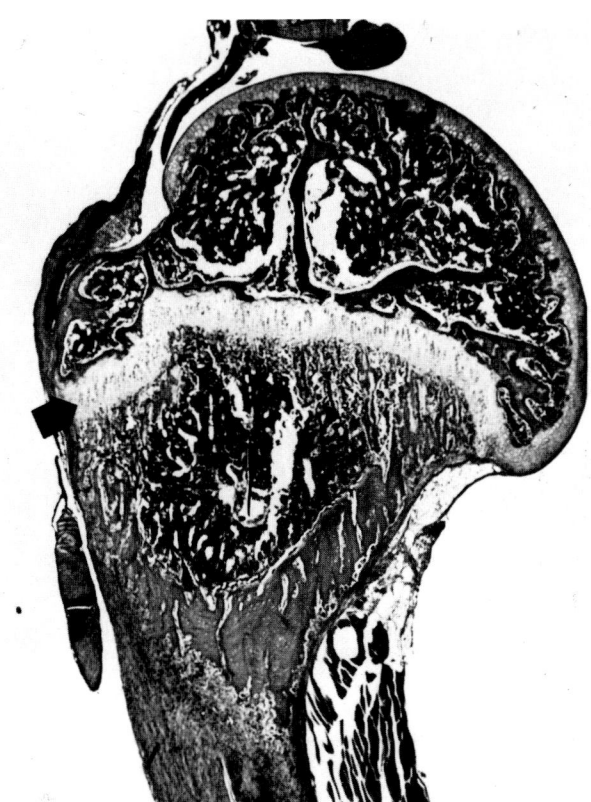

Fig. 14.10 Advanced stage of secondary ossification center development. The growth plate (*arrow*) is a synchondrosis. X3.

he minerals stored in the matrix. The availability to calcium and phosphorus stores is essential. Calcium is required in numerous cellular activities, whereas phosphorus is essential for the energy-producing aspects of cellular respiration. The vascular bed of bone supports the cellular activites associated with internal remodeling, modeling and growth. Because of the intimate association of blood-forming tissues with bone, a good blood supply is necessary to support this activity as well as insure the availability of blood cells to the rest of the body. Lastly, an adequate blood supply is essential for the proper healing of osseous tissues.

The primary sources of blood supply to a typical long bone are the *nutrient artery*, *metaphyseal arteries*, *epiphyseal arteries*, *periosteal arteries*. The relationships of some of these vessels vary slightly but significantly in growing and mature bones (Fig. 14.11).

The *nutrient artery* and vein enter the shaft of the long bone through an oblique canal. This relationship was established during development when periosteal buds invaded the primary ossification center. Upon entrance into the marrow cavity, proximal and distal divisions branch throughout this cavity. This vessel and its branches are the primary blood supply to the marrow cavity contents—red and/or yellow bone marrow. However, some of these branches are incorporated into the cortical endosteum, penetrate the cortex and become osteonal vessels

of the inner two-thirds of the cortex. Proximal and distal branches of the nutrient artery eventually anastomose with the metaphyseal arteries.

Metaphyeal arteries and veins gain access to the marrow cavity through numerous small foramina located in the compact bone of the proximal and distal metaphyses. These vessels anastomose with nutrient arterial branches and form capillary loops in association with the osseous replacement which is characteristic of endochondral ossification in the metaphyses.

The capillary loops (branches of anastomotic nutrient and metaphyseal vessels) are one-half of the *dual circulation to the growth plate*. This vasculature supports the osseous replacement activity of the primary ossification center but does not supply the nutritional needs of the cartilage of the growth plate. The latter function is fulfilled by the other half of the dual circulation—the epiphyseal arteries.

Numerous *epiphyseal arteries* and veins enter the epiphyses (secondary ossification centers) through numerous small foramina in the compact bone that delimits this structure. These vessels mimic the supportive role of the anastomotic vessels of the primary ossification center. Additionally, this vascular bed supplies the nutritional needs of the proliferative zone of the growth plate cartilage. It is the second half of the dual circulation to the growth plate. Before clo-

sure of the growth plate, the two vascular beds are independent of each other. Upon closure of the growth plate these vessels anastomose with the vessels of the primary ossification center.

The method of entry of epiphyseal vessels into the epiphyses varies with the disposition of the articular cartilage over the epiphyses (Fig. 14.12). Epiphyseal vessels generally enter the epiphyses at the junction between articular cartilage and growth plate cartilage. In those epiphyses in which there is a discontinuity between the articular cartilage and the growth plate, the epiphyseal arteries perforate the area of discontinuity to gain access to the epiphysis. The first configuration may subject the epiphyseal region to vascular compromise when trauma results in a fractured growth plate.

The *periosteal arteries* and veins supply the vascular needs of the outer one-third of the compact bone of the diaphysis. Although this vasculature is prominent especially during growth, it is maintained in the adult.

The described pattern and relationship of the vessels is generally typical of those bone which develop from endochondral ossification and have more than one ossification center. Minor deviations from this pattern occur in specific bones.

The venous drainage of bone is not as well understood as the arterial supply. Most of the venous drainage is achieved through the epiphyseal-metaphyseal-periosteal veins.

The presence of lymphatic vessels within bone has never been demonstrated satisfactorily; however, lymphatics occur within the periosteum.

Similarly, the innervation of bone remains an enigma. Nerves have been demonstrated within the marrow cavity and within osteonal canals. These poorly myelinated fibers probably are post-ganglionic vasomotor fibers of the sympathetic nervous system. The modality of pain is associated with the nerve endings that occur in the fibrous coverings of bones (periosteum, fibrous joint capsule). But clinical evidence and impressions do not support this distributional pattern of pain sensibility. Human patients complain of pain during bone marrow biopsies. Also, equine surgeons claim that horses exhibit pain when articular cartilage is removed from the underlying subchondral bone during the fusion of a joint (arthrodesis). Additional research is required before definitive statements about the nerve supply to bones are made.

Vascular Relationships—Functional Correlates. The integrity of the blood supply to bone is essential for the maintenance of normal structure and function. Alterations to the venous drainage can have profound effects upon these organs also.

Muscular activity is an important component of the mechanisms of osseous vascular integrity. The contraction of muscles temporarily occludes venous channels and

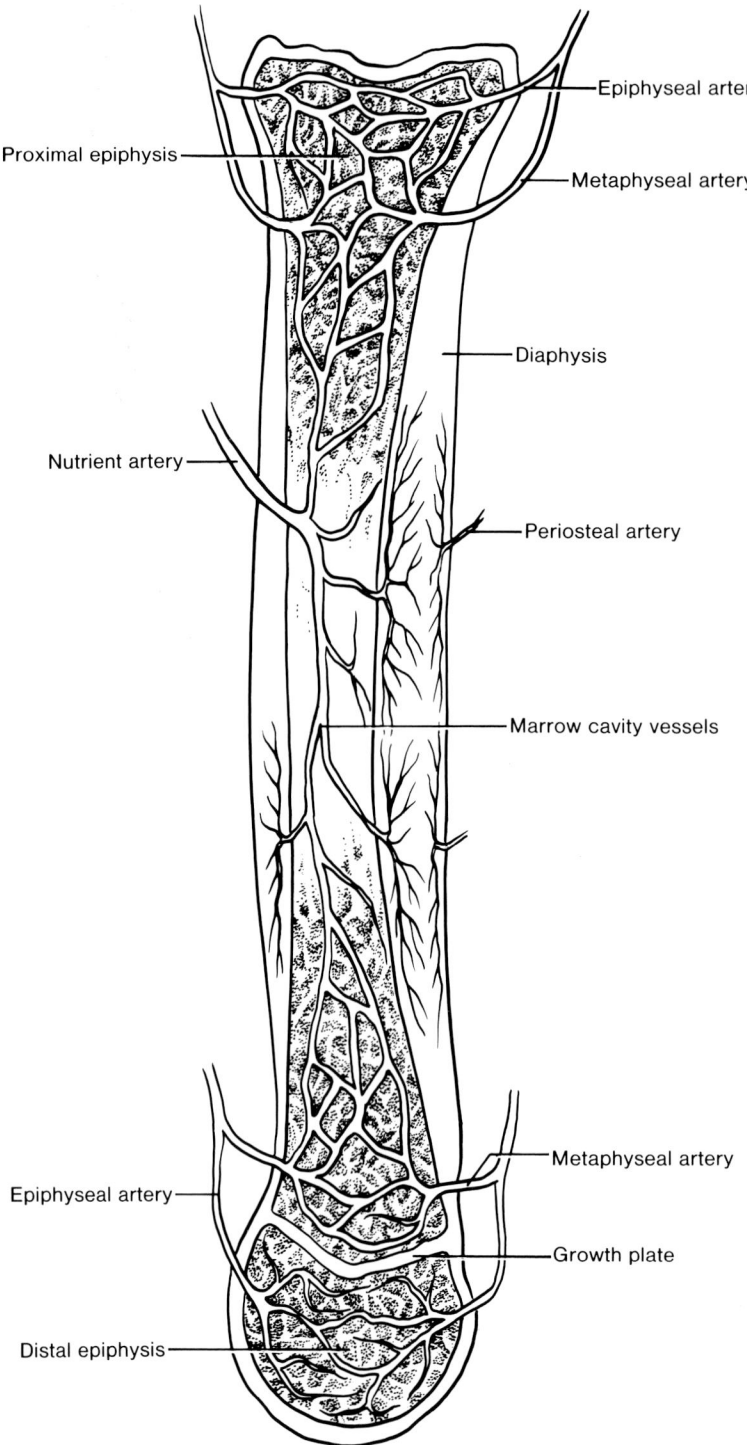

Fig. 14.11 Diagram of the typical blood supply to a long bone. Before growth plate closure, the epiphyseal and metaphyseal vasculature is separate. After closure, these vessels anastomose.

elevates bone marrow vascular pressure. This pump-like action of muscles is important to vascular drainage and bone structure. Prolonged immobilization of limbs during fracture repair is associated with a reduction in bone mass (quantitative osteopenia) proximal and distal to the fracture site.

The removal of the periosteum, either naturally or during surgical intervention, can result in the necrosis of the outer third of the compacta. The revascularization of

the region from adjacent regions in which the periosteal vessels remain intact assures that eventual replacement of damaged cortical bone will occur.

In adult bones, the epiphyseal-metaphyseal-nutrient arterial anastomoses insure that damage to one of these components has no untoward effects upon the bone. Because of the anastomosis of the metaphyseal and nutrient arterial supply, few problems are anticipated when one or the other of these

vessels is disrupted during growth. Disruption of the epiphyseal vessels during growth, however, can result in premature closure of the growth plate or avascular necrosis (death from insufficient blood supply) of the epiphysis.

Joints

The means by which two or more bones are joined together are referred to as joints or articulations. These structures are modified morphologically to serve various functions, all of which relate directly or indirectly to locomotion and/or stability.

Composition, Classification and Function. Bones are held together or connected by a variety of connective tissues. Some joints may consist only of a single connective tissue type, whereas others may consist of more than one connective tissue. The following tissues may comprise articulations: hyaline cartilage, fibrocartilage, dense white fibrous connective tissue, loose connective tissue, bone and adipose tissue. Articulations are referred to as organs, suborgans or complex tissues.

The classification of articulations is predicated most commonly on the type of movement permitted by the joints or their morphology. A morphologic classification of joints includes five types of structures:

1. Syndesmosis
2. Synchondrosis
3. Synostosis
4. Symphysis
5. Diarthrosis

The following functions are ascribed generally to joints:

1. Stabilize and unite two or more bones.
2. Facilitate movement between two or more bones.
3. Facilitate the growth of bones.
4. Permit weight-bearing.

Joints may subserve one, a combination of or all of these functions simultaneously.

Syndesmosis. A *syndesmosis* is the union of bone surfaces by dense white fibrous connective tissue. This is typical, as in the skull, when bones develop from separate ossification centers. The edges of the bones, which grow by appositional growth mechanisms, mark the limits of the *fontanelles*. The fontanelles contain the connective tissue of the joint, as well as the cells responsible for appositional growth. Progressive closure of the fontanelles results in a *suture*. A cranial suture, therefore, is an example of a syndesmosis. However, because all of the cells necessary for the continued deposition of bone are present, syndesmoses of the skull are commonly replaced by synostoses. At this point, the bones cease to grow.

Synchondroses. A *synchondrosis* is the union of two bones by hyaline cartilage (Fig. 14.10). The most common example is the rowth plate of the long bones. This joint ermits a unidirectional growth of diaphyseal bone while it permits fusion of both diaphyseal and epiphyseal bone. Some synchondroses, however (not those of the growth plate), permit a two-dimensional growth of fused bones. The ultimate fate of a synchondrosis is conversion to a synostosis.

Synostoses. A *synostosis* is the fusion of bones by bone. It may occur through syndesmoses or synchondroses. Whereas these two types facilitate growth, a synostosis ensures stability and immobility.

Symphyses. In a *symphysis*, the bones are joined through cartilage, fibrocartilage and/or dense white fibrous connective tissue. The ends of the bones are covered by hyaline cartilage. A dense white fibrous connective tissue or fibrocartilage connects the hyaline cartilage of the adjacent bones. The symphysis pubis and intervertebral joints are different examples of symphyses (Fig. 14.13).

Diarthoses

The diarthoidal joints are also called *synovial joints.* They are the commonest form of bone-to-bone articulation and permit the greatest latitude of motion. The maintained integrity of these joints is essential for normal musculoskeletal function. Unfortunately, they are subject to numerous disease processes and trauma that significantly affect locomotor function. Because of their significance in clinical medicine and surgery, they are discussed in greater depth than the other types of joints.

Origin and Nature. The synovial joints are established early during the development of the skeletal mass. When the presumptive bone centers form, they are separated from each other by mesenchyme. As elongation of presumptive bone-forming sites occurs, a gradual reduction in the intervening mesenchymal mass occurs. Eventually, the bulk of the intervening mesenchyme dissolves, and the remaining mesenchyme forms the contributing components of the synovial joint (Fig. 14.14). (Coincidentally, at this stage of development the perichondrium of the articular cartilage is lost.) Although the joint space develops from a cavitation process within the mesoderm, this process should not be confused with that associated with the formation of the celomic spaces. Mesothelial cells are not developed in association with a synovial joint. Rather, the synovial space is lined by cells which are not separated from the surrounding connective tissue by a basal lamina.

The basic components of diarthroses are *articular cartilage* and *articular capsule* (Fig. 14.15). All of the tissues mentioned previously as components of joints are either involved directly with synovial joints or are closely associated with them.

Histologic Structure. The articular surface is composed of hyaline cartilage (Fig. 14.16). The hyaline cartilage in these loci accounts for the bulk of this tissue in the adult body (Plate IV.9). It is devoid of a perichondrium. The articular cartilage is divisible into four poorly defined but functionally significant subdivisions (Fig. 14.17).

1. Superficial zone
2. Intermediate zone
3. Deep zone
4. Mineralization zone

ig. 14.12 A diagram of two different patterns of blood supply to an epiphysis. A. When the rticular cartilage covers the articular surface entirely and is continuous with the growth plate, the piphyseal vessels enter the epiphysis by traversing the perichondral ring at the periphery of the hysis (*arrow*). Fractures of the physis or neck can disrupt the vascular supply. B. When an piphysis is covered partially with articular cartilage, the epiphyseal vessels enter the epiphysis t the gap (*arrow*). These vessels are less apt to be disrupted from growth plate fractures. Redrawn and modified from Dale, G. G. and Harris, W. J.: Prognosis of epiphyseal separation. J. one Joint Surg.*40(B):*116, 1958).

The *superficial (surface) layer* is composed of small, flattened chondrocytes, the long axes of which are oriented parallel to the articular surface. An *intermediate (transitional) zone* is characterized by round cells

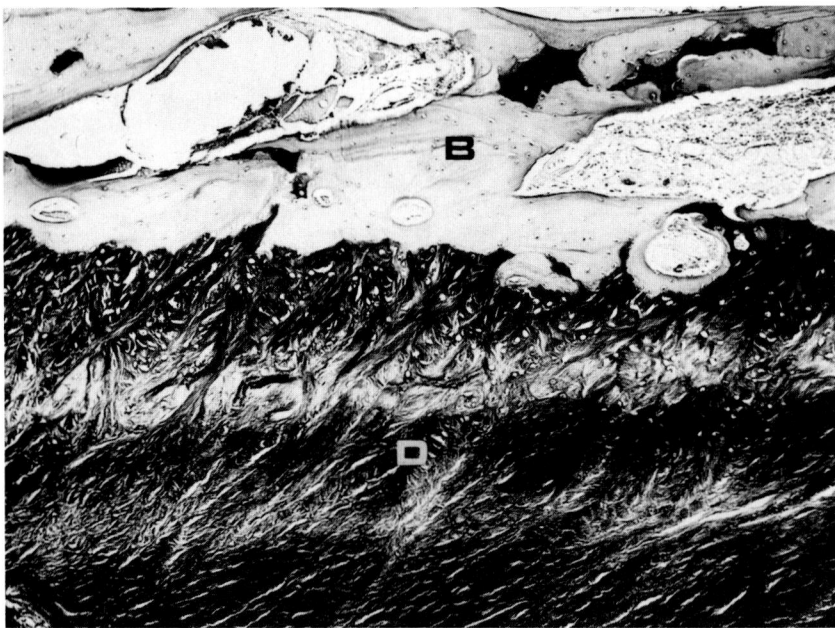

Fig. 14.13 A portion of an intervertebral joint. The bone (B) of a vertebral body is connected to an adjacent vertebral body by an intervertebral disk (D) which is composed of fibrocartilage. X160 (periodic acid-Schiff).

in various stages of maturation. These cells may be arranged in columns that are oriented perpendicular to the articular surface. The *deep zone* characteristically consists of mature and hypertrophic cells. The *mineralization zone* is present at the point of union of the articular cartilage with the underlying compact bone of the epiphysis (*subchondral bone*). The superficial edge of the mineralization zone is demonstrable histologically by the presence of *tidemarks* (Fig. 14.18). Developmentally, the tidemark represents the advancing wave of mineralization.

During development, interstitial growth of the articular cartilage occurs from the cellular region at the interface between the superficial and intermediate zone (Fig. 14.19). This region supplies cells superficially to the articular surface and to the deeper portions of the articular cartilage to support endochondral ossification. The attainment of the adult configuration marks the end of mitotic activity of the articular cartilage.

The *articular capsule* consists of a *fibrous layer* (*fibrous capsule*) and *synovial membrane* (Figs. 14.15 and 14.16). The fibrous layer is composed of dense white fibrous connective tissue which contains some elastic fibers. This fibroelastic tissue blends with the proper ligaments of the joint (medial collateral ligaments, lateral collateral ligaments, etc.). The fibrous capsule and some ligaments attach circumferentially at a *transition zone* between the fibrous periosteum and the articular cartilage of the contributing bones called the *perichondral ring*. The inner surface of the fibrous capsule is lined by the synovial membrane (Fig. 14.20). The

synovial membrane is reflected upon, blends with and is attached to the nonweight-bearing portion of the articular surface. The membrane forms and delimits the closed space of the joint cavity.

The synovial membrane consists of lining cells and subsynovial connective tissue (Fig. 14.21). The connective tissue blends imperceptibly with the fibrous capsule. The lining cells are flattened or rounded cells that form a layer that varies from one to four cells thick. These cells are fibroblasts; no basal lamina lies between them and the associated subsynovial connective tissue. Macrophages and lymphocytes are components of this lining also.

Prominent infoldings of the synovial membrane into the synovial space are called *synovial folds*, whereas slender projections are called *synovial villi*.

Types of Synovial Membranes. Synovial membranes are classified on the basis of the type of tissues with which they are associated. *Fibrous, areolar* and *adipose* synovial membranes exist. The *fibrous type* is associated with the fibrous capsule, proper ligaments and tendons that cross the joint. The thin cellular lining of this membrane rests upon the fibroelastic tissue of these components. The *areolar type* of synovial membrane is separated from the fibrous capsule by an extensive amount of loose connective tissue. This relationship permits extensive mobility of the synovial membrane. The *adipose synovial membrane* is associated with deposits of adipose tissue that are integral components of some synovial joints.

Perichondral Ring. The *perichondral ring* was described previously as a *transition zone*

between the periosteum of the diaphysis and the articular cartilage (Fig. 14.22). It is the site of attachment of the fibrous capsule and many ligaments of diarthroidal joints. It is, in fact, a perichondrium. In growing bones, it is positioned as a belt or ring at the peripheral margin of the growth plate. In adult bones, it retains its cartilage-producing potential in its same relative position to the closed growth plate. Stimulation of this area in growing bones is followed by some development anomalies characterized by excessive lateral deposition of cartilage and/or bone by endochondral ossification.

Adults bones and joints are subject to various types of trauma. If such trauma involves the tearing of the fibrous capsule and/or the ligaments at their points of attachments at the perichondral ring, then cartilage and/or bone formation can be expected. This new bone formation generally proceeds via endochondral ossification and is an attempt to re-incorporate the Sharpey's fibers that were torn as a result of the trauma. These bone spurs are called *osteophytes* or *periarticular osteophytes*.

Sharpey's fibers are collagenous fibers that are components of the fibrous capsule and ligaments that anchor these structures to bone by being incorporated in bone during developmental processes. The relationship is established by bone (or cartilage) growing around the fibers. *Periarticular osteophytosis* then, is an attempt by the perichondral ring to re-establish the relationship. Unfortunately, this process leads to compromised joint function. (Sharpey's fibers also occur in the attachment of tendons to bones. See Muscles and Tendons, Chapter 14.)

Synovial Fluid. *Synovial fluid* forms principally as a transudate from the extensive vascular network associated with synovial joints. Additionally, glycosaminoglycans, principally *hyaluronic acid*, are added to the synovial fluid by the secretory activity of the synovial lining cells. The viscosity of synovial fluid, which derives primarily from the hyaluronic acid, is one of its most conspicuous features. Low molecular weight proteins that are electrophoretically and immunologically identical to plasma proteins are present in this fluid in low concentrations. Lysosomal enzymes and proteoglycan degradation products derived from lining cells and cartilage matrix, respectively, are components of this fluid. The "weeping" properties of the articular cartilage also add some components to synovial fluid.

The turnover and absorption of synovial fluid is not understood completely. Substances may pass between or through the lining cells to be returned to the vascular bed or accompanying lymphatic vessels in a manner similar to the mechanism that accounts for the turnover of extracellular fluids.

Three functions are ascribed to the synovial fluid: lubrication of the joint surfaces; nutrition of the articular cartilage; and protection of the joint surfaces.

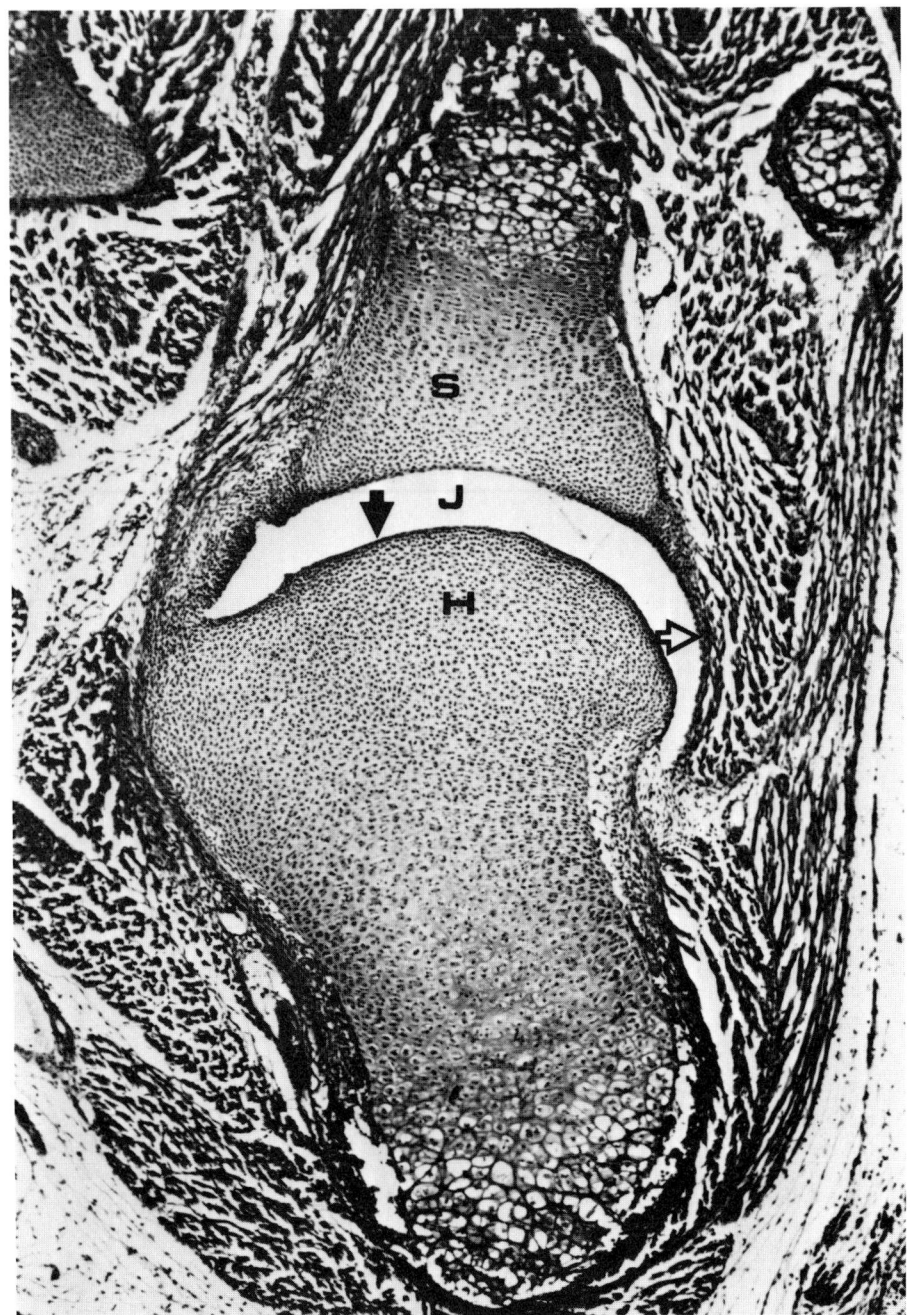

Fig. 14.14 Developing scapulo-humeral articulation in a fetal dog. The scapula (S) and humerus (H) are separated by the joint space (J). The synovial membrane (*open arrow*) has been formed. Note that the articular cartilage (*solid arrow*) is devoid of a perichondrium. X10.

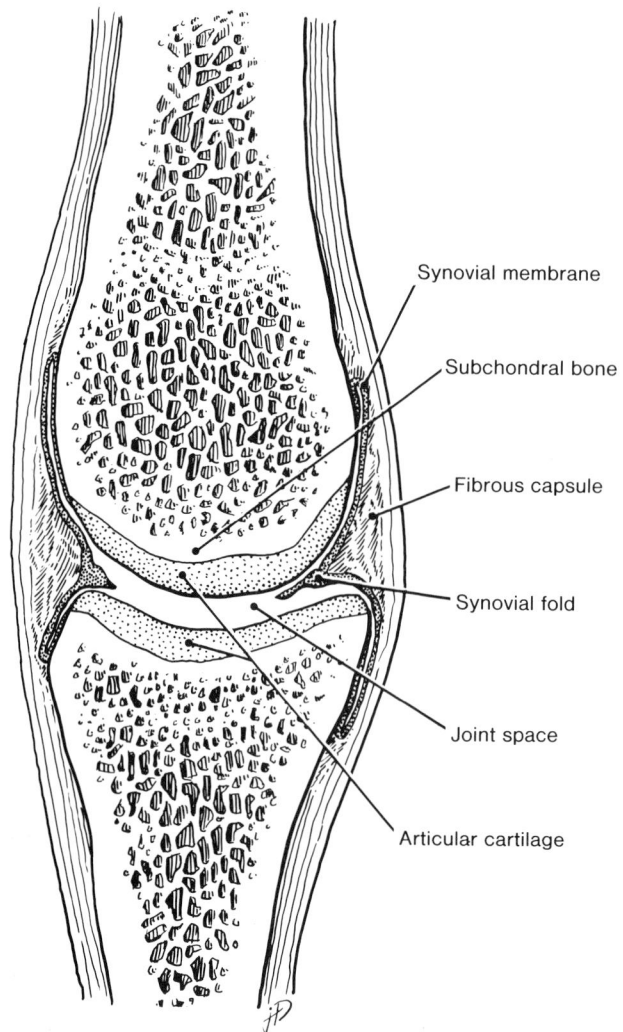

Synovial membrane

Subchondral bone

Fibrous capsule

Synovial fold

Joint space

Articular cartilage

Fig. 14.15 An idealized drawing of a synovial joint. The primary components are labeled.

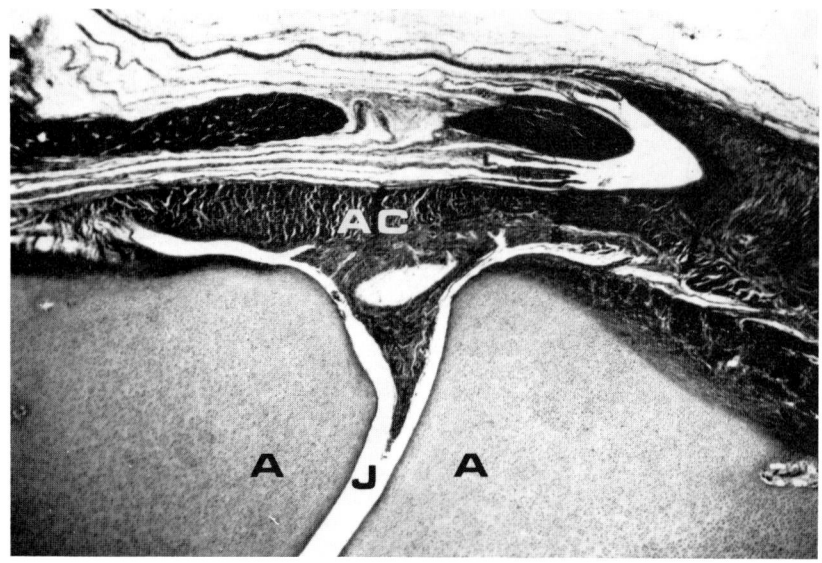

Fig. 14.16 A portion of a developing synovial joint. The ligaments and muscles traverse the lateral aspects of the joint in the upper part of the micrograph. The articular capsule (AC) surrounds the joint and projects into the joint cavity (J). The articular surfaces (A) are composed of hyaline cartilage. X10.

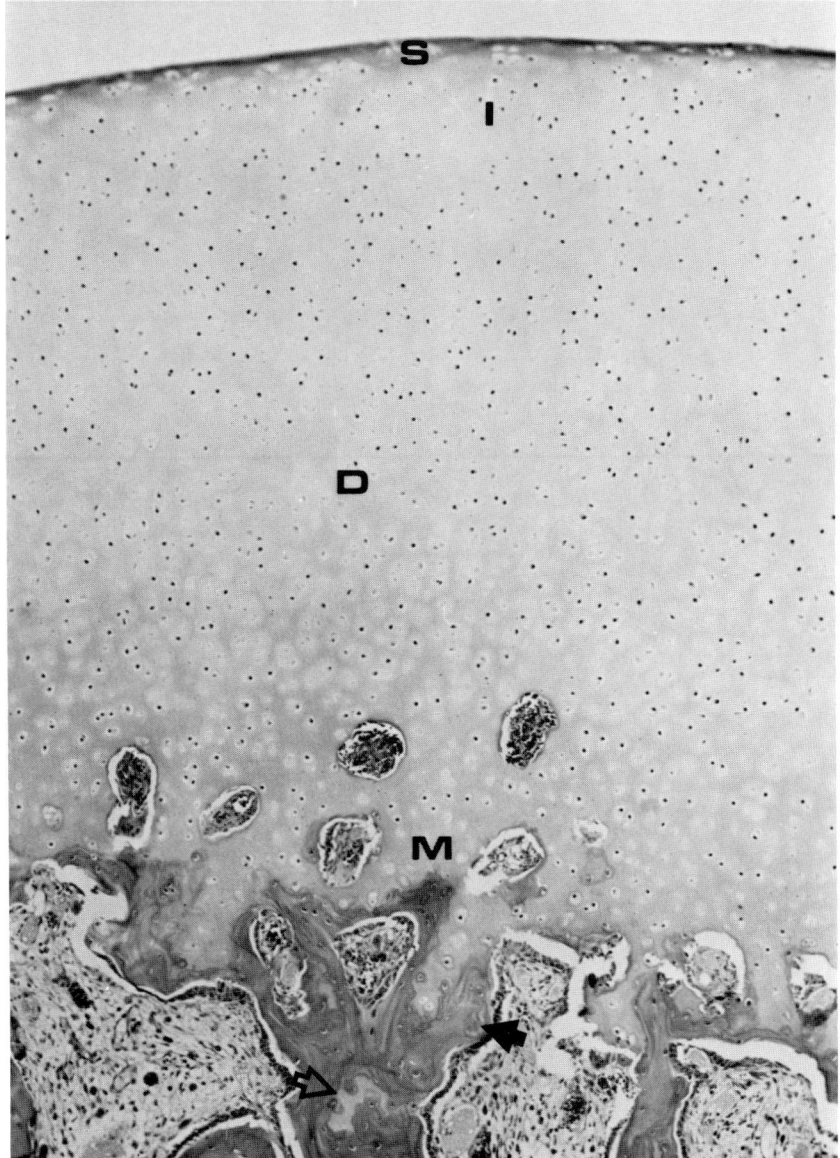

Fig. 14.17 A longitudinal section through young articular cartilage. S, superficial zone; I, intermediate zone; D, deep zone; M, mineralization zone. Woven bone (*solid arrow*) comprises the subchondral bone that underlies and supports the articular surface. Isolated foci (*open arrow*) of calcified cartilage comprise the core upon which woven bone is deposited. Note that the columnation of cells and tunnels of bone and calcified cartilage that characterize the growth plate are not apparent in the epiphyseal ossification center. X16.

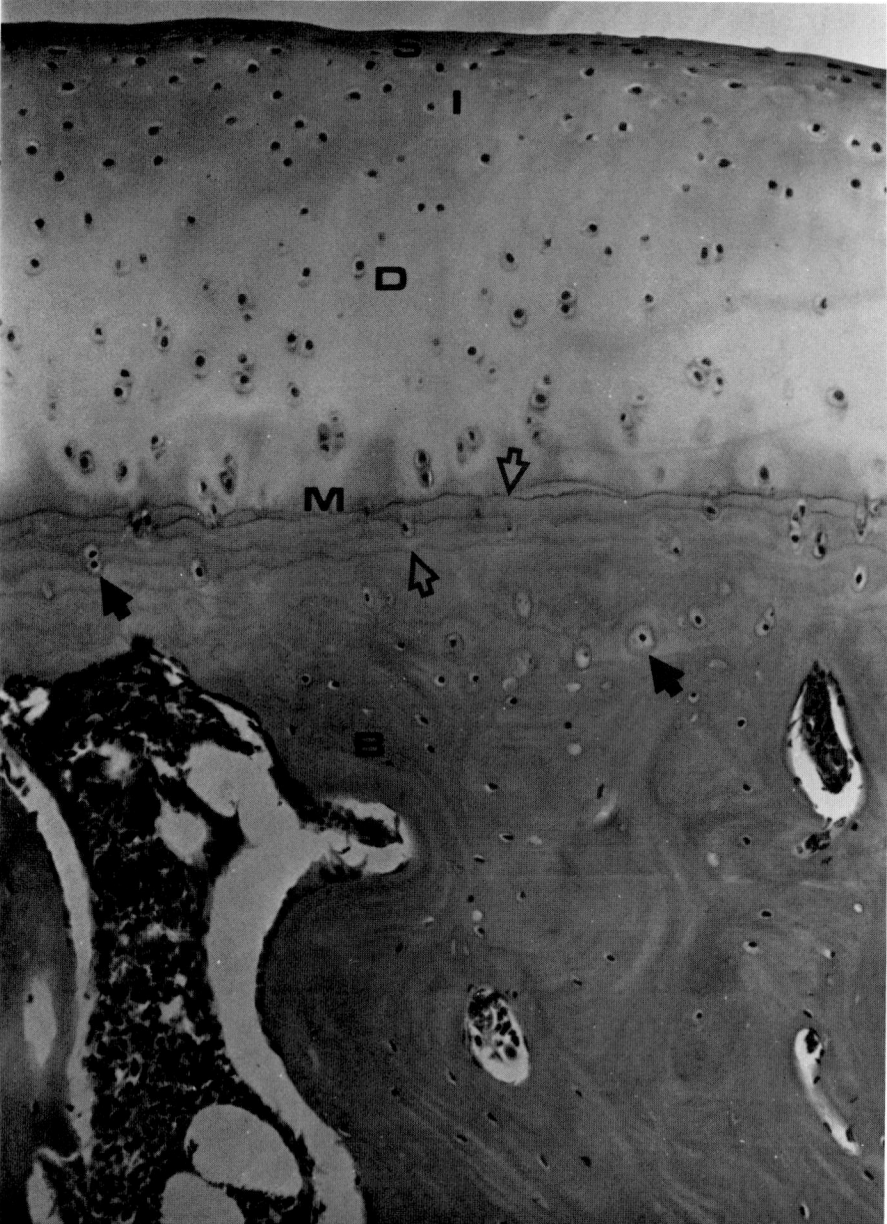

has lubricating properties equal to the entire synovial fluid. Removal of this glycoprotein from the synovial fluid significantly reduces the lubricating properties of the synovial fluids. Apparently, this glycoprotein functions as a boundary lubricant during high-load interactions.

Fluid lubrication of the joint is achieved by several mechanisms. One of these involves the weeping of cartilage when it is loaded. Small molecules pass from the cartilage into the synovial fluid during articular surface compression and return to the matrix when the load is removed. This self-pressurized hydrostatic property aids in lubrication and probably accounts for the intrinsic slippery quality of articular cartilage.

As a modified transudate of the blood, synovial fluid contains all of the essential elements to support the nutritional requirements of articular cartilage. *Nutrition* of the articular cartilage is an important function of this fluid. There is little evidence to substantiate the metabolic support of articular cartilage from the vascular beds of the sub-

Fig. 14.18 Mature articular cartilage and subchondral bone from the head of a feline femur. The superficial (S), intermediate (I), deep (D) and mineralized (M) zones of the articular cartilage are evident. The tidemarks (*open arrows*) represent the advancing wave of mineralization of cartilage. Pockets of calcified matrix (*solid arrows*) occur deep to the tidemarks adjacent to subchondral bone (B). Note the relatively smooth interface between subchondral bone and articular cartilage. Compare with Figure 14.17. X40.

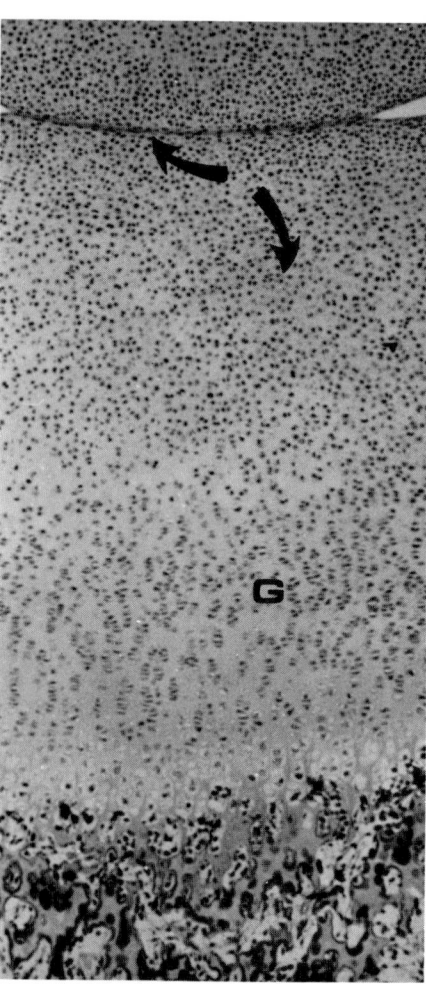

Fig. 14.19 Articular and growth cartilage of a developing bone. Interstitial mechanisms provide cartilage for the future growth plate and endochondral ossification (*arrows*). Note the columnated cells in the region of the presumptive growth plate (G). X16.

The *lubrication* of the joint surface has been attributed to the high viscosity of the synovial fluid. Because hyaluronic acid is the primary contributor to this viscosity, it has been assumed intuitively that this compound is responsible for reducing friction between the joint surfaces. However, the lubrication of the joint surfaces is a complex and dynamic process that cannot be explained simply by the presence of hyaluronic acid. *Boundary lubrication* and *fluid lubrication* principles apply to diarthroses. Boundary lubrication or *thin-film lubrication* is similar to the reduced friction that occurs

when the surfaces of bearings are coated with oil or graphite. Boundary lubrication is effective in a low load interaction or friction and is attributed to hyaluronic acid in the joint. Fluid lubrication or *thick-film lubrication* occurs when friction surfaces are separated by a thick film of lubricant. High-load interaction is characterized by boundary and fluid lubrication principles. The removal of hyaluronic acid from the synovial fluid does *not* reduce the boundary lubrication properties of the fluid. A hyaluronic acid-free glycoprotein fraction of synovial fluid has been isolated recently that

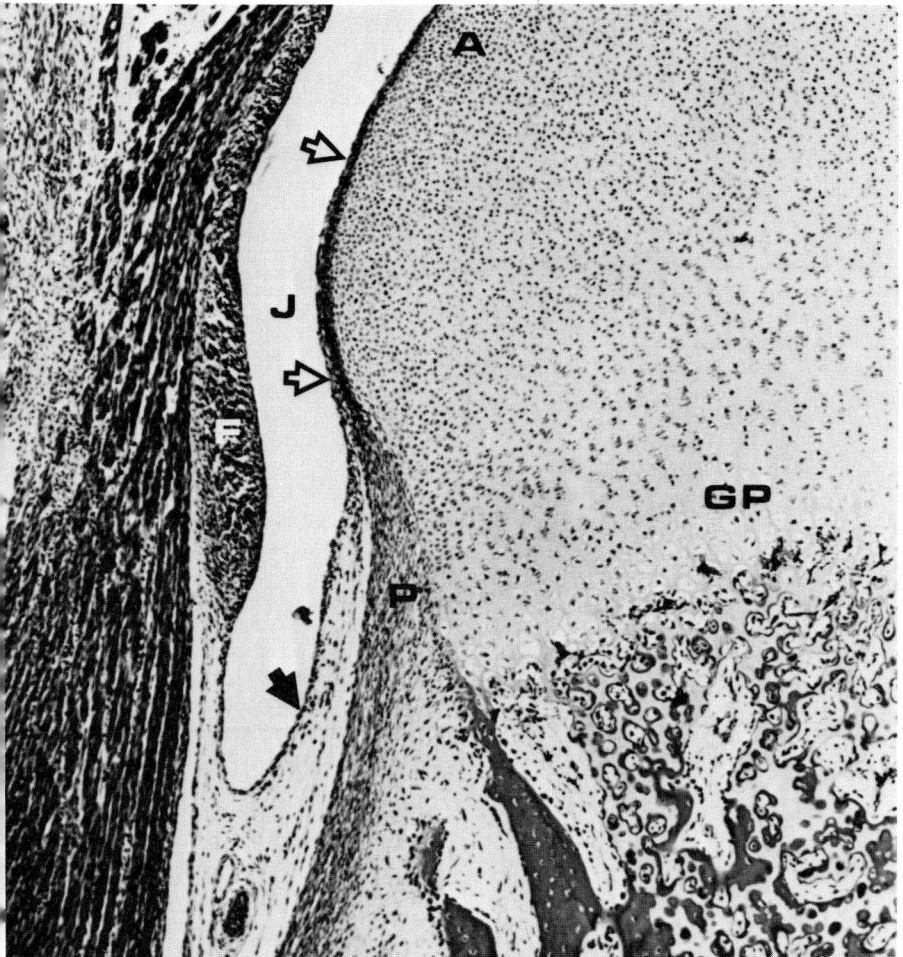

Fig. 14.20 Periarticular relationships in a developing bone. The joint space (J) is outlined by the synovial lining (*solid arrow*) and the articular cartilage (A). The fibrous capsule (F) is peripheral to the synovial lining cells. The synovial lining cells are reflected on to the non-weight-bearing surface of the articular surface (*open arrows*). The presumptive growth plate (GP) is bounded peripherally by the perichondral ring (P). X16.

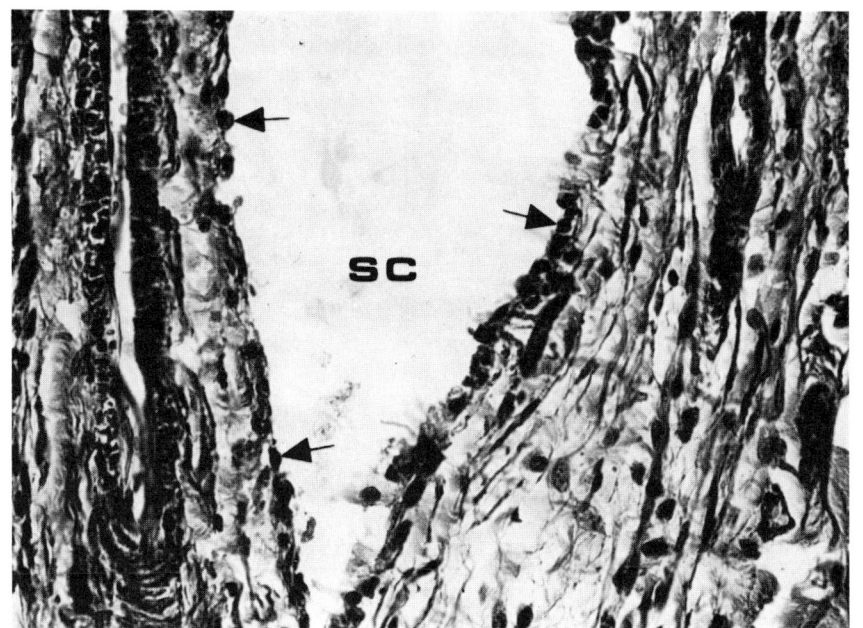

Fig. 14.21 Synovial membrane. The synovial cavity (SC) is delimited by a fibrous synovial membrane. Flattened fibroblasts (*arrows*) are the predominant lining cells. X100.

chondral bone. Rather, the weeping properties of articular cartilage probably provides a mechanism for the movement of nutrients and waste products through this avascular tissue. The cells of articular cartilage, all cartilage cells as well, are suited ideally for anaerobic metabolism. High concentrations of lactic dehydrogenase in the cells of articular chondrocytes supports this conclusion.

The *protection* of the articular cartilage by the synovial fluid is manifested in a number of ways. Its lubricating qualities protect the surfaces against mechanical damage. The presence of lysosomal enzymes as components of synovial fluid, as well as phagocytic cells being components of the lining membrane, protects against foreign bodies and microbes. Synovial fluid is a good growth medium for microbiologic agents. Additionally, the synovial cells and/or the articular chondrocytes may secrete an activator of the plasminogen system which prevents the formation of clots within the synovial fluid or on the articular surfaces.

Functional Correlates. The synovial tissues are extensively vascularized. The large capillaries, many of which are fenestrated, insure a rapid exchange of tissue fluid. Despite the slight alteration of tissue fluid by the secretory activity of the lining cells, it is reasonable to consider the joint space as an expanded portion of the connective tissue. The mechanisms governing the exchange of tissue fluid, as discussed in Chapter 6, are applicable to the exchange of synovial fluid. Extensive lymphatic capillaries are characteristic of this region also.

The fibrous capsule and associated ligaments are well innervated. Pain and proprioception are the important modalities transmitted by the nerve processes. Stretch is undoubtedly the significant stimulus for both of these sensations. Postganglionic fibers of the sympathetic nervous system, as vasomotor nerves, are present also.

The characterization of the synovial fluid is an invaluable aid when attempting to diagnose various joint abnormalities. Normal synovial fluid parameters described in Table 14.1 are compared with selected disease conditions to demonstrate the diagnostic value of synovial fluid analyses.

Joints are evaluated commonly with radiology. However, the articular cartilage is radiolucent. The radiographic interface between the two joint surfaces actually represents the mineralized cartilage and the subchondral bone of each surface. The subchondral bone is an important structural component for the articular cartilage. Also, many changes in the articular cartilage are accompanied by changes in the subchondral bone. Therefore, an evaluation of the subchondral bone is useful in the diagnosis of joint problems.

Repair of Articular Cartilage. The repair of articular cartilage was discussed in-depth in Chapter 7. The significance of the repair

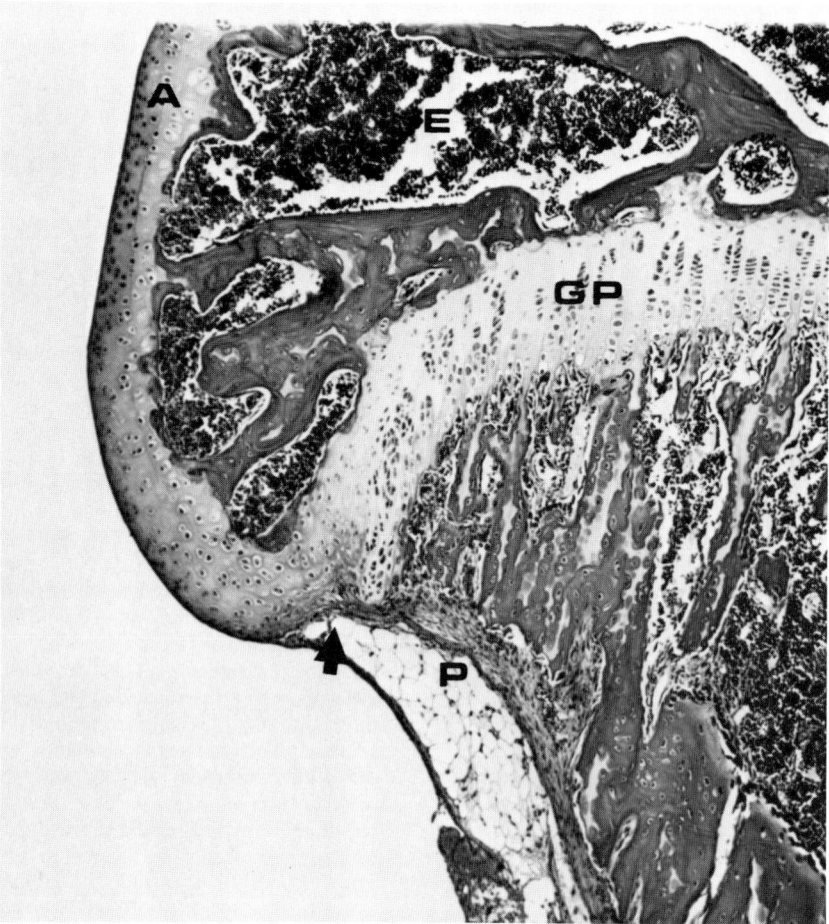

Fig. 14.22 Perichondral ring of a developing humerus. The perichondral ring (*arrow*) surrounds the peripheral limits of the growth plate (GP) at the transition point between articular cartilage (A) and periosteum (P). E, epiphyseal ossification center. X16.

Table 14.1
Synovial Fluid Analysis of Selected Conditions

Parameters	Normal	Trauma	Sepsis
Clarity	Clear	Clear-Bloody	Cloudy
Color	Straw	Straw-Xanthochromic-Bloody	Pink-Grey-Green
Viscosity	High	High	Low
Mucin clot	Good	Good	Poor
Fibrin clot	0	0-slight	minimal-marked*
pH	7.0–7.8	7.0–7.8	Decreased
Total protein	1.0–1.5	Variable	Increased
RBC's	0	+†	+
WBC's	500–3000‡	Normal-slight increase	30,000
Cytology	Healthy cells	Healthy cells	Toxic/degenerative
Monocytes	90%	70–80%	10–20%§
Neutrophils	10%	20–30%	80–90%§

* Varies with the types of agent.
† + if acute, O if chronic.
‡ Some species variation: horse-500; dog-3000.
§ Varies with the type of agent.

properties to joint integrity can not be overstated. The difference in potential between growing and adult articular cartilage is important. A review of these processes at this time would be worthwhile.

Muscle as an Organ

Muscle Organization. Although the muscles of the body, at a gross level of examination, assume varied configurations, their microscopic organizational pattern is quite similar. The components of these organs include skeletal muscle, loose and dense connective tissues, vessels, lymphatics and nerves.

Individual muscle fibers comprise the structural units for gross muscle masses. Grossly, skeletal muscle masses are distinct entities which are separated from each other by a dense white fibrous connective tissue called *fascia*. Fascia may be considered to be the capsule of the organ and is called *epimysium* by histologists (Fig. 14.23). This outermost covering extends into the muscle mass and forms a covering around individual bundles of muscle fibers, the *perimysium* Individual fibers of the bundles or *fascicle* are separated from each other by a delicate network of loose connective tissue, the *endomysium*. The endomysial connective tissue is continuous with the more densely organized perimysial connective tissue These connective tissue investments not only bind these components as a single morphologic unit, but this organizational scheme allows nerves and vessels to reach all of the muscle fibers (Fig. 14.24). Additionally, the investments are continuous with the dense white fibrous connective tissue of the tendons of origin and insertion Lymphatic vessels are present in the epimysial and perimysial connective tissue but are not components of the endomysium.

Muscles and Tendons. The connective tissue investments of muscles are continuous with the connective tissues to which they are anchored. This continuity is the means by which the mechanical activity of contraction is converted to work. The *muscle-tendon junction* is also the point wherein the actin filaments within the muscle cell are attached to the sarcolemma (Fig. 14.25). The collagen of the tendon is attached to the basal lamina at invagination points along the sarcolemma. The increased length of muscle during growth occurs by the addition of new sarcomeres at this junction.

A *tendon*, which is composed of dense white fibrous connective tissue (regularly arranged), connects muscles to their points of attachment (Fig. 14.25). They are structures which have tremendous tensile properties. Whereas the tensile strength of muscle is in the range of 80 pounds per square inch, the tensile strength of tendons may be 225 times as large. Thus, heavy muscle masses may function effectively through their small tendinous attachments. The ability to perform work is dependent upon tendons moving or gliding great distances through the associated soft tissues. Tendons consist of bundles of collagenous fibers that are bound together by perimysial-like connective tissue called *endotenon*. Blood vessels and nerves are also present within tendons. The entire tendon is surrounded by a connective tissue sheath, *epitendineum* (*epitenon*), that is similar to the epimysium Areolar connective tissue, adipose tissue or synovial sheaths between tendons and their fibrous sheaths are called *paratendon* (*paratenon*). Tendons are enclosed within *tendon sheaths* (*synovial sheaths*) at points of friction along their paths. The tendon sheaths are composed of two layers of flattened cells The inner layer is intimately associated with the epitendineum and provides a smooth surface for movement. The outer layer is attached to surrounding paratendinous tissues. The intervening space between the two layers is filled with a lubricating fluid that is similar to synovial fluid. The synovial membranes of joints may establish similar relationships to tendons such that the intervening space between the layers of the sheath is continuous with the joint space. The *mesotendon* is an elongated zone of continuity and contact between the inner and outer layers. Blood vessels and nerves enter the tendon through the mesotendon. The relationship between the tendon and the tendon sheath is similar to that estab-

lished when a cylinder is laid upon a slightly inflated balloon and then pushed into the balloon (Fig. 14.26). The cavity of the balloon is comparable to the lubricating space between the layers of the sheath. Note that this relationship is similar to that established between visceral organs, the celomic space and the mesothelial lining therewith associated.

Although some muscles do not originate and/or insert in bone, the tendinous attach-

ments to bones are the most common anchoring relationships. Fibrocartilage is often the tissue interface between a tendon and its osseous or cartilaginous attachment (Fig. 14.27). It serves to strengthen the point of origin or insertion. The actual attachment of the tendon to the bone or cartilage is achieved by *Sharpey's fibers* which are embedded in the bone or cartilage and are continuous as the collagenous fibers of the fibrocartilage and/or the tendon (Fig. 14.28). The same re-attachment problems exist as were described for the perichondral ring and its Sharpey's fibers. Attempts by the body to re-attach Sharpy's fibers to bone are characterized generally by *periosteal new bone growth* (*exostosis*).

Repair of Tendons. Classically, the healing potential of tendons was considered to be minimal. Tendons were considered to be unreactive and inert structures that were so specialized that they were unable to repair themselves. Accordingly, tendon repair was considered to be mediated by paratendinous tissues. Although the contribution of paratendinous tissues, fibroblasts and capillaries, is significant, tendons do have the ability to undergo *intrinsic* repair.

Two functional requirements must be met if repair phenomena are to return tendons to normal function. The tensile properties of the tendon must be restored and the ability to glide over great distances must be maintained. Proliferation of fibroblasts and the secretion of tropocollagen that polymerizes subsequently to collagen is essential for the restoration of tensile properties. Unfortunately, the contribution of fibroblasts from the paratendinous tissues can impair the necessary gliding property. *Extrinsic repair* is an essential component of tendon restoration, but it can lead to *adhesions* (collagenous connections) between the tendon and the surrounding tissues.

The sequence of events in the repair of a tendon can be considered to occur in distinct yet interrelated stages: *Insult (Impact), Induction, Inflammatory, Fibroblastic (Reparative), Maturation (Remodeling)*. The stages in the process correspond to those described for second intention healing of bone (Chapter 9).

The partial or complete severing of a tendon during the *insult stage* not only results in damage to the tendon proper but is accompanied by other soft tissue damage that results in the devitalization of the associated soft tissues. Hemostasis, an essential part of this stage, may exacerbate the devitalization of these soft tissues. Because the blood supply to tendons within synovial sheaths has been shown to be segmental, the location and extent of the lesion in relation to the blood supply may be an important factor in the amount of devitalization. Because the synovial fluid contained within the synovial sheath is also a source of nourishment, its disruption can complicate repair.

The *induction stage*, as described previously for bone, is probably an artificial sep-

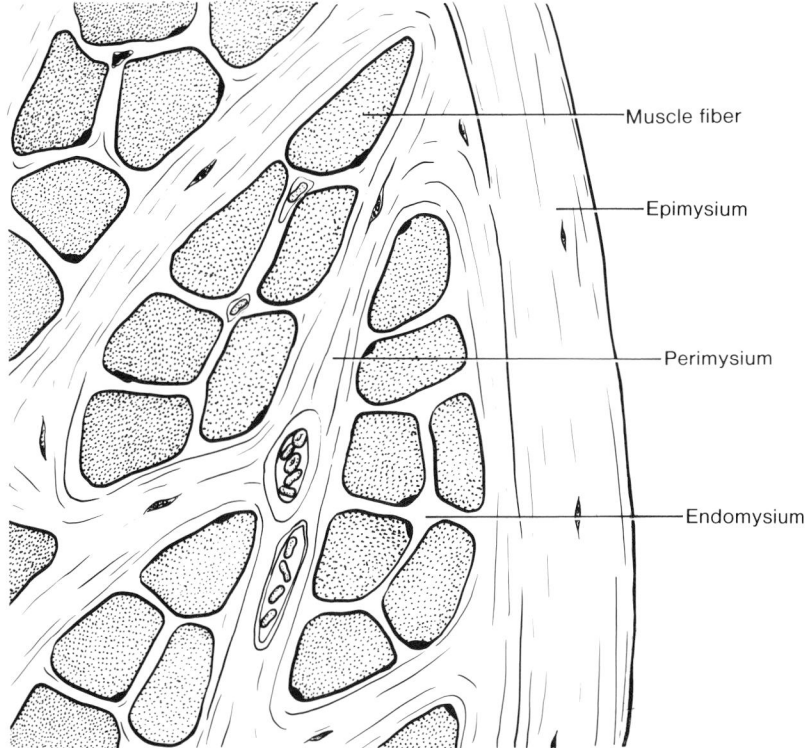

Fig. 14.23 A diagram of the connective tissue investments of skeletal muscle.

Muscle fiber

Epimysium

Perimysium

Endomysium

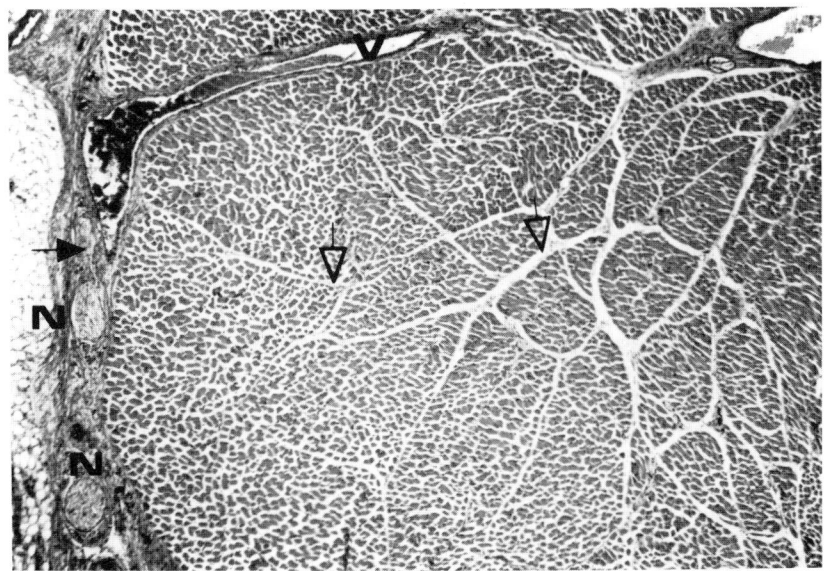

Fig. 14.24 A cross section of a skeletal muscle. Groups (fascicles) of fibers are surrounded by the perimysium (*open arrows*). This connective tissue is continuous with the epimysial (*solid arrows*) and endomysial connective tissues. Nerves (N) and vessels (V) are visible within the perimysium. X10.

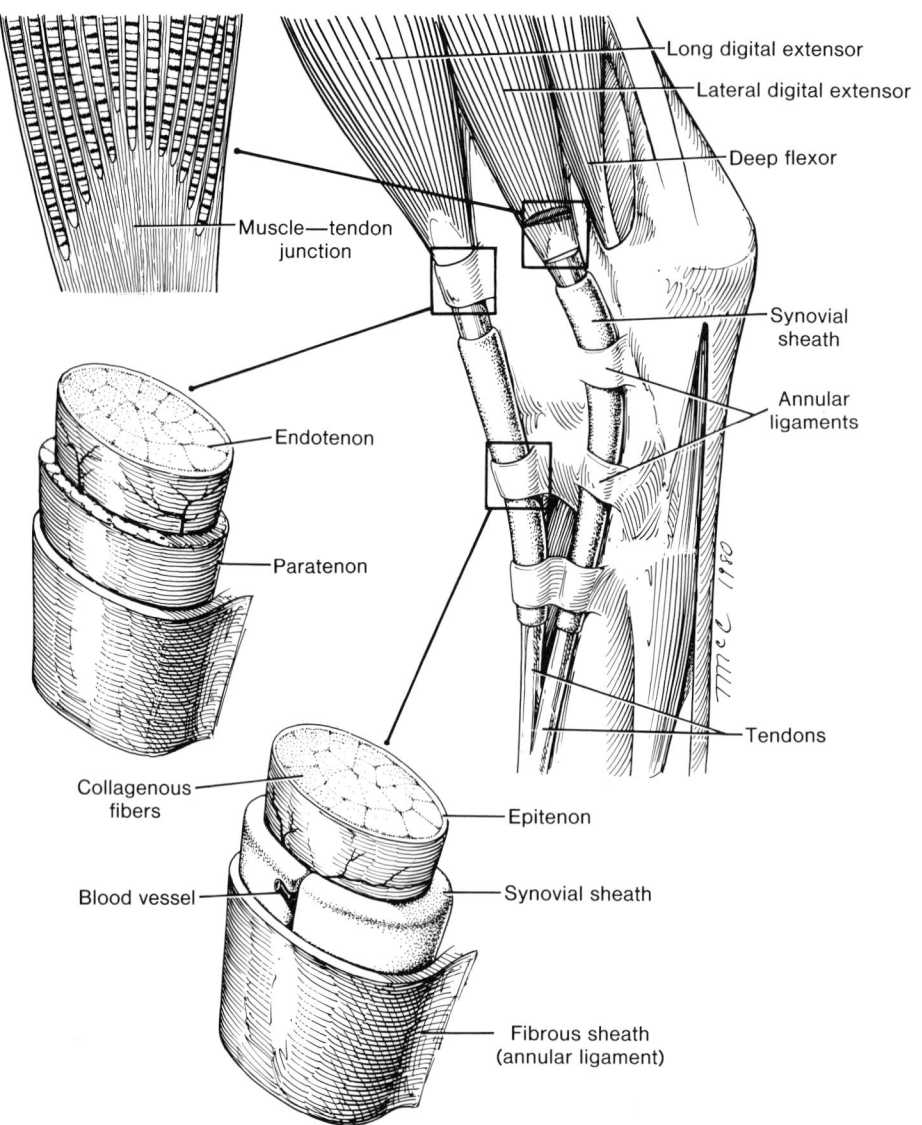

Fig. 14.25 An illustration of the superficial muscles and tendons associated with the equine tarsus. The components of these structures are labeled.

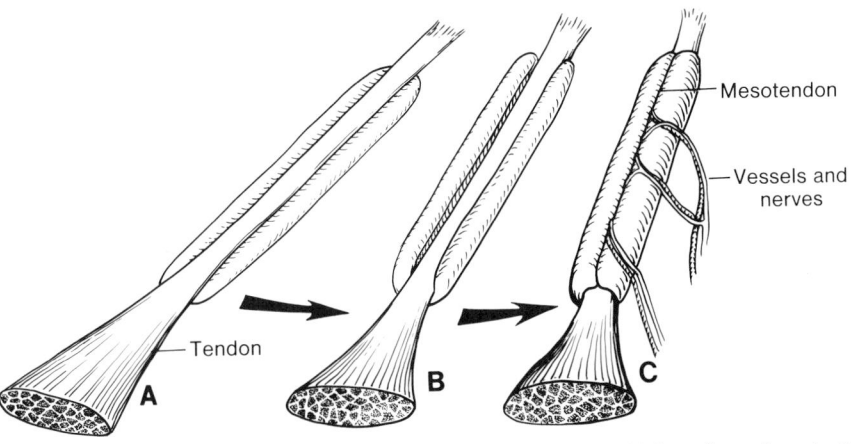

Fig. 14.26 A stylized diagram of the development of a tendon sheath around a tendon. A, initial tendinous invagination into sheath; B, continued invagination and encirclement of tendon; C, established relationship.

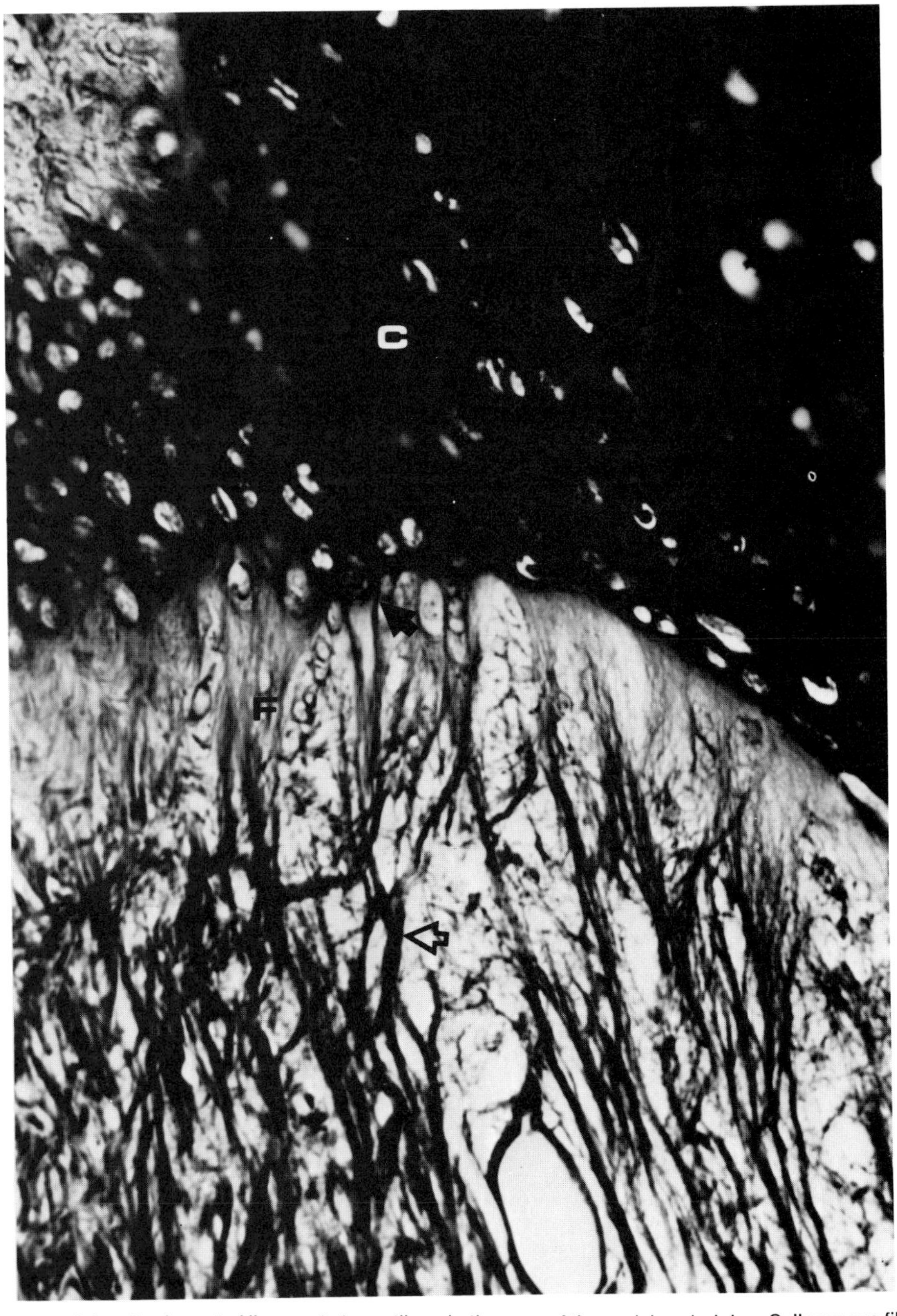

Fig. 14.27 Fibrocartilage and the attachment of ligaments to cartilage in the area of the perichondral ring. Collagenous fibers (*open arrow*) continue through the fibrocartilage (F) to become anchored in cartilage (C) as Sharpey's fibers (*solid arrow*). X100 (Aldehyde fuschin).

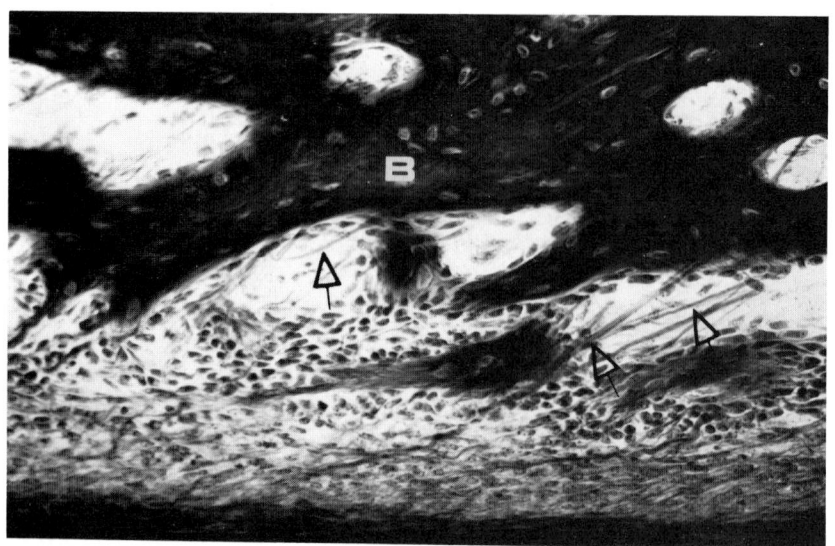

Fig. 14.28 Attachment of muscle to bone through dense white fibrous connective tissue. Sharpey's fibers (*arrows*) anchor the connective tissue to the bone (B). X40.

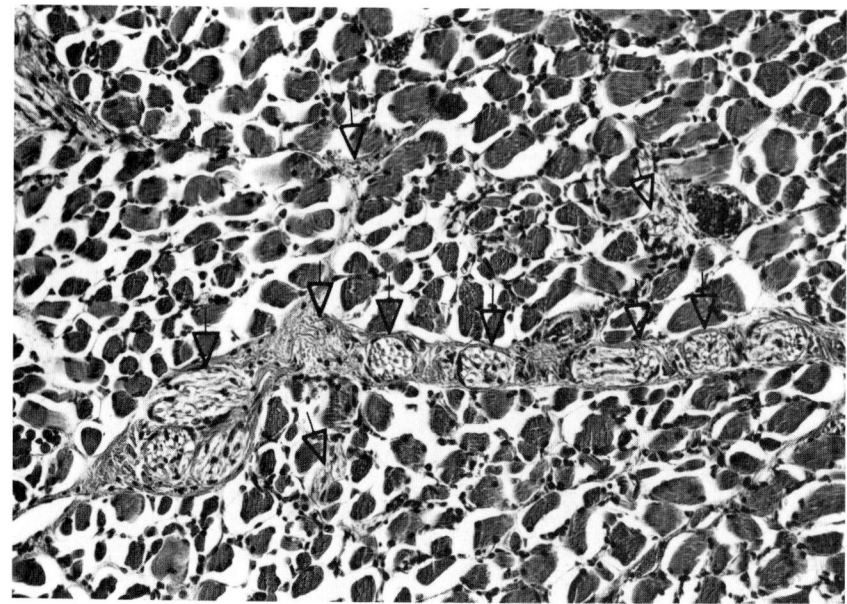

Fig. 14.29 Nerves and muscle. The nerves (*arrows*) which are associated with muscle are indicated. Branches from the nerve fibers innervate the adjacent musculature. X40.

aration of events that occur throughout the repair process. The stimuli for induction of new cells during tendon repair is unknown. Tissue hypoxia, however, may be an important factor. Fibroblasts proliferate rapidly within and adjacent to the tendon and new capillaries rapidly invade the tendon from the paratendinous tissues.

The *inflammatory stage* occurs as a sequel to the tissue damage and the amount of inflammation depends upon the extent of the damage. The cardinal signs of inflammation are apparent throughout this stage. An excessive amount of inflammation can result in an excessive amount of collagen formation (*fibrosis*) at the repair site.

The *fibroblastic stage* is characterized by proliferation of fibroblasts and their secretion of tropocollagen. The cells of the epitenon and endotenon are responsible for the intrinsic repair process. These regions become hyperplastic, and an extensive amount of collagen is deposited randomly within the repair site. The synovial sheath and paratendinous tissues also contribute cells and collagen. Their contribution constitutes the extrinsic aspect of the repair process.

During the *maturation stage*, the collagenous fibers become oriented to the long axis of the tendon, fuse and interdigitate with other fibers. The tendon eventually separates from the surrounding paratendinous tissues. The degree to which this separation is accomplished determines the extent to which normal pre-injury function is attained. Collagenous fibrous adhesions from the tendon to the paratendinous tissues can limit functional gliding.

Numerous factors influence the successful repair of a tendon. Careful management procedures of these histologic events can result in a good repair process and a return to normal function.

The events responsible for the repair of a tendon that has been torn from its attachment to bone are similar to those described. The important difference is the necessity to re-establish the attachment of Sharpey's fibers. Naturally, this requires the contribution of bone or the placement of a mechanical device (e.g., screw) to substitute for the Sharpey's fibers.

Myoneural Junction. Large nerve fibers enter the epimysial connective tissue, branch throughout the perimysium and send fine terminals into the endomysium (Fig. 14.29). A single nerve may innervate numerous muscle fibers (coarse movers of the body) or

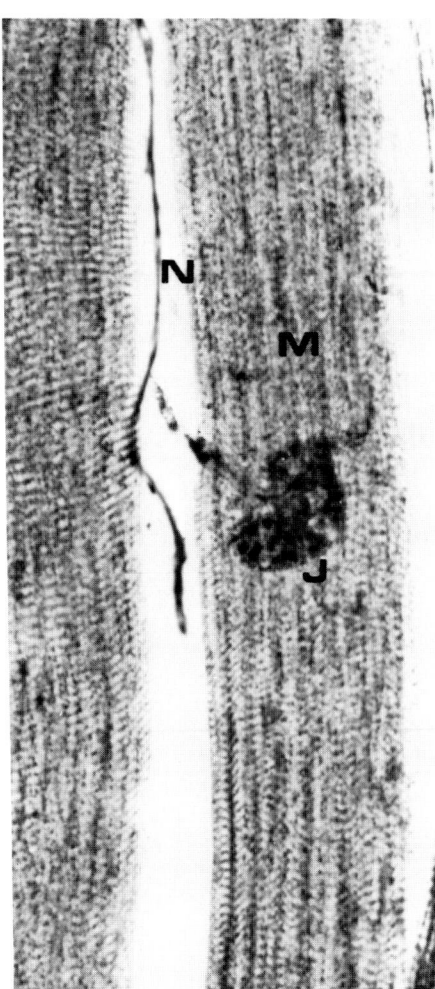

Fig. 14.31 Neuromuscular junction. A branch of a nerve fiber (N) terminates as a neuromuscular junction (J) upon a muscle fiber (M). X100 (gold impregnation).

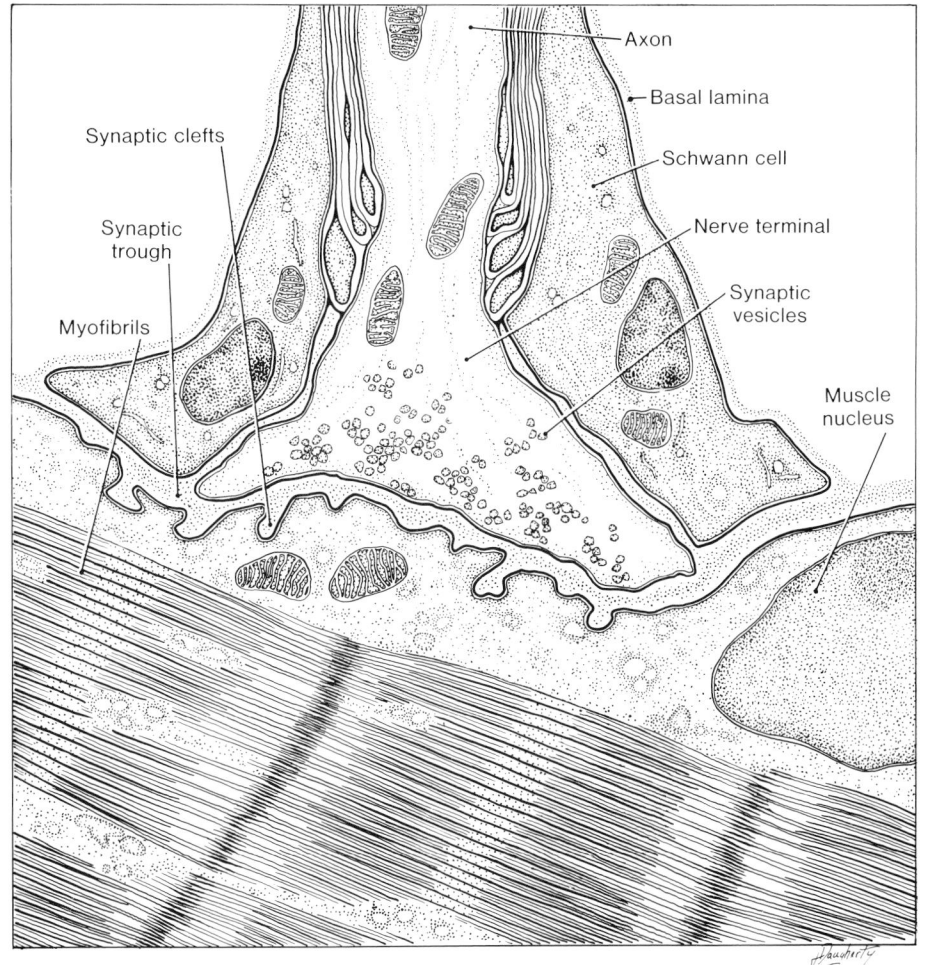

Fig. 14.30 A diagram of a myoneural junction. The components have been labeled. Compare with Figure 11.12.

each muscle fiber may be innervated by a single nerve (fine movers of the body). The muscle fibers and the nerve that innervates them are called a *motor unit*. The point of junction between the nerve terminal and the muscle fiber is referred to as the *motor endplate* or *myoneural junction* (Fig. 14.30). This relationship is demonstrable with silver and gold impregnation techniques (Fig. 14.31).

As the axon of a nerve approaches a muscle fiber, the myelin sheath terminates (Fig. 14.30). The Schwann cell, however, continues toward and covers the point of contact with the muscle fiber. The terminal aborization of the axon (*telodendrion*) continues into recesses in the muscle cell called *synaptic troughs* (*primary synaptic clefts*). The *subneural apparatus* consists of modifications to the sarcolemma which include numerous infoldings of the plasmalemma and the basal lamina, the *secondary synaptic clefts* (Fig. 11.12). Although the axon and plasma membrane are associated intimately within the synaptic troughs, they are always separated by the intervening basal lamina.

The telodendria of the axons contain numerous small vesicles and mitochondria. The vesicles, *synaptic vesicles*, contain the neurotransmitter substance, acetylcholine, which is released into the synaptic trough when the nerve is stimulated. Acetylcholine binds to receptor sites of the subneural apparatus and a motor endplate potential is generated. Subsequent depolarization spreads from this site and activates the muscle cell. The motor endplate or myoneural junction is similar to a synapse and is the means by which a nerve stimulates a muscle cell to contract.

Neuromuscular Spindle Apparatus. More complex neuromuscular relationships exist than those described previously. *Neuromuscular spindles* are scattered throughout muscle and are responsible for maintaining the tone of a muscle, as well as minimizing the possibility of damage by excessive stretching of muscles. Spindles mediate their activity through a *stretch reflex* that involves two neurons at the level of the spinal cord.

Spindles consist of muscle fibers, nerve endings and connective tissue (Fig. 14.32). A loose connective tissue capsule separates the smaller, *intrafusal* fibers of the spindle from the ordinary and larger, *extrafusal* fibers of the muscle mass. Intrafusal fibers vary in length from 2 to 10 mm and are approximately 200 µm in diameter. Two types of intrafusal fibers are present, a *nuclear bag fiber* (Fig. 14.33) and a *nuclear chain fiber* (Fig. 14.34). Of the 20 fibers that may comprise a spindle, the nuclear chain fibers outnumber the nuclear bag fibers by a ratio of 2 or 3 to 1. Both types of fibers are attached to the capsule at their poles.

Both fibers are typically striated. The nuclear bag fiber is enlarged in the center, filled with nuclei and devoid of contractile elements in this area. The smaller and shorter nuclear chain fibers are not expanded in the center, but large nuclei are prominent and contractile elements are missing in this central region. The central areas of both fibers are referred to as the *equatorial regions*.

Numerous afferent and efferent nerve endings are associated with these fibers (Fig. 14.32). Afferent endings associated with the equatorial region of both fibers are called *primary (annulospiral) endings*. When the

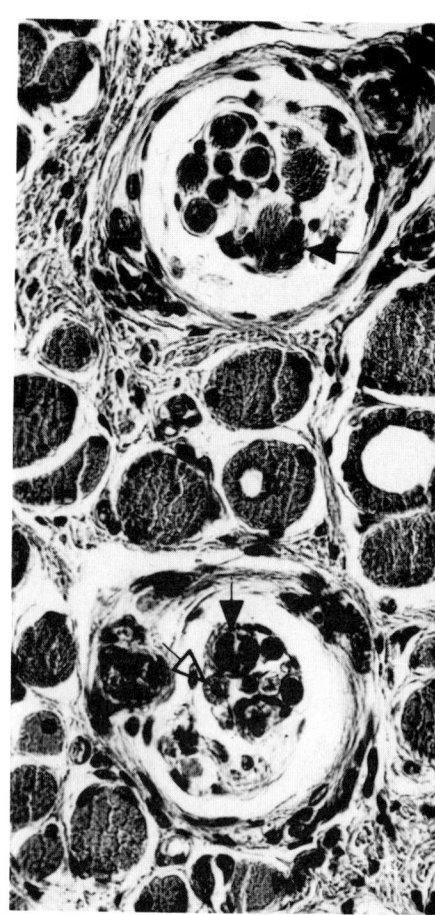

Fig. 14.33 Cross sections of two spindle apparatus from the extraocular musculature of an elk. Nuclear bag (*solid arrows*) and nuclear chain (*open arrow*) regions are apparent. Note the connective tissue capsule that separates the small intrafusal fibers from the large extrafusal fibers. X100.

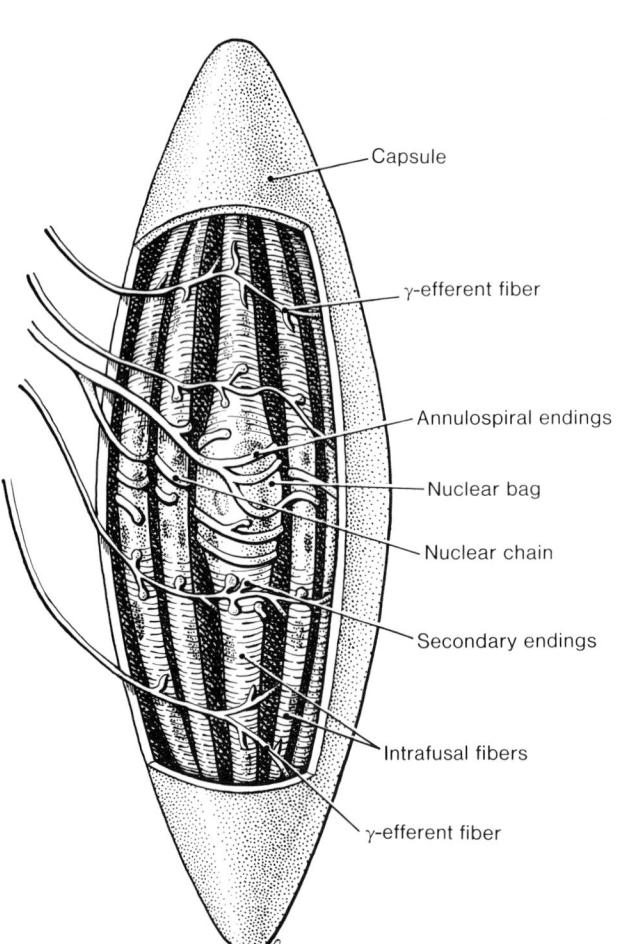

- Capsule
- γ-efferent fiber
- Annulospiral endings
- Nuclear bag
- Nuclear chain
- Secondary endings
- Intrafusal fibers
- γ-efferent fiber

Fig. 14.32 An idealized drawing of a spindle apparatus. Refer to the text for a complete description of these components.

equatorial region is stretched, these fibers transmit an impulse to the spinal cord which results in a signal to extrafusal fibers of the same muscle mass that causes a contraction. The same input signal from the primaries causes inhibition of other neurons in the spinal cord that results in a relaxation of the antagonistic muscle mass. This accounts for the stretch reflex. This type of activity explains the intuitive thought that when an extensor contracts the corresponding flexor must relax.

The input from the primaries informs the spinal cord and higher brain centers at a subconscious level about the rate of muscle lengthening or stretching and the actual length of the muscle.

Afferent *secondary endings (flower spray endings)* originate on either side of the equatorial region (Fig. 14.32). It was thought that their discharge was responsible for inhibition to the antagonistic muscle mass. Currently, they have been shown to evoke a flexor reflex pattern. Their precise function

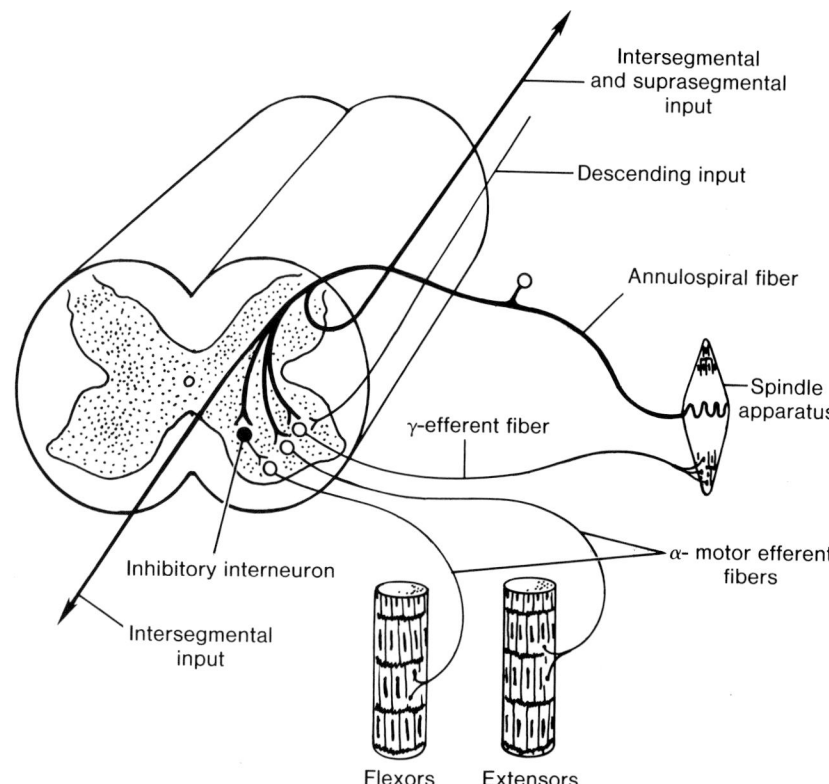

Fig. 14.35 A schematic representation of the myotatic reflex. Stimulation of the spindle apparatus by stretching induces the firing of the annulospiral afferent fibers. Collaterals synapse with α-motor neurons in the ventral gray column which cause contraction of the extensors. A synapse with an interneuron inhibits the contraction of the flexors. Collaterals from the annulospiral fibers descend and ascend the spinal cord to intersegmental and suprasegmental levels.

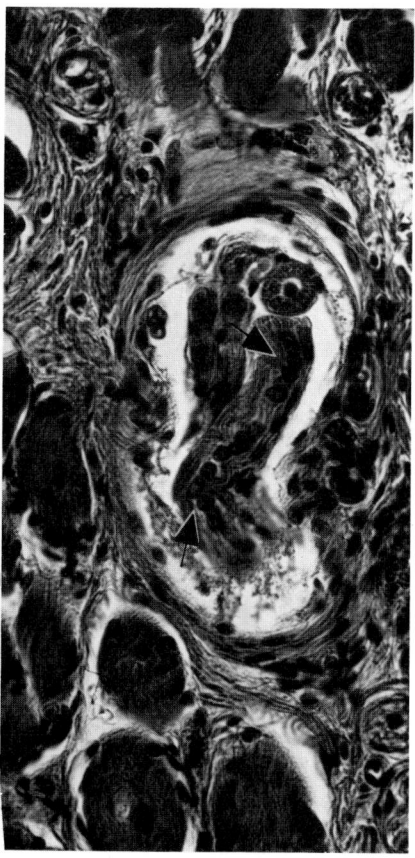

ig. 14.34 An oblique section of a spindle oparatus from the extraocular musculature of n elk. *Arrow*, equitorial regions of nuclear hain fibers. X100.

ithin the spindle is not understood. They o, however, transmit information about uscle length to the central nervous system t a subconscious level.

Small efferent fibers (*gamma efferents*) nervate the intrafusal fibers at their re- ective poles (Fig. 14.32). Rather than nctioning primarily to contract the intra- sal fibers as an end in itself, they are sponsible for establishing the degree of retch on equatorial regions. By accom- lishing this, they function to raise or lower e threshold of primary ending discharge nd thus make the spindle more or less nsitive to stretching. Once the extrafusal bers contract, the tension or stretching on e equatorial region would relax and cause collapse of these areas. By gamma efferent ischarge, tension on these regions is main- ined throughout the entire range of the ontraction. This ensures a constant infor- ational input to the spinal cord and higher rain centers about the degree of stretch or ck thereof in a particular muscle mass.

The stretch reflex or myotatic reflex is resented schematically in Figure 14.35.

eurotendinous Relationships. *Neurotendi- ous organs* (*Golgi tendon organs*) are lo- ted in the tendons close to their junction ith the muscle mass. They consist of col-

lagenous fibers that are contained within a connective tissue capsule. Numerous cells and afferent terminals are also present. They transmit information concerning the amount of stretch or tension on tendons. This type of information, therefore, also indicates the amount of contraction in a mass of muscle. With excessive tension on a tendon, the afferent discharge results in an inhibition to further contraction. Although the informational input is transmitted at a subconscious level throughout the entire range of muscular contraction, ultimately these organs minimize the possibility of ten- dons being torn from their points of attach- ment to bone or muscle.

Although the input from spindles and neurotendinous organs is at a subconscious level, conscious input is achieved through other mechanisms. Naked nerve endings (Ruffini-like) are embedded within the con- nective tissue of joint capsules. Subjected to the compression and tension associated with joint movement, they transmit information which is *kinesthetic*; i.e., information con- cerning the relative positions of various parts of the body.

References

Bone as an Organ
Arnold, J. S.: Quantitation of mineral of bone as an organ and tissue in osteoporosis. Clin. Orthop. *17:* 167, 1960.
Cooper, R. R. Milgram, J. W. and Robinson, R. A.: Morphology of the osteon. An electron microscopic study. J. Bone Joint Surg. *48A:*1239, 1966.
Elliot, H. C.: Studies on articular cartilages. I. Growth mechanisms. Amer. J. Anat. *58:*127, 1936.
Frost, H. M.: *Bone Modeling and Skeletal Modeling Errors.* C. C. Thomas, Springfield, 1973.
Frost, H. M.: New concepts of bone remodelling and of the nature of osteoporoses. J. Med. Surg. *1:*41, 1961.
Frost, H. M.: *Bone Remodelling Dynamics.* C. C. Thomas, Springfield, Ill., 1963.
Frost, H. M.: *The Physiology of Cartilaginous, Fibrous and Bony Tissue.*C. C. Thomas, Springfield, 1972.
Haines, R. W.: The development of joints. J. Anat. *81:* 33, 1947.
Hancox, N. M.: *Biology of Bone.* University Press, Cam- bridge, 1972.
Hirohata, K. and Morimoto, K.: *Ultrastructure of Bone and Joint Diseases.* Grune and Stratton, New York, 1971.
Ketchum, L. D.: Tendon Healing. In: Hunt, T. K. (edi- tor). *Fundamentals of Wound Management in Sur- gery: Selected Tissues.* pp. 121–153. Chirurgecom, Inc., South Plainfield, New Jersey, 1977.
Koch, J. L.: The laws of bone architecture. Amer. J. Anat. *21:*177, 1917.
Roy, S.: Ultrastructure of articular cartilage in experi- mental hemarthrosis. Arch. Path. *86:*69, 1968.
Silberberg, M., Silberberg, R. and Hasler, M.: Fine struc- ture of articular cartilage in mice receiving cortisone acetate. Arch. Path. *82:*569, 1966.
Sokoloff, L. and Bland, J. H.: *The Musculoskeletal Sys- tem.* Williams & Wilkins, Baltimore, 1975.
Urist, M. R. (editor): Symposium: Articular cartilage in health and disease, Clin. Orthop. *64:*3, 1969.
Wilson, F. C.: *The Musculoskeletal System.* J. B Lippin- cott, Philadelphia, 1975.

Muscle as an Organ

Bowman, J. P., Jr.: *The Muscle Spindle and Neuronal Control of the Tongue: Implications for Speech.* C. C. Thomas, Springfield, Ill., 1971.

Cohen, L. A.: Contributions of tactile musculo-tendinous and joint mechanisms to position sense in human shoulder. J. Neurophysiol. *21:*563, 1958.

Cooper, S.: Afferent impulses in the hypoglossal nerve on stretching the cat's tongue. J. Physiol. *126:*32P, 1954.

Lentz, T. L.: Development of the neuromuscular junction. J. Cell Biol. *47:*423, 1970.

Matthews, P. B. C.: Muscle spindles and their motor control. Physiol. Rev. *44:*219, 1964.

Nystrom, B.: Muscle-spindle histochemistry. Science *155:*1424, 1967.

Sokoloff, L. and Bland, J. H.: *The Musculoskeletal System.* Williams & Wilkins, Baltimore, 1975.

Spiro, A. J. and Beilin, R. L.: Histochemical duality of rabbit intrafusal fibers. J. Histochem. Cytochem. *17:*348, 1969.

Wilson, F. C. *The Musculoskeletal System.* J. B. Lippincott, Philadelphia, 1975.

Yelin, H.: A histochemical study of muscle spindles and their relationship to extrafusal fiber types in the rat. Amer. J. Anat. *125:*31, 1969.

15: Nervous System

General Characteristics

Form and Function. The nervous system is a complex grouping of organs that are comprised of the tissues described previously (Chapter 12), as well as connective tissue and vascular components. This complexity is based upon the ability of neurons to communicate with each other and all of the other tissues and organs of the body. The function of the system is perceiving stimuli, processing the information and causing appropriate response in the organism that contributes to its *homeostasis*. The neuron is the anatomic unit of the system and is the basis for the massive intercommunicating, three-dimensional network of cells and cellular processes. The essence of the anatomic organization of the nervous system is the segregation of neurons into hierarchical levels of responsibility that contribute to the interdependent functions of stimulus perception, information processing and initiation of appropriate response.

Segregated upon an anatomic basis, the nervous system is divisible into two major subdivisions, the *central nervous system* (*CNS*) and *peripheral nervous system* (*PNS*). The CNS is comprised of the brain, its extensions and the spinal cord. The units consist of numerous pools of segregated neurons that are interconnected by the dendritic and axonal processes of its constituent cells. The PNS includes the nerve trunks (cranial and spinal nerves), accumulations of peripherally-positioned nerve cell bodies and nerve terminals. The PNS receives stimuli and transduces them into useful information as action potentials and transmits this information to the CNS. Such information, upon reaching the CNS, may elicit an uncontrolled segmental or intersegmental response (reflex) and/or be transmitted to higher (suprasegmental) levels of the hierarchical organization pattern via ascending fiber pathways. These higher centers are responsible for the integration, association and interpretation of the information. The appropriate response, as an action potential transmitted over nerve fibers comprising descending pathways, is carried eventually to the effector organs (glands and muscles) by the nerve trunks of the PNS.

The PNS may be subdivided upon an anatomic basis into the *somatic nervous system* and *autonomic nervous system*. The somatic nervous system includes those nerve trunks and nerve terminals that carry information from the external environment to the CNS and subsequently carry information back to skeletal muscles. The autonomic nervous system functions similarly. Although the origination of informational input can vary, the subsequent evocation of a response involves the internal or visceral organs. The subsequent discussion of these systems will demonstrate that there are significant CNS contributions to both the somatic and autonomic nervous systems.

The conducting neuronal components of the CNS and PNS function in such a manner as to allow the organism to respond immediately and usually for a short period of time to alterations in the external and internal environment. The neurosecretory neuronal components, because of their influence on the endocrine system, permit gradual and longer term responses to environmental alterations than their conducting counterparts.

Anatomic Considerations

Development. The basic form of the vertebrate CNS is a dorsal, hollow, tubular structure which is derived from a thickened plate of ectoderm called *neuroectoderm* (Fig. 15.1). This plate of neuroectoderm, the *neural plate*, appears as a longitudinal thickening dorsal to the notochord during the presomite stage of development. The neural plate invaginates to form a *neural groove*, the lateral margins of which grow centrally and fuse along the longitudinal axis to form the *neural tube*. As these two layers of ectoderm separate from each other, a longitudinally-oriented mass of cells segregates as the *neural crest cells*.

The rostral end of the neural tube is associated with an extensive accumulation of developing nerve cells and is characterized by the development of vesicles that are destined to differentiate into various components of the brain (Fig. 15.2). This process of *cephalization* is identifiable early in development by the appearance of three vesicles: prosencephalon, mesencephalon, rhombencephalon (Fig. 15.3). The *prosencephalon* divides into two vesicles, the *telencephalon* and *diencephalon*. The telencephalic vesicles grow extensively and completely cover the rostral portions of the vesicles as the *cerebral hemispheres*. The *diencephalon* differentiates into the thalmus and its various subdivisions (*epithalamus, thalamus, metathalamus, subthalamus* and *hypothalamus*) and is associated directly with the developing eye (*optic vesicle*). Throughout

this development the rostral portion of the neural tube becomes tortuous, but the integrity of the lumen of the neural tube is maintained. The lumen associated with telencephalic development becomes the two *lateral ventricles*, whereas the lumen associated with diencephalic growth and development becomes the "donut-shaped" *third ventricle*. The third ventricle maintains its communication with the lateral ventricles through two laterally-positioned foramina (*foramina of Monro, interventricular foramina*). The *mesencephalon* does not subdivide into other vesicles but gives rise directly to the midbrain. The constricted portion of the lumen of the neural tube in the midbrain is called the *mesencephalic aqueduct*. It is the connection rostrally between the third ventricle and the *fourth ventricle* caudally that develops in association with the rhombencephalon. The *rhombencephalon* subdivides into the metencephalic and myelencephalic vesicles. The *metencephalon* gives rise to the cerebellum dorsally and the pons ventrally. The *myelencephalon* becomes the medulla oblongata which connects with the spinal cord. The continued growth and development of the brain is contingent upon the five vesicles of the neural tube (Fig. 15.3).

Cellular Differentiation, Development and Orientation. The rapid growth and development of the neural tube (especially the rostral portion) results from the marked proliferative activity of the neuroepithelial cells which comprise it. The neuroepithelium segregates into three distinct populations of cells: neural crest cells, neuroblasts and glioblasts. *Neural crest cells* separate from the neural tube and differentiate into numerous cell types scattered throughout the soma, some of which maintain their relationship with the nervous system (Fig. 15.4). Neuroblasts differentiate into the neurons of the CNS, whereas the *glioblasts* (*spongioblasts*) differentiate into the central neuroglial cells (Fig. 15.4).

Although the extent of the proliferative activity varies in different parts of the neural tube, the pattern of cellular differentiation, organization and orientation is maintained throughout the wall of this structure (Fig. 15.5). The innermost zone which lines the lumen of the tube is termed the *germinal* or *matrix layer*. It consists of actively dividing neuroepithelial cells. As these cells divide, their daughter cells migrate peripherally and form a centrally-positioned *mantle layer*. The neuroblasts of this layer may send processes rostrad and/or caudad to form the

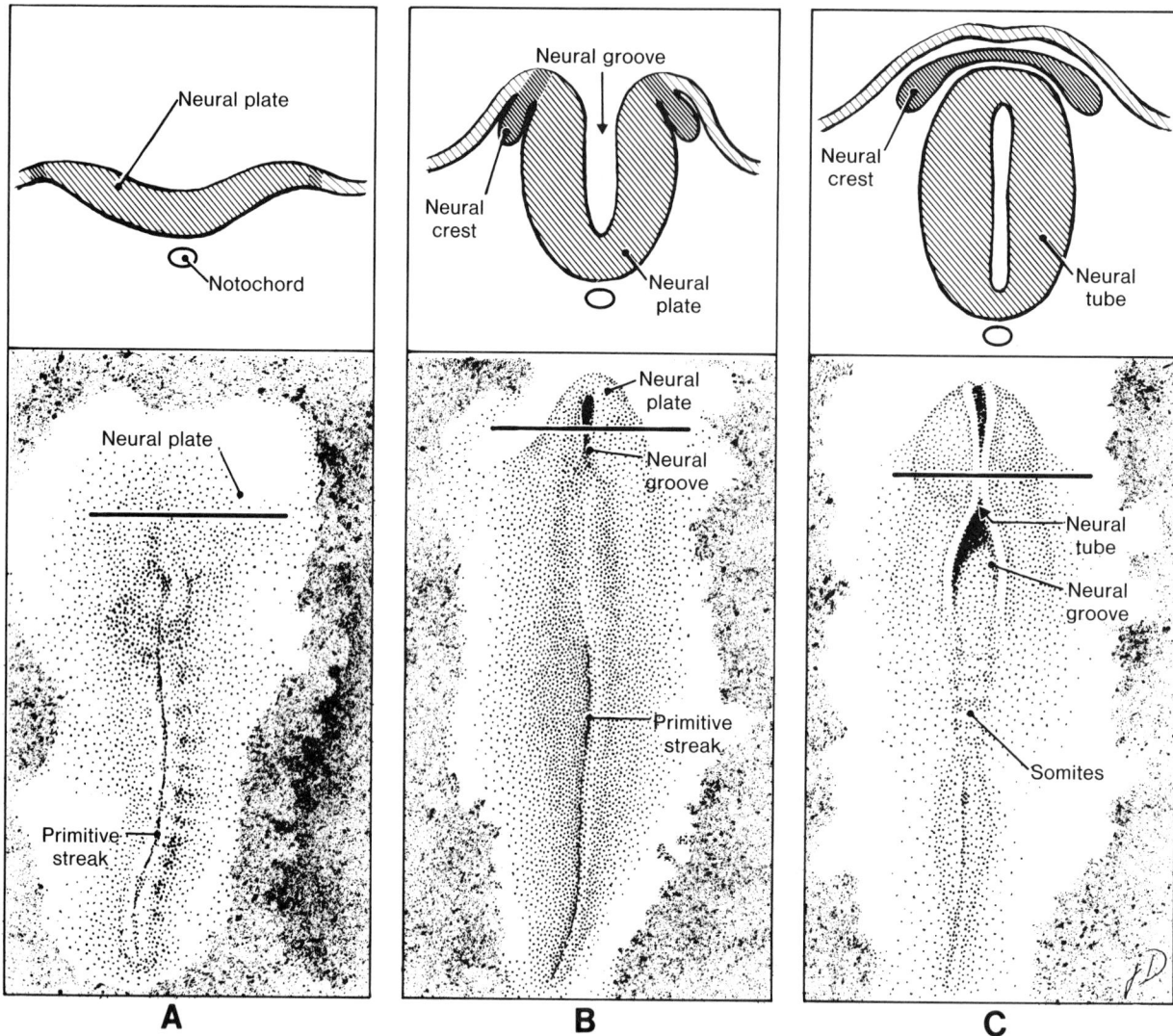

Fig. 15.1 A schematic representation of neural tube development. *Upper,* cross sections; *Lower,* dorsal views. A. The ectoderm thickens as the neural plate during the presomite stage of development. B. The neural plate continues to thicken and forms an invagination, the neural groove. C. The neural groove closes as a neural tube and neural crest cells are differentiated. All light micrographs are labeled as the magnification with the microscope before photographic enlarging. All electron micrographs are labeled as total magnification, including photographic enlarging.

outermost *marginal layer.* Or, the processes may perforate the neural tube to become motor fibers of the PNS. Glioblasts differentiate into neuroglial cells and assume their characteristic relationships to the neurons in all three layers. Upon the culmination of CNS development, the three layers of the developing neural tube will have become the white matter (marginal layer), the gray matter (mantle layer) and the ependymal layer (germinal or matrix layer). The additional proliferation of neuroepithelial cells within the vesicles of the developing brain accounts for additional neuronal pools associated with these adult structures.

A longitudinal groove, the *sulcus limitans,* is present in the wall of the neural tube from the mesencephalon caudad. A plane coincident with the sulcus limitans divides the neural tube into two distinct anatomic and functional regions (Fig. 15.6). The mantle layer of the dorsal plate, *alar plate,* is associated functionally with sensory input into the CNS, whereas the mantle layer of the ventral plate, *basal plate,* is associated functionally with motor output from the CNS. Within the spinal cord, these two plates assume the relationships described (Fig. 15.7). Within the brain stem the relative positions of these two plates is maintained; however, the altered growth pattern in this area of the neural tube accounts for the lateral positioning of the alar plate and the medial position of the basal plate (Fig. 15.7). Most importantly, the relative positioning of the neurons and neuronal pools which comprise these plates or columns is maintained in the neural tube from the mesencephalon caudally into the spinal cord.

Physiologic Considerations

Functional Organization. The PNS was described previously as consisting of nerve trunks, ganglion cells and nerve terminals. The brief discussion of the development of the CNS indicated that the motor fibers which leave the CNS to innervate various effector organs originate from the motor plate. Functionally and anatomically, these neurons are important contributors to the PNS. Similarly, the ingrowth of fibers from cranial and spinal ganglion cells from the periphery contributes significantly to both the PNS and CNS. Numerous nerve fibers, originating from various afferent nerve terminals throughout the body are essential components of these systems. The classification of the nervous system on a purely anatomic basis de-emphasizes the significant contribution both these systems make to each other. Functionally, the neurons and their fibers may be considered from different perspectives: 1) the location of the dendritic zone; 2) the location of the telodendria; 3) the type of information transmitted by the nerve fibers.

Information carried over nerve trunks is either going to or exiting from the CNS.

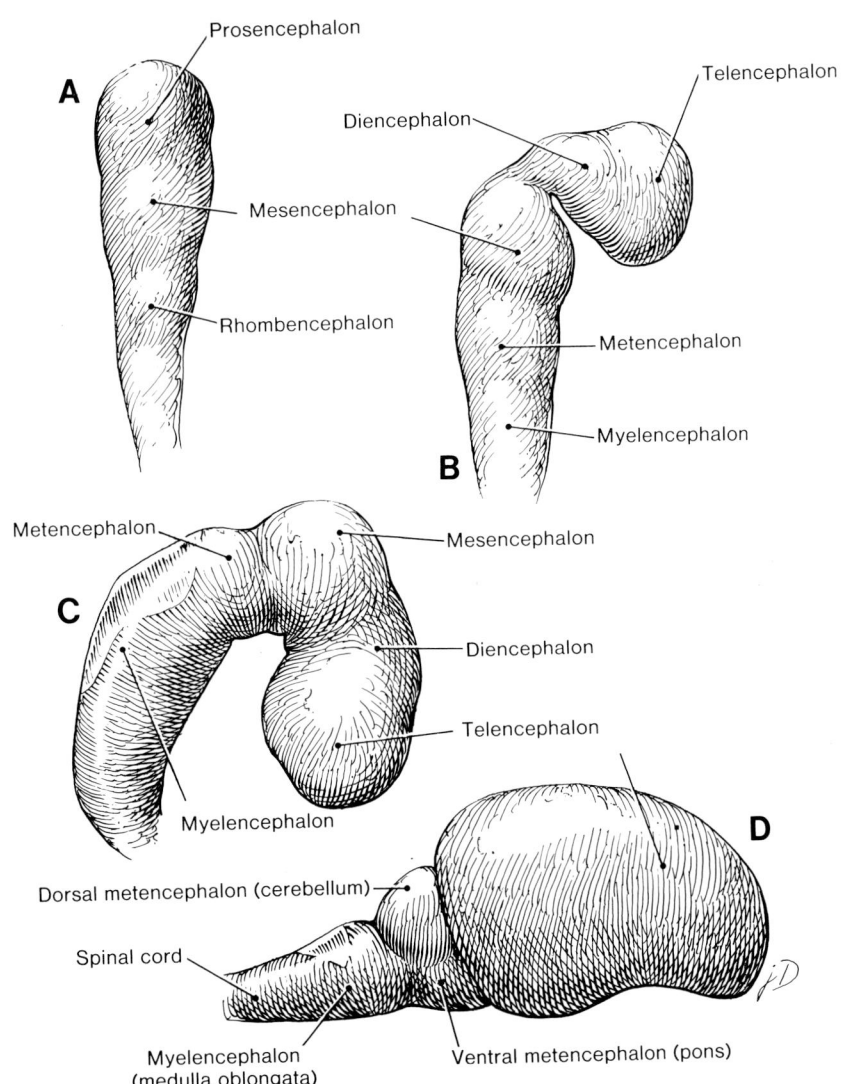

Fig. 15.2 A series of diagrams demonstrating cephalization of the neural tube. A, three vesicle stage; B, five vesicle stage; C, continued growth and development; D, telencephalic vesicles overgrow the other vesicles and the diencephalon is deep to the telencephalon.

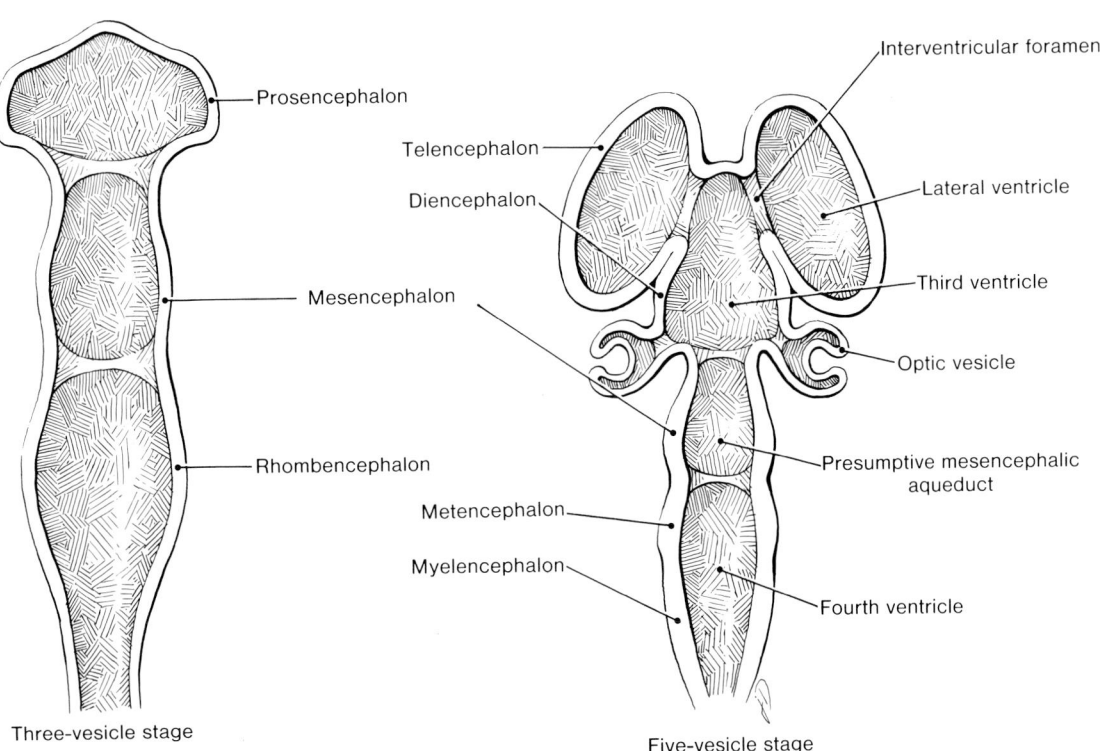

Three-vesicle stage

Five-vesicle stage

Fig. 15.3 A diagram of frontal sections through the three-vesicle and five-vesicle stage of brain development.

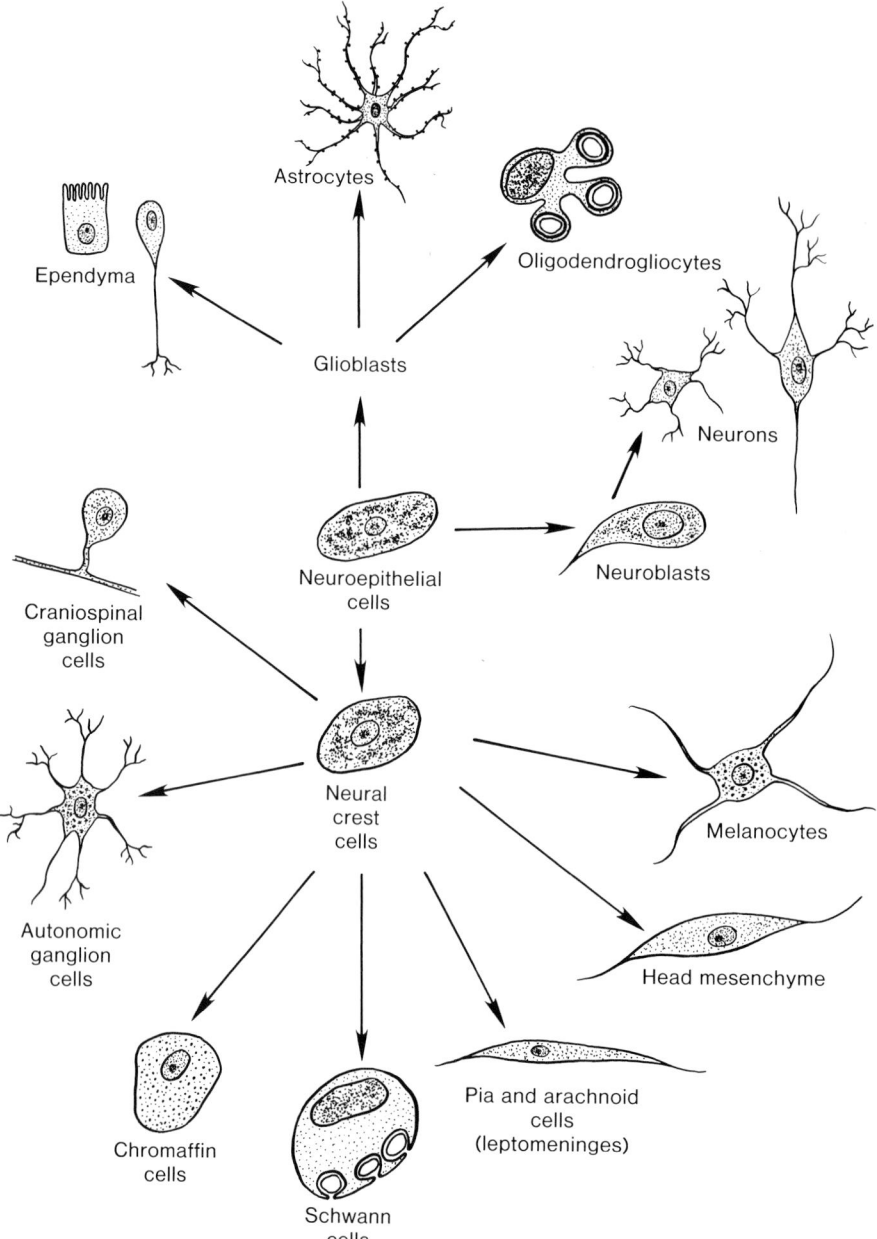

Fig. 15.4 A diagram of the cellular intermediates and derivatives of neuroepithelial cells.

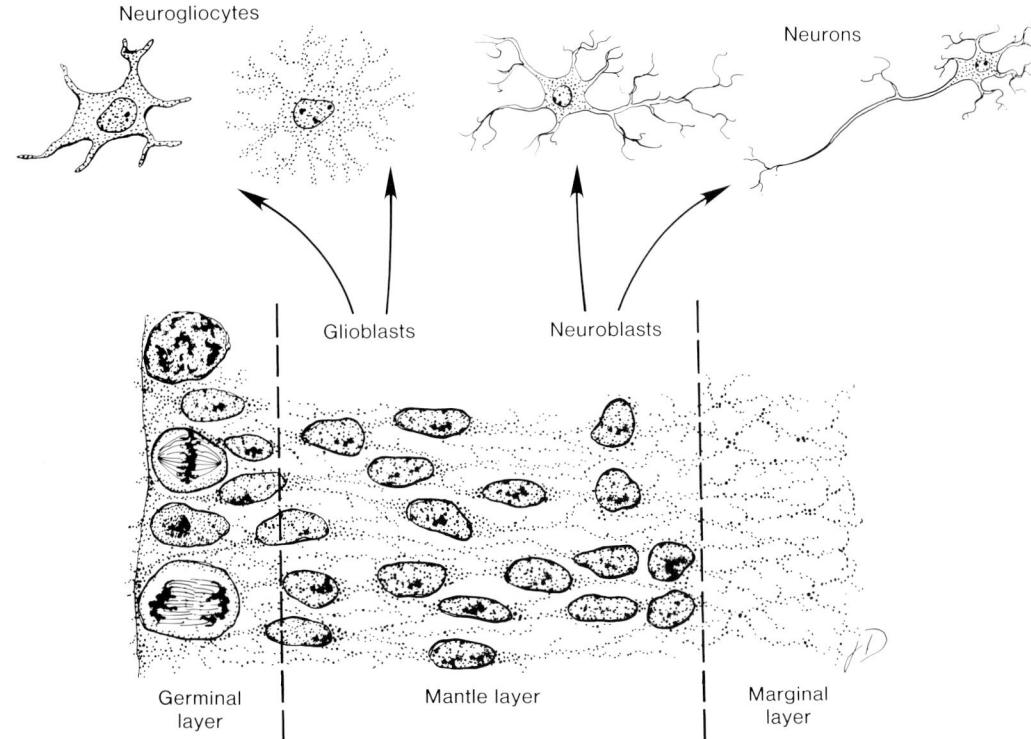

Fig. 15.5 A diagram of a cross-section through the developing neural tube. The zones of the neural tube and derivatives of the component cells are indicated.

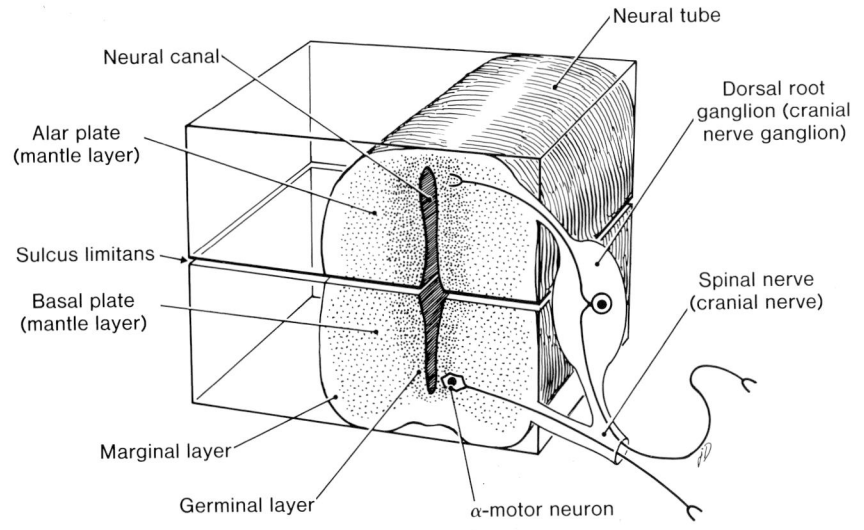

Fig. 15.6 A diagram of the relationships of the alar and basal plates in the developing neural tube.

The *motor* or *efferent fibers* innervate the effectors of the body. Their dendritic zones and cell bodies are located in the spinal cord and brain stem gray matter (basal plate). Their axonal processes comprise the cranial nerves, spinal nerves and/or the splanchnic nerves. Those neurons whose telodendria are distributed generally throughout the body to the skeletal muscle mass comprise the *general somatic efferent (GSE) system*. The neurons that form this system are called the *lower motor neurons* or *final common pathway*.

Those neurons the telodendria of which are distributed generally throughout the body to cardiac muscle, smooth muscle and glands comprise the *general visceral efferent (GVE) system*. This system is the efferent limb of the autonomic nervous system. One neuron in this two-neuron system is located within autonomic ganglia (See Autonomic Nervous System, this chapter.)

Because of the unique embryologic origin of certain skeletal muscle masses within the branchial arches, the nerve fibers that innervate them are given a special designation.

Furthermore, these skeletal muscle fibers are associated with visceral functions. Accordingly, the neurons which innervate these unique skeletal muscle cells comprise the *special visceral efferent (SVE) system*.

The *sensory* or *afferent fibers* arise from dendritic zones scattered throughout the body. These fibers carry information to the brain and spinal cord and contribute significantly to the alar plate region. The nerve cell bodies, dendritic zones and part of their axons comprise the PNS. These fibers contribute to the cranial nerves, spinal nerves and splanchnic nerves. Their telodendria, however, are located in the CNS. Those neurons the dendritic zones of which are scattered throughout the body generally and are responsive to external stimulation by pain, touch and temperature comprise the *general somatic afferent (GSA) system*. General proprioception (GP) is that system of neurons the dendritic zones of which are located in muscles, tendons and joint capsules. They respond to changes in tension and length and add valuable information, conscious and unconscious, about body position and relative position of body parts to each other. The GSA system is considered by some authors to include the GP system.

Certain organs are modified uniquely as sensory receptors that transmit information about the relationship of the organism to the external environment. The dendritic zones of the neurons that are integral components of these organs, the eye and ear, comprise the *special somatic afferent (SSA) system*. Vestibular functions of the ear are important in the static and dynamic (linear

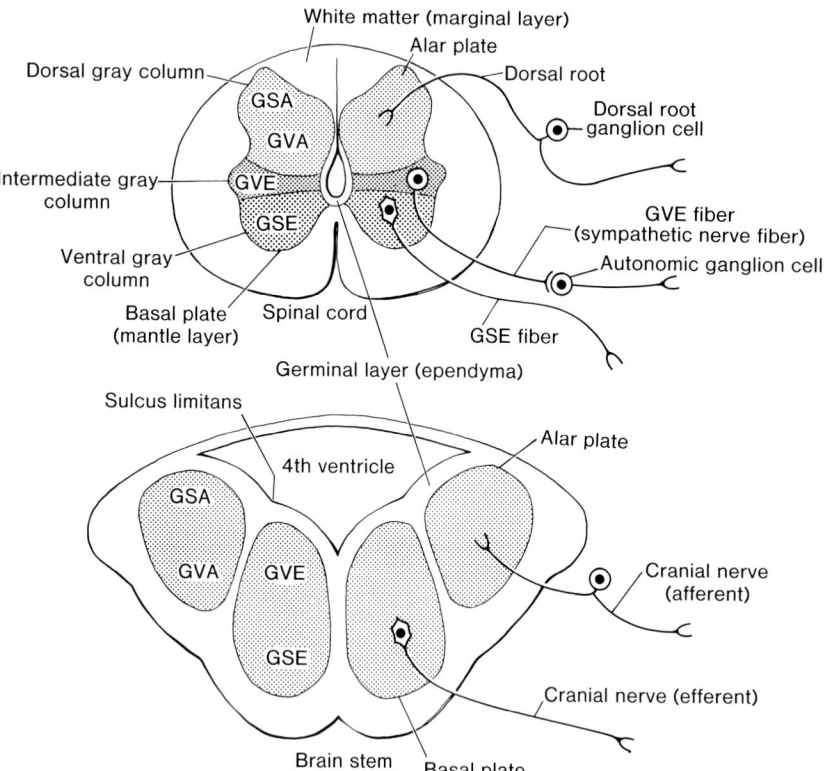

Fig. 15.7 A diagram depicting the relationships of the alar and basal plates in the spinal cord and brain stem. Refer to text for explanation of GSA, GVA, etc.

Table 15.1
Physiologic Organization of the Nervous System

System	Information carried	Location telodendria/dendritic zone	Nerves involved*
GSE	Motor	Skeletal muscle	All spinal nerves, III, IV, VI, XII
GVE	Motor	Cardiac muscle, smooth muscle, glands	All spinal nerves, III, VII, IX, X, XI
SVE	Motor	Branchial arch skeletal muscle	V, VII, IX, X, XI
GSA	Afferent (pain, touch, temp., general proprioception)	Somatopleure derivatives	All spinal nerves, V, X
SSA	Afferent (vision, hearing, special proprioception)	Retina, membranous labyrinth	II, VIII
GVA	Afferent (mechanical, chemical)	Splanchnopleure derivatives	All spinal nerves, VII, IX, X
SVA	Afferent (taste, smell)	Tongue, olfactory mucosa	VII, IX, X, I

* Roman numerals refer to cranial nerves.

and angular acceleration) relationships of the head to the external environment. These functions, comprising *special proprioception* (*SP*), are considered to be part of the SSA system by some authors.

Those neurons the dendritic zones of which are located in the walls of the visceral organs constitute the *general visceral afferent* (*GVA*) system. These receptors respond to mechanical and chemical alterations within and/or associated with these organs.

Some organs are modified uniquely for the perception of specialized visceral sensations—olfactory and gustatory sensations.

The neurons involved in this sensory input comprise the *special visceral afferent* (*SVA*) system.

These systems and the nerves with which they are associated are summarized in Table 15.1.

Reflex Arc. Although the nervous system has the ability to initiate activity seemingly independent from extraneous stimulation, the functional significance of the system is apparent when an activity is initiated in response to some sort of stimulus. Any given activity (movement of a limb, secretion of glands, increased heart rate, pupillary con-

striction) in response to a stimulus require that afferent pathways are linked to efferent pathways. The involuntary activity that results from this linkage is called a *reflex*. The afferent and efferent limbs, as well as the interneurons which may contribute, comprise the *reflex arc*. The reflex, generally, is a short term, stereotypic response to a stimulus that serves the immediate needs of the organism.

Reflexes are not uniform involuntary events that occur in response to stimuli. Anatomically, they may vary from *monosynaptic* (involving only two neurons) to *polysynaptic* (involving more than two neurons). They may involve a simple knee jerk in response to increased patellar tendon tension (patellar reflex), constriction of the pupil in response to increased light intensity (pupillary reflex), increased cardiac rate in response to decreased blood pressure (arterial pressoreceptor reflex) or a decreased cardiac rate in response to deep visceral pain during surgery (vago-vagal reflex). Although reflex activity is elicited easily with the proper stimulus, such motor activity does not occur as an event that is isolated from the rest of the nervous system. Reflexes, invariably, involve segmental, intersegmental and suprasegmental contributions.

Despite the complexity and diversity of reflexes, there is value in understanding them in the context of seemingly occurring alone: 1) It affords insights into the interconnections between neurons of the nervous system; 2) It permits an evaluation of the afferent and efferent limbs of the reflex arc; 3) It is important in the clinical evaluation of a patient.

The simplest arrangement of neurons in a reflex arc is the *monosynaptic reflex*. An example of this type of reflex (*stretch reflex*) is illustrated in Figure 15.8. A pseudounipolar nerve cell with its cell body located in the *dorsal root ganglion* has an axonal process that extends to a stretch receptor which receives general proprioceptive information. The axon is a component of the *spinal nerve* and *dorsal root* and extends into the *dorsal gray column* of the spinal cord. Its telodendrion synapses with the dendritic zone of nerve cells located in the *ventral gray column*. Upon sufficient stimulation, the excitatory postsynaptic potentials (EPSP) result in an action potential in these α-*motor neurons* (*lower motor neurons, final common pathways*). The axons of the nerves exit the spinal column and form the *ventral root* and continue to the periphery in the *spinal nerve*. The telodendria of the GSE fibers innervate the skeletal muscle that is responsive to the proprioceptive stimulation. The *stretch reflex* or *myotatic reflex* is the simplest form of reflex. Two neurons are necessary to complete the circuit. The excitation of one muscle group requires the inhibition of the antagonistic muscle group. Inhibition is achieved by the interposition of another neuron in the circuit, the *interneuron*.

branches of the telodendria of the proprioceptive fibers synapse with an interneuron. The EPSP's generated result in the activation of this neuron. It synapses with an α-motor neuron which innervates the antagonistic muscle mass. However, the synapse between the interneuron and this α-motor neuron is characterized by the generation of inhibitory postsynaptic potentials (IPSP). The α-motor neuron becomes hyperpolarized and the antagonistic muscle mass relaxes. At the same time branches from the proprioceptive fibers ascend the spinal cord to transmit GSA information to higher brain centers (cerebrum, cerebellum). Suprasegmental transmission is complemented by branches from the fibers ascending and descending to other spinal cord segments (intersegmental). Similarly, descending fiber tracts from higher brain centers exert an inhibitory influence upon the α-motor neurons involved in this type of reflexive activity. Loss of an inhibitory influence because of an upper motor lesion or long tract disease results in *hyperreflexia*. Although the reflex activity described seems to be mediated by simple circuitry, the reflex is a complex interaction between segmental, intersegmental and suprasegmental neurons. In the knee jerk (patellar) reflex, the afferent information (proprioceptive) involves the femoral nerve which originates from spinal cord segments L_3, L_4 and L_5. The efferent limb requires the activation of the stifle extensors via the femoral nerve. The flexors of the stifle must be relaxed during the reflex. Relaxation requires the inhibition of nerve fibers which originate from spinal cord segments L_6, L_7 and S_1, those fibers which comprise the ischiatic nerve.

A *multisynaptic reflex* involves more than two neurons in the reflex arc (Fig. 15.8).

The *withdrawal reflex* is a good example of a multisynaptic reflexive pathway. The application of excessive pressure (pain) to the forelimb of a dog results in the withdrawal (flexion) of the forelimb. The GSA information is transmitted as described previously; however, an additional neuron is added to the circuit. The excitation of the α-motor neurons which innervate the flexors must be complemented by the inhibition of the extensors as described previously. Segmental, intersegmental and suprasegmental relationships described previously also pertain to the reflex. If extensive interdigital pressure were applied between digits 3 and 4 of the forelimb, then this information would be transmitted to spinal cord segments C_7, C_8 and T_1 via the GSA fibers of the radial nerve. The excitation of the flexors of the scapulohumeral joint, elbow joint and carpal joint requires the involvement of the axillary nerve (C_7, C_8), musculocutaneous nerve (C_6, C_7, C_8) and median and ulnar nerves (C_7, C_8). The simultaneous inhibition of the extensors involves the inhibition of GSE fibers of the radial nerve (C_7, C_8, T_1).

The withdrawal reflex and myotatic reflex demonstrate the principle of *reciprocal innervation*. Excitation of the flexors requires the inhibition of the extensors. The converse is true also.

This pattern of reflex activity associated with, but not limited to the spinal cord, also occurs with the cranial nerves and visceral nerves. Autonomic reflex activity is discussed with the autonomic nervous system. The reflex activity associated with cranial nerves follows the same basic pattern described previously; however, such activity may involve more than one cranial nerve. One cranial nerve may serve as the afferent

limb and another may serve as the efferent limb. Naturally, they are connected by interneurons. Although the spatial arrangement of cranial nerve reflexes is different from the spinal nerve reflexes, they are logical if the relationships between the alar plate (sensory plate) and basal plate (motor plate) are kept in mind. A V–VII reflex arc is an example of this type of relationship. Noxious stimulation to the head (cornea, palpebra, muzzle) is transmitted as GSA information to the sensory region (alar plate) of the trigeminal nerve (V). An interneuron connects this sensory region to the motor nucleus (basal plate) of cranial nerve VII (facial nerve). The GSE fibers of the cranial nerve VII innervate the skeletal muscles responsible for the response (squint, blink, menace).

Peripheral Organizational Components

Ganglia. Accumulations of nerve cell bodies outside the CNS are referred to as *ganglia*. Corresponding accumulations within the CNS are referred to as *nuclei*. Two main types of ganglia are distinguished, *craniospinal ganglia* (sensory) and *autonomic ganglia* (motor). The craniospinal ganglia include the *dorsal root ganglia* of the spinal nerves and the *cranial ganglia* of the cranial nerves. The autonomic ganglia include the *paravertebral* and *prevertebral ganglia* of the sympathetic nervous system and the *terminal ganglia* of the parasympathetic nervous system. The latter may be close to, upon or within the wall of various organs. Those within the wall of organs are called *intramural ganglia*.

Ganglia, although variable in size, are usually surrounded by a connective tissue capsule the fine collagenous and reticular fibers of which are scattered throughout the organ as a fine reticulum or stroma (Fig. 15.9). Blood vessels, axons, dendrites, peripheral neuroglia and nerve cell bodies are enmeshed within the supportive framework. Amphicytes are intimately associated with the nerve cell bodies. The amphicytes and the neurons of ganglia are of neural crest ectodermal origin.

The *dorsal root ganglia* are representative of craniospinal ganglia (Fig. 15.9). These globular structures are encapsulated and the connective tissue extensions of the capsule are scattered throughout the ganglia. The predominant neuronal type is pseudounipolar (Plate II.11). Their size is quite variable. Each of the neurons is surrounded by amphicytes (Fig. 15.10). These flattened or cuboidal cells are in such intimate contact with the perikaryon that an indentation in the nerve cell body is often apparent. These cells are continuous with the neurolemmal sheath of the nerve fibers. Nerve fibers, usually in distinct fascicles, comprise the remainder of the organ.

The *autonomic ganglia* include those associated with the autonomic nervous system.

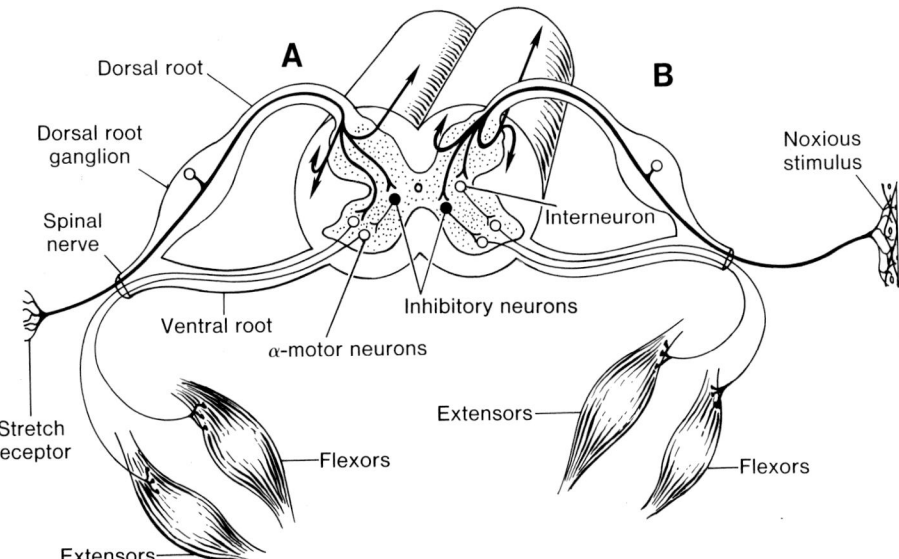

Fig. 15.8 A schematic diagram of the stretch reflex (A) and withdrawal reflex (B). The stretch reflex is monosynaptic; the axon of the afferent fiber synapses with the α-motor neuron to the extensors. The withdrawal reflex is multisynaptic; the axon of the afferent fiber synapses with an interneuron. The interneuron synapses with the α-motor neuron to the flexors.

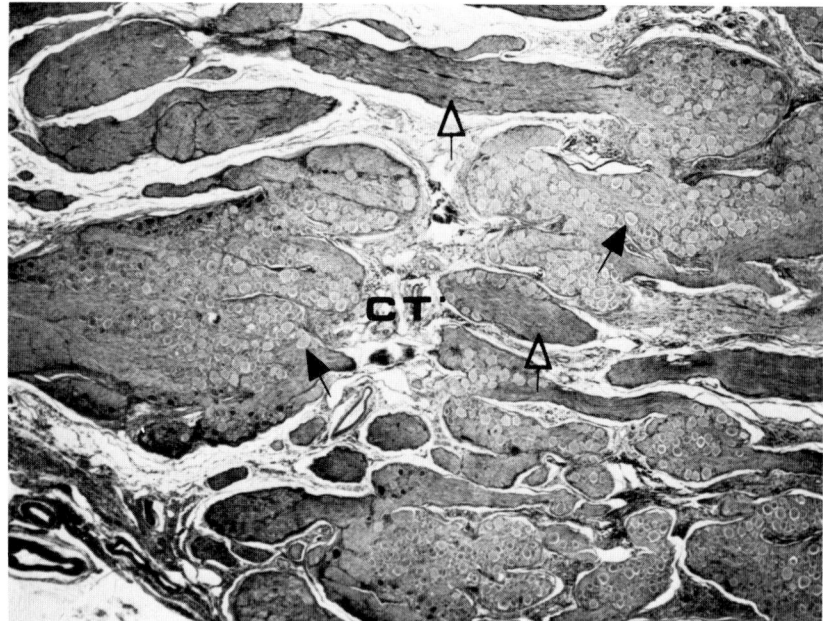

Fig. 15.9   Dorsal root ganglion. The organ consists of nerve cell bodies (*solid arrows*), nerve cell processes (*open arrows*) and connective tissue (CT). X4.

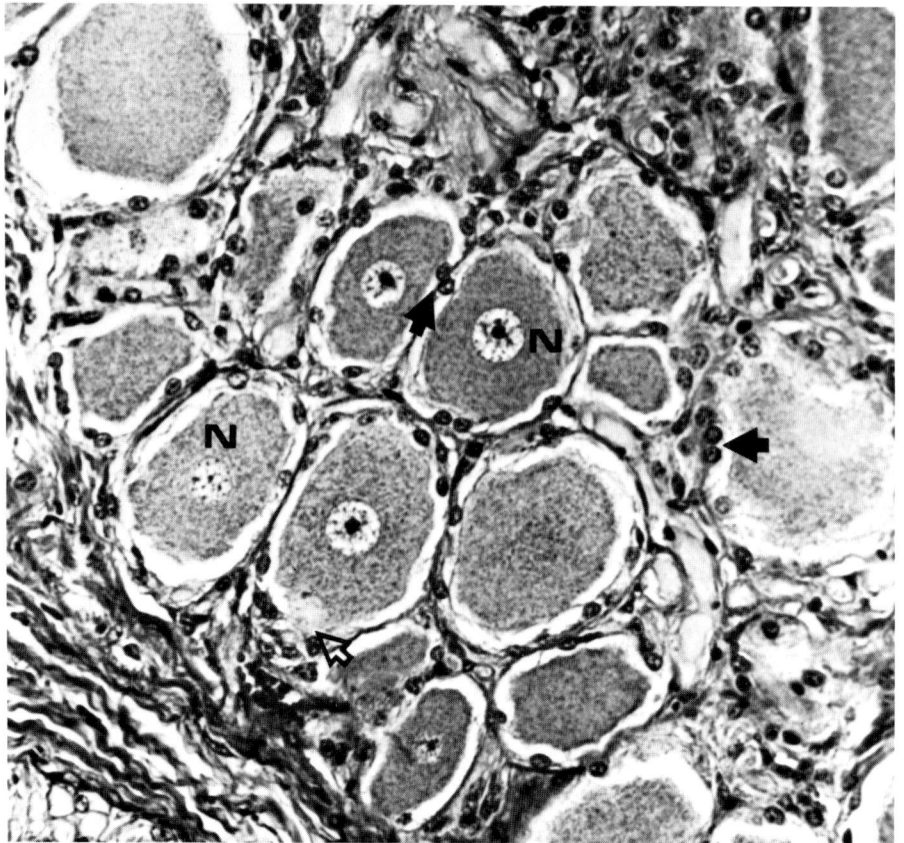

Fig. 15.10   Cells of a dorsal root ganglion. The neurons (N) are surrounded by amphicytes (*solid arrows*). Note the axon hillock of one neuron (*open arrow*). Compare with Figure 12.22. X63 (iron hematoxylin).

The *sympathetic ganglia* and the neurons that comprise them are smaller than dorsal root ganglia. Also, the former are comprised primarily of multipolar neurons. The nerve fibers are more diffusely scattered through-

out this type of motor ganglion than in the craniospinal ganglion.

Parasympathetic ganglia, away from the visceral organs, are similar to sympathetic ganglia. Those located within the organs

(*intramural ganglia*), however, are not as structured as those described previously (Fig. 15.11). They consist of a few multipolar nerve cell bodies and fibers. In most instances, these perikarya are devoid of amphicytes. However, small and flattened fibroblasts may replace them.

Nerve Trunks. The organization of peripheral nerve fibers into large trunks follows the basic pattern described for the organization of solid organs. It is almost identical to the pattern of muscle organization. The organizational scheme of nerve trunks and their relationships to central and peripheral elements are detailed in Figure 15.12.

The nerve trunks or peripheral nerves are those structures composed of axons that connect the brain, brain stem and spinal cord to the peripherally-positioned dendritic zones and/or telodendria of neurons. The *spinal nerves*, formed by the dorsal and ventral roots, are mixed nerves containing afferent and efferent fibers. The types of fibers which comprise them were detailed in Table 15.1. All spinal nerves contain GSA, GSE and GVE components. The *visceral nerves* which supply the visceral organs of the thoracic, abdominal and pelvic cavities are similar to the spinal nerves. They consist of GVA and GVE components and are discussed with the autonomic nervous system.

The cranial nerves are organized in a slightly different pattern. Dorsal and ventral roots are not apparent. They consist of single nerve trunks which may be sensory only (I, II, VIII), motor only (III, IV, VI, XI, XII) or sensory and motor (V, VII, IX, X). The mixed (sensory and motor) cranial nerves are similar to the spinal nerves. Cranial ganglia are present and these nerves carry afferent and efferent information. The sensory cranial nerves deviate slightly from the basic pattern. The olfactory, optic and vestibulocochlear nerves consist of axons of ganglion cells located in the olfactory bulbs, ganglionic layers of the retina and vestibular and spiral ganglia, respectively. The cranial nerves which are motor only may be considered similar to the ventral roots and efferent components of the spinal and visceral nerves. The cell bodies of these nerves are contained within specific nuclei of the motor column (basal plate) of the brain stem.

The nerve trunks (peripheral nerves) consist generally of bundles (*fascicles*) of nerve fibers which are invested with connective tissue elements. The outermost covering of peripheral nerves is the *epineurium* (Plates V.7, V.9) (Figs. 15.13 and 15.14). The epineurium may be considered the capsule of these organs and consists of dense white fibrous connective tissue, irregularly arranged. The outermost covering of a single fascicle is epineurium. When numerous fascicles are joined together, as is the usual case, the epineurium not only covers the entire nerve but the individual fascicles are bound by epineural connective tissue. Then, portions of the epineurium assume connective tissue septal relationships to the individual bundles.

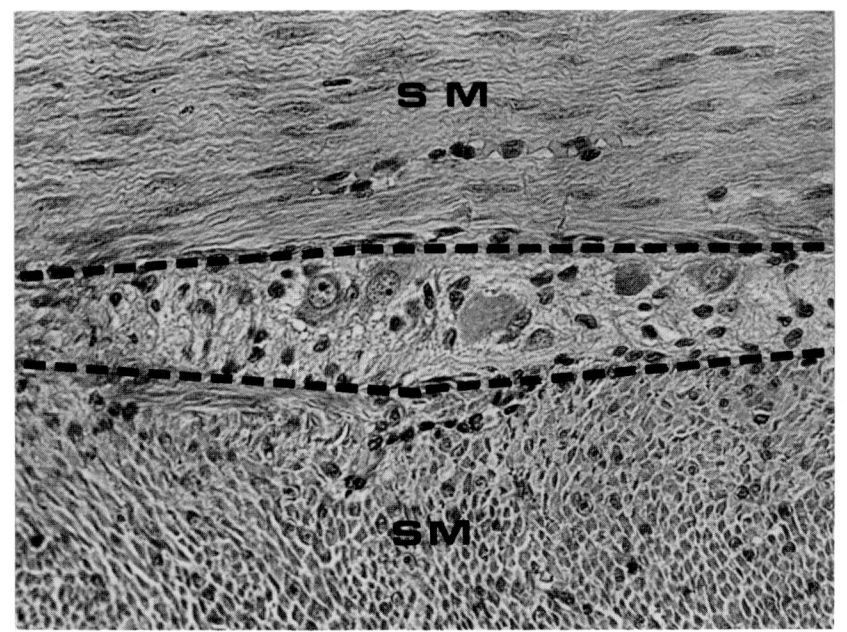

Each fascicle of a nerve trunk is invested with delicate investment of connective tissue which is continuous with the epineurium, the *perineurium* (Figs. 15.13, 15.14 and 15.15). Immediately subjacent to the perineurium is an investment of cells, *perineural cells*, which may vary from one to three layers thick. They are not connective tissue cells, because each is invested with a basal lamina. Fine collagenous and reticular fibers as well as fibroblasts may be present between the layers of perineural cells. These continuous layers of epithelioid cells serve as effective barriers between the connective tissue and the endoneurial compartment. The exact function and origin of perineural cells has not been determined. They may be continuous with, derived from or similar to the leptomeningeal investments of the CNS. The perineural cellular investments terminate before the end of the nerve.

The *endoneurium* is a connective tissue space between the perineural cells and the neurolemmal sheaths of individual nerve fibers (Figs. 15.14 and 15.15). Fine reticular fibers, an occasional fibroblast and capillaries occur within this compartment.

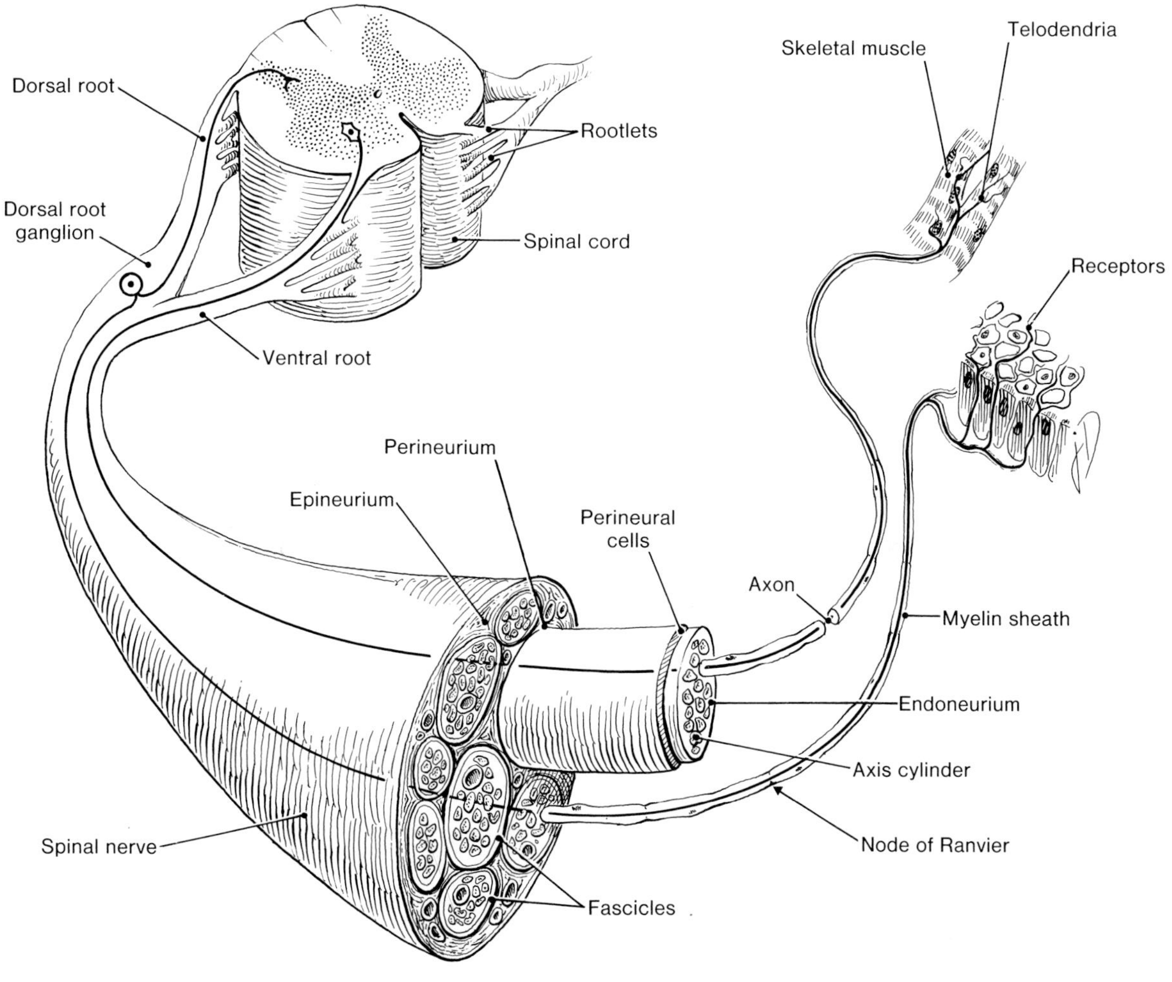

Fig. 15.11 Intramural ganglion from the myenteric plexus. *Dashed lines*, approximate limits of the ganglion. The ganglion is interdigitated between two masses of smooth muscle (SM) of the tunica muscularis. X100.

Fig. 15.12 A diagram depicting the investments of a spinal nerve and the relationship of the nerve to the CNS. Spinal nerves are mixed nerves.

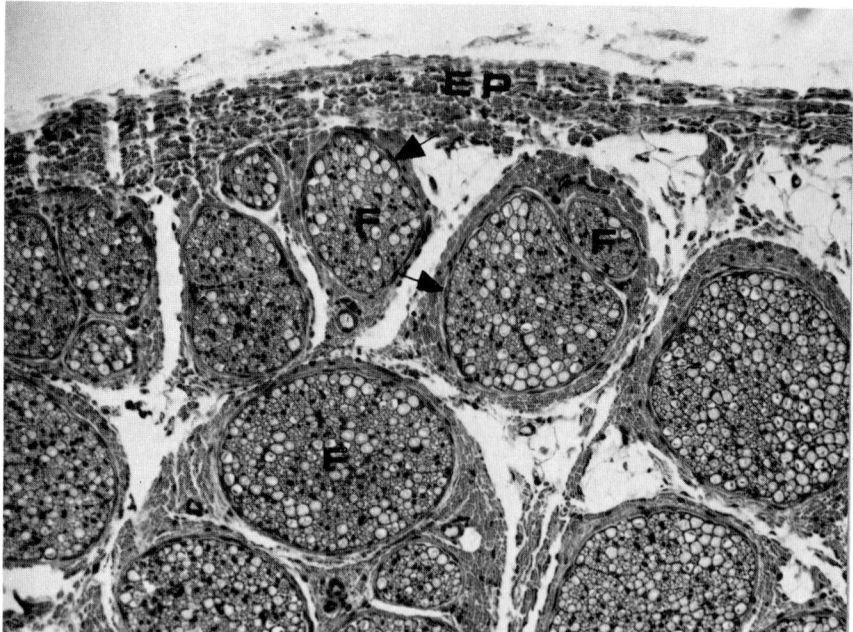

Fig. 15.13 Organization of a nerve trunk. The epineurium (EP) surrounds all the fascicles (F). Individual fascicles are surrounded by perineurium. *Solid arrows* indicate the perineural cell sheath which surrounds individual fascicles deep to the perineurium. (Compare with Figure 15.15). The endoneurium surrounds individual nerve cell processes. X40.

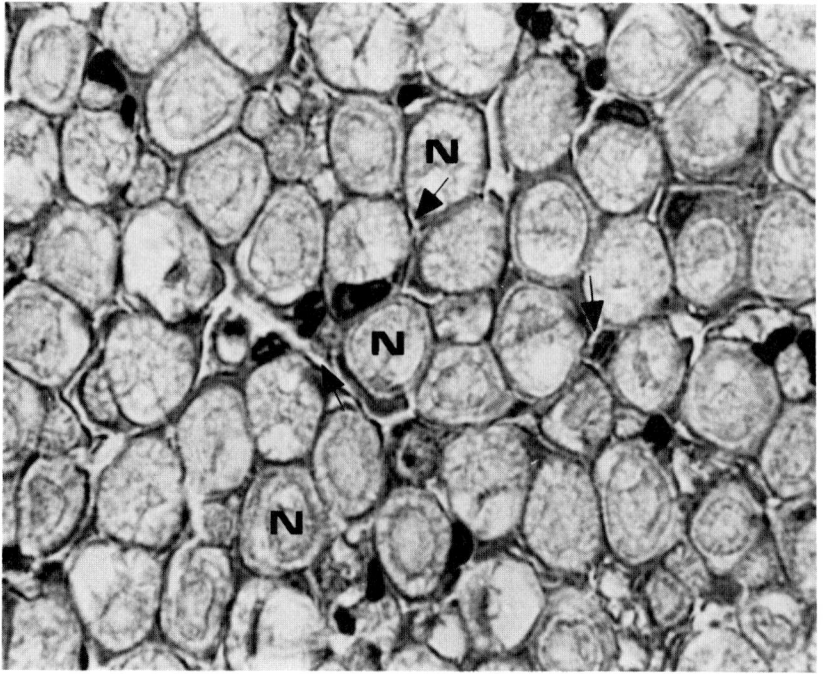

Fig. 15.14 Endoneurium. Individual nerve cell processes (N) are surrounded by the endoneurium (*arrows*). Note the axis cylinders and neurokeratin of the altered myelin sheaths. X320.

Afferent Nerve Terminals. The afferent nerve terminals (dendritic zones) are the means by which an organism perceives various stimuli from its external and internal environment. The reception of varied information once transmitted to the CNS is the basis upon which an integrated response (or lack thereof) is initiated (or not).

These receptors are transducers that convert various types of modalities (pain, touch, warmth, pressure, etc.) into a form usable by the nervous system. Although receptors have been classified in numerous ways, no is totally satisfactory and others overlap varying degrees. The following is the bas for the different classifications:

1. Source of the stimuli and location of th receptors.
2. Types of modalities transduced by the ceptors.
3. Form of the stimuli required to stimula the receptors.
4. The structure of the receptors.

Although not perfectly satisfactory, th structural basis of classification will be use

On an anatomic basis, two main subdiv sions are used to classify receptors: *free an diffuse, encapsulated.*

The *free and diffuse nerve endings* are th most ubiquitous of the body. Although the are most numerous in the epidermis, the are also found in mucous and serous men branes, muscles, joints and the connecti tissue of the viscera. The extensively arbo ized fibers may be myelinated or unmyeli ated and may terminate as flattened or bult like endings scattered among epithelial connective tissue cells (Fig. 15.16). They a usually considered touch receptors.

Merkel's disks are modified free nerv endings which are associated with deep ep dermal cells. The terminal branches are fla tened or disklike and in contact with thes modified cells. They generally occur in hai less skin. These receptors are associated wit tactile stimulation which is pain associate

The *encapsulated receptors* vary fro slight to heavy encapsulation. These includ *Meissner's corpuscles, Krause's endbulb Golgi-Mazzoni corpuscles, genital corpuscle Vater-Pacinian corpuscles, Herbst corpuscle Ruffini corpuscles, neuromuscular spindle* and *Golgi tendon organs* (Fig. 15.16).

Meissner's corpuscles are one of the mos ubiquitous encapsulated receptors of hai less skin (Fig. 15.17). They occur in th dermal papillae of the soles and palms. Th corpuscles are about 100 μm long and ap proximately 25 μm wide. They are slightl encapsulated and contain the terminals one or more nerves arranged in a helica order around a mass of cells similarly ar ranged. The overall form is that of an im bricated fir cone. These corpuscles are re ceptors for tactile discrimination. Merkel disks may be rudimentary forms of thi corpuscle.

Krause's endbulbs are slightly encapsu lated, spherical receptors which are locate in the skin and associated mucous mem branes (especially the conjunctiva). In on type, the nerve terminal enters the granula mass within the capsule and terminates a the opposite pole in a slightly expande ending. In a second type, the nerve enter the granular mass within the capsule, un dergoes arborization and terminates in ex panded endings. This type of corpuscle is cold receptor.

Golgi-Mazzoni corpuscles are similar to Meissner's corpuscles. They are, however, smaller and more thickly encapsulated than Meissner's corpuscles. They are believed to be pressure receptors which occur in the connective tissue of hairless skin and asso-ciated mucous membranes. They also occur in the dermis of the glans penis, the digital pads of carnivores and the connective tissue associated with the hoof.

Genital corpuscles are similar to Golgi-Mazzoni corpuscles. However, the former are larger and more thickly encapsulated than the latter. They may also be lobulated. The number of nerves entering the capsule varies from one to ten. They arborize and form a spiral, interlacing network of naked nerve terminals. These corpuscles occur in

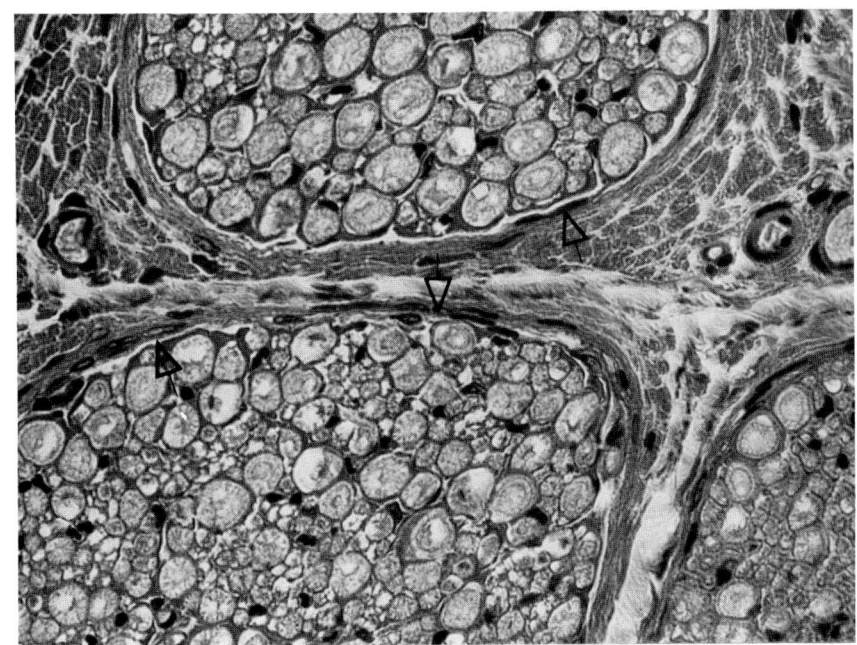

Fig. 15.15 Perineural cells. Layers of perineural cells (*arrows*) surround individual fascicles deep to the perineurium. X160.

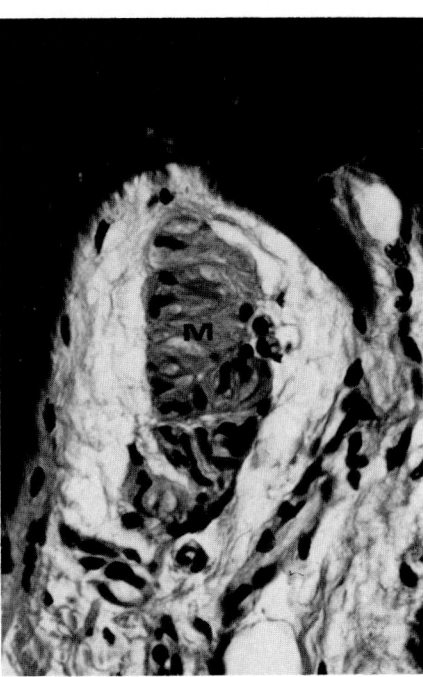

Fig. 15.17 Meissner's corpuscle. The corpuscles (M) occur in dermal papillae. X115.

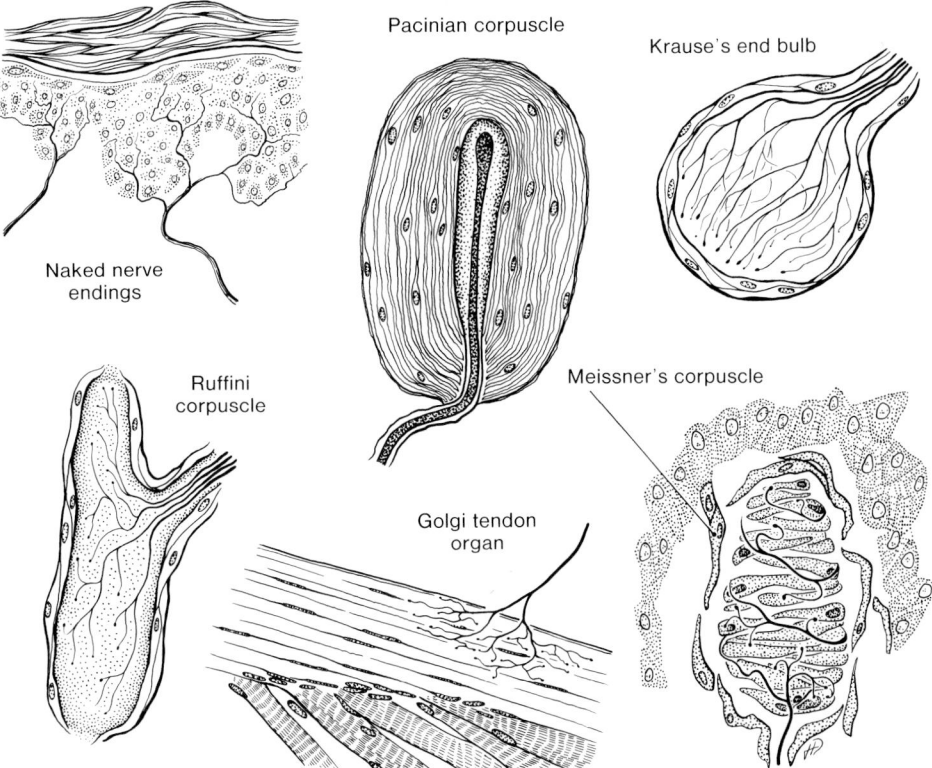

Naked nerve endings

Pacinian corpuscle

Krause's end bulb

Ruffini corpuscle

Golgi tendon organ

Meissner's corpuscle

Fig. 15.16 A diagram of various types of receptors.

the clitoris and glans penis. They are considered to be pressure receptors.

The *Vater-Pacinian corpuscles* are the largest encapsulated nerve endings of the body (Fig. 15.18). They may be 3 to 4 mm long and thus observable with the unaided eye. A single nerve enters the corpuscle and terminates in a bulbous enlargement surrounded by a mass of granular material. Concentric layers of epithelial cells (similar to perineural cells), connective tissue cells and capillaries impart an onion-like appearance (Fig. 15.19). These corpuscles are pressure receptors and are extremely unbiquitous. They occur in the deep connective tissue, mesenteries and serous membranes, as well as the connective tissue of visceral organs, muscle and that associated with tendons and ligaments.

Herbst corpuscles are smaller versions of Pacinian corpuscles. These are pressure receptors and occur in the tongues and beaks of birds.

The *Ruffini corpuscles* are composed of an arborization of nerve fibers interlacing throughout a granular mass which is enclosed by a connective tissue capsule. These corpuscles are believed to be heat receptors, but Ruffini-like receptors are associated with kinesthetic sensations (Chapter 14).

Neuromuscular spindles and *Golgi tendon organs* were described with the musculoskeletal system (Chapter 14).

Although numerous receptors and their associated modalities have been described, there is some question relating to the specificity of given afferent terminals for a specific modality. The distinctness of some corpuscles is also questioned. Meissner's corpuscles, Merkel's disks, Golgi-Mazzoni corpuscles, Krause's endbulbs and genital corpuscles are closely related and may be modified forms of one another. Similarly, Pacinian and Herbst corpuscles may be closely related. There is also evidence that receptors continuously break down and reorganize throughout life.

Central Organizational Components

Meninges. The central nervous system is well protected by its placement within the bones of the skull and spinal column. Further protection is afforded by the association of dense and loose connective tissue with the CNS (Fig. 15.20). These tissues are disposed as three fibrous membranes totally enclosing the system: *dura mater, arachnoidea* and *pia mater*. The dura mater is also referred to as the *pachymeninx*; the arachnoid and pia mater are referred to as the *leptomeninges*. Besides the protection by virtue of the connective tissue, these membranes are intimately associated with *cerebrospinal fluid*. Also, the vascular supply gains access to the CNS via these membranes.

The *dura mater* is a tough dense white fibrous connective tissue covering of the brain and spinal cord which consists of collagen, some elastic fibers and blood vessels (Fig. 15.20). In association with the brain, it consists of two layers. The outer layer is the fibrous periosteum of the inner surface of the cranial bones. This layer contains a number of blood vessels associated with the cranial bones. An inner, poorly vascularized layer blends insensibly with the outer or periosteal layer. These layers become distinct in specific areas of the brain where they separate and form the *dural sinuses*. These sinuses are responsible for the collection of cerebrospinal fluid and its return to the vascular system. The dura is separated from the arachnoid membrane by a *subdural space*.

Because the bones of the skull are not continuous as a unit with the bones of the vertebral column, the periosteum of the inner skull surface is reflected as the periosteum of the outer skull surface at the *foramen magnum*. The dura of the spinal cord, therefore, is a single layer (the inner layer of the cranial dura) and is separated from the periosteum that lines the vertebrae by an extensive space called the *epidural space*

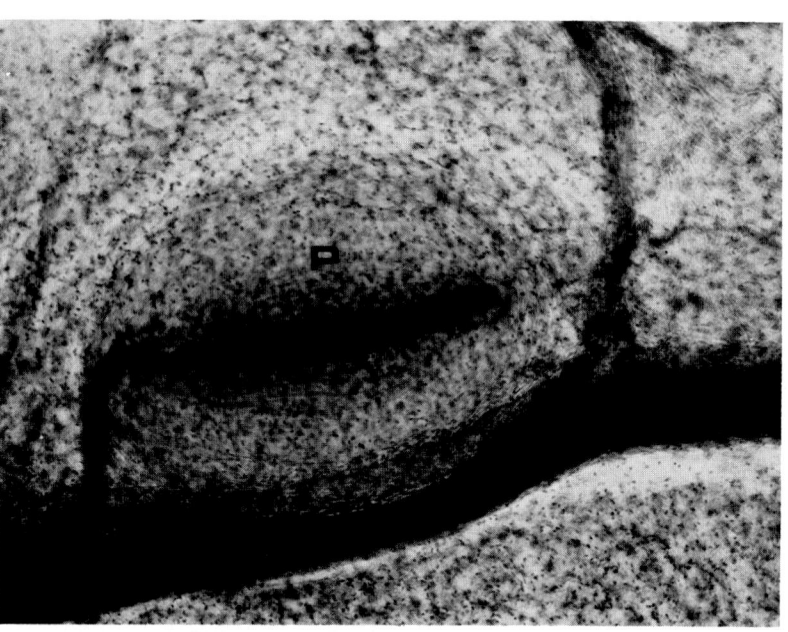

Fig. 15.18   A whole-mount preparation of a Vater-Pacinian corpuscle (P) from a mesentery. X16.

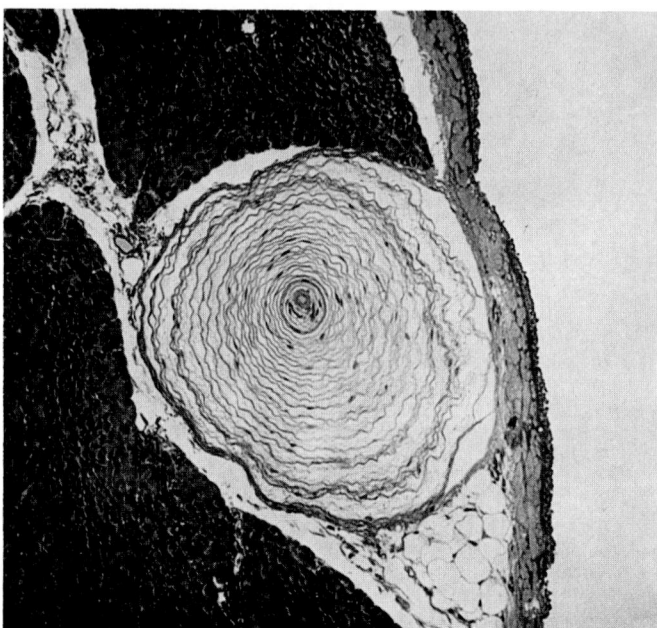

Fig. 15.19   A cross-sectioned Vater-Pacinian corpuscle in the connective tissue of the feline pancreas. The concentric layers of components impart an onion-like appearance. X25.

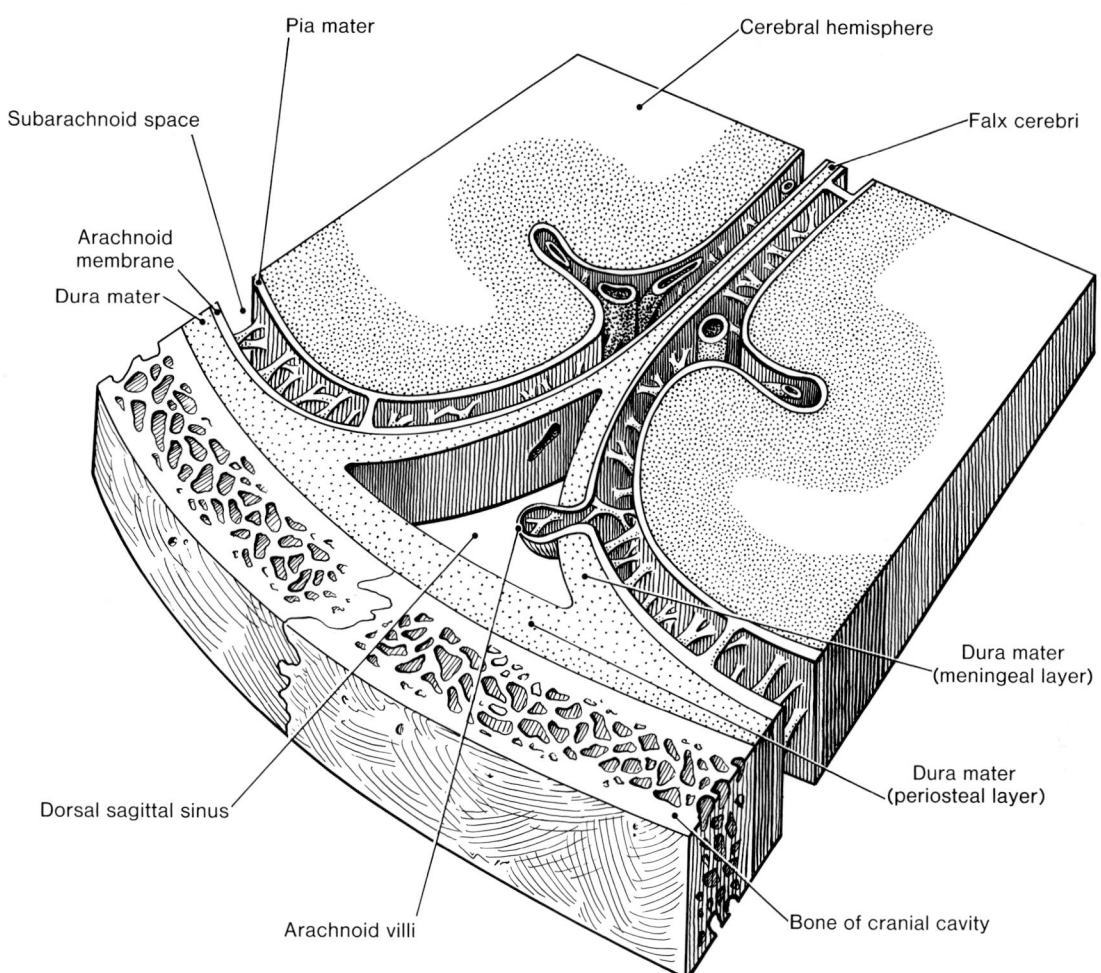

Fig. 15.20 A diagram depicting the relationships of the cranial meninges in cross section. The separation of the two layers of the dura mater forms the dorsal sagittal sinus and falx cerebri.

(Fig. 15.21). This space is filled with loose connective tissue, adipose tissue and extensive veins and venous sinuses. The epidural space is used for the administration of some anesthetics (*epidural anesthesia*).

The *arachnoidea* consists of a distinct membrane and numerous fibrous trabeculae on its inner surface (Fig. 15.20). Both are composed of fine collagenous and elastic fibers. The extensive network of trabeculae which extends to the pia mater comprises the supportive framework for the *subarachnoid space*. This space is occupied by cerebrospinal fluid that mechanically protects the central nervous system. Blood vessels, also, are scattered on the floor of this space in the pia mater. Protrusions of component tissues from the subarachnoid space extend through the inner layer of the dura mater and form *arachnoid villi* (*arachnoid granulations*) which project into the sinuses of the dura. Through this association, cerebrospinal fluid from the subarachnoid space is returned to the blood vascular system.

The *pia mater* is the most intimate protective membrane of the brain and spinal cord (Fig. 15.20). It extends into the numerous depressions and fissures that characterize the CNS. This membrane is composed of

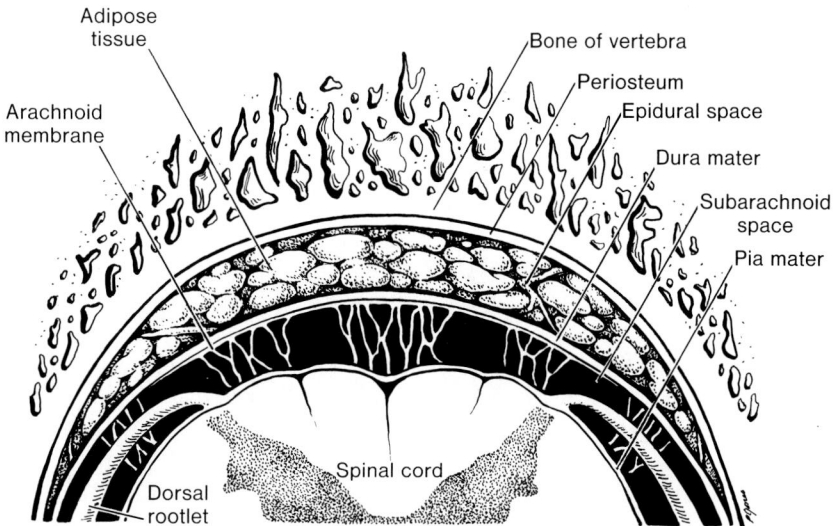

Fig. 15.21 A diagram depicting the relationships of the spinal meninges in cross-section. The dura mater of the spinal cord is separated from the periosteum by an epidural space.

very fine collagenous and elastic fibers, as well as small vessels. It is covered by a continuous membrane of flattened cells which are quite similar to the mesothelial lining cells of serous membranes. As blood

vessels enter the depths of the nervous tissue they carry with them some of the fine connective tissue components of the pia matter.

Choroid Plexus. The embryonic, tubular nature of the CNS is not lost in the adult, but it is extensively modified. The simple tube of the embryo is converted to large ventricles and a canal in the brain that is continuous with a central canal in the spinal cord. The ependymal lining of this modified tube is also retained in the adult. In specific areas (roof and walls of the ventricles) the ependyma is closely associated with the vascular pia mater, the vessels of which form the *choroid plexuses* (Fig. 15.22). Although the term "choroid plexus" refers specifically to the vascular network of the pia mater, this term is used to refer to all of the tissues that invaginate into the ventricular system of the brain and brain stem. Actually, the so-called "choroid plexus" consists of three distinct yet interrelated components: ependyma, tela choroidea and choroid plexus (Fig. 15.23). The *ependyma* is a thin layer of epithelial cells, *lamina epithelialis*, which lines the ventricular space and is associated intimately with the peripherally-positioned pia mater (Fig. 15.24). The cuboidal or columnar cells

of this lamina have well-developed brush borders and are joined along their lateral margins by tight junctions which serve as an effective seal between the ventricular and extracellular fluid space of the pia matter. The thin, web-like connective tissue of the pia mater is termed the *tela choroidea*. The vessels which comprise the *choroid plexus* are contained within the delicate connective tissue. These elements project into the ventricular system and are thrown into extensive folds (villi).

Cerebrospinal Fluid. The *cerebrospinal fluid* (*CSF*) is a clear, colorless fluid which fills the ventricular system and the central canal of the spinal cord. The CSF also occupies the subarachnoid space in association with the brain and spinal cord. The fluid is in continuity with both these spaces through two laterally-positioned foramina in the roof of the fourth ventricle, the *foramina of Luschka*. The CSF is not confined to these spaces. Rather, it penetrates into and per-

meates all of the tissues of the CNS as well. The fluid serves as a hydraulic protection and support mechanism as well as a medium for the nutrition of neural tissue of the CNS.

Although the formation of CSF is attributed generally to the "choroid plexuses" of the lateral, third and fourth ventricles, as much as 40% of this fluid may be produced at other sites. These other sites include the ependymal lining cells of the ventricular system, leptomeningeal coverings and blood vessels of the brain and spinal cord.

Cerebrospinal fluid is produced as an *ultrafiltrate* or *dialysate* of the blood and by *active secretion* by the ependymal cells. The principles of tissue fluid formation discussed previously (Chapter 6) apply generally to CSF formation. Although CSF formation normally continues at a constant rate, its production rate is independent of blood hydrostatic pressure but is influenced by the colloid osmotic pressure of the blood. The selective permeability and active secretion of the ependymal cells account for significant differences between CSF and tissue fluid. The CSF contains less calcium, potassium, glucose and protein and more magnesium, sodium and chloride than tissue fluid. Thus, an effective *blood-CSF boundary* exists that consists of diaphragmed, fenestrated capillary endothelial cells, basal lamina, delicate connective tissue, basal lamina of ependymal cells and ependymal cells.

The bulk of the CSF produced is elaborated by the plexuses of the lateral ventricles. The fluid flows into the third ventricle through the lateral ventricular foramina and additional fluid is added by the choroid plexus of the third ventricle. The fluid continues its flow caudad through the cerebral aqueduct into the fourth ventricle where more CSF is added by the choroid plexus of the fourth ventricle. Although some fluid continues caudad into the central canal of the spinal cord, this flow pattern is not dynamic. Cerebrospinal fluid gains access to the subarachnoid space via the foramina of Luschka. Once within this space, the CSF bathes and covers all aspects of the brain and spinal cord. The fluid is returned to the vasculature by passing through the *arachnoid villi* (*granulations*) which project into the *dural venous sinuses*. The arachnoid villi appear to function as pressure-dependent, unidirectional flow valves. Whereas the formation of CSF seems to be independent of vascular hydrostatic pressure, the return of CSF to the dural sinuses is dependent upon CSF/blood pressure gradients. Excessive pressure in the dural sinuses can collapse the villi and shut down the return of CSF.

Although the most obvious function of CSF is the hydraulic cushioning of the CNS, the CSF functions in the nutrition of neural tissue. CSF seeps into the neural tissue and bathes all of the constituent cells. It is, therefore, a transport medium for the ingress and egress of metabolites.

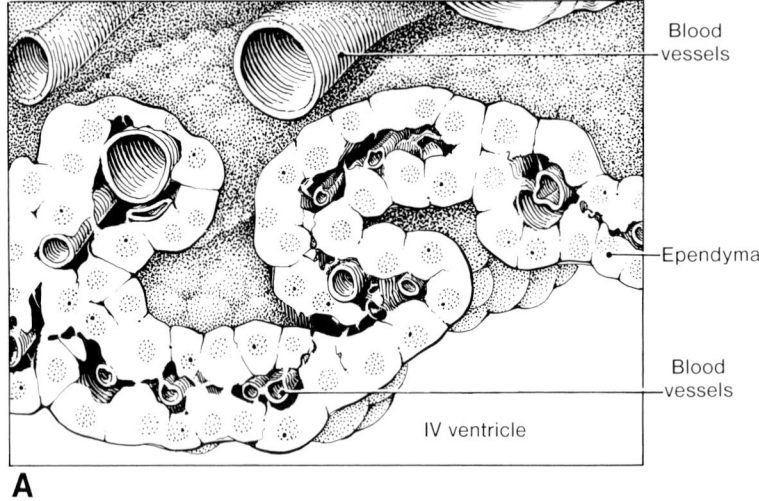

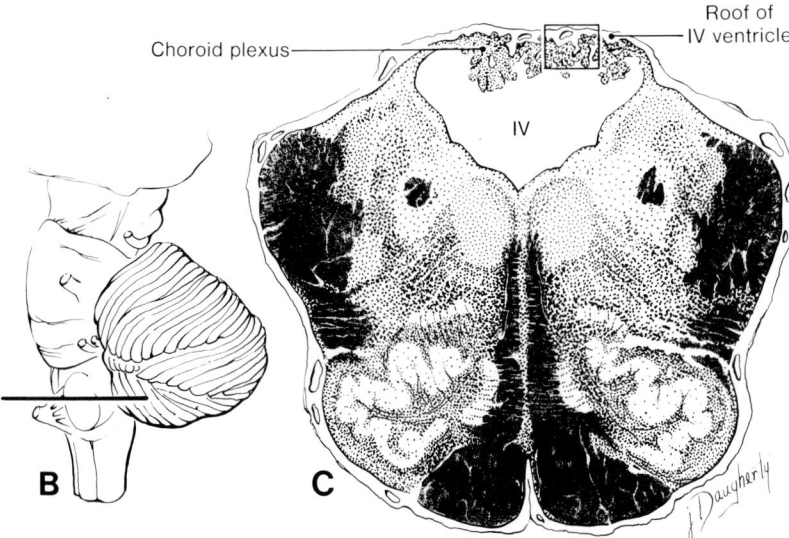

Fig. 15.22 A composite diagram depicting the choroid plexus and its relationship to the fourth ventricle. A, an artist's interpretation of a scanning electron micrograph of the choroid plexus; B, the relationship of the choroid plexus to the fourth ventricle in cross-section; C, the level from which the section was drawn.

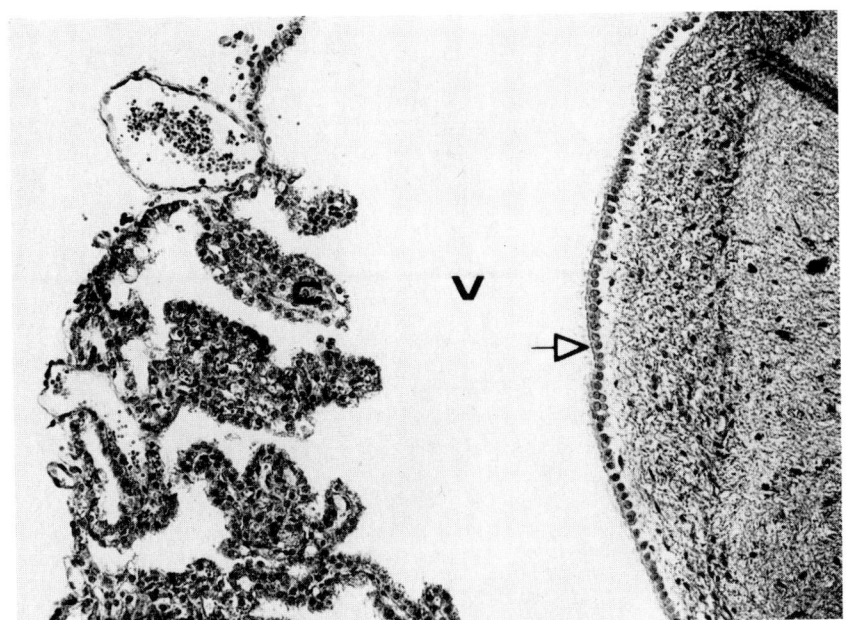

Fig. 15.23 The choroid plexus of the fourth ventricle. The choroid plexus (C) is suspended from the roof of the fourth ventricle (V). Ependymal cells are integral components of the choroid plexus. The ependymal cells (arrow) also cover the nervous tissue adjacent to the fourth ventricle. X40.

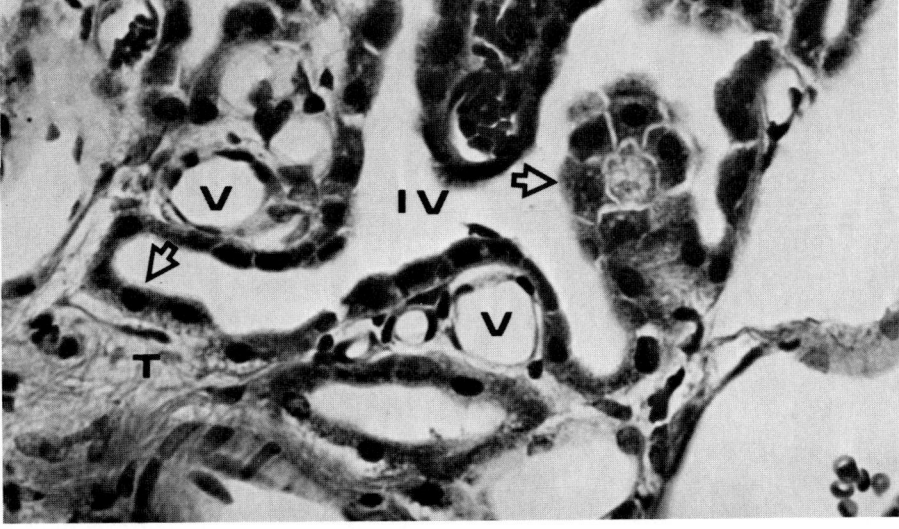

Fig. 15.24 Components of the choroid plexus of the fourth ventricle (IV). The ependymal cells (arrows) are associated intimately with the vessels (V) of the choroid plexus. Connective tissue components of the tela chordoidea (T) are evident. X125.

Blood-Brain Boundary. The blood vessels located within the subarachnoid space are bathed by CSF and are separated from the neural tissue by the pia mater (Fig. 15.25). As large blood vessels penetrate the substance of the neural tissue of the CNS they are separated from the pia mater by a perivascular space. This perivascular *space of Virchow-Robin* becomes progressively smaller and eventually is obliterated when the capillaries become juxtaposed to the neuroglial cells (astrocytes) that form the *outer glial limitans.* The juxtaposition of neuroglial cells between the capillary bed

and the neurons anatomically establishes what has been referred to as the *blood-brain barrier (blood-brain boundary).* The astrocytes which form this barrier have foot-like processes which are associated intimately with the basal lamina of the endothelial cells. Astrocytes were considered the cells through which materials passed between the capillary bed and neurons. Current evidence has established clearly that the neurons and neuroglia are bathed continuously by the CSF (Fig. 15.25). Moreover, some materials move readily from the capillary bed between neuroglial cells and gain access to the neu-

rons. It is probably most reasonable to consider the only true blood-brain barrier to be the endothelial cells and their associated basal lamina.

Spinal Cord. The spinal cord varies in configuration at the cervical, thoracic, lumbar and sacral levels. The following pattern, however, is similar at all levels of examination before the termination of the spinal cord.

The cord is generally round to oval and is surrounded by the pachymeninx (inner layer) and the leptomeninges in a pattern described previously (Fig. 15.26). The bulk of the cord is divided into two distinct areas, *gray matter* and *white matter*. The gray matter is arranged in a pattern often described as an H or butterfly. The *gray matter* consists of nerve cell bodies, unmyelinated fibers, some myelinated fibers, protoplasmic astrocytes, oligodendrogliocytes, microgliocytes, some blood vessels and associated fine connective tissue fibers. Although neurons are aggregated or scattered throughout the gray matter, they are especially distinct in the *ventral columns*. These large multipolar neurons give rise to axons carrying information to effector organs of the body. Neurons of medium size are located in the *lateral columns* of the thoracolumbar segments. These neurons give rise to axons which connect with autonomic ganglia. Small neurons characterize the *dorsal columns*. Their axons project up and down the spinal cord. The spinal canal (lined by ependyma) is contained within the *central intermediate substance* or *gray commissure*.

The *white matter* is composed of myelinated and unmyelinated fibers, scattered neuroglial elements and blood vessels. A *dorsal funiculus* occupies the region between the dorsal columns; a *lateral funiculus* is between two adjacent dorsal and ventral columns; and a *ventral funiculus* is between the two ventral columns.

The diameter of the spinal cord is not uniform from the cervical to sacral regions. Because most of the thoracic limb is innervated by the cervical segments of the spinal cord, there is a corresponding enlargement at this level. The *cervical (brachial) enlargement* or *intumescence* occurs between the levels C_6–T_1. A similar enlargement, the *lumbar intumescence*, occurs in the caudal aspect of the spinal cord in relation to the pelvic limb between segments L_4–S_2. The enlargements result from greater quantities of white and gray matter in these portions of the spinal cord than in other segments.

The white matter of the spinal cord is divisible into specific regions characterized by ascending and descending fiber tracts. Some of these tracts are diagrammed and stereotyped in Figure 15.27. Species differences exist in the distribution, size and relative positions of these tracts within the spinal cord. Major ascending tracts on each side include the fasciculus gracilis, fasciculus cuneatus, dorsal and ventral spinocerebellar

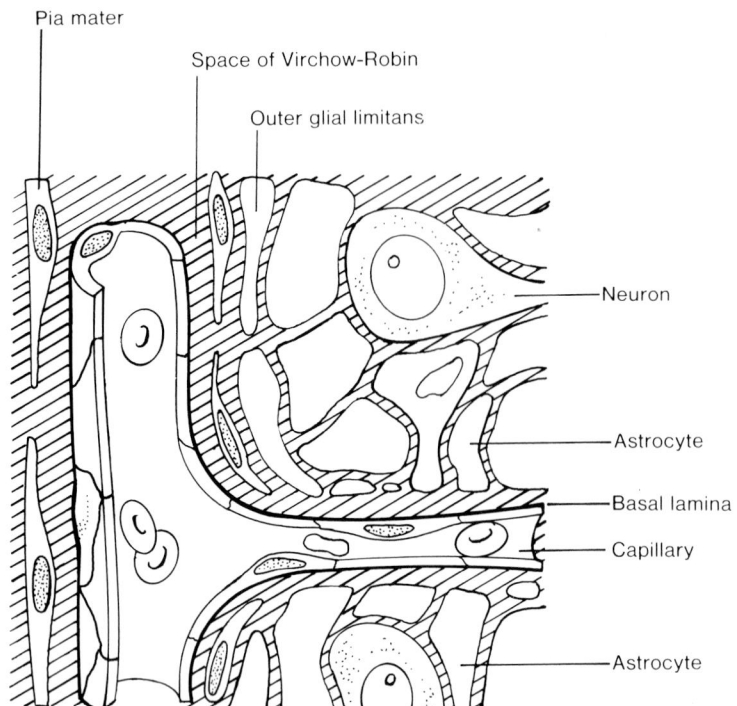

Fig. 15.25 A diagram of the blood-brain barrier. Cerebrospinal fluid in the subarachnoid space continues into the perivascular space of Virchow-Robin. Discontinuities in the outer glial limitans permits the movement of CSF between the astrocytes and around the neurons. The oblique lines are intended to demonstrate the ubiquitous nature of CSF within the brain.

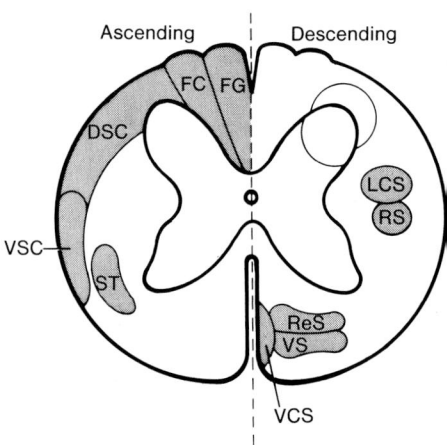

Fig. 15.27 A tracing of the spinal cord in Figure 15.26 to demonstrate ascending and descending tracts. FG, fasciculus gracilis; FC, fasciculus cuneatus; DSC, dorsal spinocerebellar tract; VSC, ventral spinocerebellar tract; ST, spinothalamic tract; LCS, lateral corticospinal tract; RS, rubrospinal tract; ReS, reticulospinal tract; VS, vestibulospinal tract; VCS, ventral corticospinal tract. The relationships depicted vary between species.

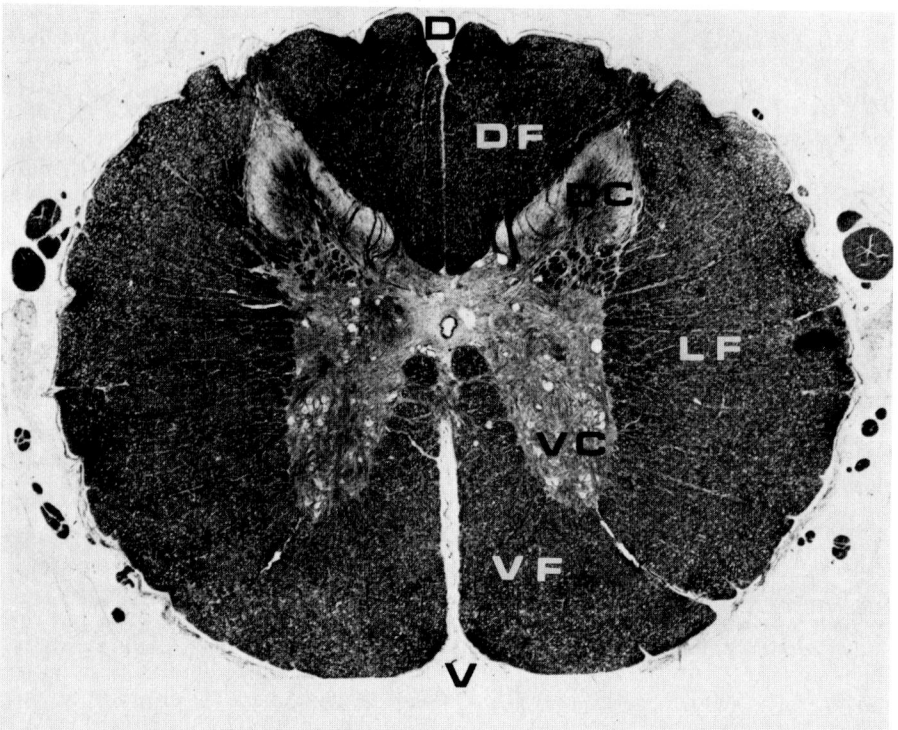

Fig. 15.26 A typical section through the cervical region of the spinal cord. The dorsal (DC) and ventral (VC) columns are prominent gray matter components. The dorsal (DF), lateral (LF) and ventral (VF) funiculi comprise the white matter of the spinal cord. D, dorsal; V, ventral. X4 (myelin stain).

tracts and the spinothalamic tract. Major descending tracts include the lateral corticospinal tract, rubrospinal tract, ventral corticospinal tract, reticulospinal tract and vestibulospinal tract. Other textbooks are suggested for an in-depth discussion of these tracts. (See references.)

Brain Stem. The brain stem is a complex structure which is continuous with the spinal cord caudally and higher brain centers rostrally. The structures which comprise the brain stem are those derived from the myelencephalon, metencephalon, mesencephalon and diencephalon. The organizational constituents are similar to the spinal cord; however, these constituents are distributed differently. Various nuclei and tracts are distributed in a specific manner throughout the brain stem (Plate V.10) (Fig. 15.28). The general pattern of nerve cell body and tract distribution for the cranial nerves rostral to the myelencephalon follows the general relationships described for the alar and basal plates. Additional nuclei occur within the region, and numerous ascending and descending tracts occur.

Cerebellum. The cerebellum is also divided into gray and white matter (Fig. 15.29). The white matter is covered by a thin layer of gray matter. Three distinct zones of gray matter are apparent: an *outer molecular layer*, a *central layer of large cells* (*Purkinje cells*) and a *deep granular layer*. The granular layer is contiguous to the white matter (Plate I.4, I.5).

The outer molecular layer consists of some small neurons and numerous unmyelinated fibers. The Purkinje cells of the central layer are large, pyramidal cells which are very prominent (Figs. 15.30, 15.31). *Do*

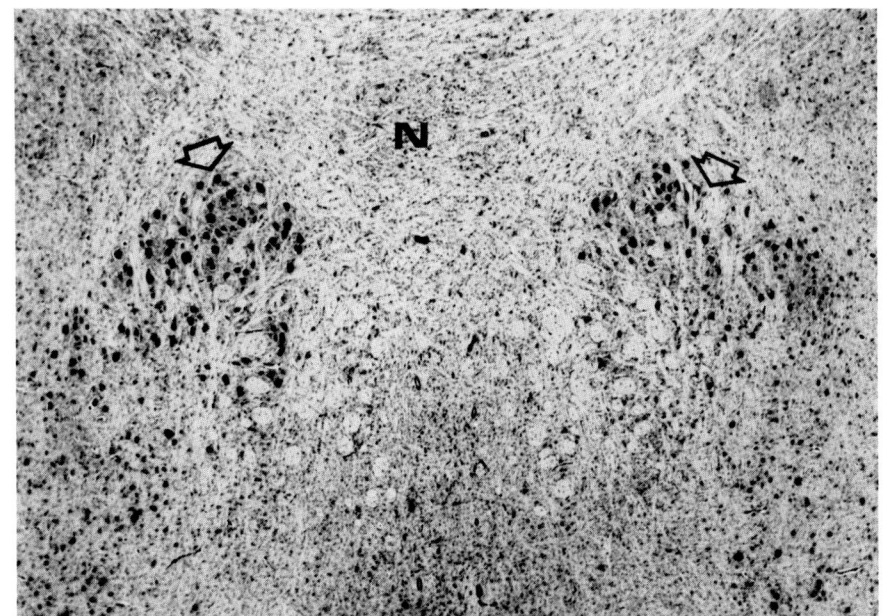

Fig. 15.28 A frontal section through the brain stem of a pig. The nerve cell bodies of two prominent nuclei (*arrows*) are apparent within the other nervous tissue (N) of the organ. X4.

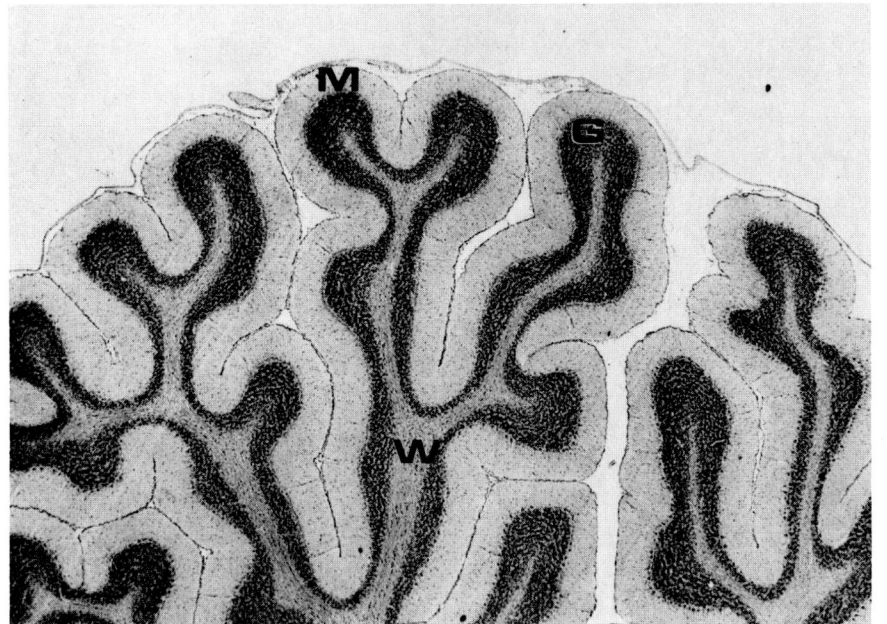

Fig. 15.29 A section through the cerebellum. The molecular layer (M) and granular layer (G) are peripheral to the white matter (W). X4.

not confuse Purkinje cells with Purkinje fibers! The neurons of the granular layer are small and tightly packed within this region. The details of the connections among these cells, as well as connections with *mossy* and *climbing fibers*, are available in texts of neuroanatomy (See references).

Cerebrum. Considering the diverse and complex functions of this portion of the brain, it is not unreasonable to assume that its cytoarchitecture reflects this diversity as well as this complexity. Although six layers of cells have been described, the degree of development of each layer varies with the section of cerebral cortex being studied (Fig. 15.32). The gray (outer) area of the cerebral cortex consists generally of the following cellular regions: *molecular layer, outer granular layer, pyramidal cell layer, inner granular layer, ganglion* or *inner pyramidal cell layer* and *polymorphic cell layer*. Throughout these areas are neuroglial elements, myelinated and unmyelinated nerve fibers and vessels. The student is referred to a text of neuroanatomy for further discussion of the cerebral cortex.

Autonomic Nervous System

Introduction. The regulation of a constant and optimal internal environment (*homeostasis*) is the function of the autonomic nervous system (ANS). It is complemented in its activity by the endocrine system. Together, these systems function to provide the fine control of the numerous parameters that permit the normal expression of cellular life.

The regulatory effects of the ANS are manifested via its influence on four types of effector systems: 1) smooth muscle (e.g., intestines, urinary bladder, blood vessels); 2) cardiac muscle; 3) exocrine glands (salivary, sweat, mucous); 4) some endocrine glands (adrenal medulla). The ubiquitous distribution of smooth muscle and exocrine glands exemplifies the broad influence of this system upon the body. The effect of cardiac function, under autonomic regulatory mechanisms, manifests broad bodily influences. Similarly, the primary hormone of the adrenal medulla (epinephrine), again under autonomic regulation, has broad bodily effects, especially in emergency situations. It is important to note that the ANS, indirectly through the effectors under its control, manifests a significant influence upon visceral bodily functions.

Organizational Components. Often the ANS is presented as an efferent (motor) system which links the central nervous system to the aforementioned effectors. The efferent portion of this system may be the most obvious, but the autonomic regulation of visceral function requires more than efferent pathways. The ANS consists of *sensors, afferent pathways, central integration* and *control centers, efferent pathways* and *effectors*. Together, these function in the maintenance of the internal environment.

The generalized pattern of organization of the autonomic nervous system is depicted in Figure 15.33. It consists of centrally and peripherally located components. The receptors (sensors) for the ANS are located throughout the viscera of the body. The common modalities monitored by the receptors are 1) stretch, 2) distention, 3) pressure, and 4) chemical changes.

Impulses from these receptors course over nerves toward the central nervous system. The nerves, carrying generalized sensory information from the viscera, are referred to as *general visceral afferent (GVA)* nerves. Upon entry into the spinal cord a reflex pathway may be established through the *internuncial neuron (interneuron)*. Similarly, a synapse will occur resulting in the ascent of the impulse to higher centers (suprasegmental). This may be at the conscious level (e.g., visceral pain) or the unconscious level. The impulses, directly or indirectly, reach the *hypothalamus*, the integration center of the autonomic nervous system. The hypothalamus, then, influences metabolic centers in the midbrain, pons and medulla. Efferent

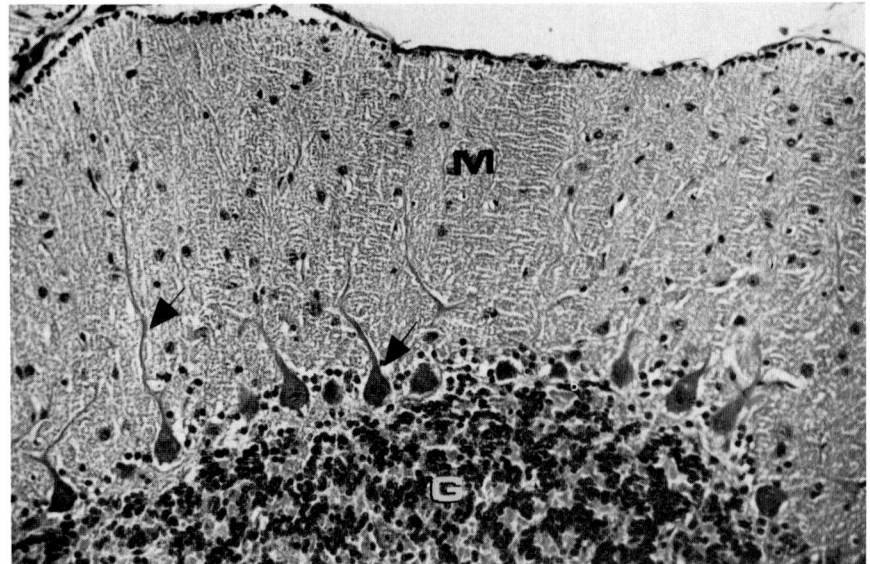

Fig. 15.30 Purkinje cells of the cerebellum. The Purkinje cells (*arrows*) occur at the interface between the molecular (M) and granular (G) layers. X40.

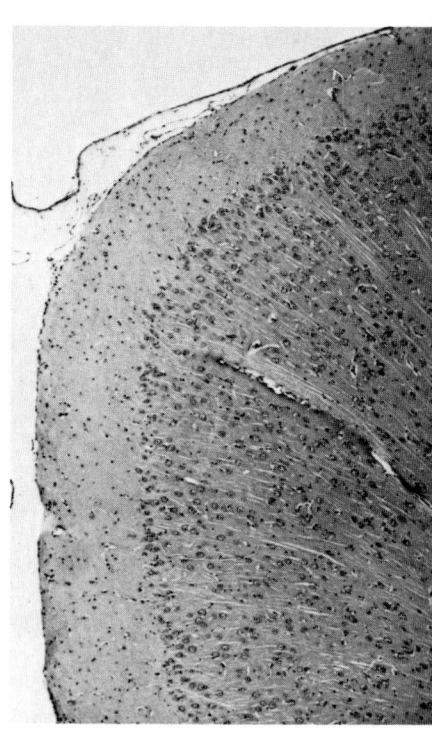

Fig. 15.32 Section through the cerebrum. The occurrence and distribution of layers of the gray matter differ in various regions of the cerebrum. X10.

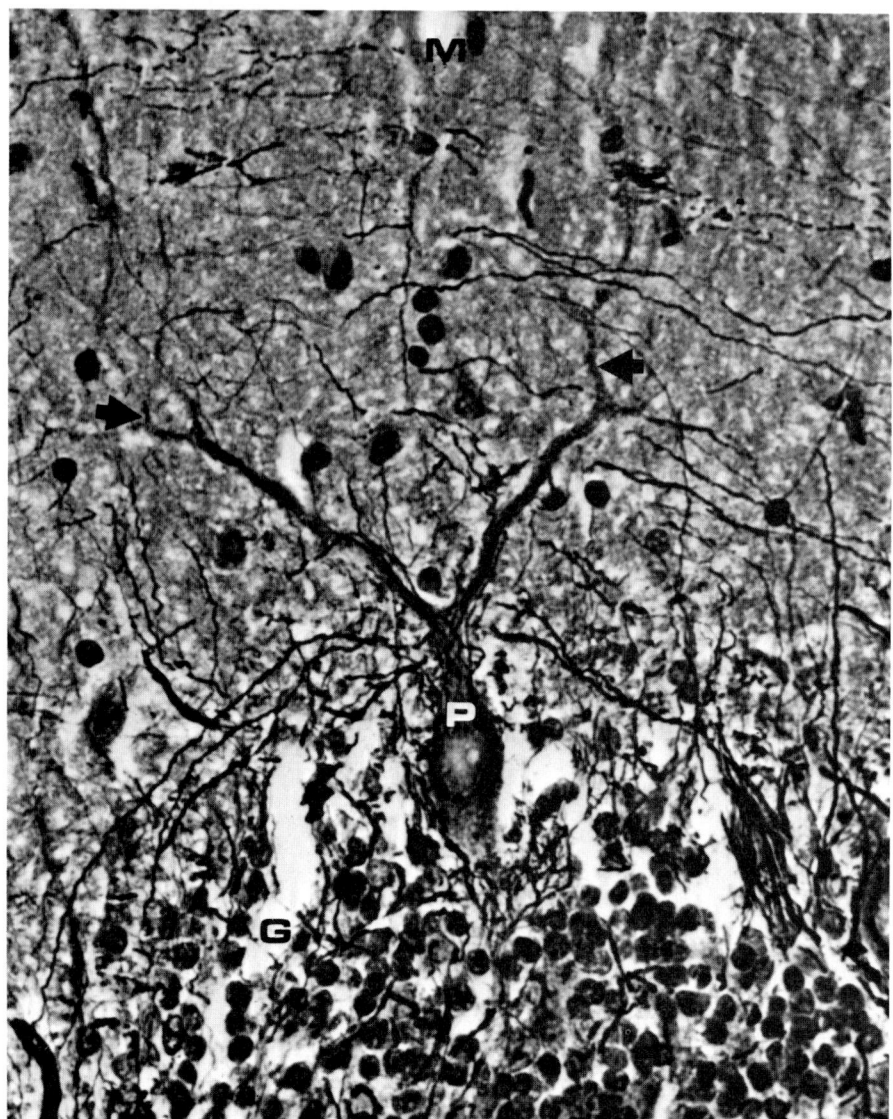

Fig. 15.31 Purkinje cell of the cerebellum. The purkinje cell (P) has dendritic processes (*arrows*) extending into the molecular layer. The axon of the cell extends through the granular layer (G) and synapses with neurons in the cerebellar nuclei. X100 (silver stain).

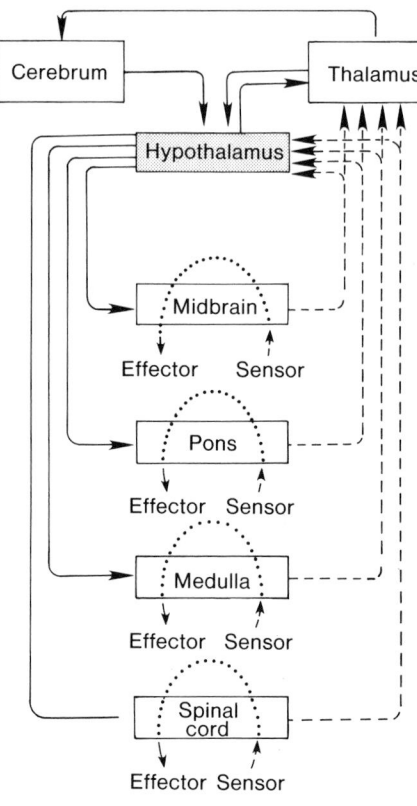

Fig. 15.33 A schematic diagram of the components of the autonomic nervous system. *Solid lines*, efferent pathways; *dashed lines*, afferent pathways; *dotted lines*, reflex pathways through midbrain, pons, medulla oblongata and spinal cord.

ibers originate in these centers, as well as the spinal cord, and innervate visceral effectors via specific cranial nerves, spinal nerves and splanchnic nerves. These fibers, carrying general motor impulses to the visceral effectors, are referred to as *general visceral efferent (GVE)* nerves.

The autonomic nervous system, then, consists of peripheral and central components that are responsible for the reception, transmission, integration, control, and subsequent initiation of an effector response. The system, therefore, consists of components that are identical to those associated with somatic sensation and response.

The autonomic nervous system is a system designed to function spontaneously or independently of volition. The *reflex arc* is central to such an organizational scheme. The higher centers, specifically the hypothalamus, serve to modulate the response. Through the integrative function of the hypothalamus, the effectors of the autonomic nervous system manifest a basic level of normal activity (*tone*) which may be modified by afferent input and efferent output. (Such control may be considered analogous to the activity of a thermostat in the regulation of house temperature.)

An understanding of the organization of the GVE component is best achieved by a discussion and a comparison of an autonomic reflex arc with a somatic reflex arc. (See Figure 15.34.)

In a polysynaptic somatic reflex: 1) afferent impulses (GSA) reach the *dorsal root* from the spinal nerve and enter the *dorsal gray column*; 2) a synapse occurs with an *interneuron*; 3) the interneuron then synapses with a neuron in the *ventral gray column* (*α-motor neuron, lower motor neuron, final common pathway*); 4) these efferent impulses (GSE) enter the *ventral root* and *spinal nerve* and subsequently reach the skeletal muscle effector. In the typical autonomic reflex: 1) afferent impulses (*GVA*) reach the *dorsal root* and enter the *dorsal gray column*; 2) a synapse occurs with a neuron (*preganglionic neuron*) located in the *intermediate grey column*; 3) this axon

courses out of the spinal cord and synapses with a second neuron (*postganglionic neuron*) which is located in a ganglion; 4) these GVE impulses are transmitted over postganglionic fibers (axons) to the visceral effectors.

Some authors refer to the neuron in the intermediate gray column as the interneuron, whereas others refer to it as the lower motor neuron. It is the author's opinion that it is consistent with the terminology applied to a somatic reflex to refer to the first neuron (preganglionic) as the interneuron and second neuron (postganglionic) as the lower motor neuron.

The myelinated axons of preganglionic neurons always synapse with a second neuron which is located outside the central nervous system. The cell bodies of the second neurons (postganglionic) may be located in *vertebral (paravertebral)*, *prevertebral (collateral)* or *terminal (peripheral) ganglia*. The unmyelinated axons of postganglionic neurons terminate on visceral effectors.

The autonomic reflex, then, always consists of at least three neurons: an afferent neuron, a preganglionic neuron, a postganglion neuron.

The specific location of these cell bodies varies with the divisions of the ANS (*sympathetic* or *parasympathetic*).

Sympathetic and Parasympathetic Divisions

Introduction. The ANS is divided into two subdivisions: *sympathetic* and *parasympathetic nervous systems*. Part of the rationale for these subdivisions is predicated upon the anatomic location of the first neuron (preganglionic neuron). These neurons are located in three regions of the central nervous system—*brain stem, thoracolumbar spinal cord* and *sacral spinal cord* (Fig. 15.35).

In the sympathetic nervous system, the cell bodies of the preganglionic neurons are located in the intermediate gray column of the *thoracolumbar spinal cord*. These neurons extend from approximately the first thoracic to the fifth lumbar segment of the

spinal cord. For this reason this portion of the ANS is referred to as the *thoracolumbar system*.

In the parasympathetic nervous system, the cell bodies of the preganglionic neurons are located in the *brain stem* in *nuclei of cranial nerves III, VII, IX, X* and *XI* and in the *sacral segments of the spinal cord*. This outflow pattern is the basis for referring to this system as the *craniosacral system*.

The Sympathetic Nervous System. Figure 15.36 is a simplified and stylized diagram of the GVE and GVA fibers of the sympathetic divisions of the ANS. This drawing completely ignores the relationship of higher centers upon the system. Rather, the reflex activity is emphasized. Moreover, not all the distributional relationships are represented. The figure is intended to demonstrate basic patterns rather than all of the pathways and associations that are characteristic of all segments.

The distributional pattern of the axons of the preganglionic neurons is variable once they enter a paravertebral ganglion via the rami communicantes:

a. A synapse may occur with a postaganglionic neuron, the unmyelinated fibers of which enter the ramus communicans and are distributed with the spinal nerves to peripheral visceral structures (Fig. 15.36A).

b. The preganglionic fibers enter the sympathetic trunk and may synapse with a postganglionic neuron at that segmental level and exit the trunk at the same level (Fig. 15.36B).

c. The preganglionic fibers enter the sympathetic trunk and may ascend or descend before synapsing with a postganglionic neuron at a different segmental level within the sympathetic trunk (Fig. 15.36C).

d. The preganglionic fibers enter the sympathetic trunk, passing through it without synapsing, and exit same via the splanchnic nerves. A synapse then occurs with a postganglionic neuron located in one of the prevertebral ganglia (Fig. 15.36D).

e. Finally, the preganglionic fibers proceed through the paravertebral and prevertebral ganglia without synapsing and innervate the adrenal medulla (Fig. 15.36E).

Numerous other patterns characterize the distribution of pre- and postganglionic sympathetic nerve fibers. Notably, the postganglionic fibers are long. The synapses between the pre- and postganglionic neurons occur some distance away from the effectors innervated.

Although specific nerves may be identified after a careful dissection of the sympathetic nervous system, invariably, the distributional pattern of these nerves follows that of the arteries. These nerves and associated prevertebral ganglia form extensive plexuses that are intimately associated with major arteries.

Generally, preganglionic fibers originating cranial to T_5 are distributed cranially, whereas those nerves originating caudal to T_5 are distributed caudally. Moreover, the extent of the ganglionated sympathetic

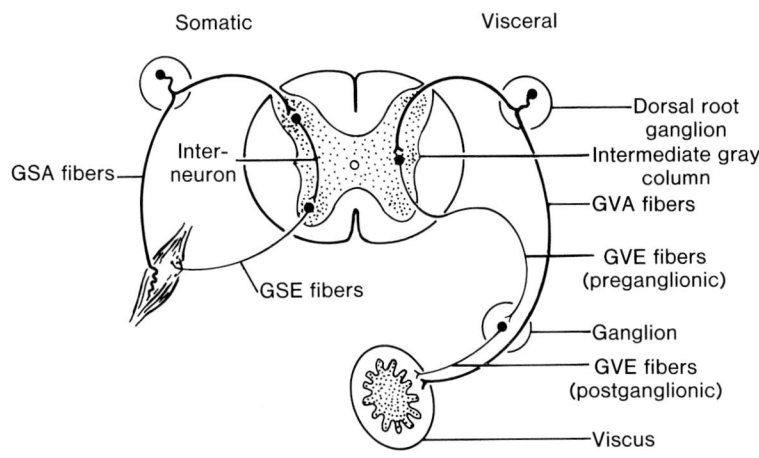

Fig. 15.34 A diagrammatic comparison between a somatic and visceral reflex. Note the additional neuron located in a ganglion in the visceral reflex.

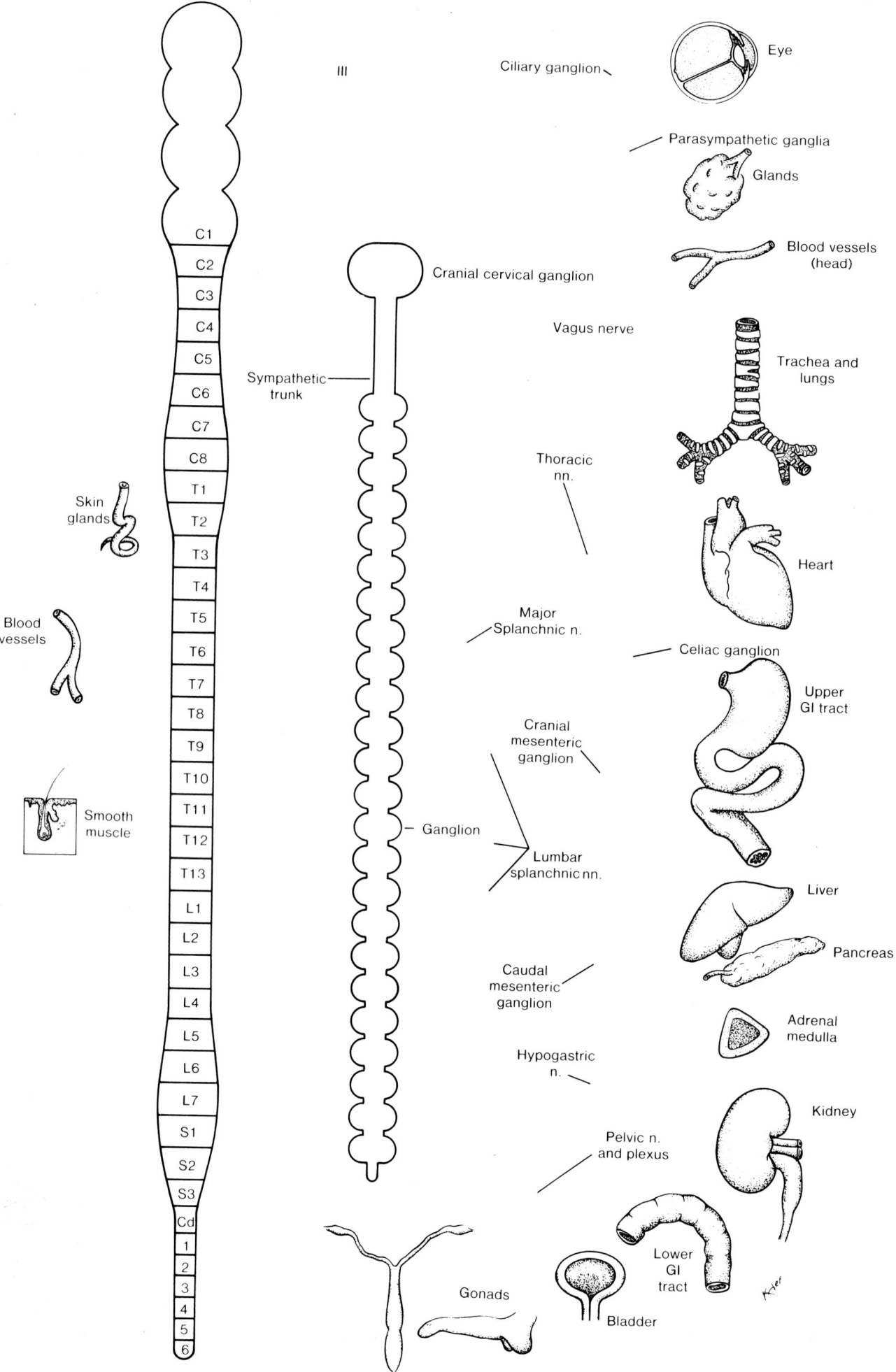

III

Ciliary ganglion — Eye

Parasympathetic ganglia

Glands

Blood vessels (head)

Cranial cervical ganglion

Vagus nerve

Trachea and lungs

C1
C2
C3
C4
C5
C6
C7
C8
T1
T2
T3
T4
T5
T6
T7
T8
T9
T10
T11
T12
T13
L1
L2
L3
L4
L5
L6
L7
S1
S2
S3
Cd
1
2
3
4
5
6

Sympathetic trunk

Skin glands

Blood vessels

Smooth muscle

Thoracic nn.

Heart

Major Splanchnic n.

Celiac ganglion

Upper GI tract

Ganglion

Cranial mesenteric ganglion

Lumbar splanchnic nn.

Liver

Pancreas

Caudal mesenteric ganglion

Adrenal medulla

Hypogastric n.

Kidney

Pelvic n. and plexus

Gonads

Bladder

Lower GI tract

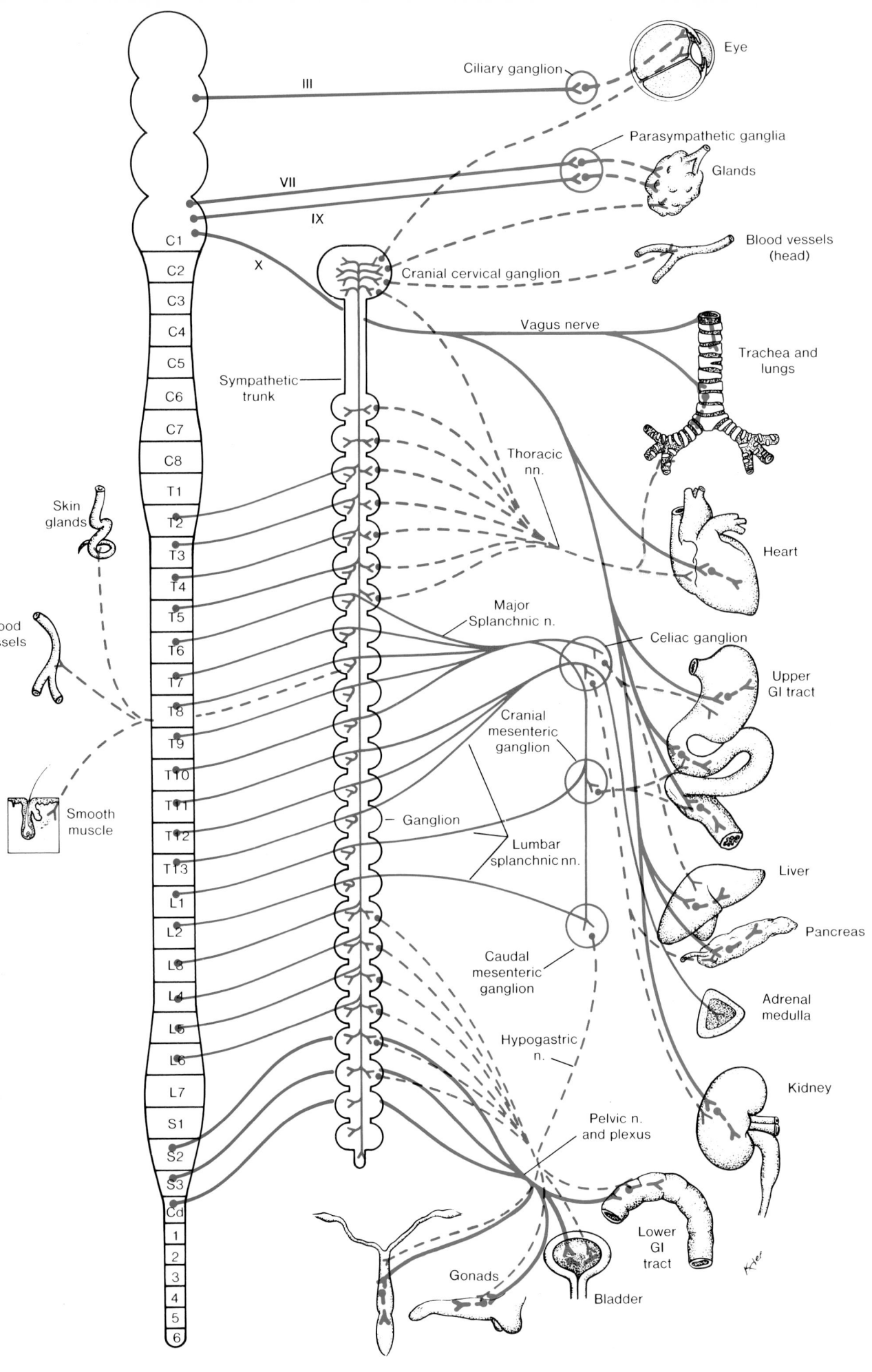

Eye

Ciliary ganglion

III

Parasympathetic ganglia

VII

Glands

IX

Blood vessels
(head)

C1

X

Cranial cervical ganglion

C2

C3

Vagus nerve

C4

Trachea and
lungs

C5

C6

Sympathetic
trunk

C7

C8

T1

Thoracic
nn.

Skin
glands

T2

T3

T4

Heart

T5

T6

Blood
vessels

T7

Major
Splanchnic n.

Celiac ganglion

T8

T9

Upper
GI tract

T10

Cranial
mesenteric
ganglion

T11

Smooth
muscle

Ganglion

T12

Lumbar
splanchnic nn.

Liver

T13

L1

L2

Pancreas

L3

L4

Caudal
mesenteric
ganglion

Adrenal
medulla

L5

L6

Hypogastric
n.

Kidney

L7

S1

S2

Pelvic n.
and plexus

S3

Cd

1

2

3

Lower
GI tract

4

Gonads

5

Bladder

6

ERRATUM

Figure 15.35 on page 296 was incorrectly reproduced in black and white only. The correct version, printed in color, appears on the reverse of this page.

The Publisher regrets any inconvenience.

trunk is greater than the site of origin of preganglionic fibers. The trunk extends from the cranial cervical region to the cranial coccygeal region. In the cervical region, the sympathetic trunk is enclosed within a common sheath with the vagus nerve, forming the *vagosympathetic trunk.*

The Parasympathetic Nervous System. Figure 15.37 is a simplified and stylized drawing of the GVE and GVA fibers associated with the parasympathetic division of the ANS. This diagram does not include all of the relationships of higher centers with the components of this system. Also, not all of the distributional patterns are represented. The intention of the diagram is to present representative pathways rather than those characteristic of all segments.

The spatial relationships between GVA fibers and the GVE fibers of the sacral portion of the parasympathetic nervous system follow the basic pattern expanded upon earlier. Afferent information reaches the spinal cord via the pelvic and splanchnic nerves. The cell bodies for the fibers, as described previously, are located in the dorsal root ganglia. These neurons synapse with the preganglionic neurons located in the intermediate horn. Preganglionic fibers are then distributed to the viscera via the pelvic nerve and plexus. Their terminal ganglia are the sites for synapses with the postganglionic neurons. These synapses, generally, occur within the walls of the organs innervated. Accordingly, they are referred to as intramural ganglia. The postganglionic fibers are very short.

Afferent information at the level of the sacral cord also ascends the spinal cord to higher brain centers. Also, afferent information may be carried via the splanchnic nerves to the vagus nerve and then to higher centers.

The reflex pattern for the cranial portion of the parasympathetic nervous system is organized in manner slightly different than described previously for the autonomic spinal reflexes. These organizational differences are related to the different embryologic events characteristic of spinal cord and brain stem development.

The parasympathetic nuclei of cranial nerves III, VII, IX, X and XI are homologous to the intermediate gray columns of the spinal cord (thoracic, lumbar and sacral segments). These nuclear areas are the sites of origin of the preganglionic fibers of these parasympathetic nerves. Synapses with postganglionic neurons occur in terminal ganglia that are located close to or within the organs innervated.

The accompanying diagram (Fig. 15.37) shows that afferent information may enter the brain stem in a variety of ways and from

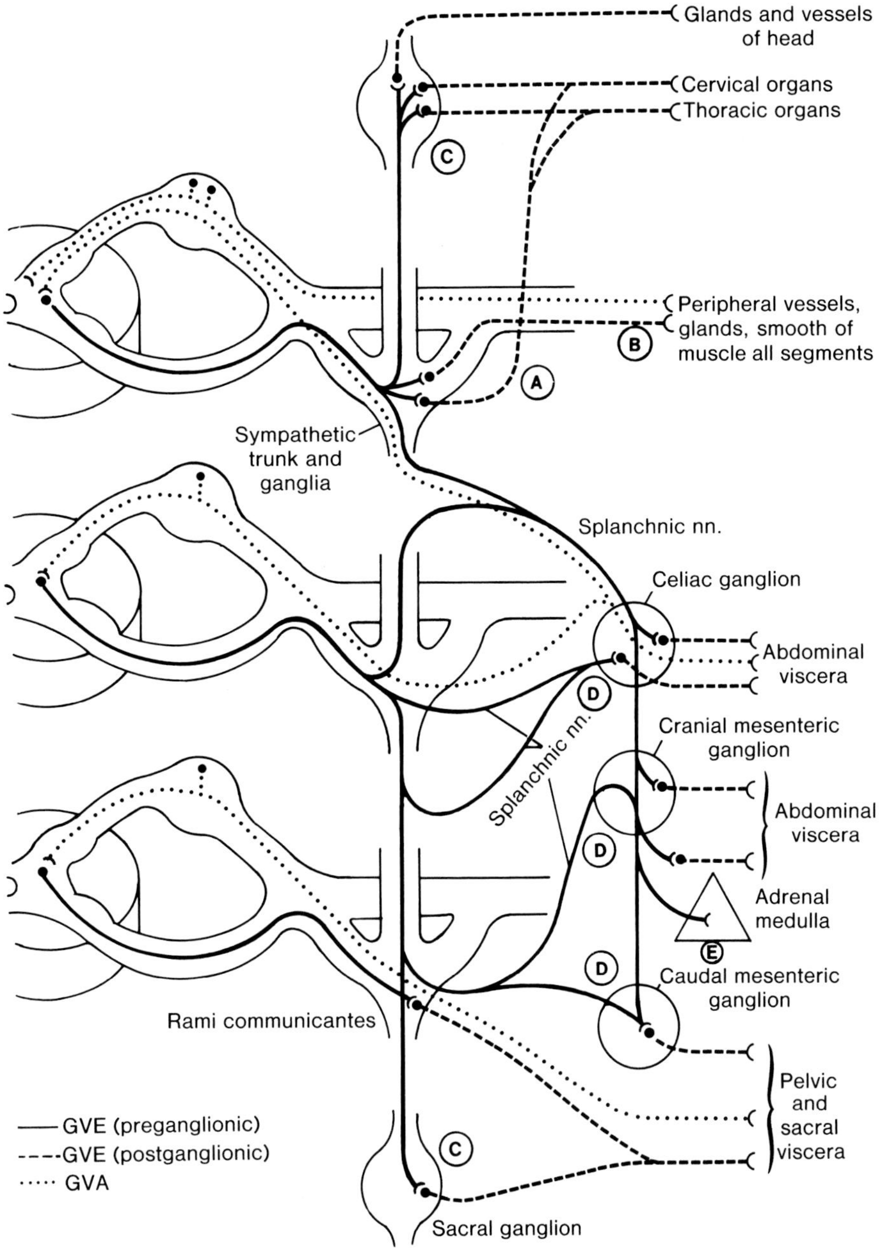

Fig. 15.36 An idealized drawing of the sympathetic nervous system that shows afferent and efferent pathways. The various patterns of efferent fiber distribution are shown. Refer to text for complete description.

various sources. The cell bodies of these afferent fibers are located in specific sensory ganglia that are homologous to the dorsal root ganglia of the spinal cord. (One exception to this is the use of special somatic afferent (SSA) information.) Upon entry into the brain stem these afferent fibers project rostrad and caudad in the *solitary tract.* These fibers terminate on interneurons of the *nucleus of the solitary tract,* the fibers of which synapse (directly or indirectly) with the preganglionic neurons of cranial nerves III, VII, IX, X and XI. Despite the altered

organizational patterns, all of the components necessary for an autonomic reflex are present.

Anatomic and Physiologic Correlates

Functional Relationships. Most of the visceral organs of the body have a dual innervation, and the functional influence of the sympathetic and parasympathetic innervation upon these organs has been described as antagonistic. One system, in fact, may enhance and/or accelerate visceral func-

Fig. 15.35 An idealized drawing of the autonomic nervous system. The diagram is simplified for clarity. The sympathetic innervation of the integument (arrector pili muscles, blood vessels, glands) is only indicated for one segment to the *left*. The innervation of the other visceral organs is shown on the *right*. Sympathetic nerves are red, parasympathetic nerves are *blue*. Preganglionic fibers are *solid*, postganglionic fibers are *dashed*.

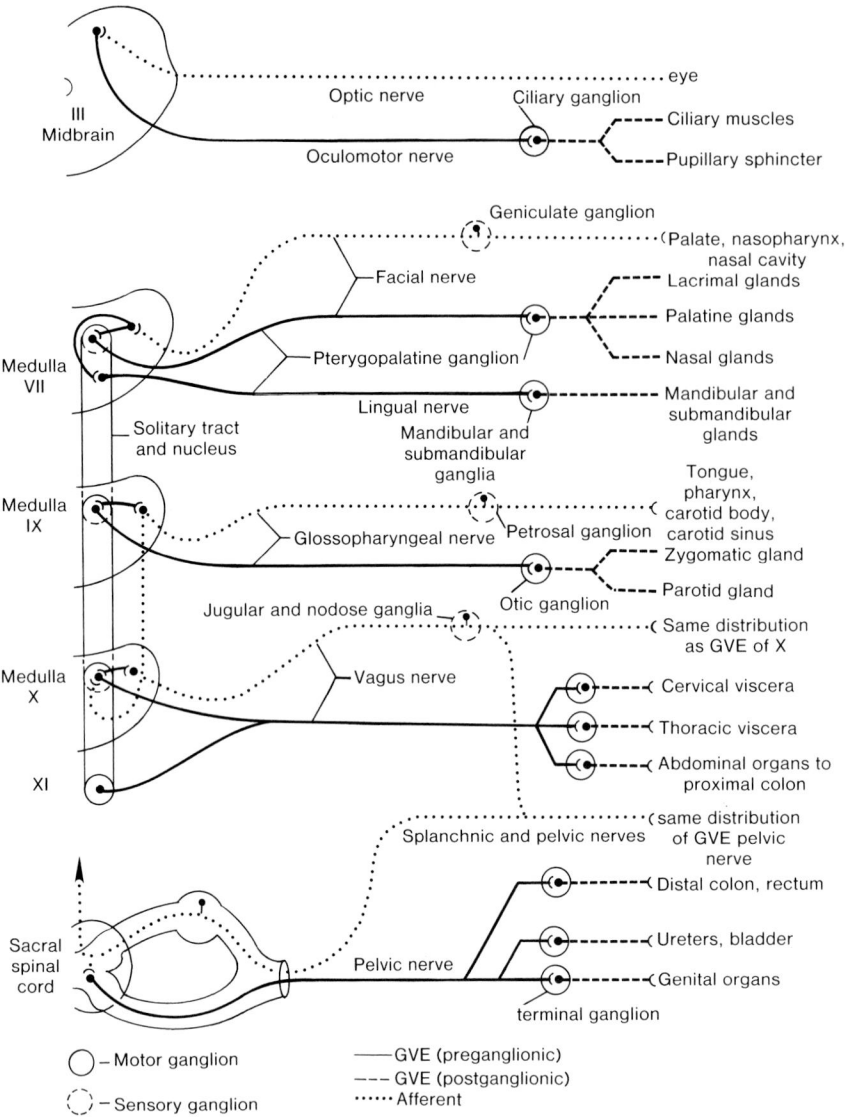

Fig. 15.37 An idealized schematic representation of the afferent and efferent constituents of the parasympathetic nervous system. Refer to the text for complete description.

tions, whereas the other may inhibit and/or decelerate visceral functions. Importantly, they manifest a synergistic effect upon visceral function to achieve a desired end—homeostasis.

There are notable exceptions to the previous generalities. Both divisions seem to stimulate salivary and pancreatic secretion. Moreover, not all organs have a dual innervation. The adrenal medulla, spleen, pilomotor muscles, sweat glands and probably all of the blood vessels of the body are innervated exclusively by the sympathetic division. The parasympathetic division provides the exclusive innervation for the ciliary and pupillary sphincter muscles, whereas the sympathetic division innervates the pupillary dilator. (Functionally, however, the pupil of the eye is controlled by dual innervation.)

The dual innervation of most organs provides for a wide range of control upon the tone, basal level of activity, of the visceral organs. The control of heart rate is a good example of how these systems complement each other. (This is a simplification of complex control mechanisms.) An increased heart rate (tachycardia) may result from a decreased parasympathetic tone or an increased sympathetic tone. A decreased heart rate (bradycardia) may result from an increased parasympathetic tone or a decreased sympathetic tone. The functional relationships of these divisions in terms of control of cardiac rate are applicable to the other visceral organs.

For those organs that are innervated exclusively by the sympathetic nervous system, tone variations are still possible. Normally, most vessels are constricted partially by the basal level of activity of this system. An increased level of activity constricts the vessels (vasoconstriction), whereas a decreased level of activity permits dilation of the vessels (vasodilation).

The preganglionic fibers of the autonomic nervous system are myelinated and relatively slow-conducting B fibers. Each preganglionic fiber potentially may diverge to numerous postganglionic neurons that give rise to mostly unmyelinated C fibers. By comparison to the somatic system, the autonomic output is diffuse and slow.

The two systems manifest differences in the degree of response. These differences may be explained, in part, on the basis of the different *innervation ratios* in the two systems. The relatively short preganglionic fibers of the sympathetic nervous system synapse with numerous neurons some distance from the organs innervated, permitting a diffuse response over the long postganglionic fibers to the organs innervated. This innervation ratio of preganglionic axons to ganglion cells may be 1:20 or more. The relatively long preganglionic fibers of the parasympathetic nervous system synapse with numerous neurons close to or within the organs innervated, permitting a more discrete and limited response than its sympathetic counterpart. In some organs, the innervation ratio seems to be 1:1. However, estimates of the ratio of preganglionic vagal fibers to ganglion cells of the submucosal plexus are as high as 1:8000. The distinction between the two systems based upon discreteness of response does not apply to all sites.

Transmitters. Transmission at the synapses between the pre- and postganglionic neurons and between the postganglionic neuron and effector organs is chemically mediated. The chemical mediators (*neurotransmitter substances*) act upon receptors to effect a response, either in the postganglionic neuron and/or the effector organs. The principal neurotransmitters of the ANS are *acetylcholine (ACH)* and *norepinephrine* (Fig. 15.38).

The preganglionic fibers of the sympathetic and parasympathetic divisions release *acetylcholine* as the neurotransmitter. These fibers are referred to as *cholinergic* fibers. The postganglionic fibers of the parasympathetic nervous system also release acetylcholine; they, too, are *cholinergic* fibers. The neurotransmitter secreted by the postganglionic fibers of the sympathetic nerves, however, is *norepinephrine*; they are referred to as *adrenergic* fibers. Nerves that release *acetylcholine* are called *cholinergic*, whereas nerves that release *norepinephrine* are called *adrenergic*.

In summary, the cholinergic nerves include *preganglionic* fibers of the *parasympathetic* nervous system, *preganglionic* fibers of the *sympathetic* nervous system, *postganglionic* fibers of the *parasympathetic* nervous system and motor fibers to voluntary skeletal muscle. The postganglionic fibers of the sympathetic nervous system secrete norepinephrine. These fibers are the adrenergic nerves of the ANS.

The nature, synthesis, release, effects and degradation of neurotransmitters was discussed in-depth in Chapter 12.

Cholinergic Receptors. These types of receptors were discussed in Chapter 12; additional information is required now as it relates to the ANS. Nerves which secrete ACH are termed *cholinergic nerves*. Drugs which mimic the effects of ACH are termed *cholinergic drugs*. ACH receptor sites are termed *cholinergic receptors*. Although ACH is released by preganglionic sympathetic and parasympathetic nerves and postganglionic parasympathetic nerves, the properties of the preganglionic and postganglionic receptor sites are different. These two sites manifest a differential responsiveness to two plant alkaloids, muscarine and nicotine.

Muscarine, a mycotic alkaloid, has little effect upon autonomic ganglion cells; however, it does mimic the stimulatory effect of ACH upon effector organs innervated by postganglionic parasympathetic nerves. These specific ACH-receptors sites are termed *muscarinic receptors*. Drugs which act in the same manner as muscarine are termed *muscarinic drugs*.

Certain drugs have the ability to block the effects of ACH at its receptor sites, preganglionic or postganglionic. These types of drugs are called *anticholinergic drugs*. Anticholinergic drugs that specifically block the receptor sites of postganglionic parasympathetic nerves are termed *antimuscarinic drugs*. Atropine, glycopyrrolate and scopolamine are examples of antimuscarinic drugs.

Nicotine, a plant alkaloid, mimics the effect of ACH on autonomic ganglion cells and on the receptors of the motor end plates of skeletal muscle. Nicotine in small amounts, as with ACH, stimulates these receptor sites, although in large doses, nicotine blocks autonomic ganglion cell transmission and the stimulation of skeletal muscle. These receptor sites are referred to as *nicotine receptors* and the drugs that manifest these effects are called *nicotinic drugs*. Because the neuromuscular junction receptors respond to certain drugs differently than receptors on autonomic ganglion cells, the former are considered to be slightly different nicotinic receptor sites.

The uniqueness of the receptor sites at the postganglionic parasympathetic synapses is important clinically. The selective blockage of muscarinic sites can be achieved by the judicious use of antimuscarinic drugs.

While all cholinergic receptors respond to ACH, not all of these receptors result in the activation of the effector organs. Activation of specific receptor sites can manifest excitatory or inhibitory effects upon the effector organ by the generation of EPSP's or IPSP's. (See Chapter 12, Neurotransmitters and Receptors.) Cholinergic stimulation of the heart results in a decreased heart rate; similar stimulation of the pupillary sphincter muscle and smooth muscle of the gastrointestinal tract results in smooth muscle contraction. Generally, the muscular sphincters of the alimentary canal relax or decrease tone upon cholinergic stimulation.

Adrenergic Receptors. The adrenergic receptors were discussed in-depth in Chapter 12. The distinction between α and β receptors is predicated upon their differential responsiveness to norepinephrine and epinephrine. Norepinephrine is a strong α receptor and weak β receptor stimulant, whereas epinephrine is a strong α and β stimulant. The stimulation of α receptors by epinephrine and norepinephrine results in vasoconstriction and pupillary dilation; however, the receptors of the smooth muscle of the gut wall are inhibitory. The β receptors, generally, result in inhibition or relaxation of the organ innervated. The notable exception is the β_1 receptor that is excitatory to the heart muscle and has a positive chronotropic and positive intropic effect upon the cardiac muscle mass. The receptors of intestinal smooth muscle, however, are inhibitory. The β_2 receptors of the smooth muscle of bronchioles and vascular beds are inhibitory, while those of the uterus have variable effects. Although β receptors are stimulated by epinephrine and to a lesser extent by norepinephrine, the identification of β_1 and β_2 receptors is predicated upon the differential responsiveness of the sites to these and other drugs.

Whereas most organs contain either α and β receptors and react accordingly, some organs contain both α and β receptors. The vessels of the dermis, mucosa, kidney and other visceral organs have more α than β receptors; the vessels of the heart and skeletal muscle have more β than α receptors. In the smooth muscle of the gut wall, the α and β receptors are both inhibitory. The vessels of some organs do not have vasomotor (sympathetic) innervation. Accordingly, they are devoid of α and β receptors. The vessels to the brain are a good example. Other mechanisms are used to insure an adequate blood supply to this organ.

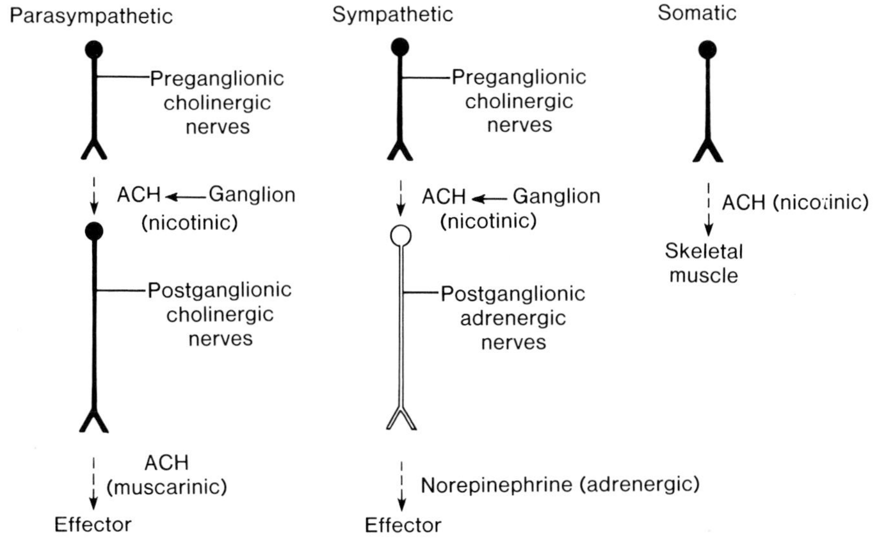

Adrenal Medulla

Relationship to the ANS. A discussion of the relationship of the adrenal medulla to the ANS is useful for several reasons: 1) it has a unique innervation pattern; 2) it demonstrates the link between the nervous and endocrine systems; 3) it is a useful model in understanding the relationships, distribution and effects of various receptors, and 4) it is important for an understanding of stress and "fight or flight" reactions.

The adrenal medulla is a unique organ that is innervated by *preganglionic sympathetic nerves*. The anatomic basis for this is simple. The cells of the adrenal medulla (as well as others such as dorsal root ganglion cells, autonomic ganglion cells and extraadrenal medullary tissue) are derived from neural crest ectoderm. The chromaffin cells of the adrenal medulla, therefore, are *postganglionic neurons*. These cells secrete epinephrine and norepinephrine ($\cong$ 85:15). The adrenal medulla is an important but nonessential component of the sympathetic nervous system. It is the means by which generalized sympathetic overflow manages to affect all cells of the body (Fig. 15.39). Adrenal medullary secretions, primarily epinephrine, affect the following processes: facilitate adrenergic transmission, increase heart rate (β_1), increase cardiac contraction strength (β_1), increase glycogenolysis (diabetogenic), release free fatty acids from adipose tissue. These effects ready the animal body for stress, such as that accompanying violent muscular activity, hypotension, hypoxia, fear, anger, anxiety. Simultaneously, blood is shunted from the vessels of the skin (α receptors) and viscera ($\alpha > \beta$) to the vessels of skeletal muscle ($\beta > \alpha$). This reactivity or sudden surge of adrenal medullary activity is described as the "fight or flight reaction." Rather, it is better described as a reaction that prepares the animal for stressful circumstances that threaten its physical well-being and/or homeostasis. The examining room is a good place to observe the effects of the adrenal medulla.

As the rest of the sympathetic nervous system, the adrenal medulla is not essential for life, as long as emergencies are minimized. In fact, demonstration of the deficiencies of complete sympathectomy is difficult if nonstressful conditions are maintained.

Fig. 15.38 A diagram of cholinergic and adrenergic nerves. Refer to text for a complete description.

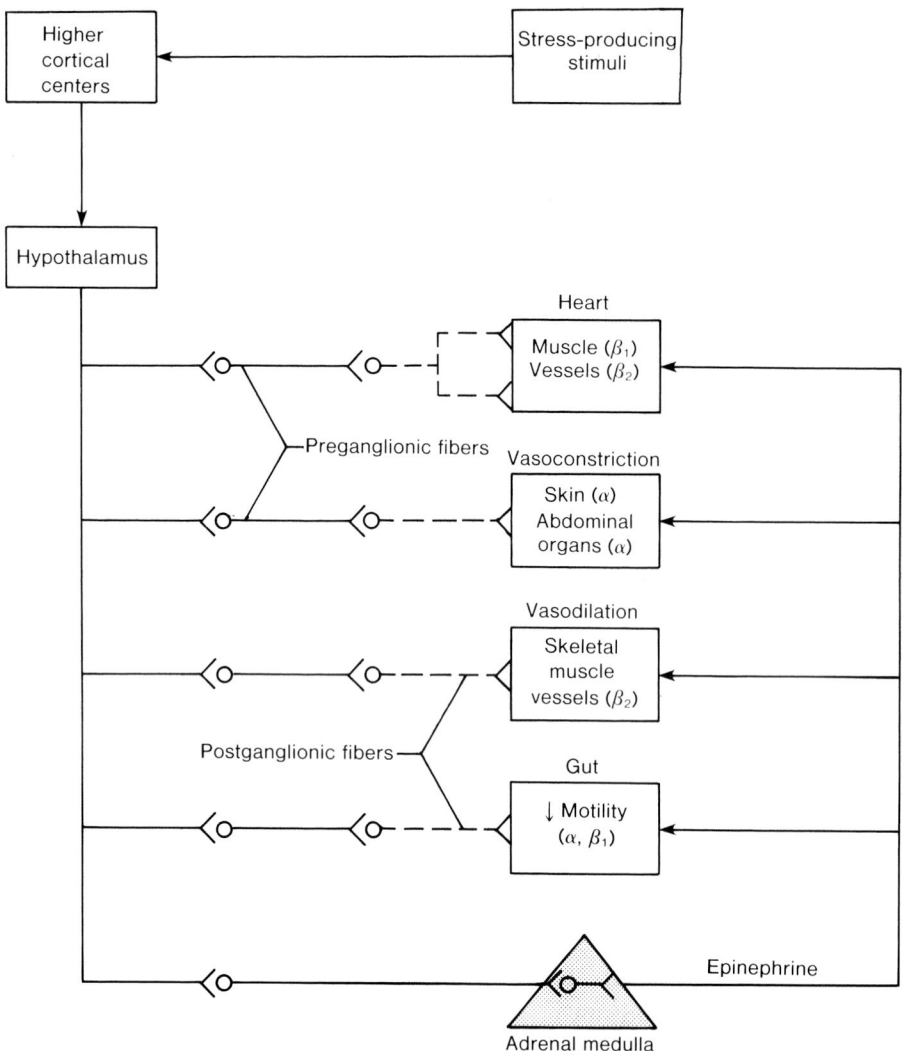

Fig. 15.39 The adrenal medulla and the sympathetic nervous system. The innervated organs react to neural stimulation as indicated. The release of epinephrine complements the neural stimulation.

Pharmacologic Considerations

Introduction. The rational use of autonomic drugs is predicated upon a thorough understanding of the autonomic nervous system and the drugs used. Knowledge of the action, mechanism, metabolism, indications, contraindications and adverse reactions of drugs used on the autonomic nervous system are essential considerations of rational use. This section, however, is not intended to be a comprehensive discussion on autonomic drugs. Rather, it is intended as an introduction to the terminology, actions and mechanisms of some autonomic drugs.

The autonomic drugs are those that act primarily on the ANS and includes those chemicals which mimic, intensify or block the effects of the neurotransmitters of the sympathetic and parasympathetic divisions of the ANS. Autonomic drugs may manifest their mimetic effects by several mechanisms. Some drugs (*congeners*) are sufficiently similar to the neurotransmitter that they are

able to *combine with the receptor site* and elicit the effector response. The similarity between epinephrine, norepinephrine and dopamine is apparent in Figure 12.15. Some drugs may *cause the release of the neurotransmitter* from the telodendria. Other drugs *inhibit the enzyme activity* responsible for the degradation of the neurotransmitter, causing it to accumulate and prolong the effector response.

The blocking effect of certain autonomic drugs can be achieved in several ways. Certain compounds are sufficiently similar to the neurotransmitters that they bind with receptor sites and *competitively inhibit* the normal neurotransmitter-receptor site reaction. Others prevent the synthesis or release of the neurotransmitter substances.

Drugs that act in the manner described are classified into four general categories: parasympathomimetic, parasympatholytic, sympathomimetic, sympatholytic.

Parasympathomimetics. Parasympathomimetic drugs mimic the effects of parasympathetic neuronal stimulation of the effector

organs. Drugs in this category are also called *cholinergic* drugs. They are effective at sites in which ACH is the chemical mediator. Some cholinergic drugs are choline esters which act directly on the postganglionic neurons and the effector organs. They are resistant to hydrolysis by cholinesterase and manifest relatively fewer sympathomimetic actions than the cholinergic alkaloid nicotine. The *cholinomimetics* are effective at ganglionic synapses (parasympathetic and sympathetic), parasympathetic postganglionic neuro-effector junctions and neuromuscular junctions of skeletal muscle.

Choline esters that are functional parasympathomimetic drugs are acetylcholine, methacholine, carbachol and bethanechol. Their similar chemical structures are demonstrated in Figure 15.40. Although acetylcholine is the sterotypic cholinergic drug, the others are sufficiently similar to it to manifest parasympathomimetic effects. These effects may be muscarinic or nicotinic. Muscarinic and nicotinic effects are manifested by acetylcholine and carbachol, the latter is dose-dependent. Methacholine and bethanechol are muscarinic drugs; the CH_3 group on the β-carbon effectively eliminates nicotinic effects. Carbachol is a strong muscarinic used for gastrointestinal atony; bethanechol is used for the stimulation of the gastrointestinal and urinary tract.

Other cholinergic drugs are inhibitors of acetylcholinesterase (ACHase). They bind with the ACHase and reduce the hydrolysis and subsequent inactivation of ACH. Some of the important ACHase inhibitors are physostigmine, neostigmine and the organophosphates. Physostigmine is an important topical agent used in the treatment of glaucoma. Neostigmine is an effective treatment for myasthenia gravis. Organophosphates are used as insecticides and their potential effect upon the body after accidental ingestion should be recognized.

The cholinergic effects of the plant alkaloids, muscarine and nicotine, were discussed previously.

Parasympatholytics. Drugs that block the effects of the parasympathetic nerves are termed *parasympatholytics* or *anticholinergic*. The drugs in this category actually block the muscarinic receptors and are best referred to as *antimuscarinic drugs*. (Some effector organs, sweat glands and some blood vessels in skeletal muscle have muscarinic receptors but are innervated by sympathetic postganglionic cholinergic nerves. Some smooth muscle cells have cholinergic receptors but lack cholinergic innervation.)

Atropine is the typical antimuscarinic drug. The antimuscarinic effects of atropine and similar compounds (scopolamine, glycopyrrolate) are manifested through a competitive inhibition of ACH. Atropine competes with ACH for receptor sites and the effectiveness of this antimuscarinic drug is dependent upon the concentration of ACH and atropine at these sites. The effects of an

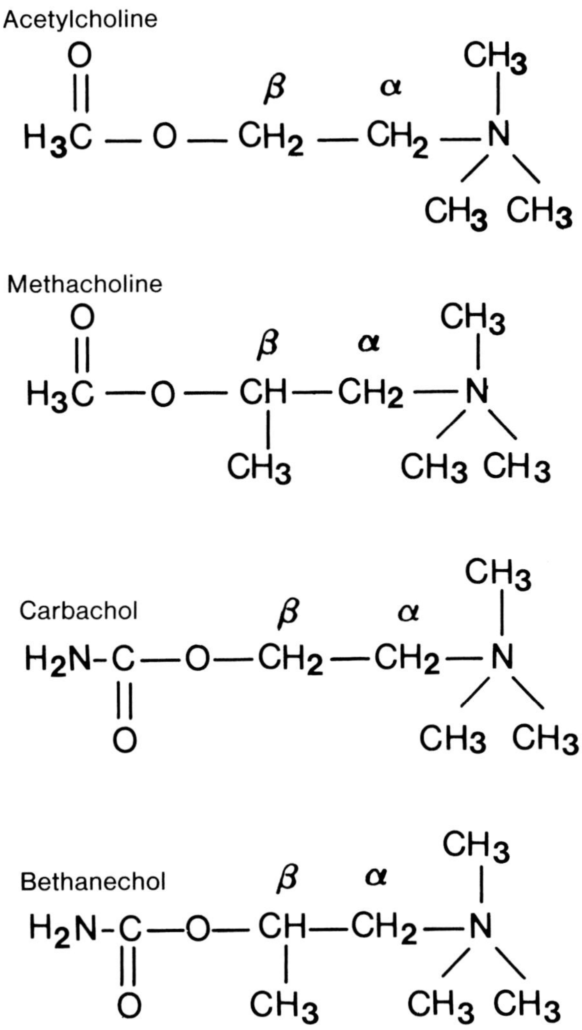

Acetylcholine

Methacholine

Carbachol

Bethanechol

Fig. 15.40 The chemical structure of four cholinergic drugs. Note their similarities and subtle differences.

antimuscarinic drug are expressed generally as sympathetic effects. This points out the significance of a balanced parasympathetic and sympathetic input to establish the tone of an organ.

Sympathomimetics. The catecholamines and other compounds comprise a complex group of drugs that may partially or completely mimic the effects of sympathetic postganglionic nerve discharge. These drugs are called *sympathomimetics* or *adrenergics*. The differential reactivity of tissues to these drugs, remember, has been part of the basis for defining different adrenergic receptors. Accordingly, these drugs are classified on the basis of their ability to affect these receptors.

The α and β *stimulators* include epinephrine and ephedrine. Epinephrine is used effectively for anaphylaxis and cardiac arrest, whereas ephedrine, a noncatecholamine, is a strong vasopressive agent which has good decongestant effects.

An effective, noncatecholamine β_1 and β_2 *stimulator* is isoproterenol. This drug is a more potent β agonist than epinephrine and

norepinephrine. It has instantaneous positive inotropic and chronotropic effects upon the heart, causes vasodilation and bronchodilation.

Selective β_2 *stimulators* were developed primarily for the treatment of bronchial asthma. Salbutamol is an effective β_2 stimulant; it is a bronchodilator which has minimal cardiac side effects.

Sympatholytics. Sympatholytic drugs are also called *antiadrenergics*. All of these drugs generally function as competitive inhibitors of norepinephrine and epinephrine. The α-adrenergic blocking agents include phentolamine, phenoxybenzamine and the ergot alkaloids. Propanolol is an effective β-adrenergic blocking agent.

Neuronal Response to Injury

Introduction. The anatomic and physiologic unity of the neuronal cell body and its processes, as well as the dependency of neuronal processes upon the cell body, are basic precepts of the neuron doctrine. Posttrauma alterations in neuronal processes

and cell bodies demonstrate this unity and dependency.

The high degree of specialization characteristic of neurons is accompanied by the loss of mitotic potential. Among the numerous complexities that relate to neuronal function, and is yet to be explained, is the dynamic interaction that occurs among neurons and between neurons and their effector organs. The death of a neuron results in the irreplaceable loss of that cell and its processes. Neurons or neuronal pools which lose their innervation are subject to *transneuronal degeneration*. Neuroglial cells, especially astrocytes, fill in the space which had been occupied by the neuron or neuronal pools. Neuron-effector organ relationships function in a similar manner. The denervation of a skeletal muscle mass results in its atrophy, which is reversed upon reinnervation. The disruption of an axonal process results in the degeneration of the myelin sheath. Similarly, the loss of the myelin sheath that results from demyelinating disease processes affects the functional integrity of the axis cylinder. The exact trophic relationships and influences between and among these components has not been clarified, but they have an *obligatory symbiotic relationship* (*obligatory symbiosis*).

Neuronal process damage within the PNS results in degenerative and regenerative alterations of the cellular process and may involve the nerve cell body. Neurons within the CNS react similarly to damage; however, the time frame for regeneration is slower than their peripheral counterparts. The changes in neurons in response to injury are referred to as *primary* and *secondary degeneration*.

Response to Injury. The transection of a nerve results in damage proximal and distal to the site of injury (Fig. 15.41). Proximally, this *primary degeneration*, which may include disintegration of the myelin sheath and loss of part of the axis cylinder, extends over a few internodal segments (Fig. 15.41B). The nature of the injury dictates the degree of proximal involvement. The proximal portion of the axon, maintaining its continuity with the nerve cell body, soon begins to undergo regeneration and new branches of the axon (*neurities*) radiate from the stump (Fig. 15.41C).

After the separation of the distal segment from the nerve cell body, complete disintegration of the myelin sheath, axis cylinder and telodendria occurs. This process, *secondary* or *Wallerian degeneration*, is characterized by progressive degenerative changes in the distal segment. The axis cylinder, separated from the trophic influence of the nerve cell body, assumes a beaded appearance, breaks up into irregular fragments and eventually disintegrates. The myelin sheath undergoes similar alterations in association with the fragmented axis cylinder. All of these changes occur within the limits of the endoneurium. The periph-

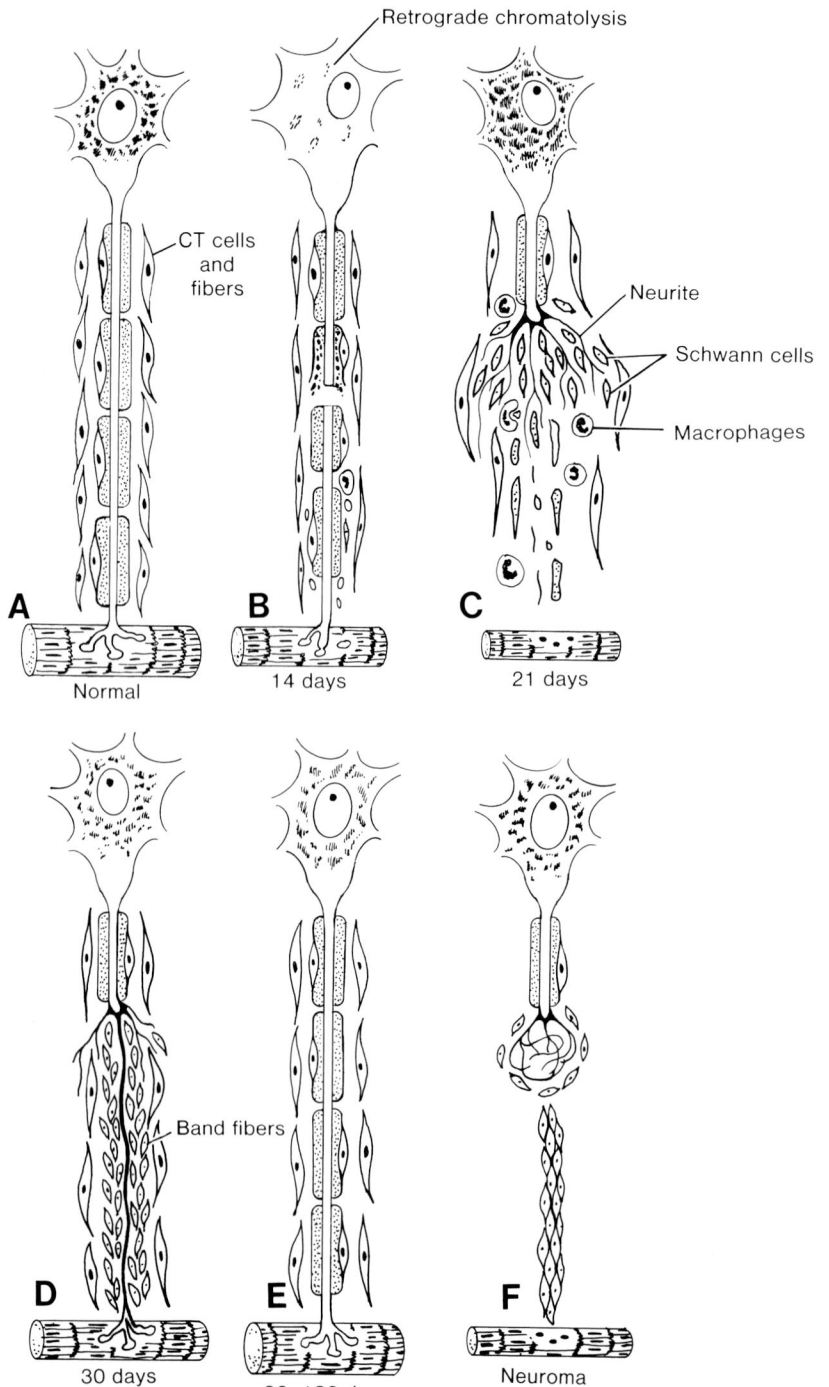

Fig. 15.41 A diagram depicting the degeneration and regeneration of a nerve fiber. A, normal neuromuscular relationship with normal muscle size. B, primary degeneration with muscular atrophy. C, reactive Schwann cells and macrophages are present and neurites have begun to grow. Distal degeneration is apparent. Muscle atrophy is progressing. D, band fibers form a tubular framework for the neurites. E, innervation re-established. Muscle mass restored. F, neuroma formation in the proximal segment. (Redrawn, modified and combined from Junqueira, L. C.: *Basic Histology*, Lange, Los Altos, 1975 and Quarton, G. C., Melnechuk, T. and Schmitt, F. O. (editors): *The Neurosciences*. Rockefeller University Press, New York, 1967).

plasmic bands) along the length of the disintegrated distal segment (Fig. 15.41D). Band fibers are important as a guiding tubular framework for the neurities of the proximal segment into the distal fragment and eventually to the neuron or effector organ. When a neurite establishes contact with the pathway supplied by the band fibers the remaining neurites are lost (Fig. 15.41E).

The changes which occur in the axis cylinder are accompanied by alterations of the cell body. *Retrograde chromatolysis* occurs within the cell body very rapidly (Fig. 15.41B). The significance of chromatolysis was discussed in Chapter 12. Eventually the nerve fiber is restored to its original relationship and regeneration will have been achieved (Fig. 15.41E).

The transection of a nerve may result in the opening of a large gap between the proximal and distal segments or the distal segment may be missing, as would result from an amputation. In either case, the neurites and associated cells may form a large, painful nodule called a *neuroma* (Fig. 15.41F). Neuroma formation is not a problem in the dog but is a significant problem in the horse. Neuromas can be a significant complication of posterior digital neurectomies that may be used as a salvage operation for navicular disease. The folding and suturing of the epineurium over the transected proximal fragment (*epineurial capping*) significantly decreases the occurrence of these neuromas in the horse.

The regeneration of nerve fibers within the CNS occurs at a much slower rate than within the PNS. The absence of band fiber formation from oligodendrogliocytes may account for the slow progression of repair. Peripheral regeneration may occur at a rate of 2–4 mm/day, whereas complete disintegration and phagocytosis of severed distal segments within the CNS may take six months. Importantly, functional regeneration within the CNS probably does not occur.

References

General

Chrisman, C. L. (editor): Symposium on advances in veterinary neurology. Vet. Clin. North Amer. 10:1, 1980.

DeLahunta, A.: *Veterinary Neuroanatomy and Clinical Neurology*. W. B. Saunders, Philadelphia, 1977.

Ettinger, S. J. (editor): *Textbook of Veterinary Internal Medicine: Diseases of the Dog and Cat*. Vol. I. W. B. Saunders, Philadelphia, 1975.

Hoerlein, B. F.,: *Canine Neurology: Diagnosis and Treatment*. 3rd edition, W. B. Saunders, Philadelphia, 1978.

Quarton, G. C., Melnechuk, T. and Schmitt, F. O. (editors): *The Neurosciences*. Rockefeller University Press, New York, 1967.

Peripheral Nervous System

Bradley, W. G.: *Disorders of Peripheral Nerves*. Blackwell, Oxford, 1974.

Cauna, N.: Structure of digital touch corpuscles. Acta Anat. 32:1, 1958.

erally-positioned connective tissue fibers form a cylindrical envelope around the reacting nerve fiber.

During the degenerative process, Schwann cells enlarge and proliferate. Reactive Schwann cells as well as macrophages are responsible for removing cellular detritus and myelin fragments from the area. Schwann cell proliferation results in the formation of *band fibers* (*cellular tubes, proto-*

auna, N. and Mannan, G.: The structure of human digital pacinian corpuscles (corpuscula lamellosa) and its functional significance. J. Anat. *92*:1, 1958.

ernand, V. S. V. and Young, J. Z.: The sizes of the nerve fibers of muscle nerves. Proc. Roy. Soc. (Biol.) *139*:38, 1951.

amble, H. J. and Eames, R. A.: An electron microscope study of the connective tissue of human peripheral nerve. J. Anat. *98*:655, 1964.

riffiths, I. R., Duncan, I. D. and Lawson, D. D.: Avulsion of the brachial plexus. 2. Clinical aspects. J. Small An. Prac. *15*:177, 1974.

rillo, M. A.: Electron microscopy of sympathetic tissues. Pharmacol. Rev. *18*:387, 1966.

ess, A.: The fine structure of young and old spinal ganglia. Anat. Rec. *123*:399, 1955.

ones, L. M., et al.: *Veterinary Pharmacology and Therapeutics.* Iowa State Univ. Press, 4th edition, 1977.

unos, G.: Adrenoceptors. *In:* George, R. et al. (editors): *Annual Review of Pharmacology and Toxicology.* Vol. 18. Annual Reviews, Inc., Palo Alto, 1978.

Kuntz, A.: *The Autonomic Nervous System.* Lea and Febiger, Philadelphia, 1953.

Meyers, F. H.: *Review of Medical Pharmacology.* 5th edition. Lange, Los Altos, 1976.

Ortiz-Picon, J. M.: The neuroglia of the sensory ganglia, Anat. Rec. *121*:513, 1955.

Schanthaveerappa, T. R. and Bourne, G. H.: The "perineural epithelium," a metabolically active, continuous, protoplasmic cell barrier surrounding peripheral nerve fasciculi. J. Anat. *96*:527, 1962.

Spencer, P. J. and Schaumburg, H. H.: Central-peripheral axonopathy. The pathology of dying back polyneuropathies. Prog. Neuropathol. *3*:253, 1977.

Central Nervous System

Barringer, J. R.: A simplified procedure for spinal fluid cytology. Arch. Neurol. *22*:305, 1970.

Elliott, H. C.: Studies on the motor cells of the spinal cord. Amer. J. Anat. *70*:95, 1942.

Globus, E. G. and Scheibel, A. B.: Pattern and field in cortical structure. J. Comp. Neurol. *131*:155, 1967.

Hartley, W. J.: Lower motor neuron disease in dogs. Acta Neuropathol. *2*:334, 1963.

Herndon, R. M.: The fine structure of the Purkinje cell. J. Cell Biol. *18*:167, 1963.

Maxwell, D. S. and Pease, D. C.: Electron microscopy of the choroid plexus. Anat. Rec. *124*:331, 1956.

Palmer, A. C.: Pathogenesis and pathology of the cerebellovestibular syndrome. J. Small An. Pract. *11*:167, 1970.

Weed, L. H.: Meninges and cerebrospinal fluid. J. Anat. *72*:181, 1938.

Wright, J. A.: Evaluation of cerebrospinal fluid in the dog. Vet. Rec. *103*:48, 1978.

Yeo, J. D.: A review of experimental research in spinal cord injury. Paraplegia. *14*:1, 1976.

16: Cardiovascular System

General Characteristics

Form and Function. The cardiovascular system consists of moieties to pump, transport and distribute required elements to the cells and tissues of the soma. These cardiovascular elements include the heart, arteries, veins and capillaries as well as the lymphatic vessels. The heart is a highly muscularized tube the contractions of which supply the force to move the blood through the system. The arteries carry the blood away from the heart to the capillaries. The capillaries mediate the exchange of materials between the vascular bed and the extravascular tissues. The venous system returns the blood to the heart (Fig. 16.1). Lymphatics arise in the tissue space and return extracellular fluid as lymph to the blood vascular system.

Although a basic scheme of organization is common to all these entities, there are modifications and deviations from the basic pattern to permit a diversity of functional adaptations. Of prime consideration in the construction of the walls of these organs are the following factors:

1. Velocity of the blood moving through the vascular channel.
2. The pressure with which blood is being propelled.
3. The volume of the blood being moved.
4. The requirements for pumping, transportation and distribution.

Some of the morphologic factors that must be considered to fulfill the functional aspects mentioned previously are:

1. The size of the lumen of the organ.
2. The thickness of the vessel wall.
3. The resistance and/or elasticity of the vessel wall.
4. The specific function of the organ as reflected in the relationships of mural elements.

A comparison between the anatomic and physiologic features of vascular components is presented in Table 16.1.

The histologic aspects of vessel construction cannot be separated from the hemodynamic role they fulfill. The arterial side of the system carries a low volume of blood under high pressure at a high velocity. The capillary system carries a large volume of blood under an appreciably diminished pressure and velocity. The venous system carries high quantities of blood at very low pressures and velocities.

Mural Organization

Basic Organizational Scheme. Although various patterns in mural morphology are observed to accommodate the pressure-volume relationships, the basic scheme consists of *tunica intima*, *tunica media* and *tunica adventitia* (Figs. 16.2, 16.3).

The *tunica intima* is composed of three distinct subdivisions: *endothelium, subendothelial coat* and *internal elastic membrane* (Figs. 16.2, 16.3, 16.4). The endothelium consists of typical squamous cells which line the lumen of the organ. This cellular layer is a common and consistent feature of all blood vessels and the heart. Typically, the nucleus is prominent and may bulge into the lumen, whereas the marginal cytoplasm is difficult to discern with the light microscope. The cells reside upon a basement membrane which separates the endothelium from the peripheral fibroelastic connective tissue and fibroblasts of the *subendothelial coat*. For the most part, these elements are oriented longitudinally (parallel to the long axis of the vessel). Smooth muscle fibers may be present, as well as cells that normally occupy connective tissue spaces. The *internal elastic membrane* is a condensation of elastic fibers that separates the tunica intima from the tunica media.

The *tunica media* consists of a mixture of smooth muscle cells, collagenous fibers, elastic fibers and fibroblasts (Figs. 16.2, 16.3, 16.5). The smooth muscle cells are arranged in a circular pattern around the lumen. They are in intimate association with collagenous and elastic fibers. *Nervi* and *vasa vasorum*, the nerve and blood supply of the vessels, may be observed within this tunic of large vessels.

At the junction between the tunica media and tunica adventitia, an *external elastic membrane* may be present. It, too, is a condensation of elastic fibers. This membrane demarcates the media from the adventitia. The *tunica adventitia* is formed of this membrane and dense fibroelastic connnective tis-

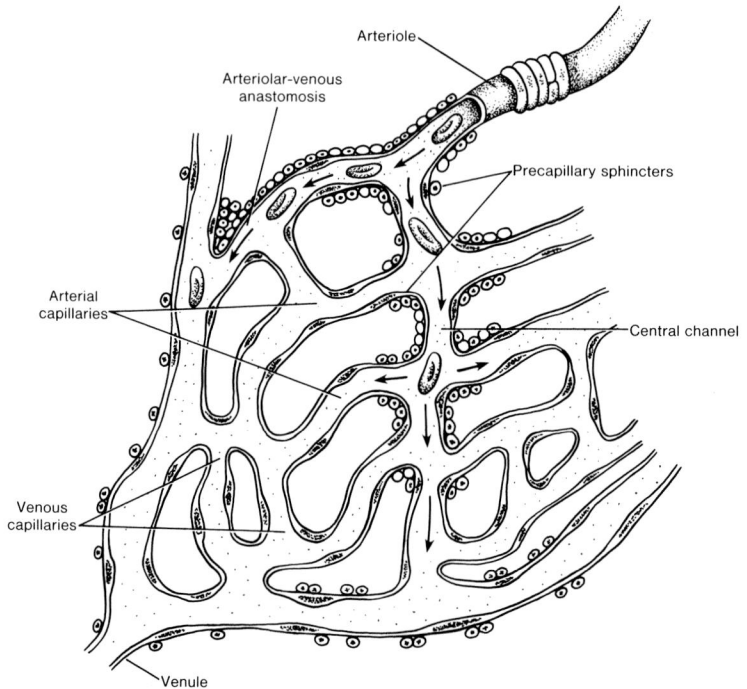

Fig. 16.1 A diagram demonstrating the relationship of capillaries to arterioles and venules. The central channel, surrounded by smooth muscle, has been named the metarteriole. Contraction of the smooth muscle shunts blood through the capillary bed. All light micrographs are labeled as the magnification with the microscope before photographic enlarging. All electron micrographs are labeled as total magnification, including photographic enlarging. (Redrawn and modified from Copenhaver, W. M., Kelly, D. E. and Wood, R. L.: *Bailey's Textbook of Histology*. Williams & Wilkins, Baltimore, 1978.)

Table 16.1
Structural and Functional Features of Vascular Components*

Parameter	Aorta	Artery	Arteriole	Capillary	Venule	Vein	Vena Cava
Luminal diameter	20,000 (2 cm)	4000 (4 mm)	4 (30 μm)	1 (8 μm)	5 (40 μm)	5000 (5 mm)	30,000 (3 cm)
Wall thickness	2,000 (2 mm)	1,000 (1 mm)	20 (20 μm)	1 (1 μm)	2 (2 μm)	500 (0.5 mm)	1500 (1.5 mm)
Ratio-wall thickness to luminal diameter	1:10	1:4	2:3	1:8	1:20	1:10	1:20
Endothelium	+	+	+	+	+	+	+
Elastin	+3	+2	+1	0	0	±†	+1
Internal elastic membrane	+	+	+2	0	0	+1	+
Smooth muscle	+0.8	+1.3	+1.3	0	+1	+1.5	+1.3
Collagen	+2	+1.5		0			+2.5
Cross-sectional area (cm²)	4.5	20	4,000	4,500	4,000	40	18
% of blood‡	2	8	1	5	10	54	
Systolic pressure (mm Hg)	120	115	60	20		8	5
Average velocity (cm/sec)	40	35	18	3	4	5	10

* Modified from Selkurt, E. E.: *Physiology*, 4th edition, Little Brown Co., Boston, 1976 and Ganong, W. F.: *Review of Medical Physiology*. Lange, Los Altos, 1975.
Based upon human data.
† Present in large veins.
‡ Does not include volume in cardiac chambers (12%) and pulmonary circulation (18%)

sue (Figs. 16.2, 16.3, 16.5). Generally, it is difficult to distinguish the end of the adventitia and the beginning of the surrounding connective tissue. Nervi and vasa vasorum ramify in the tunica adventitia.

It is of utmost importance to realize that the aforementioned entities represent generalizations concerning mural structure. Not all vessels will contain all of the aforementioned moieties; nor, if present, will all of them be represented equally in all vessels. However, the endothelium is a constant feature of all vascular components. Distinctions between vessels are made on the basis of the variations of mural elements from the generalized scheme.

Exchange System

Capillaries. *Capillaries* are the simplest members of the vascular system, but their function, by virtue of their simplicity, is extremely important. They are the means by which metabolities gain access to and waste products leave the connective tissue space. Capillaries are simple endothelial-lined tubes with a diameter of 7–9 μm. Due to this size limitation, they are able to accommodate a single red blood cell (RBC) at a time. Peripherally, this tube is covered by a basement membrane (Fig. 16.6).

In section with light microscopy a thin rim of acidophilic cytoplasm delimits the extent of the capillary (Fig. 16.7). The dark nucleus of the endothelial cell occurs along the margin of the lumen and may bulge into the lumen. Capillaries are accompanied along their entire length by connective tissue cells, thin collagenous fibers and reticular fibers. Among the many cells closely associated with them, fixed macrophages, mesenchymal cells and Rouget cells are especially prominent.

All capillaries appear somewhat similar with the light microscope. However, there are two basic types. Capillaries may be *continuous*; i.e., there are no interruptions in the continuity of the endothelial cells (Fig. 16.8). This type occurs typically in muscle, lungs, nervous system and other organs. The second type is *fenestrated*; i.e., pores are scattered throughout the walls of the endothelium (Fig. 16.9). These pores may be covered by a diaphragm or not. Fenestrated (*perforated*) capillaries occur in the endocrine glands, intestines, kidneys and other organs. Whether a capillary is continuous or fenestrated, the associated basal lamina is uninterrupted.

Various cells assume intimate relationships with the endothelial cells of capillaries. They are called *pericapillary cells* (*perivascular cells*) and include *histiocytes*, *fibroblasts*, *mesenchymal cells*, *mast cells* and *Rouget cells*. The histiocytes probably represent fixed macrophages of the connective tissue space, while the fibroblasts are typical components of the connective tissue space juxtaposed intimately to the endothelial

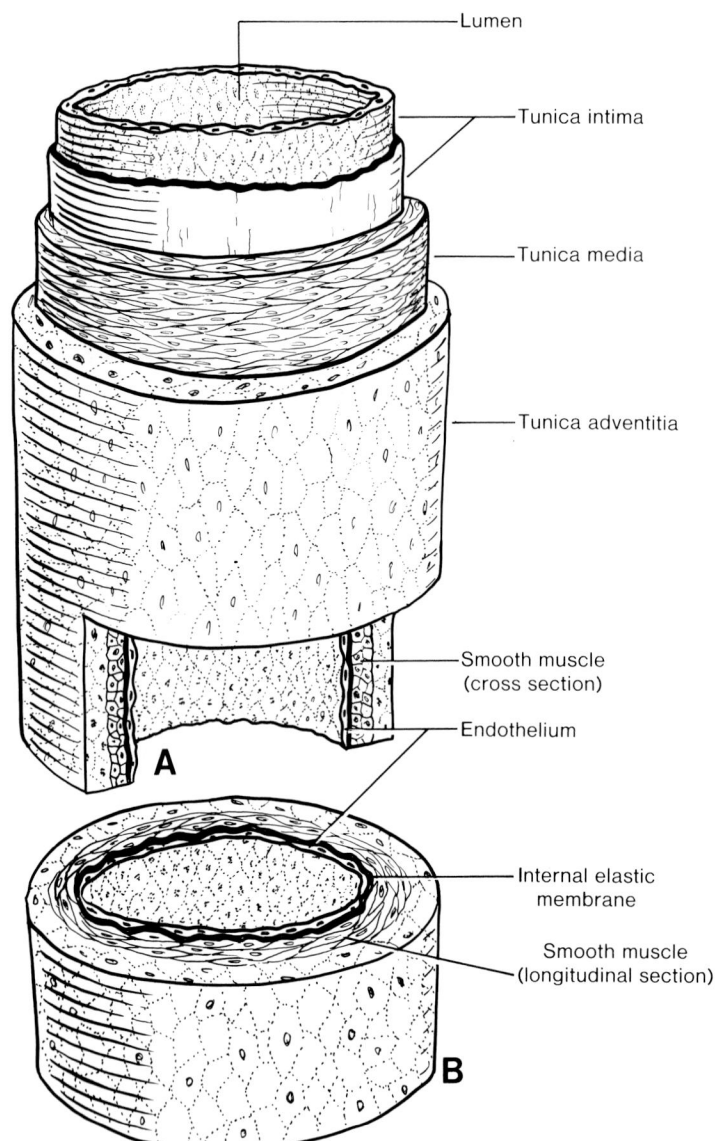

Fig. 16.2 A diagram of the mural organization of an artery. When sectioned longitudinally (A), the smooth muscle of the tunica media is cross-sectioned. When the vessel is cut in cross section (B), the smooth muscle is cut in longitudinal section.

cells. Mesenchymal and mast cells, although scattered throughout the connective tissue space, are especially obvious in pericapillary positions (Figs. 6.22, 6.31). Rouget cells (Figs. 6.29, 6.30) are smooth muscle cells intimately associated with the capillary endothelium. These cells are probably the smooth muscle cells of *metarterioles* and *precapillary sphincters* (Fig. 16.1).

Sinusoids. *Sinusoids* components of the vascular bed which are lined by endothelial or endothelial-like cells (*littoral cells*). They are similar to capillaries but are larger and irregularly shaped. A basal lamina may be present, incomplete or absent. Some of the lining cells are phagocytic, while others are not. (Refer to Fig. 6. 50 for the distribution of phagocytic cells). The phagocytic lining cells, members of the reticuloendothelial system, appreciably broaden the function of

these vascular channels. If the lining cells of the sinusoids are not phagocytic, then these channels may be considered similar to very large capillaries. Sometimes these nonphagocytic sinusoids are referred to as *sinuses*. Various types of sinusoids may be observed, but their identification requires the electron microscope. Three types of sinusoids have been described: *continuous, discontinuous* and *fenestrated. Continuous sinusoids* have a complete basal lamina and may be phagocytic or nonphagocytic. *Discontinuous sinusoids* have either an incomplete or no basal lamina and are phagocytic (Fig. 16.10). *Fenestrated sinusoids* are fenestrated, have a continuous basal lamina and are nonphagocytic. Continuous sinusoids occur in the liver of some species, while discontinuous sinusoids are characteristic of the liver, spleen, and bone marrow of most species.

Fenestrated sinusoids occur in the pituitary gland and adrenal cortex.

The organization of capillaries and sinusoids is simple compared to the previously described general plan. Actually, these structures represent the two innermost regions of the tunica intima, the *endothelium* and *subendothelial coat.* Increased organization and complexity is achieved by peripheral addition to these elements.

High Pressure System

Arterioles. There is a gradual transition from capillaries to arterioles. A *metarteriole* is a branch of an arteriole that has some smooth muscle fibers surrounding it (Fig. 16.1). These vessels function as sphincters and control the amount of blood flowing through the *central* or *thoroughfare channel* which courses through the capillary bed and joins the venous side of the circulation. *Precapillary sphincters* are capillaries with some smooth muscle fibers that control blood flow through the arterial capillaries into the capillary bed proper. The disposition of smooth muscle with metarterioles and capillaries permits the regulation of blood flow through the capillary beds of organs or parts of organs. A capillary bed by-pass may be achieved by arteriolar-venular anastomoses (Fig. 16.1).

Arterioles have a diameter less than 100 μm (Fig. 16.11). The smallest arterioles consist of a tunica intima devoid of a subendothelial coat. The only recognizable elements are the endothelium and thin internal elastic membrane the latter of which appears as a bright scalloped line (Fig. 16.12). The tunica media consists of one to three layers of smooth muscle among which are scattered some fine collagenous fibers and elastic fibers. An external elastic membrane is not present and the loose connective tissue of the tunica adventitia blends insensibly with the surrounding connective tissue.

It is not unusual to observe a scalloped endothelial layer, the individual cells of which appear to protrude into the lumen (Fig. 16.13). This, naturally, is reflected in the internal elastic membrane. It is probably due to excessive contraction of the vessel at the time of fixation. This type of change may be observed in larger vessels of the high-pressure system as well.

Small and Medium-sized Arteries. There is no sharp line of distinction between arterioles and small arteries. Rather, there is a continuum of quantitative change from the smaller to larger vessels.

The small and medium-sized arteries are also referred to as *muscular* or *distributing arteries* (Fig. 16.3). The tunica intima of these vessels is typical and consists of three layers. The tunica media consists of circularly oriented smooth muscle cells among which are scattered some collagenous fibers, reticular fibers, elastic fibers and fibroblasts. An external elastic membrane is often well-

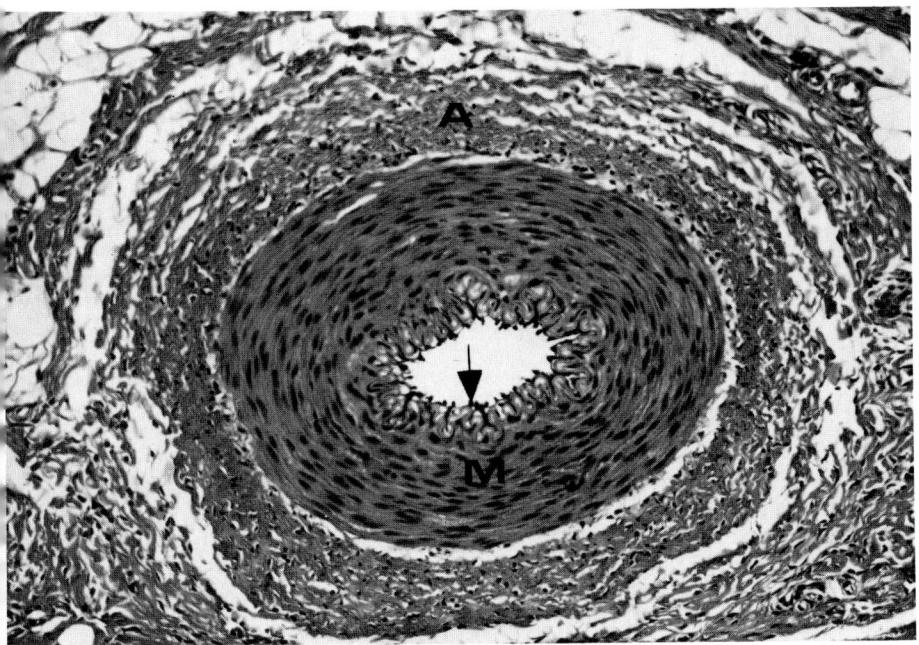

Fig. 16.3 Mural elements of a muscular artery. The three components are tunica intima (*arrow*), tunica media (M) and tunica adventitia (A). X40.

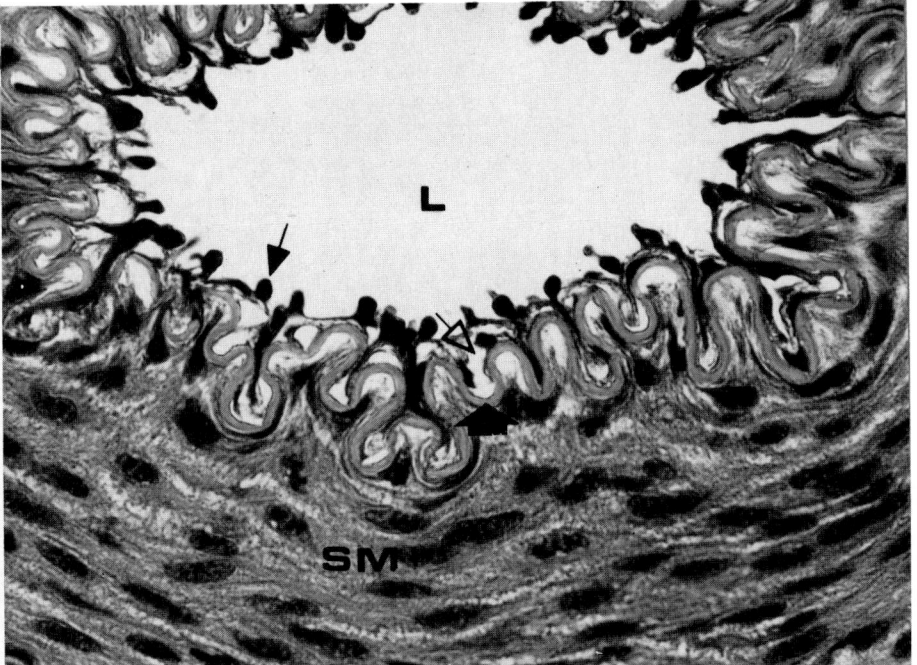

Fig. 16.4 Tunica intima of a muscular artery. The lumen (L) of the vessel is lined by endothelium (*solid arrow*), the cells of which protrude into the lumen. The protrusion results from agonal contractions of the tunica media during sample acquisition. The subendothelial space (*open arrow*) is accentuated by the vascular contraction and is artifact. The internal elastic membrane (*large solid arrow*) is adjacent to the smooth muscle (SM) of the tunica media. X160.

defined, while the tunica adventitia consists of heavy collagenous fibers, some elastic fibers, and vasa and nervi vasorum.

Elastic Arteries. The *elastic arteries* are the largest arteries in the body (Fig. 16.14). Compared to their luminal volume, they have a rather thin wall.

All the elements of the tunica intima are present. The endothelial layer consists of polygonal cells rather than the expected flattened cells. The subendothelial layer consists of collagenous fibers, elastic fibers, fibroblasts and smooth muscle cells in a loose connective tissue. An internal elastic mem-

brane is present; however, it is not always distinct because the tunica media consists of large quantities of elastic fibers that are oriented in such a manner as to be interpreted as repeating elastic membranes. Between the coarse elastic fibers are fine collagenous fibers, fine elastic fibers, fibroblasts and smooth muscle cells. A distinct external elastic membrane is not present. The connective tissue of the tunica adventitia is thin and blends insensibly with the surrounding connective tissue.

Low Pressure System

Venules. The transition from capillaries to venules is a gradual one. *Venous capillaries* attain large diameters (up to 20 times those of capillaries) and gradually become associated with other mural elements. In distinction to arterial capillaries, venous capillaries usually become associated with connective tissue first and later develop smooth muscle within their walls.

Venules usually consist of a simple endothelial tube surrounded by a loose connective tissue (Fig. 16.11). Smooth muscle cell investment occurs as the venules become small veins. The tunica adventitia of these vessels is quite thick compared to the tunica media.

Small and Medium-sized Veins. These vessels are lined by a thin tunica intima which consists of polygonal endothelial cells and a very small subendothelial connective tissue layer (Fig. 16.15). The tunica media is thin and consists of circularly-oriented muscle cells, collagenous fibers and fine elastic fibers. The tunica adventitia is well-developed and comprises the bulk of the wall.

Many of these veins are equipped with *valves* (Fig. 16.16). These are invaginations of the tunica intima into the lumen of the vessel. Valves are lined by flattened endothelial cells and contain a core of subendothelial connective tissue (Fig. 16.17). These intimal modifications are especially prominent in vessels located below the heart.

Large Veins. These vessels represent quantitative changes from the smaller ones. The tunica intima is thicker than observed in smaller veins and an internal elastic membrane may be present. The tunica media consists primarily of collagenous and elastic fibers, while the smooth muscle component is reduced or even absent. The tunica adventitia is well-developed and is the thickest part of the wall. Scattered bundles of smooth muscle may be present within this coat and oriented parallel to the long axis of the vessel. Valves are absent in the venae cavae and the hepatic portal vein.

High and Low Pressure Systems Compared

As their high-pressure counterparts, the mural organization of veins is quite variable. However, these vessels occur as companion

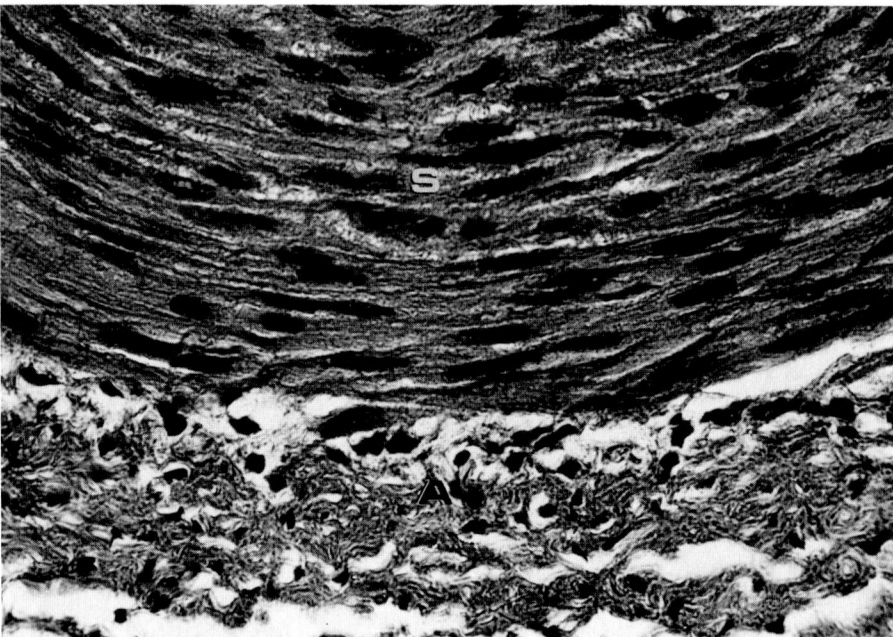

Fig. 16.5 Tunica media and tunica adventitia of a muscular artery. The tunica media contains smooth muscle cells, whereas the tunica adventitia (A) consists of fibroelastic connective tissue. X160.

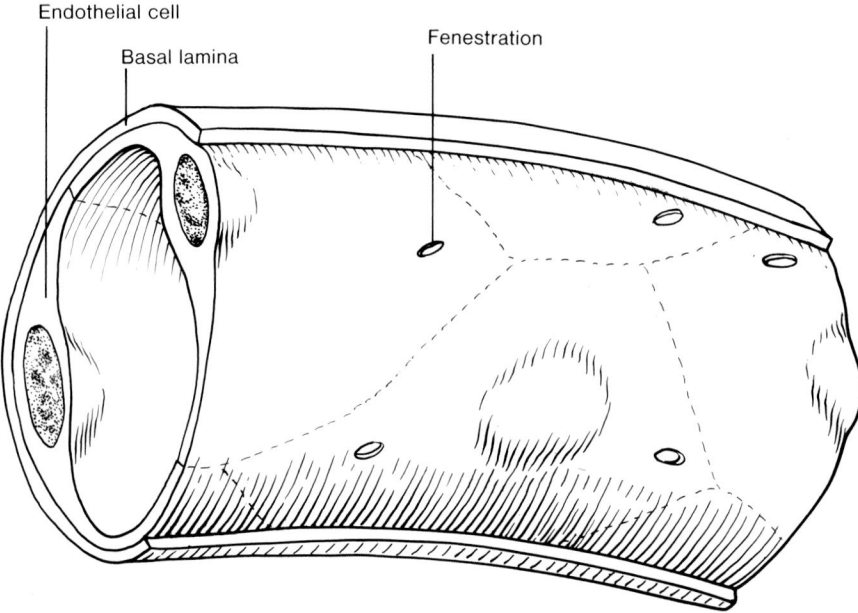

Fig. 16.6 A diagram of a fenestrated capillary. The basal lamina completely covers the abluminal surface of the endothelium.

vessels and comparisons are made easily. Generally, the mural elements of a vein of a given size, when compared with the companion artery, are less distinct. The following distinctions will assist in distinguishing these entities from one another in section:

1. Blood is rarely found in sectioned arteries, but it is typically present in veins.
2. The tunica media is well-developed in arteries, whereas the tunica adventitia is well-developed in veins.
3. Luminal diameters are greater than mural thicknesses in veins, while luminal diameters of arteries are smaller than mural thicknesses.

4. During agonal changes, veins are subject to irregular contractions, while arteries contract more regularly.
5. Internal elastic membranes may be present in arterioles, but these are usually confined to large veins.
6. The tunica adventitia of veins is usually the thickest coat of the wall.

Heart

The heart of endotherms (mammals and birds) consists of four separate chambers: two *atria* and two *ventricles*. The heart is a thick-walled, highly muscularized tube which propels the blood through the body. Two distinct, yet interconnected, circulatory patterns are apparent. Venous blood low in oxygen is returned to the *right atrium* whence it passes through the *right atrioventricular valve* (*tricuspid valve*) into the *right ventricle*. Upon contraction, blood is propelled through the *semilunar valve* of the *pulmonary artery* and carried to the lungs where it is oxygenated. Oxygenated blood returns to the *left atrium* via the *pulmonary vein*. Upon passing through the *left atrioventricular valve* (*bicuspid valve*) into the *left ventricle*, it is propelled through the *semilunar valve* of the *aorta* for distribution throughout the soma.

The mural elements of the heart are organized in a manner similar to the peripheral vessels. The heart consists of three coats: an inner coat, *endocardium*; a middle coat, *myocardium*; an outer coat, *epicardium* (Fig. 16.18).

Endocardium. The endocardium is the cardiac counterpart of the tunica intima. The endocardium consists of: *endothelium* and a *subendothelial coat*. Deep to this there is a *subendocardial coat* (Fig. 16.19). The endothelium consists of polygonal cells that reside on a basement membrane. This lining is continuous with the endothelial lining of the peripheral vessels. The *subendothelial coat* consists of fine collagenous and elastic fibers. This coat is continuous with a deeper or more peripheral *subendocardial coat* of loose connective tissue. It contains collagenous and elastic fibers, adipose cells, smooth muscle fibers, blood vessels, nerves and, in the ventricles, Purkinje fibers. Besides attaching the endocardium to the myocardium, this coat also contains the impulse conducting system of the heart (Purkinje fibers) in the ventricles.

Myocardium. The *myocardium* is comparable to the tunica media (Fig. 16.20). It consists, primarily, of cardiac muscle. Connective tissue fibers, nerves and blood vessels are also present (Chapter 11).

Epicardium. The *epicardium* is functionally similar to the tunica adventitia (Fig. 16.21). However, the epicardium is actually a serous membrane—the *visceral pericardium* of gross anatomy. The mesothelial lining resides upon a thin layer of loose connective tissue. It is continuous with a loose connective tissue layer that contains variable deposits of adipose tissue, blood vessels and nerves—the *subepicardial coat*.

Cardiac Skeleton. The cardiac muscle and valves are supported by a skeleton of dense white fibrous connective tissue (DWFCT). Some components of this skeleton may also be cartilaginous or osseous. The following elements comprise the cardiac skeleton:

1. Four fibrous rings (*annuli fibrosi*).
2. A fibrous triangle (*trigonum fibrosum*).
3. A fibrous and membranous septum (*septum membranaceum*).

The *annuli fibrosi* are dense white fibrous connective tissue rings that surround the *semilunar valves* of the pulmonary artery and aorta and the two atrioventricular valves. These rings are continuous, directly or indirectly, with the *trigonum fibrosum.* This is a mass of DWFCT between the atrioventricular canals. Similarly, it is continuous with the DWFCT of the interventricular septum—the *septum membranaceum.* These skeletal elements serve as points of attachment for the cardiac muscle mass.

Cartilage and/or bone may occur in the fibrous rings. In the ox, especially, ossification of the fibrous ring associated with the semilunar valve of the aorta is common, resulting in the formation of an *os cordis.*

Cardiac Valves. The cardiac valves are invaginations of the endocardium into the lumen of the heart (Fig. 16.22). The connective tissue of the annuli fibrosi is continuous as a supportive core in the valves between the two layers of endocardium. The connective tissue of the atrioventricular valves is continuous with the collagenous fibers of the tendinous cords (*chordae tendineae*) which are attached to the ventricular surfaces of the valves. Naturally, a thin layer of endocardium is reflected over these tendinous cords and is continuous with the endocardium of the papillary muscles. Elastic fibers are more numerous on the side of the valve facing the back pressure.

The semilunar valves are similar to the atrioventricular valves. A dense nodule of collagen or cartilage may be present on the edge of the three cusps. This is referred to as the *nodule of Arantius.*

Cardiac Conduction System. The myocardial muscle mass is modified uniquely for contractile and conducting functions. Despite the ability of cardiac muscle cells to generate and conduct impulses throughout the myocardial mass, a specialized impulse-generating and impulse-conducting system has been developed that insures the proper origination of impulses and the subsequent proper sequencing of atrial and ventricular contractions. The generating and conducting system consists of the sinoatrial node, atrioventricular node and the atrioventricular bundle (Fig. 16.23). Purkinje fibers are the histologic components of this system.

The *sinoatrial node* (*SA node*) is positioned within the wall of the right atrium at the point of confluence with the major vessels which enter the right atrium. The SA node contains Purkinje fibers which are described as *pacemaker cells.* Their spontaneous depolarization establishes the rate at which the myocardial mass depolarizes and contracts. The wave of depolarization and subsequent contraction spreads radially throughout the atrial myocardial mass and is eventually conducted to the *atrioventricular node* (*AV node*). The AV node consists of an interwoven mass of Purkinje cells located in the septal wall between the atria close to the orifice of the coronary sinus and the septal cusp of the right atrioventricular valve. This ill-defined mass of Purkinje fibers and connective tissue converges as the *atrioventricular bundle* (*bundle of His*) close to the ventricles. The atrioventricular bundle courses craniad and ventrad through the trigonum fibrosum and extends into the septum membranaceum where it divides into the *right* and *left bundle branches.* The more distinct right bundle branch courses along the interventricular septum of the right ventricle in the subendocardial coat and eventually ramifies in the myocardial mass and papillary muscles of this chamber (Fig. 16.24). The left bundle branch follows a similar course and position in the left ven-

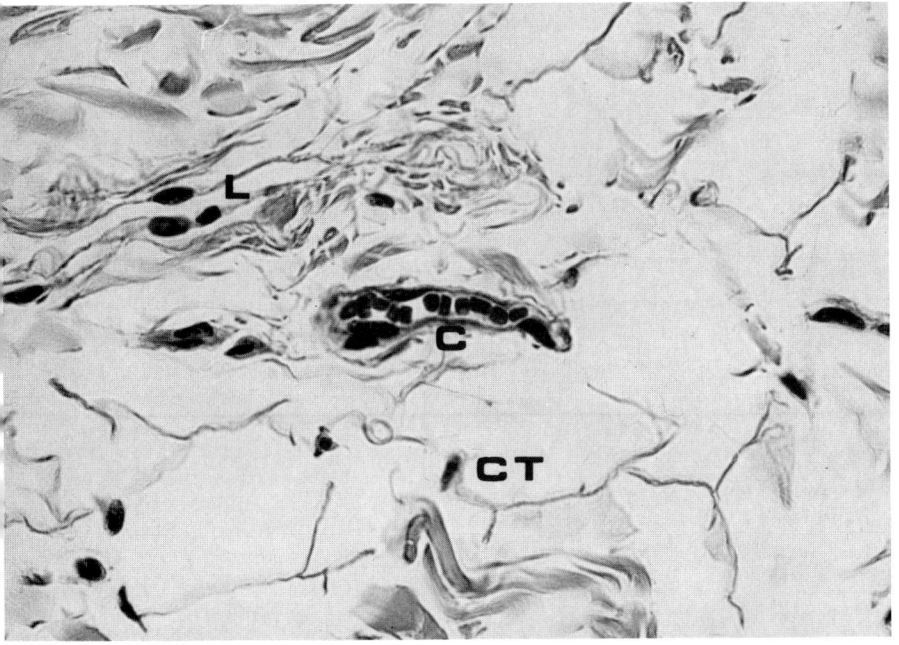

Fig. 16.7 Capillaries in loose connective tissue. The connective tissue (CT) contains a blood capillary (C) and a lymphatic capillary (L). X160.

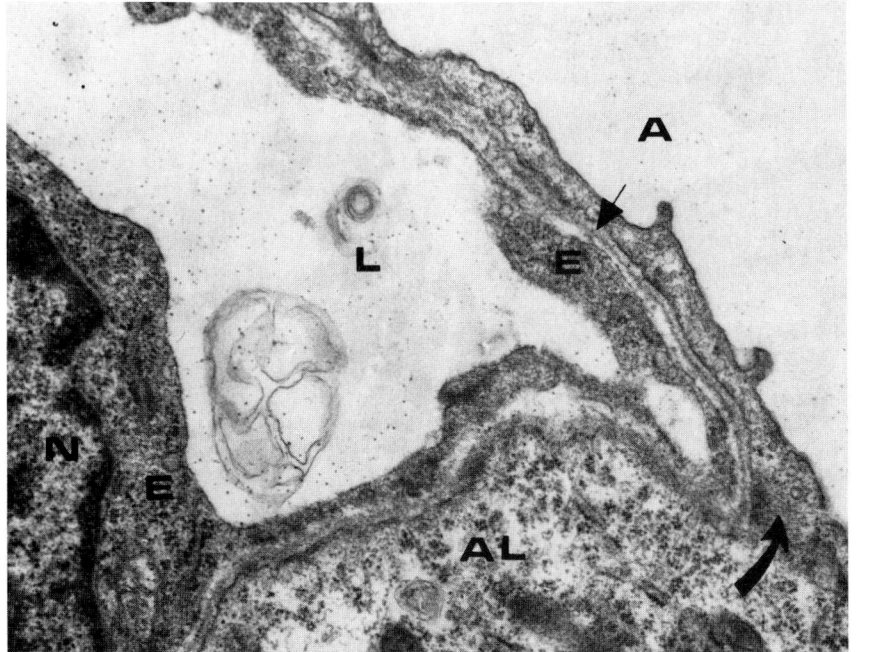

Fig. 16.8 An electron micrograph of a continuous capillary from a bovine lung. The alveolus (A) is defined by the perikaryon of the alveolar lining cell (AL) and the attenuated cellular process of the lining cell (*curved arrow*). The lumen of the capillary (L) is delimited by the endothelial cell (E) and its nucleus (N). The basal lamina (*small arrow*) is complete and the endothelial lining is continuous. X20,000.

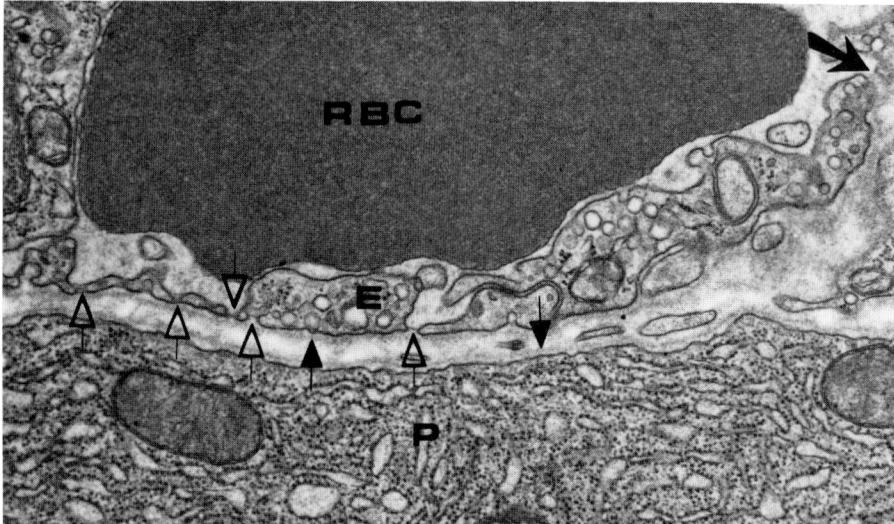

Fig. 16.9 An electron micrograph of a discontinuous capillary. The endothelium (E) of the capillary is separated from a pancreatic acinar cell (P) by two basal laminae (*small solid arrows*). The capillary contains a *RBC*. Numerous fenestrations (*open arrows*) are covered by diaphragms, while one fenestration (*large solid arrow*) is not. X25,000.

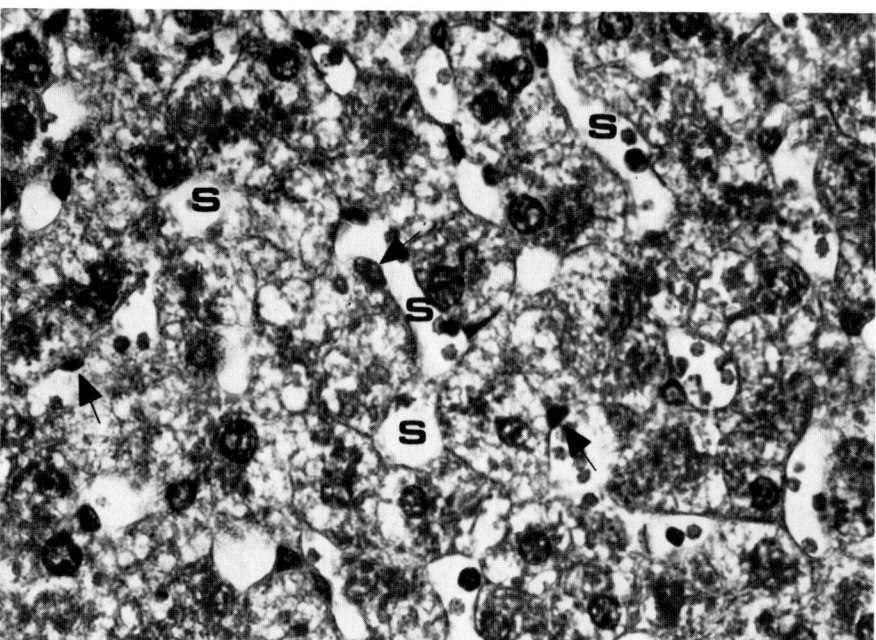

Fig. 16.10 Discontinuous sinusoids of the liver. The sinusoids (S) are lined by some phagocytic cells (*arrows*). X160.

tricle; however, it is more diffuse along its course to the outer left ventricular wall than is the right bundle branch.

The impulse originating and conducting system affords a number of advantages to the myocardial mass. The cells of the SA node, because of their relatively more rapid rate of depolarization and repolarization, assume a pacemaker function which normally precludes *ectopic foci* from assuming that role. The initial spread of excitation over the atrial musculature permits the contraction of this musculature to fill the ventricles. The AV nodal delay facilitates max-imal ventricular filling before the initiation of contraction. The atrioventricular bundles speed the impulses toward the apex and permit the wave of contraction to proceed from the apex back to the base of the heart. This sequence of contraction represents an efficient means of ejecting blood from the ventricles into the pulmonary and aortic circulations.

Cardiac Blood Vessels, Lymphatic Vessels and Nerves. The heart is richly vascularized through its coronary arteries. These vessels originate from the aortic arch immediately distal to the aortic valve. The extensive cap-illary network throughout the myocardial mass is an obvious feature of the histology of this organ.

Lymphatic vessels are present in the three coats of the heart. Numerous nerve fibers from the autonomic nervous system inner-vate the myocardial mass, nodes and smooth muscle of the coronary vessels. This inner-vation is discussed subsequently.

Regulation of Cardiac Activity

Introduction. Because the cardiovascular system is a significant contributor to home-ostasis, its activity is the object of autonomic regulation. The regulation of this system is complex and is subject to the influence of numerous factors, which include myogenic, neurogenic, humoral, chemical, metabolic, barometric and volumetric influences. Car-diovascular regulation is the sum of the regulation of the peripheral circulation and the heart. Although the regulation of each component affects the other, cardiac regu-lation is emphasized.

The essence of cardiovascular regulation is to insure an adequate amount of blood to the tissues of the body, *tissue perfusion* (Fig. 16.25). Proper tissue perfusion is dependent upon an adequate volume of blood being presented to the capillaries under appropri-ate pressure (Chapter 6, Tissue Fluid Dy-namics). Tissue perfusion is affected by nu-merous and varied influences upon the heart and peripheral vessels.

The *myogenic* influence upon the heart stems from the automaticity of the pace-maker cells. *Neurogenic* influences from the sympathetic or parasympathetic nerves can increase or decrease the rate of depolariza-tion of the cells of the sinoatrial node. Epi-nephrine from the adrenal medulla exerts an *hormonal influence* upon the α and β receptors of the cardiovascular system. A *chemical influence* is exerted by special re-ceptors which are sensitive to P_{CO_2}, P_{O_2} and pH. Appropriate stimulation of these recep-tors initiates neurogenic cardiac regulation. Pressure receptors are sensitive to alterations in blood pressure. This *barometric influence* is manifested also as neurogenic cardiac reg-ulation. The heart is capable also of ejecting a given stroke volume against an increased aortic pressure (*homeometric autoregula-tion*). *Volumetric influences* are manifested as an integral part of regulation, because the heart tends to eject whatever is returned to it. This stroke volume-diastolic filling rela-tionship constitutes *Starling's law of the heart* and is dependent upon changes in myocardial fiber length (*heterometric auto-regulation*). *Pain* may have a stimulatory or inhibitory effect upon cardiac activity. A transient tachycardia is associated with in-spiration. Added to the above are numerous local autoregulatory mechanisms that affect tissue perfusion. These include the kinins, lactate, histamine, carbon dioxide and oxy-gen.

Specialized Chemoreceptors. The *carotid bodies* and *aortic bodies* are specialized chemoreceptors which, through their responsiveness to blood levels or partial pressures (P) of carbon dioxide (P_{CO_2}) and oxygen (P_{O_2}), exert a significant influence upon the cardiovascular and respiratory systems.

The *carotid bodies* are small nodules of cell which are positioned in association with the common carotid artery. They are highly vascularized structures that consist of parenchymal cells enclosed by a capsule of connective tissue. The epitheloid cells are divisible into two distinct groups. *Type I cells* (*glomus cells*) are large, contain a round nucleus and are usually clumped together in small groups. Numerous nerve fibers ramify throughout the carotid bodies and terminate on Type I cells. The glomus cells are surrounded by Type II cells (*sustentacular cells*) which are believed to serve a supporting role. Although the Type I cell is believed to be the receptor cell which is responsive to P_{CO_2} and P_{O_2}, the precise mechanism by which it functions has not been determined. These cells have ultrastructural features of sensory and effector (secretory) cells, and their innervation appears to be both afferent and efferent. During periods of normal P_{O_2} and P_{CO_2}, the Type I cells apparently secrete dopamine and the afferent terminals (dendritic zones) associated with them discharge spontaneously. This discharge has a negative feedback control on centers located within the brain stem. During periods of low P_{O_2} and elevated P_{CO_2}, the spontaneous discharge of afferent terminals decreases, resulting in a release of central inhibition, and efferent terminals (telodendria) become active. The carotid bodies are innervated by GVA and GVE fibers from the glossopharyngeal nerve.

The *aortic bodies* are structures similar to the carotid bodies. Generally, the right aortic body is located at the junction of the right common carotid and right subclavian arteries, whereas the left aortic body is positioned at the origin of the left subclavian from the aorta. Although these structures have not been studied as extensively as the carotid bodies, they probably function in a similar manner. The bodies are innervated by fibers from the vagus nerve.

Specialized Baroreceptors. The *carotid sinus* and *aortic sinus* are specialized receptor areas that are responsive to alterations in blood pressure. The carotid sinus is a dilation of the internal carotid artery as it originates from the common carotid artery. The tunica media of the carotid sinus has fewer smooth muscle fibers and more elastic and collagenous fibers than adjacent portions of the artery. Numerous afferent terminals from the glossopharyngeal nerve ramify in the tunica adventitia of this structure. The vagus nerve innervates the aortic sinus. These receptors, which are responsive to the stretch imposed by the blood pressure upon the wall, cause a stimulation of central control centers that results in a reflex bradycardia, dilation of splanchnic vessels and a fall in systemic blood pressure.

Neuroregulation

Central Components and Afferent Input. The hypothalamic nuclei serve as the central integration centers for autonomic function (Fig. 15.33). The regulatory influence of the hypothalamus upon the cardiovascular system is mediated through various "autonomic nerve centers" that include the vasomotor centers, motor nuclei of cranial nerves and the lateral gray column of the thoracic and lumbar spinal cord. The control of this system by the hypothalamus is manifested as a basic level of normal activity or tone which is altered in response to varied types of afferent input. The diverse afferent input

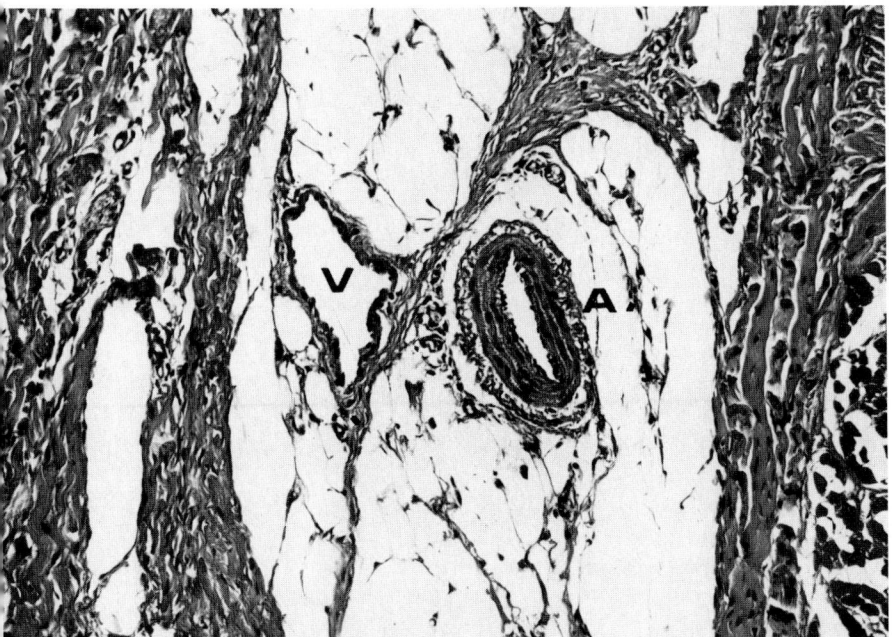

Fig. 16.11   An arteriole and companion venule. The arteriole (A) has three layers of smooth muscle in the tunica media. The companion venule (V) does not contain smooth muscle. X40.

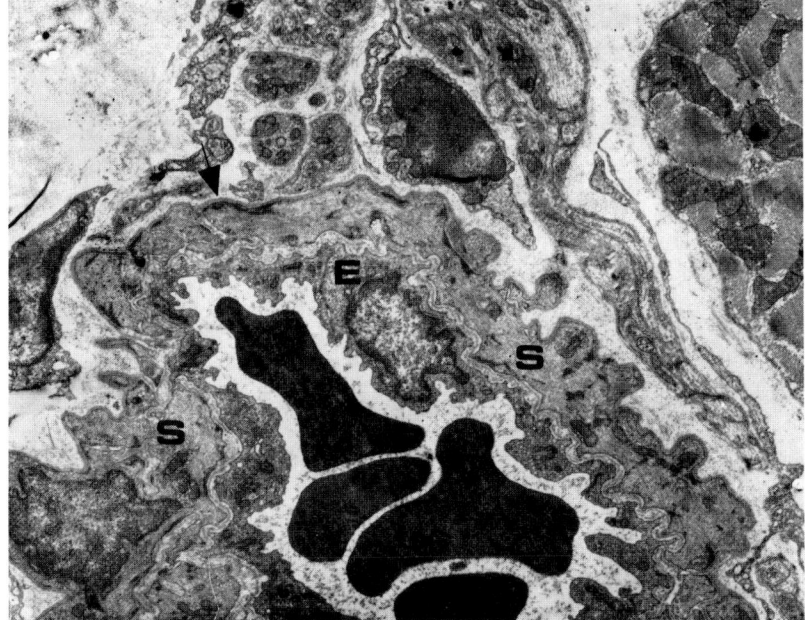

Fig. 16.12   An electron micrograph of an arteriole. The smooth muscle (S) surrounds the endothelial cell (E). A basal lamina (*arrow*) is apparent at the peripheral border of the smooth muscle cell. X14,000. (Courtesy of G. P. Epling).

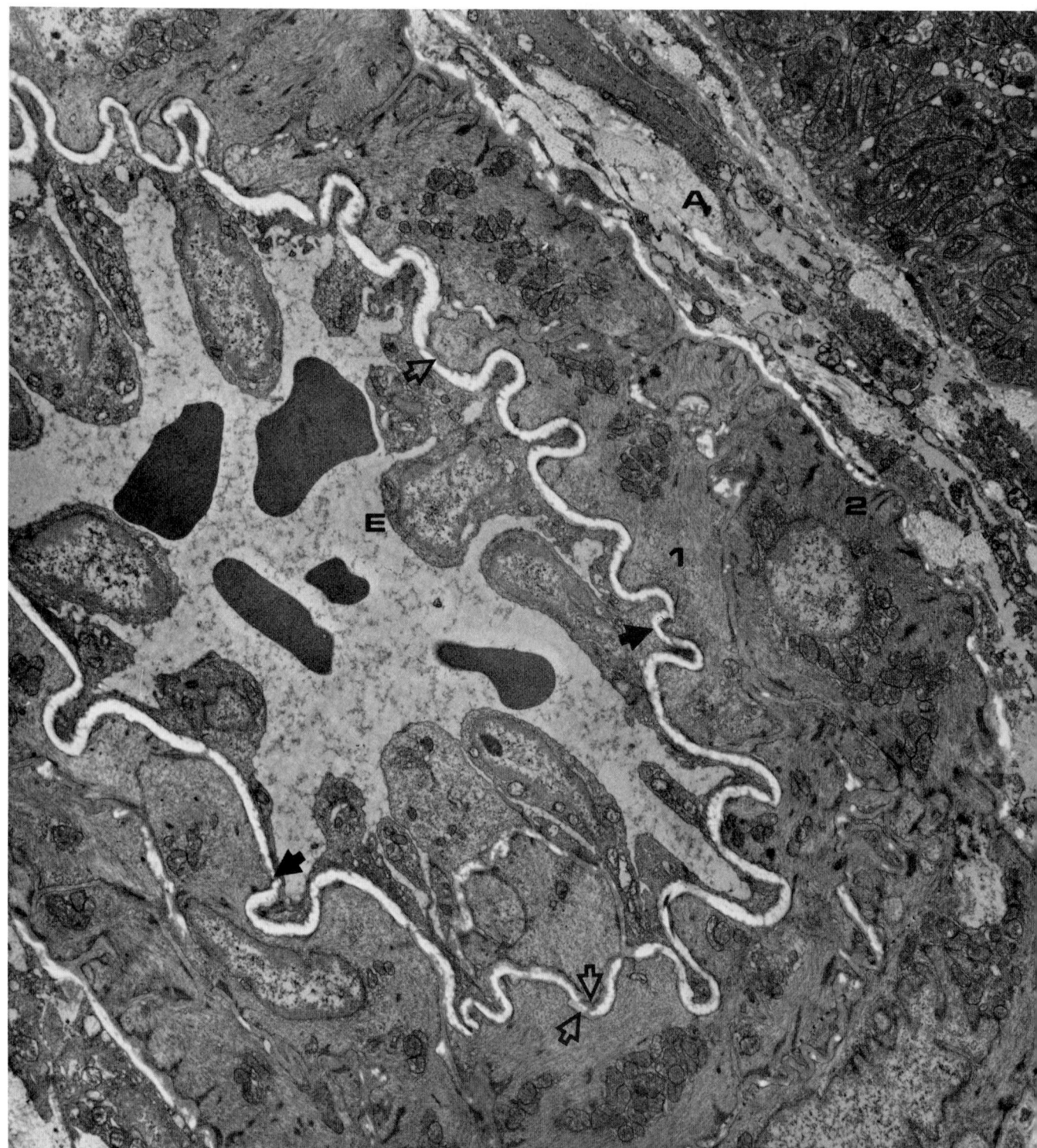

Fig. 16.13 An electron micrograph of an arteriole with a scalloped endothelial border. The contraction of the vessel has caused the protrusion of the endothelial perikaryons into the lumen of the vessel (E). The internal elastic membrane is folded for the same reason (*solid arrows*). Two smooth muscle cells (1,2) comprise the tunica media. Portions of the basal lamina are apparent on the luminal and abluminal surface of the internal elastic membrane (*open arrows*). Elastic fibers, collagen and fibroblasts are apparent in the adventitial connective tissue (A).

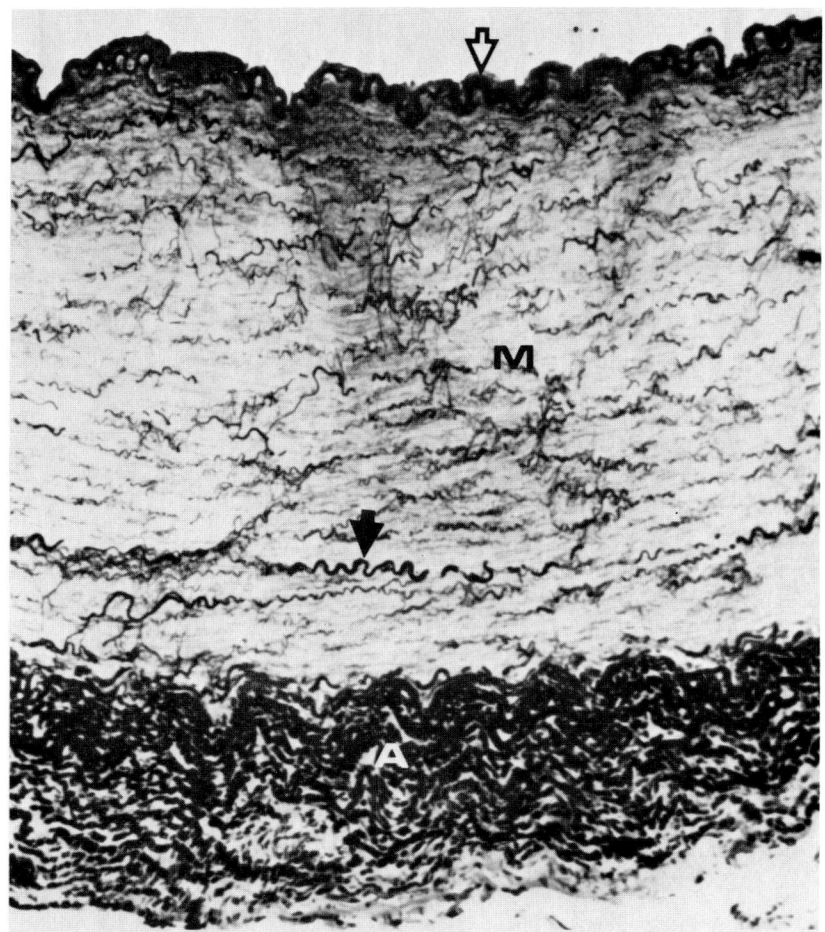

Fig. 16.14 An elastic artery. The section of aorta is stained for elastic fibers. The tunica intima contains a well-defined internal elastic membrane (*open arrow*). The tunica media (M) consists of smooth muscle (not stained) and elastic fibers (*solid arrow*). The tunica adventitia (A) has numerous elastic fibers also. X25 (orcein stain).

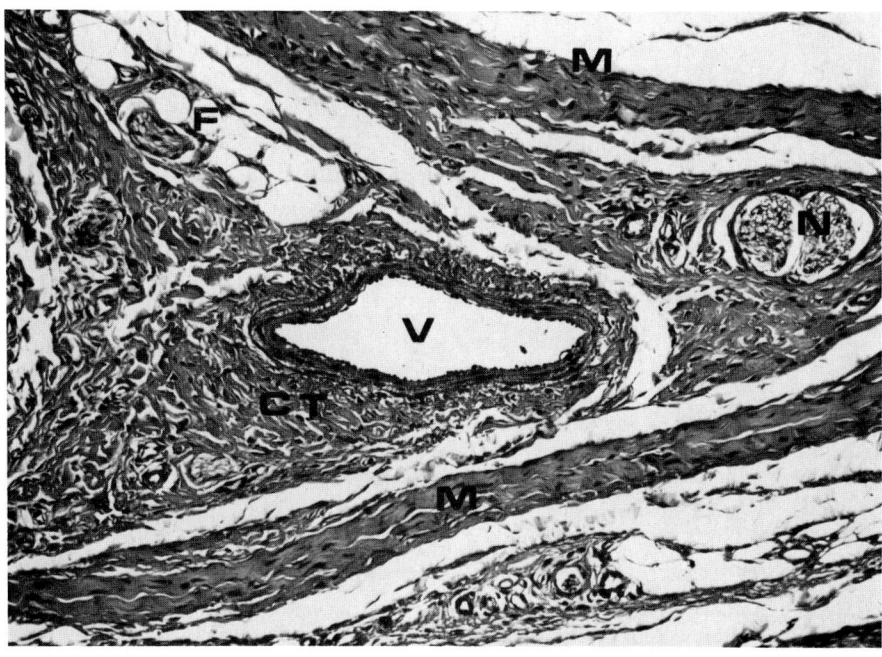

Fig. 16.15 A small vein. The small vein (V) is surrounded by connective tissue (CT). Adipocytes (F), nerves (N) and skeletal muscle (M) are present also. X40.

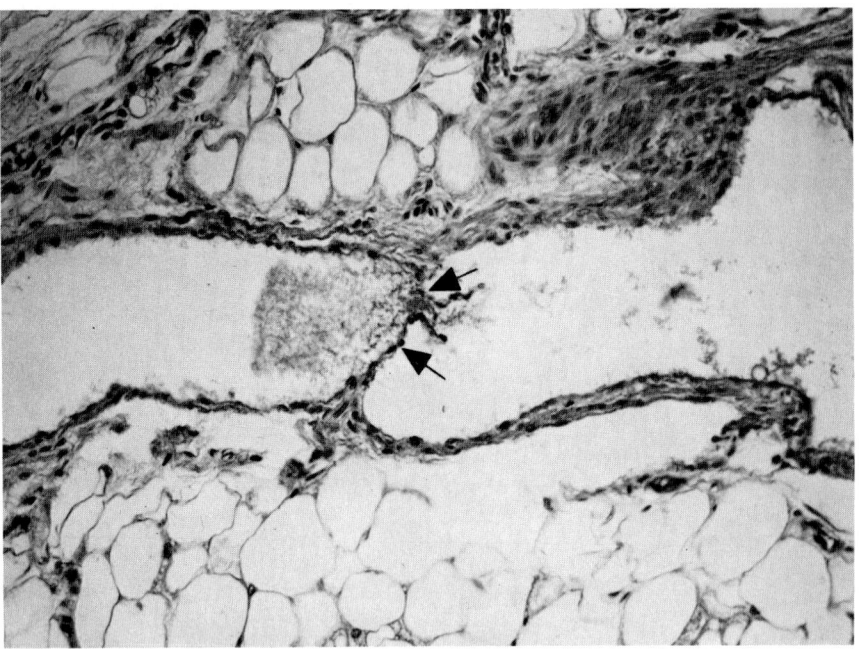

Fig. 16.16 A valve in a vein. The cusps (*arrows*) are modifications of the tunica intima that prevent the reversal of blood flow. X50.

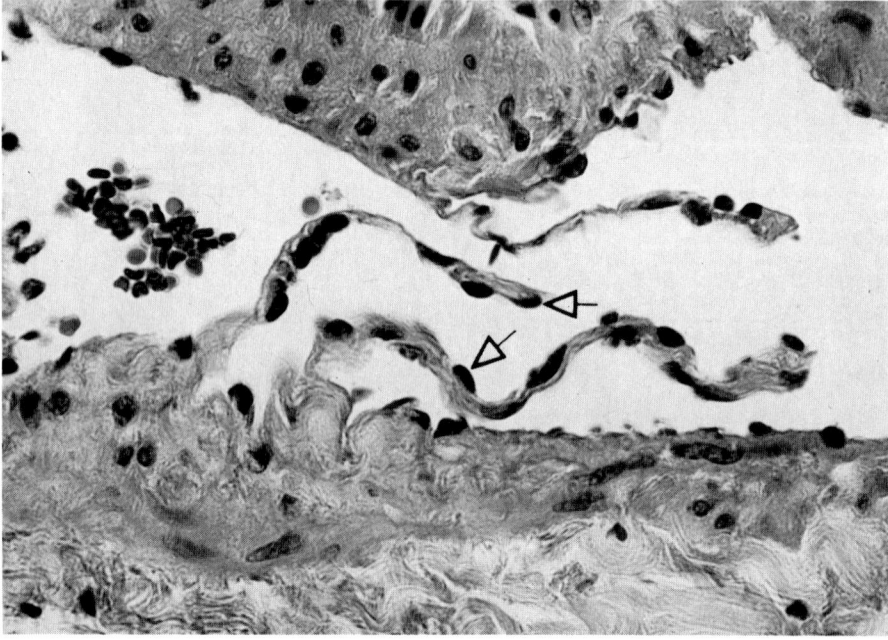

Fig. 16.17 Components of a valve. The cusps are composed of endothelial cells (*arrows*) which surround a core of subendothelial connective tissue. X160.

the peripheral components of the regulatory system. The sympathetic fibers originate as preganglionic fibers in the lateral gray column of thoracic segments one through five. Postganglionic fibers of these nerves, the cell bodies of which are located chiefly in the stellate ganglion, are distributed to the heart and coronary vessels. *Cardiac accelerator nerve fibers* are distributed to the SA node, AV node and ventricular myocardium. *Vasomotor nerves* innervate the smooth muscle of the coronary vessels.

The vagus nerve is the parasympathetic nerve concerned directly with the innervation of the heart. Preganglionic fibers originate in the dorsal motor nucleus of the vagus nerve. The fibers of the vagus nerve join the sympathetic trunk (*vagosympathetic trunk*), enter the thoracic inlet and emerge from the caudal cervical ganglion as the right and left vagal nerves along the lateral margins of the trachea. Preganglionic vagal fibers are distributed to the SA node, AV node, atrioventricular bundle and atrial musculature. The right vagus predominately innervates the SA node, while the left vagus is distributed predominately to the AV node. Numerous intramural ganglia are located within the epicardium.

Physiologic Correlates. The dual innervation of the myocardium provides an effective and precise means for the regulation of cardiac activity. Cardiac activity is determined by the balance exerted between the inhibitory cholinergic nerves of the vagus and the stimulatory adrenergic fibers of sympathetic nerves.

The stimulation of the heart by the sympathetic nerves results in a *positive chronotropy* (increased heart rate), a *positive inotropy* (increased strength of contraction) and a *positive dromotropy* (increased velocity of conduction). An increased vagal tone results in negative chronotropy, negative inotropy and negative dromotropy.

The heart rate of a resting animal is primarily under the inhibitory influence of the vagus nerve that exerts a braking effect upon the resting heart rate. Bilateral vagotomy or the use of antimuscarinic drugs results in tachycardia. Massive vagal stimulation or the use of muscarinic drugs can reduce the heart rate (bradycardia) to the point of sinus arrest. Sympathectomy or the use of β_1 blocking agents results in bradycardia, whereas sympathetic stimulation or the administration of β-stimulators results in tachycardia. The chronotropic effects upon the heart are mediated through an alteration of the depolarization rate of nodal tissue (Fig. 16.27). A change in the slope of the prepotential determines the rapidity of nodal firing.

The inotropic effect of these nerves upon the heart is not equivalent. Although the sympathetic nerves exert a marked positive inotropy upon the ventricular myocardium, the negative inotropic effect of the vagus nerve is not equivalent. The mechanism by

to central centers includes GVA (pressure, chemical), GSA (pain, temperature), SSA (optic) and SVA (olfactory through the limbic system) information. Although GVA information may be the most common and obvious input, cardiovascular alterations occur in response to the other types of information. The ANS utilizes a variety of information in its regulation of cardiovascular activity.

Figure 16.26 is a stylized diagram of the

cardiac and vasomotor centers that are located in the reticular formation of the medulla oblongata. The *vasopressor region* and *cardiac stimulator center*, as well as the *vasodepressor region*, are large, diffuse regions within the medullary reticular formation. The *cardiac inhibitory center* or *dorsal motor nucleus of the vagus nerve* is a discrete nucleus within this region.

Sympathetic and Parasympathetic Innervation. The GVE fibers of the ANS represent

which these nerves exert their inotropic effects is not clear. The positive inotropy exerted through β_1-receptor activity is mediated through cAMP. Many xanthines, which decrease the breakdown of cAMP by the inhibition of phosphodiesterase activity, are positive inotropes also. The cardiac glycosides and other antiarrhythmic drugs are believed to exert their positive inotropy upon the myocardium by the inhibition of Na^+-K^+-dependent ATPase. The increased intracellular Na^+, followed by an influx of Ca^{++} ions, causes an enhanced excitation-contraction coupling.

The dromotropic effect is manifested as an alteration in atrial and ventricular conduction speeds, as well as an alteration to nodal delay.

The dromotropic effect complements the chronotropic effect. These factors plus the inotropic effect determine cardiac performance or cardiac *output*. *The cardiac output is the heart rate multiplied by the stroke volume.*

The adrenergic receptors located in the smooth muscle of the coronary vessels are β_2 receptors. The heart is required to do more work under sympathetic stimulation. Coronary vessel dilation via these receptors insures an ample blood supply to the myocardium commensurate with the increased work demands imposed upon it.

Autonomic Reflex Activity

Arterial Pressoreceptor Reflex. Arterial baroreceptors are located throughout the body as integral components of the mural elements of these vessels. They are responsive to alterations in the stretch of blood vessels that accompanies alterations in blood pressure. The carotid sinus and aortic sinus receptors are typical; however, receptors are located also in the left and right atria, left ventricle and pulmonary arteries.

An increased blood pressure stretches the wall of the vessel and results in an increased rate of discharge (Fig. 16.28). This information reaches the vasomotor centers and stimulates the vasodepressor area while blocking the vasopressor area. This effectively decreases the sympathetic tone to the cardiovascular system. Concomitantly, these afferents reach the cardiac inhibitory center (dorsal motor nucleus of the vagus nerve) and the vagal tone to the heart is increased. Thus, an increased blood pressure reflexively results in a decreased cardiac output and peripheral vasodilation. This combination effectively lowers the blood pressure.

A decreased blood pressure has the reverse effect upon the cardiovascular system (Fig. 16.28).

The specific arterial pressoreceptor reflex involving the carotid sinus is called the *carotid sinus reflex*, *baroreceptor reflex* and *depressor reflex*. It is an important negative feedback loop that is significant in cardiovascular homeostasis. Generally, stimulation of baroreceptors inhibits the cardiovascular system. One notable exception to this generality exists. When the heart is operating under the influence of increased vagal tone, stretching of the right atrium results in an increased heart rate (*Bainbridge reflex*).

Chemoreceptor Reflexes. These reflexes utilize the carotid and aortic bodies. Medullary receptors on the floor of the fourth ventricle near the obex are involved also. The receptors for chemical reflexes are sensitive to P_{O_2}, P_{CO_2} and pH.

The carotid body, as an example, consists of a glomus of cells which is one of the most vascularized organs of the body. It receives approximately 200 times more blood than the rest of the body on a ml/min/gram basis. The mechanism of action was discussed previously (*specialized chemoreceptors*). Note that an increased discharge, as in the baroreceptor reflex, results in a release of central inhibition. The primary effects, however, are mediated through the respiratory centers. Minimal cardiac effects are noted, because peripheral hypoxia depresses cardiac activity whereas a central hypoxia stimulates cardiac activity. Chemoreceptors help to coordinate pulmonary and cardiac

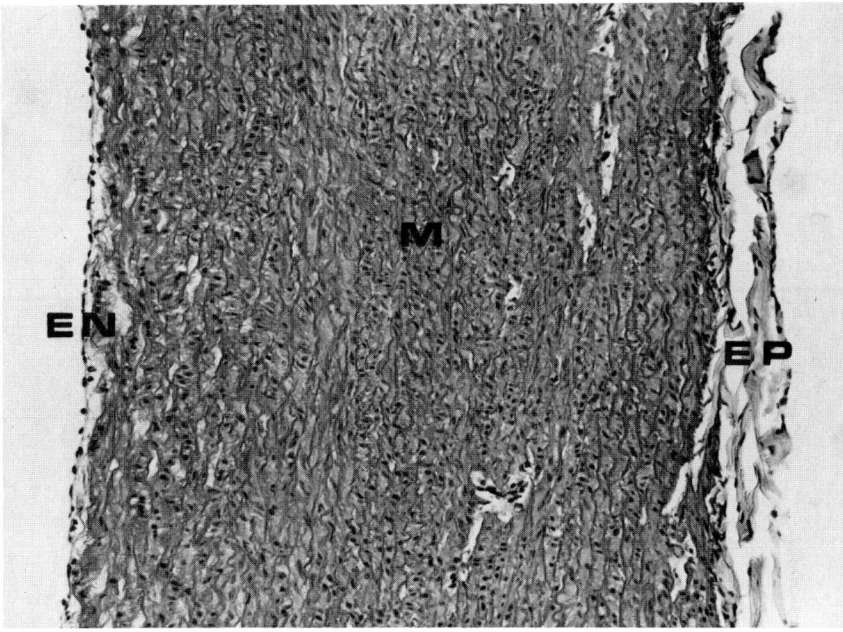

Fig. 16.18 A section of the wall of the atrium. The wall consists of endocardium (EN), myocardium (M) and epicardium (EP). X40.

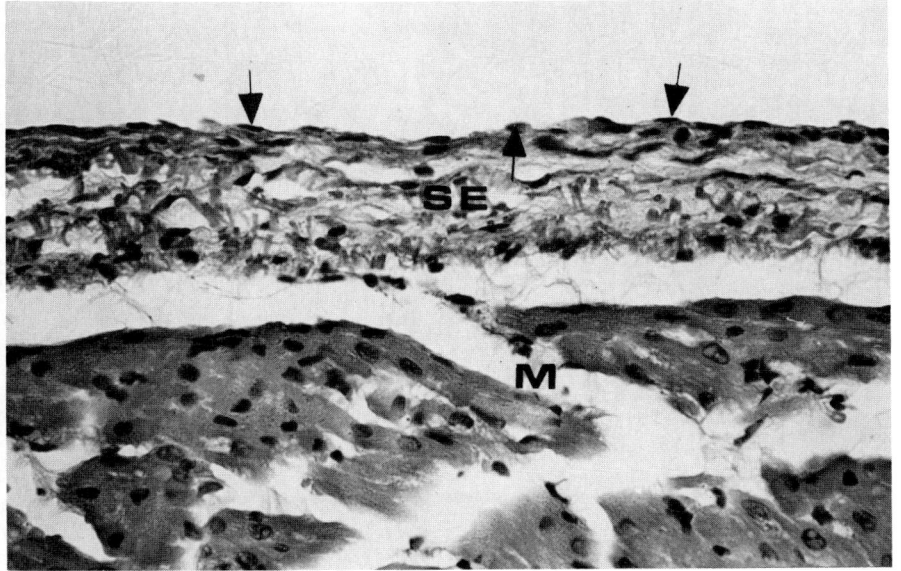

Fig. 16.19 Atrial endocardium. The endothelium (*arrows*) is underlaid by subendothelial connective tissue (SE) which is adjacent to the myocardium (M). X100.

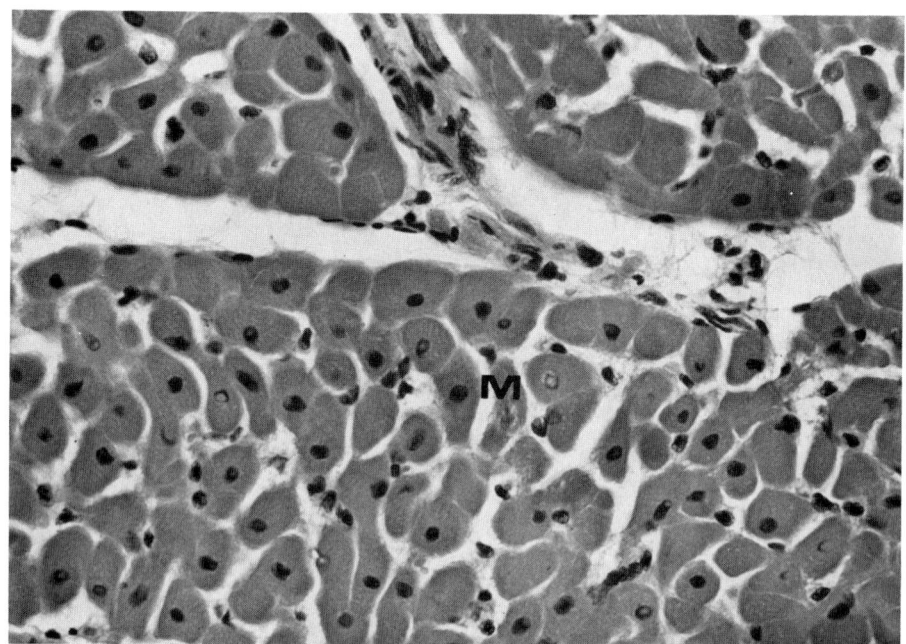

Fig. 16.20   Ventricular myocardium. The myocardium (M) consists of cardiac muscle cells separated by a well-vascularized endomysium. X100.

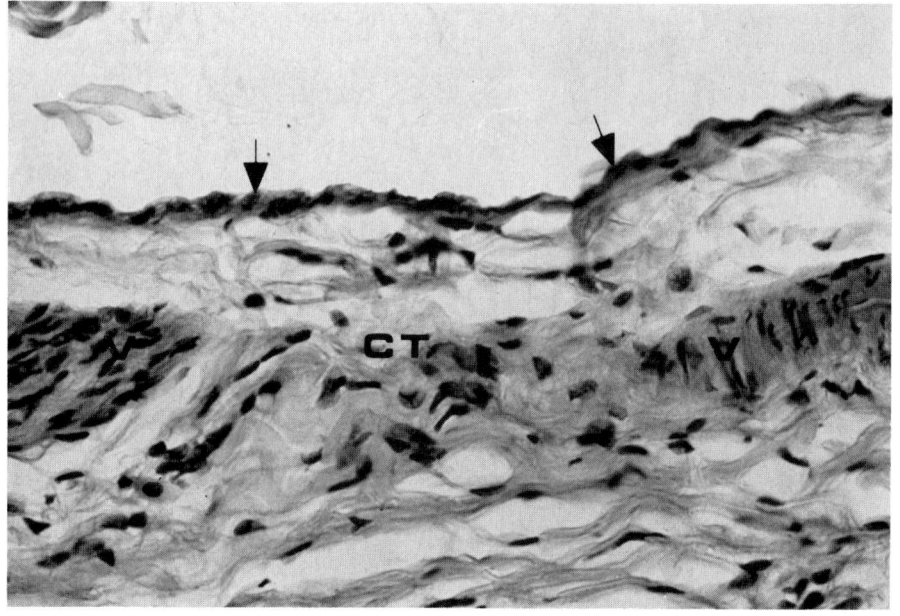

Fig. 16.21   Atrial epicardium. The mesothelial lining (*arrows*) resides upon a layer of connective tissue (CT). The smooth muscle is part of vessels (V) which have been sectioned obliquely. X100.

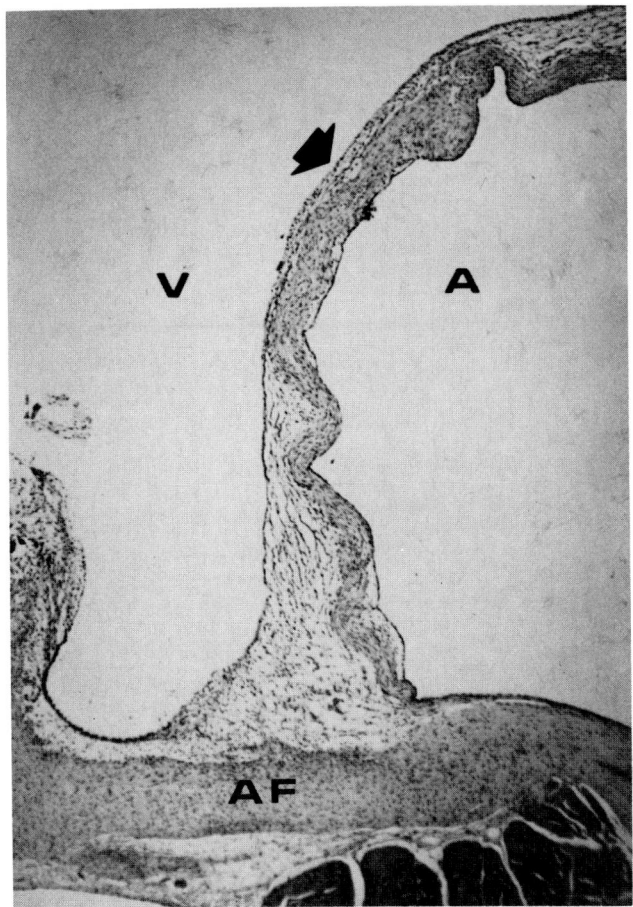

Fig. 16.22 Part of an atrioventricular valve. The valve (*arrow*) separates the ventricle (V) from the atrium (A). The connective tissue of the fibrous ring (AF) is continuous with the connective tissue core of the valve. The valve is covered by endothelium. X10.

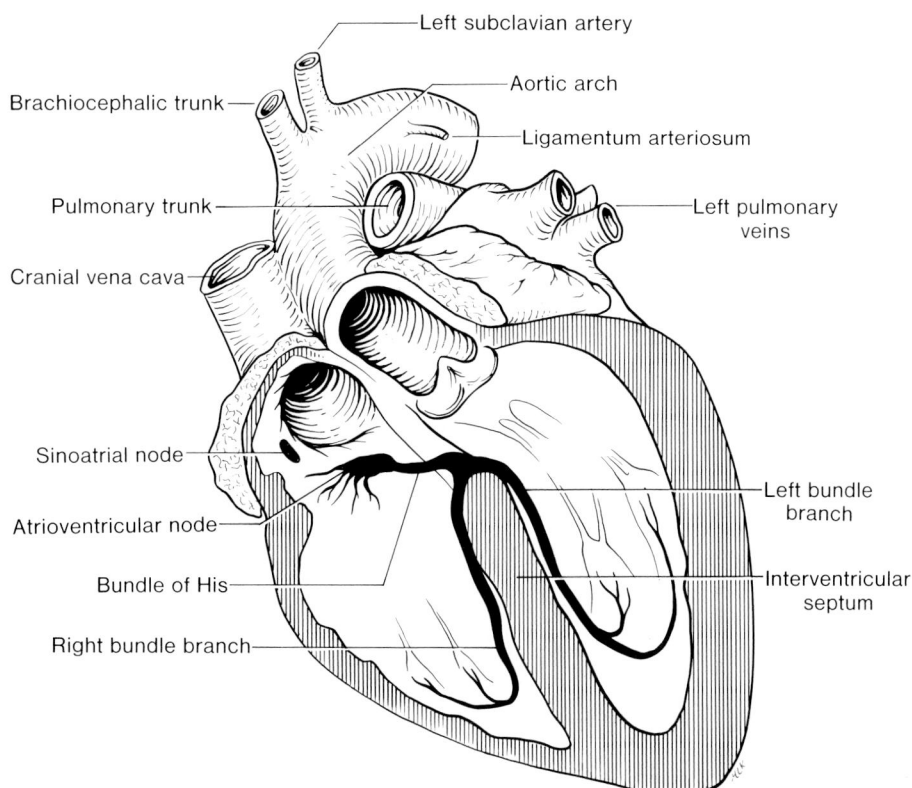

Fig. 16.23 A cut-away diagram of the canine heart. The conduction system and major components of the heart are indicated.

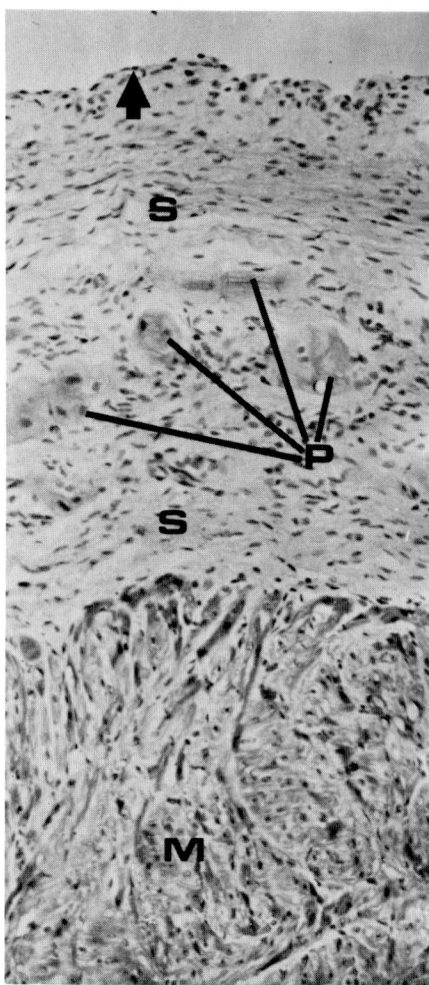

Fig. 16.24 Subendocardial Purkinje fibers of a porcine heart. *Arrow*, endothelium; S, sub-endothelium; P, Purkinje fibers; M, myocardium. The Purkinje fibers are part of the bundle branches of the ventricles. X40.

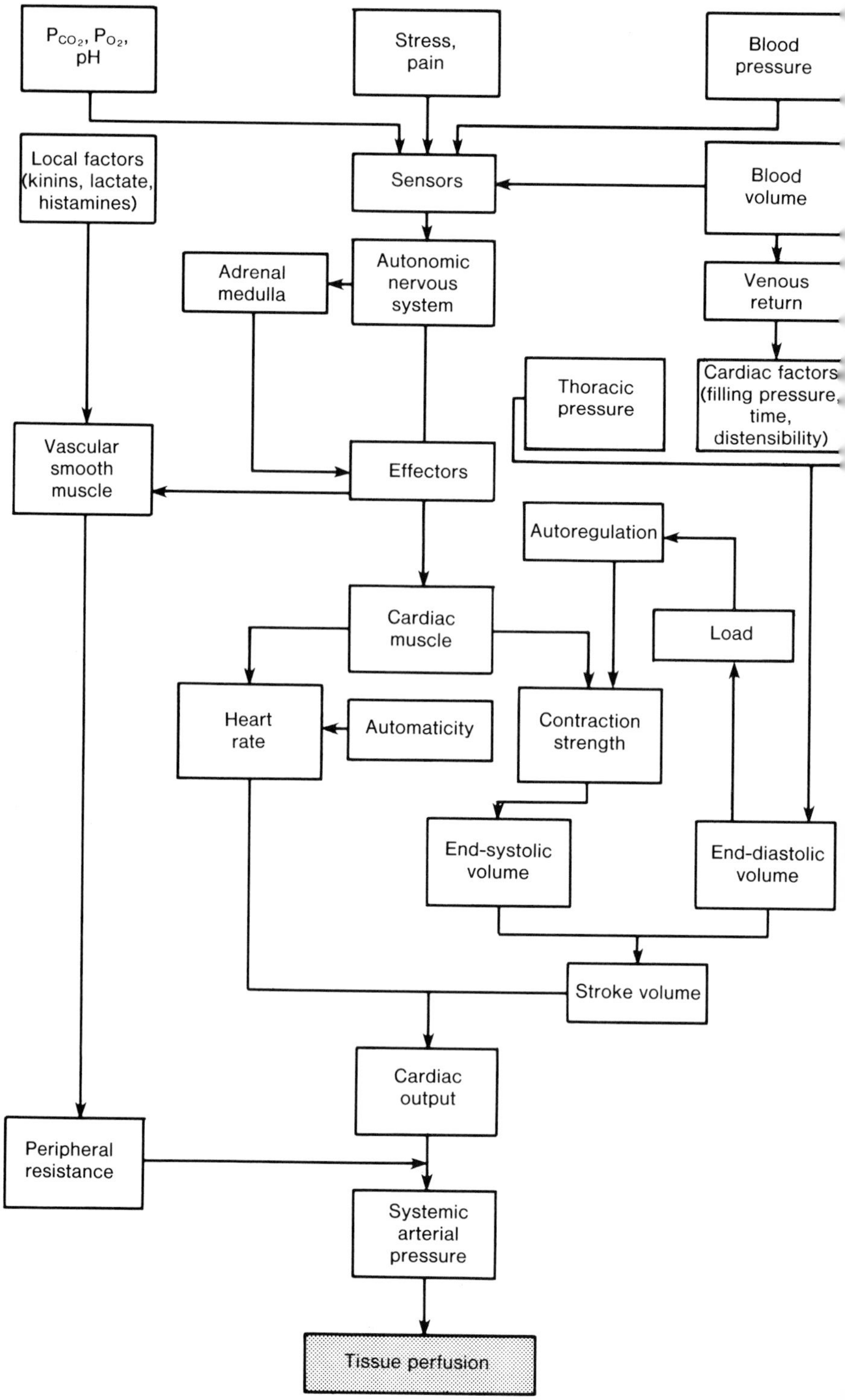

Fig. 16.25 A flow chart demonstrating the various influences upon the cardiovascular system that affect tissue perfusion.

activity to insure proper ventilation/perfusion ratios.

It is possible that blood flow to the brain could be impaired without stimulation of the carotid or aortic receptors. Under these circumstances the medullary receptors are important monitors of P_{CO_2} and pH. Cerebral ischemia, then, would result in increased activity in the cardiovascular and respiratory systems.

Sinus Arrhythmia. *Sinus arrhythmia* is an alteration of the cardiac rate coupled with respiratory activity. The sinus rhythm of normal animals is "regularly irregular;" i.e., a tachycardia accompanies inspiration that is followed by a bradycardia during expiration. The precise mechanism of this reflex tachycardia is not known; however, its disappearance during exercise, excitement and after the administration of atropine affords some insights. The following explanation of this phenomenon is plausible: As the lung

inflates there is an increased rate of discharge from stretch receptors within the lung. This information ascends the vagus nerve, inhibits the firing of the cell bodies of the cardioinhibitory center, decreases vagal tone and results in tachycardia. Subsequent deflation of the lung causes a decreased discharge rate of pulmonary stretch receptors. This releases the inhibition upon

the dorsal motor nucleus of the vagus, increases vagal tone and results in bradycardia.

Pain. Most of the sensory modalities are involved in the reflex activity associated with cardiovascular regulation. Pain manifests diverse influences upon the system. Generally, a painful stimulus results in a rise in blood pressure through an increased

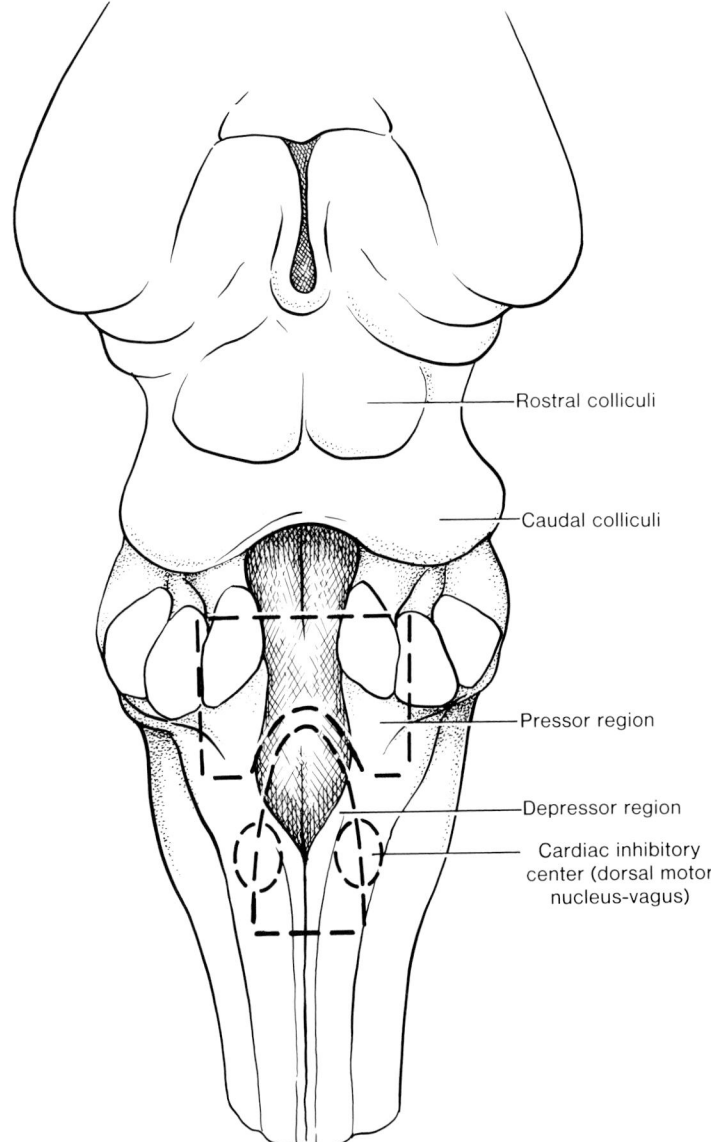

Fig. 16.26   A stylized drawing of the cardiac and vasomotor centers of the medulla oblongata.

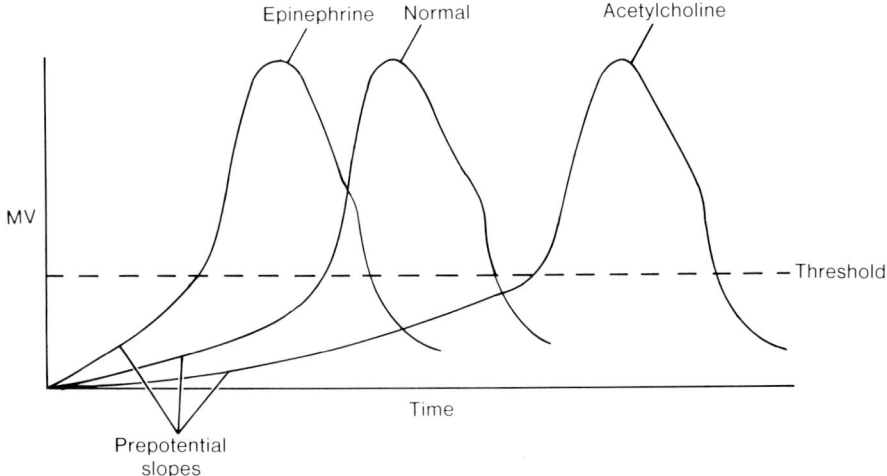

Fig. 16.27   A diagram showing the effect of epinephrine and acetylcholine upon the slope of the prepotential of cardiac nodal cells. Increasing the slope results in a more rapid firing; decreasing the slope slows the rate of firing.

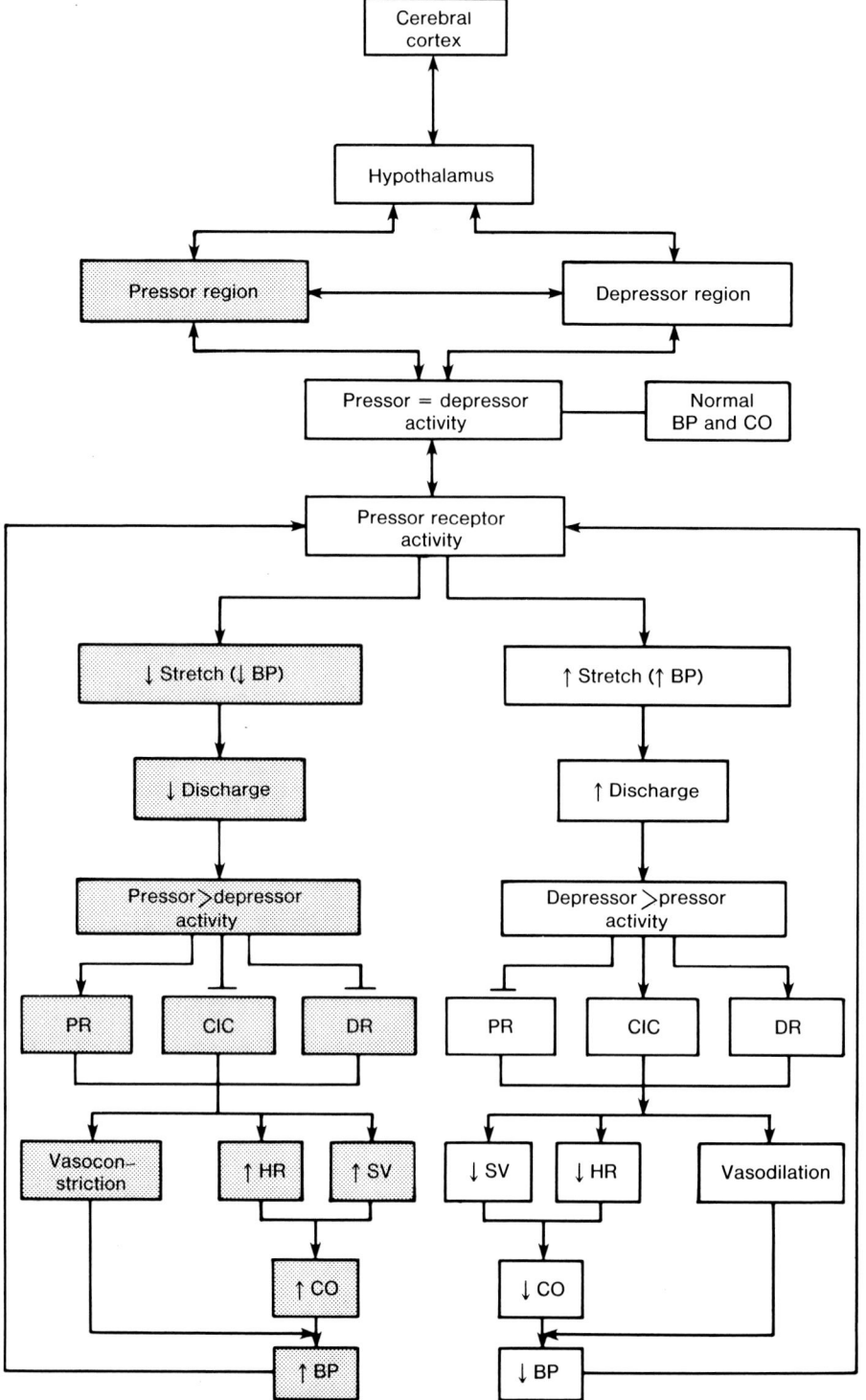

Fig. 16.28 A flow chart showing the effects of the arterial pressoreceptor reflex upon blood pressure. PR, pressor region; CIC, cardiac inhibitory center; DR, depressor region; SV, stroke volume; HR, heart rate; CO, cardiac output; BP, blood pressure. *Arrows* indicate direction of flow and/or stimulation; *bars* indicate inhibition. An increased discharge inhibits the PR but stimulates the CIC and DR; a decreased blood pressure results. The reverse occurs when a decreased blood pressure causes a decreased receptor discharge.

Hormonal Influence

Adrenomedullary and ADH Influence. The effects of the adrenal medullary secretions were discussed with the ANS (Chapter 15). The release of catecholamines from the adrenal medulla provides a long lasting adjunct to the sympathetic influence upon the cardiovascular system (Fig. 15.39). The stimulatory effects of its secretions upon α and β receptors can be anticipated.

Antidiuretic hormone (ADH) is released from the nerve fibers of the neurohypophysis at neurohemal organs. Volume receptor stimulation in the left atrium influences the release of ADH. This hormone is also released after hemorrhage. Beside the advantage of water retention, ADH may have a direct pressor effect upon the blood vessels. This effect may be significant in the long term adjustments of blood volume after minor blood loss.

Lymphatic Vessels

Capillaries and Larger Vessels. Lymph capillaries are very similar to continuous blood capillaries and are most difficult to distinguish from one another in section (Fig. 16.7). Three features generally may be used to make the distinction. Lymph capillaries are partially or completely devoid of a basement membrane. Their abluminal surfaces may have microvilli which anchor the vessel in the connective tissue space. Also, they are generally devoid of formed elements; however, agranulocytes may be encountered.

The larger vessels are not well-organized. Although the three mural regions may be present, they are not well-defined. Generally, the lymphatics have thinner walls than the veins of a corresponding size. Valves occur in lymph vessels of a smaller size than the corresponding appearance of valves in veins.

References

Vasculature

Abramson, D. I.: *Circulation in the Extremities.* Academic Press, New York, 1976.

Ahmed, M. M.: The fine structure of endothelium in coronary arterioles. Acta Anat. *69:*327, 1968.

Bennet, H. S., Luft, J. H. and Hampton, J. C.: Morphological classification of vertebrate blood capillaries. Amer. J. Physiol. *196:*381, 1959.

Bruns, R. R. and Palade, G. E.: Studies on blood capillaries. I. General organization of blood capillaries in muscle. J. Cell Biol. *37:*244, 1968.

Cliff, W. J.: *Blood Vessels.* Cambridge University Press, Oxford, 1976.

Fernando, N. V. P. and Movat, H. Z.: The capillaries. Exp. Molec. Pathol. *3:*87, 1964.

Hayes, J. R.: Histological changes in constricted arteries and arterioles. J. Anat. *101:*343, 1967.

Keech, M. K.: Electron microscope study of the normal rat aorta. J. Biophys. Biochem. Cytol. 7:533, 1960.

Leak, L. V. and Burke, J. F.: Fine structure of the lymphatic capillary and the adjoining connective tissue area. Amer. J. Anat. *118:*785, 1966.

Rhodin, J. A. G.: Fine structure of vascular walls in mammals with special reference to smooth muscle component. Physiol. Rev. *42:*447, 1962.

Wood, J. E.: *The Veins: Normal and Abnormal Function,* Little, Brown, Boston, 1965.

activity of the vasopressor centers. Vasoconstriction and increased cardiac output account for the rise in blood pressure.

Severe cutaneous pain and deep visceral pain usually have the opposite effect—bradycardia and decreased blood pressure. A vagovagal reflex involving the visceral organs occurs under a variety of circumstances but may be especially significant during abdominal surgery.

Heart

Bolton, G. R.: *Handbook of Canine Electrocardiography.* W. B. Saunders, Philadelphia, 1975.

Eckner, F. A. O., Brown, B. W., Overll, E. and Glagov, S.: Alterations of the gross dimensions of the heart and its structures by formalin fixation: A quantitative study. Virchow Arch. Path. Anat. *346:*318, 1969.

Ettinger, S. J. and Suter, P. F.: *Canine Cardiology.* W. B. Saunders, Philadelphia, 1970.

Ghidoni, J. J., Liotta, D. and Thomas, H.: Massive subendocardial damage accompanying prolonged ventricular fibrillation. Amer. J. Pathol. *56:*15, 1969.

Hogan, P. M. and Davis, L. D.: Evidence for specialized fibers in the canine right atrium. Circ. Res. *23:*387, 1968.

James, T. N. and Sherf, L.: Ultrastructure of myocardial cells. Amer. J. Cardiol. *22:*389, 1968.

James, T. N., Sherf, L. and Urthaler, F.: Fine structure of the bundle branches. Br. Heart J. *36:*1, 1974.

Langer, G. A. and Brady, A. J.: *The Mammalian Myocardium.* John Wiley and Sons, New York, 1974.

Merkin, R. J.: Position and orientation of the heart valves. Amer. J. Anat. *125:*375, 1969.

Mitomo, Y., Nakao, K. and Angrist, A.: The fine structure of the heart valves in the chicken: I. Mitral valve. Amer. J. Anat. *125:*147, 1969.

Muir, A. R.: Observations on the fine structure of the Purkinje fibers in the ventricles of the sheep's heart. J. Anat. *91:*251, 1957.

Nabors, C. E., and Ball, C. R.: Spontaneous calcification in hearts of DBA mice. Anat. Rec. *164:*153, 1969.

Rhodin, J. A. G., Delmissier, P. and Reid, L. C.: The structure of the specialized conducting system of the steer heart. Circulation *24:*349, 1961.

Regulation

Aars, H.: The baroreflex in arterial hypertension. Scand. J. Clin. Lab. Invest. *35:*97, 1975.

Armour, J. A. and Randall, W. C.: Functional anatomy of canine cardiac nerves. Acta Anat. *91:*510, 1975.

Denn, M. J. and Stone, H. L.: Autonomic innervation of the dog coronary arteries. J. Appl. Physiol. *41:*30, 1976.

Feigl, E. O.: Sympathetic control of coronary circulation. Circ. Res. *20:*262, 1967.

Feigl, E. O.: Carotid sinus reflex control of coronary blood flow. Circ. Res. *23:*223, 1968.

Feigl, E. O.: Parasympathetic control of coronary blood flow in dogs. Circ. Res. *25:*509, 1969.

Granger, H. S. and Guyton, A. C.: Autoregulation of the total systemic circulation following destruction of the central nervous system in the dog. Circ. Res. *25:*379, 1969.

Gross, D.: Pain and autonomic nervous system. Adv. Neurol. *4:*93, 1974.

Osborne, M. P. and Butler, P. J.: New theory for receptor mechanism of carotid body chemoreceptors. Nature *254:*701, 1975.

17: Lymphatic System and Immunity

General Characteristics

Form and Function. All of the basic tissues of the body contribute, directly or indirectly, to the composition of the lymphatic system. The lymphatic system and the vascular system form an important functional unit called the *hemic-lymphatic system*. The hemic-lymphatic system is a *secondary defense system*. The *primary defense system* consists of the skin and the mucous membranes. These covering and lining structures are barriers essential for the integrity of the body. The defensive aspects of the lymphatic system are manifested in various ways: *production of defensive cells, transport of materials via lymphatic vessels, filtration of lymph and blood through constituent organs, phagocytosis and production of immunoglobulins.*

The filtration function, which is complemented by phagocytosis, is an important mechanism of the lymphatic system that is achieved in various ways. Some lymphatic tissues, tonsils and similar aggregates of lymphatic nodules, remove foreign substances from the tissue and lymphatic fluid. Others, spleen and hemal node, remove substances from the blood.

The phagocytic function is achieved through the phagocytic activity of cells that line or are associated with sinusoids (Fig. 6.49). These cells are the *macrophage (reticuloendothelial) system.*

Classification of Lymphatic Tissues. The tissues and organs of the lymphatic system may be grouped into morphologically distinct subdivisions accordingly:

1. Diffuse, unencapsulated lymphatic tissues (subepithelial lymphatic tissue associated with somatic orifices and tracts of the respiratory, digestive and urogenital systems).

2. Dense, unencapsulated lymphatic tissue (subepithelial accumulations of lymphatic tissue associated with the respiratory, digestive and urogenital tracts).

3. Dense, encapsulated tissues scattered throughout the body (lymph nodes, spleen, hemal nodes, hemolymph nodes, thymus, bursa of Fabricius).

Diffuse Lymphatic Tissue

Generalized Distribution of Lymphoid Cells. The generalized distributional pattern of lymphocytes, plasma cells and monocytes (histiocytes or macrophages) is described

typically as accumulations of cells that form recognizable histologic aggregate structures, but lymphoid cells can occur within any locus of the body. Most generally, the connective tissue of the lamina propria is replete with these defensive cells. They may occur with sufficient frequency to impart a hypercellular nature to this connective tissue (Fig. 17.1). In those organs that are subjected continually to insult or potential insult from foreign materials (respiratory, digestive and urogenital systems), these cells may be considered part of the resident population of the connective tissue associated therewith. They function as an effective and readily available second line of defense for the body in these loci.

Dense Lymphatic Tissue

Solitary Lymph Nodules. These accumulations of lymphatic tissue are scattered throughout the body. These solitary nodules, with prominent germinal centers, are associated with the digestive, respiratory and urogenital tracts (Fig. 17.2). The lymphocytes from the corona migrate into the surrounding lamina propria mucosae. These solitary nodules are not intercalated into the lymphatic drainage by specific efferent vessels but are surrounded by vessels that function similarly. Some of these nodules may be encapsulated. They occur in the lamina propria mucosae, tunica submucosa and occasionally in the tunica adventitia.

Avian Lymphatic Tissue. Most avian species do not possess lymph nodes, with the exception of swamp, sea and shore birds. Solitary accumulations of lymphatic tissue as nodules characterize the walls of the digestive tract, serous membranes and skin (Fig. 17.3).

Aggregated Lymph Nodules. Accumulations of lymph nodules are encountered in scat-

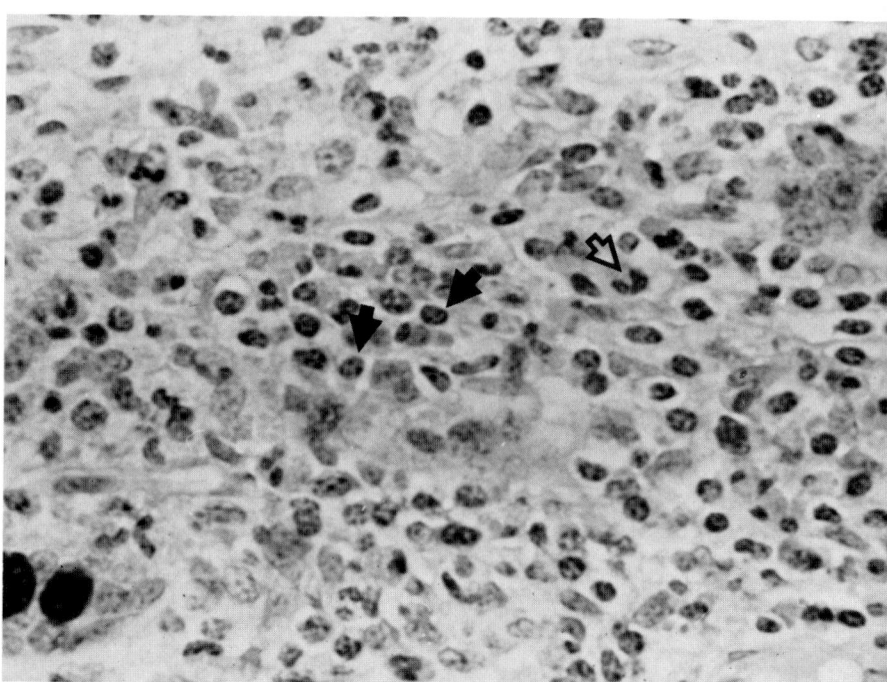

Fig. 17.1 A section of lamina propria associated with the gastrointestinal tract. The tissue is hypercellular. Numerous plasma cells (*solid arrows*), macrophages (*open arrow*) and other mononuclears are present. X160. All light micrographs are labeled as the magnification with the microscope before photographic enlarging. All electron micrographs are labeled as total magnification, including photographic enlarging.

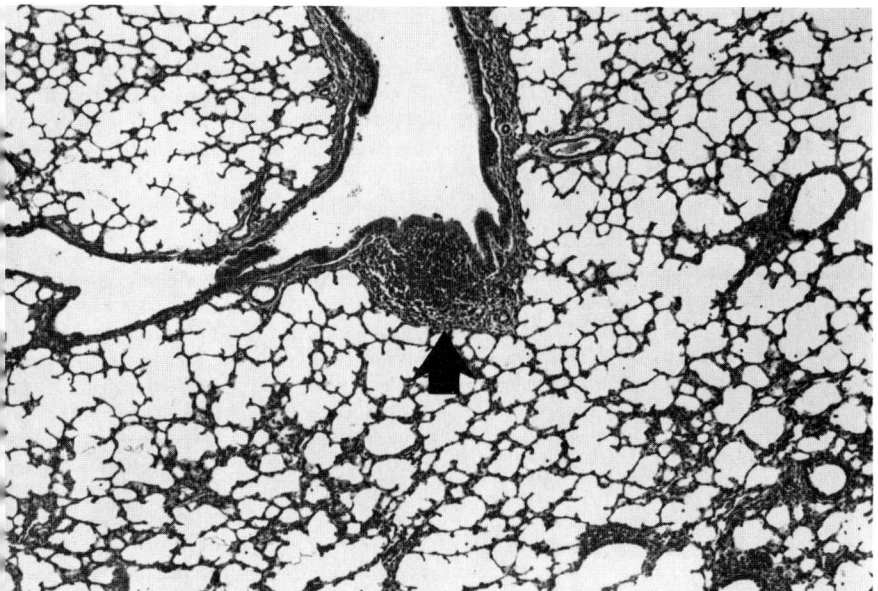

ig. 17.2 A solitary lymph nodule in the lung. The lymph nodule (*arrow*) is associated closely ith a bronchiole. X16.

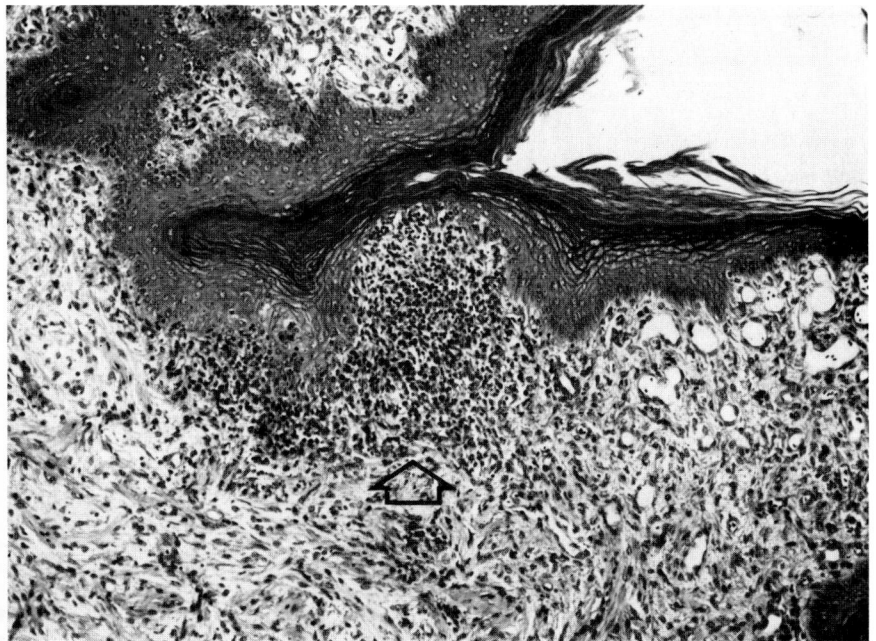

ig. 17.3 The comb of a bird. The dermis contains a lymphatic nodule (*arrow*) and loose ymphatic tissue. X40.

and *tonsils without crypts.* The *crypt* is a blind and sometimes branched invagination of the surface epithelium. A crypt and the associated lymphatic tissue is referred to as a *tonsillar follicle* (Fig. 17.6). A group of follicles constitutes a tonsil of this type. A *tonsil without crypts* is formed by a single lamina of lymphatic tissue which may be secondarily bulged outward or slightly folded to increase surface area (Fig. 17.5).

The invaginations of the tunica mucosa are significant because they serve as foci of infection and corresponding inflammatory processes.

The morphologic features and specific sites of tonsillar tissue vary among domestic species.

1. Tonsils with crypts (follicular tonsils): palatine tonsils in man, horse, ruminant, swine; lingual tonsils in man, horse, ruminant, swine; tubal tonsils in swine; paraepiglottic tonsils in sheep, goat, swine.
2. Tonsils without crypts: palatine tonsils in carnivores; pharyngeal tonsils in all domestic animals except carnivores; tubal tonsils in ruminants.

Tonsils do not possess afferent lymphatic channels. Rather, material is either filtered into the organ or carried to it by cells from the surrounding connective tissue space. Efferent lymphatic channels exist.

Lymphatic Organs

Lymph Node

Histologic Structure. These organs are dense, encapsulated components of the system that are scattered throughout the body.

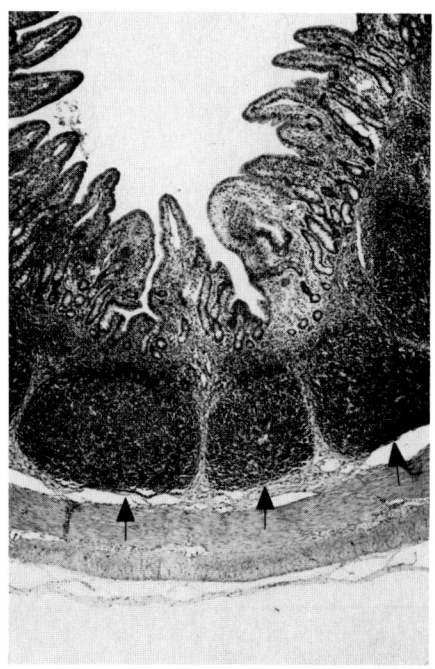

Fig. 17.4 Peyer's patches in the wall of the ileum. Peyer's patches (*arrows*) are aggregates of lymphatic nodules. X8.

ered foci throughout the soma (Fig. 17.4). n some instances the nodules are quite large nd may even become confluent. The 'eyer's patches of the intestinal wall are a ood example of these. Often, aggregated ymph nodules are referred to as tonsils, in /hich case Peyer's patches may be considered "intestinal tonsils."

'onsils. Tonsils are formed of solitary or ggregated nodules and diffuse lymphatic issue (Fig. 17.5). They form a "pharyngeal ing" along the tract from the mouth to the harynx in the lamina propria mucosae in

close association with the epithelial lining. They are basically accumulations of dense, encapsulated lymphatic tissue similar to the nodules of lymph nodes. The germinal centers are large, the cortices are dense and there is extensive infiltration of lymphocytes into the surrounding connective tissue and associated epithelium.

Although all tonsils are similar, there are two distinguishable groups that are defined on the basis of tonsillar tissue relationships with the surface epithelium with which they are associated. These are *tonsils with crypts*

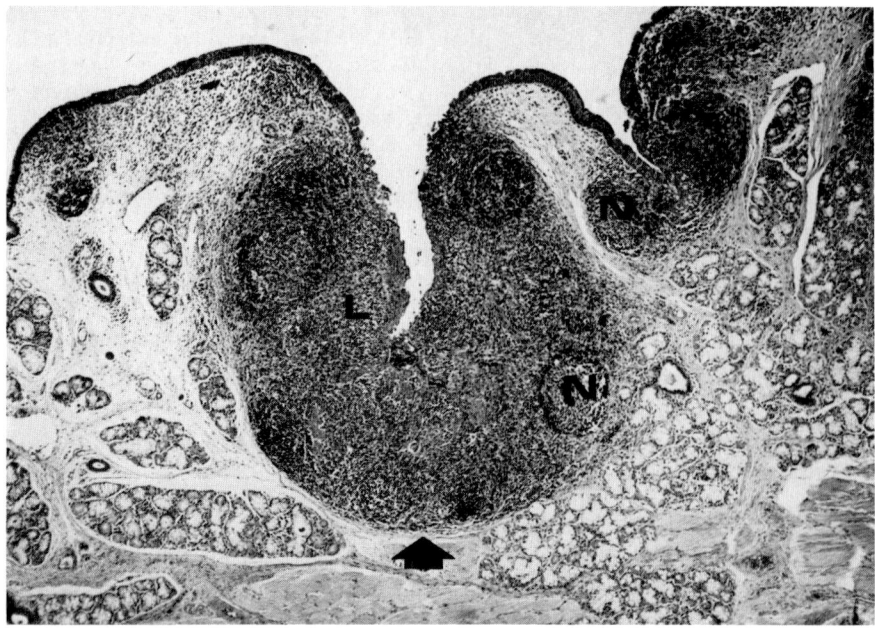

Fig. 17.5   A tonsil without crypts. The tonsil (*arrow*) is composed of nodular (N) and loose (L) lymphatic tissue. The tunica mucosa is folded slightly. Extensive infiltration of lymphocytes into the lamina propria and lamina epithelialis is evident. X10.

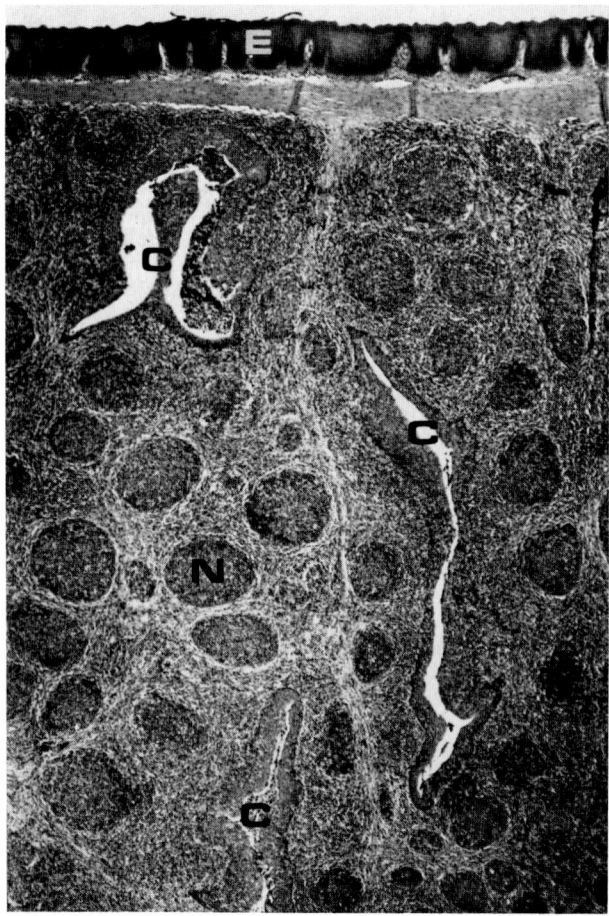

Fig. 17.6   A tonsil with crypts. Nodular (N) and loose lymphatic tissues are the primary components. The lamina epithelialis (E) is highly folded and forms extensive crypts (C) or invaginations. X10.

Although their precise location is variable, they occur constantly in specific regions of the body. Lymph nodes are usually bean-shaped and vary in size from about 1 mm to several centimeters. The nodes, sometimes called glands, consist of a *capsule, stroma, cortex, medulla, nodules and hilus* (Fig. 17.7).

The capsule consists of dense white fibrous connective tissue (DWFCT) which is continuous with trabeculae of the same tissue. The latter subdivide the organ into smaller compartments. Smooth muscle and elastic fibers are rarely present as stromal components. The fine stromal elements of the organ are reticular fibers (Fig. 17.8).

Two distinct regions of the organ are apparent, an outer *cortex* and an inner *medulla*. The cortex consists of nodules, trabeculae, fine stromal elements and lymph sinuses (Fig. 17.9). The *medulla* consists of cellular aggregates, a cellular and fine fibrous stroma and sinuses. This lymphatic tissue is arranged as aggregates of cells in cords (*medullary cords*) which are separated by connective tissue and lymph sinuses (Fig. 17.10). The hilus is a connective tissue space which contains efferent lymphatic vessels. The connective tissue of the capsule is continuous with that of the hilus through the trabeculae.

An immunologically competent and active nodule (*secondary nodule*) consists of a *germinal center* and outer *corona* (Fig. 17.11). The germinal center contains various mature and immature cellular forms. Most reticular cells are large cells with pale nuclei and long cytoplasmic processes, but some lack processes. The *dendritic cells*, reticular cells with long cytoplasmic processes, form a cellular reticulum. The enigmatic nature of reticular cells was discussed in Chapter 6. Mature lymphocytes and lymphoblasts are the dominant cell types, although plasma cells and macrophages are present also. The lymphoblasts and their progeny of lymphocytes are B cells. These centers are paler than the peripheral corona due to the presence of fewer cells as well as to their pale-staining characteristics. As lymphocytes are produced, they migrate peripherally to form the corona or *cortex of the nodule*. After a period of activity, the germinal center regresses and the nodule returns to its original configuration as a *primary nodule* devoid of a germinal center. Immunologically incompetent animals do not possess germinal centers. After antigenic insult, however, germinal centers appear.

The region subjacent to the lymph nodules of the cortex is termed the *paracortical* or *subcortical zone*. It is occupied primarily by T lymphocytes.

The *medullary cords* contain accumulations of plasma cells and their progenitors, some B lymphocytes and macrophages. In ideal preparations, these regions are clearly delimited by large medullary sinusoids.

Lymph Circulation. Although the lymph nodes may be likened to a sponge, large

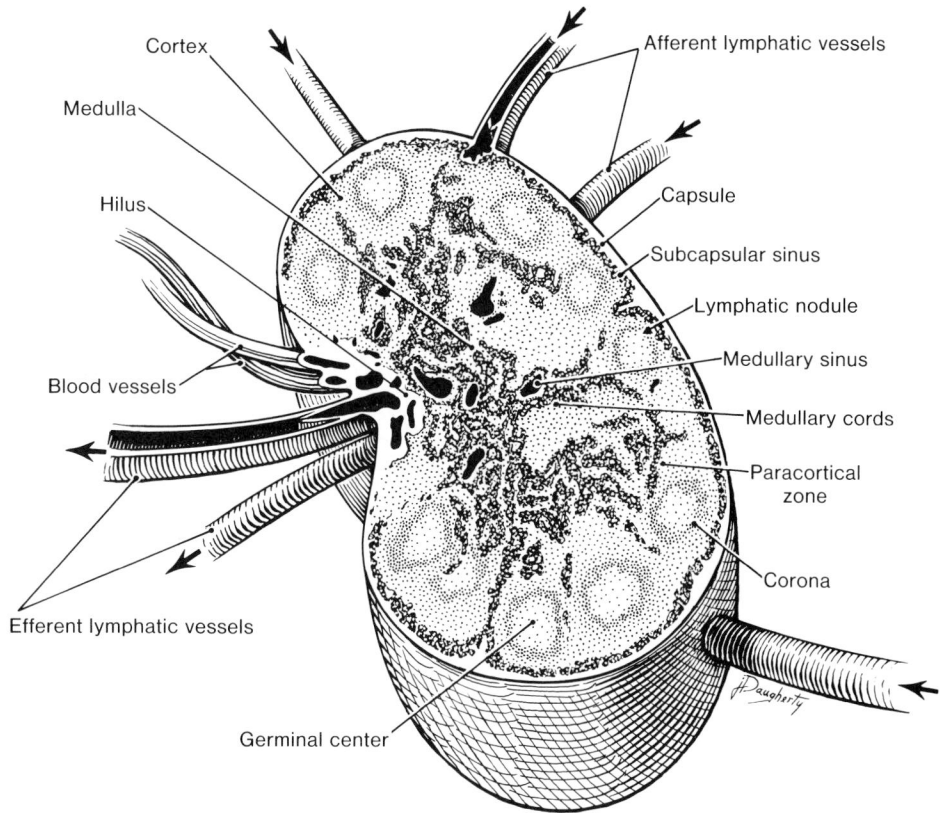

Fig. 17.7   A diagram of a typical lymph node.

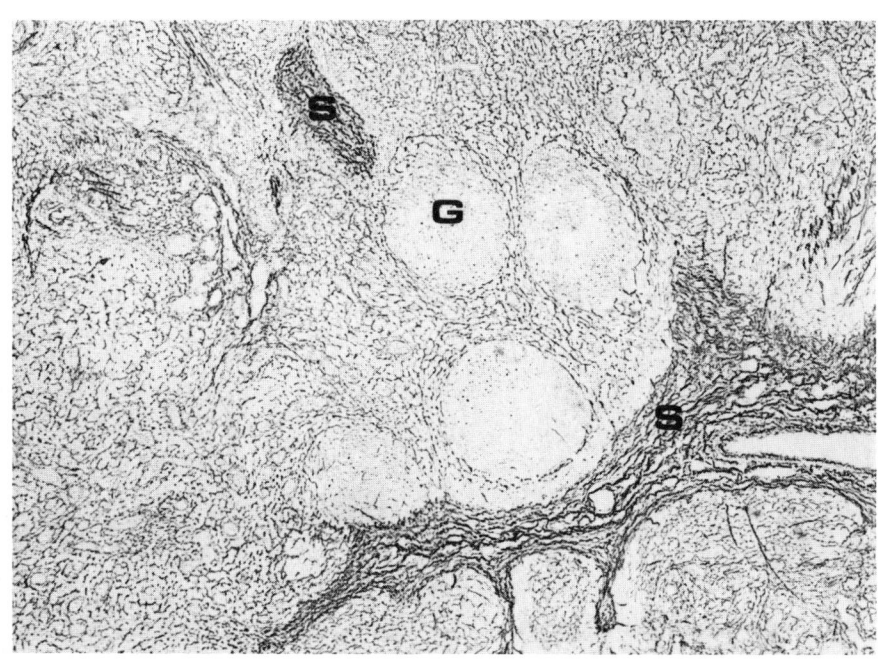

Fig. 17.8   Stromal elements of a lymph node. The trabecular stroma (S) consists of reticular and collagenous fibers, whereas other interstitial regions of the lymph node are composed of reticular fibers exclusively. The germinal centers of the nodules (G) contain a paucity of fibrous elements. X16 (reticular stain).

spaces are present which clearly delineate the flow of lymph through the organ. *Afferent vessels* enter at the capsule and empty into a prominent *subcapsular* or *marginal*

sinusoid which separates the capsule from the underlying cortical parenchyma. Percolation of lymph continues through the *cortical sinuses* and nodules into the *medullary*

sinusoids. The latter are confluent with *efferent lymphatic vessels* at the hilus of the organ. Flow through a lymph node is unidirectional—capsule to hilus.

Blood Vessels and Nerves. The arteries enter the lymph node at the hilus and continue throughout the lymph node through the trabecular connective tissue. Some continue their course through the trabeculae to the capsule of the organ, whereas others enter the medulla and supply the medullary cords and cortex. The venous drainage is typical; however, the *postcapillary venules* of the paracortical region are unique morphologically and functionally. These vessels are lined by thickened endothelial cells and are important in the *recirculation* of lymphocytes from the blood.

The nerves also enter at the hilus with the blood vessels. Most of these are probably vasomotor nerves. Some nerves, which are independent of the vasculature, occur within the trabeculae, capsule and medullary cords.

Species Differences. The porcine lymph node has the reverse pattern of that observed in other species (Fig. 17.12). Lymphatic nodules are located in the central or medullary regions of the organ, whereas the medullary cords and related aggregates of cells are located at the peripheral or cortical region. Flow of lymph, similarly, is the reverse of other domestic species; i.e., it enters at the hilus and emerges at the capsular area. Because of this particular arrange-

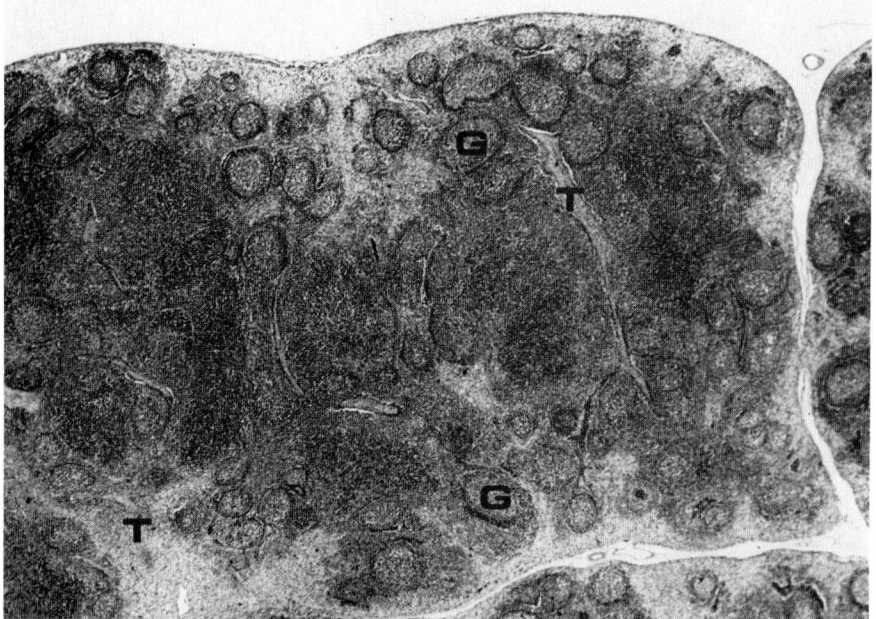

Fig. 17.9 A section of an equine lymph node. The cortex consists of nodules with germinal centers (G), trabeculae (T) and sinusoids. X4.

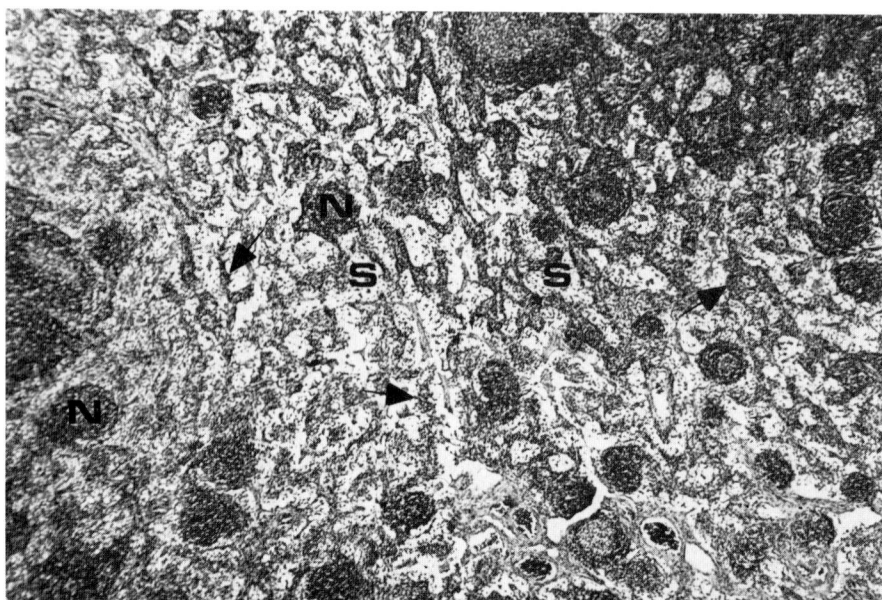

Fig. 17.10 The medulla of a canine lymph node. Nodules (N) are apparent at the periphery of the medulla. Medullary cords (*arrows*) and sinusoids (S) are the primary constituents of the medulla. X10.

ment, it is both tempting and probably correct to refer to the primary constituents as medullary nodules and cortical cords. Because most histologists are aware of this structural difference, as long as the species is specified it is unnecessary to reverse the terminology.

Important variations in lymph nodes occur in many species. In the horse, a fusion of cortical nodules is common. The ox possesses very large germinal centers. In swine, the nodules are inverted and extremely nu-

merous. The age and physiological state of the organism appreciably alter the lymph node morphology in all species.

Functional Correlates. The primary functions of lymph nodes are to *produce lymphocytes, filter lymph, phagocytose foreign materials* and *produce antibodies.*

Extensive mitotic activity, especially within the germinal centers of lymph nodules, is responsible for the production of B lymphocytes. Although the production of lymphocytes within these organs partially

accounts for the high numbers of lymphocytes in the efferent lymphatic channels, the recirculation phenomenon contributes significantly to the egress of a larger lymphocytic population in the efferent channel than enters via the afferent channels.

The walls of lymphatic capillaries are readily permeable to foreign materials (macromolecules, particulate matter, microbial agents) and connective tissue cells (Fig 17.13). The obvious result of this property is the ability of these vessels to transport various materials and cells to the lymph nodes wherein filtration and phagocytosis can occur. The permeability of the endothelial lining of the lymphatic channels within the lymph node facilitates these basic protective functions. However, the free movement of materials, microbial agents and cells from the lymphatic channels to the lymph node with subsequent access to blood vessels and efferent lymphatic vessels, also facilitates the spread of infectious agents and the metastasis of cancer cells (Fig. 17.14).

The production of antibodies is an important function of the B cell component of the lymph node. Antigenic materials that reach the lymph nodes are subjected to processing and/or degradation by macrophages. Macrophages contribute to the processing of particulate matter or large molecules of antigens. The processing results in the blastoid transformation of B lymphocytes into plasma cells. The intimate relationships of lymphoid cells within the lymph node permits the interactions that lead to humoral antibody production.

Hemal Nodes and Hemolymph Nodes

Histologic Structure. The sinusoids of *hemal nodes* are filled with blood rather than lymph (Fig. 17.15). Also, lymph vessels are not demonstrable. The capsule and trabeculae contain smooth muscle fibers. Otherwise, the organ looks much like a typical lymph node. These organs, however, have been described as miniature spleens.

Hemal nodes occur in ruminants in retroperitoneal positions along the vertebral column and in association with some of the visceral organs. They also occur in the jugular furrow.

Hemolymph nodes, as believed by some, are simply hemorrhagic lymph nodes. However, there is evidence that these are separate and distinct entities. These organs receive blood and lymph supplies that intermix in the sinusoids. Thus, they represent an intermediate form of lymphatic organ between the two aforementioned extremes.

These occur in the perirenal region of the sheep and goat and have been observed in the lumbar area of the ox.

Because of the significance of lymph nodes in diagnostic histopathology, it is important to be aware of the aforementioned variations. These, otherwise, may be mistaken for hemorrhagic lymph nodes.

Spleen

Histologic Structure. The spleen is related to other blood-forming organs and is the largest mass of lymphatic tissue in the body (Fig. 17.16). Despite its size and multiplicity of function, it is not essential for life. Among its numerous functions are *blood cell formation, hemoglobulin and iron metabolism, red blood cell destruction, blood filtration, blood storage, phagocytosis* and the *immune response.*

The capsule of the organ is covered by a thin layer of mesothelium. The associated connective tissue of this serous membrane blends with the DWFCT of the capsule. In a manner similar to that of lymph nodes, trabeculae of DWFCT extend into the parenchyma and effectively subdivide it into smaller compartments (Fig. 17.17). Smooth muscle fibers and elastic fibers are important structural components of the capsule and trabeculae of this organ (Fig. 17.18). These are continuous with the primary stromal elements, the reticular fibers. The arrangement of the capsular and trabecular

smooth muscle is species variable. These components allow for large volume changes, whereas the contraction of smooth muscle fibers discharges the blood from the organ.

Blood vessels enter the spleen proper by following trabecular pathways. Because of the nature of the mural elements and the trabeculae, it is very difficult to define clearly the typical mural divisions as outlined previously. A prominent hilar region of DWFCT extends along the length of the organ.

Like other lymphatic organs the spleen is a mixture of phagocytic sinusoids, reticular fiber stroma and a very cellular parenchyma. There is, however, no distinct cortex or medulla. The parenchyma consists of two distinct regions which are arranged in a random pattern. These regions are termed the *white pulp* and *red pulp.* Lymph nodules (*splenic corpuscles*) and *periarterial sheaths* of lymphocytes comprise the white pulp (Figs. 17.16, 17.17). However, careful examination will reveal the presence of an arteriole, mistakenly called the *central artery,* which occupies a central or paracentral position. It is sometimes referred to as the *nodular arteriole* (Fig. 17.19). It is not observed in all sections because the plane of section may parallel its course. The presence of nodules is dependent upon the same factors that influence germinal center development or regression in lymph nodes.

White and Red Pulp. The *white pulp* consists of dense lymphatic tissue which is associated intimately with branches of the trabecular arteries. This compact lymphatic tissue comprises the *periarterial sheaths* of lymphatic tissue (Fig. 17.20). Nodular enlargements, *splenic corpuscles,* are randomly distributed along the course of the arteries of the white pulp and are intercalated with the periarterial sheaths. The composition, nature and distribution of cellular components within a splenic corpuscle are similar to those of a lymphatic nodule; however, each germinal center of a splenic nodule is surrounded by a *mantle layer* (*mantle zone*) which is continuous with the periarterial sheath. The peripheral limits of the white pulp are interfaced with the red pulp by a *marginal zone* which consists of sinuses, a sheath of reticular cells and a layer of lymphatic cells. The periarterial sheath and mantle layer are thymic-dependent regions which are occupied by T cells; the splenic corpuscle produces B cells.

The areas between the splenic corpuscles and trabeculae are the areas of the *red pulp,* so named because of the extensive vascularity. The red pulp consists of splenic sinusoids and splenic cords (Fig. 17.21). The splenic sinusoids are discontinuous and are lined by phagocytic cells. These sinusoids open into the splenic cords. The cords are composed of granulocytes, granulocyte progenitors, reticular cells and phagocytic cells. In some species smooth muscle fibers also occur (Fig. 17.22). The sinusoids and cords are an integral filtration and phagocytic unit

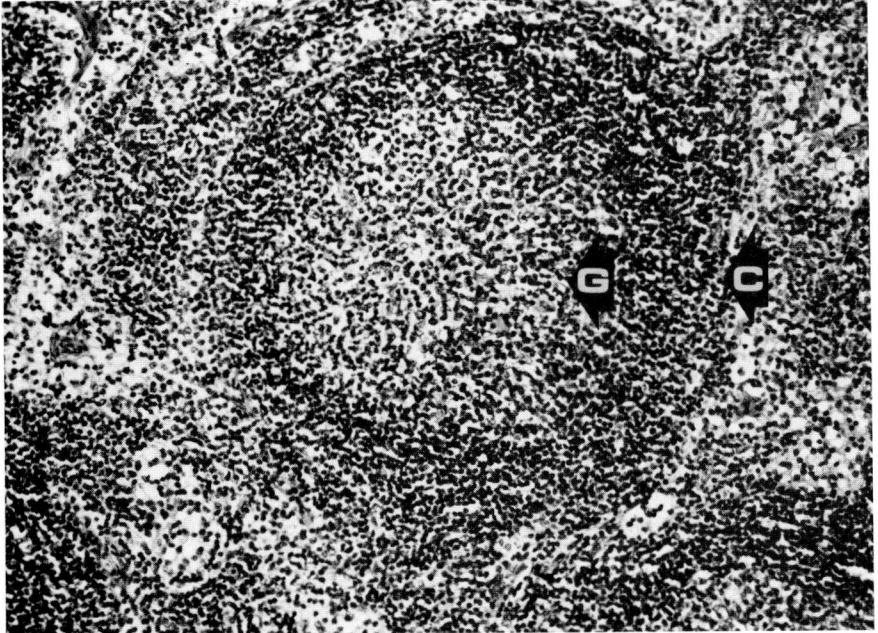

Fig. 17.11 A lymphatic nodule from a lymph node of an immunologically competent animal. The nodule consists of a central germinal center (G) and an outer corona (C). X40.

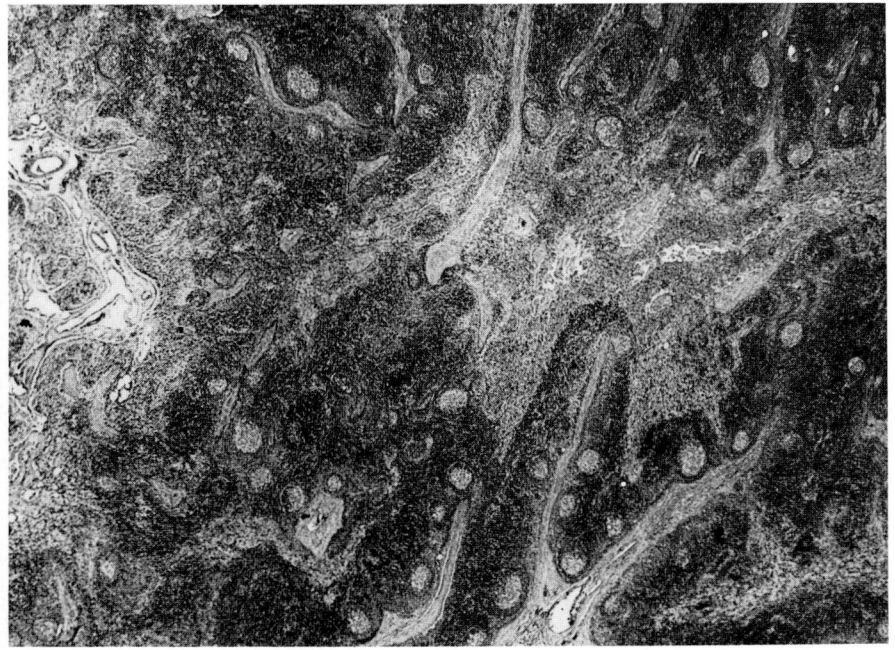

Fig. 17.12 A section of a porcine lymph node. The organization of the lymph node is the reverse of that which occurs in other mammals. X10.

with many fixed and wandering macrophages. These phagocytic cells, of course, are responsible for the removal of cellular detritus and foreign substances from the blood. A yellow-brown pigment, *hemosiderin* (a breakdown product of hemoglobin), is usually present in the phagocytic cells of the sinusoids and cords (Fig. 17.23). The three-dimensional relationships of splenic components are illustrated in Figure 17.24. **Splenic Circulation.** An understanding of the circulatory pattern through the spleen is essential for a general comprehension of its function (Fig. 17.25). *Splenic arteries* enter at the hilus and divide into *trabecular arteries*. These arteries leave the trabeculae and enter the splenic parenchyma. Upon entering the parenchyma lymphocytes accumulate in the adventitia of the vessels. This sheath of lymphocytes is continuous with splenic nodules. The vessel is then referred to as the *nodular arteriole*. Branches from this vessel supply capillaries in the white pulp and marginal region of the white pulp. They empty into the *red pulp sinuses* or into *pulp veins*. The nodular arteriole emerges from the white pulp and divides into several smaller branches, the *penicillar arterioles*. The penicillar arterioles are divisible into three regions: *red pulp arterioles*, *sheathed arterioles* and *terminal arterial capillaries*. The sheathed arterioles are branches of the red pulp arterioles and have thickened walls (*sheath of Schweigger-Seidel*), composed of concentric laminae of reticular cells and reticular fibers (Fig. 17.26). The termination of the arterial capillaries is a subject of much controversy. In the *closed theory*, the blood from the terminal arterial capillaries opens directly into the venous sinuses. This presumably occurs in man, rat and dog. In the *open theory*, the arterial capillaries terminate

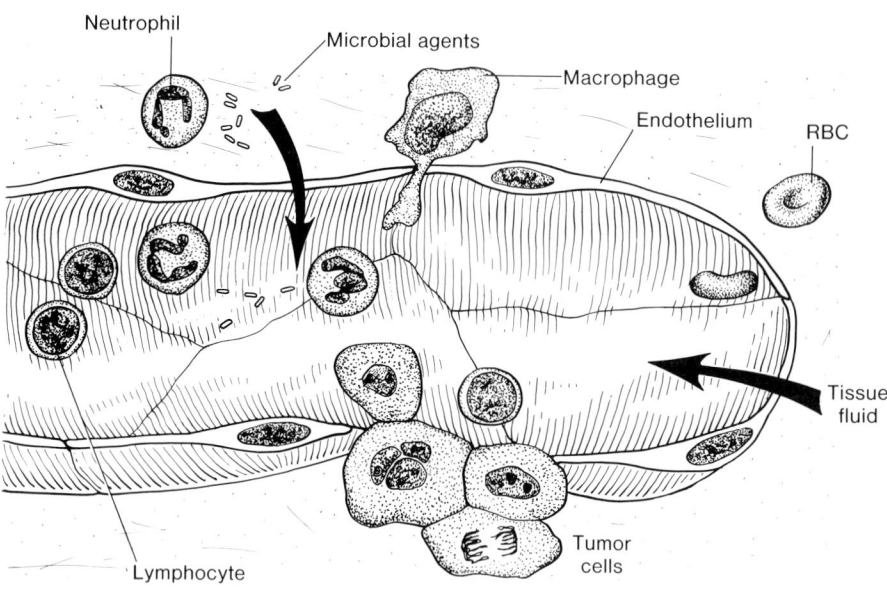

Fig. 17.13 A diagram of the terminal (initial) portion of a lymphatic capillary. White blood cells, some red blood cells, proteins, particulate matter, parasites, microbial agents and certain tumor cells gain access readily to the lymphatic vessels. Whereas such access serves as a method of involving the lymph nodes in the defense of the organism, infections may spread via the lymphatic vessels and tumor cells can spread (metastasize) to other organs of the body via the lymphatic vessels.

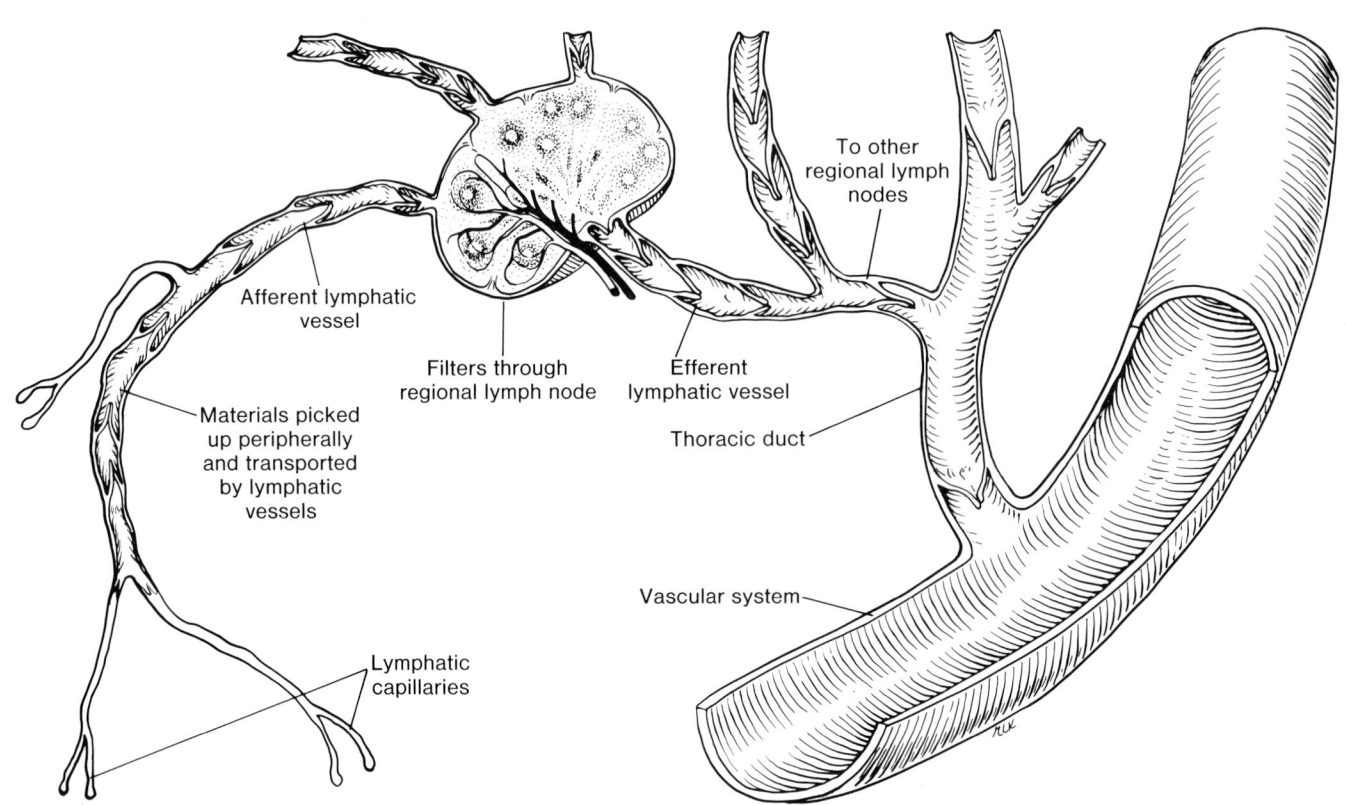

Fig. 17.14 An idealized schematic drawing of the flow of lymph to a lymph node and the return of the lymph fluid to the general circulation.

n the open reticulum of the red pulp and ilter into the venous sinuses. This is supposedly characteristic of the mouse, cat, norse, ox and swine. Some authors claim that both methods are utilized, whereas others claim that the circulation may change between both extremes. The question is academic: both methods achieve blood filtration.

Species Differences. Two basic types of spleens have been described, *defensive* and *storage* types. The first type has few trabeculae and muscle fibers but abundant lymphatic tissue (lagomorphs, man). The storage type has many trabeculae and smooth muscle fibers. It is relatively large and has less white pulp than the other form (horse, dog, cat). Intermediate forms are typical of ruminants and swine. Although red blood corpuscular destruction is typical of all spleens, it is especially well demonstrated in horses and swine.

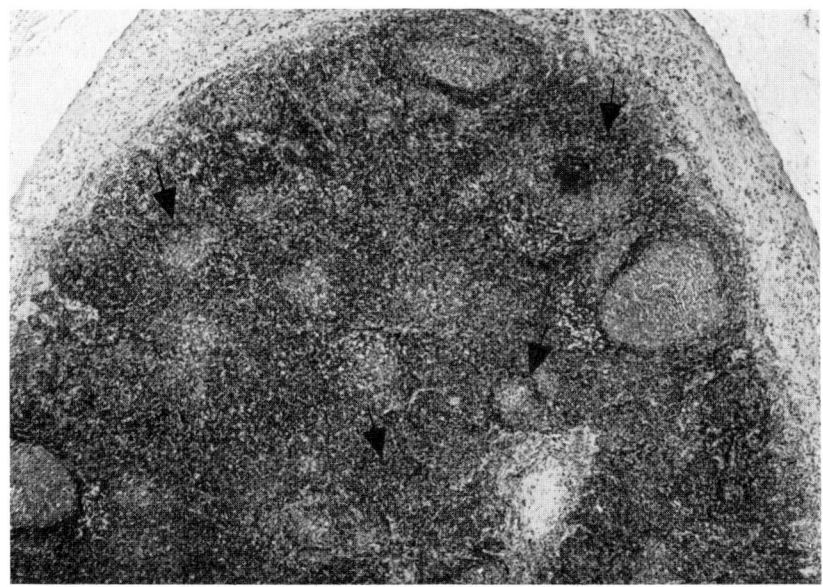

Fig. 17.15 A bovine hemal node. The organ is similar to a lymph node. Sinusoids (*arrows*), however, are engorged with blood. X10.

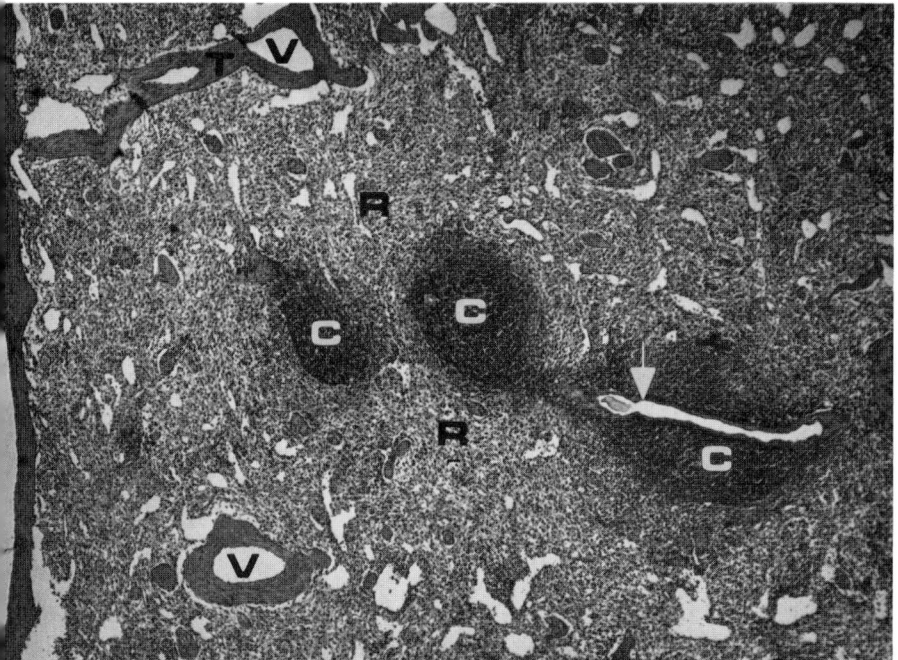

Fig. 17.16 General organization of the spleen. Trabeculae (T) invaginate into the parenchyma from the capsule. Trabeculae contain arteries and veins (V). The parenchyma consists of splenic corpuscles (C) that contain nodular arterioles (*arrow*). The corpuscles are surrounded by red pulp (R). X10.

Lymph Vessels. The spleen does not receive afferent lymph vessels from other portions of the body. Lymphocytes filter through the spleen from the blood. Only efferent lymphatic vessels occur in the white pulp; the predominant efferent channels occur in the trabeculae, capsule and hilus of the organ.

Innervation. Some myelinated nerve processes occur in the spleen: these are probably sensory nerves. The predominant nerves are postganglionic sympathetic fibers which are distributed to the smooth muscle of vessels (vasomotor), capsular smooth muscle, trabeculae and pulp regions.

Physiologic Correlates. Although the spleen performs important functions, it is not essential for life. After splenectomy other organs, especially the bone marrow and other myelolymphoid organs, assume some of its functions.

The filtration of blood by the spleen is significant in the removal of foreign particulate matter, microbial agents and old or degenerating blood cells from the circulation. Filtration and removal of blood-borne materials is achieved by splenic architecture and the macrophage system components, respectively. Sluggish blood flow through the splenic cords and marginal zones enhances phagocytosis by the perivascular macrophages of the splenic cords. Although other organs (lung, liver, bone marrow) contribute to this cleansing function, the spleen has the greatest capacity for it. The ability of the spleen to separate blood cells from plasma complements the cleansing function. The sympathetic stimulation of splenic veins increases pressure within the spleen and forces plasma into the lymphatic channels. Additionally, this separation results in a concentration of RBC's within the splenic cords.

The storage function of some spleens is enhanced by the separation phenomenon. The spleens of horses and carnivores may have a reservoir capacity for red blood corpuscles that approximates one-third of the circulating blood volume. Sympathetic discharge and the release of adrenomedullary secretions in response to stress (physical examination, venipuncture) can cause splenic capsular contraction. Contraction of the spleen results in the discharge of a concentrated mass of RBC's into the circulation with a corresponding increase in the packed cell volume. Similarly, some drugs (anesthetics, tranquilizers) may cause a splenic engorgement that is manifested as a decreased packed cell volume.

The storage function of the spleen is extended to platelets also. The spleen may store as much as one-third of the total circulating platelets. Splenectomy may result in a thrombocytosis, whereas an enlarged spleen may be associated with a decrease in peripheral thrombocytes (thrombocytopenia).

The sluggish flow of blood through the spleen facilitates the removal of aged or

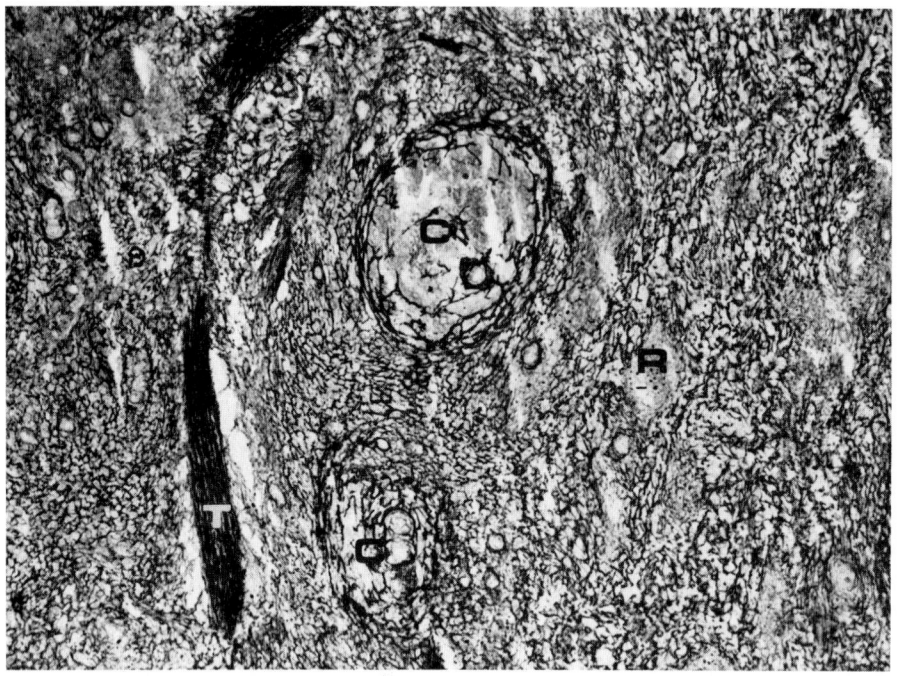

Fig. 17.17 Stromal elements of the spleen. The trabeculae (T) consist of DWFCT while the remaining stromal elements are reticular fibers. Splenic corpuscles (C) are delineated by red pulp (R). The germinal centers contain a paucity of fibrous stromal elements. X40 (reticular stain).

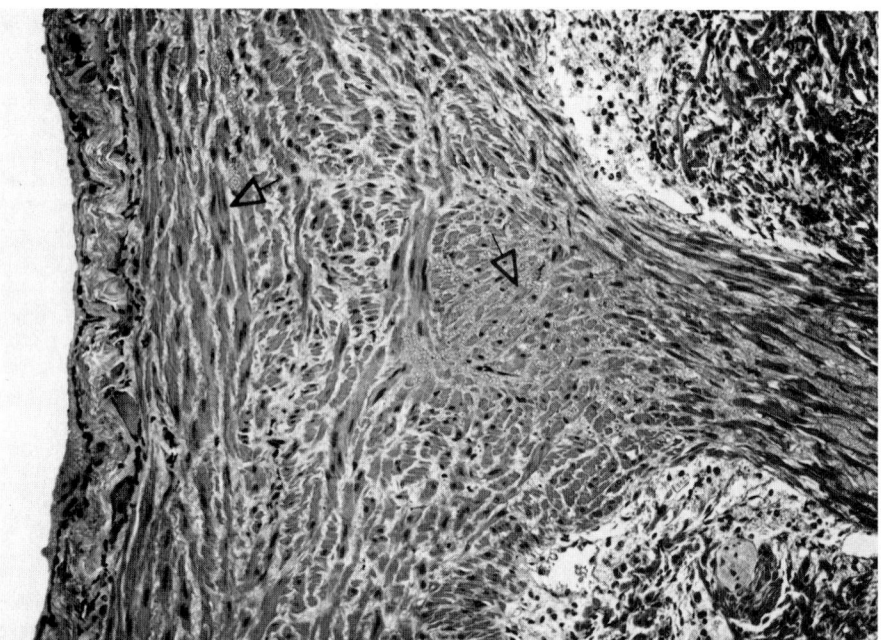

Fig. 17.18 Smooth muscle of the capsule and trabeculae of a cervine spleen. The smooth muscle (*arrows*) is a prominent splenic feature. X40.

damaged erythrocytes by this organ. The macrophages of the spleen are extremely sensitive to the surface characteristics of the erythrocytes. Cells that are incapable of surface deformation as they move through the spleen, such as the spherocytes of autoimmune hemolytic anemia, are subject to erythrophagocytosis. Similarly, the spleen is capable of removing particulate matter (HJ

bodies, Heinz bodies) and parasites from the surface of erythrocytes.

The fate of the components of the RBC, hemoglobin specifically, was discussed in Chapter 10.

Although the spleen functions as a hematopoietic organ during fetal and neonatal life, it is not a significant contributor to this function in the adult. However, the hema-

topoietic potential is retained throughou adulthood. The spleen may function as storage depot for immature RBC's durin which time they mature.

The spleen does assume an important rol in cell-mediated immunity and humoral an tibody responsiveness by virtue of its B an T lymphocyte populations within the whit pulp.

Thymus

Embryologic Origin. The thymus is derive from the endoderm of the third and fourt pharyngeal pouches in accompaniment wit the parathyroid derivative of the sam pouches. The pouches grow mediad an ventrad, separate from the pharyngeal wal join on the midline with their counterpar from the other side and continue cauda into the ventral cervical and thoracic regior The thymic anlagen, eventually separate from the parathyroid derivatives, occup part of the cranial mediastinum, thoraci inlet and ventral cervical region.

Although most endodermally-derive structures (liver, pancreas and other glands assume a parenchymatous configuration i which the epithelial component is the mos obvious cellular constituent, the thymus characterized by a uniquely different mor phogenesis. The densely packed mass o epithelial cells becomes more loosely ar ranged as a cellular reticulum coinciden with vascularization. Subsequent invasio by lymphocyte progenitors from the bon marrow converts the gland into a *lympho epithelial organ* in which the predominat feature is the presence of *thymocytes*. Thes lymphocytes comprise the parenchyma o the organ. As the gland continues to grow the epithelial cells—*epithelial-reticula cells*—become stellate cells that are attache to each other by desmosomes and form th peripheral limits of a system of labyrinth occupied by thymocytes and reticular cells The deep portion of the gland, *medulla*, ha fewer thymocytes and more reticular cell than the outer portion of the gland, th *cortex*, which has more thymocytes an fewer reticular cells. The lobules of the gland, containing cortical and medullar components, form as a consequence of vas cular invasion during development.

Histologic Structure. Both lobes of the or gan are covered by a capsule of loose con nective tissue from which septa of similal tissue arise and subdivide the organ int lobules (Fig. 17.27). These septa extend t the corticomedullary junction. The incom plete septation results in the lobules bein continuous with each other. In some sec tions, however, some lobules will appear t be completely encased by the capsular an septal tissue. Reticular connective tissu comprises the bulk of the stroma.

The organ is composed of a distinct *corte* and *medulla* (Fig. 17.27). Lymph nodules d not occur. The *cortex* consists of dense ac cumulations of small lymphocytes (*thymo*

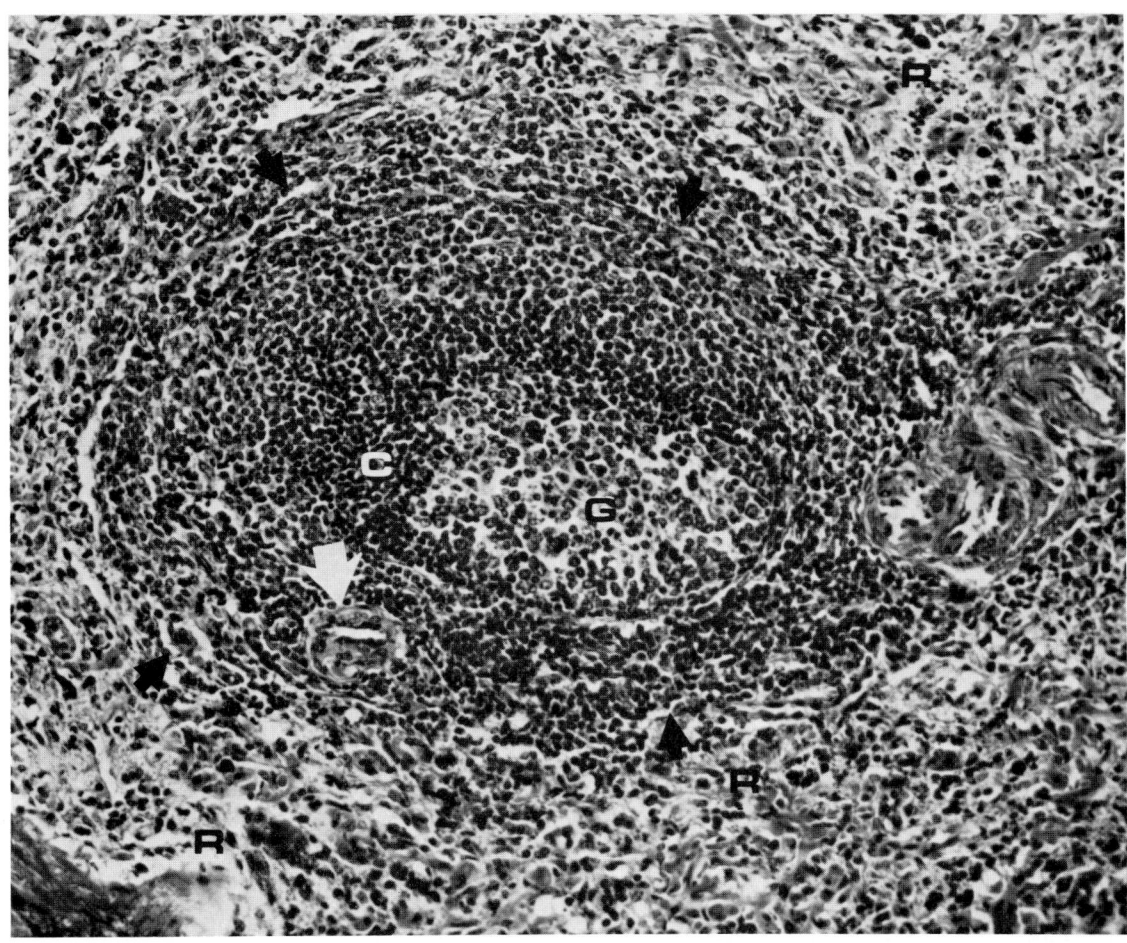

ig. 17.19   Splenic corpuscle and red pulp of a canine spleen. A germinal center (G), corona (C) or mantle layer and paracentral arteriole (*white rrow*) are apparent. The marginal zone (*black arrow*) separates the nodule from the red pulp (R). X40.

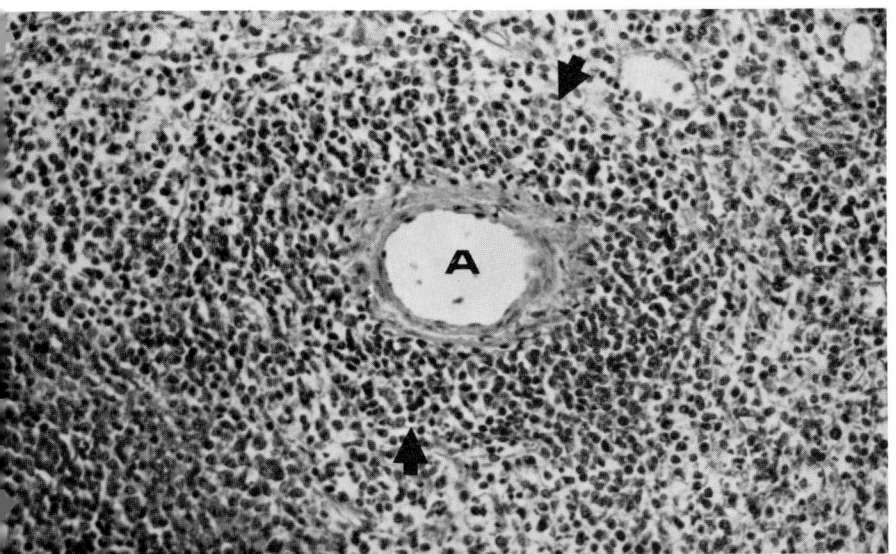

ig. 17.20   Periarterial sheath of lymphatic tissue. A condensation of white pulp constituents *rrows*) surrounds an arteriole (A). T lymphocytes occur in these loci. X40.

tes) which obliterate the reticular cells and *ticular* fiber stroma. Endodermally deved reticular cells are intercalated between *ie* blood capillaries and the cortical parenhyma. These *epithelial-reticular cells* conibute to the blood-thymus barrier.

The *medulla* of the organ consists of a cellular and fibrous stroma similar to the cortex (Fig. 17.28). The thymocytes of this region are not as dense; thus, the reticular cells are readily observed. The definitive feature of the organ, however, is the pres-

ence of *thymic corpuscles* (*Hassall's corpuscles*) which occur in the medulla (Fig. 17.29). These acidophilic bodies vary in diameter from 20 μm to more than 100 μm. They are concentric whorls of cells (probably reticular cells) in various stages of degenerative change. The hyaline-appearing cells can undergo keratinization and even mineralization. Pyknosis and karyolysis are common. They are often observed in advanced stages of involution. The peripherally located reticular cells of the bodies are continuous with the cellular stroma. Despite their being rich in gamma globulins, their exact role in immunity is unknown.

Blood Vessels and the Blood-Thymic Barrier. The arteries to the thymus ramify in the interlobular connective tissue and enter the substance of the organ at the corticomedullary junction of the lobules. Arterial capillaries penetrate and traverse the cortex to the periphery of the cortical parenchyma. Although some of these vessels are confluent with thymic venules within the capsule, most of them reverse their direction, forming arcades within the cortex and drain into venules of the corticomedullary junction and medulla. The capillaries of the cortex are impermeable to macromolecules.

Arteriolar branches from the cortico-

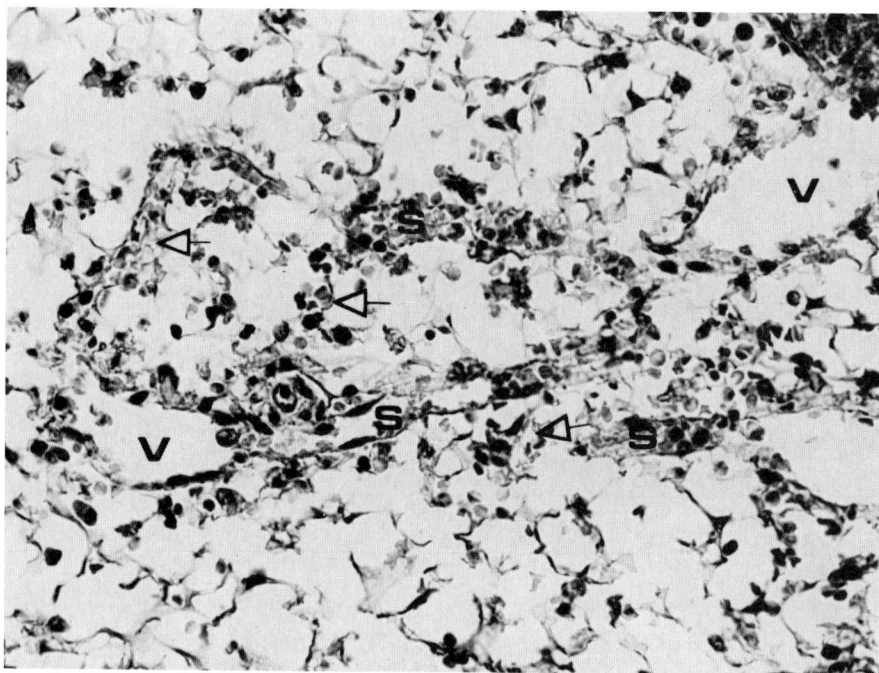

Fig. 17.21 Red pulp of the canine spleen that was flushed with physiologic saline during acquisition. Most of the free cells within the red pulp have been removed. Splenic cords (*arrows*), splenic sinusoids (S) and venous sinuses (V) are evident. X100.

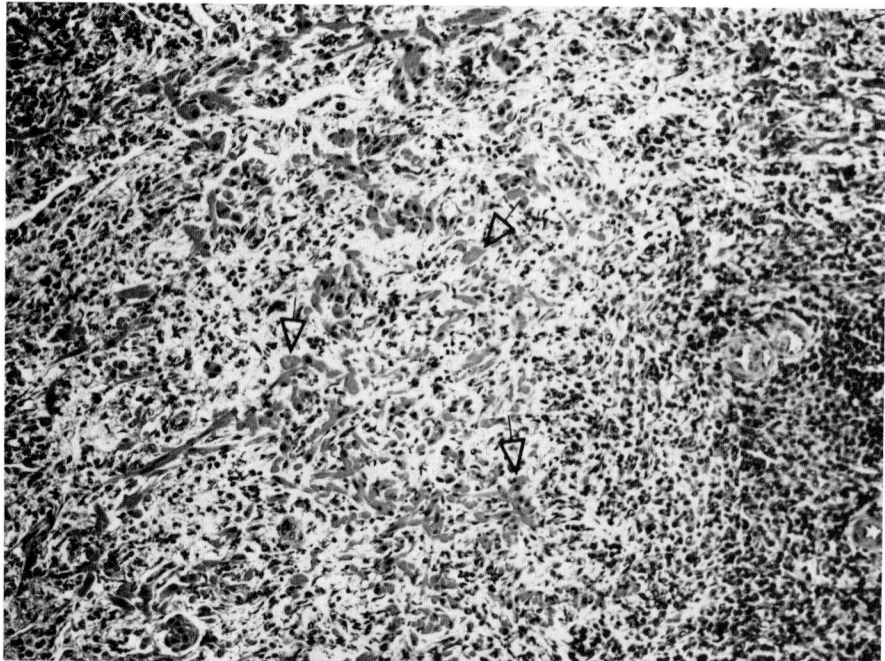

Fig. 17.22 Red pulp of a cervine spleen. The smooth muscle fibers (*arrows*) are prominent constituents of the red pulp in this organism. X40.

medullary vessels extend into the medulla, branch into capillaries and return as medullary veins to the corticomedullary junction. Postcapillary venules are permeable to macromolecules and lymphocytes.

The *blood-thymic barrier* consists of epi-thelial-reticular cellular investments of the vascular beds within the thymic parenchyma. Actually, the permeability characteristics of the cortical region limits the applicability of the term barrier to the cortical vessels. The medullary vessels are suffi-ciently permeable to macromolecules and lymphocytes that the postcapillary venule of the medulla and corticomedullary junction function in a manner similar to those vessels described with lymph nodes. Accordingly, these postcapillary venules do not contribute to a blood-thymic barrier.

Lymphatic Vessels and Innervation. Afferent lymphatic vessels are not associated with the thymus. Efferent lymphatic vessels occur as components of the connective tissue peripheral to the lobules.

Although some nerve fibers may occur freely within the parenchyma of the thymus, most of the nerve fibers of the gland, which are derived from the vagus and sympathetic nerves, are distributed to mural elements of the blood vessels.

Physiologic Correlates. The thymus is the primary lymphatic organ of mammals. Lymphocytes (thymocytes) which differentiate in the thymus leave the organ and populate secondary lymphatic organs (lymph nodes, spleen, tonsils, bone marrow and other aggregates of lymphatic nodules scattered throughout the body) with T cells. The specific distribution of T cells within secondary lymphoid organs was described previously. The movement of thymocytes through postcapillary venules to secondary lymphatic organs, *peripheralization*, is a significant aspect of cell-mediated immunity.

The thymus is an active organ during the development of the neonatal and postnatal animal and throughout adolescence. A gradual and continued involution of the thymus is accelerated after puberty and is characterized by a decrease in organ weight, a loss of cortical lymphocytes, infiltration by adipose cells and an increase in thymic corpuscles. Eventually, the infiltration of adipose cells completely replaces the cortical and medullary components of the organ.

The significant role of the thymus in immunity is demonstrated aptly by neonatal thymectomy in some species. Neonatal thymectomy results in an impairment of delayed hypersensitivity (cell-mediated immunity). The ability to produce an antibody-mediated response is impaired also, since some antibody production, that produced in response to T-dependent antigens, requires assistance from T cells. Congenital thymic deficiencies are characterized by identical immunologic deficiencies.

Humoral factors have been implicated in thymic function. *Thymosin* and *thymopoietin I* and *II* are hormones produced by the thymus which influence the development of progenitor cells into T cells.

Bursa of Fabricius. This structure is characteristic of birds (Fig. 17.30). It is a blind sac which opens on the dorsal wall of the proctodeum. It is often referred to as the "*cloacal tonsil*" or "*cloacal thymus.*" The wall of the organ is extensively folded and covered by a simple columnar or pseudo-stratified columnar epithelium. Lymphatic nodules are located between the folds of the

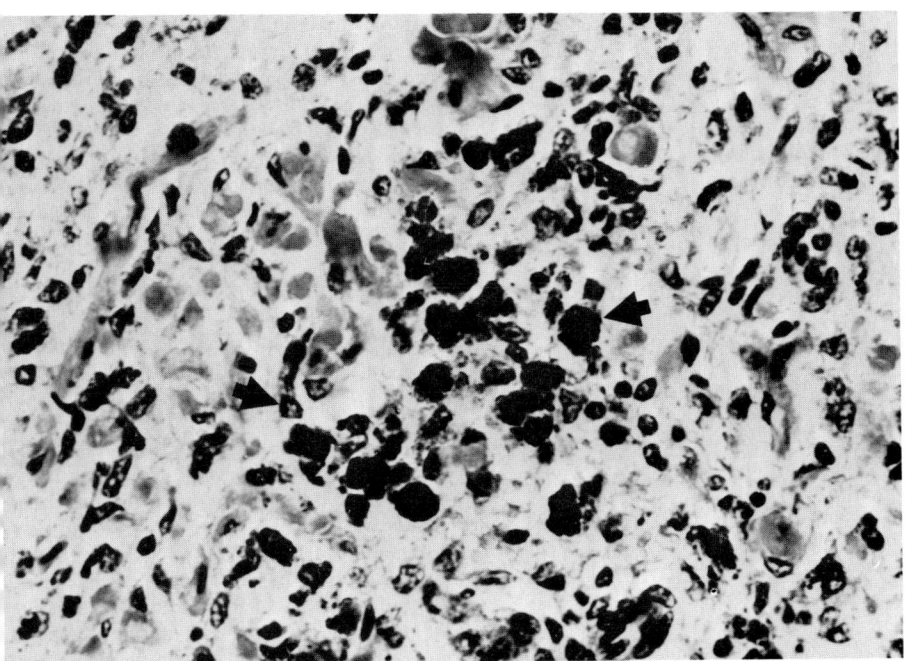

Fig. 17.23 Phagocytic cells within the red pulp of a canine spleen. Phagocytes (*arrows*) contain large quantities of hemosiderin. X100.

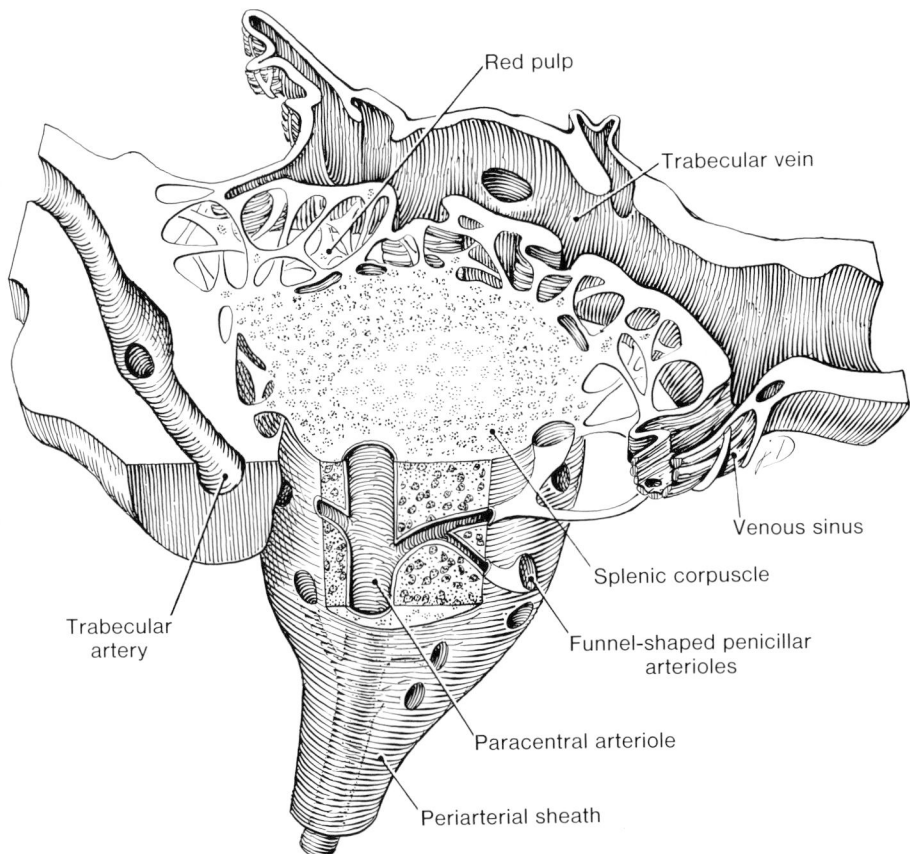

Red pulp

Trabecular vein

Venous sinus

Splenic corpuscle

Funnel-shaped penicillar arterioles

Paracentral arteriole

Periarterial sheath

Trabecular artery

Fig. 17.24 A three-dimensional drawing of a portion of the spleen.

epithelium and seem to produce follicle-like structures. Germinal centers are present. These are referred to as medullary structures, whereas the darker coronal regions are referred to as cortical areas. Although this organ resembles the tonsils and thymus, it functions in the development of B cells (Fig. 10.43).

Immunity

Introduction. Organisms of different species and individuals within a species, except for identical twins, possess a unique chemical identity. Although individuals within a species are composed of similar chemical constituents, their specific macromolecular composition is different. Moreover, various mechanisms have been developed by the body which protect it from foreign materials introduced exogenously. *The essence of these mechanisms is to maintain the chemical uniqueness by excluding all foreign materials.* The constituents that perform this protective function comprise the immune system. This system is an essential component of homeostatic mechanisms.

Nonspecific responses or *mechanisms* are integral components of the organism's resistance to exogenous macromolecules and various agents of disease. The innate genetic composition of some organisms precludes the successful invasion of a potential host by certain types of disease agents. *Similarly, specific anatomic, physiologic and biochemical factors afford non-specific protection.* The intact skin is an effective anatomic barrier to invasion by microbial agents. The elaboration of mucus and its continual rostral movement by the cilia of the respiratory tree afford an effective physiologic protection against invasive agents and particulate matter. The continual flushing of mucous membranes by fluids (lacrimation) and the continual movement of fluids (urination) and solids (defecation) from the body are dynamic defensive mechanisms. The acidity of various body secretions (urine) and the acidity of the luminal contents of some visceral organs (stomach, urinary bladder) protect against invasion by certain microbial agents. The phagocytic activity of neutrophils and macrophages affords non-specific protection. Similar protection results from the histiocytic secretion of *lysozomal enzymes* and the secretion of *β-lysins* from aggregated platelets, while the *properdin* group of serum proteins is the nonspecific activator of the complement system.

The *specific immune response* is an adaptive protective mechanism which permits the body to recognize and respond to specific foreign materials. The foreign materials that are capable of eliciting a specific immune response have a unique surface configuration (*antigenic determinant*) and are called *antigens.* Macrophages, lymphocytes and plasma cells are responsive to antigenic stimulation. The responsiveness is mani-

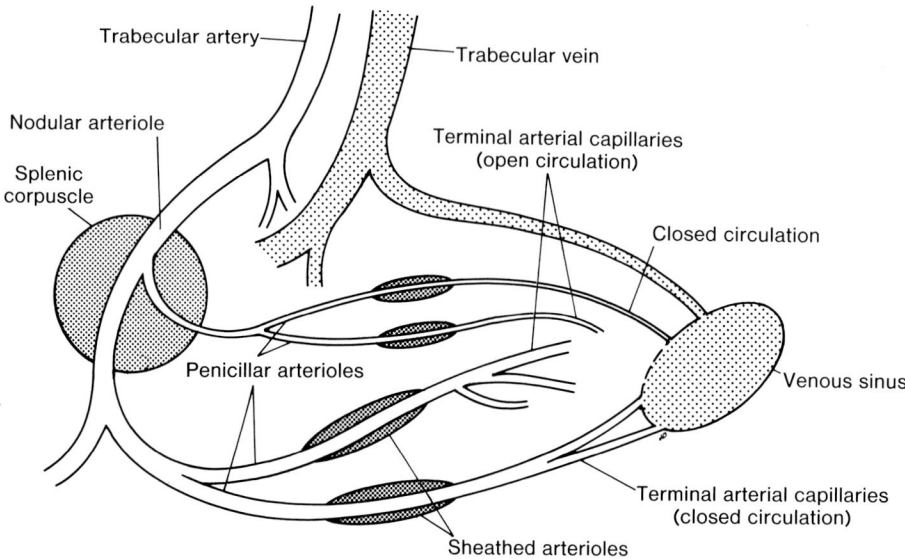

Nodular arteriole

Trabecular artery—

Trabecular vein

Terminal arterial capillaries (open circulation)

Splenic corpuscle

Closed circulation

Penicillar arterioles

Venous sinus

Terminal arterial capillaries (closed circulation)

Sheathed arterioles

Fig. 17.25 A schematic diagram of open and closed splenic circulation.

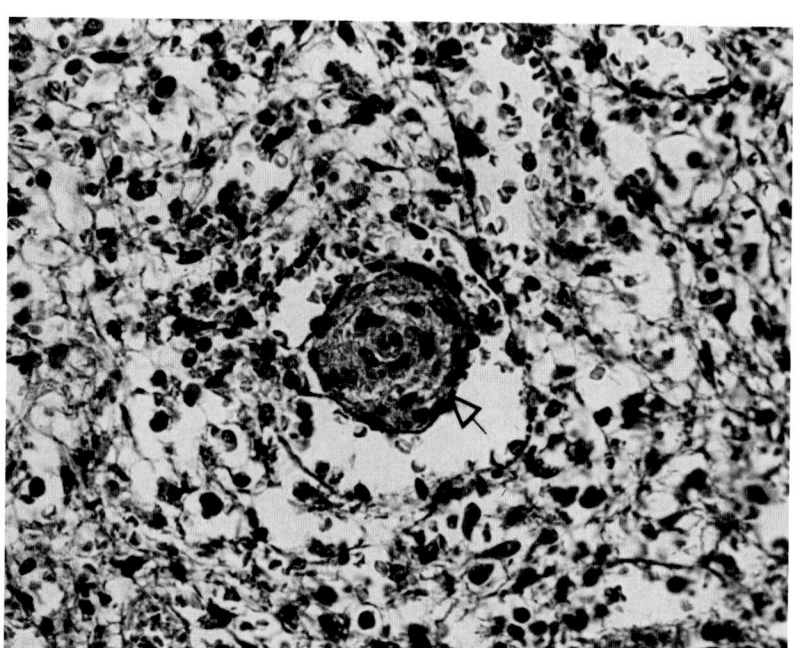

Fig. 17.26 A sheathed arteriole from the red pulp of a canine spleen evacuated and flushed with physiologic saline during acquisition. The sheathed arteriole (*arrow*) is surrounded by concentric whorls of reticular cells and fibers. X100.

fested as a *humoral antibody response* or a *cell-mediated immune response*.

Humoral Antibody Response. The humoral antibody response is a function of the B lymphocytes. Upon initial exposure to an antigen, the B lymphocyte is stimulated, becomes transformed into a blast cell, proliferates and produces a population of sensitized B lymphocytes and plasma cells (*clonal expansion*). This population includes effector cells which produce *antibodies* (*immunoglobulins*) and *memory cells* which become inactive but are capable of responding to the antigen at some future time. The initial response to an antigen, resulting in the production of antibodies, is called the

primary response (Fig. 17.31). A measurable antibody titer to the specific antigen can be determined after a variable but relatively long period of time (*latent period*). The subsequent exposure of the body to the same antigen can activate memory cells which were sensitized previously. This second exposure results in a more rapid and greater antibody-producing reaction than in the primary response and is termed the *secondary* or *anamnestic response* (Fig. 17.31).

Antibodies (Ab) bind to specific antigens (Ag) and facilitate their removal from the body. This binding may result in the precipitation of the Ab-Ag complex with subsequent *phagocytosis*; may *inhibit the uptake of*

certain antigens (viral) by cells; may induce the *lysis* of microbial agents by the activation of *complement*; or may facilitate the phagocytosis of various agents by macrophages (*opsonization*).

Antibodies (*immunoglobulins, Ig*) are plasma proteins that occur in the globulin fraction. Several classes of immunoglobulins have been identified: immunoglobulin G (IgG), immunoglobulin M (IgM), immunoglobulin A (IgA), immunoglobulin E (IgE) and immunoglobulin D (IgD).

Immunoglobulin G (*IgG*) is the most common antibody within the plasma. Approximately 85% of all immunoglobulins are IgG. Because of its small size, it leaves the vascular bed readily and enters the connective tissue. This immunoglobulin serves as the major antibody in humoral defense mechanisms and is produced in response to infections and immunizations. It is the predominant immunoglobulin of the anamnestic response. Although it is an effective *opsonin*, *agglutinin* and *precipitin* of antigens, it is not an efficient activator of complement. The half-life of immunoglobulin G is species variable (dog—7–8 days; ox—23 days).

Immunoglobulin M (*IgM*) is the second most common antibody within the globulin fraction of plasma and comprises approximately 10% of all the immunoglobulins. Immunoglobulin M is a large pentameric compound whose protective functions are probably confined to the vascular system. Although IgM is the predominant Ig of the primary response, it is also produced anamnestically; however, the level of IgM in the secondary response does not exceed the level of the primary response. This antibody functions similarly to IgG, but IgM is an efficient activator of complement. Immunoglobulin M is the first antibody formed by the fetus in response to antigenic stimulation. Immunoglobulin M has less specificity than IgG.

Immunoglobulin A (*IgA*) comprises approximately 10% of the total body immunoglobulins; however, it is not a major component of serum globulins. Rather, IgA is the major immunoglobulin in the external secretions of the body, wherein it affords primary antibody protection (first line of defense) for the mucous membranes of the respiratory, gastrointestinal and genitourinary systems and eye. Although IgA may assume polymeric forms, the most common forms of this immunoglobulin are monomers, dimers and trimers. The dimeric form of IgA passes through intestinal epithelial cells, salivary gland cells and hepatocytes. During this passage, a *secretory* or *transport piece* of protein is added to the dimeric structure, forming *secretory IgA*. The secretory piece increases the resistance of secretory IgA to proteolysis. Although secretory IgA serves as an important surface protecting compound, its mode of action is not understood precisely. It may prevent the adherence of microbial agents to epithelial surfaces. Protection of mucosal surfaces by gA may be broad-spectrum and is not characterized by an anamnestic response.

Although *immunoglobulin E (IgE)* comprises less than 1% of the total immunoglobulins, it possesses some unique characteristics that are integral components of the Type I hypersensitivity reactions.

Immunoglobulin D does not occur in domestic animals.

All of these immunoglobulins are integral components of the humoral antibody response of the organism to foreign materials. **Cell-Mediated Immune Response.** The T cells comprise the population of lymphocytes which are responsible for cell-mediated immunity (CMI). The T cells, like their B cell counterparts, are programmed to recognize and respond to specific antigens. The combination of antigen with T cell surface receptors results in a number of reactions that are not as well understood as the responsiveness of B cells to antigens. Nevertheless, the binding of antigen to T cell receptors initiates a blastoid transformation that results in cell division, expansion of this specific lymphocytic population and includes the generation of memory and effector cells. The activities of the effector cells are varied, but the response to antigenic stimulation does not include their synthesis and secretion of humoral antibodies.

Some activated or sensitized T cells become *cytotoxic lymphocytes (T killer cells)*. Upon intimate contact with the foreign cells that activated them, T lymphocytes cause lysis of the stimulating foreign cells. Although the mechanism that leads to foreign cell lysis is not understood, it probably involves a T cell-induced alteration of plasma membrane permeability.

The T lymphocytes also secrete soluble, non-antigen specific, short-lived proteins called *lymphokines*. Lymphokines, among their other activities, affect the activity of B lymphocytes and macrophages. T cells, then, exert an influence upon humoral antibody production and phagocytosis through the release of these soluble mediators.

The T cells also secrete molecules, *helper substances*, which are essential for an optimal antibody production response by the B lymphocytes. Although the precise mechanism for this influence is unknown, it probably involves macrophages and B cells. Helper substances may attach to macrophages so as to fix antigens to macrophage surfaces in a manner that permits recognition and response by the B cells. Alternatively, the helper substances may bind to the B cells in such a way as to permit their responsiveness to antigens presented by macrophages.

While some T cells serve as helper cells, others serve as suppressor cells. The *T suppressor cells* limit the humoral antibody response. Although the mechanisms are not understood, these cells may elaborate soluble factors that decrease B cell recognition of antigens, interfere with T helper cell interactions with B cells or limit the responsiveness of B cells to antigenic stimulation. Suppressor T cells may be involved in the *tolerance phenomenon*, the inability to respond to antigenic stimulation.

Cellular Interactions in Immunity. The myelolymphoid organs and the macrophage system, by virtue of their lymphocyte and macrophage populations, are essential components of normal immune responsiveness. Lymphocytes and macrophages cooperate in clearing foreign materials from the body.

The precise mechanisms of cellular cooperation in the production of humoral antibodies has not been determined; various

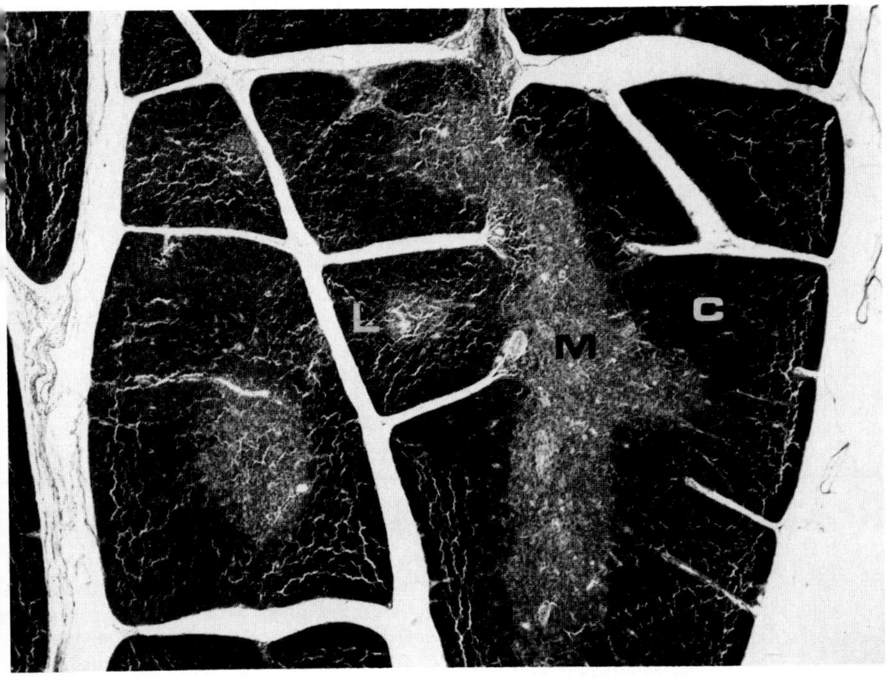

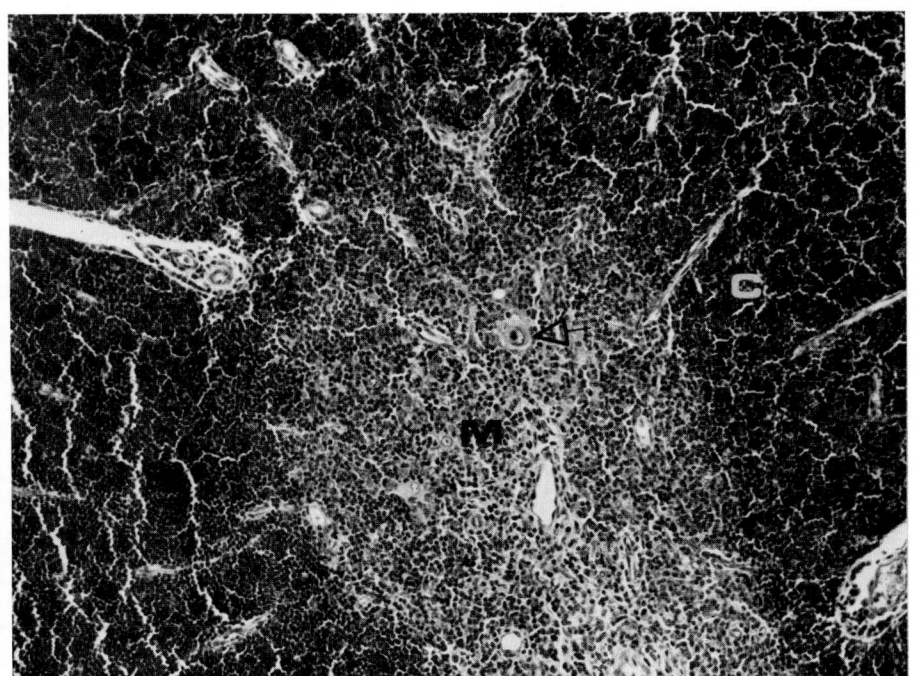

Fig. 17.27 The canine thymus gland. The loose connective tissue capsule covers the organ and divides it into distinct lobules (L). The lighter medulla (M) is surrounded by a dark cortex (C). The thymus may be considered one large nodule; individual nodules do not occur within the gland. X10.

Fig. 17.28 The cortex and medulla of a canine thymus gland. The cortex (C) contains more dense aggregations of thymocytes than does the medulla (M). A characteristic thymic corpuscle (*arrow*) is present. X40.

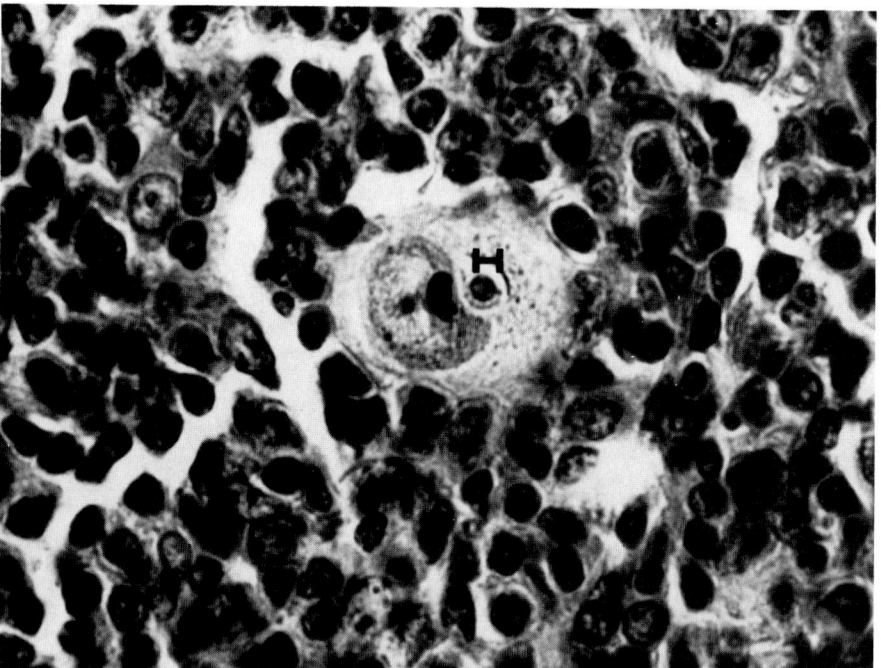

Fig. 17.29 A thymic corpuscle of a canine thymus gland. The thymic or Hassall's corpuscle (H) is a morphologic feature of the medullary portion of the organ. X320.

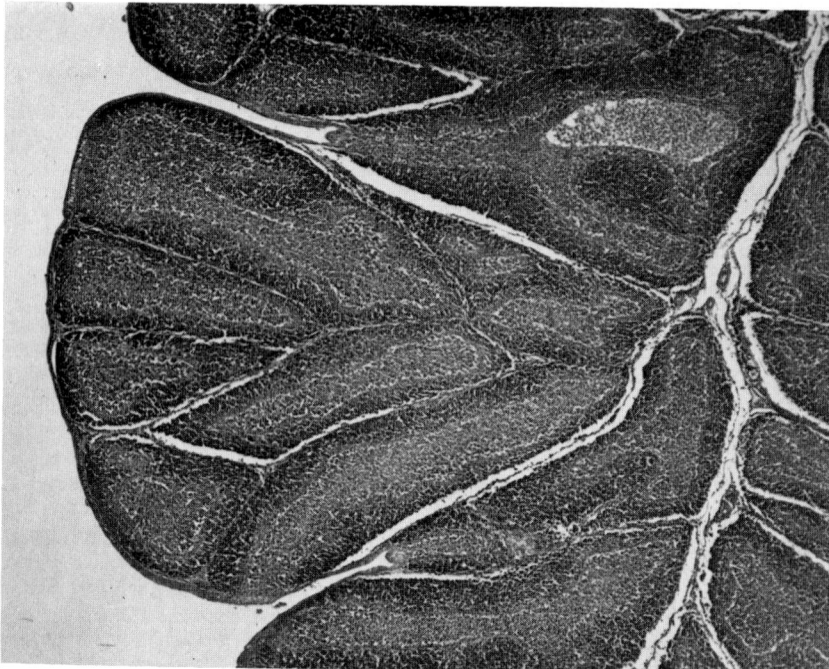

Fig. 17.30 The avian bursa of Fabricius. Lymphatic nodules are aggregated in such a way as to impart the architectural characteristics of the thymus gland. X10.

of antigen by the macrophages. Such an interaction results in a maximal antibody response to certain antigens.

Although continued research is essential to clarify the mechanisms that are operational, the macrophage plays a central role in the production of humoral antibodies. The macrophages trap and process antigens and facilitate the interaction of T cells and B cells. Whereas antigen trapping and processing is probably a nonspecific recognition activity, the subsequent cellular interactions lead to a specific antibody response.

Whereas some aspects of cell-mediated immunity are accomplished by T cells exclusively (T killer cells), macrophages, which are influenced by lymphokines, contribute to the phagocytic activity accompanying this process. The helper and suppressor aspects of this immune response were discussed previously.

The strategic positioning of wandering and fixed macrophages throughout the body insures that these cells will be exposed to foreign materials that may gain access to the body. Antigen processing and cellular interactions may occur in peripherally-positioned diffuse and nodular lymphatic tissues. Macrophage-processed and/or free antigens reach the lymph nodes by the vascular and/or lymphatic channels which enter these organs. The architecture of the lymph nodes (as well as other lymphoid organs) insures that antigens and macrophages will contact the cells responsible for specific immune responses.

Although the neutrophil performs phagocytic functions that protect the organism, these cells are not involved in antigen processing. Their entry into tissue spaces and their subsequent phagocytic activity culminates in their death and lysis within the tissue spaces.

Type I Hypersensitivity. The *type I hypersensitivities (allergies, anaphylaxis)* may be generalized or localized reactions of mast cells and basophils to certain antigens. This reactivity is mediated by immunoglobulin E. Because of the binding activity of IgE to cells, it is called a *cytotrophic antibody.* The interaction of antigen, IgE, and the reactive cells involves the release of pharmacologically active substances, the most significant of which is *histamine.* Although the type I reaction serves a protective function through its induction of an acute inflammatory response and the elimination of antigenic substances, it has deleterious side effects which can be life threatening.

Although certain antigenic substances may induce IgE production, not all individuals can produce this immunoglobulin. The production of IgE in response to antigenic stimulation (*atopy*) is determined genetically. The type I hypersensitivity response is summarized in Figure 17.32.

Upon initial exposure to the exciting antigen, the B cell population reacts by secreting IgE. Mast cells and basophils, which have specific receptors for the FC portions

theories have been proposed to explain B cell, T cell and macrophage interactions in this process. Humoral antibody production occurs as the result of macrophage and B cell interactions without the participation of T cells. This theory proposes that macrophages concentrate antigens on their surfaces or process the antigen and subsequently transfer information to B cells. Activation of B cells results from this interac-

tion. Alternatively, T cell and B cell surface interactions with antigens result in the activation of B cells and the production of humoral antibodies. The interactions involve the transfer of antigen and T cell receptors to macrophages, whereupon the subsequent or simultaneous interaction of the macrophages and B cells results in B cell activation. Finally, macrophages, T cells and B cells interact following the processing

of this immunoglobulin, bind IgE. After re-exposure to the same antigen, the antigen binds with the antigen-binding fragments of IgE. This antibody-antigen reaction causes the degranulation and/or lysis of these cells with the subsequent release of various active substances. *Histamine*, the most important of these substances, causes increased vas-cular permeability, vascular smooth muscle contraction and bronchoconstriction. Also, histamine stimulates the secretion of exo-crine glands, including those of the respira-tory tract and gastrointestinal tract. The *slow-reacting substance of anaphylaxis* (*SRS-A*) induces smooth muscle contrac-tion and an increased vascular permeability.

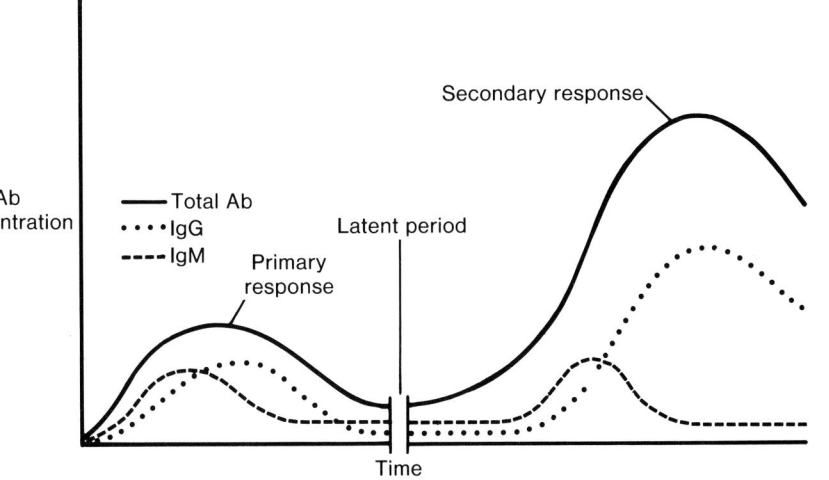

Fig. 17.31 The primary and secondary response of the body after antigenic stimulation.

Platelet aggregating factors (*PAF*) cause platelet aggregation and induces them to release their serotonin and histamine con-tent. *Serotonin* is released from mast cells and platelets. Its biologic activity is species variable. It may increase vascular permea-bility, vasoconstriction and cardiac stimu-lation. *Kininogens* are components of the α-globulin fraction of serum proteins. Kin-inogens are converted to *kinins* by the pro-teolytic activity of *kallikreins*. Kallikreins are released from the cells involved in al-lergic reactions as well as from activated platelets. *Bradykinin*, one of the important kinins, is a potent stimulator of smooth mus-cle contraction and increased permeability. The *eosinophilic chemotactic factor of ana-phylaxis* (*ECF-A*) attracts eosinophils to the area of antigen-stimulated mast cells and basophils and accounts for the localized and/or generalized eosinophilia that accom-panies such reactions. *Prostaglandin F* is released secondarily by other cells that are stimulated by the active factors from mast cells and basophils. Prostaglandin F stimu-lates degranulation of mast cells, vasocon-striction and bronchial smooth muscle con-traction.

Eosinophils are integral components of type I hypersensitivity reactions. They release factors (enzymes) which neutralize the active substances secreted by mast cells. Moreover, they secrete *prostaglandins E* (*PGE*) which are inhibitors of histamine secretion and stimulators of vasodilation. Eosinophils are important modulators of type I hypersensitivity reactions.

The clinical manifestations of type I hy-persensitivities are quite variable. Cuta-neous reactivity is manifested by the swell-ing and erythema (wheal and flare) associ-ated with insect bites. Generalized atopic reactivity (*anaphylactic shock*) may be man-ifested as cardiopulmonary distress and/or gastrointestinal upset. The type of response is species-specific, since various organs (*shock organs*) of domestic species and man have differential responsiveness to the bio-logic activity of the active substances re-leased during this reaction. Numerous anti-gens (*allergens*) are capable of inducing lo-calized and/or generalized type I reactions. **Type II Hypersensitivity.** *Type II hypersen-sitivity* is also called *cytotoxic* or *cytolytic reactivity.* This type reaction involves im-munoglobulins (IgG, IgM), complement, neutrophils, macrophages and tissue anti-gens. Type II hypersensitivity reactions are summarized in Figure 17.33.

Cytotoxic reactions are characterized by the reaction of circulating antibodies (IgG, IgM) with antigens that are attached to cell surfaces or antigens that have become inti-mate components of cell surfaces. The bind-ing of immunoglobulins with these antigens activates the complement system. The sub-sequent binding of complement at the site of antigen-antibody reaction results in the lysis of the surface-modified cell. Alterna-tively, the antigen-antibody reaction at the

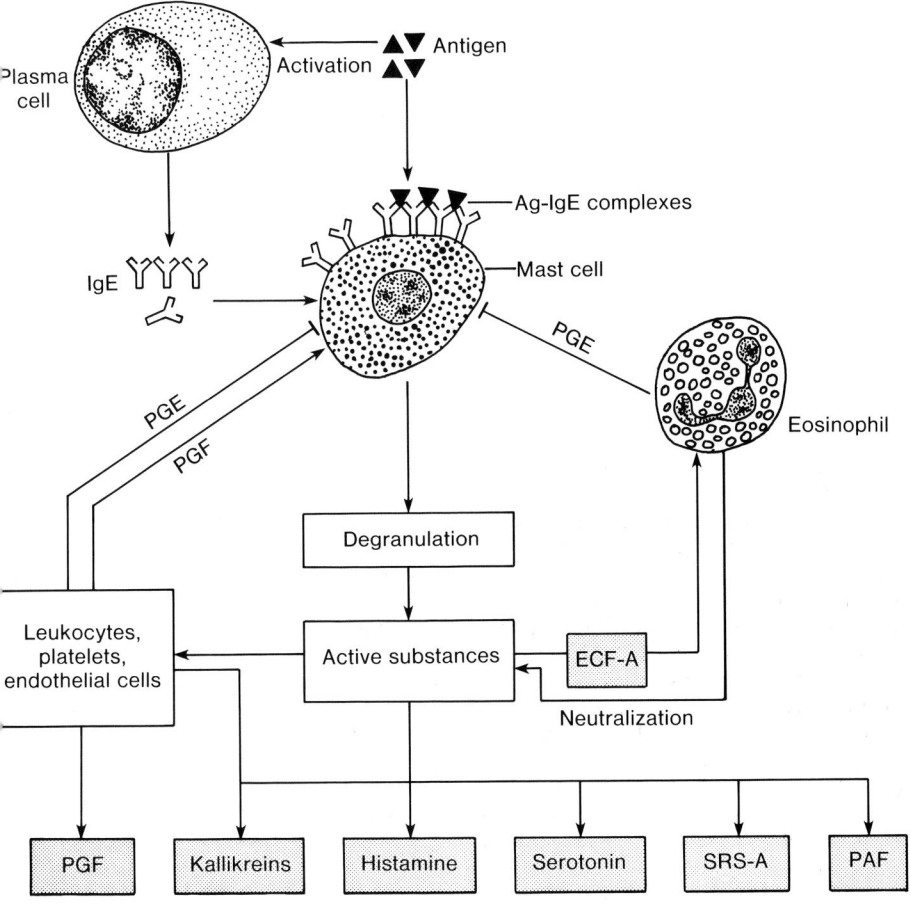

Fig. 17.32 A diagram depicting the events of the type I hypersensitivity reaction. *Arrows* represent flow or stimulation, whereas *bars* represent inhibition. Refer to the text for a complete description of this reaction.

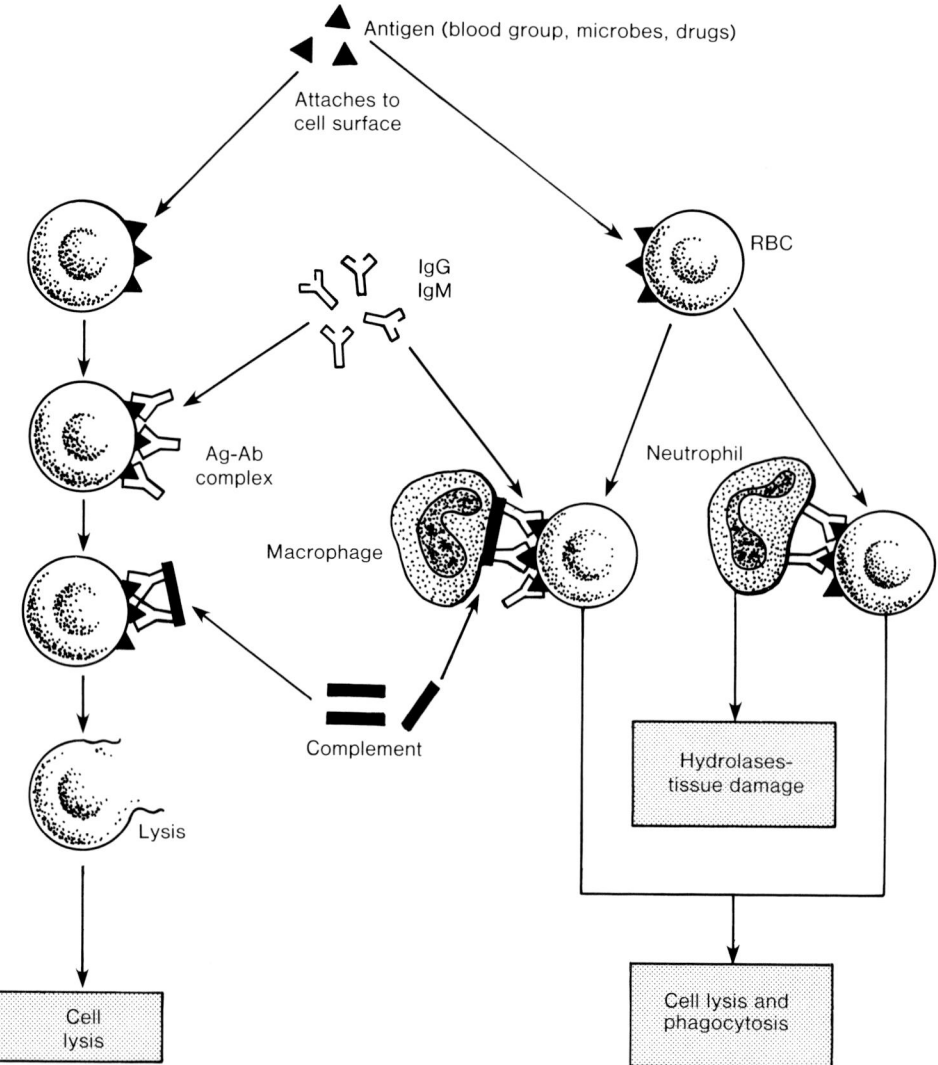

Antigen (blood group, microbes, drugs)

Attaches to cell surface

IgG
IgM

RBC

Ag-Ab complex

Macrophage

Neutrophil

Complement

Lysis

Hydrolases-tissue damage

Cell lysis

Cell lysis and phagocytosis

Fig. 17.33 A diagram depicting the events that characterize the type II hypersensitivity reaction.

cell surface permits the adherence of phagocytic cells (neutrophils and macrophages) to the cell surface. Cell lysis and phagocytosis are the consequences of this cellular responsiveness. Cellular lysis and phagocytosis are enhanced when complement is bound to the antigen-antibody complex. Additionally, the release of hydrolases by the phagocytic cells causes surrounding tissue damage.

The important characteristic of this response is the reactivity to tissue antigens. Reactions to incompatible transfusions, neonatal isoerythrolysis, RH factor incompatabilities in man (erythroblastosis fetalis), autoimmune hemolytic anemia, immune thrombocytopenia and certain other immune-mediated disease processes are characterized by type II hypersensitivity reactions.

Type III Hypersensitivity. The *type III hypersensitivity* response is also called the *toxic complex reaction.* Antigens introduced into the body result in the formation of immune complexes that activate the complement system. The initiation of the complement cascade results in the release of factors that cause platelet aggregation, mast cell degranulation and the accumulation of neutrophils. Extensive tissue damage, inflammation and necrosis result.

Type III reactions are characterized by two responses to antigens. The *Arthus reaction* is the result of the localized accumulation of immune complexes. The generalized circulation of immune complexes initiates the second type III response, *serum sickness.* Although the formation of immune complexes is the natural sequel to humoral antibody production, type III reactions may be manifested when excessive amounts of antigen-antibody complexes are formed.

The Arthus reaction may be initiated when an antigen to which the organism is able to respond is introduced into the subcutis, as might occur after a vaccination booster injection. (The Arthus reaction is diagrammed in Fig. 17.34). The antigen within the connective tissue reacts with IgG. Some controversy exists relating to the function of IgE in this reaction. The immune complexes of IgE and antigen may cause the release of vasoactive amines from mast cells. The resultant increase in vascular permeability may permit the leakage of IgG from the vascular bed and facilitate the formation of antigen and IgG immune complexes. Importantly, the immune complex involving IgG fixes complement. Various products of the complement cascade, C3a, C5a, C3b and C567, initiate helpful and damaging sequelae. The release of C567 attracts neutrophils to the local area, whereas the release of C3b facilitates the adherence of neutrophils to the immune complexes. The opsonizing influence of C3b results in the phagocytosis and clearance of the immune complexes. *Anaphylatoxins* (C3a, C5a) cause mast cell degranulation and the release of vasoactive substances. The release of hydrolases (collagenases, elastases, proteases) by the neutrophils causes the localized damage that characterizes the Arthus reaction. Vascular wall damage exacerbates the localized response by attracting more neutrophils which release more hydrolases, and damaging endothelial cells which release kallikreins and aid in the generation of kinins. The resultant hemorrhage leads to clot formation and necrosis of the tissues that have been deprived of their vascular supply (*ischemic necrosis*). The complement cascade induction of platelet aggregation also exacerbates the tissue necrosis. The severe localized inflammatory response of the Arthus reaction may be observed in dogs either infected or vaccinated with live adenovirus type I (infectious canine hepatitis virus) and is manifested as

"blue eye." Arthus reactions, however, can occur in any localized focus of antigen-antibody accumulation.

Serum sickness involves similar initiating mechanisms as those described for the Arthus reaction. The significant difference is the soluble nature of the immune and complement complex that forms. A portion of these complexes that are insoluble are cleared from the body by the macrophage system. The soluble complexes circulate throughout the vascular system and eventually deposit themselves on vascular endothelial cells. The deposition of these complexes initiates those events attributable to various complement factors described for

the Arthus reaction. Severe damage to the kidney (glomerulonephritis) can result when these complexes are deposited within the glomerulus. Although the precise mechanism of kidney damage is not understood, it occurs without the involvement of neutrophils. Mesangial cell, endothelial cell and epithelial cell proliferation, as well as basement membrane alterations cause excessive protein loss in the urine.

Type IV Hypersensitivity. *Type IV hypersensitivity* is also called *delayed hypersensitivity* and *cell-mediated immunity*. Whereas the previously-described hypersensitivities involve the immunoglobulins and are manifested within minutes or hours, the delayed hypersensitivity reaction does not require immunoglobulins and occurs initially over a period of 8–12 days. The mechanism of type IV hypersensitivity is that which was described for cell-mediated immunity. Specifically, cytotoxic lymphocytes, lymphokines and macrophages are the contributing components. The infiltration of mononuclear cells into areas of antigen concentration is the characteristic histologic feature. The rejection of foreign skin grafts, the response to intradermal injections of tuberculin, the skin reactivity to certain contact agents and the response to certain arthropods are examples of type IV hypersensitivity reactions.

Autoimmunity. The chemical uniqueness of the organism is maintained by the nonspecific and specific immune mechanisms discussed previously. The essence of these mechanisms is predicated upon the ability of the cellular components of the immune system to recognize those substances that are "self" and those that are foreign. The inability to recognize substances as self results in the formation of autoantibodies and the destruction of somatic tissues. Various mechanisms are proposed to explain this self-destructive phenomenon. Autoantibodies may be produced against body components that normally are not "seen" by the lymphocytes following damage that results in exposure to the surveillence cells. New antigens may be developed within the body as a result of viral influence and/or the incorporation of foreign materials with normal body components. These and other mechanisms may be responsible for the activation of the immune processes against "self." Autoimmunity is manifested as Type I–IV hypersensitivity reactions. Systemic lupus erythematosus, autoimmune thyroiditis, myasthenia gravis and rheumatoid arthritis are examples of autoimmune or *immune-mediated diseases*.

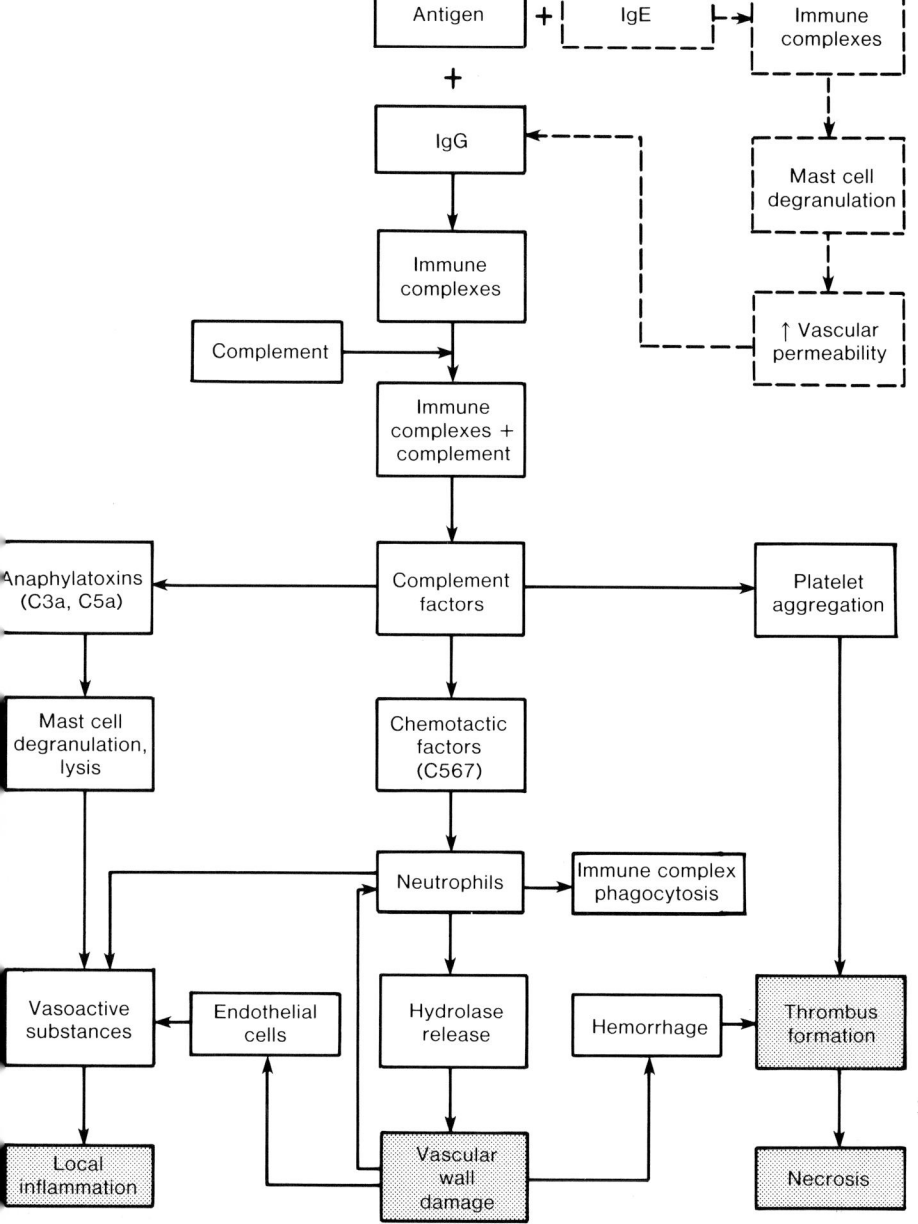

Fig. 17.34 A diagram which depicts the events associated with the Arthus reaction. The *dashed lines* and *boxes* represent controversial aspects of the reaction.

References

Burnet, F. M.: The thymus gland. Sci. Amer. *207:*50, 1962.

Clark, S. L., Jr.: The reticulum of lymph nodes in mice studied with the electron microscope. Amer. J. Anat. *110:*217, 1962.

Cohn, Z. A.: The structure and function of monocytes and macrophages. Adv. Immunol. 9:163, 1968.

Edwards, V. D. and Simon, G. T.: Ultrastructural aspects of red cell destruction in the normal rat spleen. J. Ultrastruct. Res. 33:187, 1970.

Fujisaki, S.: The fine structure of Hassall's corpuscles and reticular cells in the mouse thymus. Acta Med. Biol. 14:107, 1966.

Hayes, T. G.: The marginal zone and marginal sinus in the spleen of the gerbil. A light and electron microscopy study. J. Morphol. 141:205, 1973.

Hoshino, T., Takeda, M., Abe, K. and Ito, T.: Early development of thymic lymphocytes in mice, studied by light and electron microscopy. Anat. Rec. 164:47, 1969.

Jaroslow, B. N.: Genesis of Hassall's corpuscles. Nature 215:408, 1967.

Levin, P. M.: The development of the tonsil of the domestic pig. Anat. Rec. 45:189, 1930.

Meyer, A.: Hemal nodes in bovines and goats. Amer. J. Anat. 21:359, 1917.

Moe, R. E.: Electron microscopic appearance of the parenchyma of lymph nodes. Amer. J. Anat. 114:341, 1964.

Movat, H. Z. and Fernando, N. V. P.: The fine structure of the lymphoid tissue during antibody formation. Exp. Molec. Pathol. 4:155, 1965.

Murray, R. G., Murray, A. and Pizzo, A.: The fine structure of the thymocytes of young rats. Anat. Rec. 151:17, 1965.

Payne, F. and Breneman, W. R.: Lymphoid areas in endocrine glands in the fowl. Poult. Sci. 31:155, 1952.

Peck, H. M. and Hoerr, N. L.: The intermediary circulation in the red pulp of the mouse spleen. Anat. Rec. 109:447, 1951.

Raviola, E. and Karnovsky, M. J.: Evidence for a blood-thymus barrier using electron-opaque tracers. J. Exp. Med. 136:466, 1972.

Renston, R. H., Jones, A. L., Christiansen, W. D., Hradek, G. T. and Underdown, B. J.: Evidence for a vesicular transport mechanism in hepatocytes for biliary secretion of immunoglobulin A. Science 208:1276, 1980.

Roberts, D. K. and Latta, J. S.: Electron microscopic studies on the red pulp of the mouse spleen. Anat. Rec. 148:81, 1964.

Song, S. H. and Groom, A. C.: A scanning electron microscope study of the splenic red pulp in relation to the sequestration of immature red cells. J. Morphol. 149:437, 1974.

Tehver, J. and Grahame, I.: Capsule and trabeculae of spleens of domestic mammals. J. Anat. 65:473, 1931.

Tizard, I. R.: An Introduction to Veterinary Immunology. W. B. Saunders, Philadelphia, 1977.

Unanue, E. R.: The regulatory role of macrophages in antigenic stimulation. Adv. Immunol. 15:95, 1972.

Weiss, L.: The Cells and Tissues of the Immune System. Structure, Functions, Interactions. Prentice-Hall, Englewood Cliffs, 1972.

Yamori, T. and Mori, Y.: Electron microscopic observation of reticuloendothelial system. Tohoku J. Exp. Med. 81:330, 1964.

18: Integumentary System

General Characteristics

Form and Function. The integumentary system consists of all of the basic tissues discussed previously, as well as specific structures that are derivatives of this external body covering. The *integument* or *skin* includes the epithelial covering, its derivatives and its associated connective tissue. The outermost layer of the skin or *epidermis* is composed of stratified squamous epithelium (Fig. 5.8–5.12). The epidermis is divisible into distinct layers; the number of layers varies with different regions of the body (Plate I.1). The *dermis* or *corium* underlies the epidermis and varies from loose connective tissue to dense white fibrous connective tissue. The *hypodermis* or *subcutis* consists of loose connective tissue that connects the dermis to underlying periosteum, perichondrium, or deep fascia. The nature of the hypodermis (superficial fascia) varies with the location in the body. Some areas contain high quantities of adipose cells (footpads), whereas others have very small amounts of adipose cells (scrotum, eyelids, ears). The dermis and hypodermis contain numerous blood vessels, nerves and lymphatic vessels.

Many structures are derivatives of the skin: hair, nails, claws, feathers, horns, antlers, combs, wattles, sweat glands, sebaceous glands, mammary glands and hooves. The skin and its diversified structures perform numerous and varied functions.

The most important function of the skin is its effectiveness as a two-way *barrier* between the internal and external environment. The skin prevents the loss of water (*desiccation*), electrolytes and macromolecules into the external environment. Also, it protects against the invasion of physical, chemical and microbial agents into the body. The secretory products of tubular glands (in some animals), the hair coat and cutaneous blood supply are mediators of *temperature regulation*. The cutaneous vascular supply also contributes to alterations in *blood pressure*. The skin glands contribute to the diverse *secretory functions* of this organ (sebum, sweat). Milk is a secretory product of the mammary gland, a discrete organ of this system. In some species, the skin glands contribute an *excretory function*. The skin is involved in *calcium homeostasis* by virtue of the ultraviolet light conversion of 7-dehydrocholecalciferol to cholecalciferol within the sebaceous glands (Chapter 8); however, the ultraviolet component of solar radiation is capable of damaging living tissues. The pigmentation of the skin *protects against actinic damage*. Whereas the elasticity and strength of the skin provide for *motion* and *external form*, highly cornified structures provide for *locomotion*. *General behavioral patterns, sexual behavioral displays* and *mechanical protection* are afforded by this system, also. The skin is an extensive *sensory organ*. General somatic afferent modalities, including pain, pressure and temperature, as well as special somatic afferent information from the eyes and ears, function to integrate the organism within its surrounding external environment.

Clinically, the skin is an important organ. Besides being one of the largest organs of the body, it may reflect a variety of external and internal disease processes (ectoparasitism, immune-mediated disease, endoparasitism, endocrine disorders, nutritional problems).

Mammalian Integument

Development. The epidermis develops from ectoderm, whereas the dermis and hypodermis are derivatives of the mesoderm. Initially, the epidermis is composed of a layer of simple cuboidal epithelial cells. Proliferation of these cells results in the stratification of cells which typifies the epidermis. Basal cell layer proliferation adds progressively to the thickness of this outer covering; however, basal cell proliferation and invagination into the underlying dermis and hypodermis account for the information of hairs, feathers and glands, the cells of which are continuous with the cellular layers of the epidermis.

The dermis and hypodermis develop from typical mesenchyme. Progressive proliferation and differentiation of mesenchymal cells result in the establishment of resident cellular populations that typify loose and dense connective tissues.

Organization of the Skin

Epidermis. The *epidermis* is composed of distinct layers that comprise the outer layer of the body (Figs. 18.1, 5.8). However, the relative amounts of these layers will vary from region to region. The most basal layer is termed the *stratum germinativum* (Fig. 5.9). It varies from one to a dozen or more cell layers thick. This zone is further divisible into two distinct strata. That which abuts on the basement membrane is termed the *stratum basale* or *stratum cylindricum*. The cells of this zone vary from cuboidal to columnar. A *stratum spinosum* or *parabasal layer* is located peripheral to the basal layer (Fig. 5.10). It varies in thickness and is characterized by *apparent* intercellular bridges. The cells gradually change from a polyhedral to a squamous configuration. Pigment, when present, extends into this zone as far as the transition into the next region of the epidermis. The stratum germinativum is of variable thickness. It is usually thick in hairless regions of the body and rather thin in heavily haired regions.

The *stratum granulosum* contains flattened rhomboidal or squamous cells which possess keratohyalin granules (Fig. 5.11). The granules are also of variable occurrence and may be absent in regions where hair is abundant. The term *intermediate layer* is applicable to this zone.

The *stratum lucidum* consists of several layers of homogeneous, translucent, squamous cells that are only slightly stainable. Keratohyalin granules are no longer visible, but a substance called eleiden is present. This zone is especially prominent in very thick epidermal regions of the body, such as the footpads of carnivores.

The superficial *stratum corneum* consists of several to many layers of anucleated, squamous, cornified (keratinized) cells (Fig. 5.12). A fibrous protein, keratin, is abundant. In noncornified areas, the term *superficial layer* is used. Dead cells are sloughed from the peripheral portion of this zone.

Dermis. The *dermis* or *corium* is separated from the epidermis by a typical basement membrane. Two zones are described in the dermis, a *papillary* and a *reticular area* (Fig. 18.2). They are, however, quite similar and blend insensibly with each other. The connective tissue of the papillary region is areolar and varies to DWFCT in the reticular zone. The term reticular does not refer to the presence of reticular fibers; rather, it refers to the reticular arrangement of the collagenous fibers of the region. Elastic fibers, which usually stain a bright pink with routine hematoxylin and eosin (H and E) are prominent in both zones.

Dermal papillae extend into the epidermis (Fig. 18.2). Corresponding *epidermal pegs* are also evident in such zones. This is the means by which the epidermis and dermis become highly interdigitated. The dermal papillae probably serve to increase surface contact with the epidermis and contain numerous blood vessels and various special receptor terminals of nerves.

Lymphatic tissue, glands and smooth muscle also occur in the dermis. The cell

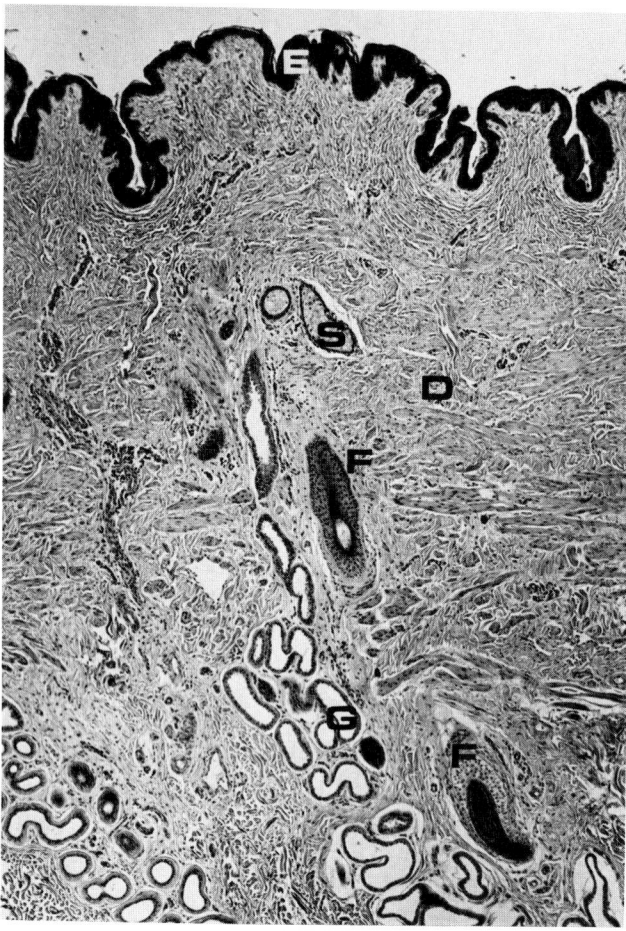

Fig. 18.1 Ovine haired skin. The epidermis (E) is underlaid by an extensive dermis (D) that contains hair follicles (F), sebaceous glands (S) and tubular glands (G). X10. All light micrographs are labeled as the magnification with the microscope before photographic enlarging. All electron micrographs are labeled as total magnification, including photographic enlarging.

population of the dermis may include all cells listed with loose connective tissue.

Hypodermis. The skin (epidermis and dermis) resides upon a *hypodermis* or subcutaneous layer of connective tissue. It is a loose connective tissue which may contain extensive quantities of adipose tissue. When the hypodermis is infiltrated by numerous adipose cells, the layer is called the *panniculus adiposus*. The hypodermis blends into the underlying dense connective tissue of the deep fascia, periosteum or perichondrium.

Blood Supply, Nerves and Lymphatic Vessels. The blood supply to the skin is extensive and is organized into three vascular plexuses: *superficial* or *subpapillary plexus,* *middle* or *cutaneous plexus, deep* or *subcutaneous plexus* (Fig. 18.3). The subcutaneous plexus is supplied by two types of arteries. *Simple cutaneous arteries* emerge from the fascial planes between muscle masses to supply the skin primarily. *Mixed cutaneous arteries* supply the muscle mass and eventually terminate in the skin. Branches from the subcutaneous plexus form the cutaneous plexus, which is intimately associated with those structures that have invaginated into the dermis (hairs, glands). Branches from the cutaneous plexus form the subpapillary

plexus. The veins of these plexuses are satellites of the arteries. Vascular patterns vary with the region of the body. Haired skin is devoid generally of extensive capillary loops into dermal papillae, whereas glabrous skin has extensive capillary loops into the papillary area of the dermis. Superficial arteriovenous anastomoses, which are effective thermoregulatory structures, are present in the superficial plexus of the pig and man but are absent in this plexus in other domestic animals. Reddening (erythema) and blister formation in response to thermal injury (burns) is characteristic only in those species with superficial arteriovenous anastomoses.

The nerves to the skin are a mixture of motor and sensory nerve fibers. General visceral efferent nerves of the sympathetic nervous system innervate the smooth muscle of the walls of blood vessels, the arrector pili muscles and the myoepithelial cells associated with tubular glands. However, the majority of the nerves to the epidermis and dermis are general somatic afferent fibers. Various sensory modalities (touch, pain, temperature, itch) are received by afferent nerve terminals (Chapter 15) and transmitted to the central nervous system by myelin-

ated and unmyelinated nerve fibers. The afferent nerve terminals are the dendritic zones of nerve cell bodies located in dorsal root ganglia or sensory ganglia of the appropriate cranial nerves. Fibers of these nerve cell bodies pass to the periphery in nerve trunks, large branches of which lie in the hypodermis. The subpapillary nerve plexus is formed by fine branches of these nerves. Sensory nerve endings of these fine branches are located in the hypodermis, dermis and epidermis (Fig. 18.3).

Branches of the cutaneous nerves innervate the hair follicles and form a *hair follicle network*. Sensory nerve endings wrap around the hair follicles and form a significant tactile receptor in mammalian haired skin. This relationship is well-developed in sinus or tactile hairs.

The sensory nerves of the dermis, *dermal network*, is more extensive in glabrous skin than haired skin.

Blind-ended lymphatic capillaries located within the dermal papillae are continuous with a network of lymphatic vessels that traverse the papillary region of the dermis. Subsequently, these lymphatic vessels, accompanying blood vessels into the hypodermis, coalesce to form large lymphatic channels that carry materials to the peripheral lymph nodes.

Specialized Skin Regions

The mammalian integument, although consisting minimally of an epidermis and dermis, is not uniform throughout its distribution over the external body surface. Some portions of the skin are haired, whereas others are glabrous. A thick epidermis may characterize some portions of the body; a thin epidermis, others. Similarly, the dermis may assume various thicknesses throughout its distribution. The dermis is the thickest part of the skin. Regional skin variations relating to amount and type of pelage, distribution and type of glands and skin thickness are functional adaptations that ideally suit the organism to its external environment.

Digital pads. The *footpads* or *digital pads* of carnivores are highly cornified, thickened, highly pigmented and hairless portions of the skin which are adaptations for locomotion. The digital pads resist abrasion and are effective shock absorbers. The epidermis of the digital pads, which is the thickest epidermis of the carnivore skin, consists of all layers described previously, as well as a stratum lucidum. The stratum corneum is a predominant feature of the epidermis; the surface is smooth in the cat and papillated in the dog. Prominent dermal papillae interdigitate with epidermal pegs. The hypodermis consists of an abundance of adipose tissue, the *digital cushion*. Coiled, tubular sweat glands (merocrine glands) are present in the dermis and hypodermis.

Scrotum. The skin of the scrotum is usually

he thinnest skin of the body. The stratum orneum is not well-developed and the der-is is not extensive. Apocrine tubular and ebaceous glands are present, but species ariations exist. Hair follicles are not abun-ant and the hairs that are present are short nd fine. Smooth muscle fibers of the tunica artos are interpersed with collagenous and lastic fibers within the dermis. The *tunica artos*, which is responsive to environmental emperatures, is responsible for the relative osition of the testes to the body wall. In igh ambient temperatures, the muscle is elaxed, the scrotum is stretched from the veight of the testes and the testes are posi-ioned away from the body wall. The con-erse is true in low ambient temperatures. This is an effective mechanism for regulat-ng scrotal temperature, inasmuch as sperm production is a temperature-dependent phe-iomenon.

Nose. Integumentary modifications charac-erize the external nose of the varied domes-ic species. The *planum nasale* of carnivores s composed of a thickened and highly cor-ified epidermis which is devoid of seba-eous glands and tubular glands. The *lanum nasolabiale* of the ox and the *planum*

nasale of small ruminants (sheep and goat) are devoid of hairs but contain tubular mer-ocrine glands that moisten the surface. The epidermis is thickened and highly cornified. The highly cornified *planum rostrale* of the pig contains many tubular merocrine glands and is covered sparsely by fine hairs. Fine hairs and sebaceous glands are characteristic of the thin skin around the nostrils of the horse.

External Auditory Meatus. The *external auditory meatus* or *external ear canal* connects the external auditory opening with the ty-panic membrane. This canal is lined by skin. Small hair follicles, sebaceous glands and modified apocrine tubular glands (cerumi-nous glands) are present. The dermis of this canal blends with the perichondrium and periosteum of the supportive cartilage and bone.

Mucocutaneous Junctions. *Mucocutaneous junctions* are points of transition between typical skin and *cutaneous mucous membranes* with which they are continuous. Cutaneous mucous membranes are moistened surfaces which are lined by stratified squa-mous epithelium (Chapter 13). Mucocuta-neous junctions occur at all body orifices.

Hairs

Hair. These modified epidermal structures are of variable occurrence in the system and serve various functions: *insulation, protection* and *sensory reception*. Hairs develop as lo-calized thickenings of the epidermis which subsequently invaginate into the underlying connective tissue and may extend into the hypodermis (Plate I. 2).

A connective tissue sheath from the der-mis is oriented circumferentially around the *hair follicle* (Fig. 18.4). A basement mem-brane (*glassy membrane*) separates the con-nective tissue from the epithelium of the follicle. The *external root sheath* is essen-tially a continuation of the *stratum basale*, *stratum spinosum* and *stratum granulosum* of the epidermis (Fig. 18.5). An *internal root sheath*, an apparent continuation of the *stra-tum corneum*, may be subdivided into three regions: a peripheral *Henle's layer*, an inter-mediate *Huxley's layer*, and an inner *cuticle of the root sheath* (Fig. 18.5). *Henle's layer* consists of a single layer of flattened cells. *Huxley's layer* consists of several layers of cells that contain *trichohyalin* granules, a substance similar to keratohyalin. The *cuti-cle of the root sheath* is a single layer of cornified cells that abuts the cuticle of the hair. These cells interdigitate with the cor-nified cells of the cuticle of the hair.

The hair consists of three regions: an outer *cuticle*, an inner *cortex* and a central *medulla* (Fig. 18.5). The *cuticle* is a single layer of enucleated, cornified cells which interdigi-tate with the cuticle of the root sheath. The *cortex* comprises the bulk of the hair shaft. It consists of several layers of flattened, cornified cells which contain "hard keratin." Pigment may be present and numerous air spaces characterize the intercellular spaces. The *medulla* may be absent in some hairs. When present, it consists of cornified, cu-boidal cells which are separated by air spaces. The cuticular, cortical and medul-lary characteristics are so specific that iden-tification to species is possible with careful examination.

The hair follicle terminates in a cone-shaped epidermal peg (*hair bulb*) that de-fines the limits of the *dermal papilla* (Fig. 18.6). The dermal papilla ensures the close association of the vascular bed to the rapidly growing epidermis in this region. Hair growth is achieved in a simple fashion. The epidermal cells at the apex of the papilla give rise to medullary cells. The epidermal cells lateral to the apex give rise to cortical cells and cuticular cells. The cells at the depths of the epidermal pegs give rise to the inner root sheath, while more laterally lo-cated cells give rise to the outer root sheath. The growth of a hair, therefore, is achieved by the simple apposition of new cells from the depths of the follicle. It is similar to typical skin growth.

A sheath of smooth muscle, the *arrector pili muscle*, attaches to the connective tissue associated with the hair follicle and the con-

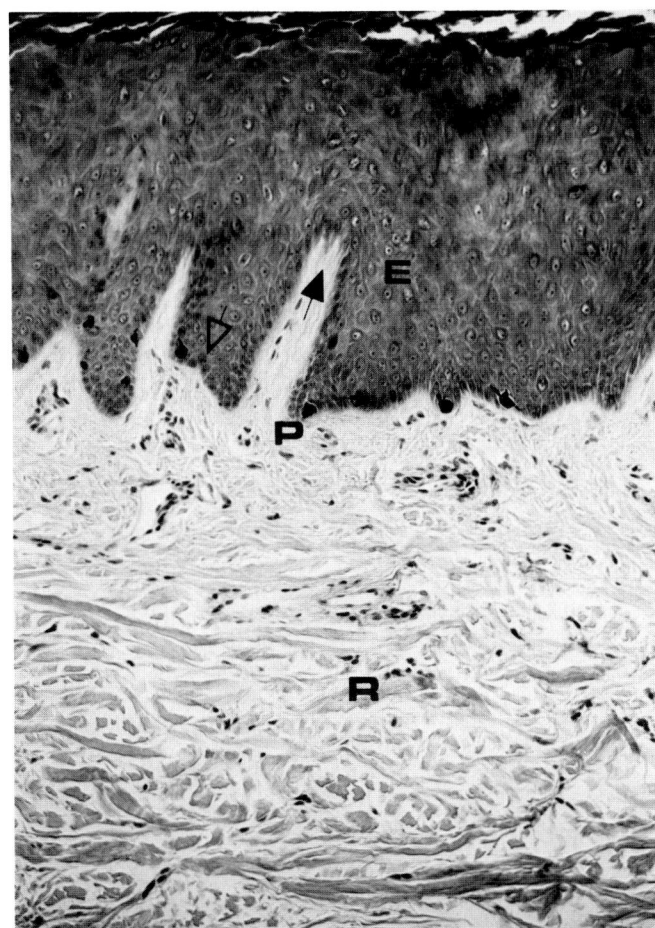

Fig. 18.2 Papillary and reticular zones of the dermis. The papillary zone (P) is immediately adjacent to the epidermis (E) and is continuous with the reticular zone (R). Dermal papillae (*solid arrow*) and epidermal pegs (*open arrow*) are well developed. X40.

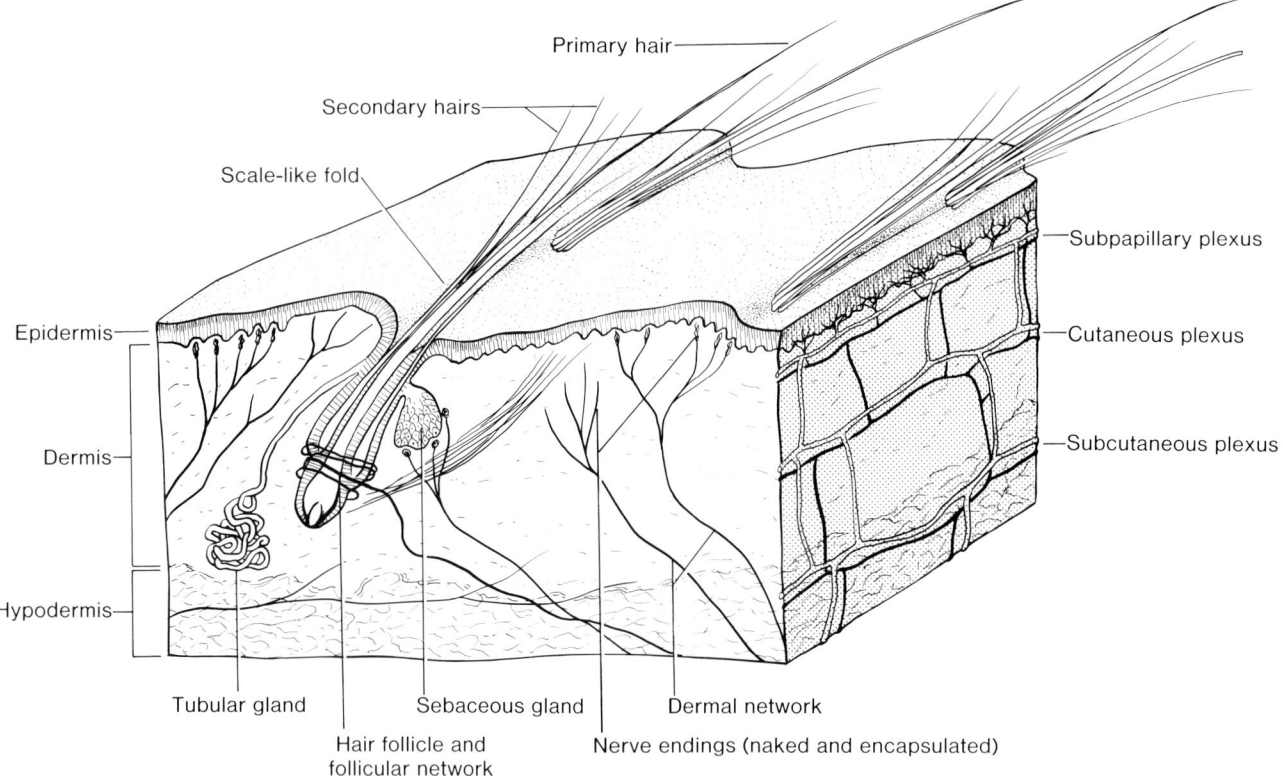

Primary hair

Secondary hairs

Scale-like fold

Epidermis

Dermis

Hypodermis

Subpapillary plexus

Cutaneous plexus

Subcutaneous plexus

Tubular gland

Hair follicle and
follicular network

Sebaceous gland

Nerve endings (naked and encapsulated)

Dermal network

Fig. 18.3 An idealized drawing of the haired skin of a dog. The face view represents major integumentary components, while the side view only shows the vasculature. (Redrawn and modified from Evans, H. E. and Christensen, G. C.: *Miller's Anatomy of the Dog.* W. B. Saunders, Philadelphia 1979).

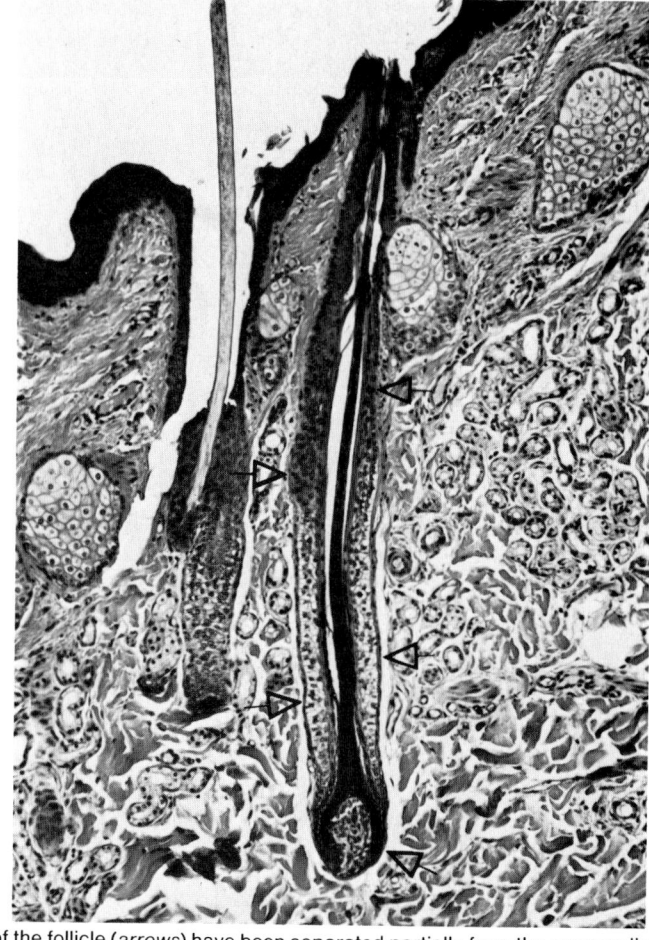

Fig. 18.4 Hair follicle. The margins of the follicle (*arrows*) have been separated partially from the surrounding connective tissue. Note the continuity of cellular components of the follicle with the surface cells. The intimate association of the dermal papilla to the hair bulb is obvious at the *lowest arrow.* X25.

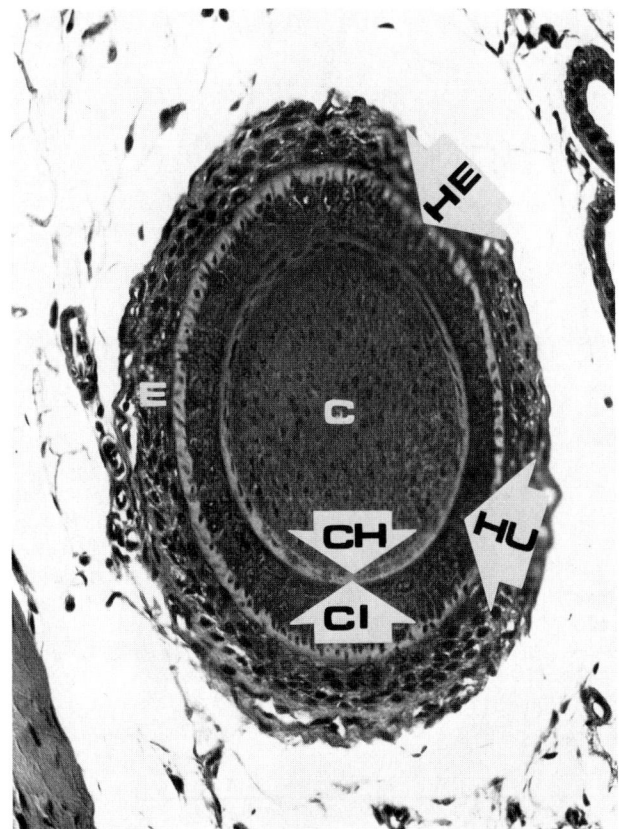

Fig. 18.5 A cross-sectioned hair follicle. The external root sheath (E) surrounds the hair and is separated from the connective tissue by a glassy membrane (not apparent). The internal root sheath consists of Henle's layer (HE), Huxley's layer (HU) and an inner cuticular layer (CI). The hair consists of a cuticular layer (CH) and cortex (C). A medulla is not present. X63.

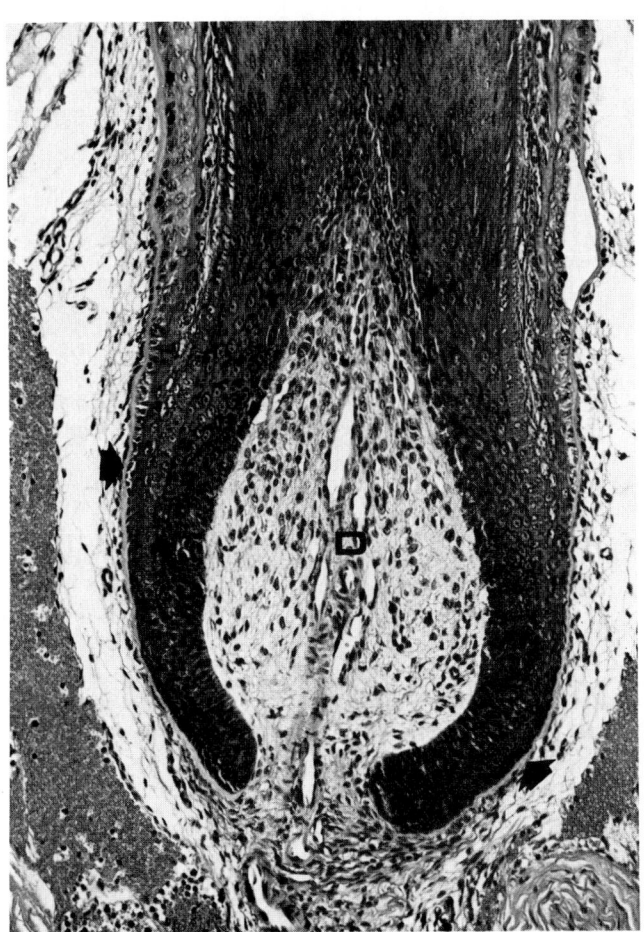

Fig. 18.6 Hair bulb and dermal papilla. The cone-shaped hair bulb surrounds the dermal papilla (D). The glassy membrane (*arrows*) is apparent. X40.

nective tissue of the papillary region associated with the skin proper (Fig. 18.7). Its contraction not only erects the hair but probably expresses the sebaceous glands which are located between the mass of muscle and the hair follicle.

Species Differences. In the horse and large ruminants, the hairs are evenly distributed on the body. In other domestic species (pig, cat, dog), the hairs are arranged in groups (*hair beds*). In the dog, a hair bed contains two to four clusters of hair follicles. Each cluster of hair follicles consists of usually one *principal* or *guard hair* and three to nine *auxiliary* (*secondary*) or *wool hairs*. A guard hair is approximately 150 μm in diameter and has a cuticle, cortex and medulla. The wool hairs are approximately 70 μm in diameter and are devoid of a medulla. Although a cluster usually has one surface opening, separate openings may be present. In the latter case they open in close association with each other. Clustering of hairs may be as exaggerated as in the chinchilla in which as many as 75 hairs may comprise a cluster with a single surface opening. The single guard hair is approximately 15 μm in diameter whereas the numerous wool hairs are maximally 11 μm in diameter.

Hair Cycle. The normal growth and shedding of hairs occur in cycles that are influenced by the photoperiod. A complete hair cycle consists of three stages—anagen, catagen and telogen. *Anagen* is the period within the cycle during which time hair growth is accomplished. *Catagen* is the transitory stage that occurs before the resting period, *telogen*.

A typical hair cycle is illustrated in Figure 18.8. The hair is produced by the mitotic activity of the constituent cells of the hair bulb during anagen. The continual apposition of new cells to the shaft of the hair results in its elongation. Termination of growth is contingent upon cessation of mitotic activity of the germinal cells within the hair bulb. The catagen period is characterized by gradual but continuous changes in the hair bulb and follicle. The hair bulb becomes a solid, keratinized mass of cells, while the distal follicle becomes thin. The club-shaped bulb that is formed is fused to the hair-shaft and migrates to the level of the sebaceous glands. These hairs, devoid of an association with distinct papillae, are called *club hairs*. A secondary germ develops deep to the club hair. This morphologic configuration marks telogen and may be maintained for weeks or months. During early anagen, the secondary germ grows deeper, forming a new hair bulb in association with a dermal papilla. Continued mi-

tosis throughout anagen results in the elongation of the shaft. The new growth eventually displaces the club hair which is shed and the cycle continues again.

Knowledge about the growth and shedding of hairs in domestic animals is incomplete. Many laboratory rodents shed their hairs in *synchronized waves* which are initiated ventrally and progress laterad and dorsad. Carnivores and man, however, have an *asynchronized mosaic pattern* of hair growth and shedding.

The hair coat of a mammal reflects the state of health and disease. Many disease conditions are characterized by a lusterless or dull hair coat in which the cuticular cells are not flattened against the cortex; thus, light is not reflected normally. The anagen stage of hair growth may be shortened in various disease states. Accordingly, many hairs in telogen may be shed synchronously.

Sensory Hairs. These structures are also referred to as *tactile hairs* or *sinus hairs* (Fig. 18.9). Although the distribution of this type of hair is rather specific, the structure of the hair and follicle is similar to normal hairs. The connective tissue sheath adjacent to the glassy membrane is thickened and separated by connective tissue trabeculae from a peripherally located connective tissue sheath. The intertrabecular spaces are filled with venous blood contained within the venous sinuses. Free nerve endings and Merkel's disks are associated with the epidermal cells and connective tissue fibers.

Special Skin Cells

Melanocytes and Langerhans' Cells. The origin, nature and function of melanoblasts and their progeny were discussed in Chapter 6. The presence of melanin bearing cells in the skin and mucous membranes (conjunctival sac, buccal cavity) imparts characteristic pigmentation. Melanin also protects the organism from harmful ultraviolet radiation. The absence of melanin increases the potential for actinic damage. Ultraviolet solar radiation may be a contributing factor in the increased incidence of ocular squamous cell carcinoma in cattle in the Rocky Mountain West. Despite their protective function, melanoblasts and melanocytes are responsible for the formation of a highly malignant tumor, malignant melanoma.

Langerhans' cells are round cells with a clear cytoplasm when processed by routine staining techniques (H and E). They occur in the peripheral portion of the stratum spinosum. Special staining techniques (gold chloride) have demonstrated these cells to have a stellate or dendritic shape. Langerhans' cells share some morphologic and histochemical characteristics with melanocytes and were once considered to be effete melanocytes. Experimental evidence, however, has demonstrated the presence of Langerhans' cells in skin grafts devoid of neural crest ectodermal elements. Moreover, Langerhans' cells appear to be distributed more

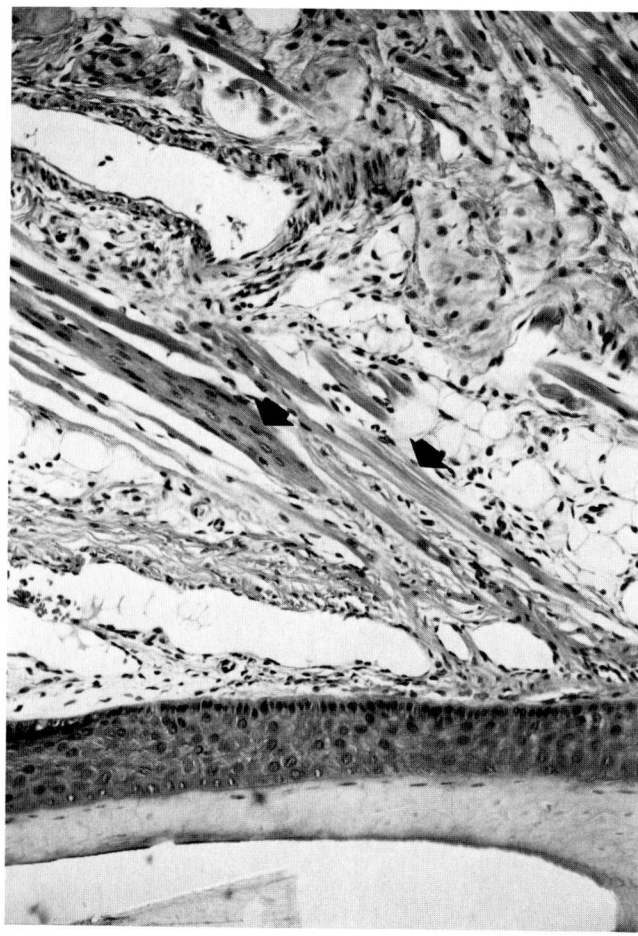

Fig. 18.7   Arrector pili muscle. The muscle (*arrows*) attaches to the hair follicle and papillary region of the dermis.

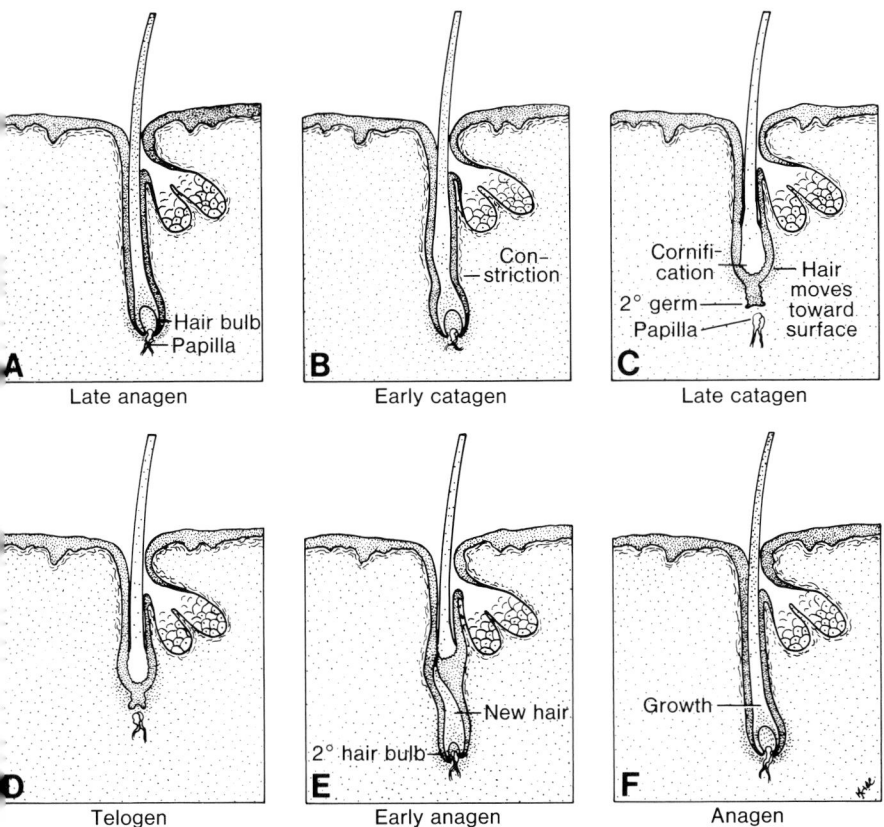

A Late anagen

B Early catagen — Con- striction

C Late catagen — Cornifi- cation / 2° germ / Papilla / Hair moves toward surface

D Telogen

E Early anagen — New hair / 2° hair bulb

F Anagen — Growth

Fig. 18.8 A diagram of the sequence of events in a typical hair cycle. A, hair growth begins to [l]ow down; B, club hair starts to form at constriction in follicle; C, club hair cornifies and secondary [g]erm forms. Club hair moves toward the surface. D, resting stage; E, secondary germ forms a [n]ew (secondary) hair bulb and club hair is pushed from the follicle as new hair growth progresses; [F], continued new hair growth and the cycle is completed.

constantly throughout the skin than mela- nocytes, the latter being subject to regional differences. Langerhans' cells also are ca- pable of phagocytosis.

Current evidence indicates that Langer- hans cells are derivatives of the bone mar- row. The cells possess surface receptors for the FC segment of IgG and C3, receptor sites similar to those that characterize the surfaces of macrophages. The Langerhans cells may belong to a group of relatively nonphagocytic macrophages that assist with the "processing" of antigen in such a man- ner as to facilitate or assist the T lymphocyte in graft rejection responses (Type IV Hy- persensitivity).

Avian Integument

Epidermis and Dermis. The epidermis of avian skin is quite thin, loose and dry (Fig. 18.10). Although much thinner than the mammalian counterpart, three strata are de- fined: *stratum basale, stratum spinosum* and *stratum corneum.* The connective tissue ad- jacent to the epidermis is composed of fine collagenous fibers; however, a papillary re- gion is not defined. The connective tissue becomes more dense in the depths of the corium and abuts on a very extensive sub- cutis. Lymphoid tissue is extensive in the corium and subcutis. The corium and epi- dermis are devoid of glands.

Feathers extend from the epidermis into the corium and assume a configuration sim- ilar to hairs. Although they are both epider- mal structures, they probably have a differ- ent phylogenetic origin.

Feathers. Feathers are of epidermal origin and, like their mammalian counterparts, de- velop within a follicle. The base of the fol- licle, however, is not continuous over the dermal papilla. Thus, the core of the feather contains remnants of vascular connective tissue (feather *pulp*).

The principal parts of the feather are the *quill (calamus)* and the *vane (vexillum)* (Fig. 18.11). The quill is contained within the follicle and contains two foramina (*proximal umbilicus* and *distal umbilicus*). As the quill grows, the dermal papilla retracts leaving behind the desiccated central *pulp.* The *vane* is the continuation of the quill above the skin surface. It consists of a *rachis*, which is actually the continuation of the quill, and *barbs.* The barbs project laterally from the rachis in an oblique and parallel manner. The barbs possess *proximal* and *distal bar- bules* that are oriented at right angles to the barbs and parallel to the rachis. The distal barbules have hooklets which engage the indentations of the proximal barbules. This

relationship establishes a relatively nonpo- rous and flexible sheet that sheds water and facilitates flight.

Down feathers have a small and thin rachis. The barbs are devoid of barbules. Thus, these feathers are loose and fluffy; they serve as good insulation.

Filoplumes are feathers with a hair-like structure. They are scattered over the body but are especially predominant structures on the head and neck.

Uropygial Gland. The uropygial gland is also referred to as the *oil* or *preen gland* (Fig. 18.12). It is the only cutaneous gland that occurs in birds, and it is especially well developed in aquatic species. It consists of numerous sebaceous adenomeres that con- tinue into a common duct or sinus and empty on the surface on a common papilla. The papilla contains smooth muscle fibers that extend around the excretory duct. The heavily encapsulated, bilobed duct is situ- ated above the last sacral vertebra. Because of its unique structure and size, this gland is considered a specialized sebaceous skin gland.

Specialized Structures. There are numerous other epidermal modifications in birds: scales, toe pads, claws, beaks, wattles, spurs and combs. Claws, spurs and beaks are sim- ilar to the mammalian claw, whereas toe pads may be compared to the pads of car- nivores. Scales are comparable to those of reptiles and occur on the legs of all birds as well as on the wings of penguins. Wattles and combs are diverticuli of the skin which contain extensive vasculature, mucous con- nective tissue and fat. In some birds (tur- key), erectile tissue may be present.

Glands of the Mammalian Skin

Sebaceous and Tubular Glands

The glands of the skin are generally those that are associated with hairs. These are the *sebaceous glands* and the *tubular skin glands.* The former deposit their excretory product into the follicle, or they may empty inde- pendently on the skin surface. The tubular skin glands are in close association with the follicles but generally open independently on the skin surface.

Sebaceous Glands. Sebaceous glands in as- sociation with hairs are evaginations of the epithelial lining of the root canal in the form of simple, branched alveolar glands (Fig. 18.13). They vary in size from 0.2–2.0 mm. The *peripheral cell layer (basal cell layer)* is either squamous or cuboidal epithelium which resides on a basement membrane (Fig. 18.14). These are the stem cells of the gland and function in a manner similar to the stratum basale of the skin. Because of the holocrine nature of sebaceous glands, this layer assures a copious supply of cells. The lumen of the alveolus is almost com- pletely filled with polyhedral cells. As they are derived peripherally they are forced to the center of the gland during which time they accumulate lipids and undergo degeneration. Numerous examples of pyknosis and karyolysis are usually present. The accumulated lipids (fatty acids, cholesterol) and the entire cell constitute the secretory product, *sebum*.

The basal cells of the alveolus are connected to the root canal by a short and wide excretory duct which is lined by a stratified squamous epithelium. Although the mechanism for the regulation of secretory activity

is not understood, it is believed that th contraction of the arrector pili muscle e presses the gland. The secretory produc therefore, enters the follicle and the spreads over the surface of the skin.

The functions of sebaceous glands a varied: sebum diminishes the possible entr of microorganisms into the skin; the secre tory product diminishes water loss; it co tains precursors to vitamin D; sebum keep the hairs and outer skin surface soft an pliable.

Some areas are devoid of sebaceou glands: foot pads, hooves, claws, horns an others.

Sebaceous glands that are not hair asso ciated are discussed with special skin gland

Tubular Skin Glands. The tubular glands the skin are simple, coiled, tubular struc tures. They are extensively developed in th horse and man and are absent in the bir There are two general types: *merocrine* an *apocrine*.

The adenomere consists of a low cuboid epithelium in the merocrine glands, wherea the epithelial lining of the adenomere apocrine glands is a low columnar typ Blebs on the luminal surface are indicativ of the apocrine secretory mechanism. Th adenomeres of both types of glands are a ranged as a *glomus* (a tuft or ball). Th glomus is connected to the surface or mo usually to the neck of the root canal abov the opening of the sebaceous gland by loosely coiled or straight excretory du which consists of a single or double layer cuboidal cells. Myoepithelial cells are asso ciated with the adenomeres.

Although the merocrine tubular gland are the primary sweat glands of man, the are usually restricted to the footpads of oth animals (Fig. 18.15). The apocrine tubul gland is the predominant sweat gland domestic animals (Figs. 18.16, 18.1). In ma these glands are usually confined to th mammary, axillary, pubic and perineal re gions. In the cat, these glands are not extensive as in other animals. They are con fined to the anal and oral regions, the low jaw and footpads. The canid has extensiv tubular glands over the entire body, b apparently they are minimally functional sweat glands.

Sweat glands serve as a cooling mecha nism for the body, as well as an excretor organ. The secretory product is mostly wate (serous) and slightly alkaline. In the hors however, it is strongly alkaline and contain albuminoids, serum globulins and som urea.

Special Skin Glands

Glands of the Anal Region. These gland may be divided into three types accordin to their association with the rectum an anus: *anal glands*, *glands of the anal sac* an the *circumanal* or *perianal glands*.

Anal glands are present in the dog, ca and pig. They are modified tubuloalveola

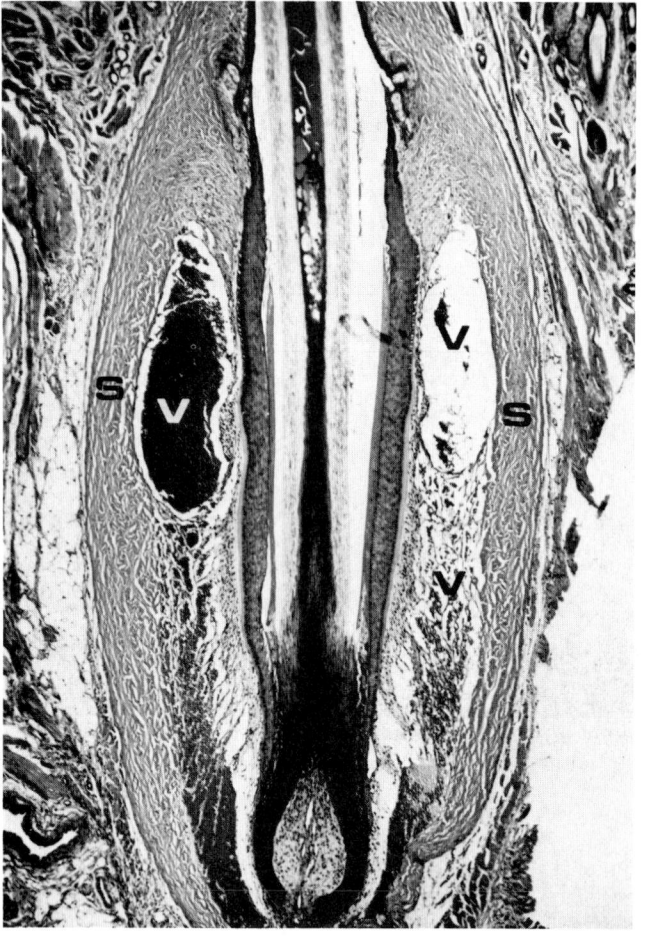

Fig. 18.9   Sinus hair from a cat. The sinus hair is surrounded by a well-developed connective tissue sheath (S) that contains venous sinuses. X10.

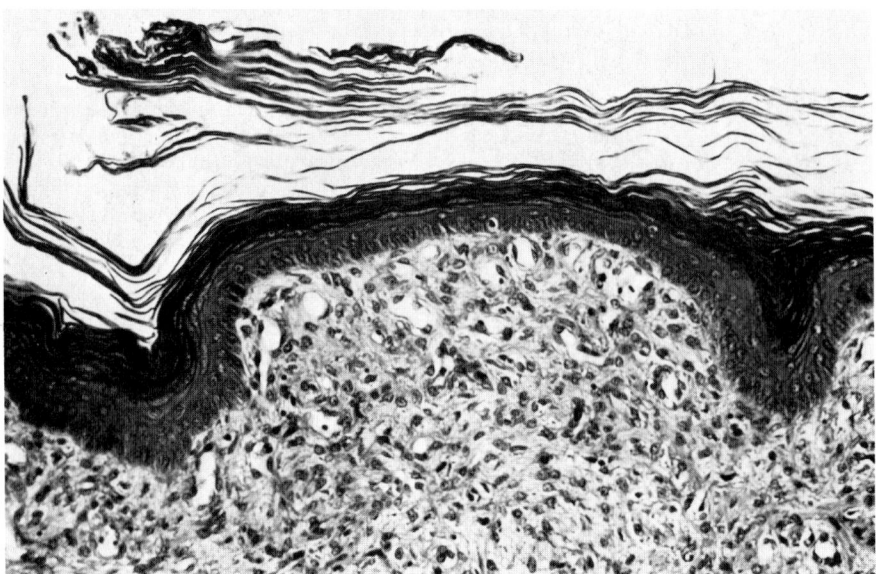

Fig. 18.10   Avian skin. The epidermis has a reduced number of layers. X63.

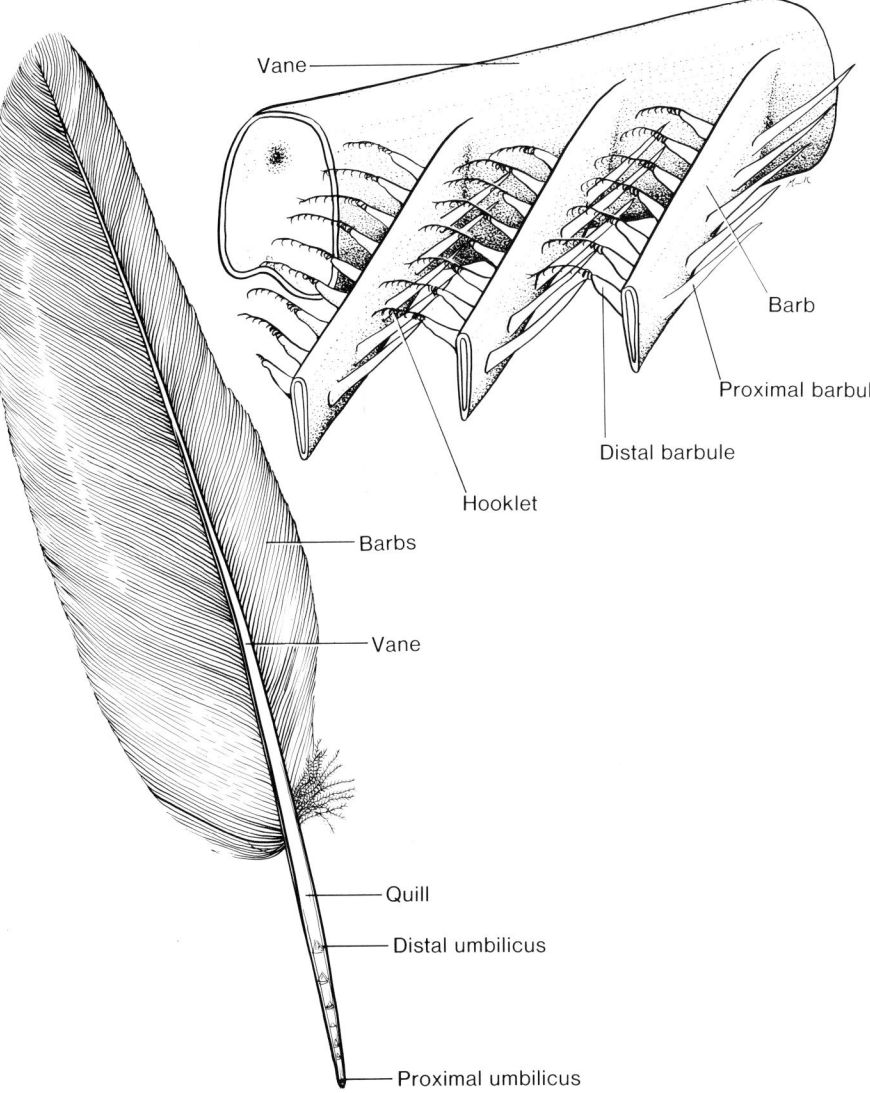

Vane

Barb

Proximal barbule

Distal barbule

Hooklet

Barbs

Vane

Quill

Distal umbilicus

Proximal umbilicus

Fig. 18.11   A drawing of the main components of a flight feather.

cyte-like (Fig. 18.21). These cells have a finely granular, acidophilic cytoplasm and pale nuclei. Numerous proteinaceous granules are present. The cells are usually polygonal, but some of them at the periphery of the organ assume a tall columnar configuration.

Nonpatent ducts from the circumanal glands have been reported to connect with the sebaceous glands of the region. It is concluded, therefore, that these glands are nonsecretory, abortive sebaceous glands. Because of the association of these solid masses of cells with sebaceous adenomeres, it is common to refer to the sebaceous and nonsecretory solid masses as circumanal glands. Many of the latter, however, are located some distance from sebaceous endpieces.

These solid masses are predisposed to neoplasia.

Mammary Gland. The following description generally applies to all species but is especially applicable to the cow.

The organ is a compound, tubuloalveolar gland which is believed to be a modified sweat gland (Fig. 18.22). Although it is normally described as being an apocrine gland, this method of secretion refers to the elaboration of lipids, whereas the protein and carbohydrate components of milk are elaborated by the merocrine method.

The mammary gland consists of the *teats* and *udder*. The udder consists of a capsule, interstitial connective tissue, secretory epithelium and a system of excretory ducts. The distribution of connective tissue and parenchyma is a function of the secretory activity of the gland. Actively lactating glands have much parenchyma and little connective tissue, while the reverse is true of nonlactating glands.

For a cow to produce 40 lb of milk per day, approximately 8 tons of blood must pass through the udder. This same amount of milk is produced, secreted, suspended and subsequently removed from the udder in a short milking period from a sac of tissue that weighs approximately 50 lb. These relationships necessitate extensive secretory tissue, blood supply and supportive connective tissues.

The following description is applicable to the lactating mammary gland (Figs. 18.22, 18.23). The secretory portions of the organ include the epithelial lining of the *alveoli* and the initial portion of the *intralobular ducts* (*secretory tubules*). During lactation, the cells assume a columnar configuration with their apical borders protruding into the lumina (Fig. 18.24). Typical apical blebs are indicative of the apocrine secretory method. The accumulation of fat droplets is manifested by the foamy appearance of the cells. These small droplets may become confluent and form a single large droplet. The lateral cell borders usually are indistinct. The nucleus may be basally displaced or may be positioned apically during the secretory process. It may even be discharged into the

veat glands that occupy the submucosa of the columnar and intermediate zones of the nal canal and open into the anus (Fig. 8.17). Anal glands of carnivores secrete pid materials whereas those of the pig se-rete mucoid substances (Fig. 18.18). Nod-lar and diffuse lymphatic tissue may be ssociated with the lamina propria of this egion. Also, venous erectile tissue may be resent.

The *anal sacs* or *perianal sinuses* are aired, lateral cutaneous diverticula of the nus that are lined by a keratinized stratified quamous epithelium. Each sac has mural lands which open into it (Fig. 18.19). The c is located between the internal and ex-rnal anal sphincters. It is supported by a ose connective tissue (lamina propria and bmucosa) which is typical of the region nd underlaid by a dense fibroelastic con-ective tissue. Because of the association ith the sphincters, much smooth and skel-

etal muscle is present in the connective tissue.

The anal sac is present in carnivores and many rodents. In the dog, the glands of the anal sac are apocrine tubular; in the cat, apocrine tubular glands and sebaceous glands are present. In both species, both types of glands open into the excretory duct or neck of the anal sac.

The excretory products of the glands of the anal sac, sloughed cells and excrement may occlude the opening of the sacs to the anus. In dogs they may have to be expressed periodically.

The *glands of the circumanal region* comprise two main types: *sebaceous glands* and *circumanal glands* (Fig. 18.20). The former are typical and may or may not be associated with hairs.

The circumanal glands of the dog are nonpatent masses of parenchymal cells which have often been described as *hepato-*

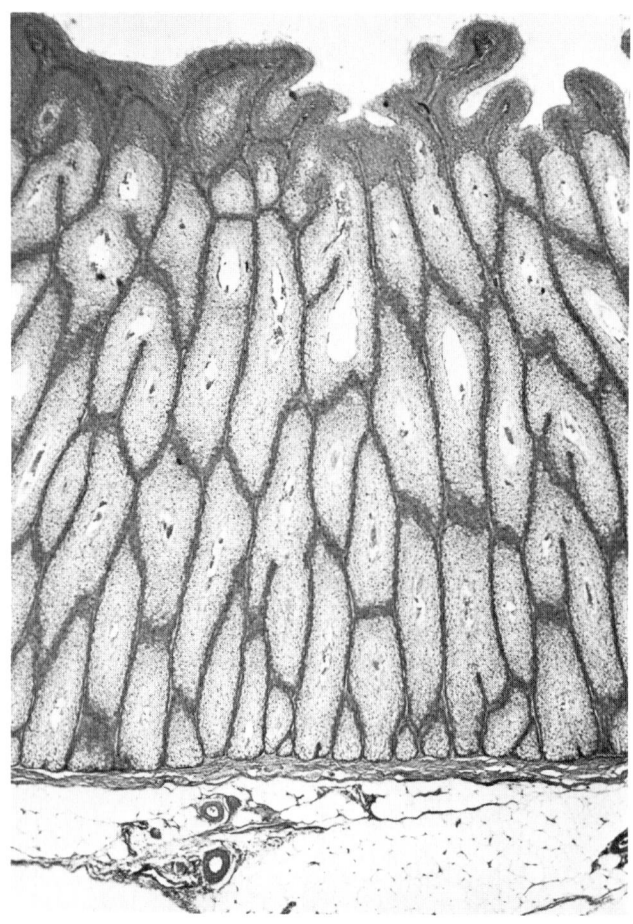

Fig. 18.12 The avian uropygial gland. Numerous sebaceous adenomeres are grouped to form this gland. X10.

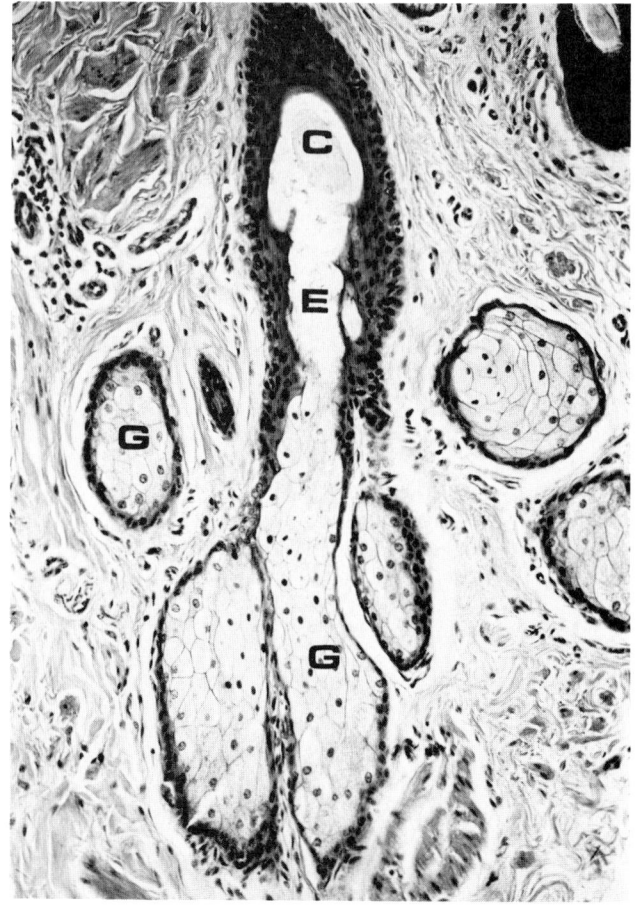

Fig. 18.13 Sebaceous glands and a hair. The sebaceous glands (G) are connected to the root canal (C) by an excretory duct (E). X40.

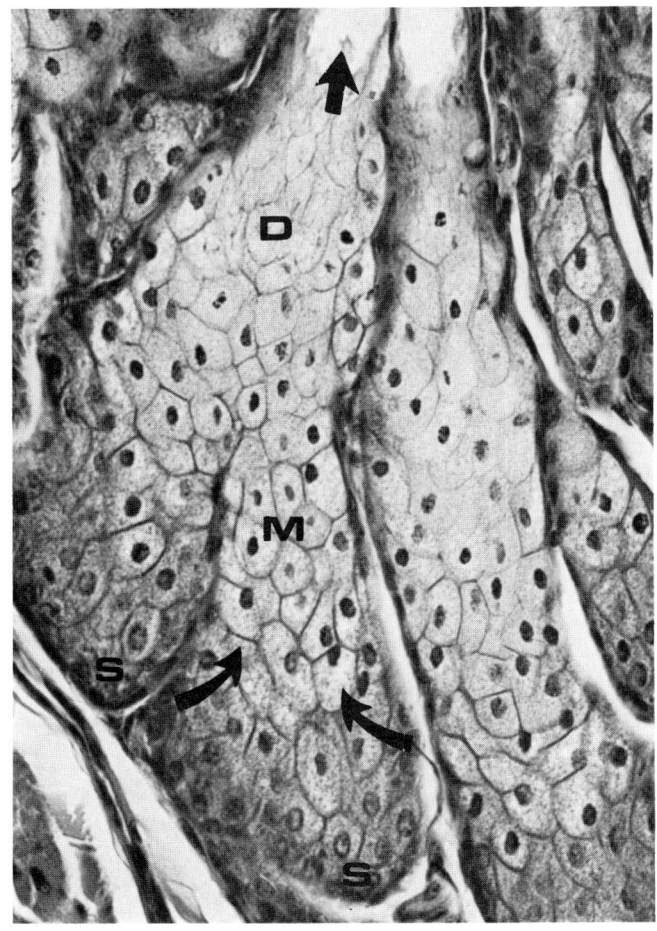

Fig. 18.14   Secretory sequence in a sebaceous gland. The stem cells (S) migrate from the periphery (*curved arrows*), mature (M), disintegrate (D) and are propelled to the excretory duct (*straight arrow*). X100.

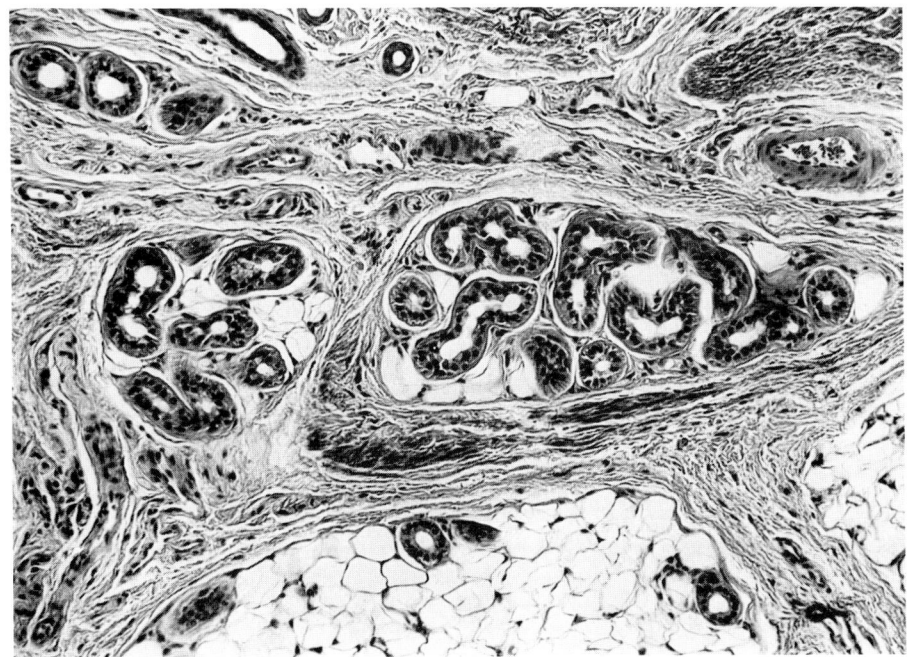

Fig. 18.15   Merocrine tubular glands of the feline footpad. These are not the typical tubular glands of domestic animals. X40.

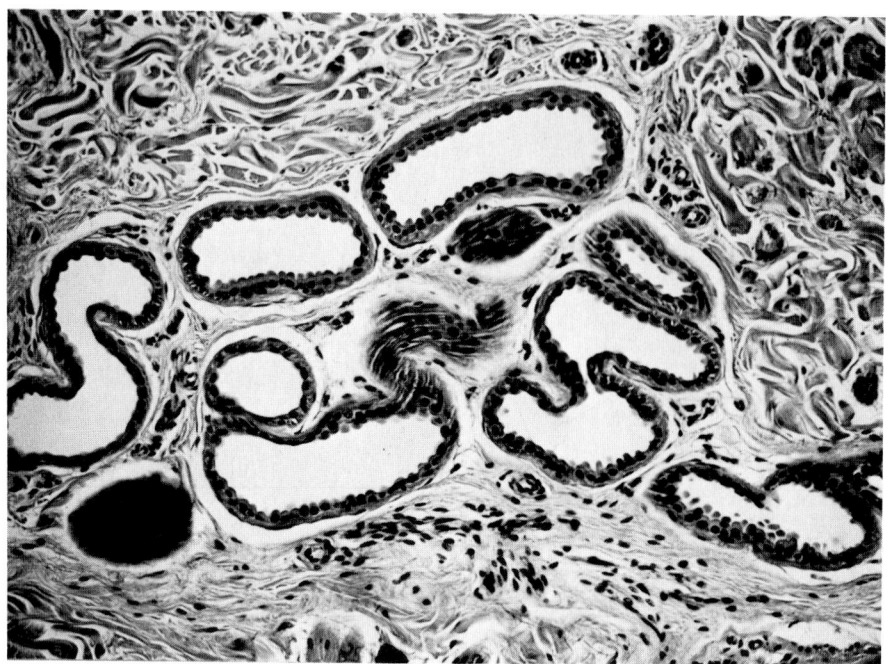

Fig. 18.16 Apocrine tubular glands of the ovine skin. These are the typical sweat glands of domestic animals. X40.

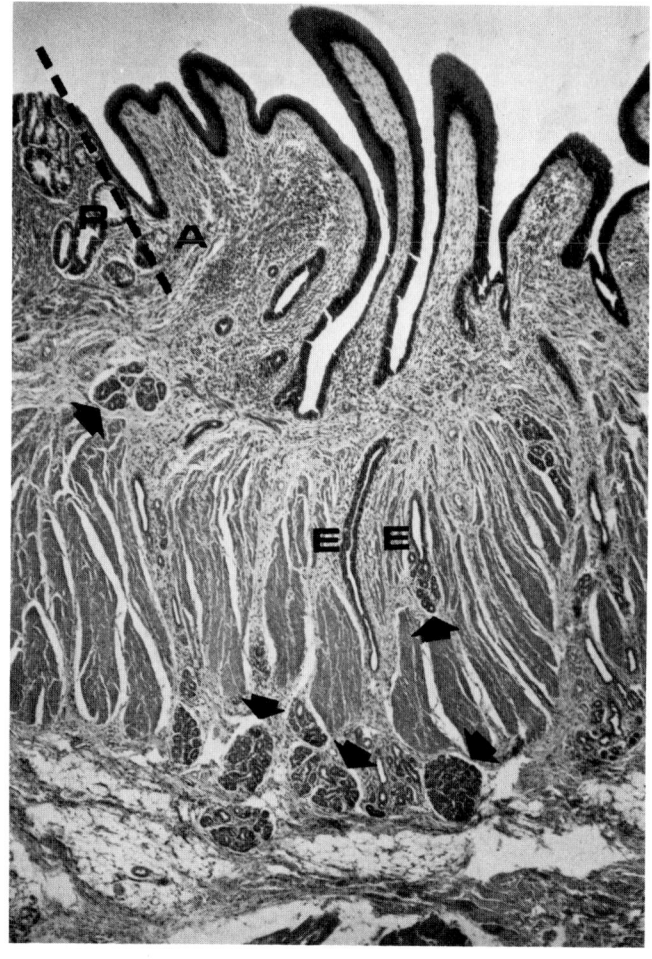

Fig. 18.17 Porcine anal glands. The anal glands (*arrows*) are located in the submucosa of the columnar and intermediate zones of the anal canal. A, anus; R, rectum; *dashed line*, anorectal junction. The excretory ducts (E) of these glands open into the anus. X10.

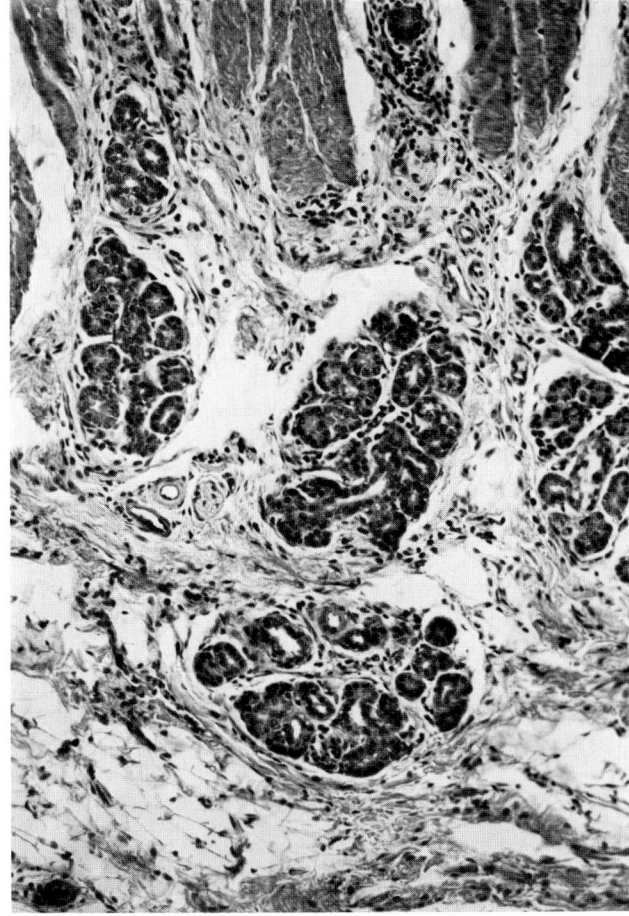

Fig. 18.18 Adenomeres of porcine anal glands. These tubuloalveolar glands of the pig secrete mucoid substances. X40.

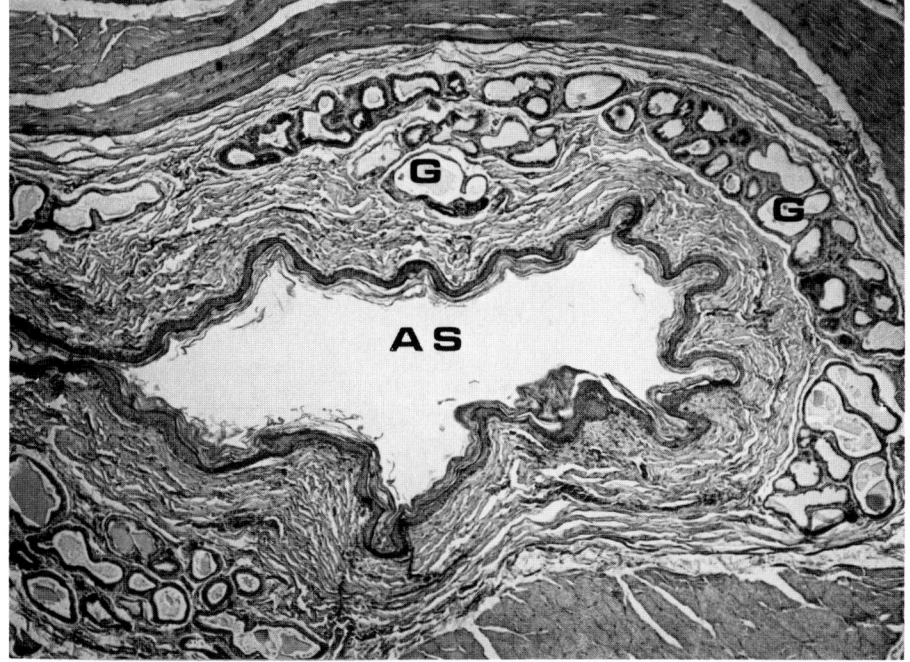

Fig. 18.19 Canine perianal sinus. The anal sacs are paired cutaneous diverticula of the anus that contain numerous apocrine tubular glands (G)
n their walls. AS, one of the anal sacs. X10.

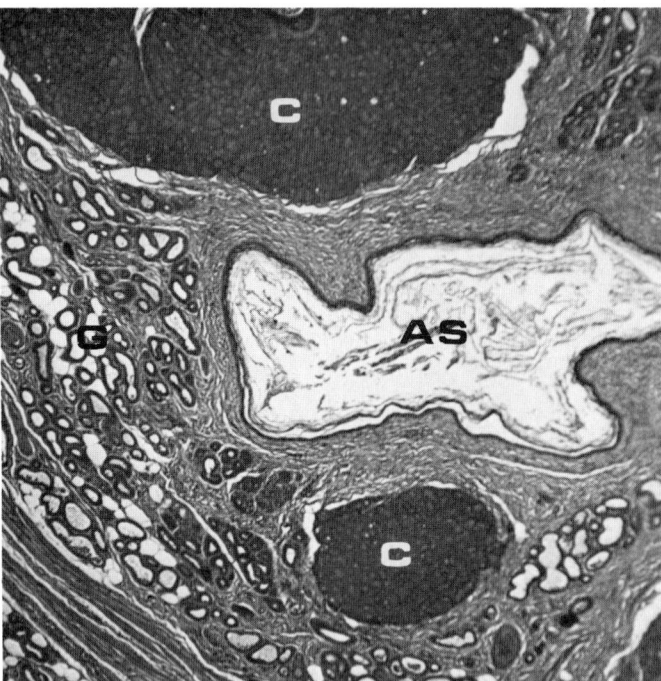

Fig. 18.20   Canine circumanal glands (C) are solid masses of cells which are in close association with the anal sacs (AS). G, apocrine tubular glands. X10.

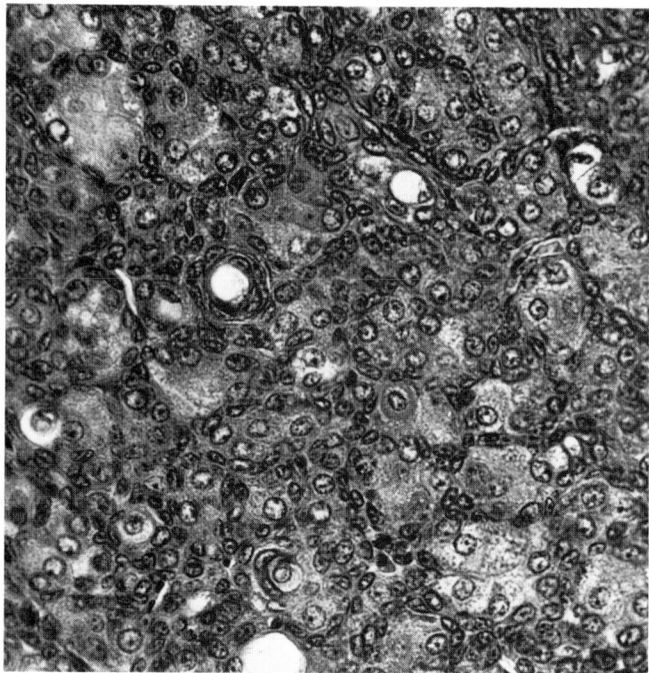

Fig. 18.21   Parenchyma of the circumanal glands. The parenchyma consists of a solid mass of polygonal cells that are acidophilic. Although ducts are present in this section, the ducts become nonpatent as they leave the gland. X100.

After the formation and secretion of milk the cells become much lower. This can be the result of a diminished or terminated secretory phase or the result of mechanical distortion due to the accumulation of the secretory product in the lumen. Not all the cells of a given secretory unit or all the secretory tubules and alveoli will be in the same state of activity at any given moment. Rather, a broad range of activity may be observed even in a highly active gland.

One or two *alveoli* drain into a single *secretory tubule*. This tubule or *intralobular duct* is lined by cuboidal epithelium, except in the initial secretory portion that is lined by a columnar epithelium. The intralobular ducts drain into a *lobular duct* that is lined by a cuboidal or columnar epithelium which is nonsecretory. The lobular duct is the primary excretory duct for a lobule and numerous lobular ducts drain into a *lobar duct*. The lobar duct is the primary excretory duct for a lobe and is lined by a bistratified columnar epithelium. Besides serving as excretory pathways for milk, the ducts may undergo expansion and serve as storage areas for milk. Numerous lobar ducts drain into the *gland sinus* (*gland cistern, lactiferous sinus*) which is lined by the same type epithelium. This is a common chamber at the base of each quarter of the udder. The volume of this cistern is quite variable. A slight constriction or *annulus* separates the *gland sinus* from the *teat sinus* (*teat cistern*); the latter is lined by a bistratified columnar epithelium. The annulus that separates the teat sinus from the gland sinus is not always apparent and is justification for referring to both sinuses collectively as the *lactiferous sinus*. The teat sinus is continuous with the outside via the *streak canal* (*papillary duct, teat canal*). The internal orifice of this canal is marked by an abrupt change to stratified squamous epithelium (keratinized). The tunica mucosa of this area is organized into longitudinal folds referred to as the *rosette of Furstenburg*. The epithelium of the teat canal continues through the external orifice and is continuous with the epidermal covering of the teat.

The connective tissue of the gland varies with its position within the organ. The sparse amount of intralobular connective tissue is areolar and contains an extensive capillary network. Numerous myoepithelial cells are intimately associated with the alveoli and secretory tubules. Interlobular (intralobar) and interlobar connective tissue is areolar. Numerous elastic and collagenous fibers, as well as blood vessels, lymphatics and nerves are present. Bundles of smooth muscle fibers are present and associated with large ducts. Helically arranged elastic fibers are also associated with large ducts.

The capsule of the organ is a fibroelastic connective tissue that is especially rich in elastic fibers. This capsule divides the organ into four quarters. The external lamina of the capsule is DWFCT and comprises the *lateral suspensory ligament*. The *medial sus-*

lumen and become part of the secretory product.

Many cells may occur in the lumina of the gland (Fig. 18.25). These may include sloughed secretory cells, macrophages and leukocytes, all of which then comprise part of the secretory product. These cells may occur in the secretory product throughout lactation. However, macrophages and leukocytes are especially prominent during early lactation when they comprise part of the *colostrum*. Colostrum functions as a laxative, but most importantly in some species it imparts a passive immunity to the nursing offspring until immunologic competency is gained.

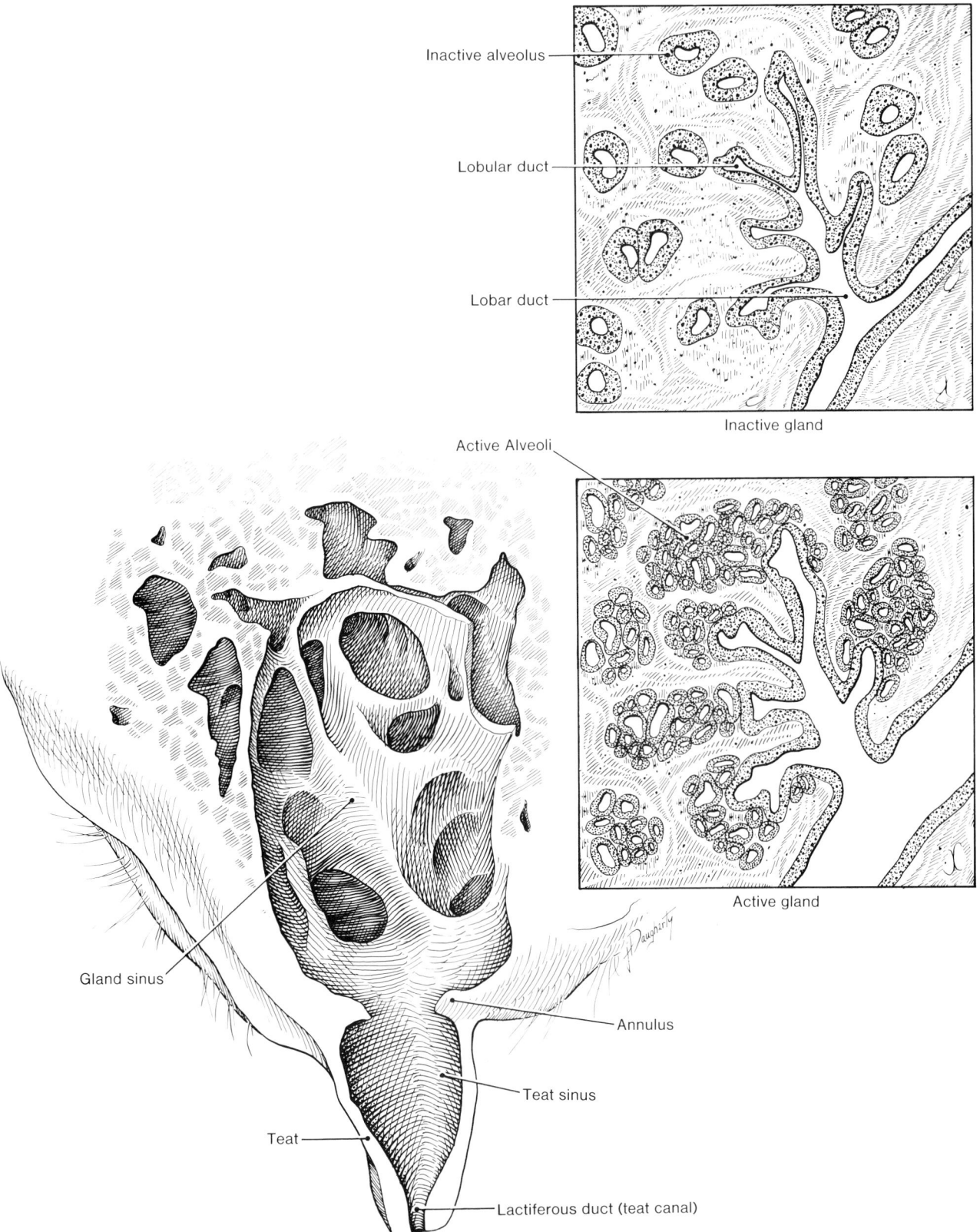

Fig. 18.22   Stylized drawing of the bovine udder. The number of alveoli is reduced greatly in an inactive gland. In an active gland, the number of alveoli increase at the expense of interstitial connective tissue.

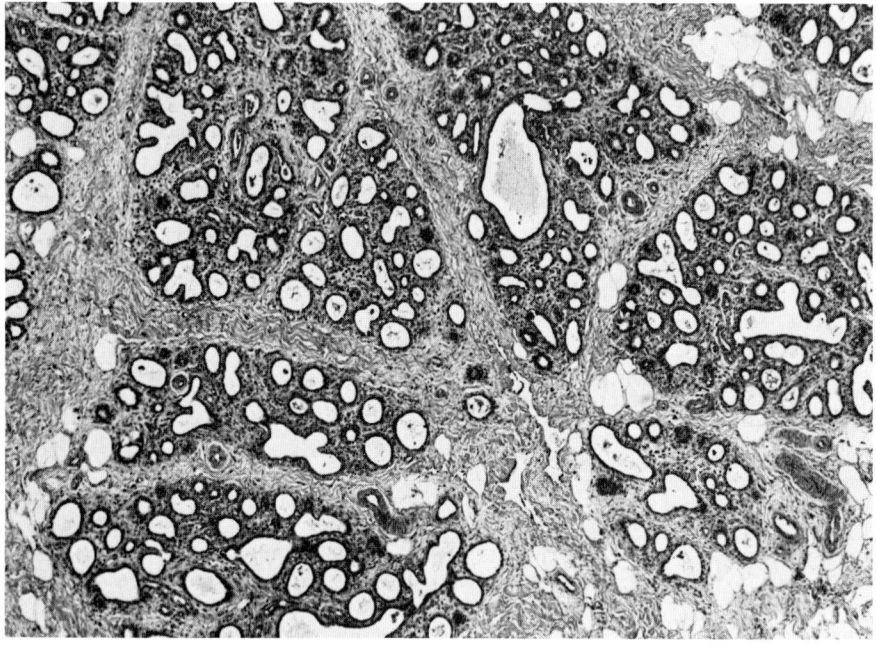

Fig. 18.23 Lactating bovine mammary gland. The parenchyma of the organ is predominant. Compare with Figures 18.22 and 18.27. X16.

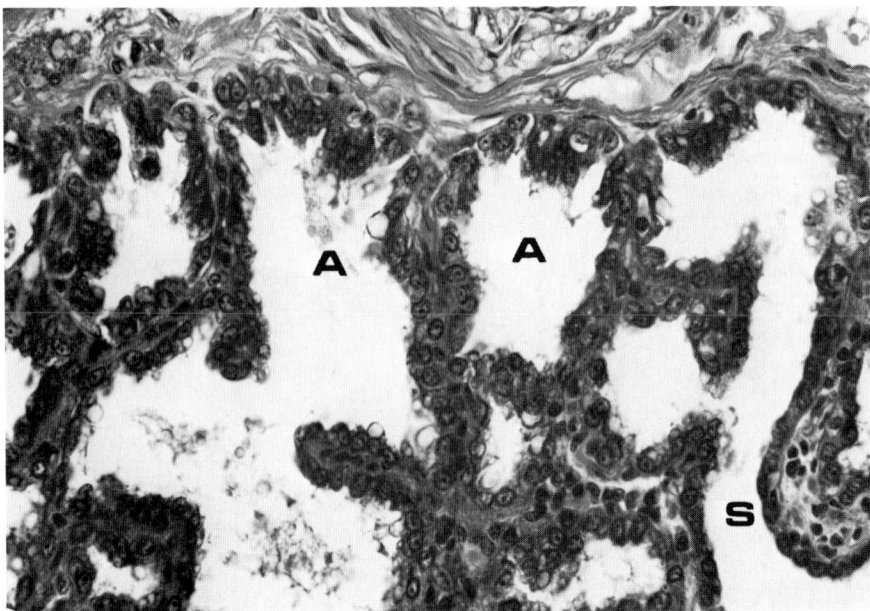

Fig. 18.24 Adenomeres of a lactating bovine mammary gland. The alveoli (A) are lined by a columnar epithelium that has blebs along its apical surface. The secretory tubules (S) are lined by a cuboidal epithelium. X100.

pensory ligament is especially rich in elastic fibers. The disposition of the capsule and connective tissue stroma is typical of solid organs.

The tunica mucosa and associated connective tissue (lamina propria and submucosa) of the teat sinus and teat canal are in close association and are actually continuous with the dermis (corium) and epidermal covering of the teat. The lamina epithelialis is bistratified columnar epithelium under-

laid with a lamina propria of areolar connective tissue which is rich in elastic fibers. There is no distinct submucosa. A tunica muscularis consists of strands of smooth muscular fibers. In the area of the internal orifice of the streak canal they are disposed as a sphincter. At the junction between the teat sinus and glands sinus this muscle also forms a sphincter. Extensive longitudinal blood vessels, thick-walled veins and lymphatic vessels are associated with the smooth

muscle layers, especially in the areas of the sphincters (Fig. 18.26). The connective tissue peripheral to the smooth muscular fibers is the corium. It is typical, except that it is especially rich in elastic fibers. The epidermal covering of the teat in the cow is hairless and nonglandular.

In the nonlactating mammary gland, the parenchyma is greatly reduced and replaced by areolar connective tissue (Figs. 18.22, 18.27). Extensive lymphocytic infiltration into the connective tissue and parenchyma is typical. Extensive adipose tissue may be present. The predominant loss of parenchyma is associated with the alveoli and secretory tubules. The remaining parenchyma is primarily the duct system. During mammary gland development, the alveoli are believed to be derived from the residual duct system.

During advanced stages of milk production, there is a gradual involution of the udder which eventually leads to a morphology associated with inactivity. Throughout lactation, but especially apparent in advanced stages, *corpora amylacea* are common (Fig. 18.28). These are concretions of casein (milk protein) and cellular detritus.

There are numerous gross and subgross anatomic differences among the mammary glands of domestic species. Although there are some histologic differences, they are academic. The number of teats, gland cisterns and teat canals per teat vary. The number of teat canals per teat in various species are: ruminants, 1; sow, 2 to 3; mare, 2 to 4; queen, 4 to 7; bitch, 8 to 20; woman, 15 to 24.

Miscellaneous Glands. Besides the previously described glands, numerous other glandular structures are localized to specific regions in different domestic species. Although these special skin glands do not possess unique histologic structural features, they do have interesting and/or unique gross relationships to other structures. However, these specialized glands are not associated with hairs.

Some of these special skin glands are comprised predominately of sebaceous glands. The *infraorbital glands* of sheep form a continuous lining around the infraorbital sinus. The sinus, located rostral and medial to the eye, is lined by thin skin, numerous sebaceous glands and a few apocrine tubular glands peripherally. The *submental organ* of cats is located within the intermandibular space and consists of accumulations of sebaceous glands. The *supracaudal gland* or *tail glands* of dogs and cats are located along the dorsal aspect of the tail. The tail glands of the cat extend along the entire length of the dorsum of the tail; excessive secretions of these glands impart a waxy appearance to the tail known as "stud tail." In the dog, the tail glands are confined to a small, raised, oval and well-circumscribed area at the base of the tail from which single coarse hairs eminate. The *preputial glands*

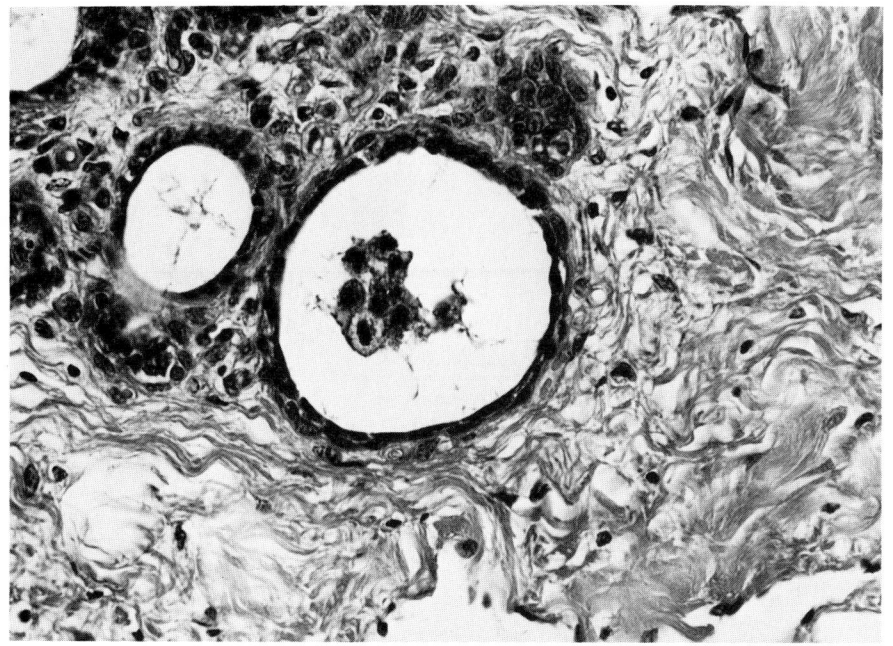

Fig. 18.25 Cells within an alveolus. The cells may be sloughed epithelial cells or migratory cells from the connective tissue. X100.

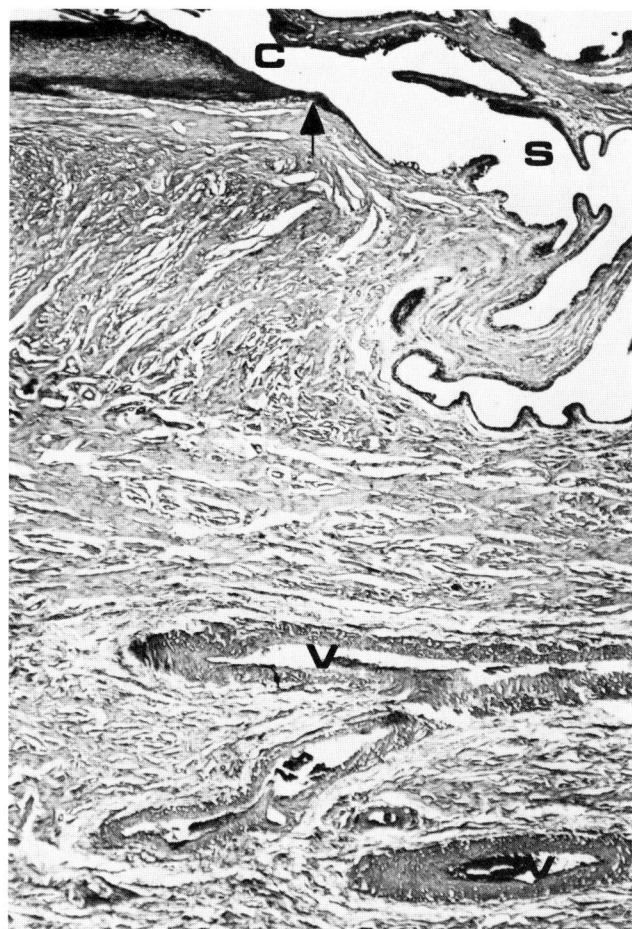

Fig. 18.26 Junction between the teat sinus and the streak canal in a bovine mammary gland. The junction (*arrow*) between the teat sinus (S) and the internal orifice of the streak canal (C) is marked by a transition from bistratified columnar to stratified squamous epithelium. Vessels (V) are oriented longitudinally in this region. X10.

of the stallion are prominent and active sebaceous glands that elaborate sebum (*smegma*). The *scent glands* or *horn glands* of the goat are modified sebaceous glands associated with hairs that are located along the caudomedial aspect of the horn base. Their secretory product, which includes caproic acid, imparts the typical odor to male goats.

Special skin glands also include accumulations of tubular glands. The *mental organ* of pigs is an accumulation of aprocrine tubular glands in the intermandibular space. Porcine *carpal glands*, aggregations of merocrine tubular glands, are located on the medial aspect of the carpus.

Also, special skin glands may include aggregations of tubular and sebaceous glands. The *interdigital glands* of sheep are located in the interdigital sinus and consist of a mixture of sebaceous and apocrine tubular glands. The lining of the ovine inguinal sinus contains inquinal glands which are constituted similarly.

Hooves and Claws

Equine Foot. The hoof is the insensitive cornified layer of the epidermis. The foot, however, includes the hoof, dermis and all the structures contained therein (Fig. 18.29). The hoof is much like any other epidermally derived structure. The unique morphology of the hoof is achieved by the different relationships between the epidermis and related dermis or corium. This is manifested in two distinct ways. In some regions, the dermis is papillated; i.e., typical but pronounced dermal papillae and corresponding epidermal pegs are present. In other regions the papillae and epidermal pegs are confluent. As a result, the adjacent epidermal and dermal regions are *laminar.*

Most parts of the hoof are formed of cornified material which is arranged in a tubular manner. Some regions, however, are nontubular. One region is laminar. The hoof, therefore, is composed of *tubular, intertubular* and *laminar horn* (keratin).

The hoof may be divided into the following distinct regions histologically: *periople, coronet, laminae, bars, sole* and *frog* (Fig. 18.30). Corresponding to these epidermal regions are areas of the corium that bear the same name. Thus, there is a *perioplic epidermis* and a *perioplic corium,* etc.

The perioplic, coronary and laminar epidermises comprise the *wall* of the hoof (Fig. 18.31). In older horses, the coronary and laminar epidermises are the primary constituents of the wall.

The *perioplic epidermis* is referrred to as the *stratum externum* or *stratum tectorium* (Fig. 18.32). It is composed of soft, thin, white, shiny and cornified material which extends over the wall and *bulbs.* The perioplic epidermis is the means by which the hoof is directly attached to the epidermis of

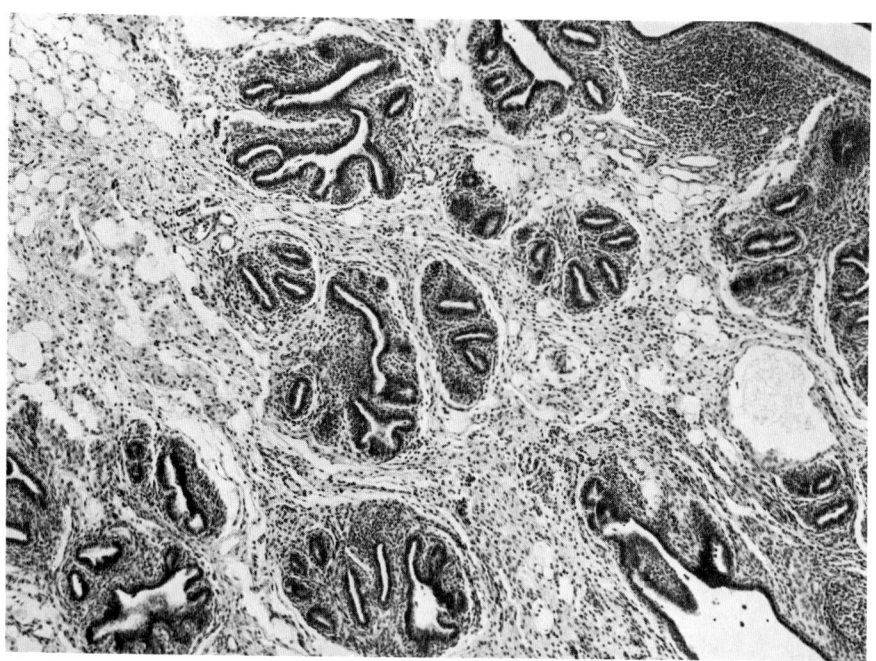

Fig. 18.27 A nonlactating bovine mammary gland. The parenchyma is reduced while the amount of connective tissue is increased. Compare with Figures 18.22 and 18.23. X16.

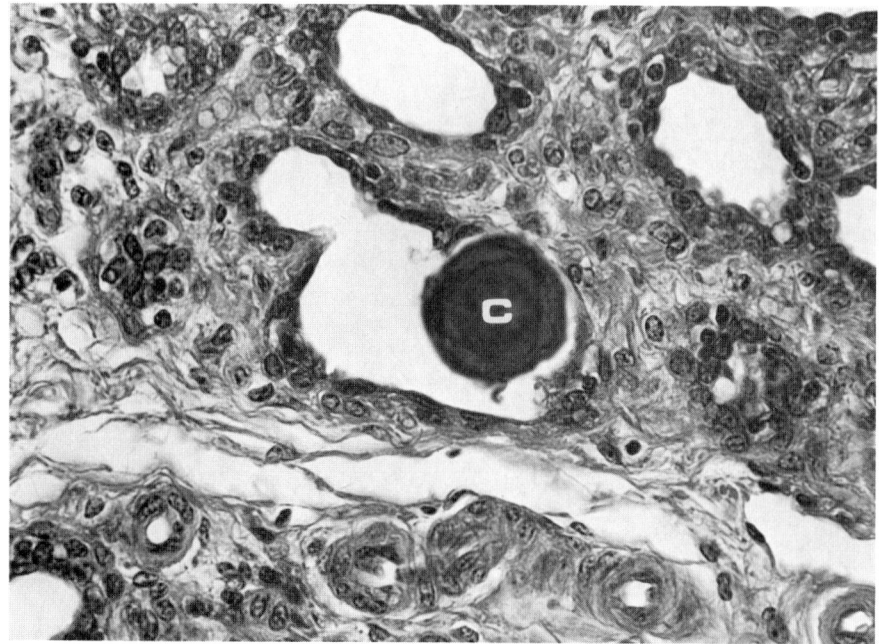

Fig. 18.28 Amylaceous corpuscle in an alveolus of the bovine mammary gland. The corpuscle (C) is a concretion of milk protein and cellular debris. X100.

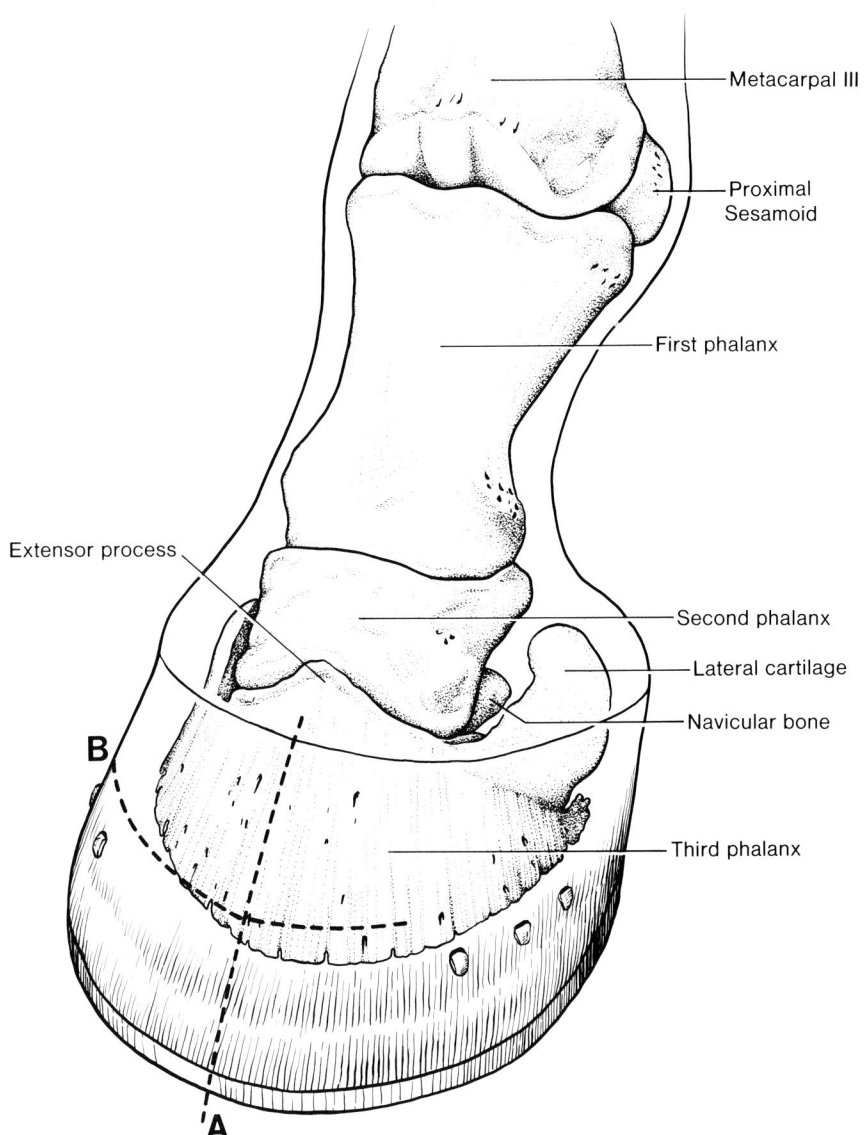

Fig. 18.29 A simplified drawing of the equine foot. The *line* at A (perpendicular to the ground surface) represents the plane of section in Figures 18.30, 18.32, 18.33, 18.35 and 18.36. The *line* at B (parallel to the ground surface) represents the plane of section for Figures 18.31, 18.34 and 18.37.

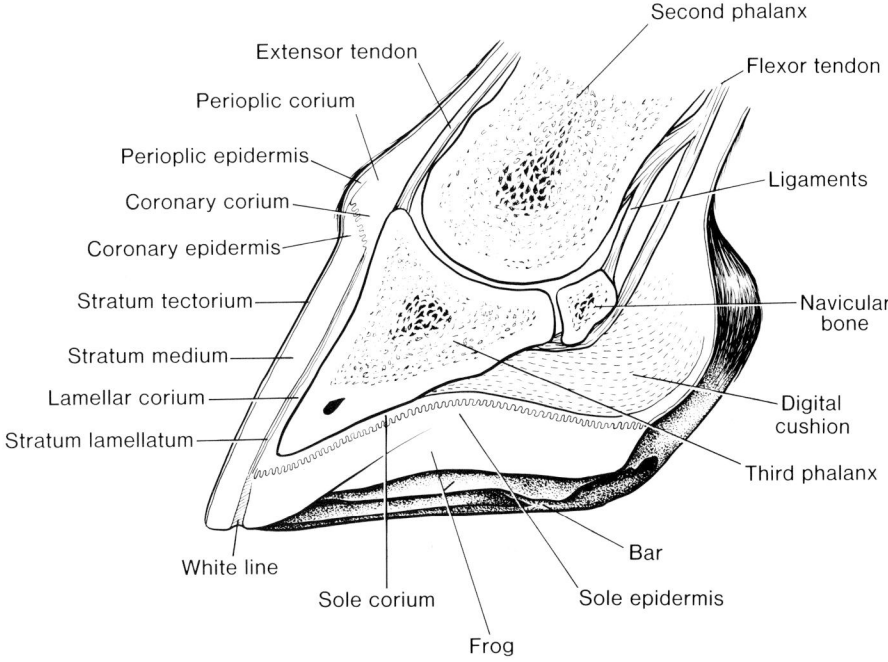

Fig. 18.30 A longitudinal section through an equine foot.

359

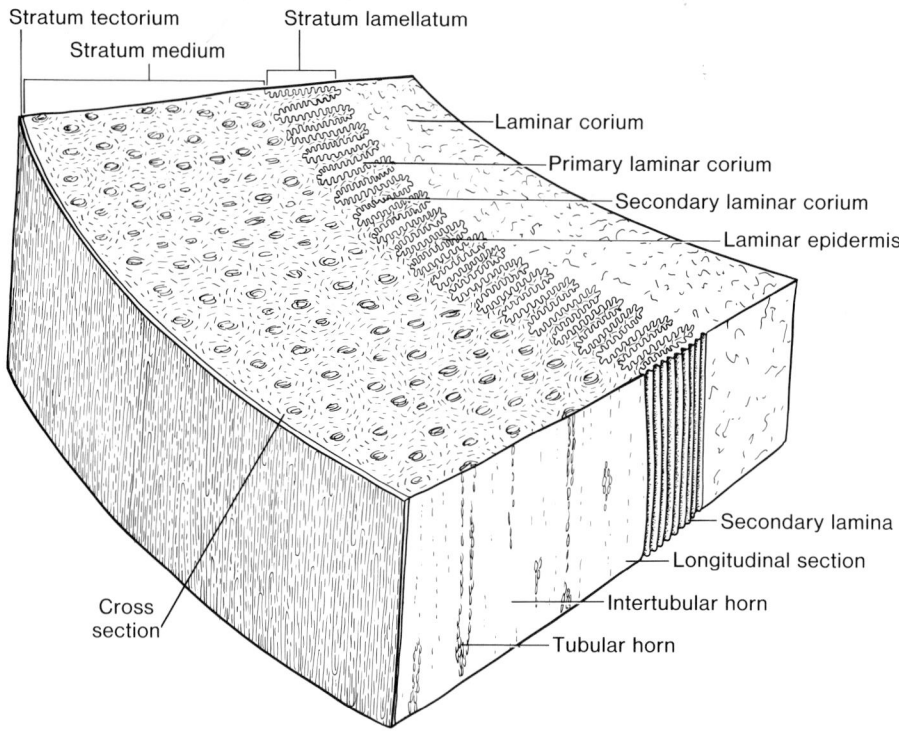

Fig. 18.31 A cross-section and longitudinal section through the wall of the equine hoof.

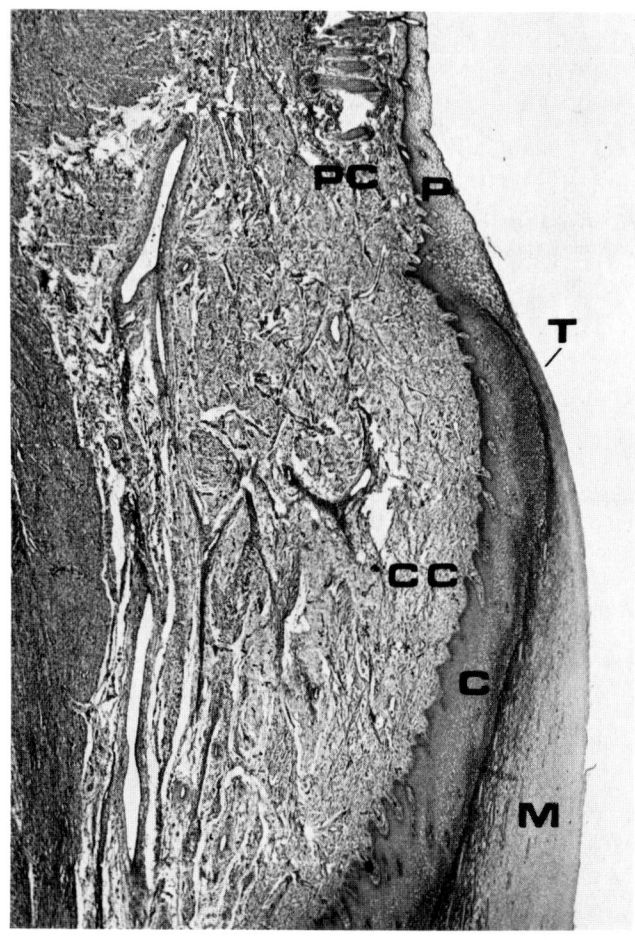

Fig. 18.32 A longitudinal section through the perioplic and coronary region of a fetal equine foot. PC, perioplic corium; P, periople or perioplic epidermis; T, stratum tectorium; CC, coronary corium; C, coronary epidermis; M, stratum medium. X4.

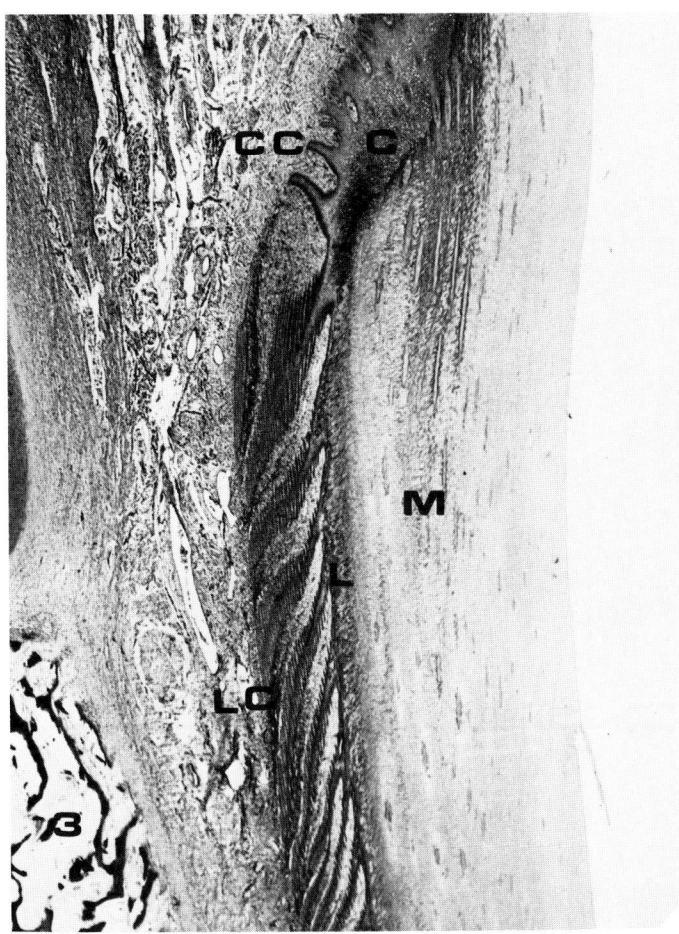

Fig. 18.33 Longitudinal section through the coronary and laminar region of a fetal equine foot. CC, coronary corium; C, coronary epidermis; M, Stratum medium; L, laminar epidermis; LC, laminar corium; 3, third phalanx. The slight obliquity of the section permits the visualization of individual laminae. X40.

the skin. It may be absent in older animals. It is probably the means by which water loss from the hoof is diminished. The associated *perioplic corium* is papillated. These papillae are highly vascularized and oriented "perpendicular" to the ground surface. This orientation results in a downward growth of the perioplic epidermis.

The *coronary epidermis*, underlaid by the *coronary corium*, is also referred to as the *stratum medium* (Fig. 18.33). Normally, it is devoid of a stratum granulosum and a stratum lucidum. This is typical of most parts of the hoof. It is composed of very prominent tubular and intertubular horn which comprises the bulk of the hoof wall (Fig. 18.34). The tubular horn is elaborated in a manner that may be compared to the growth of hairs (Fig. 18.35). The spaces between the tubular horn are filled with intertubular horn. The tubules of horn arise from the germinal epithelium that covers the lateral and distal portions of the dermal papillae. The intertubular horn is elaborated from the germinal epithelium in the depths of the epidermal pegs. The papillae of this region are elongated and are oriented "perpendicular" to the ground surface. This orientation results in the cornified cells being elaborated in a similar relationship to the ground sur-

face: i.e., the tubular horn is "perpendicular" to the ground also.

The *epidermis of the laminar region* (*stratum lamellatum*) is composed of nontubular horn (Fig. 18.36). This horn is elaborated at a very slow pace in a plane which is perpendicular to the stratum medium of coronary origin. It fuses with the stratum medium and assists in holding the wall proper to the foot. The orientation and configuration of the dermal papillae are altered in this region. The dermal papillae and corresponding epidermal pegs are converted to elongated ridges that are oriented "perpendicular" to the ground surface. By analogy, the fingers of the hand would represent dermal papillae and the intervening spaces would represent the epidermal pegs. Successive stacking of one hand upon the other converts the confluent papillae and pegs to ridges or laminae. There are *primary* and *secondary laminae* in this region (Fig. 18.37). The secondaries are oriented at an acute angle to the primaries. The primary epidermal laminae are composed of stratum spinosum and horn. Collectively, these areas are referred to as the *insensitive laminae*. The remaining secondary laminae, with the germinal epithelium and associated dermal structures, are referred to as the *sensitive*

laminae. The laminae of the epidermis (stratum lamellatum) interdigitate with corresponding projections of the *laminar corium*. The insensitive laminae continue to the ground surface as the laminae of the wall. The junction between the laminae of the wall and *epidermis of the sole* is called the *white line*.

The epidermis and corium of the laminar region are oriented "perpendicular" to the ground surface. At the white line these structures are reflected around the corner of the wall and become parallel to the ground surface. This point of reflection results in the fusion of horn material which is oriented differently. Thus, the white line is formed. The white line is an important landmark for shoeing horses. A properly oriented nail driven peripherally to the white line will not touch any sensitive structures of the foot.

The *epidermis of the bars*, *sole* and *frog* is similar to the papillated regions described previously. However, the papillae are not as elongated as those described previously and the horn material is softer than that which composes the wall.

The corium of the foot is a continuation of the connective tissue which comprises the corium of the skin. The corium of the foot, however, does contain numerous elastic fibers. In the region of the coronary corium, an extensive venous plexus is present. In most instances, the corium of the foot is intimately associated with the fibrous periosteum of the enclosed osseous structures. These relationships aid not only in shock absorption but also in attaching the hoof to the deeper structures of the foot. The laminar corium attaches the laminar region to the third phalanx and assists in the suspension of the foot within the hoof. The corium of the frog contains modified sweat glands which invaginate from the epidermis of the frog.

A *digital cushion* occupies the space between the bones and tendons of the foot and the ground surface of the hoof. This fibroelastic connective tissue, which is rich in adipose tissue, is an effective shock absorber.

Ruminant and Porcine Claws. An understanding of the complexity of the equine hoof and related structures facilitates the understanding of similar structures in other species, because the latter are more simple histologically.

Although there are many gross differences between these and the equine hoof, there are only a few significant histological differences (Fig. 18.38). The claws of these species consist of: *wall*, *sole* and well-developed *bulbs*. The laminar epidermis consists of primary laminae only (Fig. 18.39). These occur with a greater frequency than in the horse. The orientation of the papillae of the sole is more craniad than in the horse. Usually, there are more zones of the epidermis apparent.

Claws of Carnivores. The claws of carnivores consist of a wall and sole (Fig. 18.40).

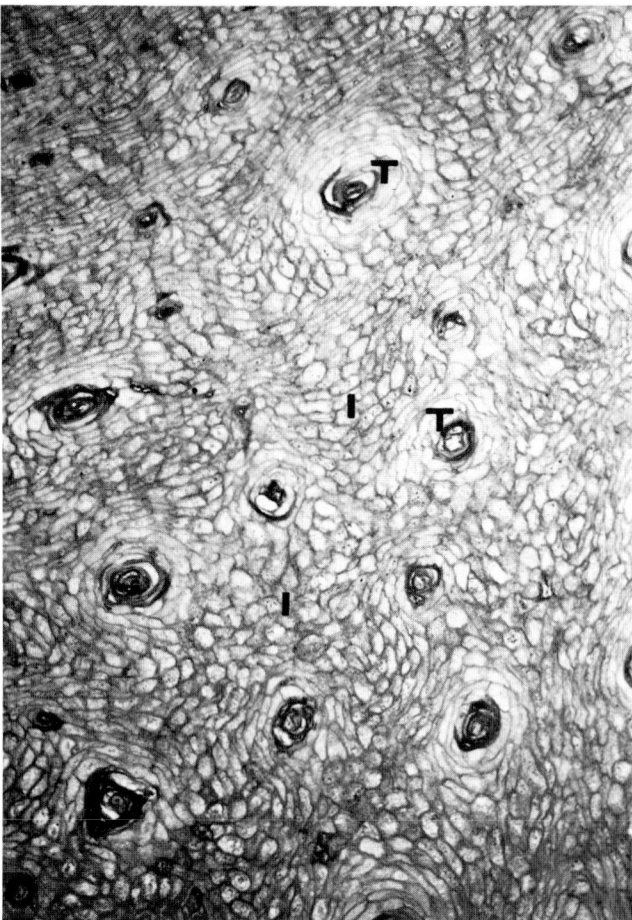

Fig. 18.34   Organization of the stratum medium of the equine hoof. The stratum medium is composed of tubular (T) and intertubular horn (I). X40.

The coronary epidermis and associated corium comprise the majority of the wall and consist of long dermal papillae and corresponding epidermal pegs. Laminar epidermis and associated corium are restricted to the dorsolateral aspects of the wall. The sole corium consists of thick papillae.

Integumentary Appendages

Horns of the Ox. The horn of the ox consists of three basic components: *os cornua, corium* and *epidermis*. The *os cornua* or *frontal process* is an outgrowth of the frontal bone. The medullary cavity of the os cornua is continuous with the diploe of the frontal bone. It is covered by typical integumentary corium which is papillated. The associated epidermis gives rise to tubular horn and some intertubular horn. At the base of the horn the epidermis gives rise to soft horn, the *epikeras*, which is similar to the perioplic epidermis of the hoof.

Cellular proliferation of the basal cells of the epidermis is slow and the horn continues to elongate at a very slow pace.

Antlers of Cervids. The antlers of deer and associated species consist of bone and velvet. These structures undergo cyclic growth, maturation and shedding which is inti-

mately associated with the seasonal breeding habits of these species. The bone develops by a modified type of endochondral ossification. During growth, the developing cartilage is located at the end of each *tine*. It mineralizes and osseous replacement occurs. Eventually, as in the growth plate, the osseous replacement occurs at a faster rate than cartilage differentiation and "closure" occurs. At that point the core of the antler is bone which is continuous with the *pedicle* of the frontal bone. Throughout development, the developing bone is covered by the integument, *velvet*. Upon maturation, the velvet becomes necrotic and is removed by rubbing. The bony protuberance remains as the mature antler. An abscission zone develops at the base of the antler (similar to that which occurs in leaves) and it is dropped. At this point, the entire process begins again.

Besides being a biologic curiosity, much information about chondrogenic and osteogenic processes may be had by the study of antler growth. Some species grow as much as 25 lb of bone during the 3-month active growing period at a rate of up to 1 cm per day at the antler tip. No mammalian growth process compares with it. Although antlers are usually confined to males, the female caribou and reindeer are antlered.

Miscellaneous Appendages. The horn of the pronghorn is very similar to the horn of the ox. However, the cornified material is shed annually.

The frontal process of the giraffe is similar to the antler. However, it is not shed.

The horn of the rhinoceros consists of matted hair.

Dewclaws, Chestnut and Ergot. *Dewclaws* of ruminants, swine and dogs represent vestigial digits covered by horn material and associated dermis similar to the horn material characteristic of the species. A bony core may or may not be present (limb and species variable).

Chestnut and *ergots* are areas of the equine epidermis that are highly keratinized and consist of tubular and nontubular horn (Fig. 18.41). They are devoid of hairs and glands. Some authorities consider these to be vestiges of some of the digits.

Repair of the Skin

Introduction. The numerous and varied functions of the skin depend upon the maintenance of mophologic integrity. Disruptions in the outer covering of the body may cause functional alterations that have profound effects upon the organism. Microbial agents may enter the body through injuries that disrupt integumentary continuity, whereas excessive fluid and protein loss may occur through large foci denuded of their epidermal coverings.

The skin is subject to various types of wounds or disruption in anatomic integrity—abrasions, contusions, lacerations, punctures and incisions. Three types of healing processes have been described for wounds in which tissues underlying the epidermis are exposed to the external environment—open wounds. *First intention healing* occurs when the skin, which has been disrupted by a clean incisional wound, is closed immediately. *Second intention healing* results when the wound, with tissue loss, is allowed to heal spontaneously without any or minimal surgical intervention. *Third intention healing* is a combination of first and second intention healing. The tissues are allowed to heal spontaneously for a period of time and then wound closure is accomplished. Injuries to the skin that result in a loss of integumentary continuity require contributions from the epidermis, dermis and hypodermis for healing to be accomplished. The vasculature, neutrophils, macrophages, fibroblasts and epidermal cells are the mediators of skin repair.

The repair of skin is a dynamic complex of cellular activity that is initiated with injury and continues through the reorganization of the tissues of the injury site. Although skin repair represents a continuum of integrated cellular activity, for discussion the repair process may be divided into distinct yet interrelated stages: *insult (wounding), induction, inflammatory, proliferative* and *maturation stages*.

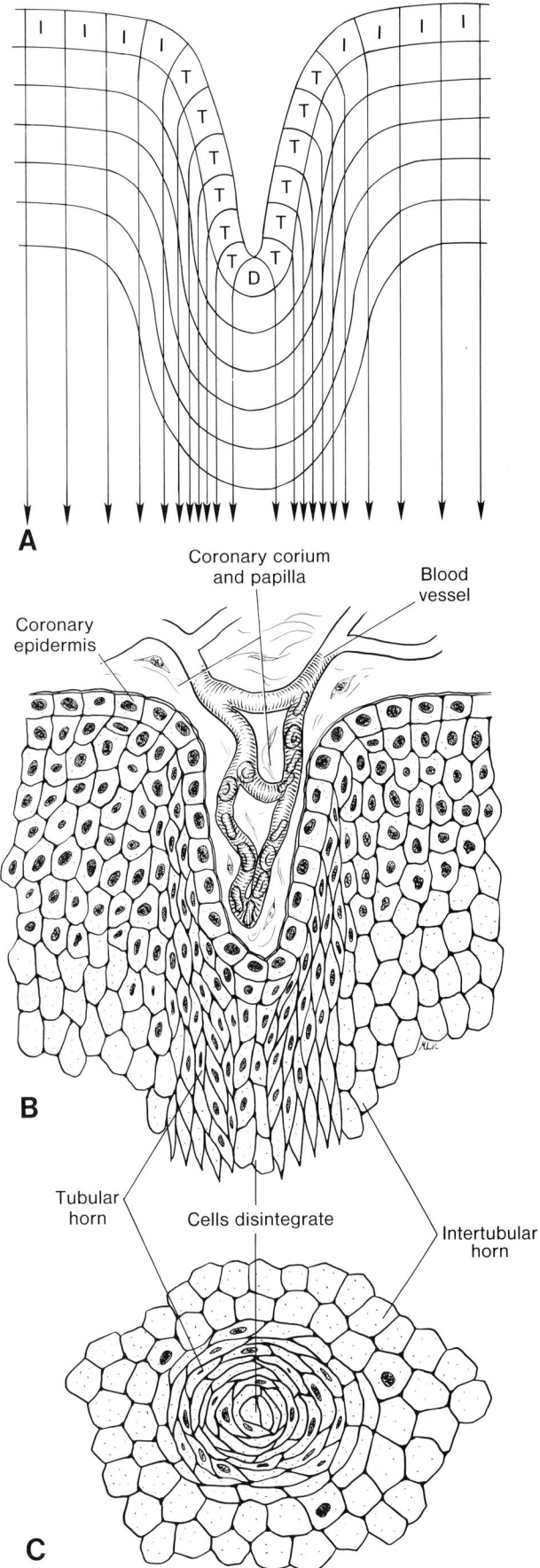

A

Coronary corium
and papilla

Blood
vessel

Coronary
epidermis

B

Tubular
horn

Cells disintegrate

Intertubular
horn

C

Fig. 18.35 Scheme depicting the elaboration of tubular and intertubular horn by the coronary epidermis. A. This scheme represents a longitudinal section through the coronary region. Cells indicated with a T line the shoulders of an epidermal peg. These cells will give rise to tubular horn. The cells indicated with an I line the apex of an epidermal peg. These cells will give rise to intertubular horn. The cells at D will disintegrate. B. This is the cellular representation of the scheme depicted in A. C. A cross-section through the tubular and intertubular horn of the stratum medium. Drawings A, B and C are in register with each other.

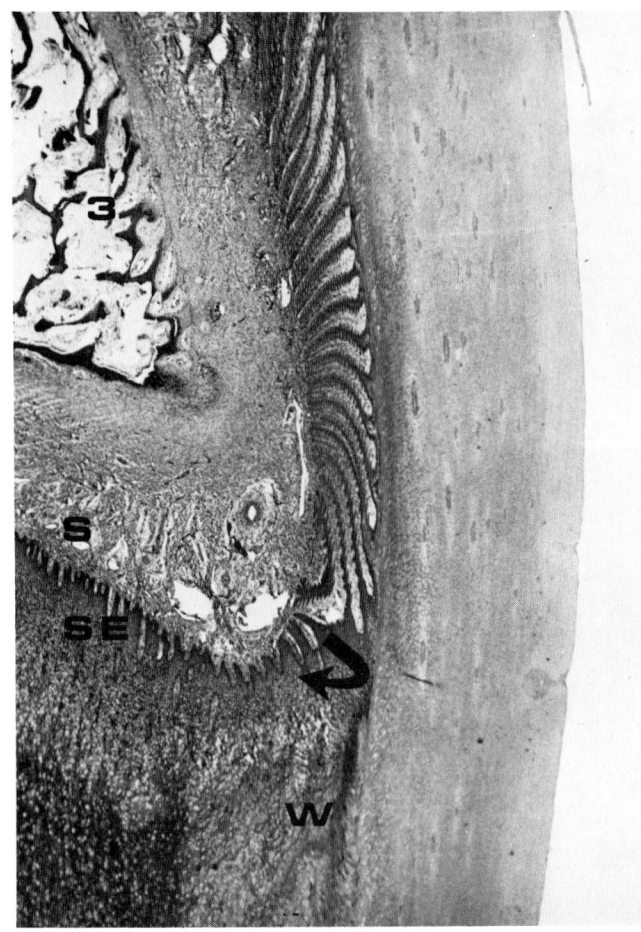

Fig. 18.36 Longitudinal section through the laminar and sole region of a fetal equine foot. The corium and epidermis of the laminar region is continuous (*curved arrow*) with the sole corium (S) and sole epidermis (SE). The point of transition or reflection of the epidermis is continued to the ground surface as the white line (W). 3, third phalanx. The change of orientation of keratinized material partially accounts for the appearance of the white line. Primarily, the white line is visible because the degree of keratinization or hardness of horn material is different in the stratum medium, white line and sole epidermis. The slight obliquity of the section permits visualization of individual laminae. X4.

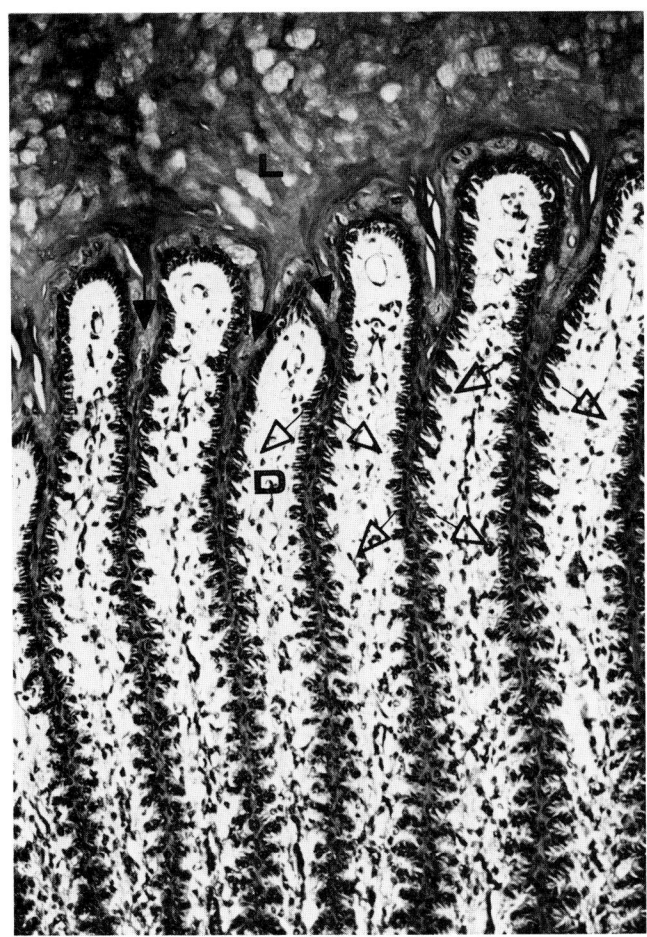

Fig. 18.37 Sensitive and insensitive laminae of the equine foot. The stratum lamellatum (L) and the primary epidermal laminae (*solid arrows*) comprise the insensitive laminae. The secondary laminae, as indicated by the orientation of *open arrows*, and the corium (D) comprise the sensitive laminae. X100.

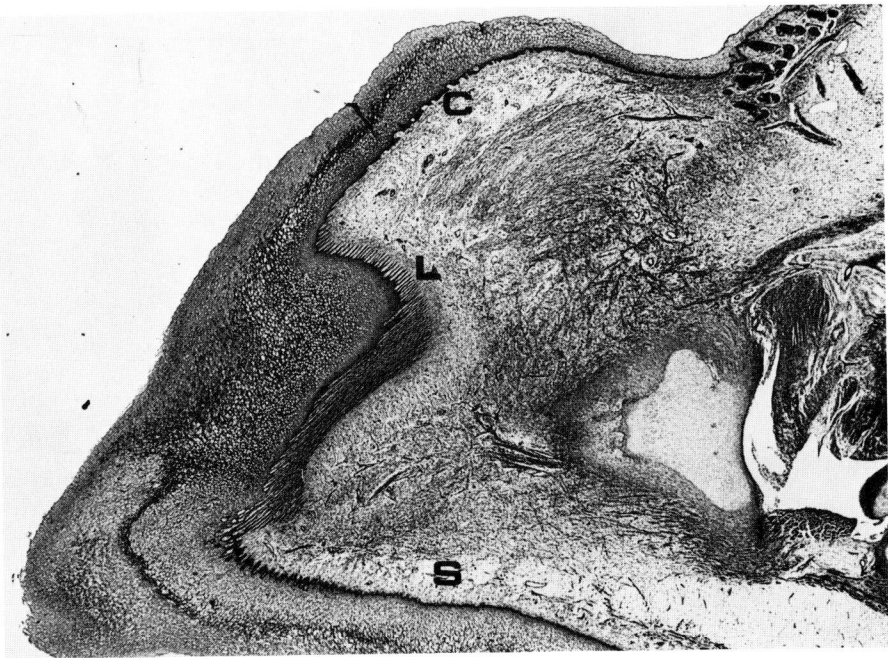

Fig. 18.38 Longitudinal section through an ovine fetal claw. The coronary (C), laminar (L) and sole (S) epidermis and corium are indicated. X4.

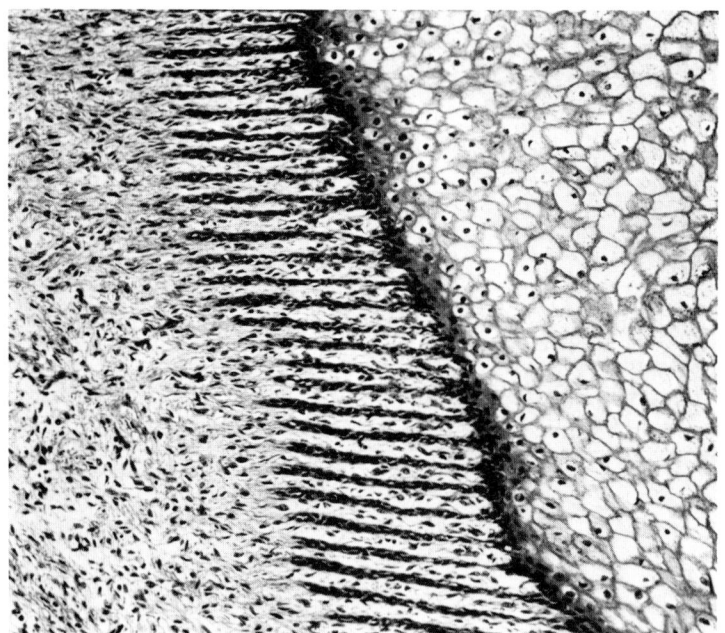

Fig. 18.39 Laminae of the fetal bovine claw. Only primary laminae are present. X40.

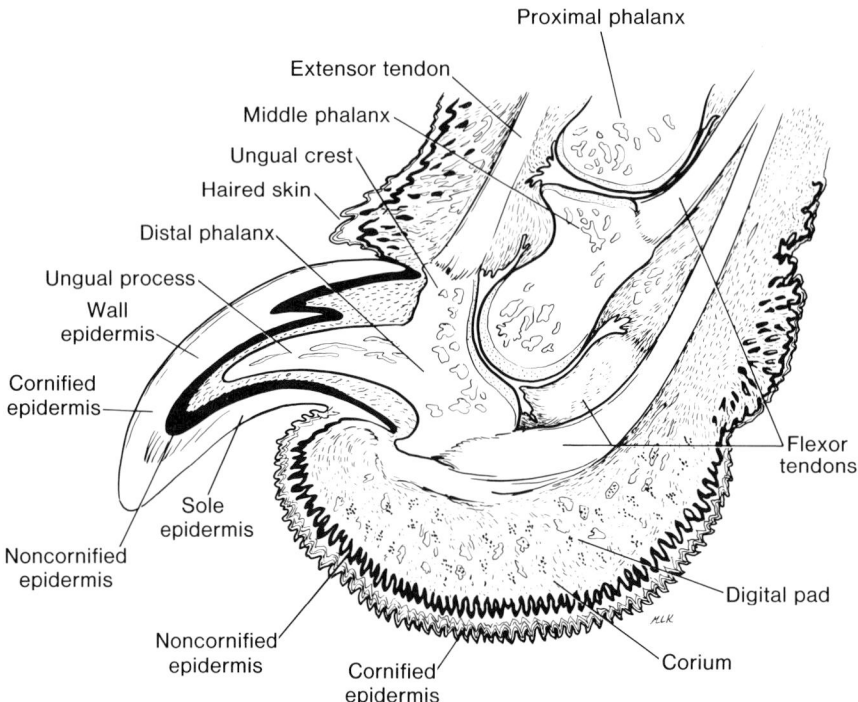

Fig. 18.40 A stylized drawing of a sagittal section through the canine foot.

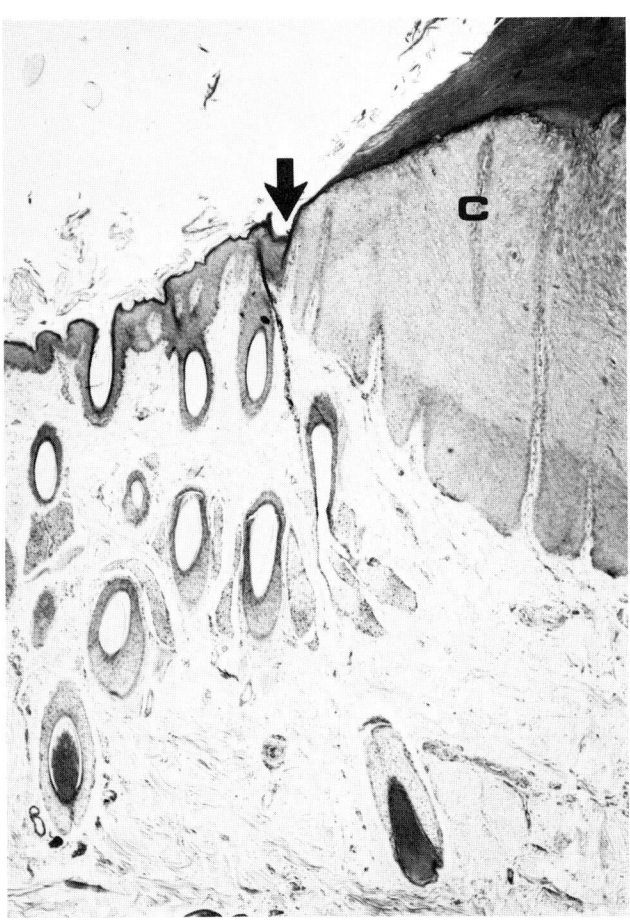

Fig. 18.41   Equine chestnut. The point of transition (*arrow*) from typical epidermis to chestnut (C) is marked by an increased epidermal thickness and increased keratinization. X10.

The events involved in skin repair—requiring epidermal, dermal and hypodermal contributions—are similar in most integumentary repair processes. The methods by which the injured sites are handled dictate alterations in the process. Minor abrasions to the epidermis without damage to the underlying dermis generally repair themselves through the mitotic activity of the stratum basale of the epidermis. Whereas first intention healing may occur at a faster rate than second intention healing, all stages of the repair process are integral components of these methods. Excisional wounds in which excessive amounts of tissue are lost are characterized by a marked proliferation of fibrous connective tissue (*granulation tissue*).

For the sake of simplicity, an incisional wound undergoing second intention healing is described subsequently. The sequence of events is illustrated in Figures 18.42–18.46.
Insult (Wounding) Stage. The initial stage of the repair process begins with the insult or wound (Fig. 18.42). Disruption of the integrity of the skin results in hemorrhage, local cell death and contamination with microorganisms. Hemostatic mechanisms are operational locally and account for clotting of the extravasated blood in the wound gap.

Similar mechanisms account for the plugging of severed blood vessels. The clot, filled with cellular debris, microorganisms and components of the clotting mechanism, fills the gap in the incised tissues. The clot minimizes further fluid loss and forms a seal over the injured area. Deprived of their normal vascular supply, the tissues at the site of injury undergo desiccation.
Induction Stage. Although the identification of this stage as a distinct entity may be artificial, induction of new cells into the area of injury is an essential initiator of repair. However, induction of new cells must occur throughout the repair process. Although various substances may serve as chemotactic factors for neutrophils, macrophages and fibroblasts, the precise stimuli for an integrated repair have not been identified. Initially, the resultant localized tissue hypoxia and acidosis may induce essential neovascularization (Fig. 18.43). Fibroblasts may respond to local lactic acid accumulations resulting from the activity of macrophages, but collagen synthesis can not occur until essential metabolites are supplied by the vasculature.
Inflammatory Stage. The inflammatory stage begins immediately after the injury (Fig. 18.43). Although vasoconstriction is

the immediate localized response to injury, it is followed by capillary dilatation with an accompanying increase in vascular permeability. The release of vasoactive substances from endothelial cells, mast cells and platelets—histamine, serotonin, bradykinin, prostaglandin E_2—inititates the localized vascular response. Chemotactic factors released at the injury site attract neutrophils and fibroblasts. Bradykinin and prostaglandin E_2 may function to attract these cells to the wound.

Neutrophils are the predominant cells at the injury site for the first 3 days after injury. They are effective phagocytes that function to control microbial contamination and remove cellular detritus. Macrophages, mast cells, eosinophils, lymphocytes and plasma cells are attracted to the injury site during the inflammatory stage. Macrophages are responsible for the phagocytosis of cellular debris and other damaged tissue components (collagen, elastin). Mast cells, by virtue of their release of vasoactive amines, contribute to the acute inflammatory response. Lymphocytes and plasma cells afford protection through their roles in cell-mediated and antibody-mediated immunity. Eosinophils may be present at the wound site in response to the formation of immune

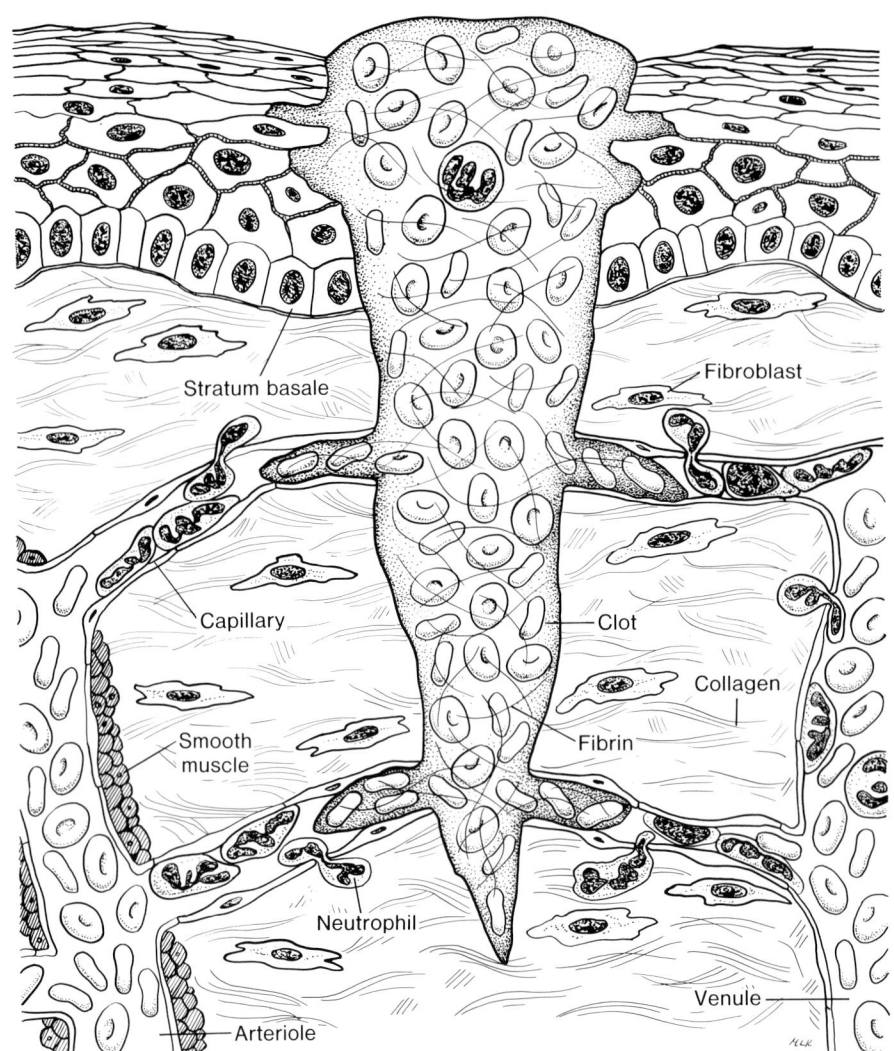

Fig. 18.42   The initial events of skin repair. Clot formation has occurred and the defect has been filled. Capillaries have been plugged. Hemostasis has been achieved. The labels on this figure also apply to Figures 18.43–18.46.

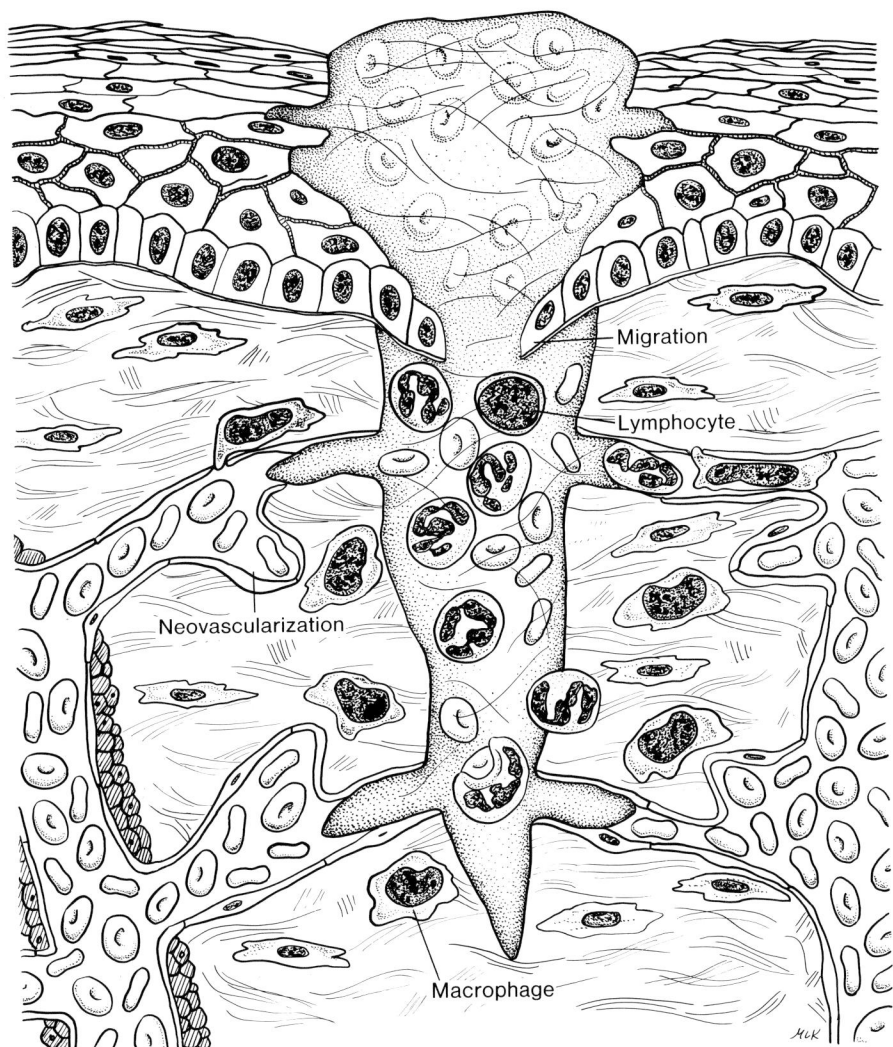

Fig. 18.43   Induction and initiation of inflammation. Inflammatory cells have invaded the wound site. Neovascularization and epidermal cell migration have been initiated.

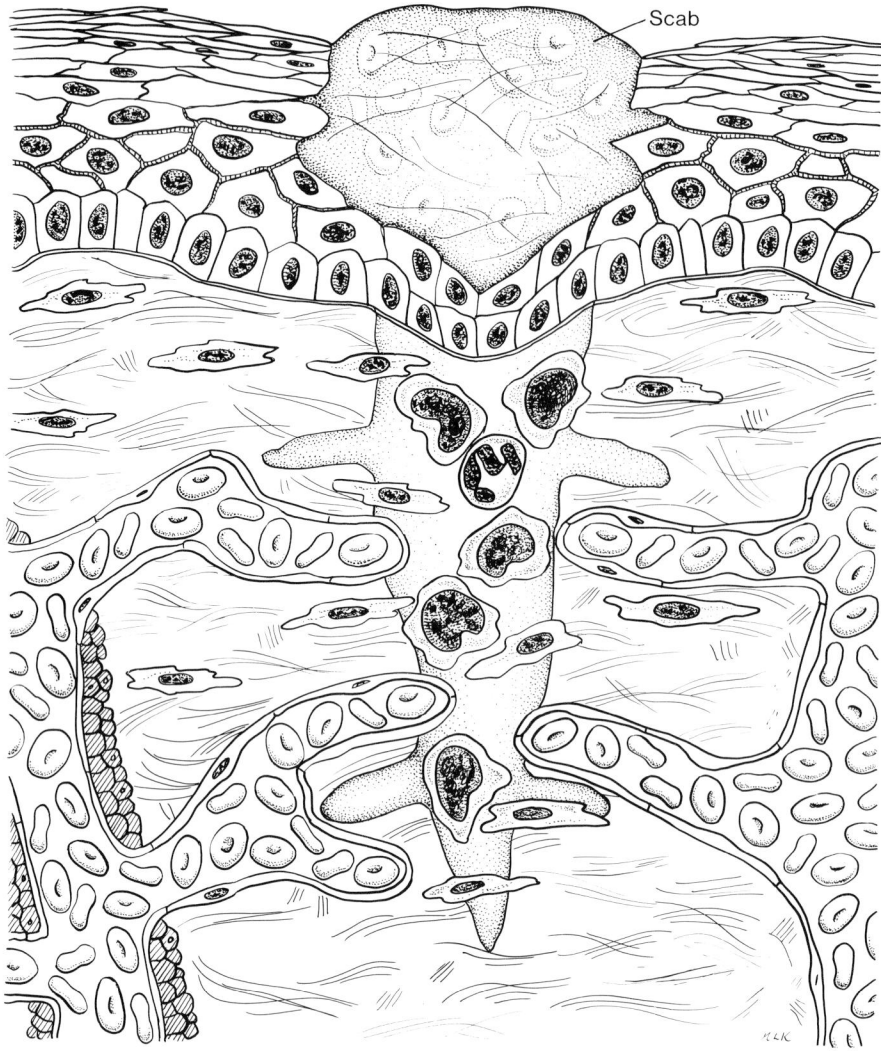

Fig. 18.44 Proliferative stage of wound repair. Inflammation has subsided and the epidermal cells have migrated over the wound site beneath the scab. Neovascularization continues and fibroblasts invade the clot with the new blood vessels.

complexes or in response to the specific activity of mast cells.

The duration of the inflammatory stage is dependent upon various factors—the amount of contamination, the extent of tissue damage and the presence of infection. A clean wound, one in which no microbial agents are present, may be characterized by a peak inflammatory response in 3–4 days. Progression of repair is accompanied by a gradual and steady diminution of the cellular populations which characterize the inflammatory stage.

Proliferative Stage. The proliferative stage, involving the mitotic activity of epidermal cells, endothelial cells and fibroblasts, extends 10–14 days postinjury (Fig. 18.44). Epidermal cells within the stratum basale along the margins of the wound migrate across the wound defect. Additionally, similar cells from cut hair follicles within the defect may migrate to cover the wound. Migration is a random process that is initi-

ated within the first 24 hours after injury but is not visible until keratinization occurs. The epidermis adjacent to the wound site subsequently proliferates to replace the migrating cells. The migrating cells, retaining their mitotic potential, proliferate and begin to replace the epidermis. The result of this migratory and proliferative activity is the re-establishment of an epidermal barrier over the underlying connective tissue of the dermis but beneath the scab. The scab sloughs in approximately 7 days.

Endothelial cell proliferation from the ends of severed vessels initiates the re-establishment of vascularity (Fig. 18.45). Fusion of these cells from arterial and venous capillaries completes the neovascularization. Perivascular fibroblasts proliferate and synthesize matrix materials in response to the improved microenvironment. Fibroblasts, moving along fibrin strands which serve as a temporary scaffold, advance into the wound site with the advancing vascular

beds. Some fibroblasts develop the ability to move along matrix materials by contractile mechanisms. These fibroblasts, which contain contractile myofilaments, are termed *myofibroblasts*. The fibroblastic cells begin to dominate the wound site as the inflammatory stage diminishes.

The connective tissue at the wound site contains numerous fibroblasts and is vascularized extensively. White blood cells are numerous also; however, the wound is devoid of nervous tissue. This newly generated tissue, *granulation tissue*, is the mediator of connective tissue repair and is responsible for *wound contraction*—the movement of full thickness skin toward the center of a defect. Wound contraction is an active process that is probably dependent upon the myofibroblast. The contraction phenomenon can be activated by smooth muscle stimulants and suppressed by smooth muscle inhibitors. The myofilaments of myofibroblasts are integral components of this

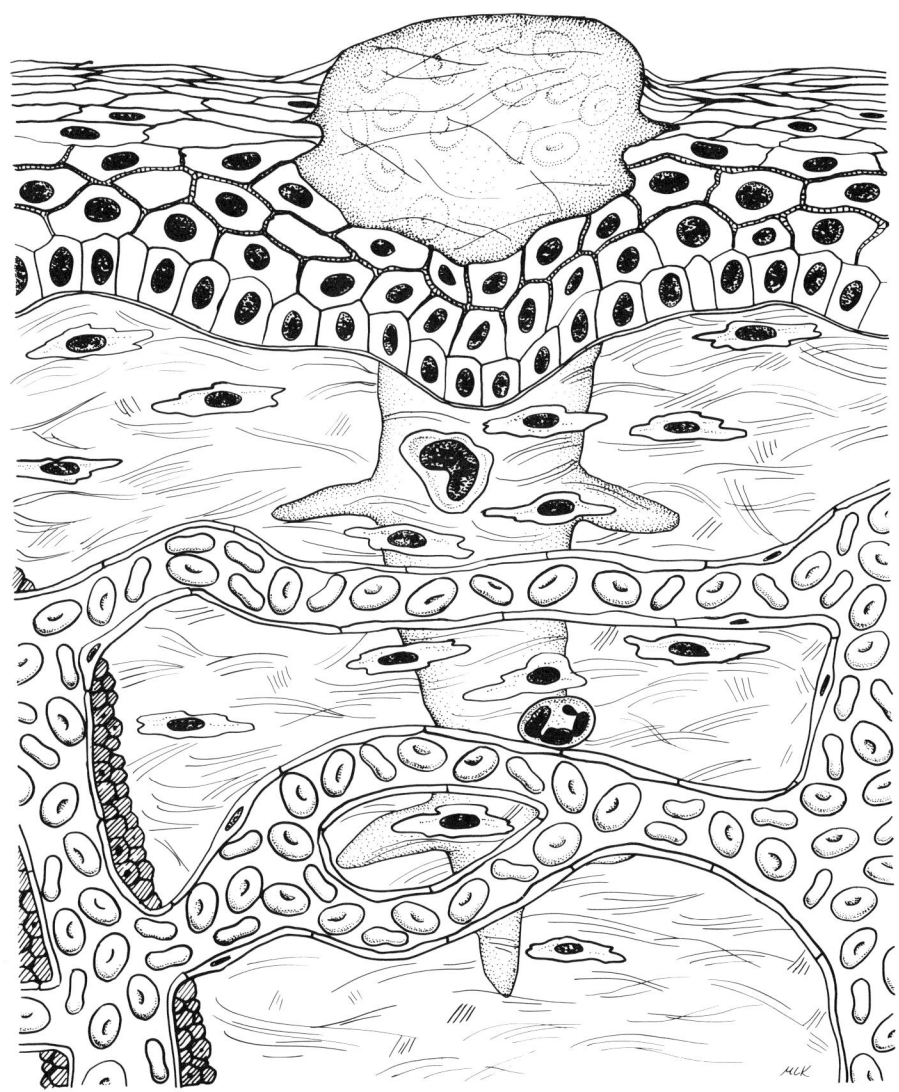

Fig. 18.45 Continued proliferation at the wound site. Neovascularization is complete. Fibroblasts continue to proliferate and produce matrix materials.

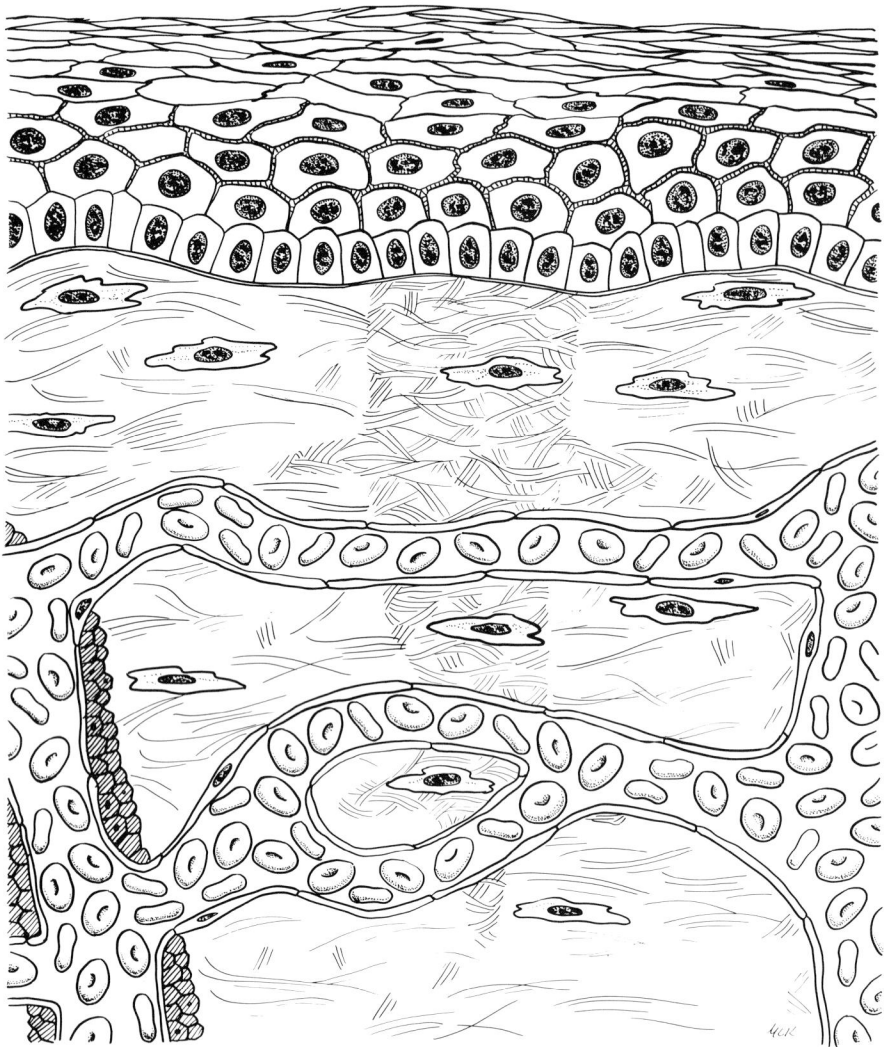

Fig. 18.46 Completion of wound repair. Continued remodeling of the wound site will increase wound strength and result in the removal of excess collagen.

process. Although mesenchymal cell differentiation accounts for the population of fibroblastic cells of granulation tissue, the determinants for the differentiation of myofibroblasts and fibroblasts is unknown. Granulation tissue, typically, contains both populations of cells.

Maturation Stage. The gradual reduction of the number of fibroblastic cells and a corresponding decrease in the number of capillaries within the wound are the histologic features of the maturation stage (Fig. 18.46).

Whereas the previous stage was dominated by fibroblasts and their synthetic activity, the maturation stage is characterized by a balanced synthesis and degradation of connective tissue components. Collagenous fibers typically align themselves along stress lines within the wound. A gradual and continual increase in wound strength can be anticipated. While wound strength may approach 25% of preinjury strength by 3 weeks postinjury, some wounds may continue to improve wound strength for two years.

Innervation of the wound site eventually reoccurs. Nerve regeneration was described previously.

References

Abercrombie, M., Flint, M. H. and James, D. W.: Collagen formation and wound contraction during repair of small excised wounds in the skin of rats. J Embryol. Exp. Morphol. *2:*264, 1954.

Adam, W. S., Calhoun, M. L., Smith, E. M. and Stinson A. W.: *Microscopic Anatomy of the Dog: A Photographic Atlas.* C. C. Thomas, Springfield, 1970.

Baker, B. B.: Epidermal cell renewal in the dog. Diss Abst. Int. *32B:*5526, 1972.

Baker, K. P.: Hair growth and replacement in the cat Brit. Vet. J. *130:*327, 1974.

Chase, H. B.: Growth of the hair. Physiol. Rev. *34:*113 1954.

Creed, R. F. S.: The histology of the mammalian skir with special reference to the dog and cat. Vet. Rec *70:*736, 1958.

David, L. T.: Histology of the skin of the Mexican hairless swine (*Sus scrofa*). Amer. J. Anat. *50:*283 1932.

Findlay, J. D. and Yang, S. H.: The sweat glands of Ayrshire cattle. J. Agric. Sci. *40:*126, 1950.

Godall, A. M. and Yang, S. H.: Myoepithelial cells ir bovine sweat glands. J. Agric. Sci. *42:*159, 1952.

Hausman, L. A.: Structural characteristics of the hair of mammals. Amer. Natur. *44:*496, 1930.

Hibbs, R. G.: The fine structure of human exocrine sweat glands. Amer. J. Anat. *103:*201, 1958.

Hunt, T. K. and Van Winkle, W., Jr.: *Fundamentals of Wound Management in Surgery—Wound Healing Normal Repair.* Chirirgecom, Inc., South Plainfield New Jersey. 1976.

Katz, S. I., Tamaki, K. and Sachs, D. H.: Epiderma Langerhans cells are derived from cells originating in bone marrow. Nature. *282:*324, 1979.

Maibach, H. I. and Rovee, D. T. (editors): *Epiderma Wound Healing.* Year Book Medical Publishers Chicago. 1972.

Moffat, G. H.: The growth of hair follicles and its relation to the adjacent dermal structures. J. Anat. *102:*527 1968.

Montagna, W.: *The Structure and Function of the Skin* 9th ed. Academic Press, New York, 1962.

Muller, G. H. (editor): Symposium on the skin and internal disease. Vet. Clin. North Amer. *9:*1, 1979.

Muller, G. H. and Kirk, R. W.: *Small Animal Dermatology.* W. B. Saunders, Philadelphia,1976.

Munger, B. L.: The cytology of apocrine sweat glands. I Cat and monkey. Z. Zellforsch. *67:*373, 1965.

Nielsen, S. W.: Glands of the canine skin. Am. J. Vet. Res. *14:*448, 1953.

Stump, J. E.: Anatomy of the normal equine foot, including microscopic features of the laminar region. J. Amer. Vet. Med. Ass. *151:*1588, 1967.

Toker, C.: Observations on the ultrastructure of a mammary ductule. J. Ultrastruct. Res. *21:*9, 1967.

Webb, A. J. and Calhoun, M. L.: The microscopic anatomy of the skin of mongrel dogs. Am. J. Vet. Res. *15:*274, 1954.

Webber, A. F., Kitchell, R. L. and Sautter, J. H.: Mammary gland studies. I. The identity and characterization of the smallest lobule unit in the udder of the dairy cow. Amer. J. Vet. Res. *16:*255, 1955.

19: Digestive System

General Characteristics

Form and Function. The digestive system consists of the alimentary canal and accessory structures such as the lips, tongue, teeth and extramural glands. The *alimentary canal (tract)* is a tubular and modified tubular structure that extends from mouth to anus and conforms generally to the basic structural pattern described in Chapter 13. The alimentary tract is divided conveniently into a number of organs—mouth, pharynx, esophagus, stomach, small intestine, large intestine, rectum and anus—on the basis of structure and anatomic location. Although the mural organization of these subdivisions varies, the specific modifications of each alimentary tract component conform to the basic organizational scheme while permitting functional uniqueness.

The epithelial lining of most of the alimentary canal is derived from endoderm; however, the rostral and caudal epithelium of the canal is derived from stomodeal and proctodeal ectoderm, respectively. Neurectodermal derivatives account for the innervation of the digestive organs, whereas the mesoderm gives rise to the muscular and connective tissue components.

Diverse functional adaptations of the component organs of the digestive system are reflected in the varied histologic modifications that are apparent from mouth to anus. The muscularized lips and tongue aid in *prehension* of foodstuffs, whereas the teeth permit *mastication*. *Deglutition* (swallowing) results from the integrated activity of the muscularized structures of the buccal cavity and pharynx. The muscularized esophagus propels the bolus of food into the stomach wherein *mechanical* and *chemical digestion* is initiated. The remainder of the tube continues digestion and *absorption*, and *propels* the luminal contents toward the anus, culminating in the *elimination* of the digested residue, feces. Some of the less obvious but essential functions of the alimentary tract and accessory glandular structures are the *synthesis and secretion of enzymes, secretion of digestive juices, vitamin production, plasma protein synthesis and secretion, detoxification of harmful substances* and *elaboration of essential body metabolites*. Numerous other functions are performed by specific organs of this system: these will be discussed with the individual organs.

The solid, fluid and semifluid luminal contents of the digestive system are outside the body. Materials do not enter or leave the body through this system until they cross the epithelial barrier of the digestive tract. Digestion is accomplished within the alimentary canal by the secretion of enzymes, bile and hydrochloric acid outside the body. The selective absorption of materials vital to the organism is a function of the lining cells of this system.

Histologic Organization. Although the mural organization of tubular organs was discussed in Chapter 13, it is presented here in outline form. The essence of alimentary tract organization is the presence, absence and/or specialization of various mural components.

Tunica Mucosa
    Lamina Epithelialis Mucosae
    Lamina Propria Mucosae
    Lamina Muscularis Mucosae
Tunica Submucosa
Tunica Muscularis
    Lamina Muscularis Interna
    Lamina Muscularis Externa
Tunica Serosa, or
Tunica Adventitia

Oral Structures

Buccal Cavity

General Characteristics. The buccal cavity is that portion of the alimentary tract that does not have a typical tubular configuration. Numerous organs of diverse function occupy this region and alter its tubular morphology; however, the mural organization of the buccal cavity conforms to the basic pattern. Generally, the buccal cavity may be described as an extension of the skin which has been modified as a *cutaneous mucous membrane*; i.e., it is lined by stratified squamous epithelium and is moistened by the secretions (mucous, serous, mixed) of the salivary glands.

Histologic Structure. The lamina epithelialis is stratified squamous epithelium with varying degrees of cornification. Large epithelial papillae with cores of connective tissue project from the surface epithelium in some species. These assist in the prehension and mastication of food (ruminants).

The lamina propria blends insensibly with the tunica submucosa. Usually, the lamina propria is described as being devoid of glands; it possesses only the excretory ducts of the submucosal glands which are generally referred to as buccal glands. These are either mucous, serous or mixed glands.

The submucosal tunic blends with and rests upon the fascia associated with the underlying skeletal muscle. If absent, the lamina propria then assumes this relationship. In some instances, the skeletal muscle is replaced by bone. Then, the lamina propria or tunica submucosa will rest upon the periosteum of the associated bony structures.

Because the general histological appearance of the buccal cavity is quite uniform, only a few of the unique or different structures will be described.

Lip

This is the mucocutaneous junction, the point of transition from the epidermis to the mucous membrane of the buccal cavity (Fig. 19.1). The external surface is covered by a thin layer of keratinized stratified squamous epithelium. Hairs, sebaceous glands and tubular sweat glands are encountered more frequently on typical skin than on the lips.

At the point of actual transition, the thin epidermis becomes the thickened cutaneous mucous membrane of the buccal cavity. It is keratinized in species whose diets contain much roughage (ruminants, horse). It is nonkeratinized in the pig and carnivores. The degree or absence of keratinization is diet-dependent.

The core of the lip is composed of fibroelastic connective tissue and skeletal muscle (*orbicularis oris*). On the integumentary side of the lip the dermis and hypodermis are typical. On the labial side the lamina propria and tunica submucosa are typical although not distinct from one another. Submucosal glands (*labial glands*) are present. They are mucous in small ruminants and carnivores and mixed in other species. These glands are branched tubuloalveolar types. They are serous glands in the bovine nasal planum. The tunica muscularis is skeletal muscle (orbicularis oris).

Cheek

The lamina epithelialis, lamina propria and tunica submucosa of the cheek are similar to the structure of the lip (Fig. 19.2). Serous or mucous *buccal glands* occupy the submucosal connective tissue space.

Hard Palate

The *hard palate* is composed of a keratinized stratifed squamous epithelium which is especially thick and highly keratinized in the *dental pad* of ruminants (Fig. 19.3). The lamina propria-submucosa is typical and is continuous with the fibrous periosteum of the bony roof of the buccal cavity. Adipose tissue and an extensive vascular bed are present. The caudal region of the hard palate of most species has numerous branched tubuloalveolar glands which may be mucous or mixed.

Soft Palate

The soft palate is a fibrous and muscular caudal extension of the hard palate. On its dorsal aspect (nasopharynx) it is covered by a pseudostratified ciliated columnar epithelium (*respiratory epithelium*), while its ventral side is covered by a typical cutaneous mucous membrane. The connective tissue core may contain glands similar to those in the hard palate. Lymphatic nodules are frequently encountered. The palatine tonsil of the pig is entirely within the soft palate.

Tongue

The tongue is a cranial projection from the ventral floor of the buccal cavity which is covered by stratified squamous epithelium and contains a core of connective tissue and skeletal muscle. Structures of significance which are part of the lingual composition are *lingual papillae* and *taste buds* (Fig. 19.4). **Histologic Structure.** The lamina epithelialis consists of epithelium which is variously keratinized. Numerous epidermal pegs and dermal papillae comprise the epithelial and connective tissue junction (*papillary body*). Extensive invaginations of the dermal papillae into the epithelium result in evaginations of the mucous membrane as *lingual papillae*. In horses and ruminants the posterodorsal aspect of the tongue has a thickened mucous membrane that gives rigidity to this structure. The lamina propria and tunica submucosa are typical and blend with the connective tissue (epimysium) of the core of intrinsic and extrinsic lingual musculature.

The *lyssa* is characteristic of carnivores. It attaches the ventral portion of the tongue to the floor of the buccal cavity. It consists of dense white fibrous connective tissue (DWFCT), some adipose tissue, skeletal muscle and occasionally some cartilage. In the pig it consists primarily of adipose tissue and some connective tissue. It is not well-developed in horses and ruminants.

Lingual Papillae. *Lingual papillae* are generally confined to the dorsal aspect of the tongue. These differ in size, form, number, distribution and function. Also, they are species-variable. The lingual papillae include the following; *filiform, lenticular, foliate, fungiform* and *circumvallate*.

Filiform papillae are the most numerous and are especially well-developed in the cat and ruminants wherein they serve mechanical functions (Fig. 19.5). These include prehension of foodstuffs and rasping activities. The keratinized papillae are shaped like rose thorns with their curvature directed caudad. The core of connective tissue is typical lamina propria.

Lenticular or *conical papillae* also serve mechanical functions (Fig. 19.6). The papillae are shaped like a double convex lens. They are especially prominent on the dorsum of the caudal one-third of the tongue.

Fungiform papillae are mushroom-shaped papillae that serve a mechanical and gustatory function (Fig. 19.7). Taste buds may be present. These papillae are not as keratinized as the previous types. The primary papillation of the lamina propria is prominent and secondary papillations may be present. The connective tissue core, which may contain diffuse lymphatic tissue, is typical.

Foliate papillae are leaf-shaped and are separated from each other or the associated mucous membrane by an invagination of the mucous membrane (Fig. 19.8). These

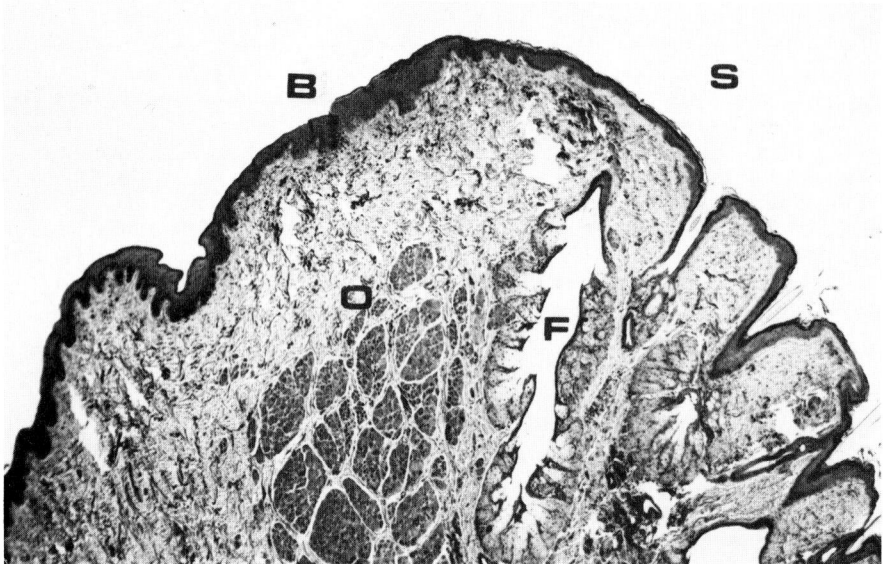

Fig. 19.1 A section through a feline lip. The buccal surface (B) is a mucous membrane. The skin (S) is typical and contains hair follicles (F) and associated sebaceous glands. The orbicularis oris muscle (O) is in the center of the structure. X10. All light micrographs are labeled as the magnification with the microscope before photographic enlarging. All electron micrographs are labeled as total magnification, including photographic enlarging.

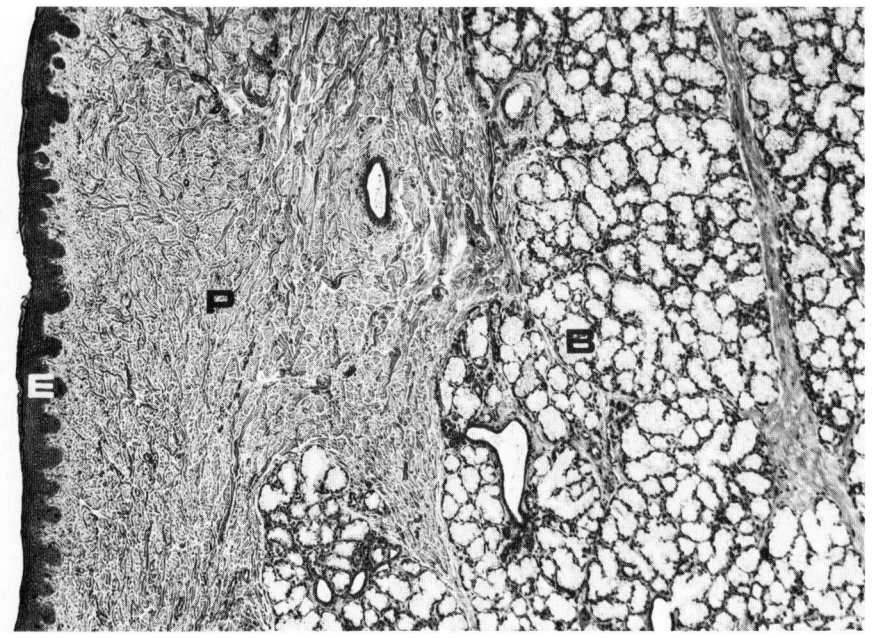

Fig. 19.2 A section through the feline cheek. The lamina epithelialis mucosae (E) is underlaid by a typical lamina propria mucosae (P). Numerous mucus-secreting buccal glands (B) are present. X16.

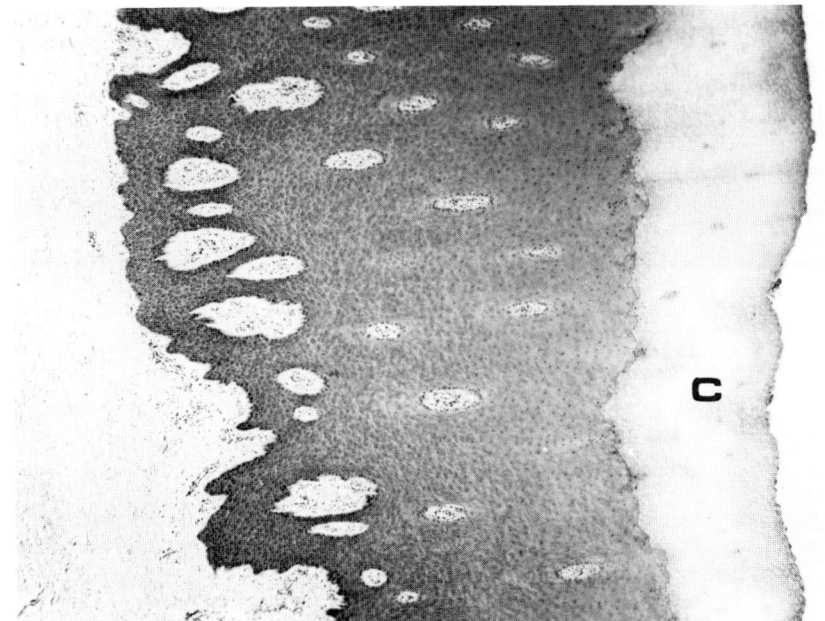

Fig. 19.3   A section of bovine dental pad. This structure replaces the upper incisors of ruminants. The pad has a thickened lamina epithelialis that is highly cornified (C). X10.

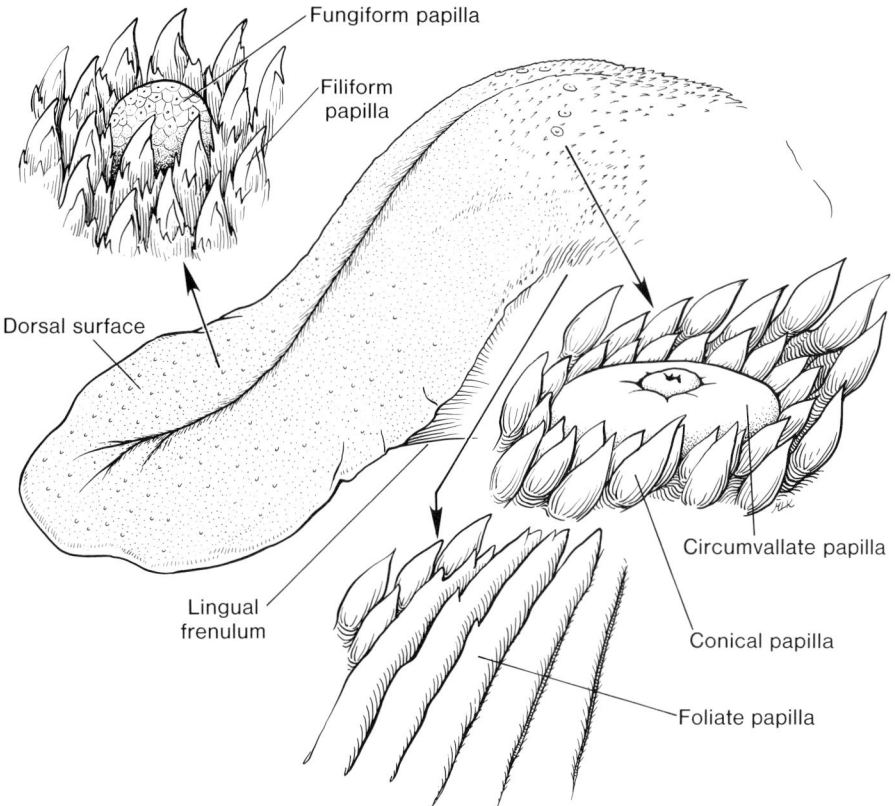

Fig. 19.4   A diagram of the canine tongue and lingual papillae. (Redrawn and modified from Evans, H. E. and Christensen, G. C.: *Miller's Anatomy of the Dog.* W. B. Saunders, Philadelphia, 1979).

papillae are gustatory. The epithelium of these papillae is nonkeratinized. Finger-like projections from the lamina propria are present. Branched, tubuloalveolar serous glands of the lamina propria-submucosa

open into the base of the *epithelial furrow.* These glands are *von Ebner's glands.* Taste buds occupy the lateal walls of the epithelial lining.

Circumvallate (vallate) papillae are the

largest papillae and those least encountered (Fig. 19.9). These papillae are not elevated above the lamina epithelialis and are surrounded by a deep furrow. Numerous taste buds are located in the lateral walls of the lamina epithelialis. The prominent connective tissue core is typical lamina propria. Branched, tubuloalveolar serous glands (von Ebner's glands) open into the base of the furrow and cleanse this region of foodstuffs.

Taste Buds. The *taste buds* of the tongue, as receptors for gustatory sensations, are intraepithelial structures located in the walls of foliate, fungiform and circumvallate papillae (Figs. 19.10, 19.11). Taste buds are ovoid masses of cells which extend from the basement membrane and open through a small canal, *taste pore,* at the surface of the epithelium. Microvillous projections of constituent cells extend into the taste pore as "taste hairs."

Two cell types can be distinguished routinely within the taste bud in light microscopic preparations of these structures (Fig. 19.12): *supporting (sustentacular) cells* and *gustatory cells.* Both of these cell types, although described as columnar cells, appear spindle-shaped. The gustatory cell, which is the sensory cell, has a dense, acidophilic cytoplasm and a vesicular, elongated nucleus. The sustentacular cell has a vacuolated, acidophilic cytoplasm and a dense, elongated nucleus. Nuclear morphology is usually the distinguishing feature. A third type of cell may be identified in the taste bud in well-fixed specimens. This cell (*basal cell*) is small and is located along the lateral and basal borders of the taste bud.

Electron microscopic studies indicate that there are four cell types (Types I–IV) in the taste bud. Precise correlation between electron microscopic and light microscopic studies has not been achieved. The type IV cell is the basally-positioned cell of light microscopy which probably functions as the stem cell for all of the other cells. Cell death and turnover within this structure are rapid. New cells may differentiate from the basal cells every 10 hours, whereas the average life span of the differentiated cells is approximately 250 hours. The maintenance of functional integrity is dependent upon new cells establishing contact with intraepithelial sensory nerve endings. Humoral substances elaborated by the nerves maintain this functional integrity.

Gustatory Sensation. Nerve endings within the taste buds (*intragemmal fibers*) terminate on sensory cells. The basic gustatory modalities of sour taste, sweet taste, salt taste and water taste have been described in the dog. The distribution of the modalities on the tongue have been mapped and have been associated with various types of lingual papillae. Sour taste is distributed evenly over the dorsal surface of the tongue, whereas salt taste is distributed along the lateral and caudal margins of the tongue,

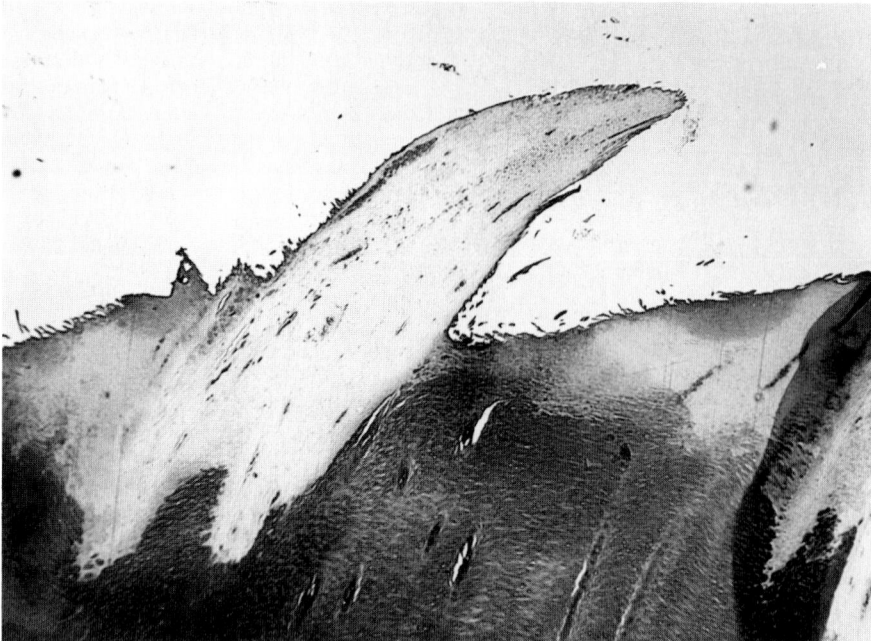

Fig. 19.5 A typical lingual papilla from a feline tongue. This papilla is entirely an epithelial structure. X10.

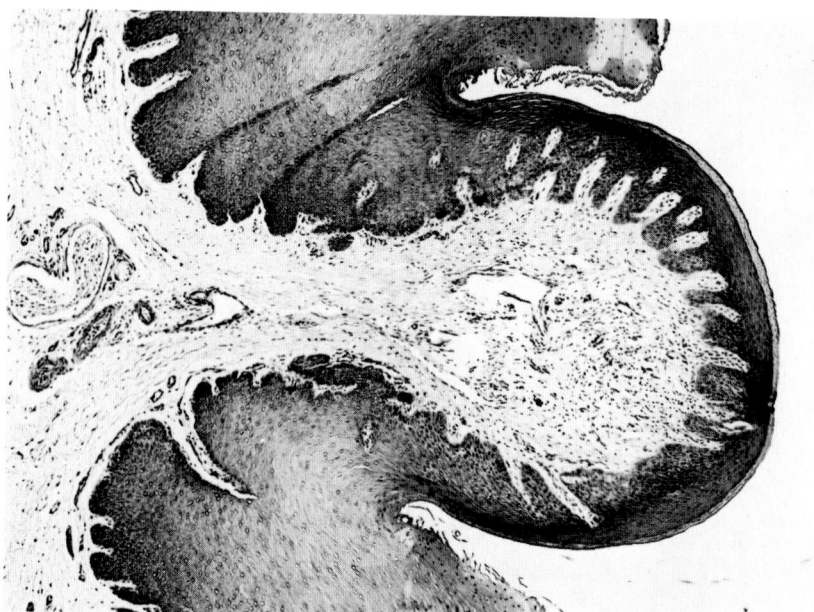

Fig. 19.6 A typical lentiform papilla from the dorsal aspect of a bovine tongue. X16.

which corresponds to the distribution of the chorda tympani of the facial nerve. Sweet taste sensitivity is distributed along the rostral and lateral margins of the tongue. Water taste is confined to the rostral border of the tongue. The rostral two-thirds of the tongue, that portion innervated by the facial nerve, may be sensitive to sweetness, saltiness, sourness and water. The caudal one-third of the tongue, that portion innervated by the glossopharyngeal nerve, may be sensitive to sourness only.

Tonsils

Because the buccal cavity and associated structures are subjected to varied insults

from foreign materials and microorganisms, numerous diffuse and aggregated accumulations of lymphatic tissue are present in the lamina propria-submucosa of this region. Invasion of lymphocytes into the lamina epithelialis from the associated connective tissue is a common occurrence in this region.

The tonsils are important, auxiliary protective organs of the caudal portion of the buccal cavity (Chapter 17).

Teeth

General Characteristics. Although mammalian teeth differ in gross and subgross appearance, they consist of the same components: *enamel, dentine, cementum* and

pulp. Teeth are either simple or complex. *Brachydont* (*simple*) teeth do not continue to grow at the completion of eruption (Fig. 19.13). Further, these teeth are divisible into a definitive *crown, neck* and *root.* The *hypsodont* (*complex*) teeth of ruminants, rodents and the horse are constantly erupting structures (Fig. 19.14). These teeth do not possess a definitive crown, neck and root. Rather they are considered to be composed of root only. The hypsodont teeth include the cheek teeth of ruminants, all of the teeth of the horse, the incisorform teeth of rodents and the canine teeth of the pig.

Different teeth are modified for various functions: tearing, shearing or crushing of foodstuffs. Also they are excellent protective devices.

Development of Simple Teeth. The development of teeth requires contributions from the epithelium and the underlying connective tissue (Fig. 19.15). An epithelial ridge, *dental lamina*, develops in the *dental arch* of each jaw and grows into the underlying mesenchymal region. Proliferation of the epithelium along the lateral border of the lamina further extends this structure into the mesenchyme. From this lateral extension, the *enamel organs* of the *deciduous teeth* (*milk teeth*) arise. At a later period, medial or lingual outgrowths of the dental lamina give rise to enamel organs of the *permanent teeth*. Proliferation of the invading epithelium as a solid mass of cells continues to the *cap stage* accompanied by a mesenchymal condensation at the base of the cap (Fig. 19.16).

By complementary growth of the epithelium and associated mesenchymal tissue of the *dental papilla*, the *bell stage* is achieved (Fig. 19.17). The epithelium is now the *enamel organ* and is divisible into distinct regions: *inner enamel epithelium, stellate reticulum* and *outer enamel epithelium* (Fig. 19.18). The *inner enamel epithelium* consists of columnar cells, *ameloblasts*, which are separated from the dental papilla by a basement membrane. This epithelium is continuous with the *outer enamel epithelium* at the lower edges (rim) of the bell. This outer epithelium is composed of small, flattened cells. The center of the enamel organ is composed of the *stellate reticulum*. The central cells, previously tightly packed, are separated by extensive intercellular spaces. These cells are stellate in appearance. The region of contact between the stellate reticulum and the inner enamel epithelium is occupied by cuboidal cells, the *stratum intermedium* (Fig. 19.18). As development of the tooth progresses, the stellate reticulum (*enamel pulp*) atrophies and the outer enamel epithelium collapses upon the inner enamel epithelium.

The dental papilla is entrapped within the confines of the enamel organ. A thin layer of columnar cells differentiates from the mesenchyme along the inner surface of the basement membrane, the odontoblasts. The remainder of the papilla becomes the pulp f the tooth. It consists of blood vessels, nerves and loose connective tissue.

A condensed mass of connective tissue circumscribes the enamel organ and the dental papilla. The connective tissue of this dental sac is continuous with the connective tissue of the dental papilla. The dental sac is of importance because it gives rise to the following:

1. It gives rise to the *alveolar bone* and periosteum surrounding the root.

2. It forms a layer of *cementum* peripheral to the dentine of the root.

3. It forms a network of anchoring collagenous fibers which connect the cementum of the root to the alveolar bone, the *periodontal membrane.*

The sequence of tooth development includes the differentiation of enamel, dentine and cementum. The deposition of enamel is achieved by the secretory activity of the ameloblasts. This appositional process proceeds from the apex of the papilla toward the gingiva and rim of the bell. This process is initiated after the deposition of secretory products from the odontoblasts. The odontoblasts secrete their products in such a way that predentine and dentine are deposited at the apex of the papilla, laterally toward the rim and in a direction opposite to enamel deposition. This process, also, is appositional. The activities of the ameloblasts and the odontoblasts result in the formation of the *crown* of the tooth.

At the point of continuity between the inner and outer enamel epithelium (the future *neck* region of the tooth) a fold of epithelium develops and grows downward as the *epithelial root sheath* (sheath of Hertwig). Dentine continues to develop in this region. Instead of enamel, however, the mesenchyme interdigitates itself between the odontoblasts and the root sheath and cementum develops. The root, therefore, consists of cementum and dentine. And, the transition from crown to root is the *neck* of the tooth.

As the aforementioned processes are occurring, the dental sac gives rise to the alveolar bone and other structures. The downward growth of the root exerts pressure against the stationary alveolar bone which results in a translation of upward movement or *eruption.*

During eruption, the crown of the tooth breaks through the enamel organ and gingiva. The ameloblast activity ceases at eruption. The continued deposition of the root during eruption, however, results in the definitive position of the tooth being achieved.

The subsequent development of the enamel organ of the permanent teeth follows the same steps outlined. As the permanent tooth bud develops, its growth exerts pressure against the root and associated structures of the deciduous tooth which results in resorption. The loss of the deciduous tooth is followed closely by its permanent tooth replacement.

Cellular and Matrix Components of Teeth. The cellular components of teeth include *ameloblasts, odontoblasts, cementoblasts* and various connective tissue cells. The matrix components include *enamel, predentine, dentine, cementum* and *periodontal membrane.*

The *ameloblasts* are columnar cells which in cross-section appear hexagonal (Fig. 19.19). These polarized cells have an elongated, basally positioned nucleus. The basal part of the cell is rich in mitochondria. The apical portion of the cell is rich in granular endoplasmic reticulum and Golgi apparatus. At the apex of the cell, *Tome's processes* (prismatic extensions of the ameloblast apical cytoplasm) are apparent. Material for enamel formation is secreted through these processes in the form of rods as a slightly mineralized substance. During the secretory processes, the ameloblasts retreat before their advancing front of secretory products. The result is an acellular enamel composed of rods and inter-rod material. Enamel consists of approximately 95–97% of inorganic material in the form of apatite crystal. It is the hardest substance in the body. Upon completion of enamel formation, the ameloblasts disintegrate. Enamel, therefore, is incapable of repair.

Odontoblasts are not as tightly packed together as the ameloblasts (Fig. 19.20). These columnar cells are also polarized. The predominant organelles are the apically disposed granular endoplasmic reticulum and a large supranuclear Golgi apparatus. The

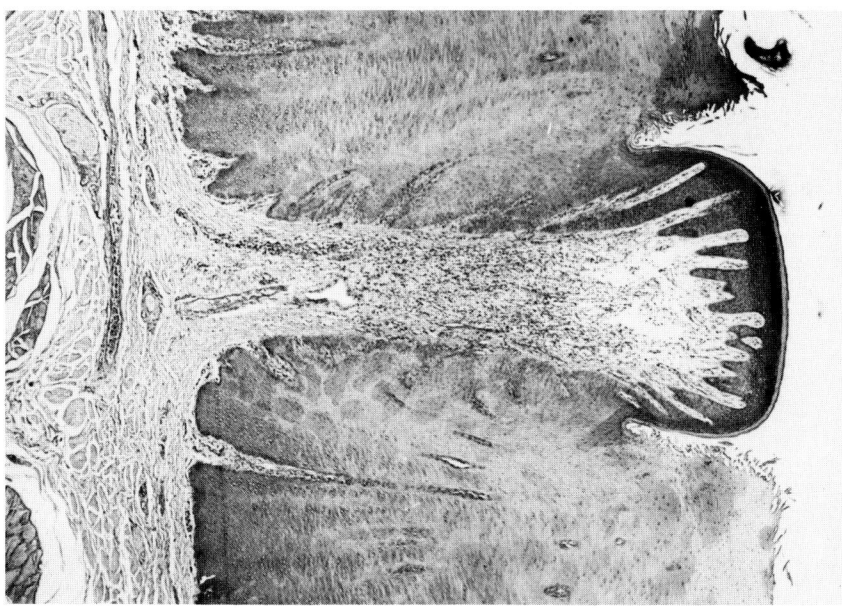

Fig. 19.7 A typical fungiform papilla from a canine tongue. This structure may be gustatory. X10.

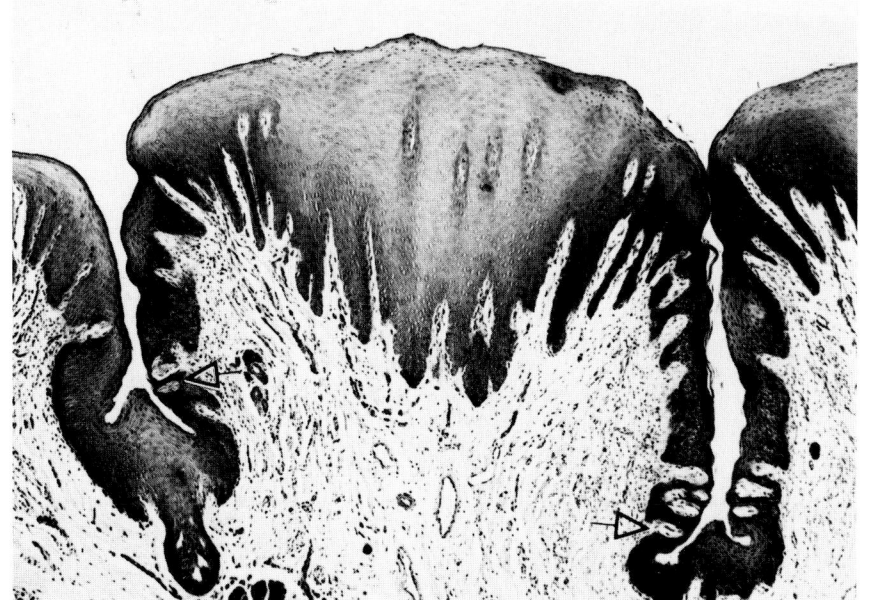

Fig. 19.8 A typical foliate papilla from a canine tongue. These papillae are gustatory. *Arrows,* taste buds. X16.

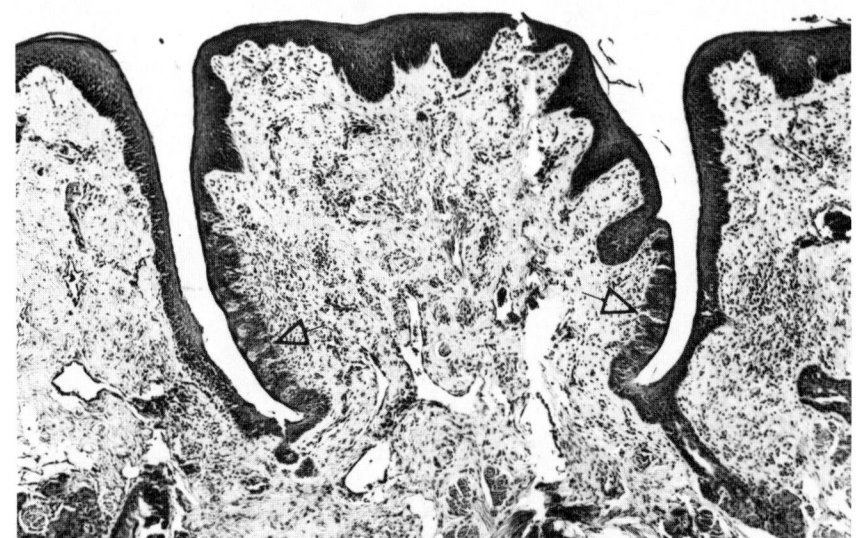

Fig. 19.9   A typical circumvallate papilla of the canine tongue. Taste buds (*arrows*) are present. X16.

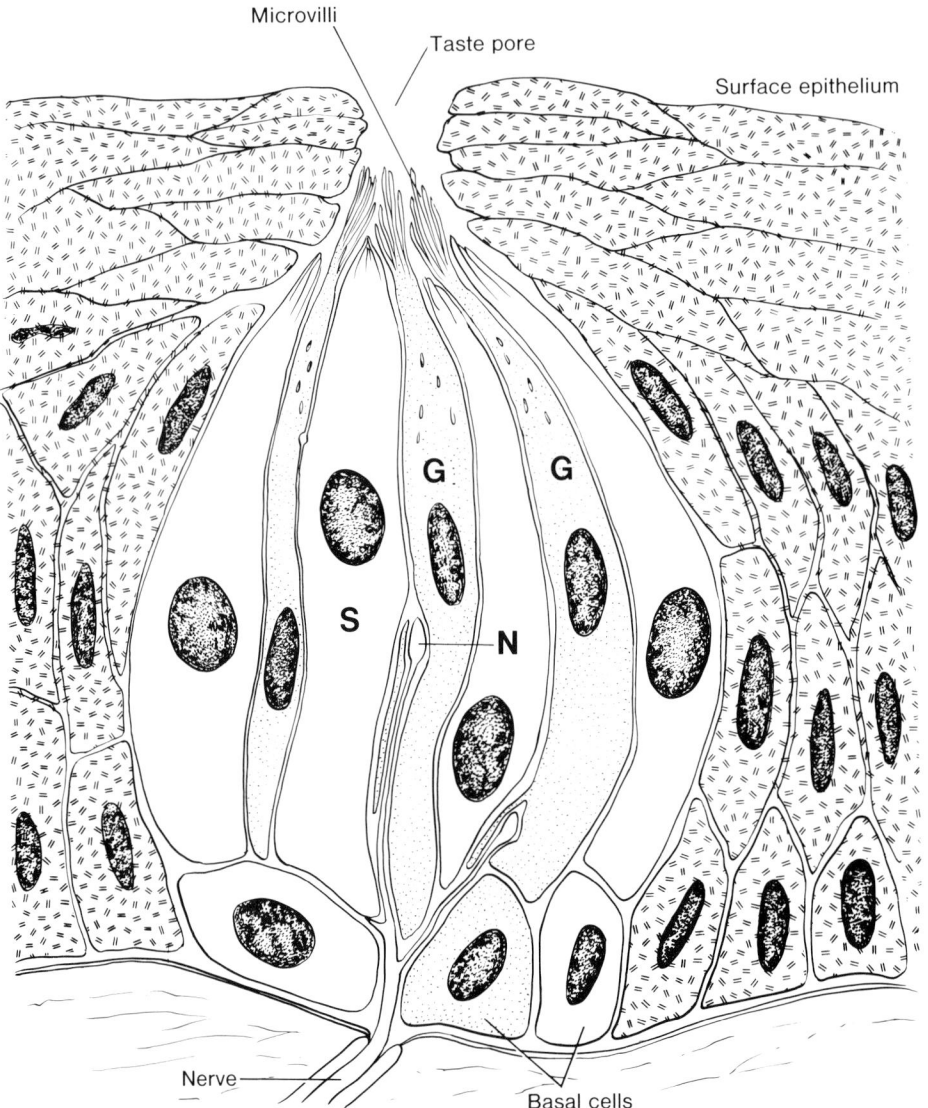

Fig. 19.10   An idealized drawing of the electron microscopic appearance of a taste bud. G, gustatory cells; S, sustentacular cells; N, nerve ending

initial secretory product of the odontoblasts is *predentine*. It is deposited initially at the dentinal-enamel junction. It is not a uninterrupted layer. Rather, it contains *odontoblastic processes* (*Tome's fibers, dentinal fibers*). As predentine is secreted the odontoblasts retreat before the advancing front, but their processes remain and are contained within *dentinal tubules*. Subsequent mineralization of predentine results in *dentine*. This method of secretion is similar to the relationship between osteoid seam and mineralizing bone. Dentine, however, contains about 69% inorganic substances.

Unlike ameloblasts, odontoblasts do not disintegrate upon the completion of their secretory activity. Rather, they are viable and potentially functional cells throughout the life of a tooth.

Cementoblasts are differentiated from the dental sac and give rise to *acellular cementum* and *cellular cementum*. This material with its contained *cementocytes* is very similar to woven or immature bone. Sharpey's fibers become embedded in this material by an appositional growth of cementum around the collagenous fibers. This process is similar to the means by which the collagen of tendons is incorporated in and attached to bone.

The *periodontal membrane* consists of coarsely bundled collagenous fibers and fibroblasts. These fibers are embedded in the cementum and associated alveolar bone as Sharpey's fibers. These fibers anchor the tooth in the *alveolus* (*socket*) and are the fibers ruptured during tooth extraction.

Brachydont Dentition. The *crown* of the tooth is covered by enamel and is that portion of the tooth visible above the *gingiva* (Fig. 19.13). The crown is composed of enamel and dentine. The dentine is visible on the surface in worn teeth from which the enamel has been removed by constant abrasion. The *neck* of the tooth is the point of transition between the crown and the root. It is, importantly, the point of *epithelial attachment* to the cementum. The *gingival crevice* or *gingival sulcus* is the depression between the tooth and gingiva above the point of epithelial attachment. The point of the gingiva adjacent to the crown is termed the *gingival crest*. The gingival sulcus and epithelial attachment are especially significant in periodontal disease. *Tartar* or *calculus* commonly accumulates on the tooth in the gingival sulcus.

The root is composed of dentine and cementum in apposition to one another. The periodontal membrane serves as the suspension mechanism between the alveolar bone and cementum of the root.

The dental pulp is a loose connective tissue rich in vascular supply and nerves. It is bounded by the dentine of the crown and root (or roots).

Hypsodont Dentition. The constantly erupting teeth are unique morphologically and

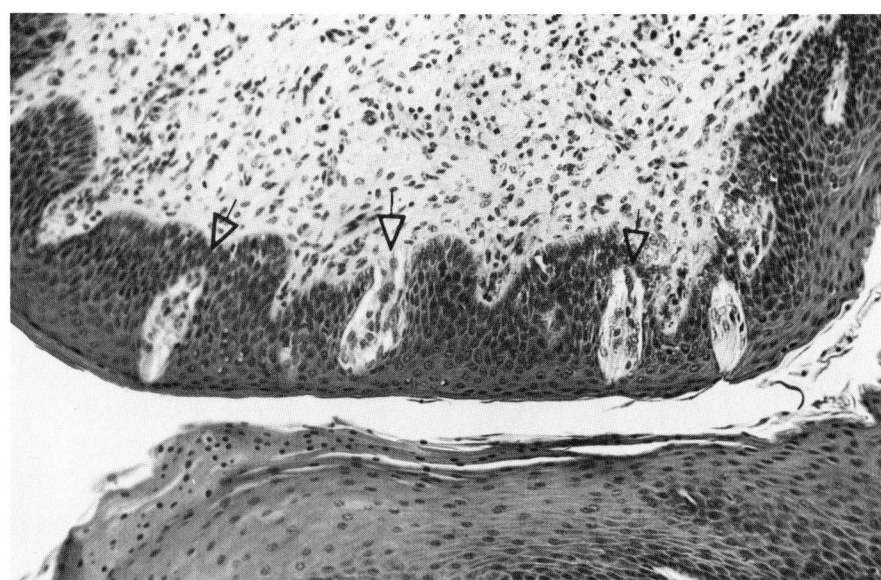

Fig. 19.11   Taste buds associated with a circumvallate papilla of a canine tongue. The taste buds (*arrows*) are intraepithelial structures. X40.

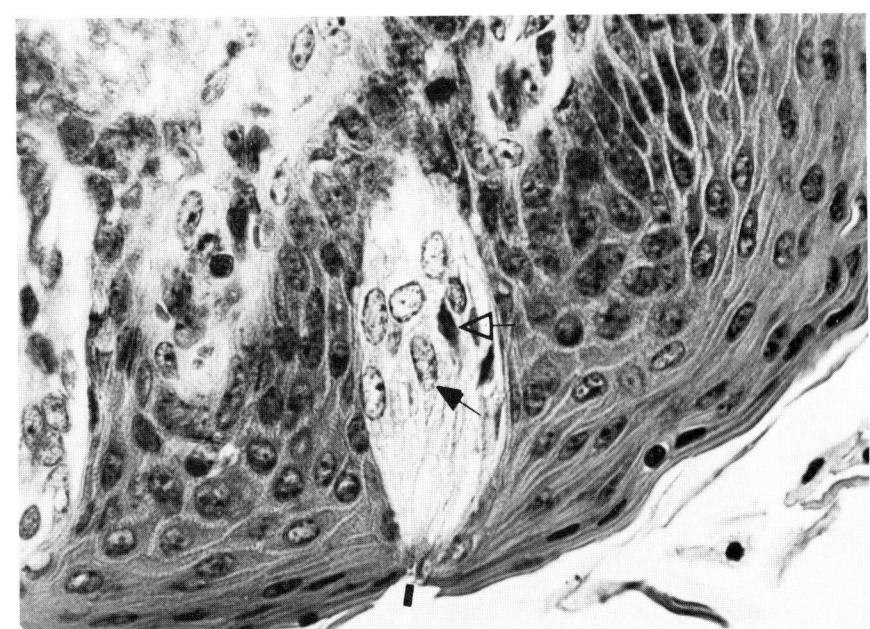

Fig. 19.12   The cells of taste buds. Sustentacular cells (*open arrow*) and gustatory cells (*solid arrow*) are spindle-shaped cells. The taste pore (*bar*) opens on the epithelial surface. X160.

differ significantly from the brachydont teeth (Fig. 19.14). This difference is based upon some alterations in the developmental sequence. In brachydont teeth the enamel organ is intact until the time of eruption. In hypsodont teeth, the enamel organ is ruptured prior to eruption. This brings the connective tissue of the dental sac in close association to the newly formed enamel. As a result, cementum is deposited on the enamel. Also, the resulting morphology of the mature hyposodont tooth, especially the *infundibular recess*, requires that the enamel

organ is more complex in surface morphology than that of simple teeth.

In brachydont teeth, the eruption of the crown is accompanied by the disintegration of the ameloblasts. In hypsodont teeth, ameloblasts do not disintegrate. They continue their activity for an extended period beyond eruption.

Although hypsodont teeth are described as root teeth without a definitive crown, neck and root, this is not entirely true. A typical root (cementum and dentine) is confined to the lower portion of the tooth.

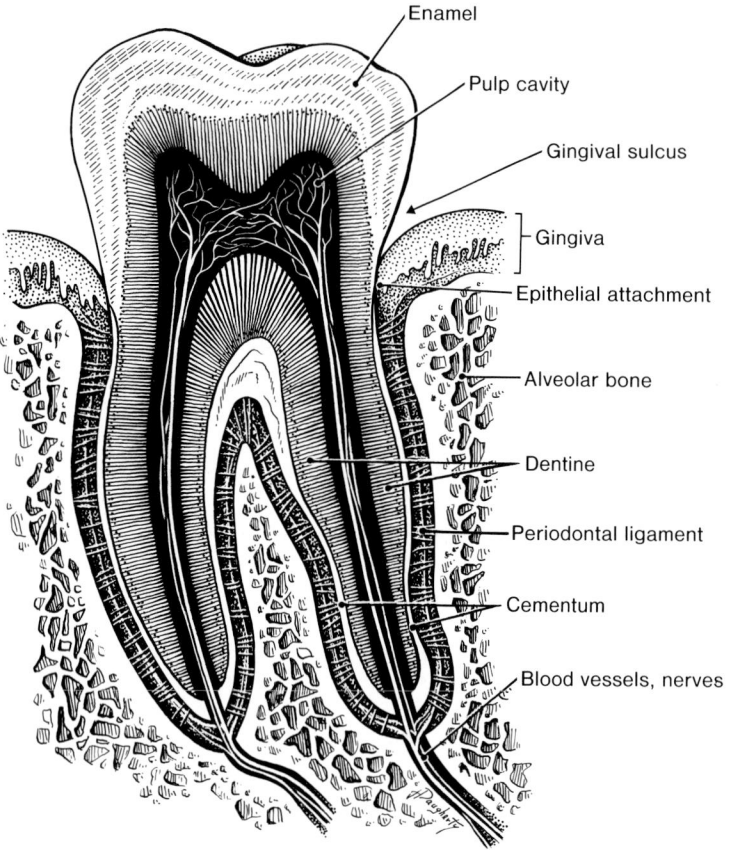

Fig. 19.13   A brachydont molariform tooth.

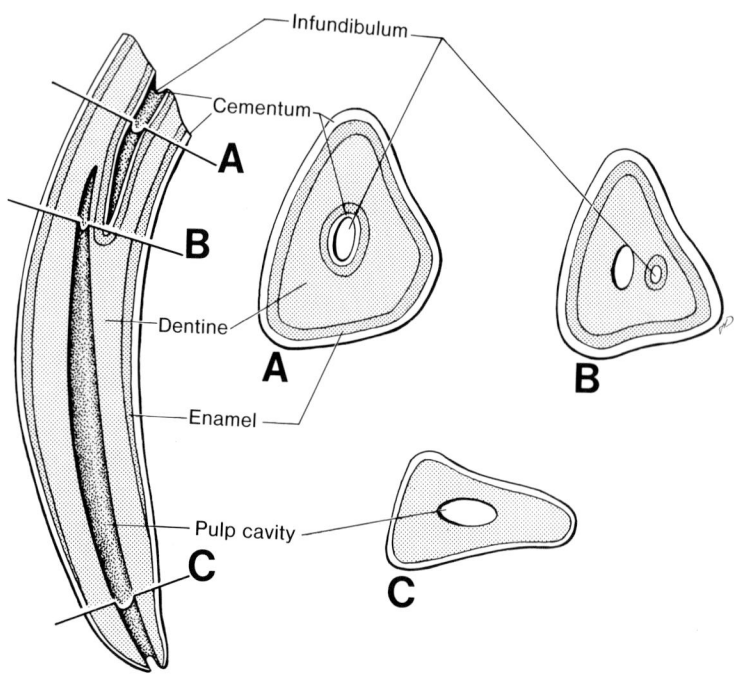

Fig. 19.14   Sections of a hypsodont incisorform tooth of a horse. The entire peripheral surface is covered by cementum.

Salivary Glands

General Morphology. The salivary gland are derived from the epithelium of the buc cal cavity which invaginates into the asso ciated lamina propria-submucosa. Althoug the adenomeres of the salivary glands a located at various distances from the epithe lial lining of the buccal cavity, all of th excretory ducts of these glands open ont the buccal epithelium. Predicated upon the size, location and proximity to the bucca cavity, the salivary glands are classified a major or minor glands. The *major salivar glands*—parotid, mandibular, sublingua zygomatic and molar glands—are larg structures that are located generally som distance from the buccal cavity; conse quently, their excretory ducts may be lon; The *minor salivary glands*—labial, lingua buccal and palatine glands—are small stru tures that are approximated closely to th buccal cavity; their excretory ducts are shor

The major salivary glands conform gen erally to the basic pattern described for com pound tubuloalveolar glands (Chapter 5 Structures unique to these salivary gland are *alveoli, intercalated ducts* and *striate ducts*. The striated duct, also called the s cretory tubule, is the intralobular duct these glands. The secretory pathway of th major salivary glands is *alveolus - interc lated duct - intralobular duct (secretory t bules) - lobular duct - intralobar duct - lob duct - excretory duct*.

The adenomeres of the major salivar glands may consist of mucous and serou cells which have a variable distribution (Fi 19.21). Some adenomeres may be mucou some serous and others may be mixed (Fig 19.22, 19.25, 19.26). The distribution of se ous and mucous cells in mixed salivar glands is variable also. Some adenomere are serous or mucous exclusively. Othe consist of single cells or groups of cells one type (e.g., serous cells) intermingle with predominant cells of the other typ (e.g., mucous cells). Additionally, *serous d milunes* may cap mucous endpieces. Th morphologic characteristics of mucous an serous cells were discussed in Chapter *Myoepithelial cells* are juxtaposed intimatel to the secretory epithelial cells of the alveol Myoepithelial cells or *basket cells* are ste late-shaped with an elongated nucleus. Th contraction of basket cells assists the mov ment of secretory products from the alveol

The *intercalated ducts* are small tubul lined by a low cuboidal epithelium (Fi 19.23). They are nonsecretory ducts whic connect alveoli to striated ducts. The *striate ducts* are lined by a columnar epitheliur The naming of the lining cells of these duc is from the infranuclear striations that resu from dense accumulations of mitochondr and numerous infoldings of the basal pla malemma (Fig. 19.24). Striated ducts do n occur in salivary glands that are exclusive mucus-secreting. In the absence of striate

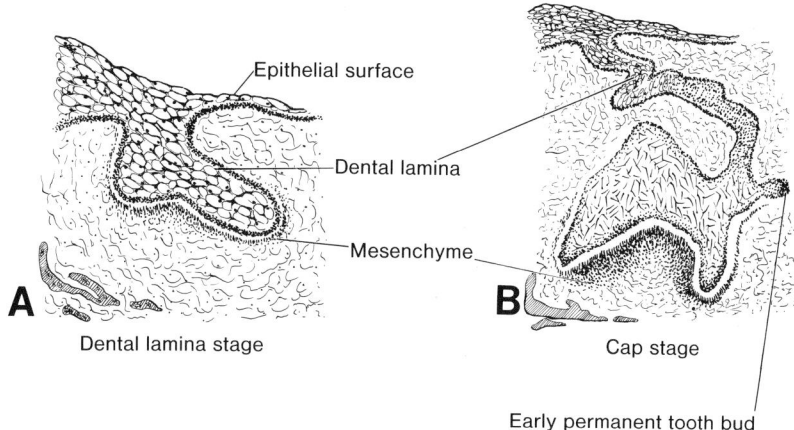

Epithelial surface

Dental lamina

Mesenchyme

A   **B**

Dental lamina stage   Cap stage

Early permanent tooth bud

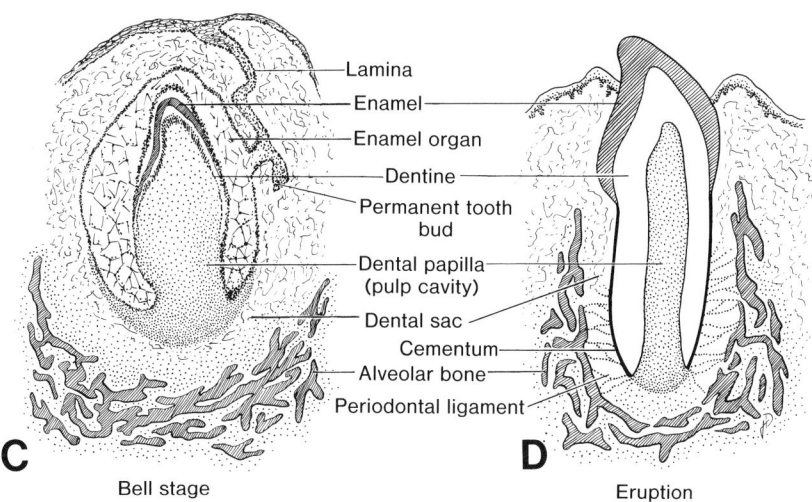

Lamina
Enamel
Enamel organ
Dentine
Permanent tooth bud
Dental papilla (pulp cavity)
Dental sac
Cementum
Alveolar bone
Periodontal ligament

C   **D**

Bell stage   Eruption

ig. 19.15   Early development of a deciduous branchydont tooth. A. The surface epithelium proliferates and invaginates into the underlying :esenchyme as the dental lamina. B. The attached epithelial mass begins to cavitate adjacent to the mesenchymal condensation. C. The enamel gan forms during the bell stage. Enamel and dentine have begun to form. D. Eruption has occurred. Dentine and cementum will be added ontinually until complete eruption is achieved.

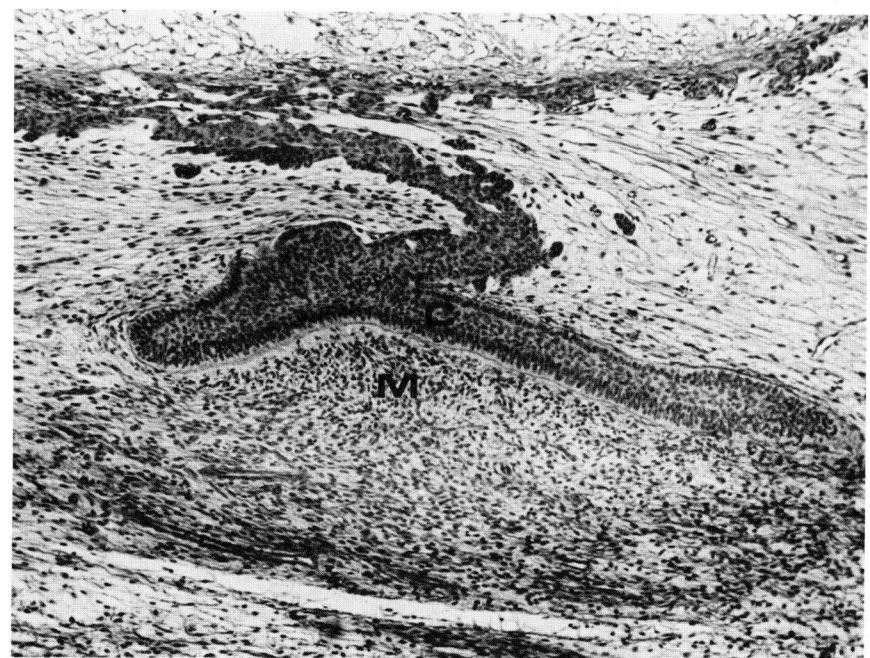

ig. 19.16   Cap stage of a secondary tooth bud. The enamel organ is still a condensed mass of epithelial cells (C) associated with mesenchyme M). X25.

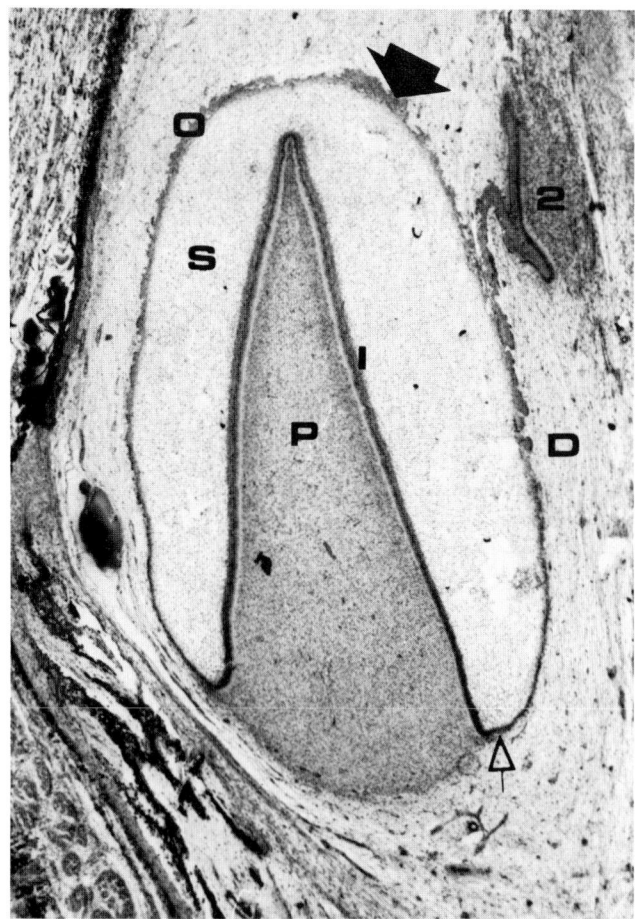

Fig. 19.17   Enamel organ in an early bell stage. The enamel organ (*solid arrow*) has a permanent tooth bud attached to it (2). The enamel organ consists of an outer enamel epithelium (O) which is continuous with the inner enamel epithelium (I) at the rim of the organ (*open arrow*). The stellate reticulum (S) is between the inner and outer epithelial layers. The enamel organ surrounds a mesenchymal condensation, the dental papilla (P). D, dental sac. X6.

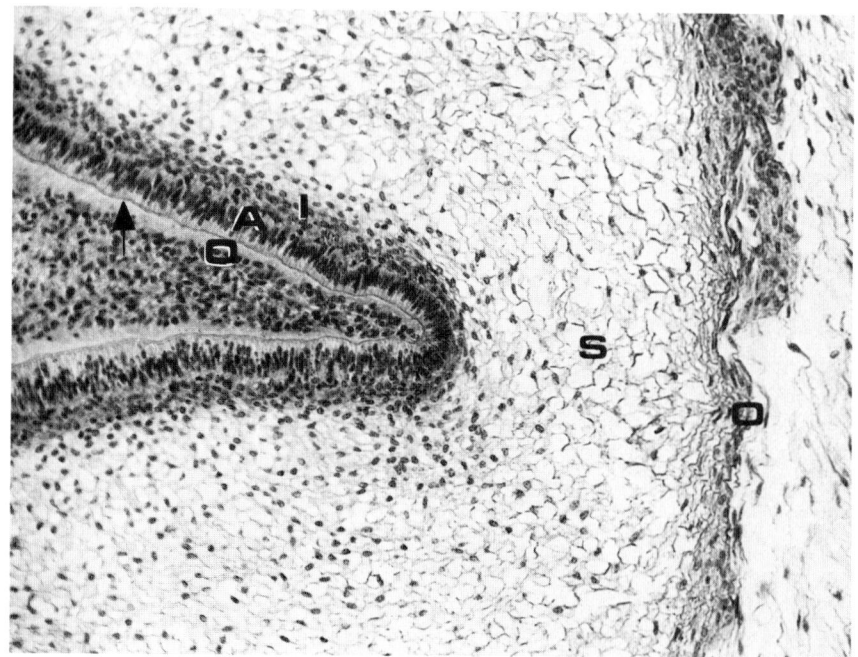

Fig. 19.18   Components of the enamel organ. The outer enamel epithelium (*O-right*) is adjacent to the stellate reticulum (S). A layer of cuboidal cell, stratum intermedium (I), underlies the inner enamel epithelium which is composed of ameloblasts (A). The ameloblasts are separated from the odontoblasts (*O-left*) of the dental papilla by a basement membrane (*arrow*). X40.

ducts, the intralobular duct is lined by simple columnar epithelium.

Bistratified cuboidal or bistratified columnar epithelium may be present at point of transition between intralobular ducts and lobular ducts (Figs. 5.14, 5.15). Portions of the larger ducts (intralobar ducts, lobar ducts) may be lined by pseudostratified columnar epithelium. Eventually, stratified squamous epithelium replaces the other lining tissues and becomes the characteristic lining of the excretory duct which is continuous with the lining epithelium of the buccal cavity.

The epithelium of the salivary glands (lining and secretory cells) is separated from the surrounding connective tissue by a basement membrane. The intralobular connective tissue, that which is associated intimately with the secretory portions of the gland, consists of reticular or areolar connective tissues. It becomes more dense in association with the larger ducts as the lobar connective tissue. The later blends with the dense white fibrous connective tissue of the capsule.

The organization of minor salivary glands, although not as extensive, is similar to that which characterizes the major salivary glands.

Parotid Salivary Gland. The *parotid salivary gland* conforms to the pattern described for major salivary glands. Although this gland is usually a serous gland in all domestic animals, man and rodents, a few mucous cells or adenomeres may be present in carnivores (Fig. 19.25). Also, it may be a mixed gland in young puppies and lambs.

Mandibular Salivary Gland. The mandibular salivary gland conforms to the pattern described for major salivary glands also. It is a mucous gland in the dog and cat (Fig. 19.26); serous in rodents; mixed in the horse, man and ruminants. The distribution of serous and mucous cells in mixed mandibular salivary glands is variable.

Sublingual Salivary Gland. The morphologic organization of the sublingual salivary gland is typical. These glands are predominately mucous in ruminants, swine and rodents; mixed in small carnivores, man and the horse (Fig. 19.27).

Unique Salivary Glands of Carnivores. The *zygomatic salivary gland* of small carnivores is located deep to the zygomatic process of the maxillary bone above the palate and beneath the orbit. Although predominately a mucous gland, some serous demilunes are present. The remainder of the gland is organized in a manner described for major salivary glands.

The *molar salivary gland* of felids is located near the commissure of the lips. The molar glands are similar to the zygomatic glands.

Miscellaneous Salivary Glands. The minor salivary glands comprise a group of small glands that are scattered throughout the buccal cavity. They are located within the

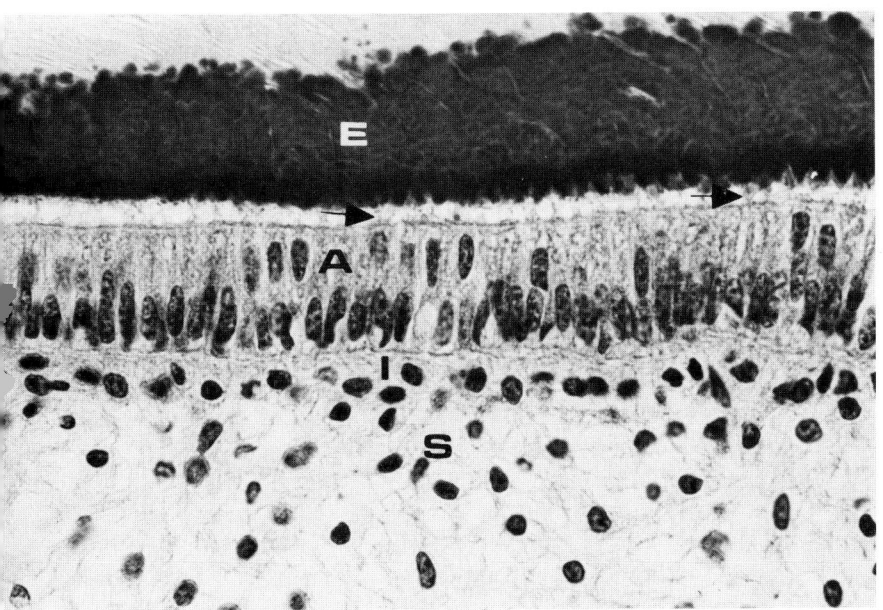

ig. 19.19 Layer of ameloblasts. The ameloblasts (A) are associated intimately with the stratum
termedium (I) the cells of which are continuous with the stellate reticulum (S). Enamel (E) has
en deposited and Tome's processes (*arrows*) are apparent. X160.

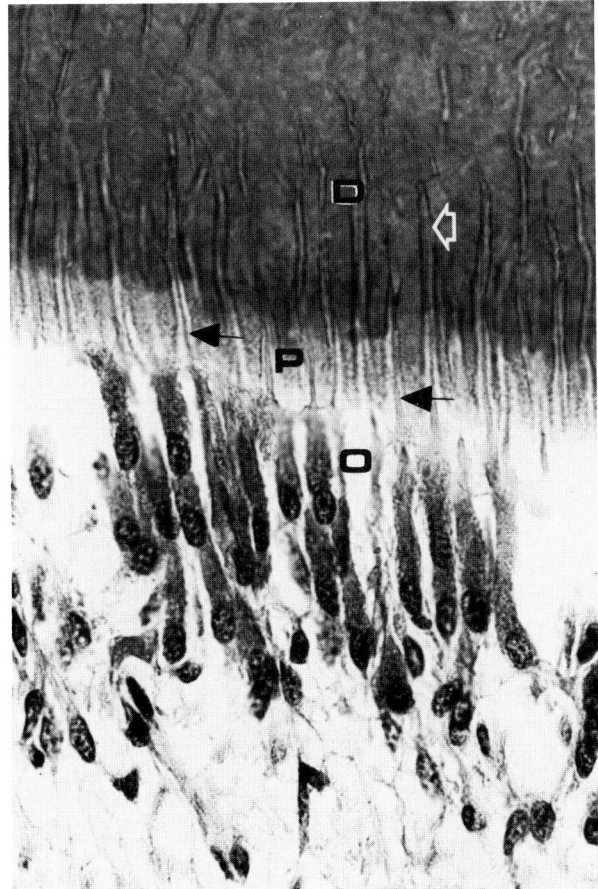

ig. 19.20 Layer of ondotoblasts. The odontoblasts (O) have apical processes, dentinal fibers
solid arrows), which extend into dentinal tubules (*open arrow*). Predentine (P) is secreted and
en mineralized as dentine (D), X160.

lamina propria-submucosa in close proximity to the lamina epithelialis. Minor salivary glands, named on the basis of location, include the labial, lingual, buccal and palatine glands. The minor salivary glands are best described as diminutive forms of those major glands described previously. Minor salivary glands are mucous, serous or mixed.

The *labial glands* are mucous in small ruminants, dogs and cats; serous in large ruminants, swine and horses; mixed in man. The *lingual glands* of large ruminants and horses are mixed, whereas those of carnivores and sheep are mucous. *Von Ebner's glands* are specialized lingual glands which secrete a serous product in association with the large gustatory lingual papillae. *Dorsal buccal glands* are mucous in large ruminants, carnivores and horses; *ventral buccal glands* of these animals are serous. The buccal glands of man and swine are mixed. Palatine glands are mixed also.

Functional Correlates. *Saliva*, the mixed secretory product of all of the salivary glands, serves a variety of functions. Besides the basic function of moistening the cutaneous mucous membrane and the foodstuffs, saliva lubricates, facilitates mastication, deglutition, and phonation. Also, saliva aids in the adjustment of the pH of the upper digestive tract, aids in the dissolution and tasting of foodstuffs and initiates a limited amount of carbohydrate digestion. However, the pig seems to be the only domestic animal that has a significant amount of salivary amylase to be of any consequence. The salt content of saliva may assist in the regulation of somatic electrolytes. Lactoperoxidase and immunoglobulin A serve protective functions as a salivary antimicrobial system.

Saliva consists of proteins, glycoproteins, electrolytes and water. It is a dilute aqueous fluid that is not an ultrafiltrate of blood, because the concentrations of hydrogen ions, chloride ions, potassium ions, sodium ions, protein and glucose differ from those within blood. The production of saliva requires energy.

Salivation is under the reflex control of medullary salivary centers of the autonomic nervous system. Afferent impulses originate in sensory receptors in the buccal cavity, pharynx, stomach and nasal cavity. The presence, odor, taste and mastication of foodstuffs are stimulatory to the sensory receptors. Parasympathetic components of cranial nerves VII, IX and X are the motor fibers to the salivary glands. Sympathetic nerves innervate these glands also. Both components of the autonomic nervous system excite salivary secretion. Parasympathetic stimulation, the dominant excitatory stimulus, results in a voluminous, dilute, watery saliva. Sympathetic stimulation brings about a diminished, viscous, mucous saliva. Antimuscarinic drugs effectively curtail salivation.

The amount of saliva secreted by an ani-

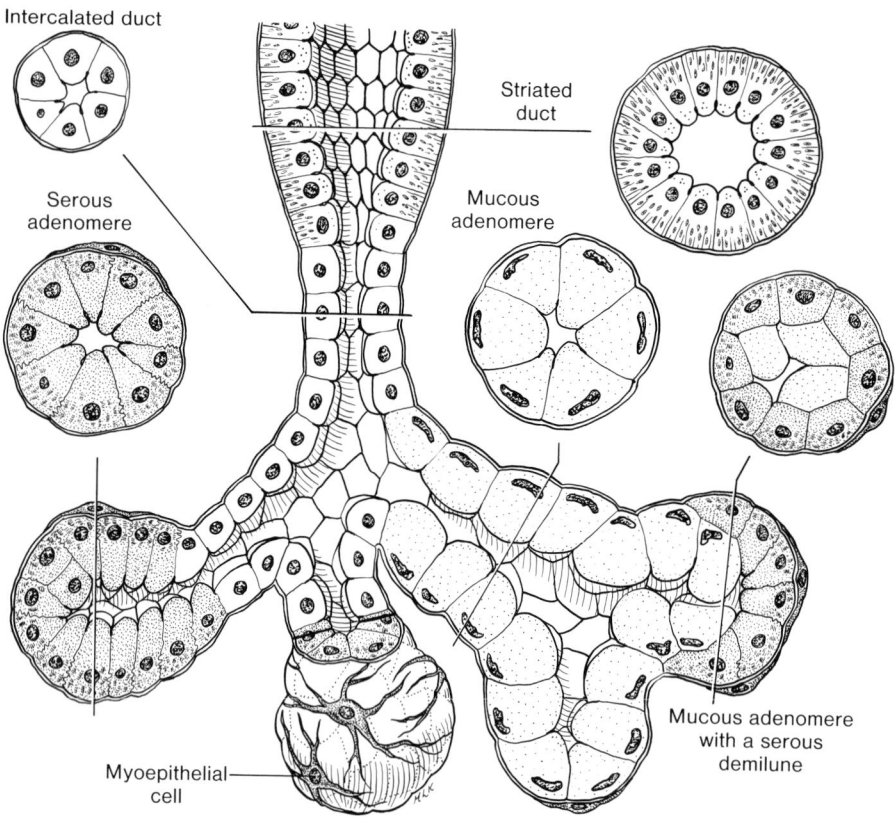

Fig. 19.21   An idealized drawing of the types of adenomeres that characterize the salivary glands.

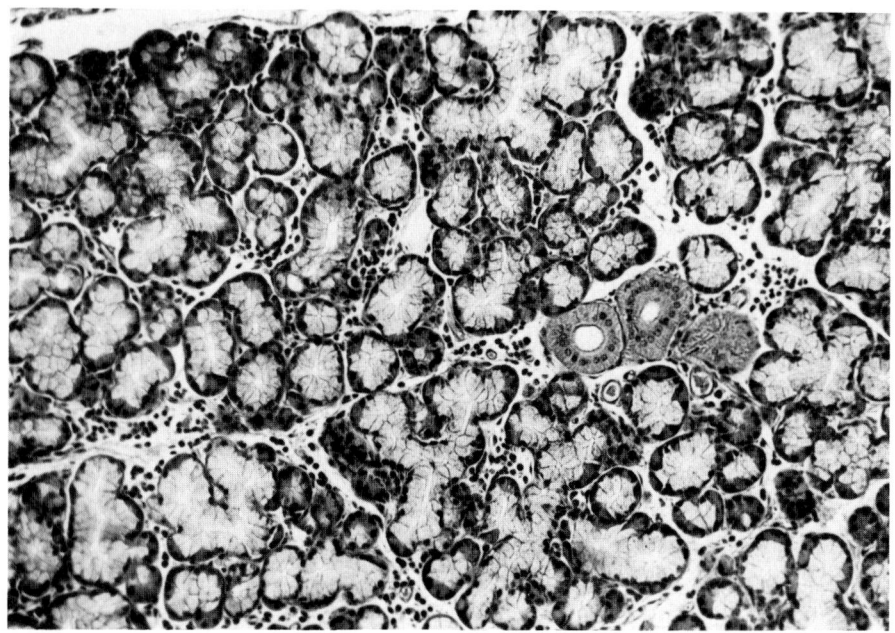

Fig. 19.22   An equine sublingual salivary gland. This is a mixed salivary gland. Note the mucous adenomeres and serous demilunes. X40.

mal varies with the species. Man may produce 1–2 liters per 24-hour period; sheep, 1 4 liters per 24-hour period; cattle, 90–19 liters per 24 hours; horses, 38 liters per 2 hours. The type of diet influences the amount and nature of the salivary secretion In the dog, a fresh meat diet stimulates the secretion of a viscous saliva, whereas a dr food preparation elicits a voluminous, watery saliva. The flow of saliva may be influenced by psychic stimulation. The sight o suggestion of food can cause a *conditione reflex flow* of saliva in dogs and swine. A *unconditioned reflex flow* of saliva occurs i response to the presence of food in th mouth. Ungulates only possess an uncon ditioned reflex secretion of saliva.

The ion content of saliva is dependen upon the type and rate of secretory activit of the salivary glands. The epithelial linin, cells of the striated ducts exert an influenc upon the ionic and water content of th secretion. The basal morphology of striatec duct epithelium represents a large surfac area for the rapid transport of fluids an ions. The juxtaposition of energy-producin mitochondria affords a readily available en ergy source. The basal morphology, wit plasmalemmal infoldings and associatec mitochondria, resembles other epithelia cells that are involved in the rapid move ment of fluid and ions (Fig. 5.49).

The juxta-alveolar connective tissue o the salivary glands contains numerou plasma cells and small lymphocytes, as wel as the usual contingent of resident cells Immunoglobulin A produced by plasma cells in these loci is transported through th alveolar lining cells during which time the secretory piece is added. Secretory IgA which is resistant to proteolysis, protects the mucous membranes of the buccal cavity from pathogenic microorganisms.

Pharynx

Histology. The *oropharynx* is an extension of the buccal cavity and connects it with th esophagus. The lamina epithelialis is strati fied squamous epithelium. Varying degree of keratinization are species-variable. The lamina propria is typical and contains ton sils, individual lymph nodules and scattered leucocytes. Numerous papillae are obviou and resemble dermal papillae of the skin Although a typical lamina mucularis is no present, a layer of elastic fibers delimits thi space from the tunica submucosa. The latter is typical and contains branched tubuloal veolar mucous glands. The tunica muscu laris is composed of striated muscle which is not oriented in any particular manner The tunica adventitia is typical and blends with the accompanying deep fascia.

Esophagus

This structure is a muscular tube that i modified for the voluntary and involuntary

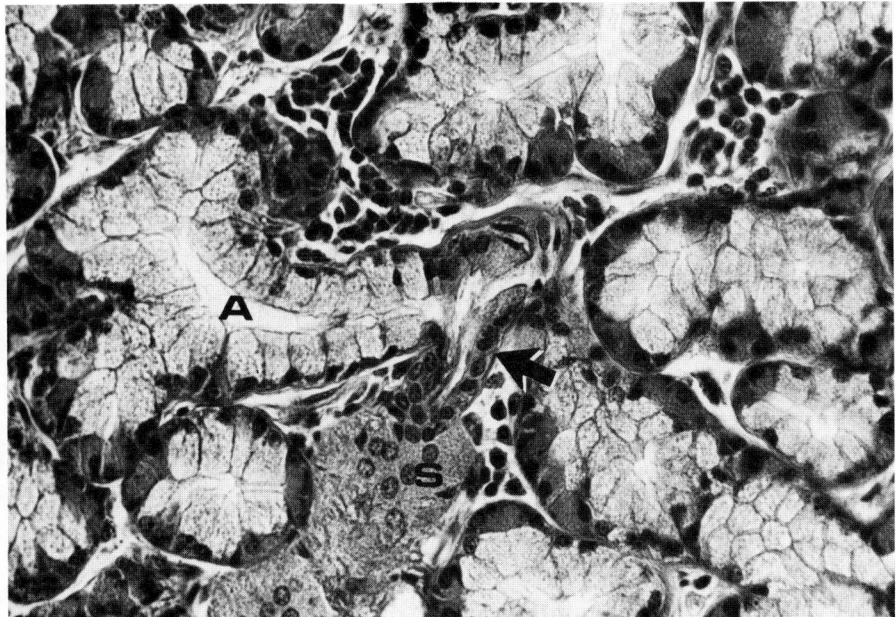

Fig. 19.23 Alveolus, intercalated duct and striated duct of an equine mixed salivary gland. The alveolus (A) is lined by mucous cells and serous demilunes. The intercalated duct (*arrow*) connects alveoli to striated ducts (S). X100.

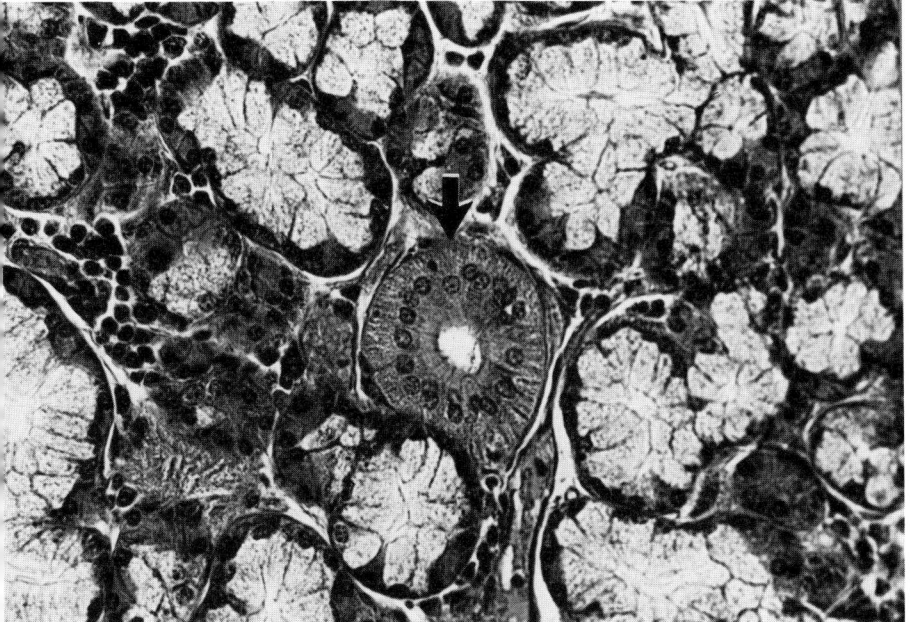

Fig. 19.24 Striated duct of an equine mixed salivary gland. The striated duct (*arrow*) is lined by simple columnar epithelium with basal striations. X100.

movement of foodstuffs to and from the stomach.

Mucosa. The lamina epithelialis is stratified squamous epithelium. Varying degrees of cornification may be apparent. It is especially apparent in those species which ingest hard, dry foodstuffs.

The lamina propria is typical and in some species may contain numerous lymph nodules and scattered lymphatic tissue (man and pig). These are especially prominent at the esophageal-gastric junction. Small blood vessels, lymph vessels and nerves are present.

The lamina muscularis mucosae is typical but of variable occurrence (Fig. 19.28). This

muscular layer is continuous with the elastic fiber layer of the pharynx. In man it is a thick and complete layer. In the horse, ruminants and the cat, it consists of scattered muscle bundles which may eventually fuse in the aboral portion of the esophagus. In the dog and pig, it is absent in the cervical portion; it may become complete near the stomach (Fig. 19.29).

Submucosa. The tunica submucosa is typical and contains numerous branched tubuloalveolar mucous glands. These glands are present the entire length of the canine esophagus; in the pig they are present in the cervical portion but sparse in the thoracic portion; in ruminants, the horse and cat they are present in the cervical portion.

The tunica mucosa and tunica submucosa have longitudinal folds that permit expansion of the esophagus.

Muscularis. The tunica muscularis consists of striated muscle, smooth muscle or a mixture of both. The inner and outer lamina may be distinct in the aboral portion. Striated muscle, smooth muscle or a mixture of both vary according to species: in ruminants and the dog it is entirely striated (Fig. 19.30); in the pig the cervical portion consists of striated muscle, the thoracic portion is mixed and the caudal portion consists of smooth muscle; in the horse and cat it consists of striated muscle to the middle portion and then consists of smooth muscle.

Serosa/Adventitia. The tunica adventitia is typical in the cervical portion. It is replaced by a tunica serosa in the thoracic portion. The tunica serosa is also typical.

Histophysiology. As a muscularized tube that connects the pharynx with the stomach, the esophagus has properties that are related directly to the distribution and type of muscle that comprises the tunica muscularis. The ease of vomition and/or regurgitation in ruminants and the dog is linked to the distribution of skeletal muscle throughout the course of the esophagus. Although emesis and regurgitation are abnormal physiologic events in the dog, regurgitation is a normal physiologic event in the digestive sequences of ruminants. The pig and cat are capable of vomiting when sufficient irritation occurs within the pharynx and stomach. Despite the distribution of skeletal muscle within the cranial two-thirds of the esophagus of the horse, vomition is rare in this species.

The junctions of the esophagus with the pharynx and stomach are not marked by anatomic thickenings that serve as sphincters. However, the pharyngoesophageal and gastroesophageal junctions serve as physiologic sphincters which are capable of maintaining intraesophageal luminal pressure higher than intragastric pressure. The "caudal esophageal sphincter" of the horse has sufficient tone that it remains closed during gastric dilation to the point of gastric rupture without vomiting occurring.

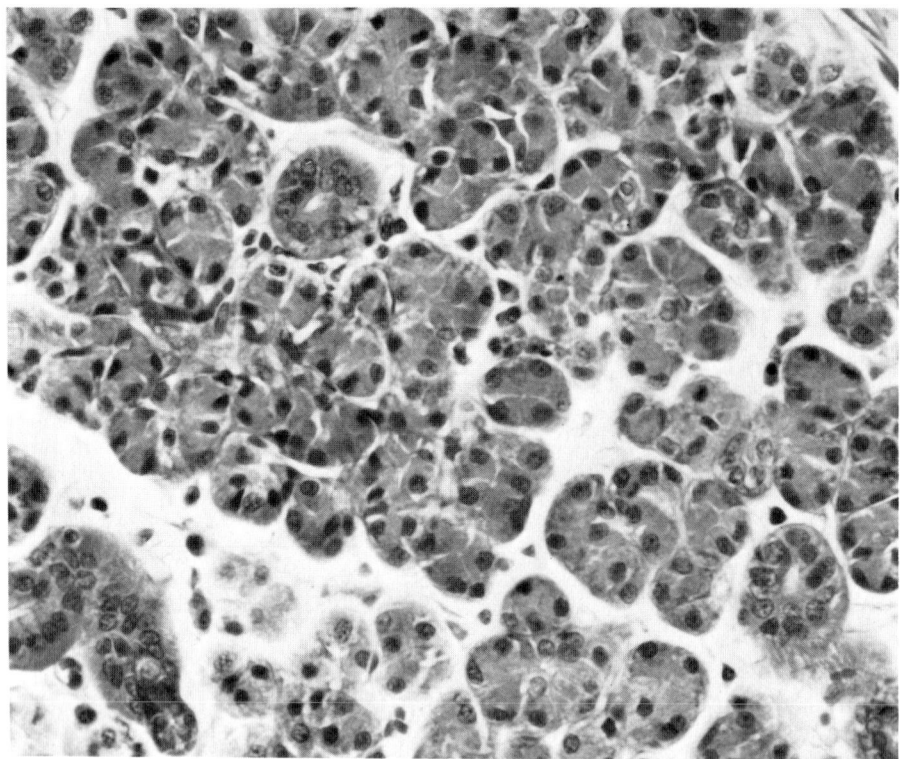

Fig. 19.25 A canine parotid salivary gland. The adenomeres are composed of serous cells. X40.

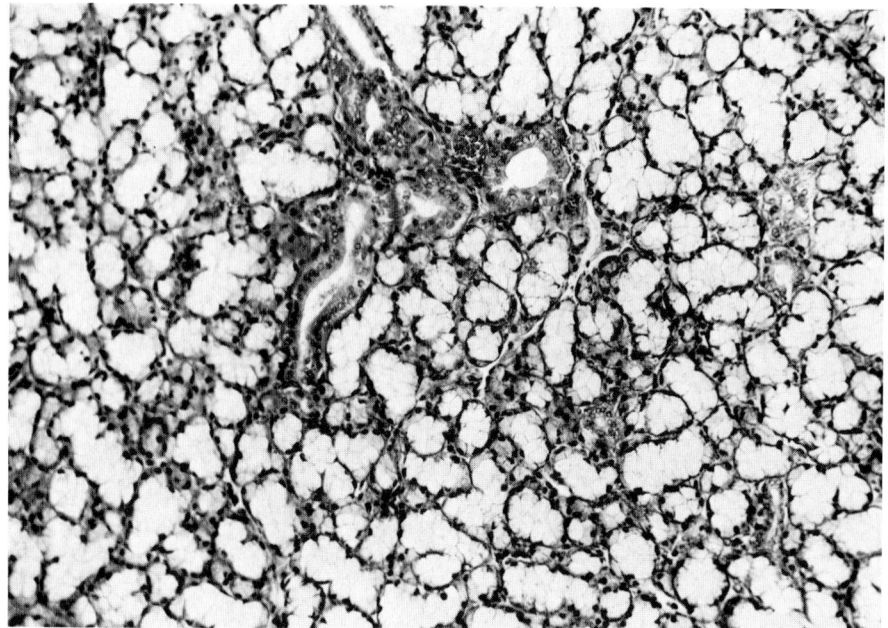

Fig. 19.26 Canine mandibular salivary gland. This is a mucous gland. X40.

During deglutition, food within the buccal cavity is propelled into the pharynx by the caudal movement of the tongue. This event initiates a series of coordinated voluntary and involuntary muscular activities that permits the food to pass the "pharyngoesophageal sphincter" and enter the esophagus. The localized distention of the cranial portion of the esophagus initiates a wave of peristalsis that moves the bolus toward the stomach. Relaxation of the "gastroesophageal sphincter" permits food to enter the stomach.

The innervation of the esophagus is described simply as being derived from parasympathetic and sympathetic branches of the autonomic nervous system. The general visceral efferent innervation of esophageal smooth muscle and glands is derived from the autonomic nervous system. Similarly general visceral afferent fibers of the esophagus are part of the autonomic nervous system. However, most domestic species, with the exception of domestic fowl, have either all skeletal muscle or a preponderance of skeletal muscle in the tunica muscularis of the esophagus. The innervation of the

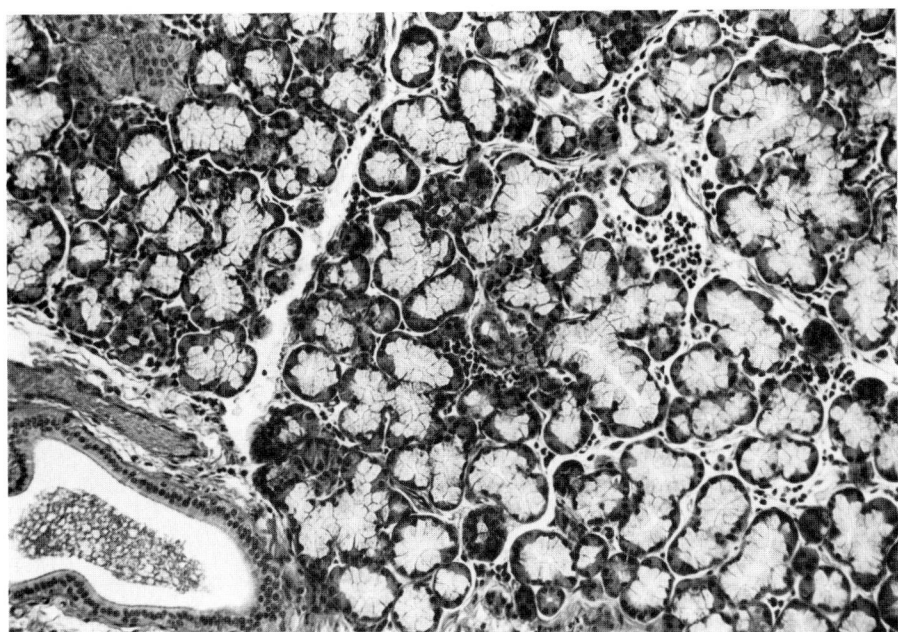

ig. 19.27 An equine sublingual salivary gland. This is a mixed salivary gland. Note the excretory duct in the lower left portion of the micrograph. 40.

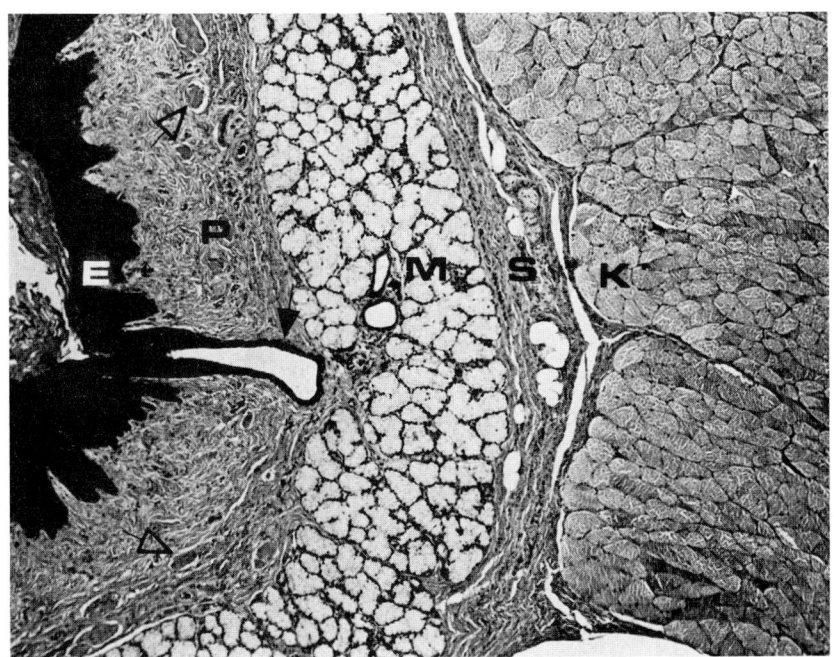

ig. 19.28 Porcine esophagus (lower cervical region). The lamina epithelialis (E) is supported by a lamina propria (P). The lamina muscularis consists of scattered bundles of smooth muscle (*open arrows*). Mucous glands (M) are continuous with the epithelial lining via excretory ducts (*solid arrow*). A tunica submucosa (S) is adjacent to the skeletal muscle (K) of the tunica muscularis. X12.

sophageal skeletal muscle fibers probably riginates as special visceral efferent fibers rom the nucleus ambiguus and are distrib- ted to the esophagus by the vagus nerve.

Esophageal dysfunction can result from number of causes in the dog (foreign body, tricture, perforation). Regurgitation of oodstuffs, not vomition, is the pathogno- nonic sign of obstructive esophageal dis-

ease. Often, surgical intervention is consid- ered in such cases. Unfortunately, the heal- ing potential of the esophagus is less than optimum and leakage into the surrounding areas is common. Poor tissue strength cou- pled with a minimal amount of adventitial or serosal connective tissue complicates the healing process. A marginal segmental blood supply and the constant movement of

thoracic organs (heart, lungs) compounds the healing process. The greater omentum of the peritoneal cavity and the tunica serosa associated with the visceral organs are effec- tive sealants. The cervical esophagus is de- void of a tunica serosa, whereas the thoracic esophagus, although juxtaposed between the mediastinal pleura, is not associated inti- mately with the tunica serosa of this region.

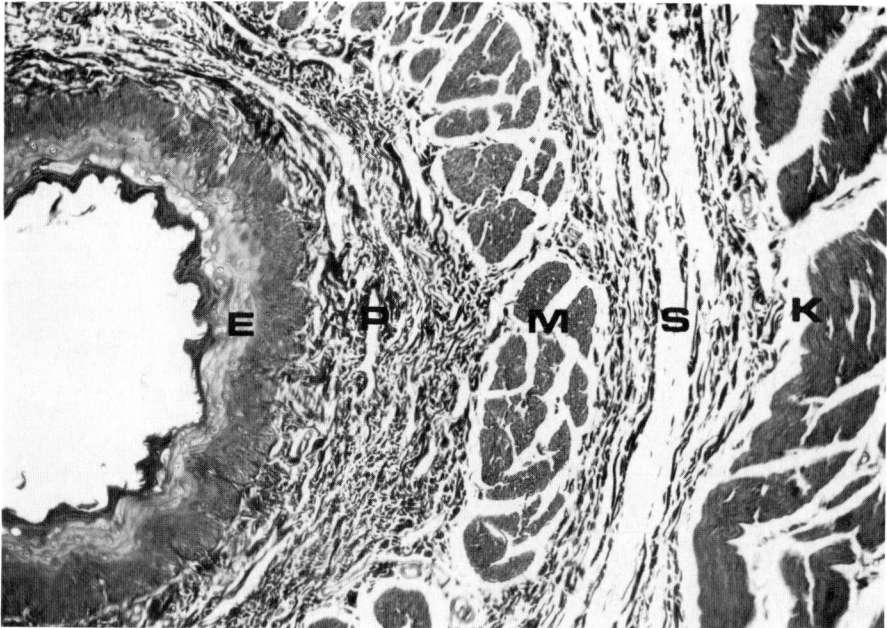

Fig. 19.29   Canine esophagus (thoracic region). The lamina epithelialis (E) and lamina propria (P) are typical. The lamina muscularis (M) is extensive. S, tunica submucosa; K, skeletal muscle of tunica muscularis. X40.

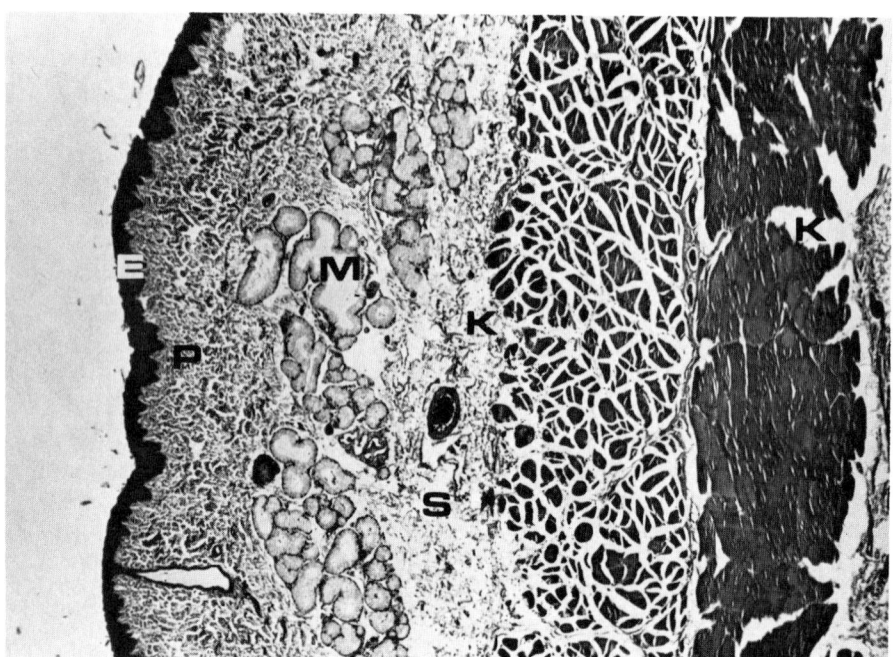

Fig. 19.30   Canine esophagus (cervical region). E, lamina epithelialis; P, lamina propria; M, mucous glands; S, tunica submucosa; K, skeletal muscle of tunica muscularis. A lamina muscularis is not present. X10.

Glandular Stomach

General Characteristics.   The *glandular stomach* is a musculoglandular organ which is the caudal continuation of the alimentary canal. The glandular stomach, modified as an enlarged tube which may assume a sac-like configuration when filled with food,

connects the esophagus to the duodenum. Foodstuffs delayed within the stomach are subjected to the enzymatic and hydrolytic action of gastic juice. The muscular wall of the organ induces the mechanical mixing and breakdown of foodstuffs. Peristaltic waves of contraction propel the mixed and partially digested foodstuffs (*chyme*) to the duodenum.

Histologic Organization

Although the mural elements of the glandular stomach conform to the pattern which typifies tubular visceral organs (Chapter 13) the organ has unique characteristics which permit its identification in histologic sections.

Mucosa.   The tunica mucosa consists of lamina epithelialis mucosae, lamina propria mucosae and lamina muscularis mucosae. The mucosa and part of the associated submucosa are thrown into tortuous folds *plicae gastricae* (*gastric folds*), which are oriented generally parallel to the long axis of the organ (Fig. 19.31). The prominence of these folds, although not completely effacable, varies inversely with the degree of gastric distention. The epithelial surface is divided into smaller irregular areas called *gastric areas* (*areae gastricae*) by numerous small grooves. The gastric areas are marked with numerous small depressions, gastric pits (*foveolae gastricae*), into the bottom of which the gastric glands open. The depth of the gastric pits varies with specific regions of the stomach.

The lamina epithelialis of the stomach including the gastric pits, is a simple columnar epithelium. The lining cells are mucus secreting; however, they are sufficiently unique as to be distinguished from the cells of the gastric glands and the rest of the lining cells of the digestive tract. Because mucinogen is not preserved by routine histologic preparations, the entire apical portion of the gastric lining cells has a clear zone (Fig. 19.32). The size and shape of the clear zone is dependent upon the amount of mucinogen that was present and the shape of the cell; however, the clear zone is a prominent feature of these cells. The shape of the nucleus, which may be oval or spheroidal, is dependent upon the shape of the cell and the amount of mucinogen that was present. The shape of the gastric lining cells as well as the chemical composition of its mucinogen, differs from that of typical goblet cells. The lining cells become progressively more cuboidal as they approach the opening of the gastric glands in the depth of the gastric pits.

The gastric lining cells are devoid of a striated border, although some microvilli are present. The absence of a striated border distinguishes these cells from the typical lining cells of the intestine. The difference between the gastric and intestinal lining cells is obvious especially at the gastroduodenal junction.

The lamina propria of the stomach is typical and consists of loose connective tissue. Usually, the connective tissue space has numerous mononucleated cells (lymphocytes, macrophages, plasma cells) which impart a distinct hypercellularity. Scattered lymphatic follicles may be encountered also.

The actual thickness of the lamina propria varies with the region of the stomach. Gas

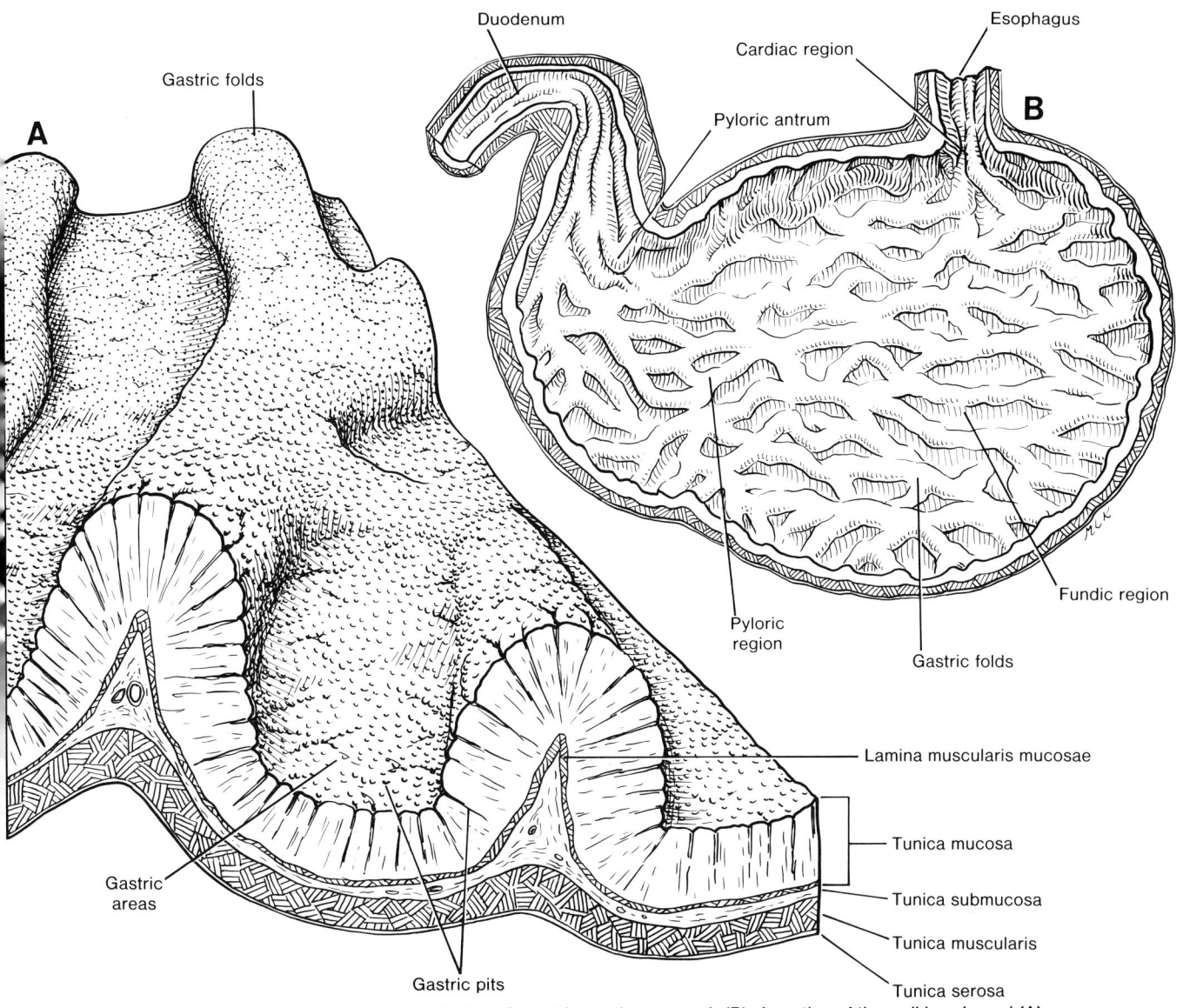

Fig. 19.31 A drawing of a longitudinal section of the canine stomach (B). A portion of the wall is enlarged (A).

tric glands, which are continuous with the gastric lining cells, penetrate variable distances into the lamina propria. Although the lamina propria may be thick, the actual connective tissue constituents are scant because they are interdigitated between the extensive gastric glands.

The lamina propria may contain a distinct zone, the *lamina subglandularis*, at the junction of the lamina propria and lamina muscularis (Fig. 19.33). The outer layer of this zone which is adjacent to the lamina muscularis consists of a condensation of dense white fibrous connective tissue and is called the *stratum compactum*. An inner layer, consisting of numerous fibroblasts, is called the *stratum granulosum*. The lamina subglandularis is especially well-developed in carnivores and is observed occasionally in the equine stomach. The layer may protect the stomach from perforation by sharp objects.

A lamina muscularis is present, but its arrangement is variable. Two to four muscle layers may comprise the lamina. The smooth muscle fibers are oriented longitudinally and circularly. Thin strands of smooth muscle extend into the lamina propria between the glands.

Submucosa. A tunica submucosa is present and typical. Adipose tissue, loose connective tissue, blood vessels, nerve processes, ganglion cell cytons and lymphatics are present. The nerve fibers and ganglion cell cytons form the *submucosal plexus (Meissner's plexus)*.

Muscularis. The tunica muscularis is present and typical. The nerves form the *myenteric plexus (Auerbach's plexus)* between the inner and outer laminae of smooth muscle.

Serosa. The tunica serosa is present and typical.

Regions and Glands of the Stomach

Regional differences in the tunica mucosa of the stomach permit the histologic identification of four distinct gastric regions:

esophageal region and *cardiac, fundic* and *pyloric gland regions* (Fig. 19.34).

Esophageal region. The esophageal region of the stomach is the nonglandular portion of the stomach which is lined by stratified squamous epithelium. Keratinization may be present but is dependent upon species and diet. The esophageal region is limited in carnivores, man and swine. In ruminants, it is extensive and is subdivided into the rumen, reticulum and omasum. These chambers will be described with the compound stomach.

Cardiac Gland Region. The cardiac gland region is not developed equally in all species (Fig. 19.34). The beginning of the cardiac gland region is marked by a transition from stratified squamous to columnar epithelium. This point of transition is called the *margo plicatus* in the horse. The histologic features of the cardiac gland region conform to those described generally for the stomach (Fig. 19.35). The cardiac glands are the distinctive histologic components of this region.

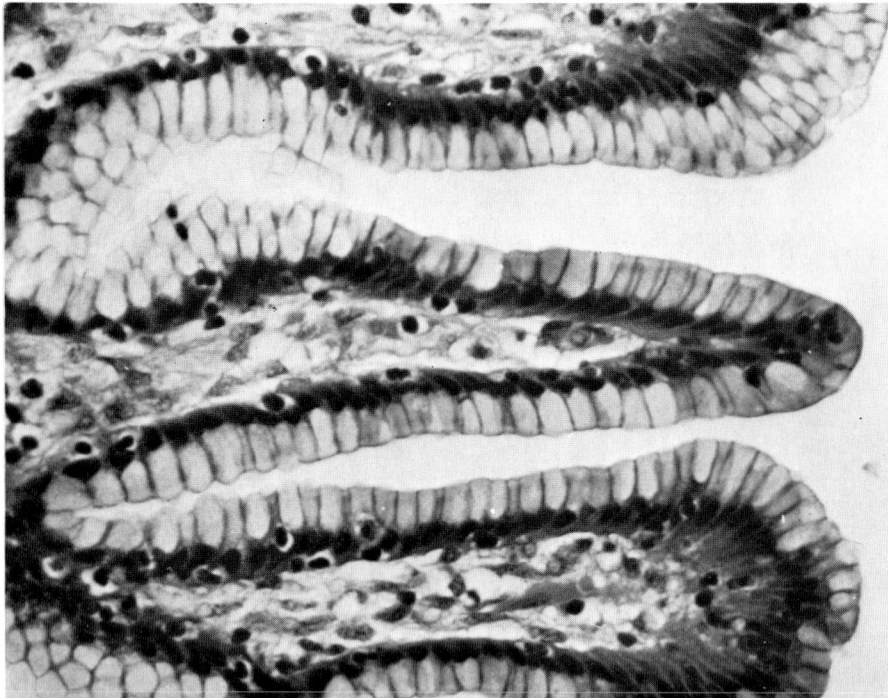

Fig. 19.32 The lining cells of the equine stomach. Note the clear zone in the apical portion of the cells. X160.

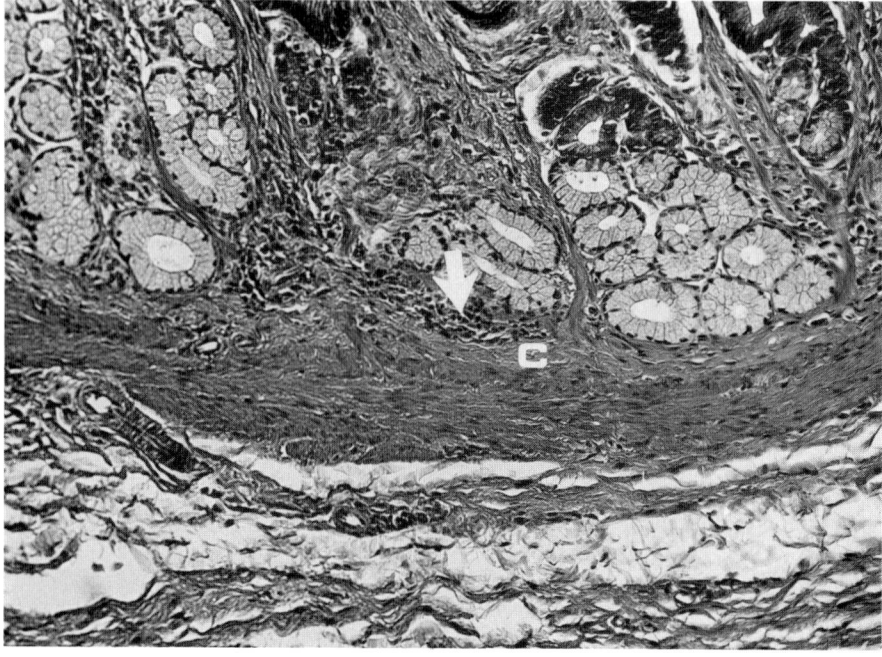

Fig. 19.33 Lamina subglandularis of the canine stomach. The lamina consists of a stratum compactum (C) and a stratum granulosum (arrow). X40.

The *cardiac glands* are branched tubular coiled glands which consist of a neck and body region (Fig. 19.36). The neck of the gland is that portion of the structure nearest the opening of the gastric pit. The body is the remainder of the adenomere. The neck and upper portion of the body are lined by cuboidal cells. The cuboidal lining cells are mucus-secreting. The remaining cells of the gland are columnar, mucus-secreting cells. Some *parietal cells* may be present in the canine cardiac gland region, whereas some *chief cells* may be present in porcine cardiac glands.

Argentaffin cells (*enterochromaffin cells*) are small, pyramidal cells with a clear cytoplasm that are located between the lining cells of the glands and the associated basement membrane. Special silver staining techniques are required to demonstrate these cells optimally. With special silver stains, numerous silver-containing granules are demonstrated in an abluminal or infranuclear position. Electron microscopic and immunocytologic techniques have been used to demonstrate as many as ten different cell types that correspond to the argentaffin or enterochromaffin cells that are scattered throughout the gastrointestinal tract.

The argentaffin cells do not secrete materials into the lumen of the organ. Rather, their products are secreted into the lamina propria and are distributed by the blood vessels. The argentaffin cells are *gastrointestinal endocrine cells* that secrete hormones. For this reason, they are referred to more appropriately as *enteroendocrine cells*. Secretions associated with these cells include *serotonin, histamine, epinephrine, gastrin* and *enteroglucagon*. The secretory and muscular activities of the gastrointestinal organs, including the pancreas and gallbladder, are controlled to a considerable extent by the release of these hormones in response to the changing properties and constituents of luminal contents.

Fundic Gland Region. The *fundic gland region* is similar to the morphology described for the cardiac region, but the extent of the fundic gland region is species variable (Fig. 19.34). The unique histologic features of the fundic region relate to the configuration of the fundic glands, the types of cells contained within the glands and the thickness of the lamina propria.

The glands of the fundic region, *fundic glands* or *gastric glands proper*, are branched tubular glands which are longer than but less frequently branched than their cardiac region counterparts (Fig. 19.37). The length of the fundic glands thickens the lamina propria (Compare the thickness of the lamina propria in Figures 19.35 and 19.37). The amount of connective tissue within the lamina propria is reduced greatly because the glands are packed tightly (Fig. 19.38).

A fundic gland is divisible into four regions: *base, body, neck* and *isthmus*. The isthmus or opening of the gland into the gastric pit is continuous with a constricted part of the gland, the neck. The body or main tubular portion of the gland continues from the neck and terminates as a slightly dilated and bent adenomere, the base.

Three cell types are distinguishable readily in routine preparations of fundic glands: *chief cells* (*zymogen cells*), *parietal cells* and *mucous neck cells*. A fourth cell type, the *enteroendocrine cells*, may be seen occasionally or may be demonstrated with special techniques. A fifth cell type, *transitional cell*, is described occasionally in the isthmus. Transitional cells are cuboidal cells which may be responsible for the replacement of lining and glandular epithelial cells.

Mucous neck cells line the constricted portion or neck of the gland and are interspersed among the parietal cells. The mu-

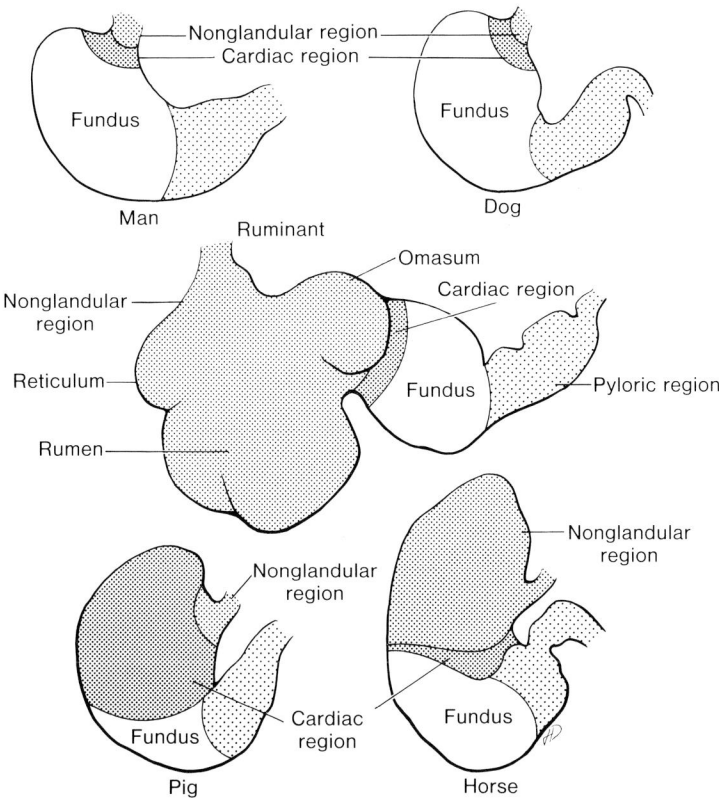

Fig. 19.34 A diagram of the distribution of glandular and nonglandular regions of the stomachs of selected animals. The organs are not drawn to scale.

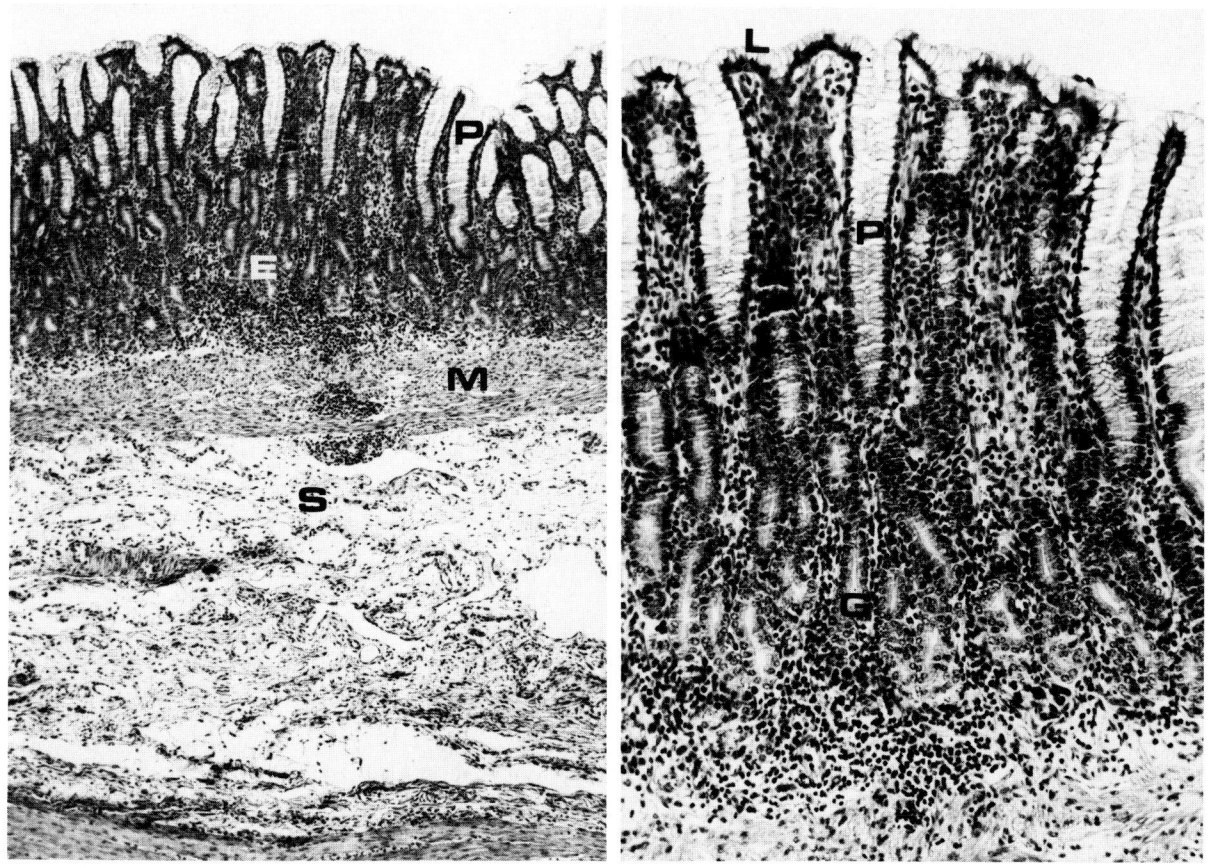

Fig. 19.35 Cardiac region of the canine stomach. A simple columnar epithelium (E) lines the surface and gastric pits (P). The lamina muscularis (M) and tunica submucosa (S) are typical. X16.

Fig. 19.36 Cardiac glands of the canine stomach. The lamina epithelialis is composed of a simple epithelium that lines the lumen (L), gastric pits (P) and cardiac glands (G). X40.

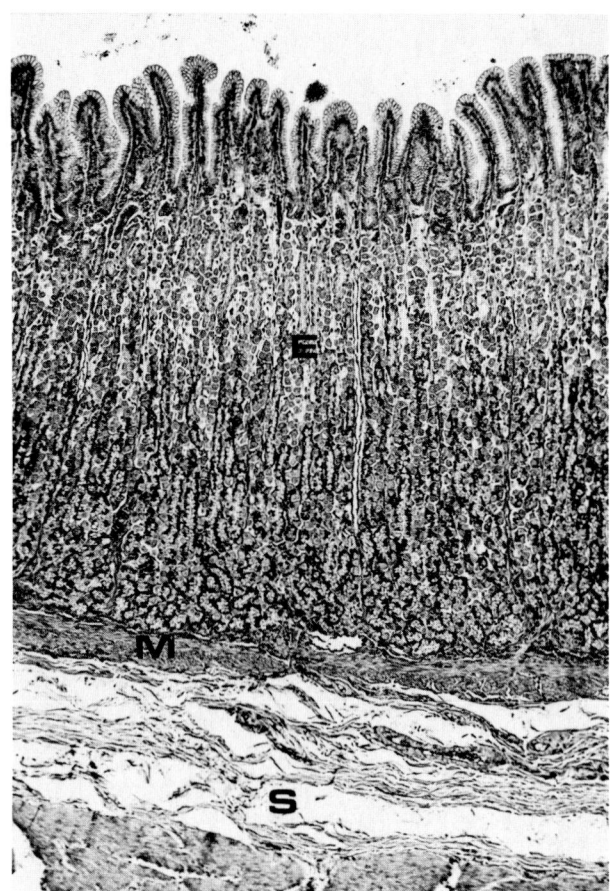

Fig. 19.37 Fundic region of the canine stomach. The lamina epithelialis (E) is highly folded. The tunica mucosa is very thick. The lamina muscularis (M) and tunica submucosa (S) are typical. X16.

cous neck cells are cuboidal or low columnar cells with a pale-staining cytoplasm (Fig. 19.39). The mucoid product of these cells differs from that of the surface lining cells but is similar to the mucoid secretion of the cardiac and pyloric glands. The mucus of the neck cells is less viscous than that of the surface lining cells and contains acid mucosubstances. The secretory product of the mucous neck cells may protect the fundic gland from the proteolytic and hydrolytic activity of the proteases and hydrochloric acid, respectively. The mucous neck cells may be capable of differentiating into surface lining and/or glandular lining cells.

The *chief cells* (*zymogen cells*) are the predominant cells of the fundic glands (Fig. 19.40). They are pyramidal-shaped cells with a basally-positioned round nucleus. Apically-positioned secretory granules (*zymogen granules*) are present in fasted animals; however, the cells are labile to fixation and the secretory granules may be leached from the cell, imparting an apical foamy appearance. A distinct polarity is evident in these cells (Fig. 19.41). The basal portion of the chief cells contain numerous rough endoplasmic reticular profiles and free ribo-

somes which impart a distinct basophilia. The chief cells are responsible for the synthesis and secretion of gastric enzymes. *Pepsinogen* is the inactive form of the proteolytic enzyme *pepsin*. Pepsinogen is activated by hydrochloric acid within the lumen of the stomach. *Prorennin* is the inactive form of the proteolytic enzyme *rennin*. The inactive form is converted to the active form by the proteolytic activity of pepsin. Rennin, which is only present in young animals, converts soluble milk protein (*casein*) to an insoluble form (*paracasein*). Paracasein is then subject to the proteolytic activity of pepsin. Gastric *lipase* is secreted by the chief cells also.

Parietal cells (*oxyntic cells*) are distinguished easily from the other cells of the fundic glands because of their bright-staining acidophilic cytoplasm (Fig. 19.40). They are large cells that are scattered throughout the gland from neck to base. Their spheroidal or pyramidal configuration with a round nucleus is a distinctive feature (Plate II.7). Parietal cells are "wedged" between the chief cells as if their placement had been an afterthought of development. Although their basal borders are in contact with the basement membrane, not all of the cells

reach the luminal surface directly. Numerous canaliculi extend from the apical plasmalemma as invaginations into the cytoplasm proper (Fig. 19.42). The canaliculi appear to be occluded by numerous microvilli projecting into these spaces. Apical microvilli also extend between the chief cells and reach the luminal surface. Although not all the cells reach the luminal surface directly, their secretory products have access to the surface through the canalicular and microvillar system. Parietal cells elaborate hydrochloric acid. Also, they may secrete *intrinsic factor*, a substance necessary for the absorption of vitamin B_{12} (*extrinsic factor*) in man. Carnivores probably do not require intrinsic factor for the absorption of vitamin B_{12}.

Enteroendocrine cells are present and typical.

Pyloric Gland Region. The extent of the *pyloric gland region* is species variable (Fig. 19.34), although the histologic organization of the pyloric region is similar to the cardiac region (Fig. 19.43). The gastric pits are deeper than in other regions of the stomach, but the pyloric glands are similar to the cardiac glands (Fig. 19.44). The pyloric glands are short, simple or branched tubular glands. The predominant cell is the mucus-secreting cell similar to those that occur in the cardiac glands.

The remaining mural elements are typical; however, a well-developed inner circular lamina of the tunica muscularis is a striking feature of this area. It forms the *pyloric sphincter* at the *gastroduodenal junction* (Fig. 19.45).

Histophysiology of the Stomach

Gastric Motility and Secretion. The musculature of the stomach is contracting continually. When emptied, mild peristaltic contraction waves begin and increase in intensity over a period of hours. When food enters the canine stomach there is an initial period of relaxation followed by slow waves of contraction (*gastric slow wave*) which originate from the longitudinal musculature along the rostral portion of the greater curvature. Food is moved toward the pylorus by these propulsive waves of contraction. Subsequently, peristaltic waves originating in the antrum, *antral peristalsis*, propel liquid contents into the duodenum while preventing solid masses of foodstuffs from gaining access to the small intestine. The gastric slow waves are the pacemakers for antral peristalsis. Chyme is gradually and continually squirted into the duodenum. The antrum, pylorus and cranial duodenum probably function as a contractile unit. Regurgitation of chyme from the duodenum back into the stomach does not occur normally because the contraction of the pylorus persists longer than that of the cranial duodenum.

Gastric emptying is achieved when antra

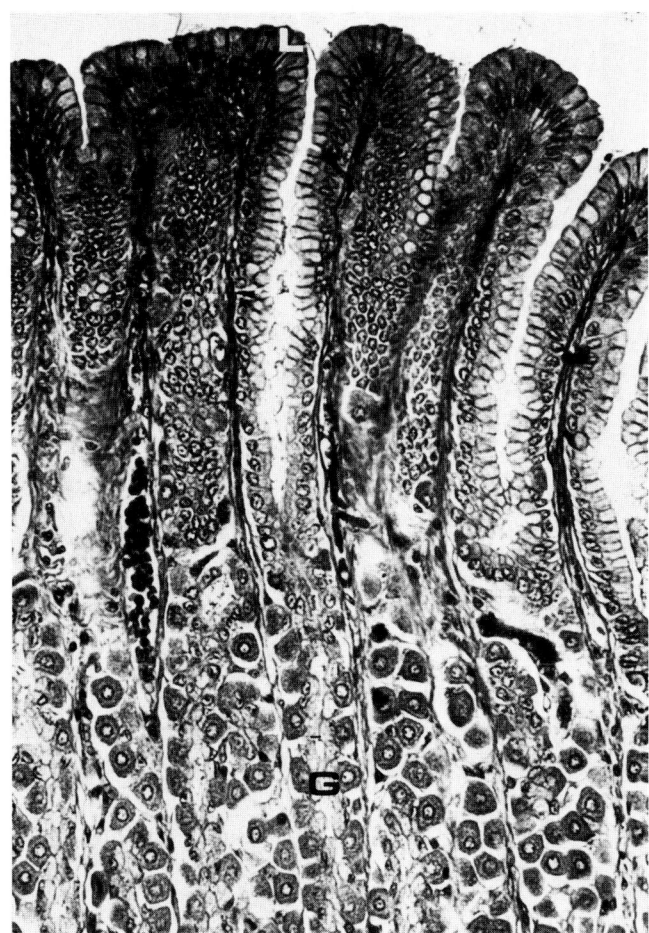

Fig. 19.38 Gastric pits and fundic glands of the canine stomach. The lining epithelium (L) is columnar, extends into the gastric pits and is continuous with the lining cells of the fundic glands (G). Note the reduced amount of connective tissue between the fundic glands. X63.

contractions overcome the resistance of the pyloric sphincter. The rate at which the stomach empties is influenced by the type of food in the diet. Carbohydrate-rich diets leave the stomach in a few hours; protein-rich diets exit more slowly; fat-rich diets exit the stomach the slowest. Gastric motility and emptying is influenced also by various duodenal factors. Duodenal distention with chyme, increased acidity and the products of proteolysis activate a neural reflex which decreases gastric motility, the *enterogastric reflex*. *Gastric inhibitory peptide* and *vasoactive intestinal peptide* are factors that have been isolated from the intestinal mucosa which have an inhibitory effect upon gastric motility and secretion. The neural and humoral regulatory mediators permit the small intestine to achieve a more complete digestion of the substances present.

Gastric juice is the combined secretory product of the lining and glandular epithelial cells of the stomach. Normal gastric juice consists of various organic and inorganic components: Na^+, K^+, Mg^{++}, H^+, Cl^-, $HPO_4^=$, $SO_4^=$, pepsin, rennin (in young animals), lipase, mucus and water. The mucoid component is predominantly the product of the lining cells of the stomach and the glandular epithelial cells of the cardiac and pyloric glands. The function of the mucus is to protect the mucosa from being irritated or digested. The hydrochloric acid and enzymes are secreted by the glandular cells of the fundic glands. The pH of gastric juice, approximately 1.0, is sufficiently strong to damage the mucosa were it not for the mucous coating of the cells.

Gastric secretion is controlled and influenced by several mechanisms and is divided conveniently into three phases: *cephalic, gastric* and *intestinal*. The *cephalic phase* represents the reflex activation of the stomach (motility and secretion) in response to the thought, sight, smell or taste of food. The cephalic secretory response is due to the vagal activation of secretory cells by the release of acetychloline at the muscarinic sites and by the vagal mediation of *gastrin* release from enteroendocrine cells within the pyloric antrum. The gastric juice secreted during the cephalic phase has a high concentration of hydrogen ion and is rich in pepsin.

The *gastric phase* of gastric secretion begins when food enters the stomach and continues until gastric emptying is accomplished. The vagus nerve and gastrin are the influencing factors during this phase. The presence of food in the stomach and the distention of this organ activate general visceral afferent fibers which ascend to higher centers via the vagus nerve. The reflex secretion is accomplished when general visceral efferent fibers of the vagus stimulate gastric secretory cells and gastrin-producing cells. The release of gastrin, however, is not dependent totally upon vagal stimulation. Antral distention also causes the release of gastrin. Similarly, various chemicals present in the partially digested food (meat extracts, amino acids, ethyl alcohol) also stimulate the release of gastrin. Gastrin release in response to local mechanical and chemical factors is probably mediated through an intrinsic reflex (Fig. 19.46). Afferent fibers within the mucosa respond to the local excitatory stimuli. The cell bodies of these fibers are probably located in the submucosal plexus. Efferent fibers from these cells synapse with postganglionic neurons of the submucosal plexus whose postganglionic fibers innervate the gastrin-producing cells. The preganglionic fibers of the vagus synapse with the same postganglionic cell body. The latter may be considered the final common pathway for vagally-induced gastrin secretion and intrinsically-induced gastrin secretion.

Gastrin has a variety of effects upon the stomach. The main effect of this hormone is the stimulation of the chief cell and the parietal cell. The activity of the chief cell with the subsequent release of chemical factors (meat extracts and amino acids) has a positive influence upon the elaboration of gastrin. Hydrochloric acid, however, inhibits gastrin secretion.

The *intestinal phase* of gastric secretion has a positive and negative effect upon gastric activity. As chyme enters the intestine its constituents function as *secretagogues*; i.e., compounds capable of causing secretion. The secretagogues cause the release of gastrin from the intestinal mucosa. The predominant effect of the intestinal phase upon gastric activity is that of inhibition. The enterogastric reflex inhibits gastric motility, while the secretagogues stimulate the release of the hormones *secretin, enterogastrone* and *cholecystokinin-pancreozymin* from the duodenal mucosa. Enterogastrone inhibits gastric acid secretion and gastric motility. Secretin stimulates the secretion of bicarbonate ions from the pancreas which neutralizes the acidity of the chyme. *Cholecystokinin-pancreozymin* (*CCK-PZ*) is an intestinal hormone that is released in response to the presence of fatty acids in the duodenum. Among its other effects, CCK-PZ also inhibits gastric emptying.

The events of the intestinal phase, while

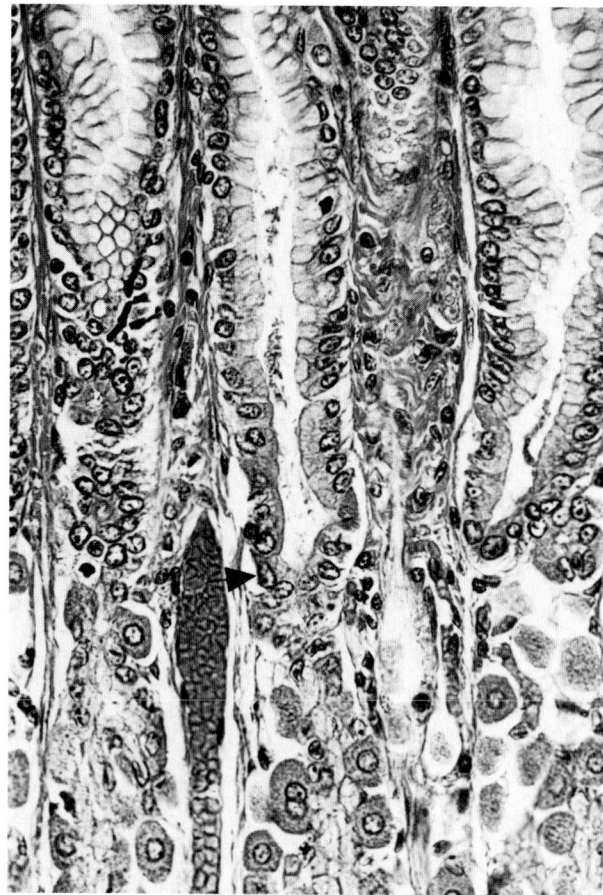

Fig. 19.39 Mucous neck cells of the fundic glands of a canine stomach. The neck of the gland is constricted (*arrow*) and is lined by mucous neck cells (*arrow*). The secretory product of these cells is mucoid; however, the mucoid product differs from that of surface lining cells. X100.

predominately inhibitory upon the stomach, insure a more complete digestion of the chyme.

The gastrointestinal hormones are discussed in more detail in Chapter 22.

Gastric Acid Secretion. The production of hydrochloric acid by the parietal cell is an efficient cellular process that requires the expenditure of energy. Hydrochloric acid is moved against a concentration gradient into the gastric lumen; the concentration of hydrogen ions in gastric juice is approximately 3 million times greater than that in plasma. The energy for this process is derived from oxidative metabolism within the parietal cell.

The precise origin of the hydrogen ion has not been settled; however, it may be derived from the ionization of water or the cytochrome system. For each hydrogen ion that is secreted, an hydroxyl ion remains. For the pH to remain constant within the cell, the hydroxyl ion must be neutralized. This is achieved by the *carbonic anhydrase* system. Carbon dioxide, which is formed within the cell as a result of normal metabolic processes or diffuses into the cell from the connective tissue, is hydrated to carbonic acid by carbonic anhydrase. The dissocia-

tion of carbonic acid into hydrogen and bicarbonate ions provides the buffer for the excess hydroxyl ions. The hydrogen ions react with the hydroxyl ions to form water, while the bicarbonate ions diffuse into the connective tissue.

The movement of ions in and out of the parietal cell occurs in an orderly and predictable manner. Chloride ions diffuse from the blood into the parietal cell. The available hydrogen ion is coupled with the chloride ion and actively transported across the cell membrane into the gastric lumen. This active transport mechanism requires energy derived from oxidative phosphorylation and is linked to the uptake of a sodium ion from the gastric lumen. Sodium is pumped actively across the basal cell membrane in exchange for a potassium ion. The potassium ion then diffuses passively out of the cell with the bicarbonate ion that was formed by the dissociation of carbonic acid. The passive and active movement of ions associated with hydrochloric acid secretion occurs in such a manner as to maintain cellular electrical balance.

The bicarbonate ion that leaves the parietal cell enters the general circulation; blood leaving the gastric circulation may be alka-

line. The elevated secretion of hydrogen ions associated with a meal is sufficiently high to cause a bicarbonate production that can raise systemic blood pH and alkalize the urine. This mechanism is a reasonable explanation for the *postprandial alkaline tide*.

The secretion of hydrochloric acid is influenced by the vagus nerve and the hormone gastrin. Additionally, *histamine* is a potent stimulator of hydrochloric acid secretion. The high histamine content of the gastric mucosa has led to the belief that histamine may be the common mediator of gastric acid secretion. Two types of histamine receptors, H_1 and H_2 *receptors*, have been identified. Antihistaminic drugs that are used commonly for the prophylactic treatment of allergies block the H_1 receptor sites. The H_2 receptor sites, the type that occur on parietal cells, are not blocked by H_1 blocking agents; specific H_2 blocking agents are required to inhibit gastric acid secretion. The precise relationships between the vagus nerve and acetylcholine, gastrin and histamine in the excitation of the parietal cell have not been determined. Separate yet functionally integrated cholinergic, gastrin and H_2 receptors may interact to modulate the activity of the parietal cells.

Excessive activity of the parietal cell with a predisposing or concomitant alteration in the protective mucous coat can lead to an erosion of the gastric mucosa, a *gastric (peptic) ulcer*. The constant hydrochloric acid secretion of human parietal cells may augment the potential for problems; the dog, although still susceptible to gastric ulceration, secretes hydrochloric acid when stimulated by food.

Renewal, Replacement and Repair. All of the epithelial cells of the tunica mucosa of the stomach are replaced continually. Surface lining cells may be replaced as often as every 3 days, whereas glandular epithelial cellular replacement may occur every 5–days. Mitotic activity is limited to the lining cells in the depths of the gastric pits. As lining cells are exfoliated from the surface, they are replaced by the luminal migration of cells from the zone of mitosis. Similarly undifferentiated cells in the isthmus migrate toward the base of the gland to replace mucous neck cells, chief cells and parietal cells. The chief and parietal cells are long lived and their replacement occurs slowly.

After a wound in the stomach, the margins of the discontinuity are characterized by epithelial cells that appear to be undifferentiated mucous-secreting cells. These cells divide and migrate over the defect similar to that described for the epidermis. Once the lamina propria has been covered, the lamina epithelialis invaginates to form new gastric pits and glands. All of the epithelium is mitotically active during this stage of healing. Eventually, typical surface lining cells are differentiated and mucous neck cells are identifiable within the glands. Chief

ells and parietal cells appear to differen-
ate from the mucous neck cell. The remainder of the mural elements (connective
issue, nerve and smooth muscle) repair
hemselves as described previously.

The healing properties of the stomach are
xcellent. The extensive anastomotic blood
upply, regenerative potential of the epithe-
ium, extensive submucosal connective tisue, well-developed serosal covering and
uxtaposition of the greater omentum all
ontribute to its repair potential.

Compound Stomach

General Characteristics. The ruminant
tomach consists of four parts: *rumen, reticulum, omasum* and *abomasum* (Fig. 19.34).
The *forestomach*, consisting of the first three
hambers, is derived from the esophageal
egion of the stomach and is lined by an
glandular stratified squamous epithelium.
The forestomach functions to break down
ngesta through mechanical and chemical
ctivity. The rumen serves as a large fermentation vat in which microorganisms
bacteria and protozoa) break down the ingested foodstuffs and produce *volatile fatty
acids*. Volatile fatty acids are absorbed

across the lamina epithelialis into the blood
vessels of the lamina propria. The mechanical action of the reticulum and omasum
converts the fermented ingesta into a mass
of fine particulate matter. Absorption of
metabolites occurs across the epithelium of
the forestomach. The ingesta is then moved
into the abomasum wherein enzymatic
digestion of the foodstuffs is accomplished.

Rumen

The rumen is also referred to as the
paunch. The characteristic feature of this
chamber is the conical papillae that project
into the lumen from the cutaneous mucous
membrane (Fig. 19.47). These papillae may
be 1.5 cm long and contain a core of highly
vascularized connective tissue composed of
fine collagenous and elastic fibers.

Histologic Organization. The lamina epithelialis is stratified squamous epithelium
which is cornified and of variable thickness
(Fig. 19.48). The layers of this epithelium
are not well-defined. The cells of the stratum
corneum are usually swollen or vesiculated.
On the apex of the papillae they are typically flattened.

The lamina propria consists of connective

tissue identical to that which occupies the
papillae. The components are continuous
with each other. The lamina propria blends
insensibly with the loose connective tissue
of the tunica submucosa. A condensation of
connective tissue fibers in the deep region
of the lamina propria-submucosa extends
into the papillae. The region may be similar
to the stratum compactum of the lamina
subglandularis and is sometimes mistaken
for the lamina muscularis mucosae. The
combined lamina propria-submucosa is generally devoid of lymphatic nodules and is
aglandular.

The tunica muscularis is present and typical. The *pillars* of the rumen are extensive
folds of the entire wall which contain a core
of muscle from the tunica muscularis. The
tunica serosa is present and typical.

Reticulum

The reticulum is also called the *honeycomb*. The morphology of the reticulum is
quite similar to that of the rumen. Only
those features that distinguish it from the
rumen are presented.

Histologic Organization. The mucous membrane has numerous, anastomotic *primary
folds* which are oriented, upon surface view,
as a reticulum or honeycomb (Fig. 19.49).
From these vertically projecting folds are
numerous *secondary* and *tertiary papillae*.
Within the lamina propria of the tips of the
primary or *reticular folds* is an isolated mass
of smooth muscle of the lamina muscularis
mucosae (Fig. 19.50). This mass extends
throughout the length of the folds and is
continuous with the lamina muscularis mucosae of the esophagus. The course of the
smooth muscle, therefore, is oriented parallel to, but above, the plane of the surface
lining. The lamina muscularis mucosae is
confined to the aforementioned region in
this chamber.

The lamina propria-submucosa, tunica
muscularis and tunica serosa are present and
typical.

The functions of this chamber are similar
to the functions of the rumen.

Omasum

The terms *many plies* and *book* are also
applied to the omasum (Fig. 19.51).

The keratinized cutaneous mucous membrane has numerous foliate *primary folds
(laminae)* as well as smaller papillae. The
laminae are covered with short, cornified
papillae (Fig. 19.52). The lamina muscularis
mucosae is present and continuous. The
lamina muscularis mucosae forms a double
layer of smooth muscle that follows the
contour of the laminae as well as that of the
unraised surface lining. Another layer of
smooth muscle is interdigitated between the
smooth muscle of the lamina muscularis
mucosae within the laminae. It is continuous

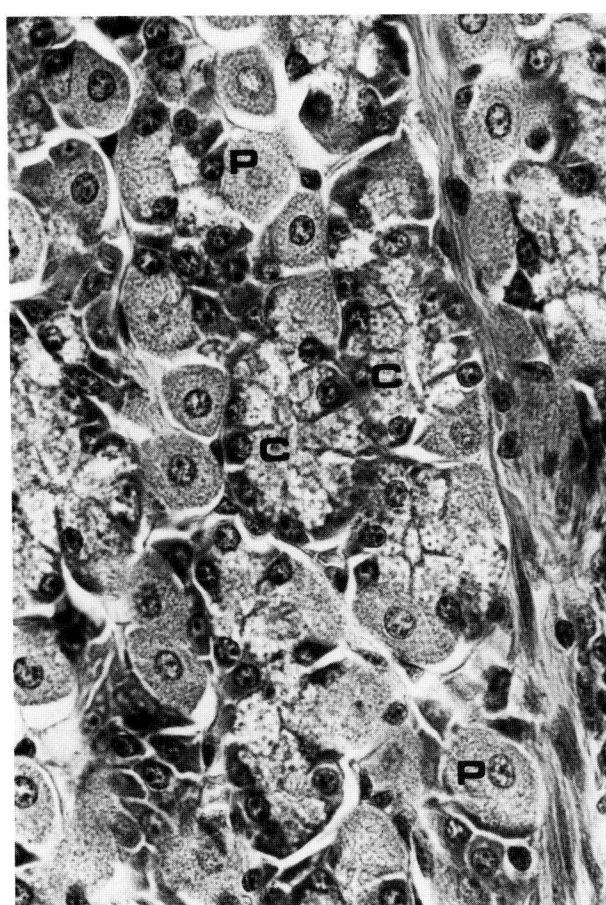

Fig. 19.40   Chief cells and parietal cells of the fundic glands of a canine stomach. The chief cells
(C) have granules along their apical borders. The parietal cells (P) are granular and acidophilic.
X160.

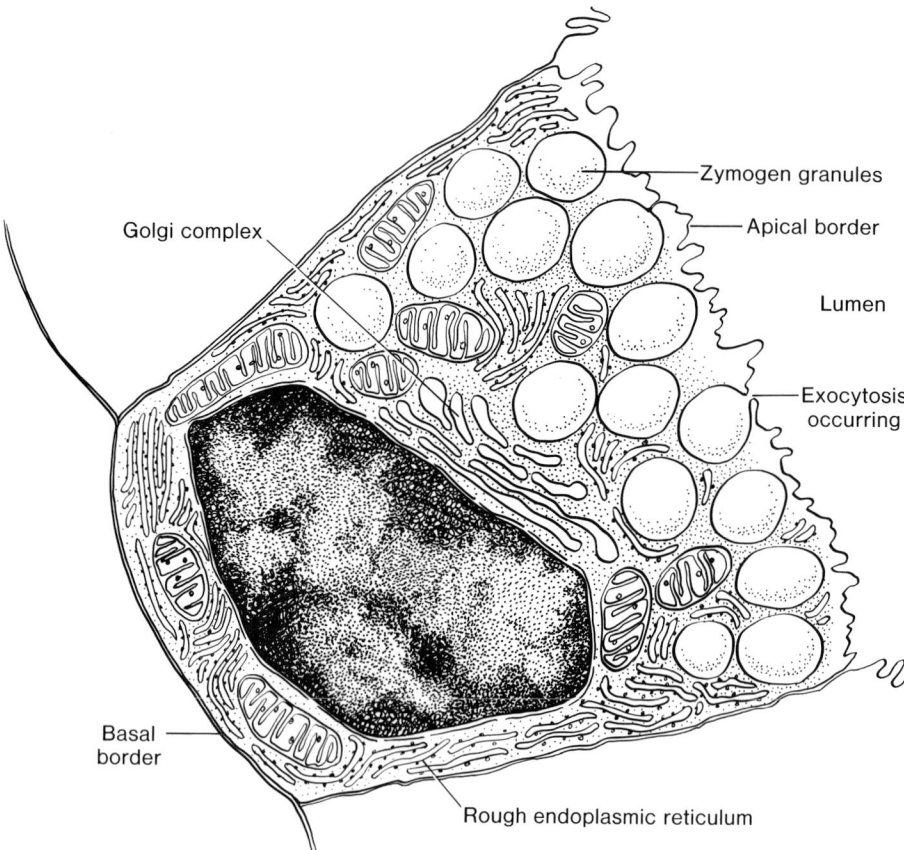

Fig. 19.41 A drawing of a chief cell as seen with the electron microscope. Note the distinct cellular polarity.

with the inner layer of smooth muscle of the tunica muscularis. At the apex of the laminae, the smooth muscle masses fuse into a thickened muscular mass.

The lamina propria, tunica submucosa, tunica muscularis and tunica serosa are present and typical. At the apices of the laminae, however, a mucous connective tissue is present.

Abomasum

The abomasum is the glandular portion of the ruminant stomach. The description of the glandular stomach applies to this organ.

Histophysiology of Ruminant Digestion

Development. The rumen, reticulum and omasum comprise approximately 89% of the total weight of the adult bovine stomach, and the abomasum contributes the remaining 11%. Whereas the four chambers of the compound stomach are evident within the embryo at approximately 60 days of gestation, the relative proportions of these chambers are not the same as in the adult. The abomasum is the predominant chamber and may comprise as much as 56% of the total organ weight at birth. The adult proportions are achieved gradually and are attained eventually at approximately six months of age. The speed with which the adult pro-

portions and chamber capacities are achieved is dependent upon the nature of the animals' diet. An increase in dietary roughage accelerates the development, whereas maintenance on milk or similarly constituted diets retards the development. Similarly, the development and growth of ruminal papillae are dependent upon roughage in the diet.

Gastric Groove. The *gastric groove* of the ruminant stomach is a series of mural folds that extend from the cardia through the abomasum. The gastric groove is divided into three segments by two internal orifices, the *reticulo-omasal orifice* and the *omaso-abomasal orifice*. The *reticular groove* (*reticular sulcus, esophageal sulcus*) extends from the cardia to the reticulo-omasal orifice; the *omasal groove* extends along the floor of the omasum from the reticulo-omasal orifice to the omasoabomasal orifice; the *abomasal groove* continues the gastric groove into the abomasum.

The reticular groove is a direct connection between the esophagus and omasum that permits the direct passage of milk in a suckling calf to bypass the rumen and reticulum and be deposited at the reticulo-omasal orifice. The reflex closure of the reticular groove and opening of the reticulo-omasal orifice and omasal groove direct milk into the abomasum. Sucking, swallowing and the chemical constituents of milk are contributory influences upon the reflex.

The lamina epithelialis and lamina propria of the reticular sulcus are similar to other portions of the forestomach. The lamina muscularis mucosae of the reticular sulcus is continuous with the same layer in the esophagus, and is especially prominent along the margins of the sulcus. The lamina propria blends insensibly with the tunica submucosa between the incomplete muscle bundles of the lamina muscularis mucosae. The tunica muscularis consists of smooth and skeletal muscle fibers. The outer longitudinally-oriented skeletal muscle is continuous with the esophageal musculature and forms the floor of the sulcus. The continuity of esophageal musculature through the reticular sulcus to its termination at the reticulo-omasal orifice insures a coordination of activity that permits the delivery of milk to the abomasum. The reflex closure of the reticular sulcus generally diminishes with age.

Motility of the Compound Stomach. Motility of the forestomach is essential to accomplish three primary functions: mixing, regurgitation and eructation. As a functional unit, the forestomach may be considered to consist of two chambers—rumen-reticulum and omasum. The neuronal regulation of their movements is achieved through control centers in the medulla oblongata. The general visceral efferent fibers of the vagus nerve are stimulatory, whereas those of the sympathetic nerves are inhibitory. Also, general visceral afferent information from stretch receptors within the forestomach modulates the activity of medullary control cells.

The *mixing contractions* of the rumen-reticulum are divided into two distinct groups—A-wave and B-wave. The *A-wave* (*primary wave, backward-moving wave*) originates in the reticulum, moves caudad over the dorsal sac through the caudodorsal blind sac, spreads over the ventral sac and terminates in the caudoventral blind sac. Ingesta is propelled caudad by the A-wave contractions. The *B-wave* (*secondary wave, forward-moving wave*) originates in the caudoventral blind sac, spreads over the dorsal rumen and terminates in the ventral sac. B-wave contractions occur independently of reticular contractions.

Regurgitation contractions, although involuntary, may be regulated and suppressed by the activity of conscious centers. Reticular contractions force coarse ruminal ingesta to the cardia. A-wave contractions follow the reticular activity. The transfer of ingesta from the rumen-reticulum to the esophagus is dependent upon one of three mechanisms: 1) the development of increased ruminal-reticular pressure; 2) a decrease in thoracic esophageal pressure; or, 3) a combination of both. Ruminal-reticular contractions may increase pressure within these chambers, whereas a simultaneous forced inspiratory movement with a closed glottis decreases intrathoracic pressure. An intraesophageal pressure decrease results and ingesta moves

Labels on figure: Zymogen granules, Apical border, Lumen, Exocytosis occurring, Golgi complex, Basal border, Rough endoplasmic reticulum

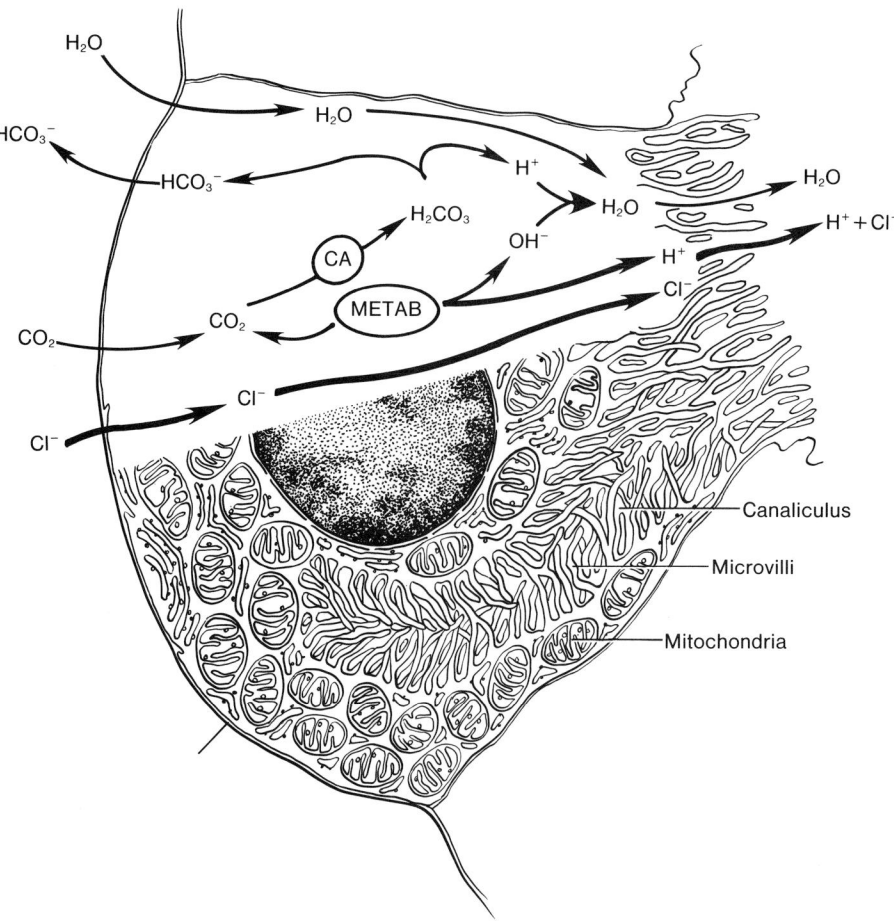

Fig. 19.42 A drawing of a parietal cell as seen with the electron microscope. The upper portion of the cell demonstrates the metabolic pathways involved in the synthesis and secretion of hydrochloric acid. Carbon dioxide (CO_2) diffuses into the cell as well as being one of the products of metabolism (*metab*). Carbon dioxide is hydrated to carbonic acid (H_2CO_3) under the influence of carbonic anhydrase (CA). Carbonic acid dissociates into hydrogen ion (H^+) and bicarbonate (HCO_3^-). Bicarbonate diffuses into the interstitium. Chloride ion diffuses into the cell, is coupled with H^+ and is transported actively into the lumen of the gland as hydrochloric acid (See Gastric Acid Secretion).

into the esophagus. Reverse peristalsis propels the ingesta to the buccal cavity where it is remasticated and eventually reswallowed. Regurgitation permits more thorough processing of the ingesta.

Eructation contractions permit the expulsion of gas from the rumen. Contraction waves initiated in the dorsal sac of the rumen move craniad and ventrad into the reticulum. Relaxation of the esophageal musculature permits the gas to pass into the pharynx and into the lungs from whence it is expired during normal exhalation. As much as 50 liters of gas/hour can be produced in the bovine rumen during fermentation processes. Eructation is essential to prevent the accumulation of the gases. Abnormally large accumulation of gas (*bloat*) within the rumen can result in death.

Fermentation, Synthesis and Absorption.
The ruminant forestomach is a remarkable complex of organs that is capable of massive fermentation through its population of bacteria and protozoa. The fermentative processes within the rumen and reticulum permit the degradation of cellulose and the subsequent enzymatic digestion of it and

other forestomach constituents within the abomasum. Thus, the ruminant is capable of converting plant materials into animal products.

The relationship between the ruminant and the population of microbes in the fermentation vat is dependent upon their mutual cooperation (*synergism*). The ruminant supplies the ideal anaerobic environment (temperature, pH) and food supply, whereas the microbes degrade plant materials (cellulose), produce volatile fatty acids, synthesize microbial proteins and produce B vitamins.

The anaerobic fermentation produces carbon dioxide, water, methane, lactic acid, acetic acid, butyric acid and propionic acid. These substances, regardless of the source or nature of the carbohydrate substrate, are the endproducts of carbohydrate fermentation.

The *volatile fatty acids* (*VFA*), acetic, butyric and *propionic acids*, contribute approximately 70% of the ruminant's daily energy needs. Although most of the absorption of volatile fatty acids occurs through the ruminal papillae, some of the acids are absorbed

by the reticulum and omasum. The amount and type of volatile fatty acids absorbed varies with the type of diet. The fate of the individual volatile fatty acids differs also. *Acetic acid*, which accounts for about 60% of the absorbed volatile fatty acids, is the primary source of acetyl-coenzyme A for the synthesis of lipids. Additionally, acetic acid is metabolized by adipose tissue, muscular tissue and the mammary gland. *Propionic acid*, comprising about 25% of the absorbed volatile fatty acids, is the most important source for the production of glucose (*gluconeogenesis*) within the liver. Because only minimal quantities of glucose are available to the ruminant from digestion, propionic acid is essential. *Butyric acid*, which comprises about 15% of the absorbed volatile fatty acids, is converted to *beta hydroxybutyric acid*, a *ketone body*, in the lamina epithelialis of the rumen. Beta-hydroxybutyric acid is metabolized in the liver. Ketone bodies (*acetoacetic acid* and *beta hydroxybutric acid*) are oxidized in skeletal muscle also. Acetone is produced from the decarboxylation of acetoacetic acid and isopropanol from the decarboxylation of the beta hydroxybutyric acid.

Proteins are an important source of amino acids for the animal organism. Those amino acids that can not be synthesized by the organism must be supplied in the diet (*essential amino acids*). Although the ruminant has essential amino acid requirements, they need not be supplied in the diet. The microbial flora are capable of metabolizing plant protein to amino acids and subsequently synthesizing microbial proteins. Similarly, the microbes are capable of converting *nonprotein nitrogen* sources to amino acids and subsequently to microbial proteins. *Urea*, a common nonprotein nitrogen source, gains access to the rumen through salivary secretions, absorption through the ruminal mucosa from the blood and dietary supplementation. The production of microbial proteins from various sources supplies the ruminant with all of the amino acids required by the animal. Microbial proteins become available to the ruminant as the microbes die and become digested.

The microbial flora also produce all of the B vitamins required by the organism. As long as cobalt is supplied in the diet, it is virtually impossible to induce a vitamin B complex dietary deficiency.

Despite the stratified squamous epithelium that lines the forestomach, extensive absorption of nutrients probably occurs in all of the chambers. Volatile fatty acids, lactic acid, ammonia, inorganic ions and water are absorbed through the ruminal lamina epithelialis. The absorption of materials from the omasum probably occurs also. Materials moving slowly through the interlaminar spaces of the omasum are probably subject to greater absorption than those that move through the chamber rapidly. Volatile fatty acids are probably absorbed by the abomasum also.

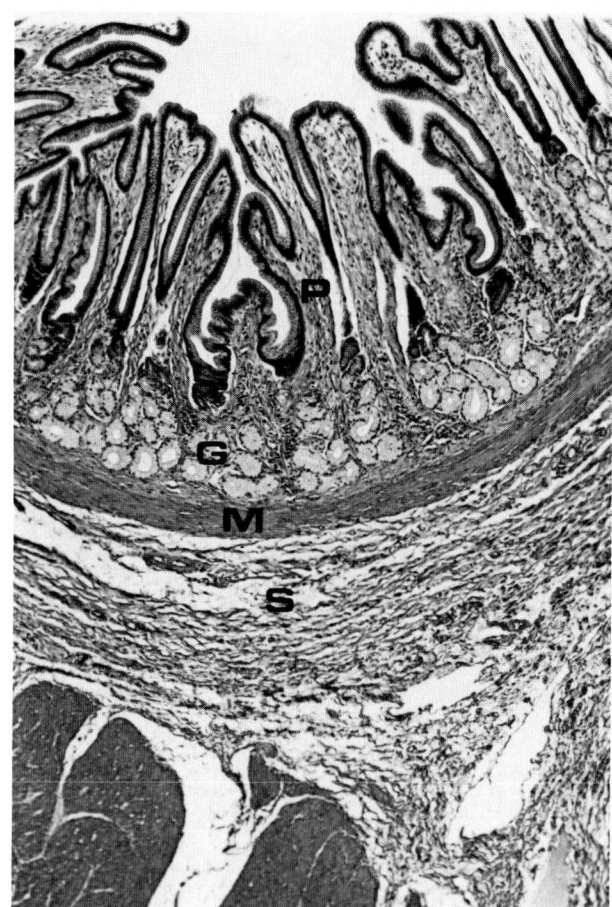

Fig. 19.43 Pyloric region of the canine stomach. The surface and gastric pits are typical. Since the tunica mucosa is not as highly folded as in other regions of the stomach, the lamina propria (P) is more visible. Pyloric glands (G) are present. The lamina muscularis (M) and tunica submucosa are typical (S). X16.

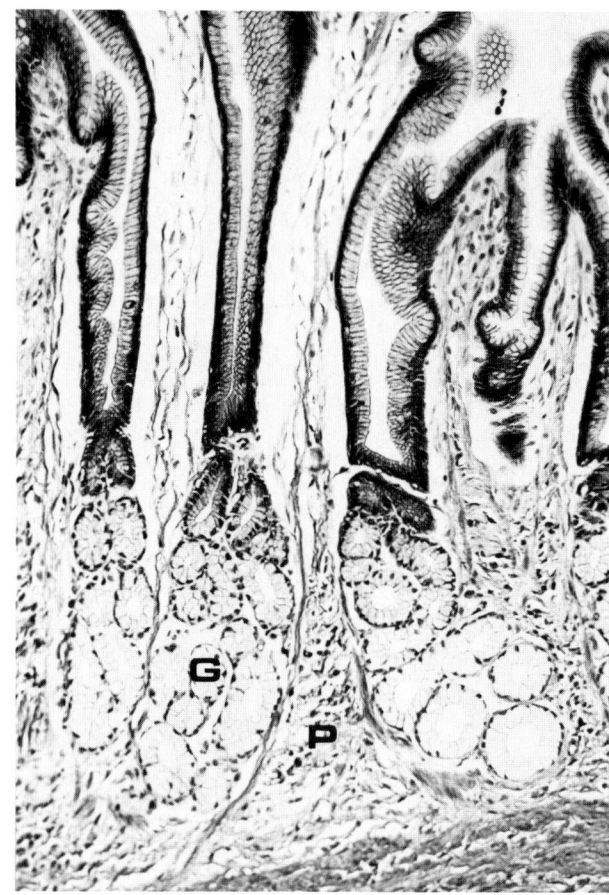

Fig. 19.44 Pyloric glands of the canine stomach. The lining of the gastric pits is continuous with the lining of the pyloric glands (G). The lamina propria (P) is extensive and typical. X40.

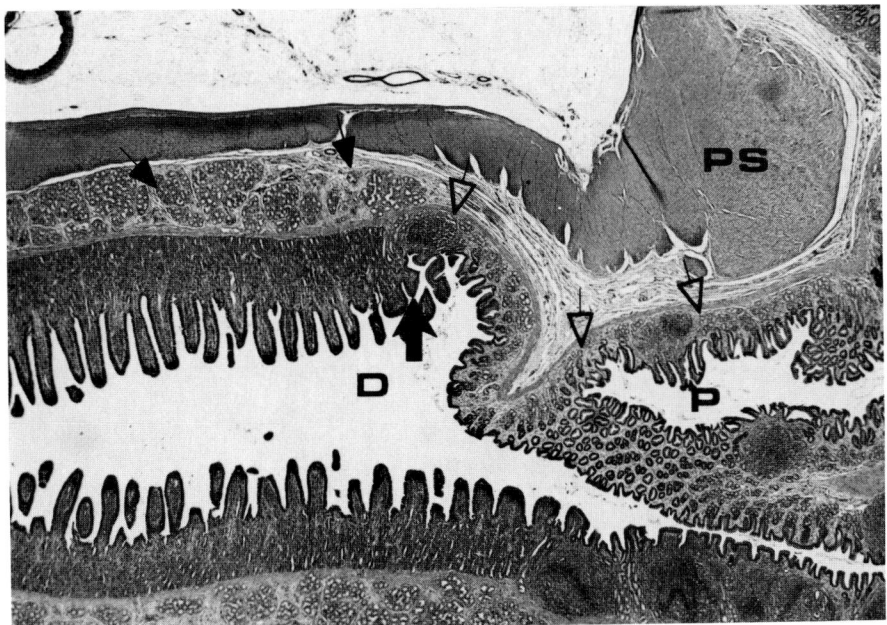

Fig. 19.45 Gastroduodenal junction (canine digestive tract). The pyloric region of the stomach (P) is continuous with the duodenum (D). The tunica muscularis is modified as the pyloric sphincter (PS). The pyloric glands (*open arrows*) are similar to the submucosal glands of the duodenum (*small solid arrows*). The latter may be the intestinal continuation of the former. *Large solid arrow*, actual point of mural reorganization. X4.

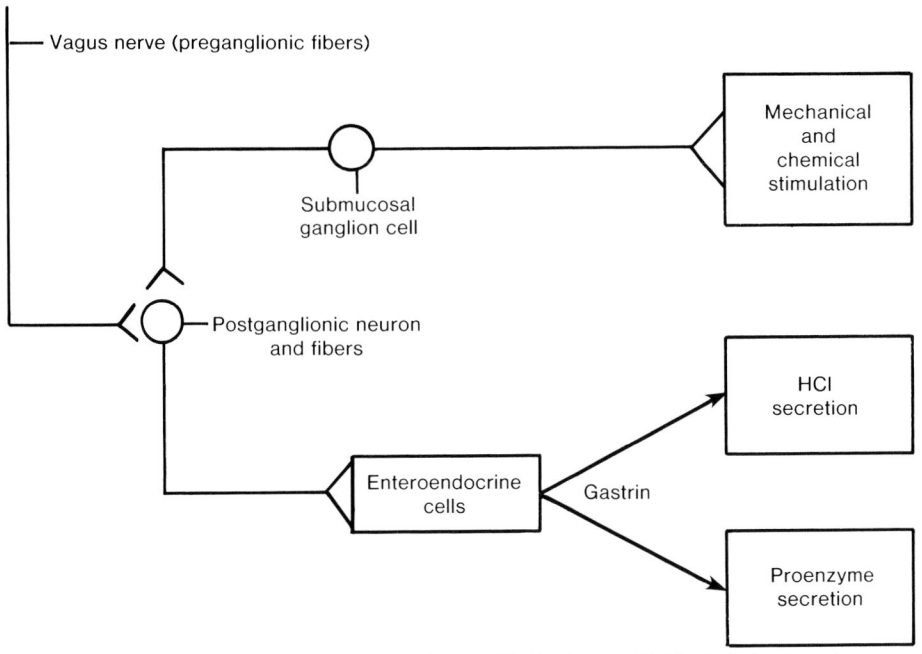

Fig. 19.46 A hypothetical scheme to explain vagal induction and intrinsic induction of gastrin secretion. The postganglionic neuron may be the final common pathway for local stimulation and/ or vagal stimulation of gastrin secretion.

Small Intestine

General Characteristics. As a continuation of the digestive tube, this region is modified highly for the secretion and absorption of materials. It has numerous modifications to increase the absorptive and secretory surface: *length, plicae, villi* and *microvilli.* Although there are distinctive features of the various regions of the intestine, these regions share many features in common. The com-

mon features will be discussed and then the distinctive features of the specific regions of the intestine will be presented.

At the gastroduodenal junction there is an abrupt change in the character of the mucous membrane. Gastric pits are replaced by finger-like projections, the *villi* of the mucous membrane (Fig. 19.53). Permanent folds, *plicae circulares* (*valves of Kerkring*) are present and have villi projecting from them. These folds also contain portions of

the tunica submucosa. At the base of the villi are openings to the *crypts of Lieberkuhn.*

Histologic Organization

Mucosa. The lamina epithelialis consists of three types of cells: *lining cells, goblet cells* and *enterochromaffin cells.*

The *lining cells* are typical columnar epithelial cells. The apical border has numerous microvilli arranged in an orderly array as a *striated border.* The finely granular, acidophilic cytoplasm contains the basally displaced, elongated nucleus. These cells are actively engaged in the absorptive process.

The *goblet cells* are typical (Plate I.12). They tend to increase in frequency toward the rectum. Their secretory product protects the lining. In the lower intestine, the mucoid layer facilitates the movement of the luminal contents toward the anus.

The *enterochromaffin cells* are typical and have been described with the stomach.

The crypts of Lieberkuhn open at the base of the villi. They are simple, branched tubular invaginations. The epithelium contains *columnar lining cells, goblet cells, argentaffin cells* and *Paneth cells.*

Paneth cells are specialized pyramidal cells of the intestine (Fig. 19.54) that contain supranuclear acidophilic granules and have a basally-displaced nucleus. The basal portion of the cell is basophilic. Paneth cells are present in ruminants, equids and man but are absent in the other domestic species. Although the Paneth cells have many of the characteristics of protein or enzyme-secreting cells that suggest a digestive function, no evidence supports this supposition. The bacteriocidal enzymes (lysozyme) that are present within the cells intimate a phagocytic function.

The lamina propria mucosae is usually described as areolar. However, the accumulation of reticular fibers, reticular cells, granulocytes and agranulocytes in this tissue has prompted some to classify it as a *reticuloareolar connective tissue.* Crypts of Lieberkuhn and lymph nodules are also present. The crypts of Lieberkuhn may occupy the bulk of this layer. The frequency of lymph nodules, however, increases caudally and may occupy the lamina propria as well as the tunica submucosa, as in the case of *Peyer's patches.*

Besides the aforementioned components, numerous lymphatic vessels (*lacteals*) are present and extend with the connective tissue into the core of the villi.

A lamina subglandularis is present in the initial part of the intestine of carnivores.

The lamina muscularis mucosae is present and typical. Strands of smooth muscle and connective tissue fibers are interdigitated between the crypts of Lieberkuhn and into the cores of the villi.

Submucosa. The tunica submucosa is present and typical. Submucosal glands are simple branched tubuloacinar glands that open into the crypts (Fig. 19.55). They may be mucous (ruminants, dog), mixed (cat) or

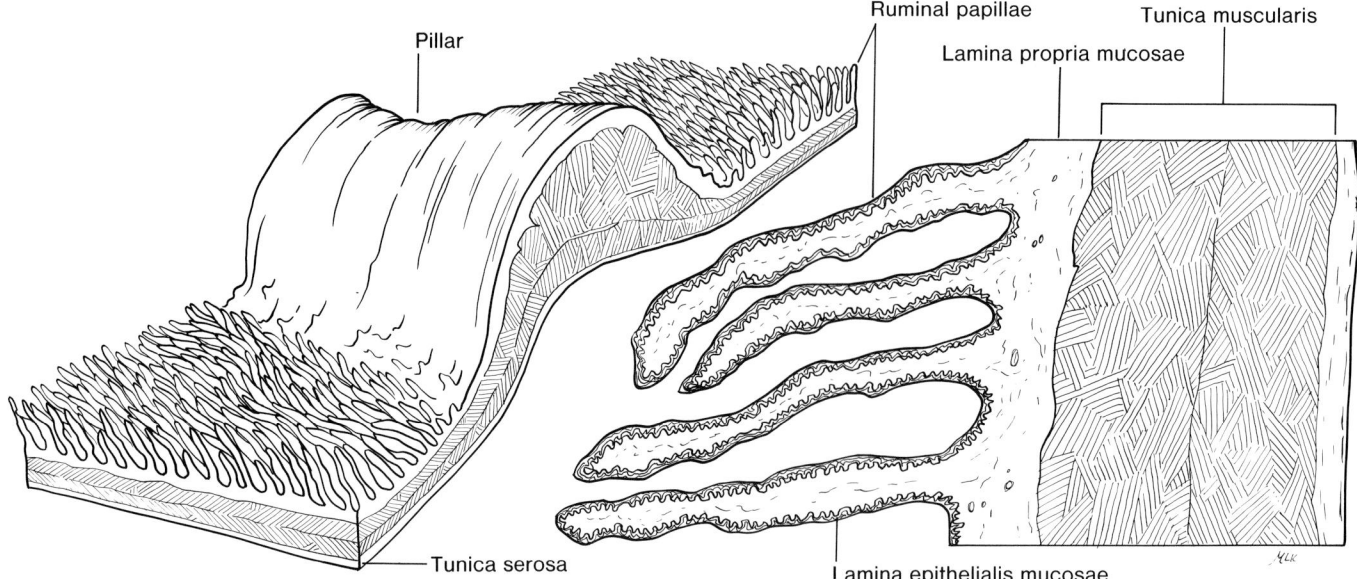

Fig. 19.47 A three-dimensional and cross-sectional drawing of the wall of the rumen. The core of connective tissue is all that is contained within the papillae.

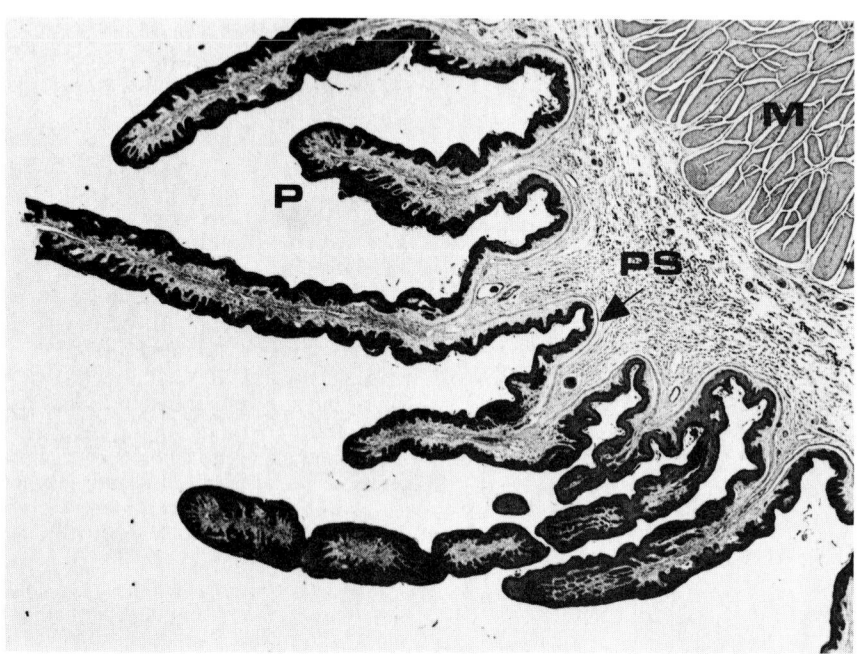

Fig. 19.48 A section of bovine rumen. Conical papillae (P) project from the luminal surface of the organ. A lamina muscularis is not present. The lamina propria-submucosa (PS) is typical and adjacent to the tunica muscularis (M). A condensation of connective tissue fibers (*arrow*) should not be mistaken for the lamina muscularis. X4.

serous (horse, pig). These glands are variously referred to as *Brunner's glands* or *duodenal glands.* They are most properly referred to as *intestinal submucosal glands.* In carnivores, man and small ruminants, they are confined to the initial or middle portion of the duodenum. In the horse, pig and large ruminants, they extend into the jejunum. These glands may represent a caudal continuation of pyloric glands which have been displaced to the submucosa.

Muscularis. The tunica muscularis with Auerbach's plexus is present and typical. The contraction of this smooth muscle is responsible for peristalsis.

Serosa. The tunica serosa is present and typical.

Regions of the Small Intestine

Duodenum. This is the fixed portion of the small intestine (Fig. 19.56). The tunica mucosa is highly folded with villi and plicae circulares. Crypts of Lieberkuhn are prominent. Intestinal submucosal glands are of variable occurrence. In man and small ruminants they extend from the initial to the middle portions of the duodenum. In the dog, they are confined to the initial part of the duodenum.

Lymphatic nodules may be present, but they are sparse.

Although variable, the villi tend to be regularly shaped, blunt and wide.

Jejunum. This mesenteric region of the small intestine is essentially similar to the duodenum (Fig. 19.57). Intestinal submucosal glands are confined to the initial portion of the jejunum in some species. The villi are slender, smaller and fewer in number than in the cranial portion of the small intestine (Fig. 19.58). Mucosal-submucosal lymph nodules are present, especially in the pig. The remaining mural elements are present and typical (Plates III.3, III.4).

Ileum. This region is similar to the jejunum (Fig. 19.59). There is an increasing number of goblet cells. Lymphatic tissue is very prominent in the mucosal-submucosal region. These aggregates are collectively referred to as *Peyer's patches.* These lymphatic nodules may become so prominent that they fill or even obliterate the villi. In such instances, the mucous membrane is flattened and interrupted by crypts. These areas look quite similar to tonsils and their associated crypts and are referred to as *lymph craters.* They are especially prominent in swine. Peyer's patches are located in an antimesenteric position; i.e., they are positioned opposite the point where the tunica serosa is reflected as the mesentery of the organ (Fig. 19.60).

The villi of this region are club-shaped. Plicae are no longer present. Actually, plicae are most prominent in the jejunum and diminish in size orad and aboard.

Histophysiology of the Small Intestine

Motility and Secretion. Intestinal motility functions: 1) to mix the chyme to insure that digestive enzymes contact the partially digested foodstuffs; 2) to move the chyme in

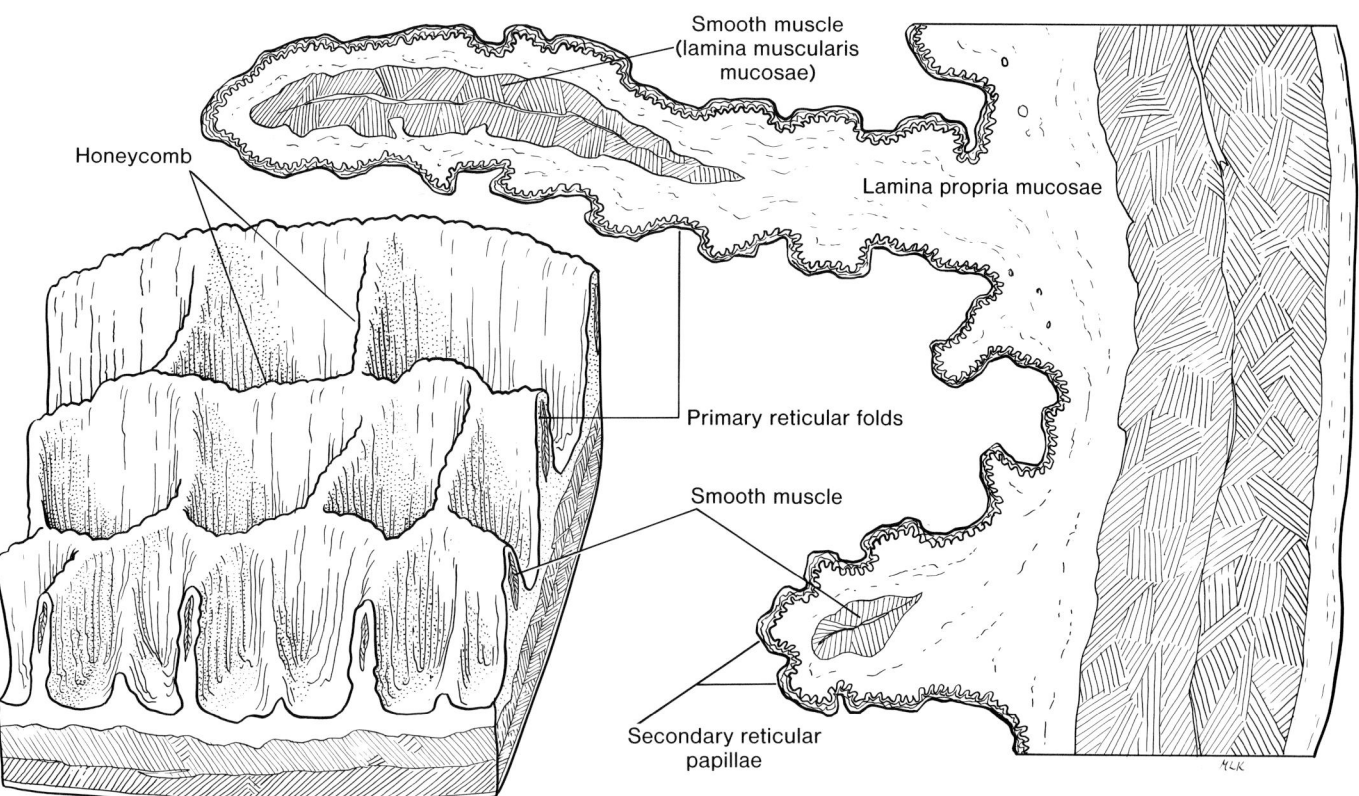

Fig. 19.49 A three-dimensional and cross-sectional diagram of the wall of the reticulum. An isolated mass of smooth muscle is located in the tip of the reticular fold.

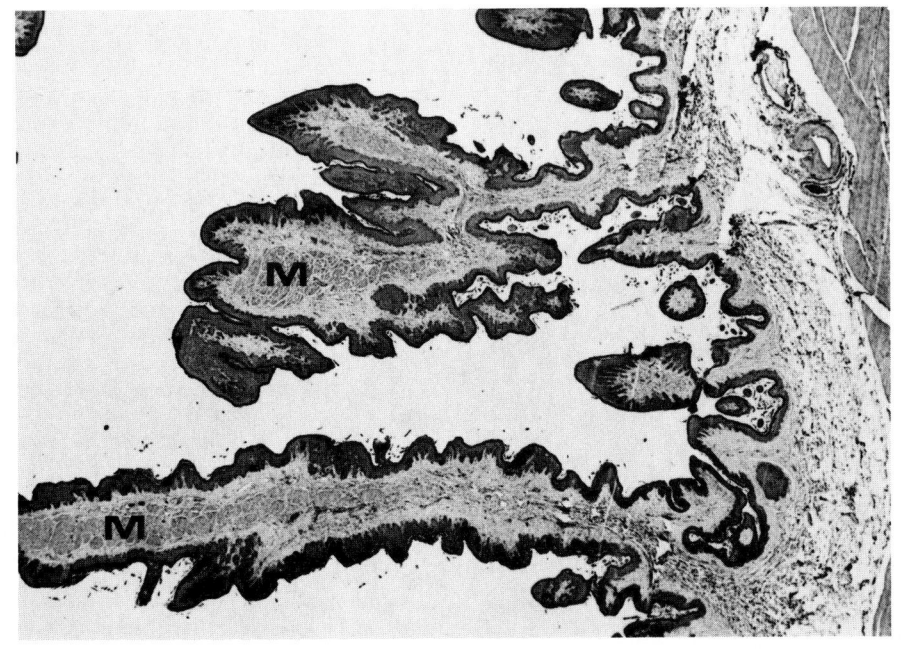

Fig. 19.50 A section of bovine reticulum. The reticulum consists of primary reticular folds from which numerous secondary and tertiary papillae project laterally. The lamina muscularis (M) is present, but it is confined to the tips of the primary reticular folds. X4.

order that it contacts all absorptive surfaces; 3) to propel the chyme through the intestine. *Segmenting contractions* are ring-like contractions that occur in the lamina interna of the tunica muscularis. Denervation does not affect these contractions; they are initiated locally in the smooth muscle. Segmenting contractions do not propel the intestinal

contents aborally but function to mix the contents to facilitate digestion and absorption. *Peristalsis (peristaltic contraction)* is a contraction which propels the contents of the lumen aborally. Peristaltic waves of contraction involve shortening of the segments (longitudinal layer) followed by ring-like contractions of the circular layer. Although

peristaltic contractions occur independently of extrinsic innervation, the intrinsic nerve supply (submucosal and myenteric plexuses) must be intact. Bipolar neurons of the submucosal plexus have one process in the mucosa, whereas the other process synapses with neurons in the myenteric plexus. Contractions of the smooth muscle respond to increased stretch of the intestinal wall. This response to stretch is called the *myenteric reflex*. Normally, peristalsis occurs slowly enough to permit absorption of materials. Rapidly propagated muscular contractions, *peristaltic rushes*, may traverse the entire intestine. The decreased transport time that results may cause a diarrhea, malabsorption or maldigestion.

The contractile activity of the intestine, similar to that of the stomach, is regulated by a pacemaker center in the longitudinal muscle of the duodenum close to the opening of the bile duct. The *slow waves* proceed aborad, pass to the inner lamina of circular smooth muscle and continue aborad as a ring of contractions. Segmenting and peristaltic contractions may occur in conjunction with slow wave contractions.

The extrinsic nerve supply influences the strength and frequency of intrinsic intestinal contraction. Vagal stimulation augments intestinal smooth muscle activity, whereas sympathetic stimulation decreases or completely inhibits it. Sensory stimulation of various regions may result in the inhibition of the intestine. Intestinal motility may cease when any part of the intestine is distended (*intestino-intestinal inhibitory reflex*).

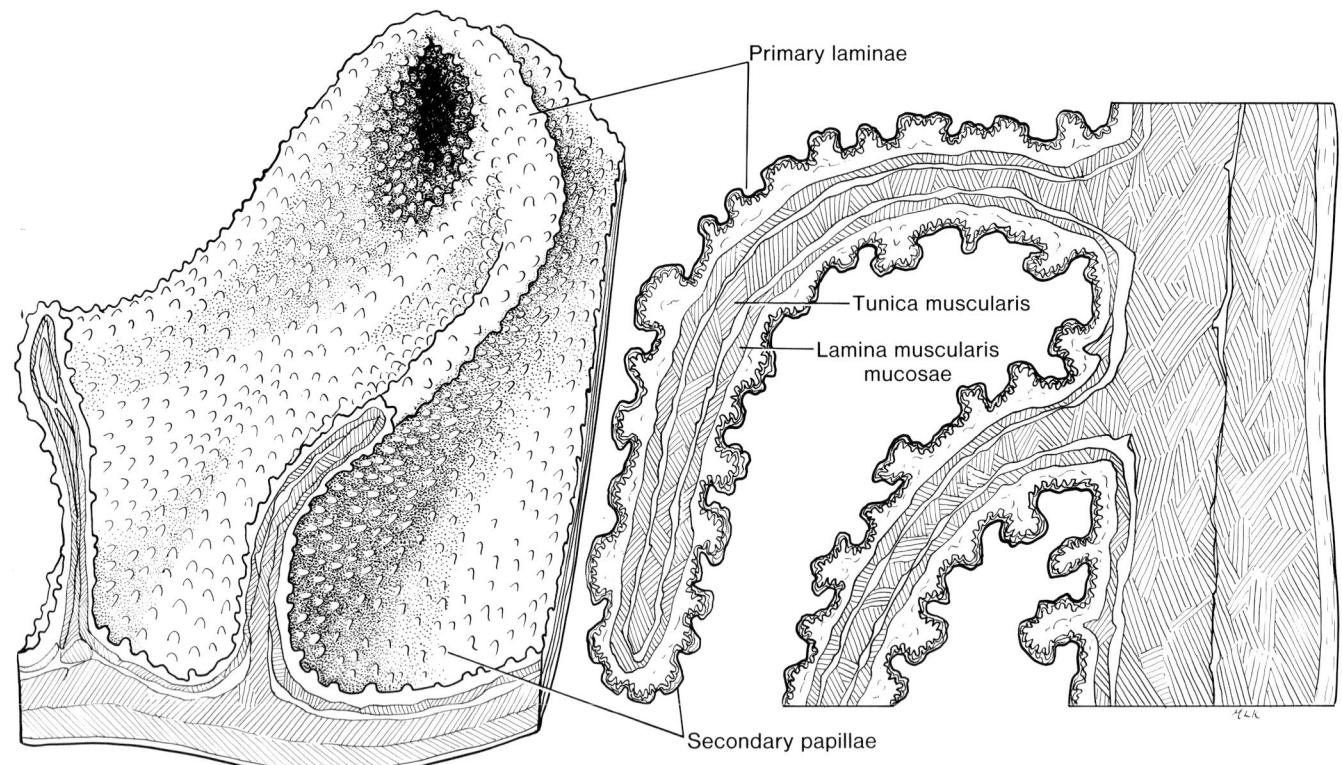

Fig. 19.51   A three-dimensional and cross-sectional drawing of the wall of the omasum. Note that the core of the laminae contains elements of the lamina muscularis mucosae and tunica muscularis.

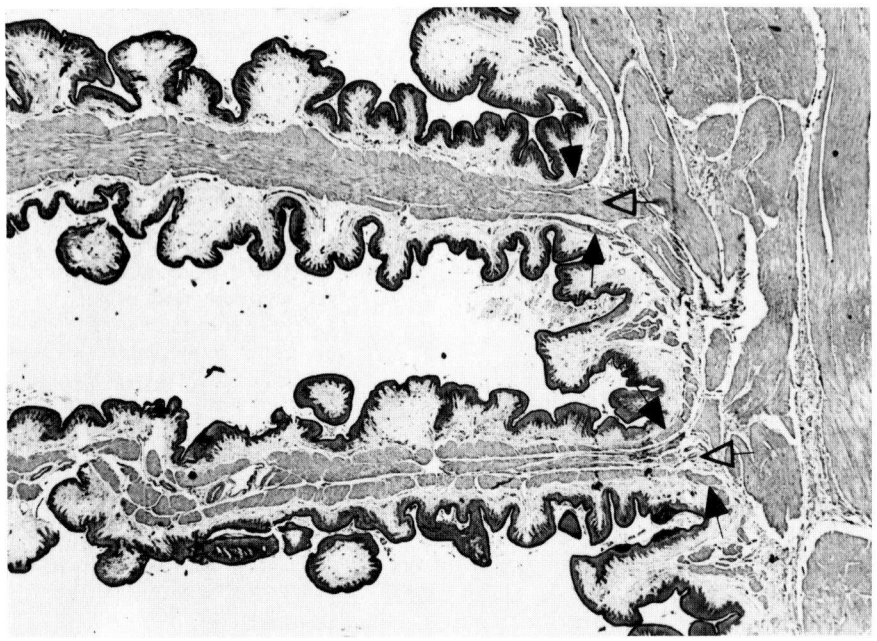

Fig. 19.52   A section of bovine omasum. The omasum has numerous laminae from which smaller papillae project. Three layers of smooth muscle occur in the laminae. The two peripheral layers are those of the lamina muscularis (*solid arrows*). The central layer is continuous with the smooth muscle of the tunica muscularis (*open arrows*). X4.

are responsible for this activity. Intestinal juice contains water, electrolytes, mucins, secretory IgA and enzymes. Many of the enzymes, intracellular in origin, become components of intestinal juice after the disintegration of cells that have been shed into the lumen. Localized mechanical and chemical stimulants are an effective means of increasing intestinal secretion. Neuronal and humoral stimulation occurs also. The precise mechanisms by which this is achieved have not been elucidated. Secretin may stimulate intestinal submucosal glands, whereas a substance contained within an extract of canine small intestine, *enterocrinin*, may stimulate the secretion of intestinal juice.

Pancreatic juice and bile, which are secreted into the cranial portions of the duodenum, are discussed subsequently in this chapter.

Digestion and Absorption. The complete digestion of foodstuffs and their subsequent absorption into the body are essential functions of the small intestine. Many enzymes, including those from disintegrated cells from the lamina epithelialis and those from the pancreas, become components of the luminal contents and contribute to digestive processes. However, some of the enzymes, which are integral components of digestion, are not secreted into the intestinal lumen but remain integral components of the plasma membrane of the striated border of intestinal lining cells. The striated border not only accounts for an increased absorptive surface but contains some of the en-

Similarly, trauma, peritonitis, obstruction and surgery can result in the inhibition of the intestine. Stimulation of the intestine occurs when food enters the stomach or when chyme enters the intestine (*gastrointestinal excitatory reflex*).

Gastrin and cholecystokinin-pancreo- zymin stimulate intestinal motility, whereas secretin inhibits it.

The proximal portion of the small intestine secretes large quantities of intestinal juice. The goblet cells of the small intestine, the lining cells of intestinal submucosal glands and the cells of the intestinal crypts

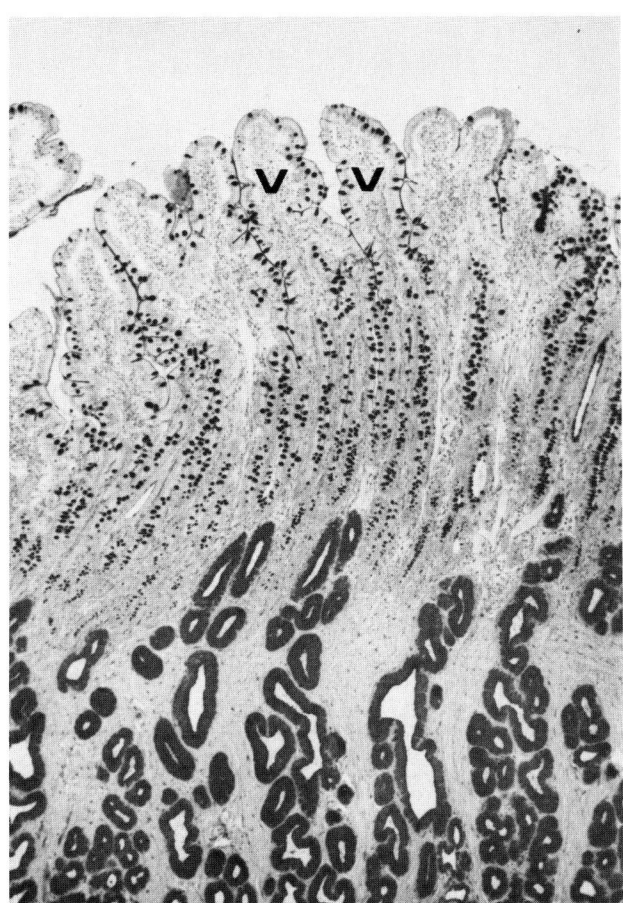

Fig. 19.53 Intestinal villi of the canine duodenum. The villi (V) project from the luminal surface of the organ. The dark-staining cells along the apices and lateral margins of the villi are goblet cells. Submucosal glands (*lower portion of micrograph*) also stain darkly. X16 (Alcian blue-periodic acid-Schiff).

zymes that are necessary for the complete digestion of nutrients before absorption. *Sucrase, maltase, lactase* and *aminopeptidase* are some of the digestive enzymes which are components of the plasmalemma.

Monosaccharides result from the enzymatic degradation of polysaccharides. The absorption of monosaccharides is by a *facilitated diffusion* in which a monosaccharide and sodium are linked to a carrier compound within the cell membrane. The entry of the monosaccharide does not require an expenditure of energy, but the sodium is subsequently transported out of the cell actively.

The digestion of *proteins* and the absorption of *amino acids* occurs in a manner similar to that described for carbohydrates. Proteins and peptides are digested by gastric enzymes, pancreatic enzymes and hydrochloric acid. *Aminopeptidases*, as plasmalemmal components, split amino acids from the peptides attached to the striated border. Amino acids and sodium are absorbed by the cell in a manner similar to that described for monosaccharides.

Ordinarily, proteins must be digested before absorption of them is possible. One unique exception to this generalization exists. Some animals, ruminants and horses, confer *passive immunity* upon their young exclusively through the immunoglobulins present in *colostrum*. Carnivores utilize *placental* and *colostral transfer* to confer passive immunity upon their young. The transfer of maternal immunity through the colostrum is dependent upon the intact absorption of the *immunoglobulins* by the intestinal absorptive cells. Although the mechanism of absorption is not well understood, immunoglobulins are probably subject to endocytosis and may be protected from cellular digestive processes by binding to a receptor molecule within the cell. Finally, the immunoglobulins are transported through the cells and released into the general circulation. The ability to absorb immunoglobulins diminishes rapidly in the neonatal animal.

Lipids comprise a large group of compounds that include *triglycerides, fat-soluble vitamins (vitamins A, D, E, K), cholesterol* and *phospholipids*. Triglycerides are a major form of dietary lipids; their digestion and absorption are summarized in Figure 19.61.

The initial digestion of dietary *neutral fats* (triglycerides) is the *emulsification* of large fat droplets with bile salts. Progressive emulsification produces small fat droplets which are then subject to the enzymatic activity of *pancreatic lipase*. Pancreatic lipase selectively hydrolyzes the triglycerides into 2-monoglyceride with the release of two fatty acids. Aggregates of monoglycerides, fatty acids, and bile salts form *micelles*. The monoglycerides and fatty acids diffuse through the plasma membrane and enter the smooth endoplasmic reticulum wherein they are reconstituted into triglycerides. Small vesicles containing triglycerides are pinched off from the smooth endoplasmic reticulum and migrate directly or through the Golgi apparatus to the lateral cell margins at the level of the nucleus. The vesicles fuse with the lateral plasma membrane and the droplets enter the intercellular space. The droplets of triglycerides, *chylomicrons*, migrate to the center of the villi where they enter the lacteals and are carried to the vascular system via the abdominal and thoracic lymph channels. Fatty acids comprised of more than 16 carbons are transported to the blood via the lymph channels, whereas those with less than 16 carbon atoms enter the portal circulation directly.

The small intestine is responsible for the absorption of other nutrients also. Water, bile salts, sodium, hydrogen ion, bicarbonate ion, calcium, phosphate, chloride, sulfate and iron are absorbed throughout the small intestine generally. The duodenum, however, does not absorb bile salts, vitamin B_{12} or hydrogen ion, while the ileum does not absorb sulfates.

Renewal, Replacement and Repair. Careful histologic evaluation of the cells that cover the intestinal villi and line the intestinal crypts reveals that the lining cells of the crypts are less differentiated than the lining cells of the villi. The striated border is better developed and the microvilli are longer toward the apex of the villi than at the base of the crypts. Moreover, numerous mitotic figures are present deep in the crypts. These facts, coupled with the evidence obtained from labeled thymidine studies, demonstrate unequivocally that the lining cells of the villi arise from cells deep in the crypts. Stem cells within the crypts divide, differentiate and migrate toward the tips of the villi from whence they are shed into the intestinal lumen. Lining cells (absorptive cells) of the villi, goblet cells and paneth cells differentiate from the primitive stem cells. Only the Paneth cells do not migrate onto the villi. Most of the intestinal epithelial cells are replaced approximately every 3 days.

The repair of the small intestine is similar to that described for the stomach.

Large Intestine

General Characteristics. The large intestine is the caudal extension of the alimentary canal. It begins at the ileocecal junction and terminates at the anus. The classic anatomic divisions include the cecum, colon, rectum and anus. Significant structural modifications characterize the cecum and colon among domestic species. The cecum is a small structure in carnivores but is a large fermentation vat in horses, those herbivores

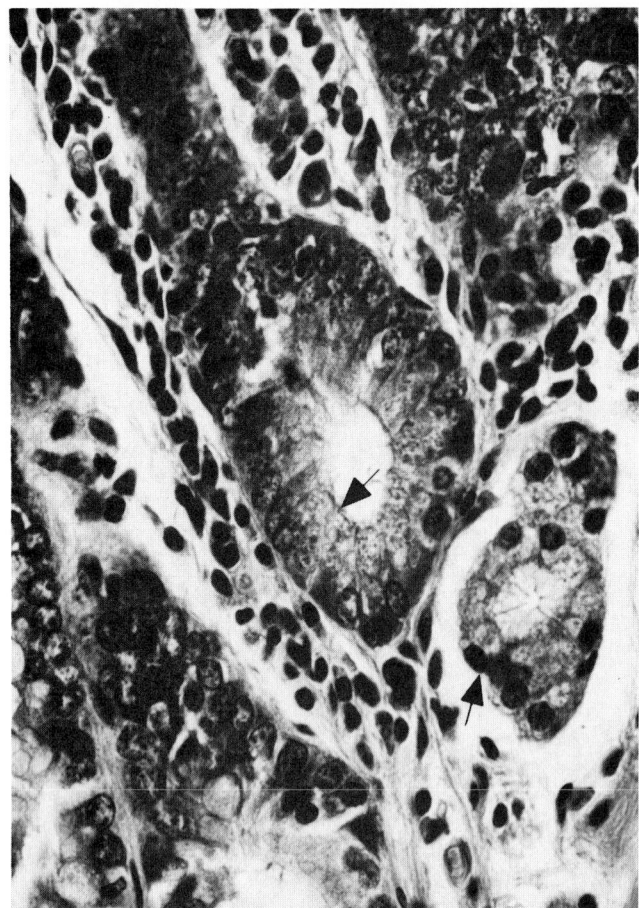

Fig. 19.54 Paneth cells of the intestinal crypts of an equine duodenum. The cells are pyramidal-shaped entities (*arrows*) with apical granules X160.

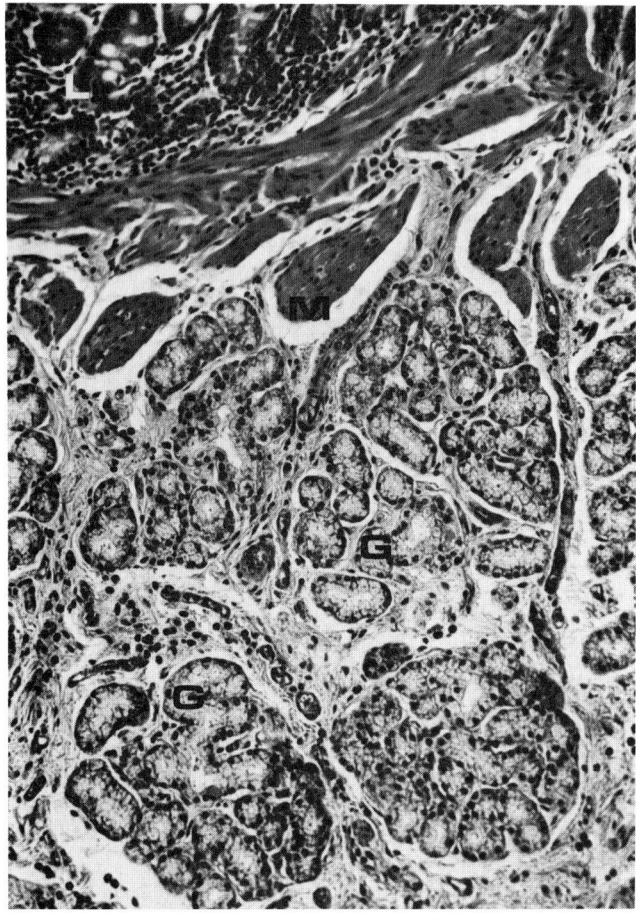

Fig. 19.55 Submucosal glands of the equine duodenum. The submucosal glands (G) are located peripheral to the tunica mucosa. The glands, however, are continuous with the intestinal crypts. L, lamina epithelialis; M, lamina muscularis. X40.

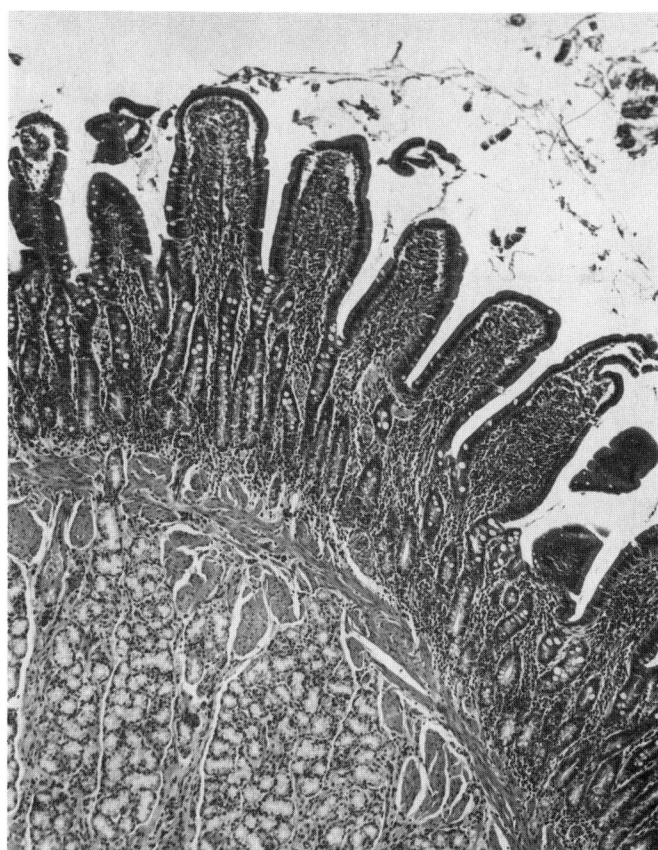

Fig. 19.56 Equine duodenum. The villi are blunt and wide. Submucosal glands are present. X16.

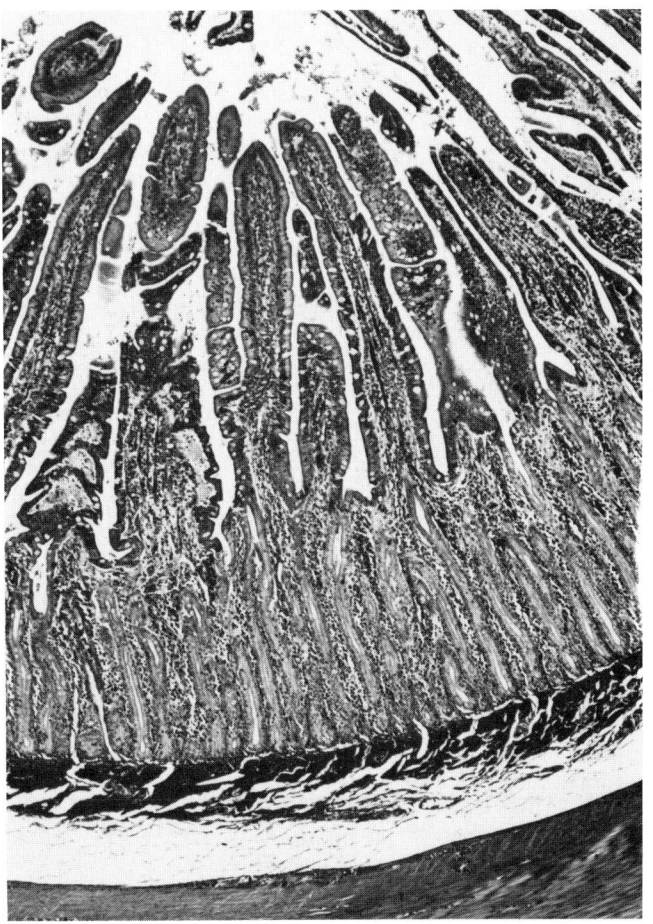

Fig. 19.57 Jejunum of a bushbaby. The villi are long and slender. X16.

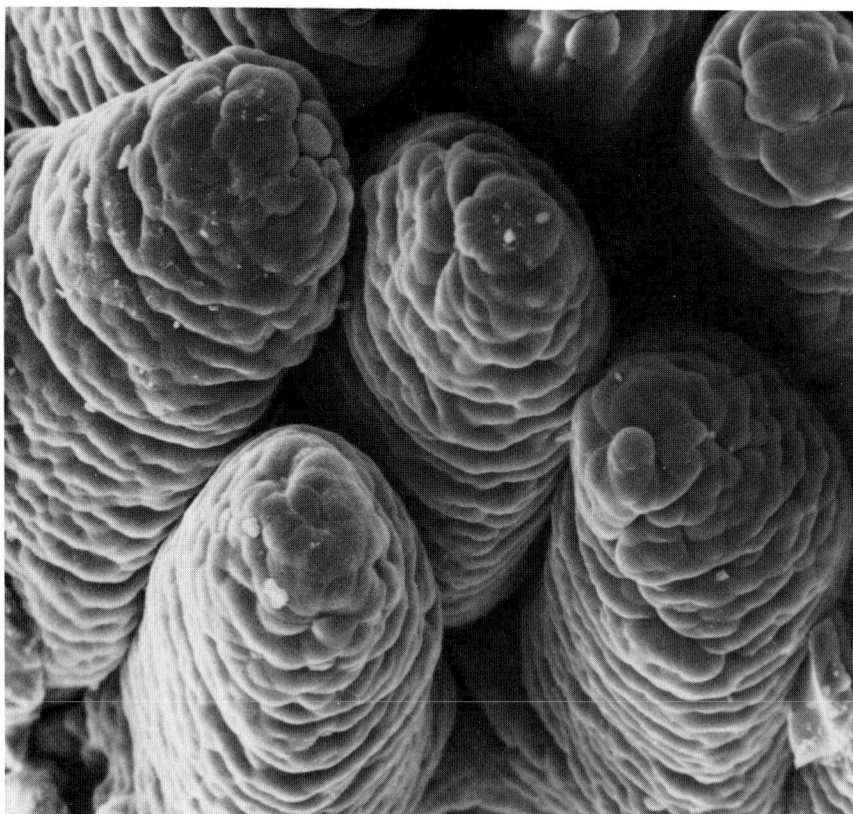

Fig. 19.58 A scanning electron micrograph of the villi from the jejunum of a young mouse. Compare with Figure 13.8. (Courtesy of D. L. Eisenbrandt).

with a simple stomach. Anatomic subdivisions of the colon are identified on the basis of their relative positions and relationship to the animal body. The *ascending, transverse* and *descending colon* form a U-shaped configuration in most mammals. The ascending colon of the horse is a large structure characterized by specific flexures and segments that connects the voluminous cecum to the small transverse colon. The ascending colon of ruminants and swine forms a complex spiral loop (ansa spiralis). Despite the numerous gross anatomic modifications of the large intestine, specific regions of the organ are difficult to identify based upon histologic uniqueness.

Histologic Organization. The organization of the mural elements of the large intestine conforms to the pattern described for the small intestine. Specific features occur in all regions of the large intestine that distinguish it from the small intestine: villi are absent; intestinal crypts, which are elongated and straight, open to the surface at the luminal margin; goblet cells are a conspicuous feature of the lamina epithelialis, although Paneth cells are absent; the plicae circulares of the small intestine are replaced by longitudinally-oriented folds; diffuse lymphatic tissue and lymph nodules are conspicuous histologic features.

Regions of the Large Intestine

Cecum. The *cecum* is an important intestinal modification in herbivores with a simple

stomach (horse, rabbit, guinea pig). The histologic features described for the large intestine generally are applicable to the cecum (Fig. 19.62). The distribution of lymph nodules varies among domestic species. Lymph nodules may be more prominent at the opening of the cecum (ruminants, swine, dog) or may be distributed more toward the distal part of the organ (horse, cat). The remaining histologic components and tunics are similar to the small intestine. The outer layer of the tunica muscularis of the pig and horse has thickened, flat, longitudinally-oriented bands of smooth muscle and elastic fibers, *taeniae ceci*. The relatively shorter length of the taeniae compared to the rest of the cecum produces segmental sacculations called *haustra*.

Colon. The diameter of the colon is greater than that of the small intestine. The mucous membrane of the colon is smooth and conforms to the general description of the large intestine (Fig. 19.63). The other tunics conform to the general pattern, except for modifications of the tunica muscularis.

The outer layer of the tunica muscularis is thickened into flat, longitudinally-oriented bands of smooth muscle and elastic fibers, *taeniae coli*, in the pig, horse and man. Haustra are apparent. A thin layer of longitudinally-oriented smooth muscle occurs between the thickenings.

Rectum. This portion of the gut is similar to other portions of the large intestine with a few exceptions. Taeniae coli are absent,

but the tunica muscularis is thicker in this region than in the colon. The lining and glandular epithelium contains many goblet cells. Also, a tunica adventitia replaces the tunica serosa. The tunica mucosa has longitudinally oriented folds in which there is a core of erectile tissue within the lamina propria.

The remaining mural elements are present and typical.

Anus. This region of the gut, a mucocutaneous junction, is marked by a transition from columnar epithelium to stratified squamous epithelium at the *rectoanal junction* (Fig. 19.64). The lamina epithelialis is similar to the lining of the buccal cavity.

At the level of the rectoanal junction, the lamina muscularis mucosae and the outer layer of the tunica muscularis end. The inner layer of the tunica muscularis continues and terminates as the internal anal sphincter.

A tunica adventitia is present and blends insensibly with the surrounding connective tissue.

In certain species the anal glands, anal sacs and circumanal glands are associated with the anus (Chapter 18).

Histophysiology of the Large Intestine

Motility and Secretion. The motility of the colon functions in a manner similar to the movement of the small intestine. Muscular contractions facilitate the mixing of ingesta and its propulsion to the anus. *Slow wave contractions,* which originate in the intermediate region of the colon, spread toward the cecum or distal colon and account for antiperistaltic and peristaltic movement of the ingesta. *Segmenting contractions* insure the mixing of ingesta also. *Mass contractile movements,* originating from the distal segment of the colon, can evacuate the colon or propel the feces toward the anal opening over a long distance.

Colonic movements in the proximal segment of the organ can occur independently of extrinsic nerve supply. Distention of the colon is sufficient to initiate its intrinsic contraction. The entry of food into the stomach or duodenum causes a reflex contraction of the colon (*gastrocolic reflex* and *duodenocolic reflex*). The effects of vagal and sympathetic stimulation of the colon are similar to those described for the small intestine.

The distal segment of the colon, rectum and anus are more dependent upon extrinsic innervation than the proximal segment. Disruption of neuronal control can result in decreased motility and incontinence. Distention of the caudal segment of the large intestine initiates general visceral afferent impulses that are carried to the sacral segments of the spinal cord. General visceral efferent fibers, originating in the sacral spinal cord, complete the reflex that results in evacuation of the large bowel. Reflex evacuation may be inhibited by higher brain centers. The continued contraction of the colon and rectum, the relaxation of the in-

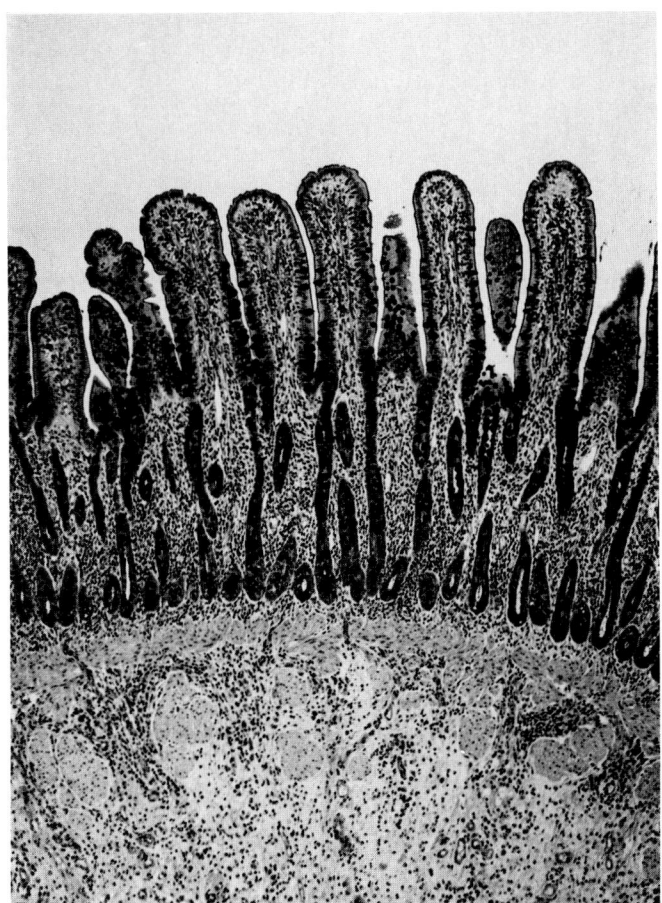

Fig. 19.59 A section of equine ileum. The villi are club-shaped. X16 (Alcian blue-periodic acid-Schiff).

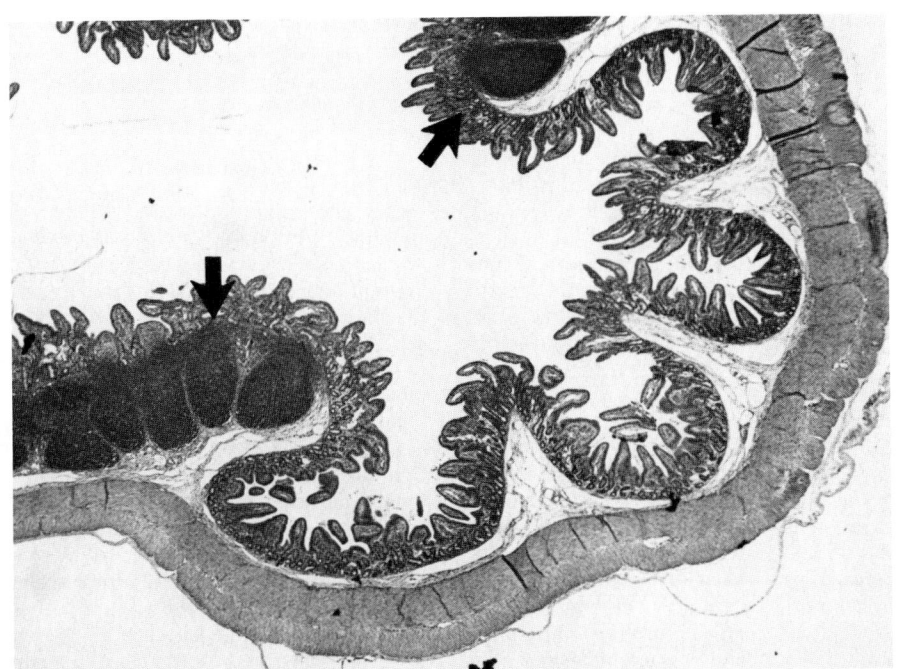

Fig. 19.60 A section of porcine ileum. Peyer's patches (*arrows*) are located in the antimesenteric portion of the ileum. The patches may be sufficiently large to obliterate the villi. X4.

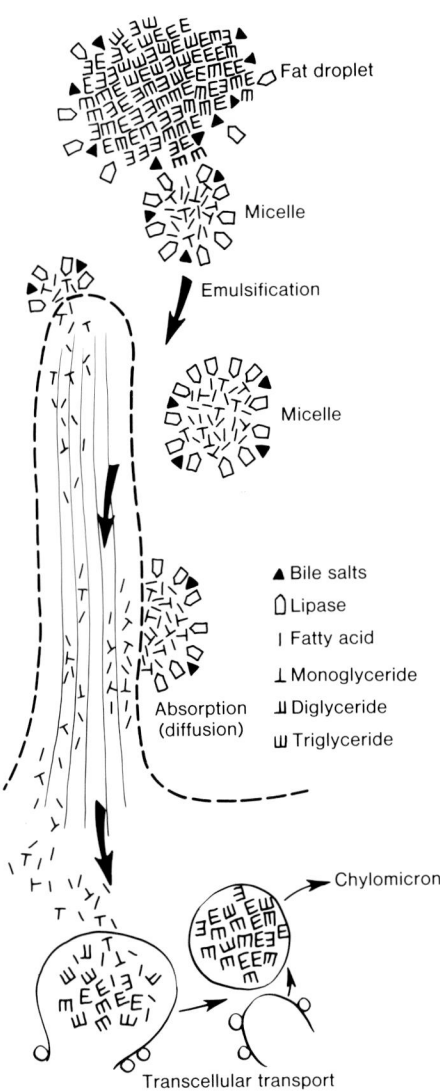

Fat droplet

Micelle

Emulsification

Micelle

▲ Bile salts

⬠ Lipase

I Fatty acid

⊥ Monoglyceride

⊔ Diglyceride

Ⅲ Triglyceride

Absorption (diffusion)

Chylomicron

Transcellular transport

Fig. 19.61 Digestion, absorption and transcellular transport of triglycerides. The emulsification and digestion of triglycerides occurs in the gut lumen under the influence of bile salts and lipase activity. Monoglycerides and fatty acids diffuse across the plasma membrane and enter the smooth endoplasmic reticulum. The monoglycerides and fatty acids are resynthesized to triglycerides within the vesicles. The vesicles are either transported through the Golgi apparatus or pass directly to the lateral cell border. The triglycerides enter the intercellular space as chylomicrons. The sequestration and subsequent resynthesis of triglycerides within the vesicles maintain a favorable diffusion gradient.

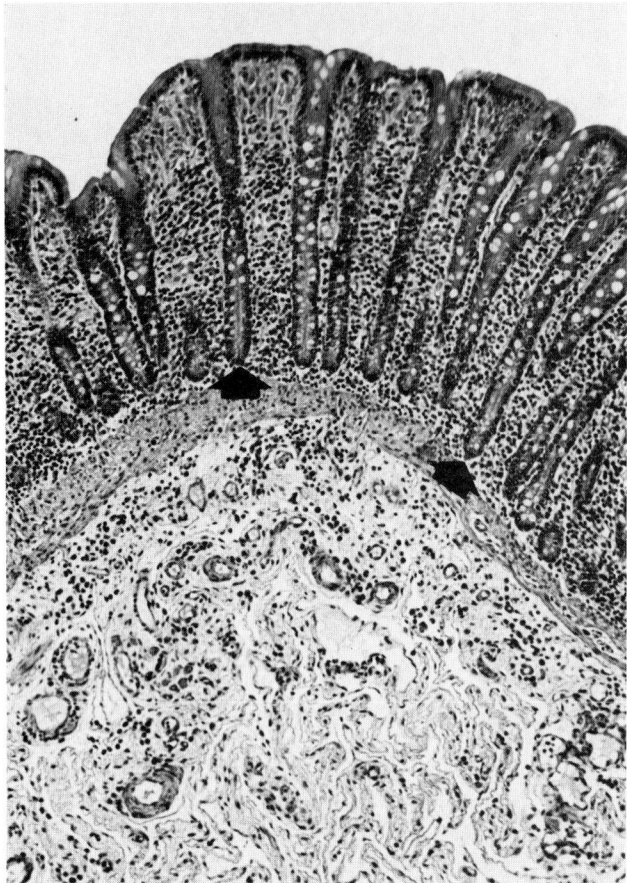

Fig. 19.62 Equine cecum. Villi are absent and intestinal crypts (*arrows*) open at the surface. X16.

ternal anal sphincter (smooth muscle) and the external anal sphincter (skeletal muscle), together with the contraction of para-anal muscles, results in defecation.

Mucus is the primary secretory product of the large intestine. The mucous secretion lubricates and facilitates the passage of feces as well as protecting the mucosa from mechanical and chemical injury. Acids produced by colonic bacteria are potentially irritating to the mucosa and are neutralized by the alkaline pH of colonic secretions. Upon appropriate stimulation, the large intestine is capable of secreting high volumes of water and electrolytes.

Synthesis and Absorption. Synthesis of various nutrients occurs to varying degrees in the large intestine of most animals and is attributed to the colonic microflora. The synthesis of vitamins B and K is especially significant. The vitamins may be absorbed by the mucosa or may be eliminated in the feces. In the latter case, *coprophagy* is a behavioral pattern that supplements daily vitamin requirements. The synthesis of many compounds is an important aspect of large intestinal digestion in nonruminant herbivores.

The large intestine absorbs water, sodium, chloride and vitamins, while adding potassium and bicarbonate; however, most of the absorption of water is accomplished by the small intestine. In man, the small intestine absorbs 20 times more water daily than the large intestine.

Digestive Function. The large intestine is a fermentation organ in nonruminant herbivores (horse, rabbit, rodents). Although the digestion and absorption of lipids, soluble sugars and proteins occurs in the glandular stomach and small intestines as it does in nonherbivorous animals, cellulose digestion and the subsequent absorption of its digestive products occur in the cecum and colon of the horse and related animals. Volatile fatty acids, produced from the anaerobic metabolism of cellulose by cecal and colonic microflora are absorbed by the large intestine. Microbial protein production and subsequent utilization by the host organism are similar to that described previously.

Renewal, Replacement and Repair. The renewal and replacement of large intestinal lining cells is similar to that described for the small intestine. Whereas dietary intake contributes to the mass of fecal material that is formed and eventually eliminated, dietary intake is not requisite for the elimination of formed feces. The passage of formed feces will occur during starvation. The exfoliated

cells of the intestinal tract contribute to this fecal volume, indicating that numerous cells are lost and replaced daily.

The repair of the large intestine is accomplished in a manner similar to that described for the small intestine. However, numerous factors diminish the healing potential. The large intestine is filled with foreign material (feces) and has a high bacterial count. The blood supply, although adequate for normal functioning, is not sufficient to insure maximal healing. Leakage from the large intestine is a common sequel to repair. That portion of the large intestine which is in the pelvic cavity is devoid of a serosal covering. As such, leakage is an especially common sequel to repair.

Intestinal Fluids

Secretory and Absorptive Balance. The absorptive load to which the gastrointestinal tract is exposed daily far exceeds just those substances that result from digestive processes. Water and electrolytes comprise a major component of the absorptive load. Oral fluids, approximately 20–30 ml/#/day in the normal dog, comprise only a fraction of the water load presented to the alimentary tract. Endogenous secretions comprise the bulk of the absorptive load presented to the intestines. They include major contributions from the salivary glands, gastric mucosa, liver, pancreas and intestinal mucosa. The normal balance requires that absorption exceeds secretion (Fig. 19.65). The less differentiated cells of the intestinal crypts, as well as goblet cells of the villi, provide most of the intestinal secretory activity. Absorption is accomplished by the differentiated and older cells which line the villi. Although large intestinal absorptive activity is critical for homeostasis, approximately 80% of the absorption of the fluid load is achieved in the small intestine, especially in the midjejunum. Disruptions in absorptive/secretory balance can cause diarrhea.

Peritoneum

The *peritoneum* is the serous membrane that lines the abdominal cavity (*parietal peritoneum*) and covers all of the abdominal visceral organs (*visceral peritoneum*). As serous membranes, these linings of the celomic space consist of two layers—mesothelium and submesothelial connective tissue. The mesothelium is typical and was described in Chapter 4. The amount of submesothelial connective tissue associated with the abdominal wall and organs is variable; it is a typical loose connective tissue with numerous blood vessels and lymphatics.

A *mesentery* is a double layer of mesothelium with intervening connective tissue that suspends organs from the abdominal wall. Mesenteries are the connections between visceral and parietal peritoneum. Some are designated by the prefix *meso-* (mesocolon,

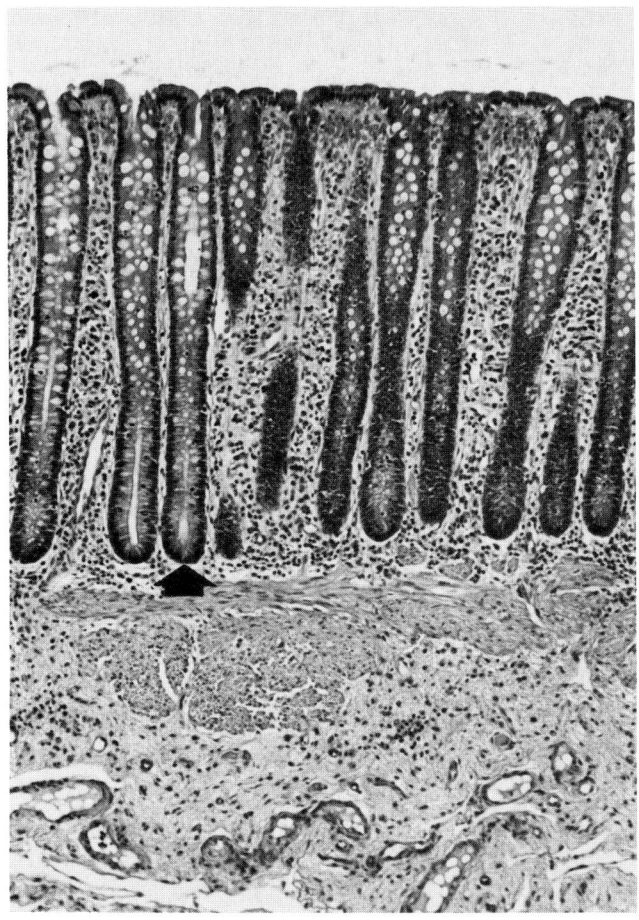

Fig. 19.63 Equine colon. Villi are absent and intestinal crypts (*arrow*) open at the surface. Compare with Figure 19.62. X16.

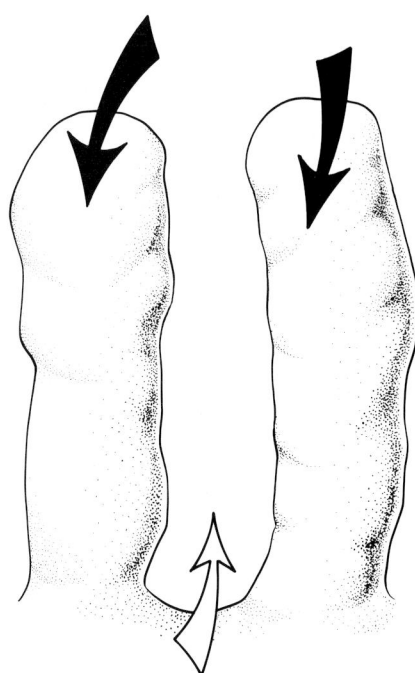

Fig. 19.65 A diagram of two villi and the intervillous space. Absorption of the fluids across the villi must exceed the secretory activity from the intestinal crypts and goblet cells in order to maintain proper fluid balance.

mesovarium, mesometrium, mesoduodenum). Specialized folds of peritoneum with few vessels are called *ligaments* (hepatogastric ligament, hepatoduodenal ligament, suspensory ligament of the ovary). They suspend organs from the abdominal wall or from other organs. Mesenteries and ligaments are special categories of *connecting peritoneum*, that serosal modification which connects organs to each other or the abdominal wall.

The *greater omentum* is a unique type of connecting peritoneum which is derived embryologically from the dorsal mesentery of the stomach (dorsal mesogastrium). Expansion and extensive growth of the dorsal mesogastrium produces the greater omentum and *omental bursa*. The greater omentum is suspended from the greater curvature of the stomach, covers the ventral aspect of the abdominal organs and is reflected upon itself to attach to the colon and pancreas. The *lesser omentum* is a connecting peritoneal modification of the ventral mesogastrium that joins the lesser curvature of the stomach and duodenum to the liver. Adipose tissue, blood vessels, nerves and lymphatics occur within the connective tissue between the enclosing layers of mesothelium of connecting peritoneum. Adipose tissue, especially prominent in the greater omentum, imparts a lacy appearance to the structure.

Peritoneal investments of abdominal organs are significant contributors to the repair process of the abdominal visceral organs. Fibrin deposition in the submesothelial and subserosal connective tissue decreases leakage after repair by sealing the

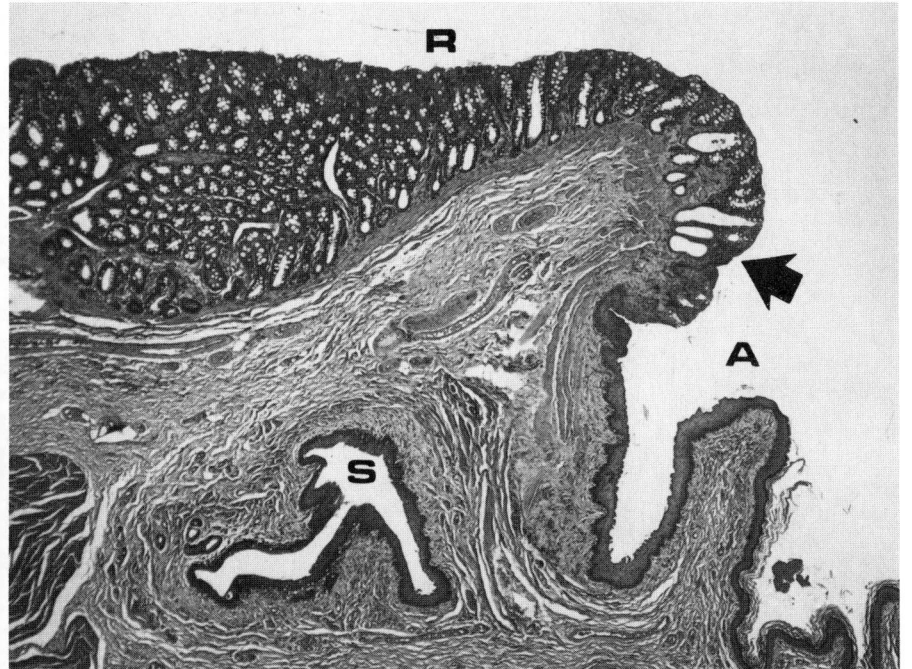

Fig. 19.64 Rectoanal junction (feline digestive tract). The columnar epithelium of the rectum (R) changes to the stratified squamous epithelium of the anus (A) at the rectoanal junction (*arrow*). An anal sac (S) is apparent in this region. X10.

wound. Excessive and/or rough handling of the peritoneum can cause fibrin deposition in focal areas. The subsequent activity of fibroblasts and the deposition of collagen in such areas are the bases for *peritoneal adhesions*.

Avian Digestive System

Regions of the Digestive System

Buccal Cavity. The buccal cavity and associated structures are quite different from those observed in mammals generally. Instead of lips and cheeks, a cornified beak is appended to the upper and lower jaw bones. The tongue is narrow, pointed, devoid of taste buds and contains a bone, the *entoglossal bone*. The anterior portion of the bone is continued by hyaline cartilage. The stratified squamous epithelium, which is variously cornified, is continuous with the mucous membrane of the buccal cavity.

Teeth are not present. However, rudimentary tooth buds are present in some birds.

Definitive salivary glands are not present. Instead, the mucosal-submucosal connective tissue of the buccal cavity is well-endowed with simple branced tubular mucous glands (Fig. 19.66). These glands are lined with extremely large cells which conform generally to the morphology of mucous cells.

Esophagus and Crop. The lamina epithelialis of these two structures is a highly cornified stratified squamous epithelium (Fig. 19.67). The lamina propria consists of areolar connective tissue which contains diffuse lymphatic tissue and some lymph nodules. The accumulation of lymphatic tissue is especially prominent caudal to the crop. The mucous membrane is arranged in longitudinal folds. The lamina muscularis mucosae consists of an undulating mass of longitudinally oriented smooth muscle. Simple branched tubuloalveolar mucous glands are present in the esophagus. The tunica submucosa, tunica muscularis, tunica adventitia and tunica serosa are present and typical.

The *ingluvies* or *crop* is an esophageal diverticulum. The lamina epithelialis of the crop is thicker than that of the esophagus. Simple branched tubuloalveolar mucous glands are present in anseriform birds, but they are absent in galliform and columbiform birds. In columbiform birds, the superficial cells of the lamina epithelialis undergo a fatty change to a substance called *crop milk*.

The enlargement of the esophagus serves to moisten foodstuffs through its mucoid secretion as well as to macerate the materials through the muscular contractions of the tunica muscularis.

The remaining tunics of the wall are similar to the esophagus.

Proventriculus. This structure is the glandular stomach of avian species (Fig. 19.68). Its mural structure conforms generally to the pattern that typifies most digestive organs. Its glands, however, are quite different from those that have been encountered thus far.

The tunica mucosa is extensively folded into flattened ridges separated by grooves or sulci. *Mucosal glands* or *rugosal glands* (simple branched tubular glands) open into the base of the sulci. Elevations in the tunica mucosa (papillae) contain the opening of the excretory duct of *submucosal glands* or *subrugosal glands* (Fig. 19.68).

The lamina epithelialis consists primarily of columnar cells. These cells extend into the sulci. The lamina epithelialis continues into the mucosal glands as a cuboidal epithelium. The nature of their secretory activity is unknown.

The lamina propria is typical and contains numerous accumulations of diffuse and nodular lymphatic tissue.

The lamina muscularis mucosae consists of an interrupted band of longitudinally oriented fibers, strands of which are interdigitated between the mucosal glands.

The tunica submucosa is typical but is seemingly displaced by the large and numerous *submucosal glands* (Fig. 19.68). These glands are compound, branched tubular glands. The adenomeres radiate 360° around a central excretory duct lined by a tall columnar epithelium which may be simple or pseudostratified. The radially oriented tubular glands are lined by secretory cells that may be cuboidal or pyramidal (Fig. 19.69). The apical portions of the secretory cells are not joined together; thus, a serrated appearance is imparted to the lining. These cells have a granular and acidophilic cytoplasm with a centrally or parabasally positioned nucleus. This is the only cell type in the gland. Because avian gastric juice is similar to the mammalian counterpart, it is assumed that this cell must secrete both zymogenic and acidic secretory products.

The tunica muscularis is slightly modified: inner longitudinal, middle circular and outer longitudinal layers are present.

The tunica serosa is typical.

Ventriculus. This portion of the digestive system, the *gizzard* or *muscular stomach*, is connected to the proventriculus by a narrow isthmus which is devoid of submucosal glands. The luminal surface of this organ is lined by a cornified secretory product that is elaborated by the mucosal glands (Fig. 19.70).

The surface lining of the tunica mucosa consists of low columnar cells with round and basally positioned nuclei (Fig. 19.71).

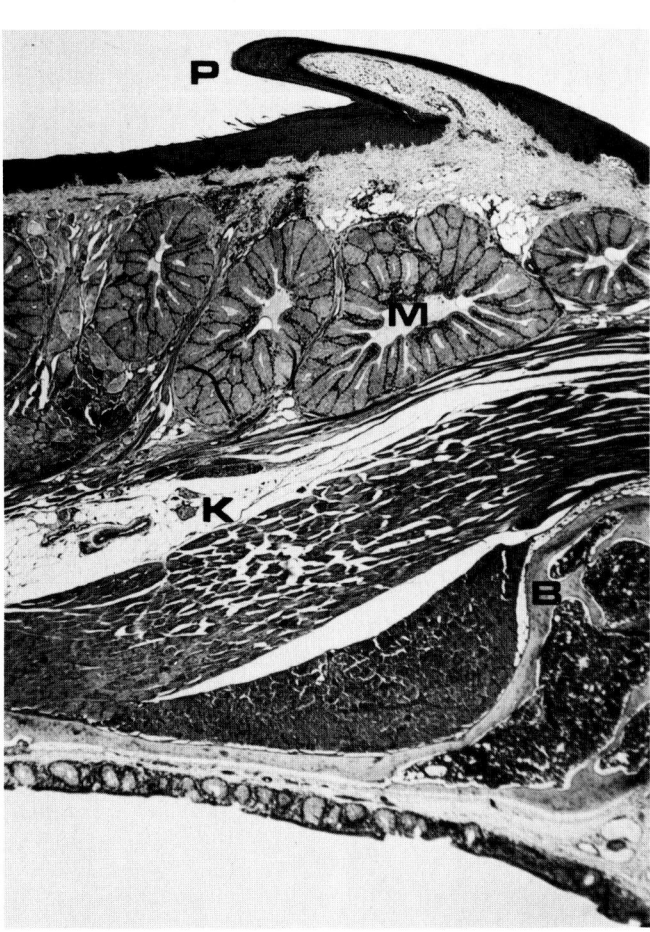

Fig. 19.66 A longitudinal section an avian tongue. A papilla (P) protrudes from the dorsal surface. The mass of the tongue consists of mucous glands (M), skeletal muscle (K) and bone (B). X10.

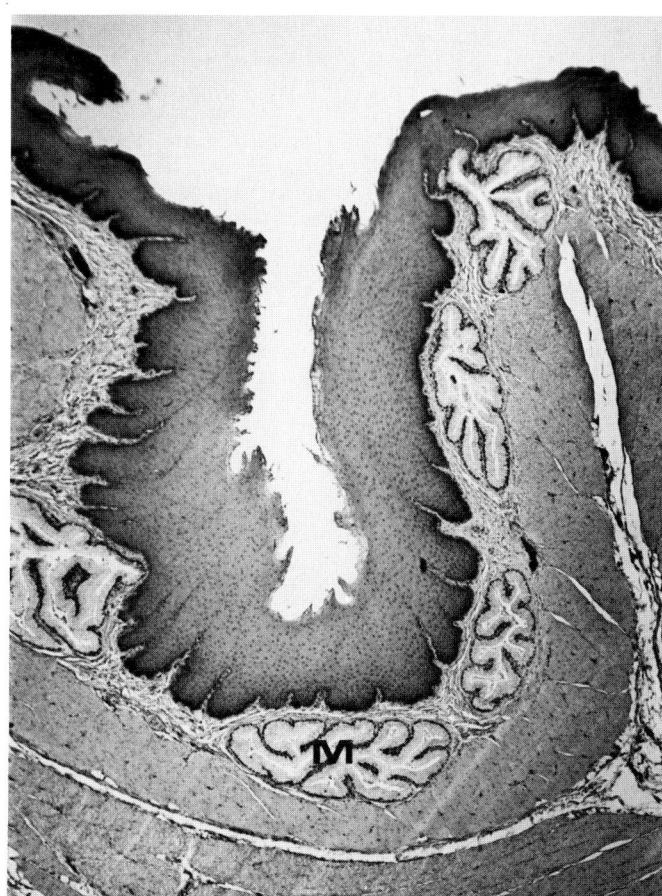

Fig. 19.67 Avian esophagus. The lamina epithelialis mucosae is stratified squamous epithelium. M, mucous glands. X10.

The surface cells continue into the glands and are replaced by a goblet-like cell. The mucosal glands are straight tubular glands.

The lamina propria-submucosa is present and typical. There is no lamina muscularis mucosae.

The tunica muscularis is present, but it is not typical. It consists of smooth muscle and DWFCT. The lateral border of the gizzard consists of regularly arranged DWFCT. From this connective tissue the smooth muscle arises and spreads throughout the muscular tunic.

The tunic serosa is present but thin.

Lower Digestive Tract. The *small intestine* is not divisible histologically into distinct regions. Except for the following exceptions, the small intestine is similar to that of mammals.

The lamina propria and tunica submucosa contain large quantities of diffuse and nodular lymphatic tissue. These may become aggregated in the caudal portion in a manner similar to that of Peyer's patches. A third layer of circular muscle may comprise the inner portion of the tunica muscularis.

The *caeca* are two blind sacs appended to the junction of the small and large intestine. Villi are present at the orifice but diminish and are lost at the end of the organ. The lamina propria and tunica submucosa contain numerous diffuse and aggregated lymphatic tissue. The accumulation of nodules at the caecal orifice is referred to as the *caecal tonsil*. The junction of this organ to the other portions of the intestne is circumscribed by a sphincter from the inner circular mass of the tunica muscularis.

Water absorption occurs in the caeca and some believe that cellulose digestion also occurs.

The *rectum* has short and thick villi and an increased number of goblet cells. Except for those differences, this area is similar to the small intestine.

The *cloaca* is the common orifice for the digestive, excretory and reproductive organs which is divisible into a *coprodaeum, urodaeum* and *proctodaeum*. It is lined by a simple columnar epithelium. The tunica mucosa is extensively folded and accounts for the compartmentalization of this structure. Lymphatic tissue is present in the associated connective tissue. The bursa of Fabricius (Chapter 14) is an evagination of the proctodaeum.

The tunica mucosa of the *anus* is highly folded and lined by a stratified squamous epithelium which is cornified. The lamina muscularis mucosae is absent and striated muscle of the tunica muscularis forms the anal sphincter.

Liver

General Characteristics. The liver, as the single largest gland of the body, accounts for 2–5% of the body weight of the organism. The ratio of liver weight to body weight is usually a constant. The liver is actually a compound tubular gland with diverse metabolic functions.

The liver is a complex organ structurally and functionally. Despite the complexity, the numerous and varied functions of the liver are accomplished by two cell types—the *hepatocyte* and the *von Kupffer cell*. Whereas other organs utilize numerous cells to satisfy varied functional demands, as well as having undifferentiated cells perform mitotic functions related to renewal and replacement, the hepatocyte retains a high mitotic potential while performing diversified functions. Hepatic functions related directly to the hepatocyte include synthesis (sugars, plasma proteins, clotting factors, lipids, urea, ketone bodies), secretion (bile salts), excretion (bile pigments), storage (lipids, vitamins, glycogen), biotransformation (toxic substances, drugs, hormones) and metabolism (lipids, proteins, carbohydrates). Hematopoiesis is a function during embryonic development, and the potential for blood cell production is retained in the adult.

The von Kupffer cell, a member of the macrophage system, lines the hepatic sinusoids and is associated intimately with the hepatocyte. The function of the cell accounts for the phagocytic activity of the liver.

The liver, although removed from the mainstream of the alimentary canal, opens to the gastrointestinal tract, and the hepatic parenchyma and ducts are derived embryologically from the endoderm of the gut lining. Although the liver is described generally as developing as a diverticulum of the gut lining, only a portion of the liver, the extrahepatic bile duct system, develops as a duodenal diverticulum. The hepatocytes develop from cells which secondarily invade the mesenchyme into which the diverticulum has advanced. The dual endodermal development accounts for the unique morphologic configuration of liver parenchyma; i.e., plates or laminae of hepatocytes interdigitated with mesenchymally-derived sinusoids are continuous with the extrahepatic bile ducts which open at the duodenum. Intrahepatic bile ducts develop secondarily from hepatocytes and eventually fuse with the extrahepatic biliary system. If the liver were to develop as a simple gut diverticulum, then the relationship of hepatocytes to ductal cells would be similar to that described for the glands of external secretion.

Histologic Organization

Connective Tissue. The disposition of connective tissue and its relationship to the

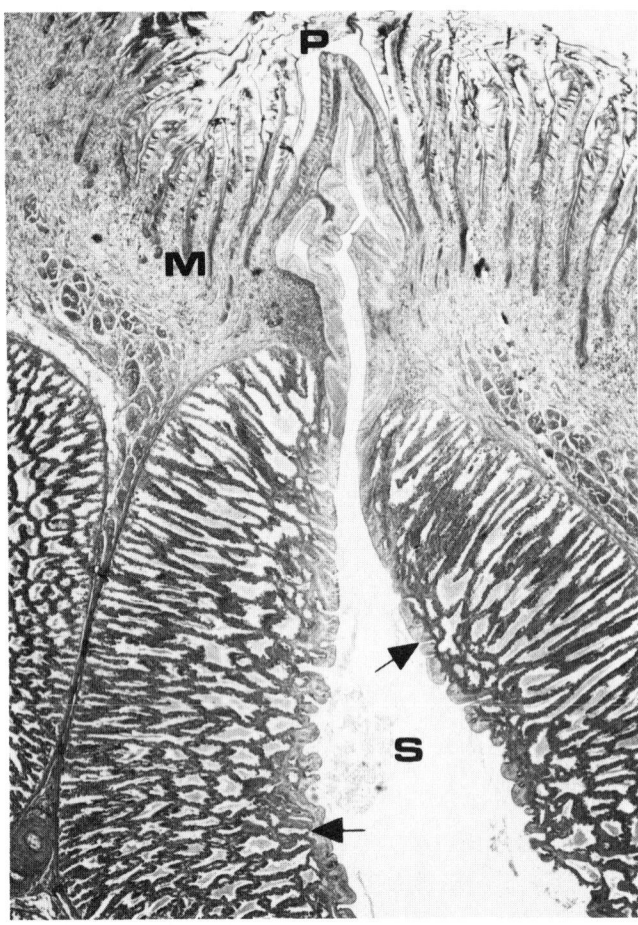

Fig. 19.68 Avian proventriculus. Mucosal glands (M) are formed by grooves or rugae on the surface of the organ. These are called rugosal glands. Submucosal glands (S) or subrugosal glands consist of adenomeres (*arrows*) which radiate from a central excretory duct. The subrugosal glands open on papillae (P) at the surface. X4.

parenchyma conforms generally to that described previously for parenchymatous organs (Chapter 13). The liver is almost completely surrounded by visceral peritoneum. The serous membrane covers the organ and is reflected over those structures—biliary duct system, arteries, veins—which exit or enter the liver. The fibrous capsule (*capsule of Glisson*), which consists of dense white fibrous connective tissue rich in elastic fibers, underlies the serous membrane (*capsula serosa*). The capsular connective tissue is continuous with the interstitial connective tissue that serves as a supportive stroma for the parenchyma. The interstitial (interlobular) connective tissue, although scant in most species, is prominent in those interlobular regions called *portal areas* and consists of a loose connective tissue; however, the lobules of the porcine liver are invested completely by loose connective tissue in such a manner that distinct lobules are evident histologically (Fig. 19.72) and grossly. Intralobular connective tissue is scant in all species. It is a reticular connective tissue confined to parts of the space of Disse.

Hepatic Lobules. *Hepatic lobules,* whether distinctly or indistinctly outlined by inter-lobular connective tissue, comprise the morphologic units of the liver. These prismatic polygonal masses of tissues are comprised of *plates* or *laminae* of hepatocytes interdigitated between anastomotic hepatic sinusoids (Fig. 19.73). The plates of cells and sinusoids appear to radiate from a centrally-positioned vessel, the *central vein* (Fig. 19.74). The concept of the hepatic lobule is based upon two simple relationships: the structural organizational pattern and the pattern of blood flow from the periphery through the sinusoids to the central vein.

Hepatocytes. The *hepatocytes,* comprising the parenchyma of the organ, are polyhedral cells the boundaries of which are usually distinct (Fig. 19.75). The vesicular nucleus contains prominent nucleoli. The centrally-positioned nucleus is surrounded by an acidophilic cytoplasm which contains basophilic material (Plate III.12). Binucleate cells may be observed. The histologic appearance of the hepatocyte depends upon the physiologic state of the organism at the time of sampling. Fasted animals have small, turbid and indistinctly outlined hepatocytes. After a feeding, the hepatocytes enlarge, become distinctly outlined and are filled with numerous glycogen and lipid inclusions, causing a foamy or honeycombed appearance.

The ultrastructural features of the hepatocyte confirm its functional multiplicity (Fig. 19.76). Numerous mitochondria are scattered throughout the cell, their shape and distribution being dependent upon the functional activity of the cell. An extensive network of clustered rough endoplasmic reticulum and free ribosomes corresponds to the basophilia of light microscopy. The smooth endoplasmic reticulum extends throughout the cytoplasm and is continuous with rough endoplasmic reticular profiles. Lysosomes, peroxisomes, lipid droplets and glycogen are present also. A prominent Golgi apparatus assumes a juxtanuclear position. The plasma membranes of the hepatocytes that are adjacent to the sinusoids have numerous, short, irregular microvilli. The cell membranes of contiguous hepatocytes have desmosomes and gap junctions. Adjacent plasma membranes of cells comprising the plates have indentations in them that are in register with each other. Small microvilli project into the indentations. The small indentations, ramifying between adjacent cells as a system of *bile canaliculi* (Fig. 19.77), are just visible with the light microscope.

Hepatic Sinusoids. The *hepatic sinusoids* are the intralobular vascular supply. Blood from interlobular vessels is transported through the sinusoids to the central veins. The sinusoids comprise a vastly anastomotic network that separates the hepatic plates from each other (Fig. 19.73). All hepatocytes have at least one surface juxtaposed to a sinusoid.

The wide lumen of the sinusoid is lined by two distinct cell types. The predominant cell is a typical *endothelial cell;* the other cell type is a phagocyte and a member of the macrophage system—*Kupffer cell.* The Kupffer cells usually reside upon the endothelial cells; however, the phagocytic cells may extend across the sinusoidal lumen or even form part of the wall of the sinusoid.

The hepatic sinusoids, which are generally devoid of a basal lamina and have numerous cellular gaps between the littoral cells, permit the free movement of materials between the plasma and hepatocytes. Despite the juxtaposition of the sinusoids to the hepatocytes, they are separated by a *perisinusoidal space (space of Disse)* which varies in width. Some cells, reticular fibers and hepatocytic microvilli occupy the perisinusoidal space (Figs. 19.76, 19.78).

Biliary System and Portal Triads. The *biliary system* of the liver consists of *bile canaliculi, intrahepatic ducts* and *extrahepatic ducts* for the conduction of bile from the hepatocytes to the duodenum (Fig. 19.79). The system of secretory cells and conducting tubules comprise the exocrine glandular components of the liver. The bile canaliculi are the smallest components of

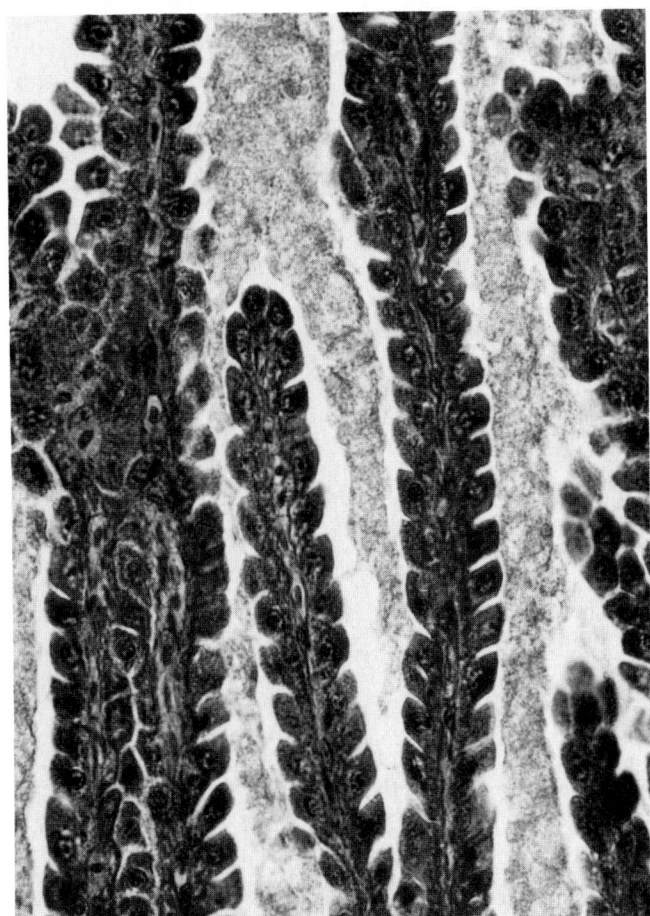

Fig. 19.69 Secretory cells of the subrugosal glands (proventriculus). The acidophilic cells are not joined at their apical surface, imparting a serrated appearance to the lining. X160.

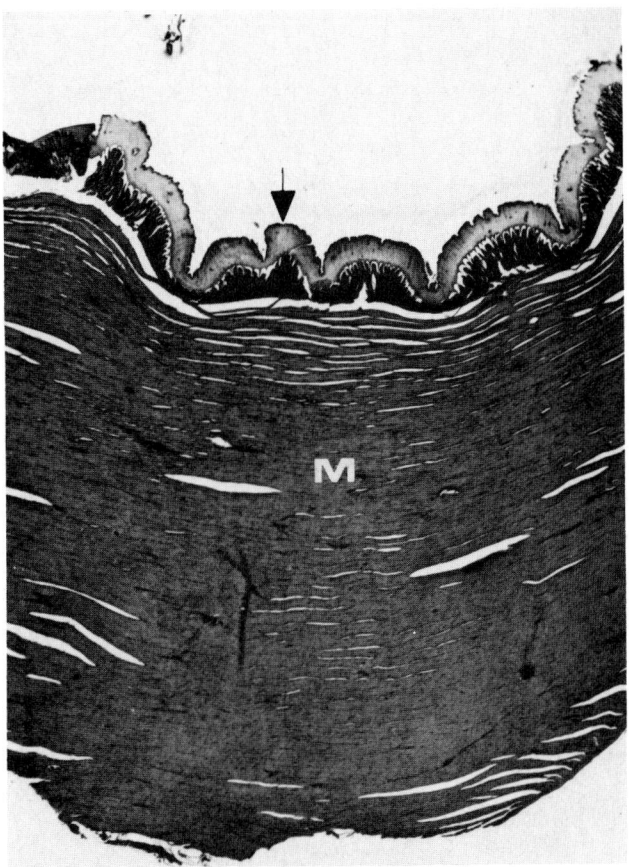

Fig. 19.70 Avian ventriculus. The lining (*arrow*) is cornified material secreted by the mucosal glands. The tunica muscularis (M) is very thick. X4.

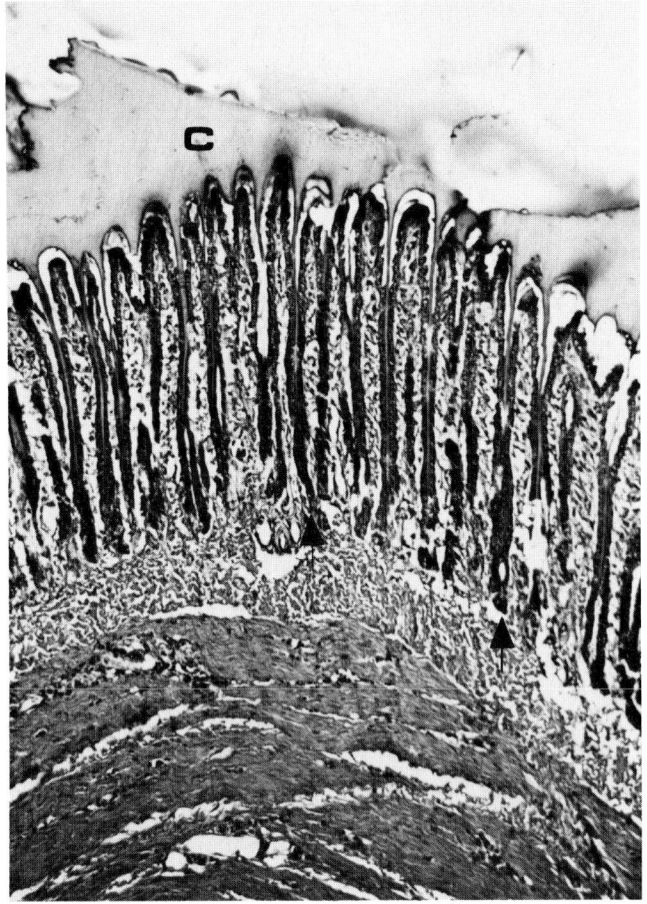

Fig. 19.71 Mucosal glands and lining of the avian ventriculus. The cornified material is the secretory product of the mucosal glands (*arrows*). X40.

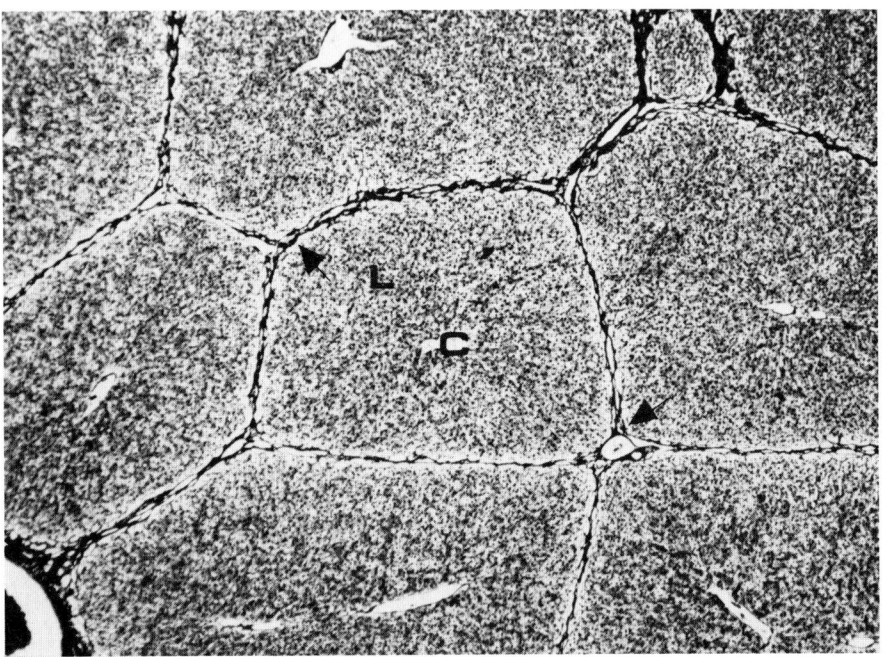

Fig. 19.72 A section of porcine liver. The lobules (L) are well defined by the interlobular connective tissue (*arrows*). A central vein (C) is located in the center of each lobule. X10 (Reticular stain).

the biliary system and are formed between adjacent hepatocytes (Figs. 19.77, 19.78). When compared to other exocrine glands, the bile canaliculi and hepatocytes that form them may be considered to be the secretory intralobular ducts of the liver. Bile canaliculi become confluent with small *interlobular bile ducts* located at the periphery of the lobule through small ductules lined by cuboidal epithelium. The small ductules (*ducts of Hering, cholangioles, terminal ductules*) are lined by small, pale-staining cells which may be modified hepatocytes. Interlobular ducts ramify throughout the interlobular connective tissue and anastomose with other interlobular ducts to form larger interlobular bile ducts. The interlobular bile ducts always ramify throughout the connective tissue in association with branches of the hepatic artery and hepatic portal vein, forming a *portal triad*.

The bile ducts, located between adjacent lobules, are lined by a low simple cuboidal epithelium surrounded by areolar connective tissue. Larger interlobular bile ducts are lined by a simple columnar epithelium. The areolar connective tissue surrounding larger bile ducts contains smooth muscle and elastic fibers. The interlobular bile ducts become confluent and form progressively larger *intrahepatic ducts*. The latter become the extrahepatic ducts, consisting of *hepatic ducts*, *cystic duct* from the gallbladder and *common bile duct* (*ductus choledochus*), which transport bile to the duodenum.

The epithelium of the duct system blends into and is actually an extension of the lamina epithelialis of the duodenum. The bile canaliculi located deep in the liver are actually spaces "outside the body."

The *portal triad*, consisting of an interlobular bile duct and branches of the hepatic artery and hepatic portal vein, are especially obvious in regions between three or more lobules in which there is an accumulation of interlobular connective tissue, a *portal canal* or *portal area*. The portal canal contains a portal triad, nerves and small lymphatic vessels, as well as interlobular connective tissue (Fig. 19.80). The branch of the hepatic portal vein is usually the most prominent structure, whereas the lymphatics are usually collapsed and inconspicuous. The portal area with its conspicuous portal triad is an important landmark in the organization of the liver and the study of the normal and abnormal livers.

Vascular, Lymphatic and Neural Relationships. The functional uniqueness of the liver is reflected in its unique dual vascular supply. The blood supply may be divided into *nutritional* and *functional* units. The nutritional arterial vasculature is supplied by the *hepatic artery*, whereas the functional venous vasculature is supplied by the *hepatic portal vein* (Fig. 19.74).

The hepatic artery divides into branches that supply the individual lobes of the liver. The lobar branches subdivide into smaller interlobular branches that ramify through

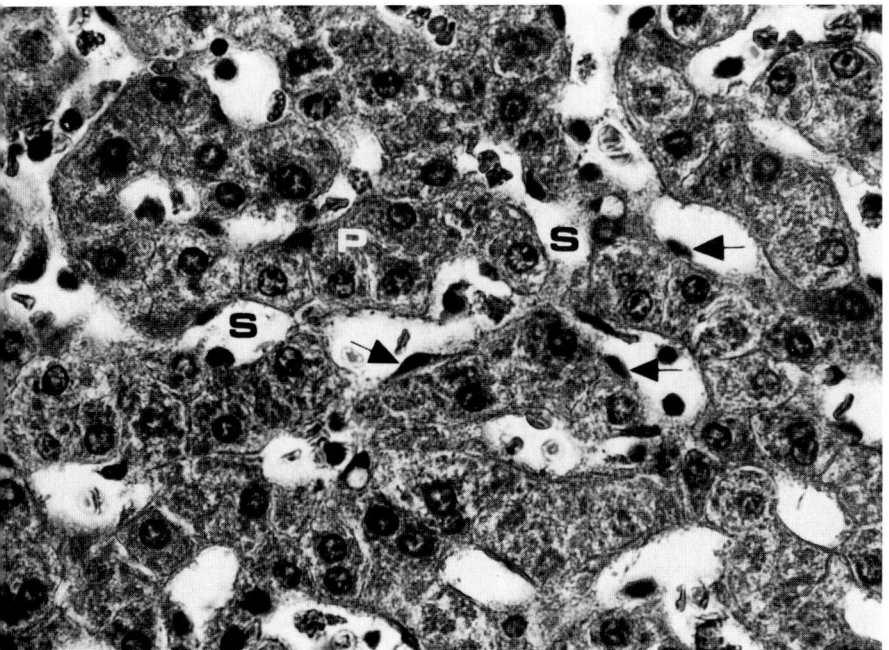

Fig. 19.73 Plates and sinusoids of the liver. The plates of hepatocytes (P) are separated from each other by sinusoids (S) that are lined by Kupffer cells (*arrows*) and endothelial cells. X160.

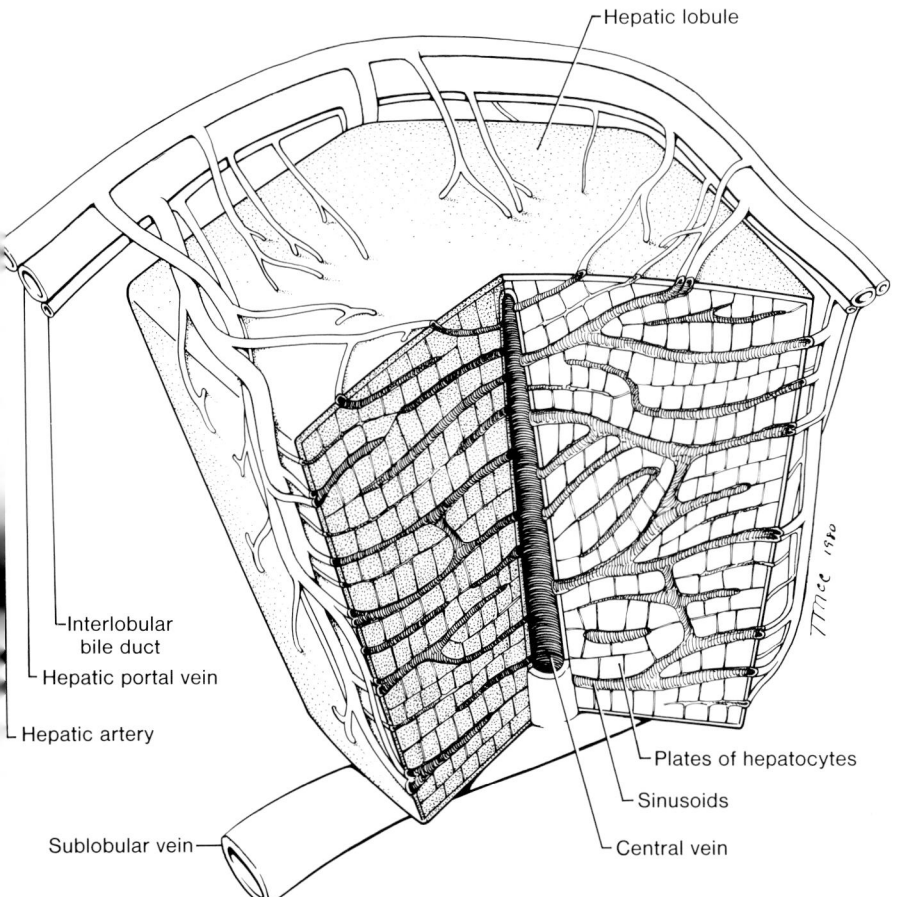

Hepatic lobule

Interlobular bile duct

Hepatic portal vein

Hepatic artery

Sublobular vein

Plates of hepatocytes

Sinusoids

Central vein

Fig. 19.74 A three-dimensional drawing of an hepatic lobule. The hepatic lobule, whether or not distinctly outlined by connective tissue, conforms to this general shape.

out the interlobular connective tissue space as components of the portal triads. The arterial blood is delivered to the lobules via the hepatic sinusoids. The hepatic arterial blood supply accounts for approximately one-fifth of the vascular supply to the liver.

The hepatic portal vein, originating from capillaries within the small intestines and spleen, supplies approximately four-fifths of the vascular supply to the liver. The hepatic portal vein enters the porta of the liver and divides into lobar and interlobular branches. The ramification of branches of the hepatic portal vein is similar to that of the branches of the hepatic artery, because both are components of the portal triad. Venous blood of the hepatic portal venules is delivered to the hepatic sinusoids via inlet venules where it is mixed with the arterial blood of the hepatic arterioles (Fig. 19.81).

Venous drainage is accomplished by a convergent sinusoidal drainage toward the *central vein.* The central vein, oriented perpendicular to the long axis of the lobule, drains into vessels in a sublobular position, the *sublobular veins.* The larger *hepatic veins* form from the confluence of sublobular venous drainage.

The dual blood supply to the liver accomplishes two interrelated functions. The hepatic artery, laden with metabolites and rich in oxygen, supports the metabolic requirements of the parenchyma and the cells of the supportive vascular and neural stroma. The hepatic portal vein, although laden with substances derived from intestinal absorption, is deficient in oxygen. The substances within the portal system, including metabolites and toxic materials, are delivered to the Kupffer cells and hepatocytes for metabolic processing. The mixture of venous (80%) and arterial (20%) blood imposes potential restrictions upon hepatocytic function. Any compromise of the arterial blood supply may deprive the hepatocytes in a centrolobular position of required amounts of oxygen, resulting in their death.

The lymph vessels form an extensive network within the interlobular connective tissue and within the connective tissue of the capsule. However, lymphatic vessels do not occur within the lobules, despite the observation that more lymph exits the liver than from any other organ of the body. The space of Disse, although not a typical lymphatic channel, has been implicated as the region in which the voluminous amount of lymph forms. Lymph formed within the perisinusoidal space probably flows retrograde to the normograde flow within the sinusoids and is picked up by the interlobular lymph vessels.

The nerve supply of the liver consists predominately of nonmyelinated fibers of the sympathetic division of the autonomic nervous system. Although most of the nerve fibers are vasomotor, some innervate the bile ducts, but none of the nerves penetrates the lobules.

Liver Units. The histologic organization

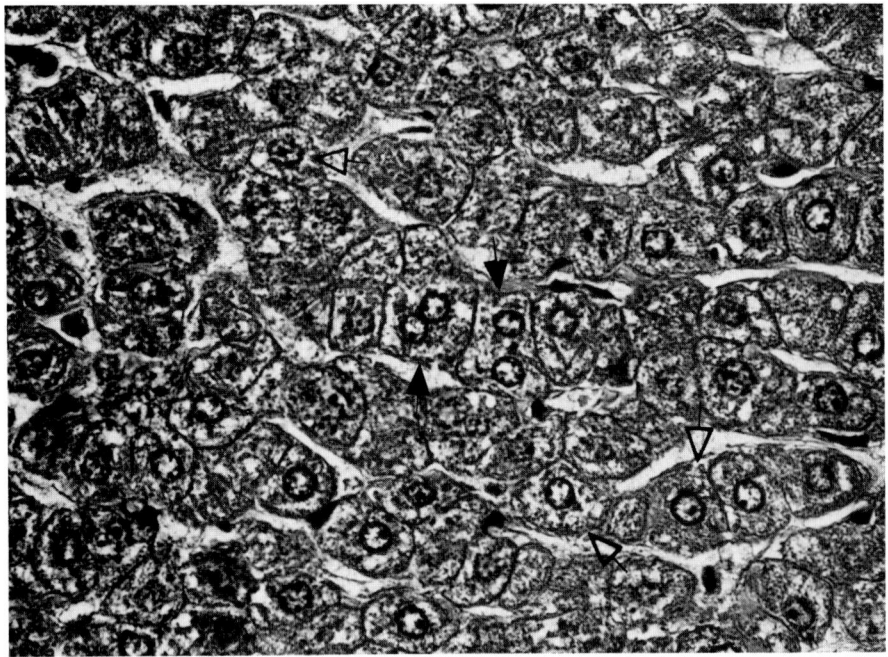

Fig. 19.75 Parenchyma of the liver. The hepatocytes may be uninucleated (*open arrows*) or binucleated (*solid arrows*). X160.

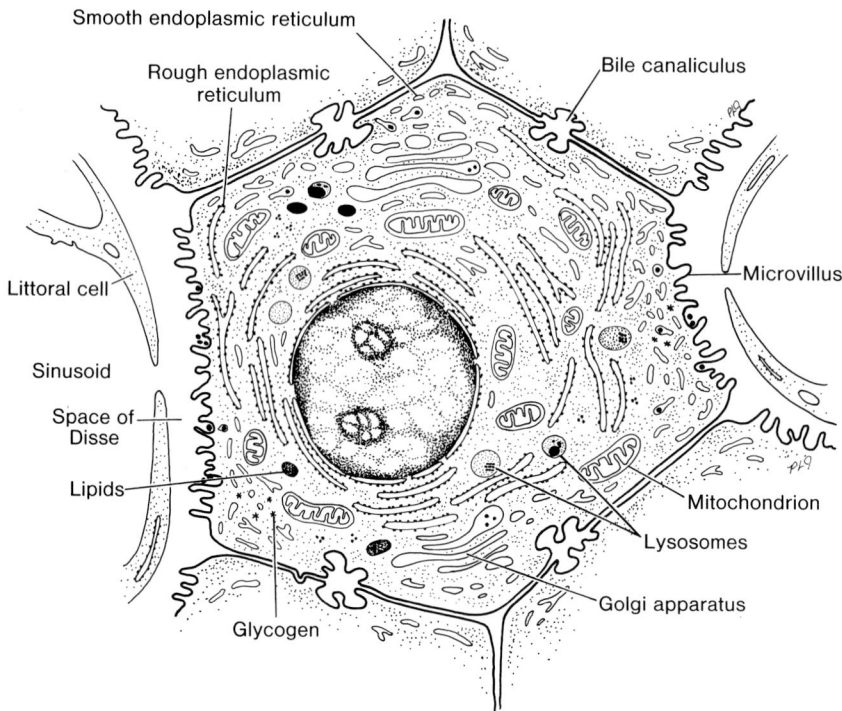

Smooth endoplasmic reticulum

Rough endoplasmic reticulum

Bile canaliculus

Microvillus

Littoral cell

Sinusoid

Space of Disse

Lipids

Mitochondrion

Lysosomes

Golgi apparatus

Glycogen

Fig. 19.76 A drawing of an electron micrograph of an hepatocyte, adjacent cells, spaces of Disse and sinusoids.

of the liver may be considered from three perspectives—morphologic, secretory and vascular. The morphologic or anatomic unit is the *hepatic lobule*; the secretory or functional unit is the *portal lobule*; the vascular unit, the *hepatic acinus.*

The *hepatic lobule*, as described previously, is that histologic entity which has a centrally-positioned vein and is bounded peripherally by varying amounts of interlobular connective tissue (Figs. 19.72, 19.74, 19.82). The hepatic lobule is especially prominent in the pig because of the extensive amounts of interlobular connective tissue. The lobulated pattern of the liver may become more prominent in all species in certain types of disease processes characterized by an increase in interlobular connective tissue.

The *portal lobule*, as the secretory or functional unit of the liver, is a consideration of the organization of the liver from the basis of its exocrine function (Fig. 19.82). All of the bile canaliculi drain into interlobular bile ducts. A single, large interlobular bile duct, located within a portal area, eventually drains the exocrine secretions from adjacent hepatic lobules. The interlobular bile duct within the portal area then becomes the central focus of the portal lobule.

The *hepatic acinus*, as the vascular unit of the liver, represents the organization of the liver from the perspective of the vascular supply to the hepatic lobules (Fig. 19.82). Branches of the hepatic portal vein and hepatic artery radiate from the portal area and extend between hepatic lobules. The end branches of these vessels open into the hepatic sinusoids. Because the axis of the hepatic acinus is perpendicular to the axis of the portal area, the sinusoids and parenchyma of two adjacent hepatic lobules as well as the interlobular blood vessels comprise the acinus. (The interlobular bile ducts follow the same pattern, but the vascular supply is the primary focus of this perspective.) Three zones (*peripheral, intermediate* and *centrolobular*) are identifiable on the basis of their proximity to the interlobular vessels. The perspective afforded by consideration of the organization in terms of the vascular supply is significant in pathology. Certain disease processes of the liver parenchyma are manifested in a zonular pattern related to the end branches of interlobular vessels.

Histophysiology of the Liver

Synthesis, Secretion and Storage. Besides synthesizing many of the substances necessary for the functional and structural integrity of the component cells, the hepatocytes synthesize many substances for export to other parts of the body. Albumin, fibrinogen, α and β globulins, lipoproteins and cholesterol are significant products of hepatocytic metabolism. Glycogen is synthesized from glucose (*glycogenesis*) and stored in the hepatocytes. The release of glucose from glycogen stores (*glycogenolysis*) within hepatocytes occurs upon somatic demand. Similarly, lipids stored in the liver are released in times of somatic need. Numerous vitamins (A, D, K, B-complex) are stored in the liver. Although protein synthesis and secretion comprise major functions of hepatocytes, proteins do not seem to be stored in the liver; they are secreted into the blood as they are synthesized.

Excretion. While the liver synthesizes, stores and secretes many products into the blood and biliary system, the excretory function of the liver relates to the synthesis and

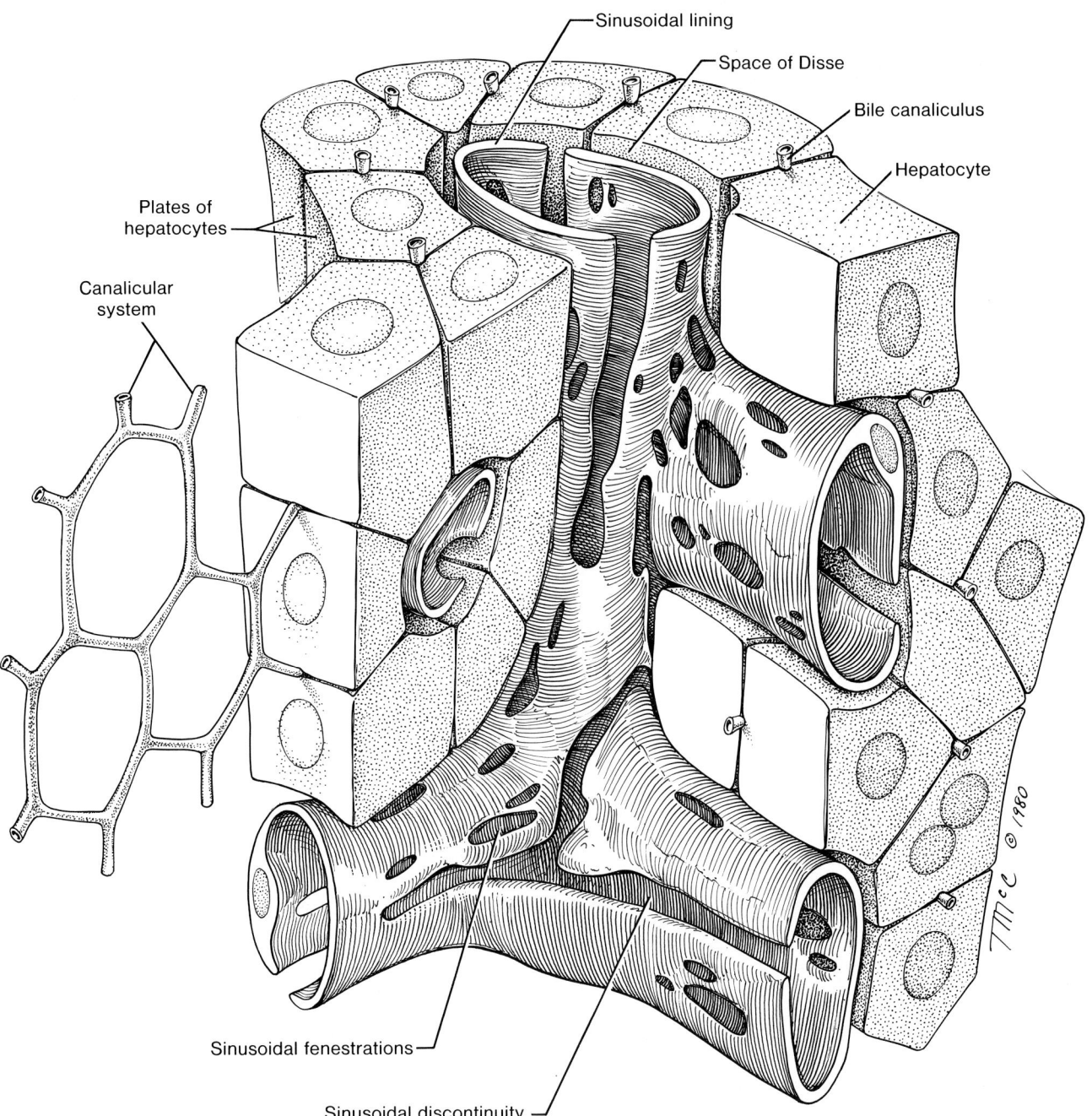

Sinusoidal lining

Space of Disse

Bile canaliculus

Hepatocyte

Plates of hepatocytes

Canalicular system

Sinusoidal fenestrations

Sinusoidal discontinuity

Fig. 19.77 A three-dimensional stylized drawing of the relationships between hepatocytes, sinusoids and bile canaliculi. The canaliculi are represented as tubules for illustrative purposes.

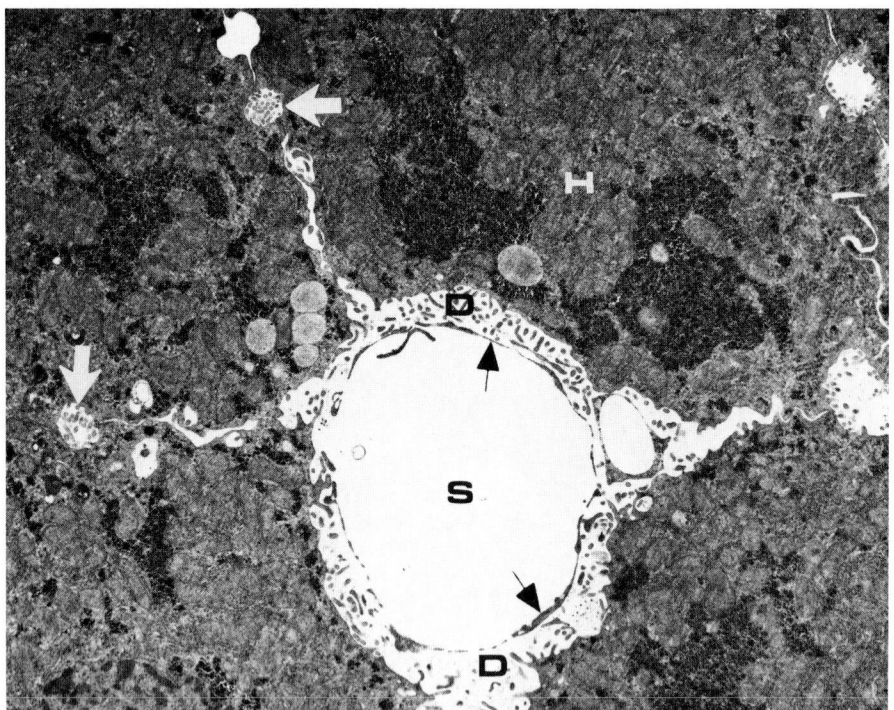

Fig. 19.78   An electron micrograph of a liver. The hepatocytes (H) form the bulk of the organ. Portions of contiguous borders form bile canaliculi (*white arrows*). The sinusoids (S) are lined by Kupffer cells and endothelial cells (*black arrows*). The space of Disse (D) separates the sinusoid from the hepatocytes. The cell processes within the space are microvillous projections of hepatocytes. X6000 (Courtesy of W. Todd).

secretion of substances that enter the bile. The secretion of bile comprises the exocrine function of the liver. The primary constituents of bile are the *bile salts*—sodium and potassium salts of *glycocholic* and *taurocholic acid. Cholic acid*, formed from cholesterol, is conjugated to glycine or taurine to form the bile salts. The bile salts function to emulsify fats in the small intestine, form water-soluble complexes with lipids (*micelles*) in the small intestine to facilitate lipid absorption and activate intestinal lipases.

Bilirubin, a bile pigment derived from the metabolism of hemoglobin, is conjugated to a glucuronide by glucuronyl transferase within the hepatocytes (Chapter 10 and Fig. 10.45). Although bilirubin constitutes the pigmentary portion of the exocine secretions of hepatocytes, the conjugation of bilirubin to glucuronic acid is an important detoxifying function of liver cells.

Cholesterol, fats, phospholipids, electrolytes and other organic compounds are components of bile. Selective reabsorption of some components of bile and their subsequent resecretion by the liver are achieved through the *enterohepatic circulation*.

Biotransformation. Many biologically active and/or toxic compounds that are produced by (hormones, metabolites), injected into (drugs) or absorbed by (toxins) the body are acted upon by the liver to alter their toxicity, to reduce their activity and to eliminate them from the animal body. These processes, often considered to be detoxifi-

cation, do not always result in the detoxification of selected substances. As a result of certain types of hepatic activity, some drugs become more toxic to the body. *Biotransformation* better describes the activity of the liver in terms of the alteration and elimination of numerous and varied chemical compounds.

The biotransformation of many chemical compounds occurs within the smooth endoplasmic reticulum, mitochondria and cytosol of the hepatocytes. Biotransformation reactions may be subdivided into two broad categories—synthetic and nonsynthetic reactions. *Synthetic reactions* or *conjugation reactions* involve the coupling of substances to several endogenous reactive compounds—glucuronide, acetic acid, sulfate or amino acids. The significance of *glucuronyl transferase*, an enzyme of the smooth endoplasmic reticulum, in bilirubin metabolism was discussed previously. Conjugation reactions occur within the cytosol also. Conjugation of compounds with acetic acid involves several *N-acetyltransferases* and *acetyl coenzyme A*. Nonsynthetic reactions involve the cytosol, smooth endoplasmic reticulum and mitochondria. Nonsynthetic mechanisms include oxidation, reduction and hydrolysis reactions.

Although the conjugation reaction is an effective means of detoxifying many substances, not all biotransformations result in detoxification. Ethylene glycol is subject to biotransformation by *alcohol dehydrogen-*

ase. The product of this oxidation reaction *oxalic acid* that chelates calcium, is toxic to the kidneys. The essence of biotransformation reactions is to increase water solubility and polarity. As a result, compounds become less lipid soluble and are unable to penetrate cell membranes. Accordingly, inactivation and elimination of the compounds are achieved. The phagocytic function of the Kupffer cell complements the biotransformation activity of the hepatocyte.

General Metabolism. Besides the specific examples of metabolism discussed previously, the liver is involved in numerous other metabolic functions that are essential to the organism. The liver is involved in all aspects of carbohydrate, protein and fat metabolism. *Gluconeogenesis*, the synthesis of glucose from *glucogenic amino acids*, citric acid cycle intermediates and lactic acid, is a significant aspect of carbohydrate metabolism in hepatocytes.

Most of the beta-oxidation of fat occurs in hepatocytes. *Ketone body formation* also occurs in the liver.

Protein metabolism includes diverse reactions. *Deamination* and the production of keto acids is important in lipid (*ketogenic amino acids*) and carbohydrate (*glucogenic amino acids*) synthesis. Ketogenic amino acids yield acetyl coenzyme A when metabolized and can form ketone bodies (acetoacetate), whereas glucogenic amino acids yield glucose precursors. The liver is able to synthesize nonessential amino acids, and the liver and other tissues are able to convert one amino acid to another through *transaminase* reactions. *Serum glutamic pyruvate transaminase (SGPT)* is a liver-specific transaminase in carnivores that is used to determine liver function. The enzyme leaks from damaged hepatocytes, and elevation of SGPT may be detected in the serum. The formation of urea within hepatocytes is the means by which the body excretes nitrogenous waste products. Urea also contributes to the countercurrent mechanism of the kidney; therefore, it is influential in the concentrating of urine.

Although the liver assumes a passive role in the storage of vitamins, hepatocytic function and bile secretion is essential for the absorption of fat-soluble vitamins (A, D, E, K) from the intestinal tract. The liver also assumes an active role in the metabolism of vitamin D (Chapter 8).

Regeneration. The mitotic potential of the hepatocytes is retained throughout the life of the organism. Surgical extirpation of part of the liver is followed by a rapid restoration of its original mass. Similarly, liver mass is restored in a short period of time after experimental surgical extirpation of threefourths of the rat liver; complete restoration of the organ is achieved in 30 days. Mitotic activity and cellular hypertrophy account for the restored mass.

Although acute damage from toxic sub-

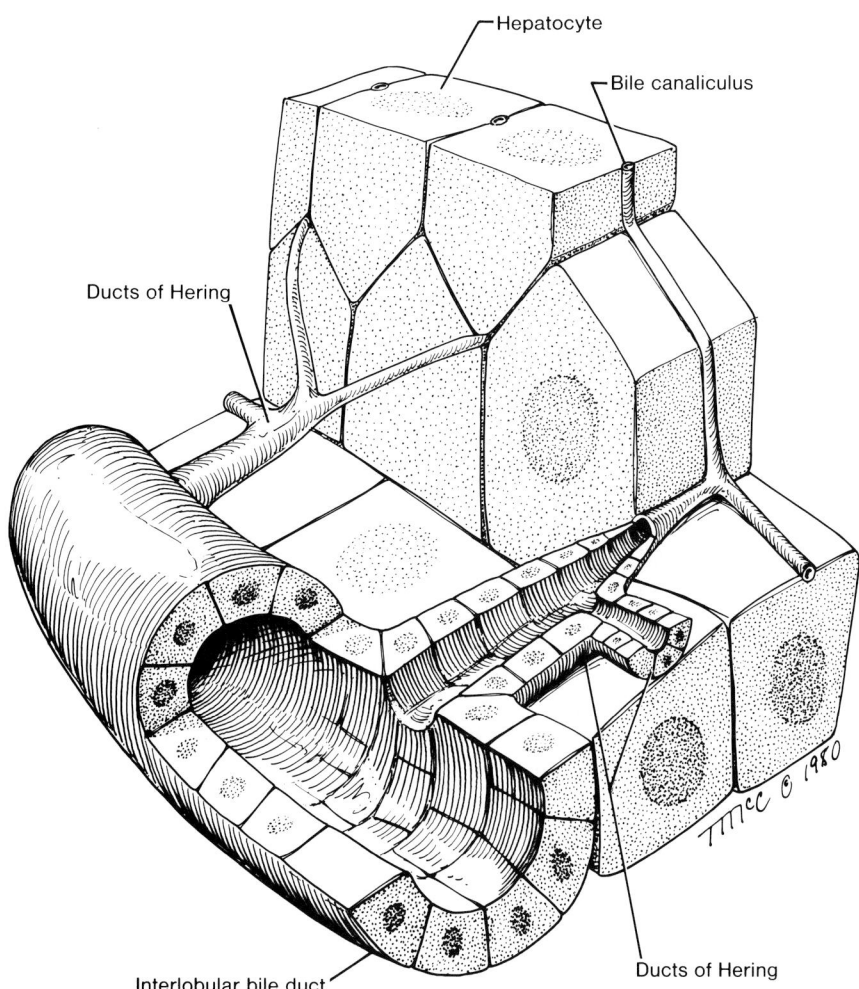

Fig. 19.79 A three-dimensional stylized drawing of the canalicular system and its relationship to intrahepatic bile ducts. The ducts of Hering are modified hepatocytes. The bile canalicular space is outside of the body. Again, the bile canaliculi are represented as tubules for illustrative purposes.

stances may be followed by complete organ recovery, chronic exposure usually results in altered organ function, decreased organ size and an increase in intrahepatic fibrous connective tissue (*cirrhosis*).

Gallbladder

General Characteristics. The *gallbladder* (*cholecyst*) functions as a storage organ for bile. It also concentrates this secretory product of the liver by the absorption of water from its lumen. It is a diverticulum of the common bile duct.

The lamina epithelialis is composed of simple columnar epithelium (Fig. 19.83). The lamina propria-submucosa consists of areolar connective tissue. The tunica muscularis consists of smooth muscle which is not oriented in any particular manner. The tunica serosa is present and typical.

The tunica mucosa is so extensively folded in the dog and cat that the invaginations are often misinterpreted as simple glands (*Rokitansky-Aschoff sinuses*). However, there are glands in the bile ducts and

gallbladder of certain species, notable the ox.

The *hepatic, cystic* and *common bile ducts* are structurally similar to the gallbladder. The mural smooth muscle is disposed as circular and longitudinal layers.

Functional Correlates. The primary functions of the gallbladder are to store, concentrate, acidify and deliver the bile to the duodenum upon demand. Bile is prevented from entering the duodenum by the *sphincter of Oddi*, a smooth muscular modification surrounding the common bile duct as it passes through the duodenal wall. The sphincter remains closed during fasting and forces bile from the hepatic ducts and common bile duct into the cystic duct and gallbladder. When food enters the mouth, the tone of the sphincter decreases. Cholecystokinin-pancreozymin is released from intestinal cells by stimulation from fatty acids, acid, protein digestive products and calcium in the duodenum. Relaxation of the sphincter of Oddi and contraction of the smooth muscle of the gallbladder and associated ducts results from CCK-PZ secretion. Substances that cause the gallbladder to contract

are challed *cholagogues*. The smooth muscle of the gallbladder and ducts is innervated by both divisions of the autonomic nervous system.

Exocrine Pancreas

General Characteristics. The pancreas is a compound tubuloalveolar gland which is a diverticulum of the epithelium of the gut (Fig. 19.84). It is an exocrine and an endocrine organ. The exocrine structure will be covered in this chapter. The exocrine portion of the organ is very similar to that described for the salivary glands. The main differences in this organ are its special glandular epithelium, the absence of striated ducts, the absence of basket cells and the presence of endocrine tissue.

The cells of the glandular epithelium are conical or pyramidal (Fig. 19.85). Although these cells resemble typical serous cells, the pancreatic glandular cells differ in the basal region. This region possesses radial striations and is basophilic (Plate II.10). This is due to the basal accumulation of numerous

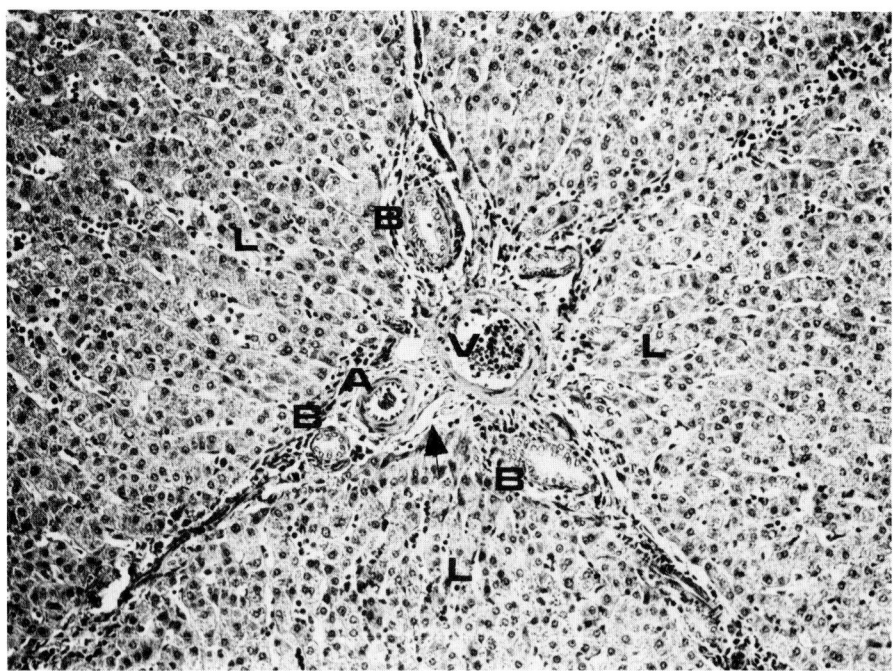

Fig. 19.80 Portal area of the liver. This region is located between lobules (L). The region contains branches of the bile duct (B), hepatic portal vein (V) and hepatic artery (A). Lymphatic vessels (*arrow*) are present also. X40.

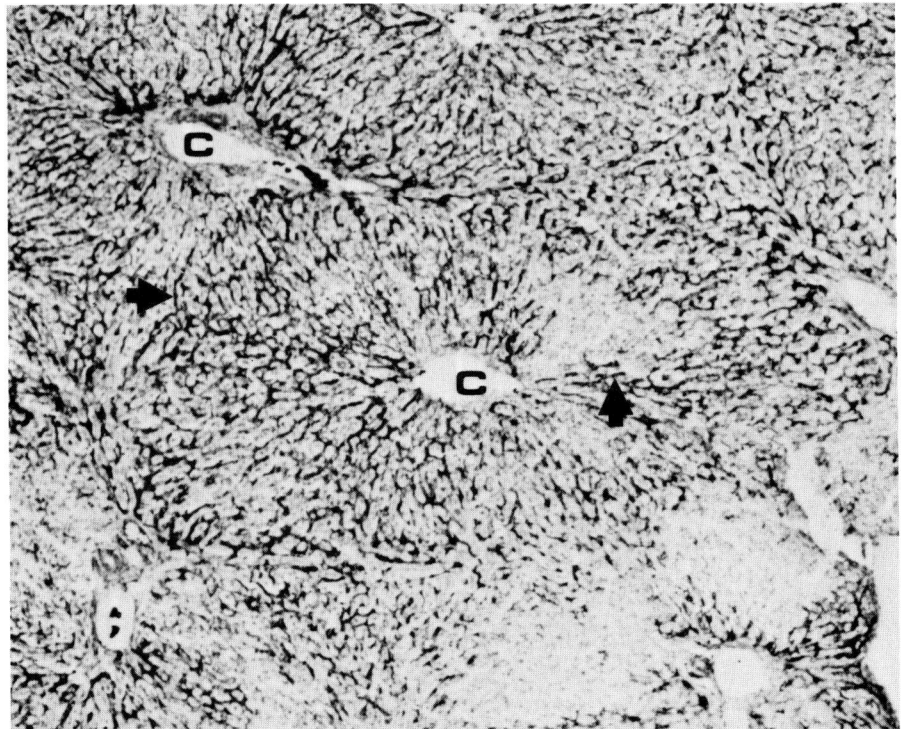

Fig. 19.81 A section of galline liver. The bird had been injected with india ink antimortem. The phagocytic cells of the sinusoids have trapped some of the india ink. The sinusoids (*arrows*) are outlined. C, central vein. X16.

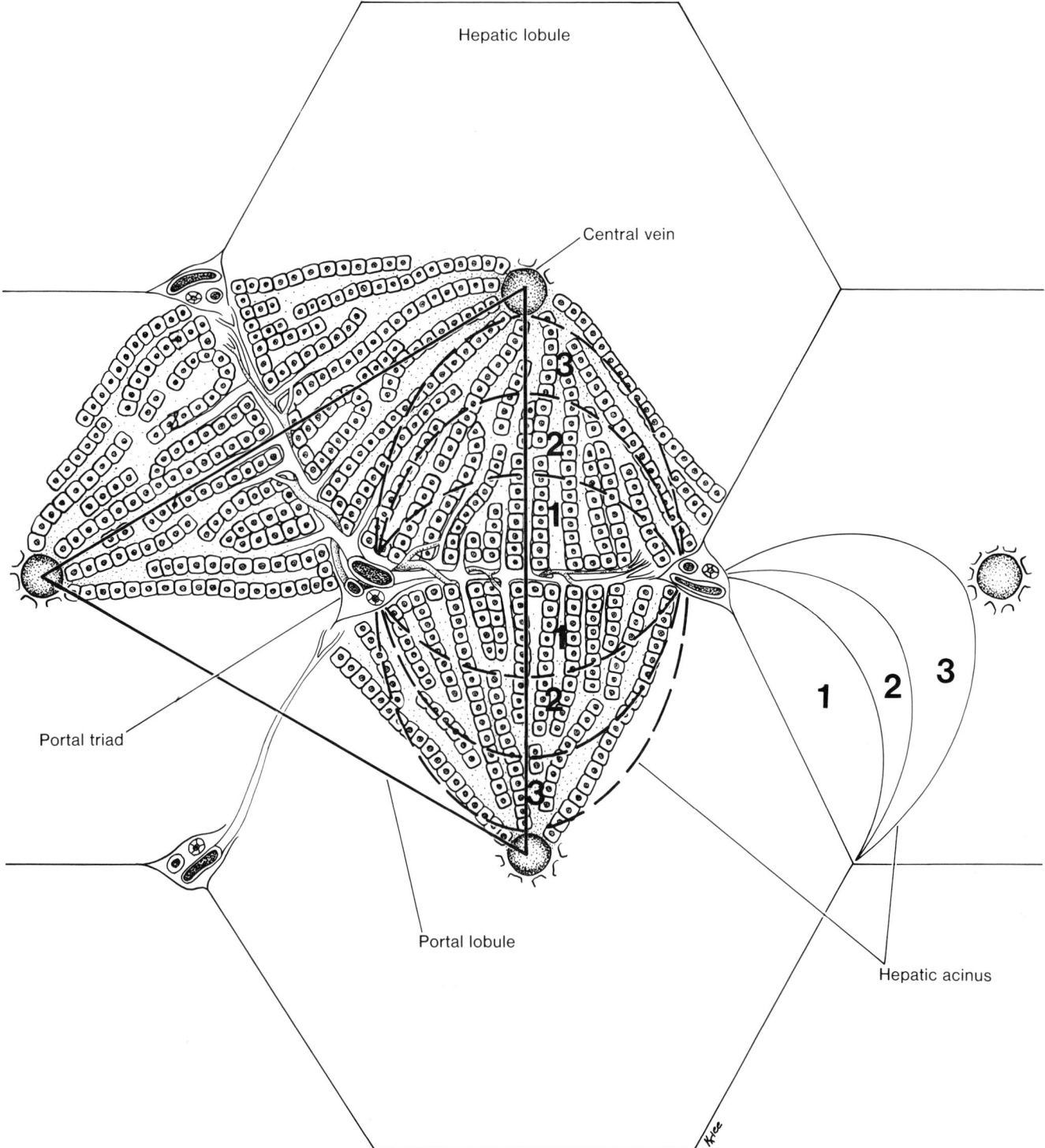

Fig. 19.82 Diagram of the organization of the liver. The organization of the liver may be considered from its structure (hepatic lobule), exocrine activity (portal lobule) and vascular supply (hepatic acinus). The hepatic lobule is the histologic structure in which the central vein is the central landmark. The portal lobule (outlined as a triangular area) has the interlobular bile duct within the portal area as the centralized landmark. The hepatic acinus represents zones of contiguous lobules that are supplied by the same interlobular vessels. The zone closest to the interlobular region (1) has the best blood supply, whereas the zone closest to the central vein (3) has the poorest blood supply.

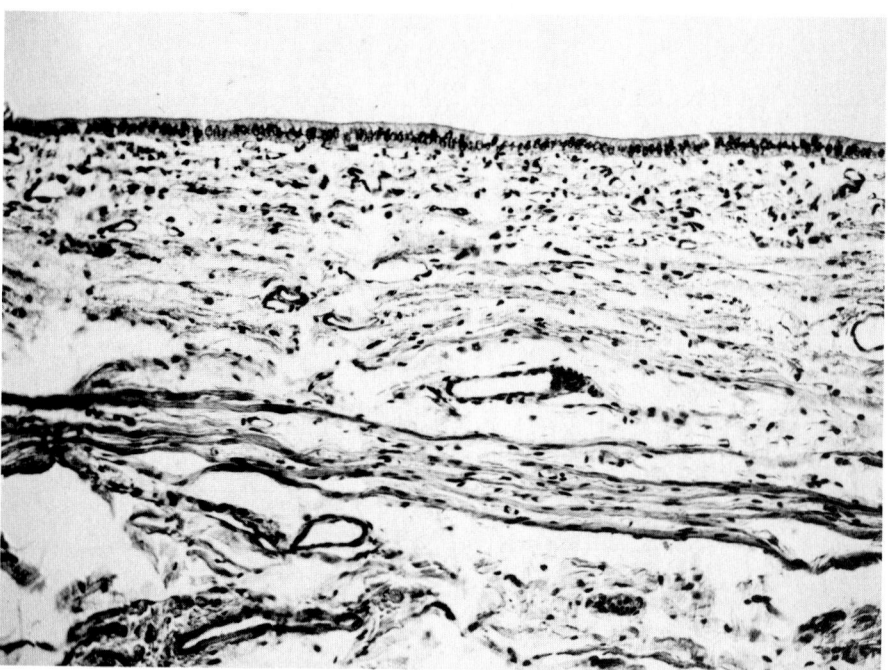

Fig. 19.83 Bovine gallbladder. The columnar epithelium is underlaid by a typical lamina propria-submucosa. X40.

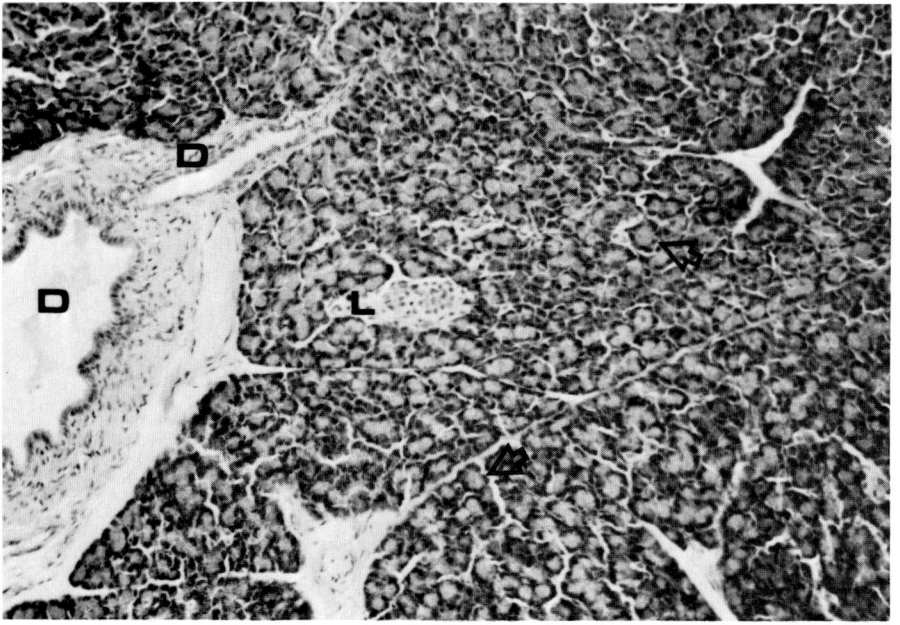

Fig. 19.84 Canine pancreas. The bulk of the gland consists of exocrine adenomeres (*arrows*) and duct system (D). L, islets of Langerhans. X40.

mitochondria and rough endoplasmic reticulum. The nucleus is usually in a parabasal position. A supranuclear pale-staining area (Golgi zone) may be apparent. The acidophilic luminal region is granular and may possess zymogen granules. Their presence or absence is related to the physiologic state of the organism. Granules accumulate during fasting and are extruded during digestion.

The adenomere opens into a small *intercalated duct* that is lined by a squamous or cuboidal epithelium. Rather than the ductular epithelium beginning at the termination of the acinar cells, a variable amount of overlap exists. As such, the lining cells of this duct reside, initially, upon the secretory cells of the acinus. The cells that line this surface are referred to as *centroacinar cells.* These cells do not seem to impair the secretory process, but their significance is not understood.

As the duct system becomes confluent, a change from cuboidal to columnar epithelium occurs. The epithelium of the larger ducts may contain goblet cells as well as simple branched tubuloaveolar mucous glands.

The DWFCT of the capsule subdivides the gland through the formation of connective tissue septa. The finest connective tissue is that which is associated with the adenomeres and smaller ducts, becoming progressively coarse and continuing with septal connective tissue.

Functional Correlates. *Pancreatic juice* is an alkaline fluid (pH = 8.0) which contains numerous enzymes that are essential in digestion. The enzymes include *trypsin, chymotrypsin, carboxypeptidase A and B, elastase, ribonuclease, deoxyribonuclease, phospholipase, esterase, collagenase,* and *amylase.* The proteolytic and lipolytic enzymes are secreted as enzyme precursors to prevent digestion of the cells in which they are synthesized. *Trypsinogen,* the inactive form of trypsin, is activated by the proteolytic enzyme *enterokinase* released from the intestinal mucosa. Once activated, trypsin can activate other trypsinogen molecules as well as *chymotrypsinogen,* the inactive form of chymotrypsin. Trypsin also activates *prophospholipase A* into the activated form, phospholipase A.

The release of activated enzymes into pancreatic tissue, as occurs in pancreatitis, can have devastating effects upon the organism. Phospholipase A splits a fatty acid from lecithin, forming *lysolecithin.* Lysolecithin causes damage to cell membranes. The activation of other pancreatic enzymes can digest cellular components, destroy the pancreas and damage other visceral organs after leakage into the peritoneal cavity. Serum elevations of lipase and amylase are suggestive of pancreatic disease.

Numerous electrolytes (Na^+, K^+, Ca^{++}, Mg^{++}, Cl^-, $SO_4^=$, $HPO_4^=$ and HCO_3^-) are components of pancreatic juice; however,

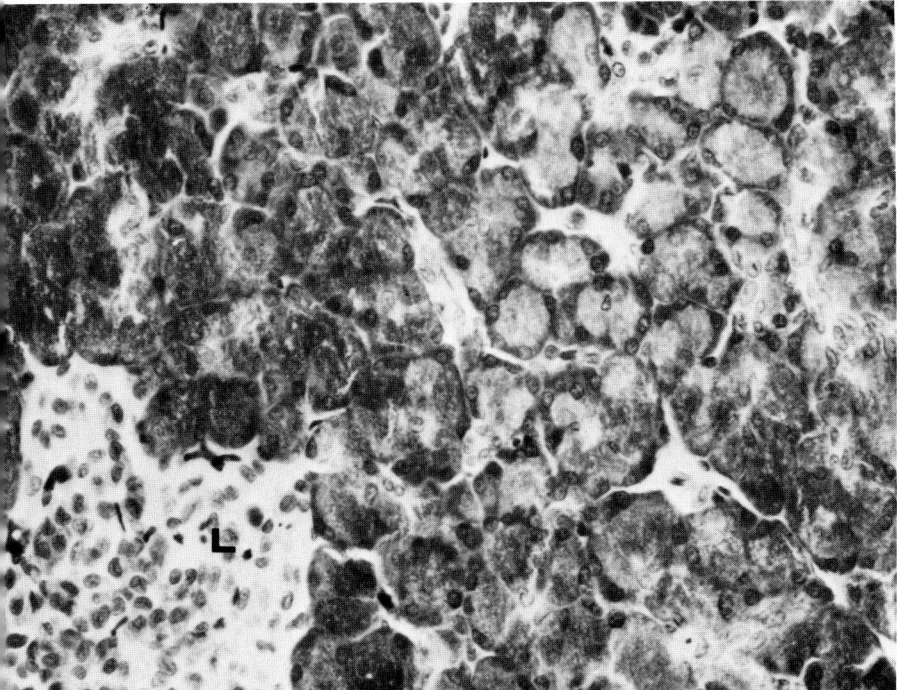

Fig. 19.85 Acini of the canine pancreas. The acini consist of lining cells that have an apical acidophilia and a basal basophilia. The apices contain zymogen granules. L, islet of Langerhans ×100.

he major salt secreted by the pancreas is sodium bicarbonate, which produces the alkalinity of pancreatic juice. Sodium bicarbonate neutralizes the acidity of the fluids entering the duodenum.

The regulation of pancreatic exocrine secretion is mediated by neural and hormonal mechanisms. Parasympathetic stimulation via the vagus causes the secretion of small amounts of pancreatic juice that is rich in enzymes. The mechanisms involved in the cephalic phase of gastric digestion may stimulate pancreatic secretion also.

The presence of acid in the duodenum causes the release of secretin from the intestinal mucosa. Secretin influences the intralobular ducts and causes the release of a thin, watery, bicarbonate-rich and enzyme-poor pancreatic secretion. The neutralization of the acidity reduces secretin release that then reduces pancreatic activity. The release of CCK-PZ from intestinal cells causes the flow of an enzyme-rich pancreatic juice. The hormonal activation of pancreatic secretion is the primary mechanism of regulation.

References

Buccal Cavity
Anderes, R. L.: Canine tooth structure, development, blood and nerve supply. North Amer. Vet. *16:*37, 1935.

Bailey, C. B. and Balch, C. C.: Saliva secretion and its relation to feeding in cattle. Brit. J. Nutr. *15:*371, 1961.

Elwood, W. K. and Bernstein, M. H.: The ultrastructure of the enamel organ related to enamel formation. Amer. J. Anat. *122:*73, 1968.

Garlick, N. L.: The teeth of the ox in clinical diagnosis. I. Developmental anatomy. Amer. J. Vet. Res. *15:* 226, 1954.

Hand, A. R.: The fine structure of Von Ebner's gland of the rat. J. Cell Biol. *44:*340, 1970.

Kallenbach, E.: Fine structure of rat incisor enamel organ during late pigmentation and regression stages. J. Ultrastruct. Res. *30:*38, 1970.

Lester, K. S. and Boyde, A: Scanning electron microscopy of developing roots of molar teeth of the laboratory rat. J. Ultrastruct. Res. *33:*80, 1970.

Murray, R. G., Murray, A. and Fujimoto, S.: Fine structure of gustatory cells in rabbit taste buds. J. Ultrastruct. Res. *27:*444, 1969.

Shackleford, J. M. and Wilborn, W. H.: Ultrastructure of bovine parotid glands. J. Morph. *127:*453, 1969.

Swenson, M. J. (editor): *Duke's Physiology of Domestic Animals.* 9th edition, Comstock, Ithaca, 1977.

Weinrab, M. M. and Sharaw, Y.: Tooth development in sheep. Am. J. Vet. Res. *25:*891, 1964.

Tubular Organs
Adkins, R. B., Ende, N. and Gobbel, W. G.: A correlation of parietal cell activity with ultrastructural alterations. Surgery *62:*1059, 1967.

Bonfanti, C.: Duodenal glands in the horse. Rev. Med. Vet. *4:*95, 1952.

Brobeck, J. R. (editor): *Best and Taylor's Physiological Basis of Medical Practice.* 10th edition, Williams &

Wilkins, Baltimore, 1979.

Brunser, O. and Luft, J. H.: Fine structure of the apex of absorptive cells from rat small intestine. J. Ultrastruct. Res. *31:*291, 1970.

Cardell, R. R., Badenhausen, S. and Porter, K. R.: Intestinal triglyceride absorption in the rat. An electron microscopical study. J. Cell Biol. *34:*123, 1967.

Demke, D. D.: A brief histology of the intestine of the turkey poult. Amer. J. Vet. Res. *15:*447, 1952.

Deveney, C. W. and Dunphy, J. E.: Wound healing in the gastrointestinal tract. In: *Fundamentals of Wound Management in Surgery: Selected Tissues.* pp. 61–95. Chirurgecom, Inc., South Plainfield, New Jersey. 1977.

Elias, H.: Comparison of duodenal glands in domestic animals. Amer. J. Vet. Res. *8:*311, 1947.

Hampton, J. C.: An electron microscopic study of mouse colon. Dis. Colon Rectum *3:*423, 1960.

Johnson, F. R. and Young, B. A.: Undifferentiated cells in the gastric mucosa. J. Anat. *101:*617, 1967.

Leeson, C. R. and Leeson, T. S.: The fine structure of Brunner's glands in the rabbit. Anat. Rec. *159:*409, 1967.

Moon, H. W.: Mechanisms in the pathogenesis of diarrhea: A Review. J. Am. Vet. Med. Assoc. *172:*443, 1978.

O'Brien, T. R., Biery, D. N., Park, R. D. and Bartels, J. E.: *Radiographic Diagnosis of Abdominal Disorders in the Dog and Cat: Radiographic Interpretation, Clinical Signs, Pathophysiology.* W. B. Saunders, Philadelphia, 1978.

Rubin, W.: Enzyme cytochemistry of gastric parietal cells at a fine structure level. J. Cell Biol. *42:*332, 1969.

Titkemeyer, C. W. and Calhoun, M. L.: A comparative study of the structure of the small intestine of domestic animals. Amer. J. Vet. Res. *16:*152, 1955.

Trier, J. S.: Structure of the mucosa of the small intestine as it relates to intestinal function. Fed. Proc. *26:* 1391, 1967.

Watson, A. G.: Structure of the canine esophagus. N. Z. Vet. J. *21:*195, 1973.

Large Digestive Glands
Burkel, W. E. and Low, F. N.: The fine structure of rat liver sinusoids, space of Disse and associated tissue space. Amer. J. Anat. *118:*769, 1966.

Caro, L. G. and Palade, G. E.: Protein synthesis, storage, and discharge in the pancreatic exocrine cell. An autoradiographic study. J. Cell Biol. *20:*473, 1964.

Ekholm, R. and Edlund, Y.: Ultrastructure of the human exocrine pancreas. J. Ultrastruct Res. *2:*453, 1959.

Elias, H. and Sherrick, J. C.: *Morphology of the Liver.* Academic Press, New York, 1969.

Loud, A. V.: A quantitative stereological description of the ultrastructure of normal rat liver parenchymal cells. J. Cell Biol. *37:*27, 1968.

Rappaport, A. M.: The structural and functional unit in the human liver (liver acinus). Anat. Rec. *130:*673, 1958.

Trotter, N. L.: A fine structure of lipid in mouse liver regenerating after partial hepatectomy. J. Cell Biol. *21:*233, 1964.

Wood, R. L.: Evidence of species differences in the ultrastructure of the hepatic sinusoid. Z. Zellforsch. *58:*678, 1963.

Yamada, E.: The fine structure of the gallbladder epithelium of the mouse. J. Biophys. Biochem. Cytol. *1:* 445, 1955.

20: Urinary System

Kidney

General Considerations. The kidney and associated urinary passages function to *filter* the blood, *remove* waste materials, *recover* useful metabolites, *store* the fluid waste and eventually *transport* the waste products to the exterior of the body. Because the kidney *regulates* fluid volume, acid/base balance and electrolyte composition within the body, it is the central organ involved in creating and maintaining an internal environment in which the constituent cells of the body can thrive. Additionally, the kidney functions as an endocrine organ through its secretion of *renin*, a proteolytic enzyme involved in the regulation of blood pressure. The secretion of *renal erythropoietic factor* (*erythrogenin*) involves the kidney in the regulation of erythropoiesis. Renal cellular constituents are active in the synthesis of active metabolites of vitamin D; thus, the kidney also influences calcium metabolism.

The kidney is composed of two distinct morphologic regions, an outer *cortex* and inner *medulla* (Fig. 20.1). The separation into two distinct regions at the *cortico-medullary junction* implies that the regions are composed of different components. Actually, elements of both regions occur in each other, but a quantitative difference of components occurs in the distinct regions.

The kidney is a compound tubular gland composed of *uriniferous tubules*. Like any compound gland, it is divided into lobes and lobules (Fig. 20.1). In some species there is only one lobe, whereas in others the lobulation may persist or secondarily fuse. A lobe consists of medullary and cortical components. The medullary portion consists of a *pyramid*, the broad base of which is in contact with the cortex. One or more pyramids may join to form a *papilla*, the rounded, apical portion of the pyramid(s) which projects into a minor calyx. The tip of the papilla is fenestrated (*area cribrosa*); the perforations correspond to the openings of the uriniferous tubules into the calyces or renal pelvis.

Among the domestic species, swine and large ruminants have kidneys described as *multipyramidal* or *multilobar* (Fig. 20.1). A papilla projects into a *minor calyx*; the calyces are continuous with the ureter.

Unipyramidal or *unilobar* kidneys are characteristic of carnivores, small ruminants and horses. The kidney consists of one lobe (cat) or one lobe that results from the fusion of several lobes developmentally. A single, broad based papilla forms the *renal crest*.

The renal crest is associated intimately with the expanded portion of the ureter, the *renal pelvis* (Fig. 20.1).

The uriniferous tubule of the kidney consists of a *nephron* and a *collecting duct system* (Fig. 20.2). The kidneys of a medium-sized dog may contain as many as 800,000 nephrons. The nephron is that portion of the uriniferous tubule which produces the urine and consists of a *capsule of Bowman, proximal convoluted tubule, loop of Henle* and a *distal convoluted tubule*. A tuft of arterial capillaries, the *glomerulus*, and *Bowman's capsule* comprise a *renal corpuscle*. The collecting duct system, which collects, concentrates and transports the urine, consists of *arched collecting tubules, straight collecting tubules* and *papillary ducts* (*ducts of Bellini*).

Two distinct regions are visible in histologic sections of the renal cortex. The cortex proper or *cortical labyrinth* is separated by *medullary rays* (Fig. 20.3). The labyrinth contains renal corpuscles, proximal and distal convoluted tubules and arched collecting ducts. A medullary ray is comprised of the descending and ascending limbs of Henle's loop and straight collecting tubules. Similarly, the medulla is divisible into an *outer* and *inner zone*. The outer zone, that region juxtaposed to the cortex, contains the loops of Henle of short nephrons and straight collecting tubules. The inner zone is comprised of Henle's loops of long nephrons, straight collecting tubules and papillary ducts.

The development of the kidney progresses through stages in which three different and overlapping renal systems are evolved. The *pronephros* is the first and most simple renal system. The regression of the pronephros is followed by the development of a more sophisticated system, the *mesonephros*. The *metanephros* or definitive kidney develops subsequently. The metanephros originates from two embryonic anlagen—the metanephric blastema and the metanephric duct. The *metanephric blastema*, a derivative of mesoderm, gives rise to the nephron. The metanephric duct, a diverticulum of the mesonephric duct, gives rise to the collecting duct system, renal pelvis, minor and major calyces and ureter. The continued induction of more nephrons by the progressive branching of the metanephric duct continues into the postnatal period of the dog. The development of the *urogenital sinus* from the divided ventral portion of the cloaca accounts for the development of the trigone of the bladder and urethra. The body and apex of the bladder develop from the initial part of the allantoic stalk. The differentiation of the urinary system is linked intimately to the organogenesis of the genital system. In the male, the *mesonephric duct* (*Wolffian duct*) is "discarded" from the urinary system and utilized as the definitive genital tract (ductus deferens and epididymis). In the female, new ducts (*paramesonephric* or *Mullerian ducts*) develop in close association with the mesonephric ducts and form the uterine tubes, uterus and vagina.

Connective Tissue and Serosa. The kidney is covered by a loosely adherent capsule of dense white fibrous connective tissue. Loose connective tissue attaches the capsule to the parenchyma. Smooth muscle may be present in the inner portion of the capsule. The capsular connective tissue is continuous with the adventitial coat of the ureter or renal pelvis at the hilus of the organ.

The connective tissue stroma associated with the renal parenchyma is scant. Reticular connective tissue forms a delicate meshwork around and between the uriniferous tubules. The adventitial tunics of blood vessels, lymphatic vessels and nerves also form part of the renal interstitium.

Uriniferous Tubules

Renal Corpuscle. The *renal corpuscle* is composed of a *tuft* or *glomerulus* of capillaries (which connects the afferent and efferent arterioles) and *Bowman's capsule*, the expanded end of the nephron (Fig. 20.4). The latter consists of a *visceral* and *parietal lining* of squamous epithelium. The glomerular capillaries are interdigitated with the visceral lining. Their relationship to one another is analogous to inserting a finger into a balloon. The finger represents the capillary bed. The surface of the balloon contacting the finger represents the visceral lining. The space between the "visceral lining" and the outer wall of the balloon ("parietal lining") represents the initial portion of the nephron into which the glomerular filtrate is pushed.

Because the lining of Bowman's capsule is simple squamous epithelium, it is difficult to distinguish the visceral lining from the capillary endothelium. This endothelial lining is fenestrated and covered by a complete basal lamina (Fig. 20.5). The relationship of the visceral lining to capillary endothelium has been clarified with electron microscopy (Figs. 20.6, 20.7). The body of the lining cells is not in direct contact with the basal lamina. Rather, cell bodies are elevated from but contact the basal lamina by cyto-

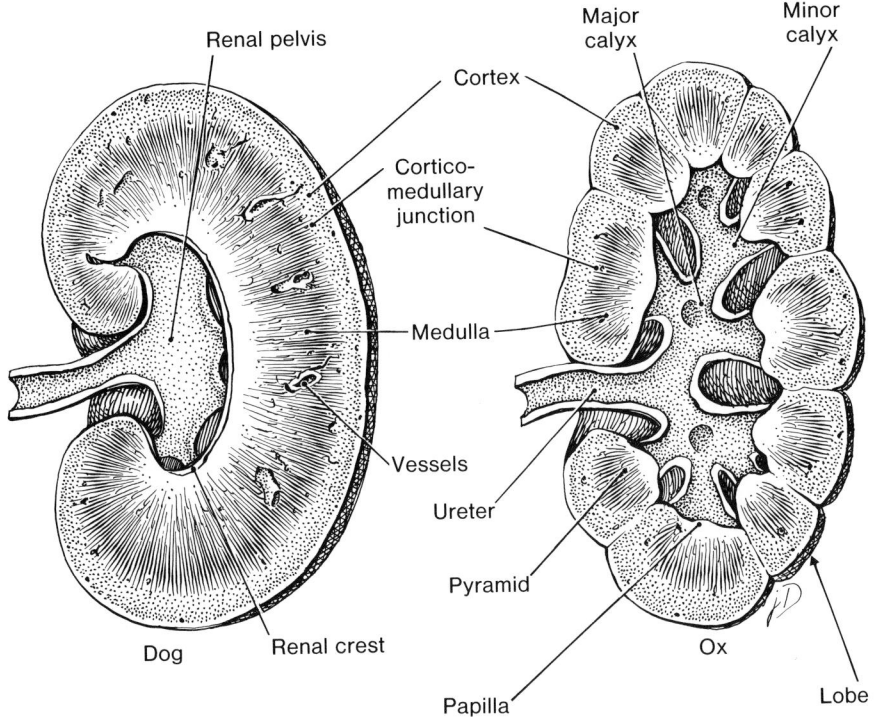

Renal pelvis
Cortex
Major calyx
Minor calyx
Cortico-medullary junction
Medulla
Vessels
Ureter
Pyramid
Dog
Renal crest
Ox
Papilla
Lobe

Fig. 20.1 A diagram of the kidney of a dog (unilobar) and an ox (multilobar). All light micrographs are labeled as the magnification with the microscope before photographic enlarging. All electron micrographs are labeled as total magnification, including photographic enlarging.

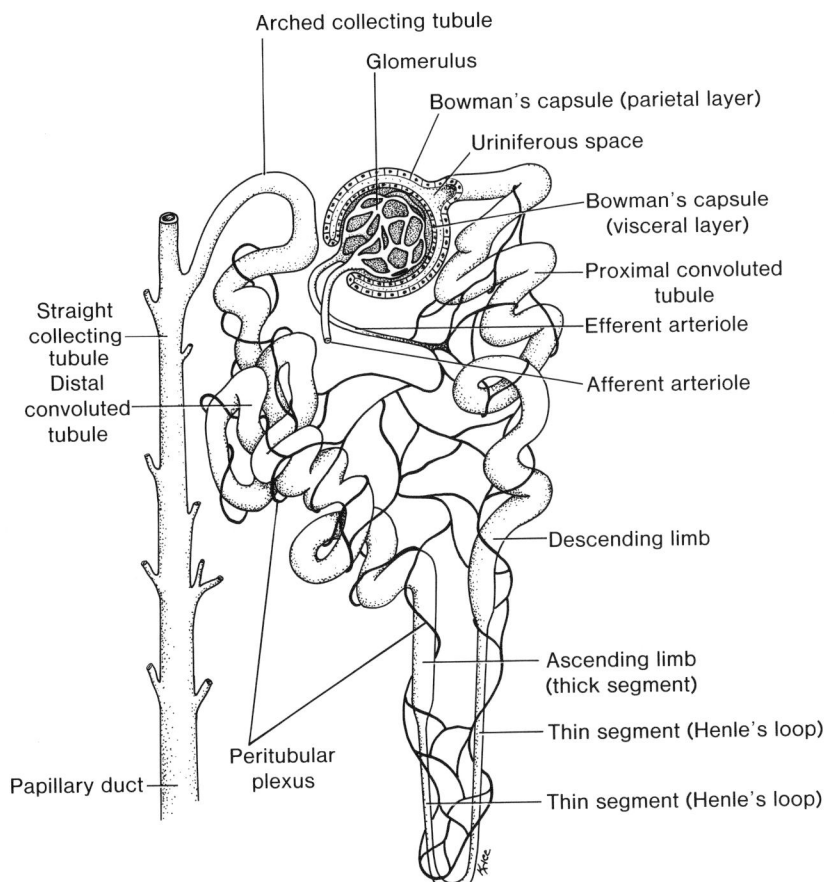

Arched collecting tubule
Glomerulus
Bowman's capsule (parietal layer)
Uriniferous space
Bowman's capsule (visceral layer)
Proximal convoluted tubule
Efferent arteriole
Afferent arteriole
Straight collecting tubule
Distal convoluted tubule
Descending limb
Ascending limb (thick segment)
Thin segment (Henle's loop)
Peritubular plexus
Thin segment (Henle's loop)
Papillary duct

Fig. 20.2 An idealized drawing of a nephron and collecting tubules.

plasmic processes (Fig. 20.8). Large cytoplasmic *foot processes* (primary) have small (secondary) foot processes (*pedicels*) radiating from them. The secondary foot processes interdigitate with each other and are separated by *filtration slits* (Fig. 20.9). A thin membrane (*filtration membrane*) extends across the filtration slits. These cells with foot processes (visceral lining cells) are referred to as *podocytes*. Although the podocytes are aligned along the periphery of the capillaries, the actual barrier to filtration is the basal lamina (Fig. 20.10).

Besides the endothelium and podocytes, a third cell type is usually encountered: *mesangial* or *intercapillary cells*. These stellate cells are located between the capillary loops of the glomerulus. The mesangial cells are mesenchymally-derived cells that are similar to pericytic cells occurring elsewhere in the body associated with capillaries. The cells are enveloped by the basal lamina. Although their precise function has not been defined, they are phagocytic cells which may remove particulate matter from the renal corpuscle.

The squamous cell configuration of the parietal layer of Bowman's capsule is readily apparent. With periodic acid-Schiff (PAS) staining, the prominent basement membrane surrounding the capsule and glomerulus is readily demonstrated (Figs. 5.46, 5.47). Two distinct regions of the renal corpuscle are apparent in ideal sections: a *vascular pole* and a *urinary pole* (Fig. 20.4). The vascular pole is the region of entry and exit of the arterioles. It is also the region in which the *juxtaglomerular apparatus* is located. The urinary pole is the point of continuity between Bowman's capsule and the proximal convoluted tubule. At this point a transition from the squamous epithelium of the parietal layer to the cuboidal epithelium of the proximal tubule occurs.

Proximal Convoluted Tubule. The *proximal convoluted tubule* is the longest, widest and most developed segment of the nephron (Fig. 20.11). Its function is extremely important, and it is the segment that is easily affected by disease processes and toxic substances. It is lined by cuboidal cells with a well-developed brush border. With routine staining (hematoxylin and eosin), the eosinophilic and granular cytoplasm does not contrast markedly with the brush border. A marked difference, however, is noted with PAS staining. The mucopolysaccharides of the cell coat on the microvilli are strongly PAS-positive. The basal portion of these cells is highly folded and contains numerous mitochondria. The mitochondria contribute to the basal striations that may be apparent. Because the lateral border of cells are highly interdigitated, they are not readily observed in light microscopic sections. The nuclei of these cells are spherical, small and located in a basal or parabasal position. Varying physiologic states contribute to an altered morphology of this segment. Generally, however, the luminal size is small and the

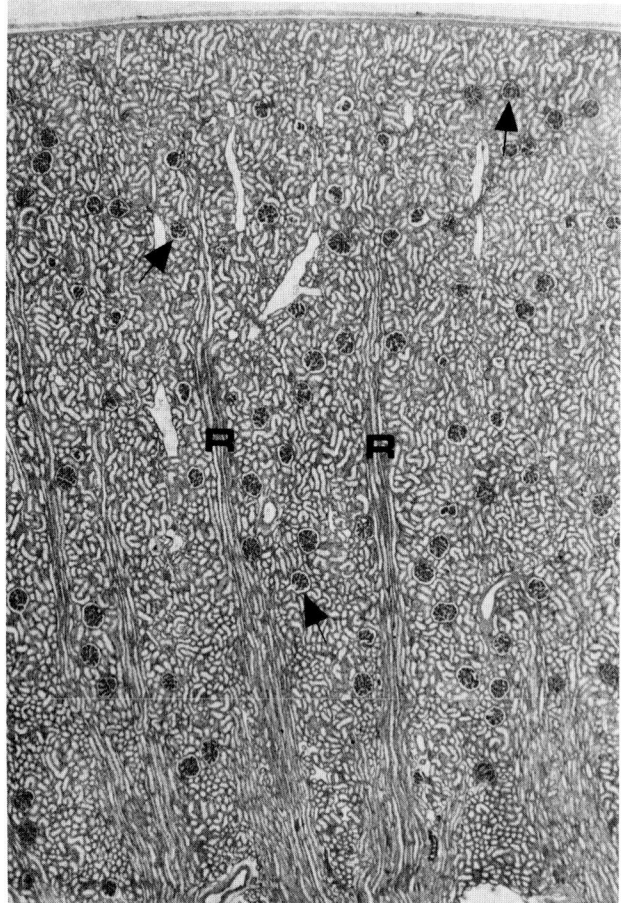

Fig. 20.3   Cortex of a canine kidney. Numerous glomeruli (*arrows*) are scattered throughout the cortex among profiles of tubules. The medullary rays (R) are prominent. X4.

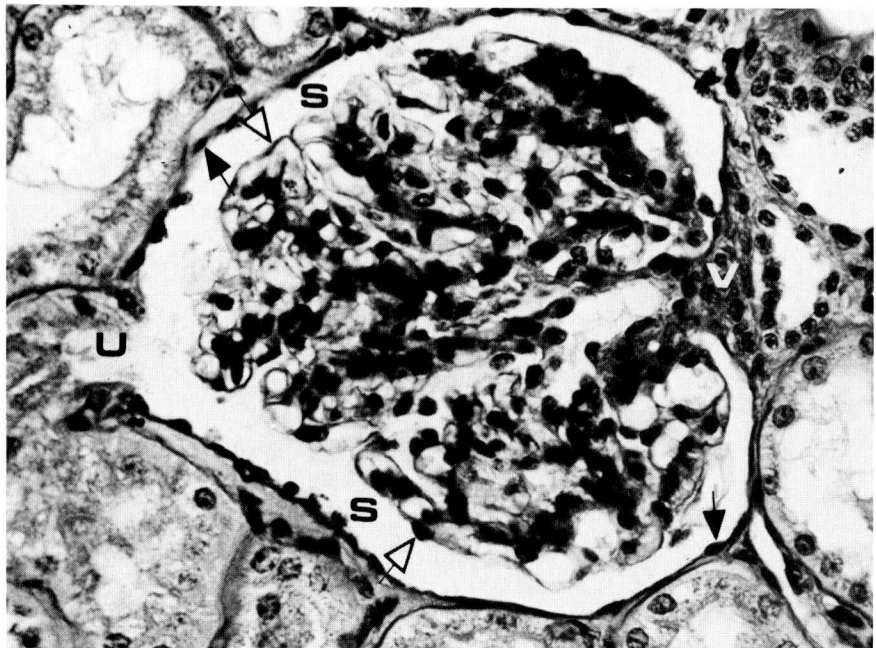

Fig. 20.4   A renal corpuscle from a canine kidney. The renal corpuscle consists of a Bowman's capsule and a glomerulus. Bowman's capsule is comprised of a parietal layer (*solid arrows*) and a visceral layer (*open arrows*) of cells separated by the uriniferous space (S). Vessels enter and leave the glomerulus at the vascular pole (V). The parietal layer of Bowman's capsule is continuous with the proximal convoluted tubule at the uriniferous pole (U). X100.

tube is composed of cells with prominer brush borders.

Loop of Henle. The proximal convolute tubule continues into the *loop of Henle.* Thi segment of the nephron is of variable lengt and the length is indicative of the ability c the organism to conserve water. The loop c Henle consists of three portions: the *straigh portion of the proximal tubule (descendin limb),* a *descending and ascending thin seg ment* and a *straight portion of the distal tubul (ascending limb).* There are some variation in the loop of Henle. Those nephrons in juxtamedullary position have long *interme diate segments* (thin segments) the apices o which are deep in the medulla and ma extend into the apices of the medullary pa pillae. Peripherally positioned nephron (subcapsular) have short loops of Henl which extend a short distance into the med ullary region. The transition from the cu boidal epithelium of the descending limb t the squamous epithelium of the *descendin thin segment* is abrupt. Because there ar numerous capillaries (blood and lymphatic in this region of the medulla, the microscop ist must look carefully to distinguish th thin segments. Usually, the thin segment have larger lumina and more nuclei tha protrude into the lumina than the capillar ies. The morphology of the actual *loop* (Fig 20.12) and *ascending thin segment* is simila to the descending thin segment. The transi tion to the cuboidal epithelium of the *as cending limb* is also abrupt. The straigh portion ascends to the region of the vascula pole of the glomerulus and is positioned between the afferent and efferent arterioles A condensation of cells in part of the wal of this tubule at this point is called the *macula densa.* The tubule continues from this point as the *distal convoluted tubule* (Fig 20.13).

Distal Convoluted Tubule. The distal tu bules are short and are not as frequently encountered in sections as their proximal counterparts. Although distal convoluted tu bules are not as large as proximal convo luted tubules, their luminal diameter to mu ral thickness ratios are greater than the prox imal convoluted tubules. More cells line these tubules and their lateral borders are more clearly defined than their proximal counterparts. These cells are less acidophilic than the cells of the proximal tubules. The nuclei of these cells are central to parabasal in position.

Collecting Duct System. The collecting duct system is composed of *arched (initial) col lecting tubules, straight collecting tubules* and *papillary ducts.* Arched collecting tubules connect the distal portions of the nephron, distal convoluted tubules, to the straight collecting tubules. Arched collecting tubules enter the straight tubules in the medullary rays of the cortex. The arched tubules are lined by cuboidal epithelial cells that stain lightly with routine staining techniques. Their nuclei are large and their cell borders

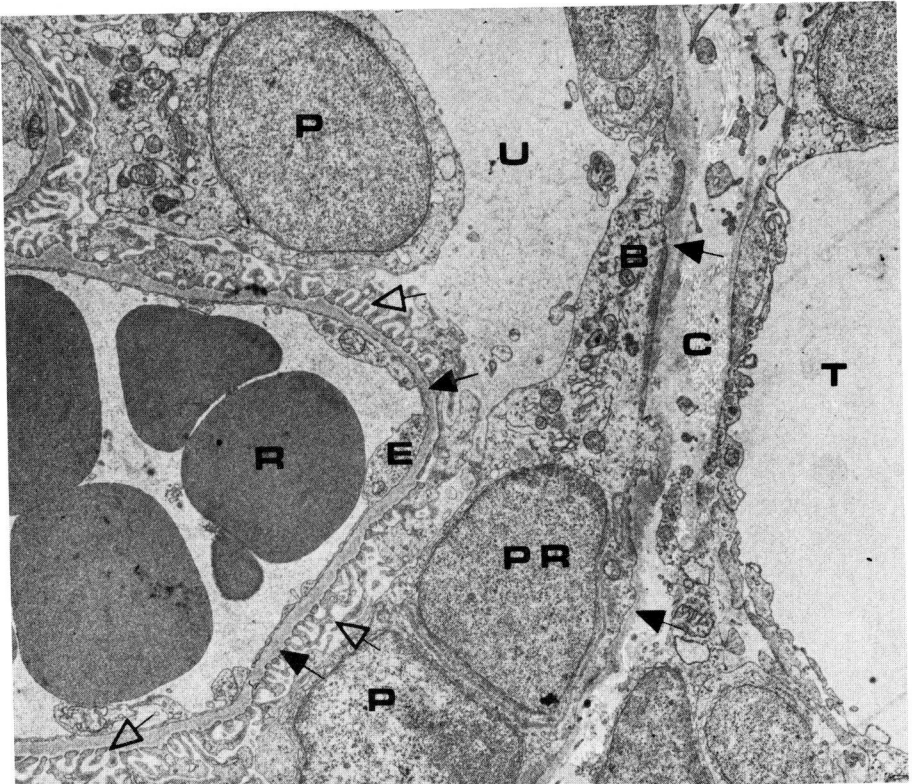

Fig. 20.5 An electron micrograph of a portion of a glomerulus. Numerous podocytes (P) are in close association with a capillary laden with erythrocytes (R). The podocyte processes, pedicles (*open arrows*), are adjacent to the well-developed basal lamina (*solid arrows*). One podocyte (PR) is reflected as the parietal layer of Bowman's capsule (B). The parietal layer is bounded by a basal lamina (*solid arrows*) and connective tissue (C). A portion of a uriniferous tubule (T) is adjacent to the renal corpuscle. E, endothelium. X6000.

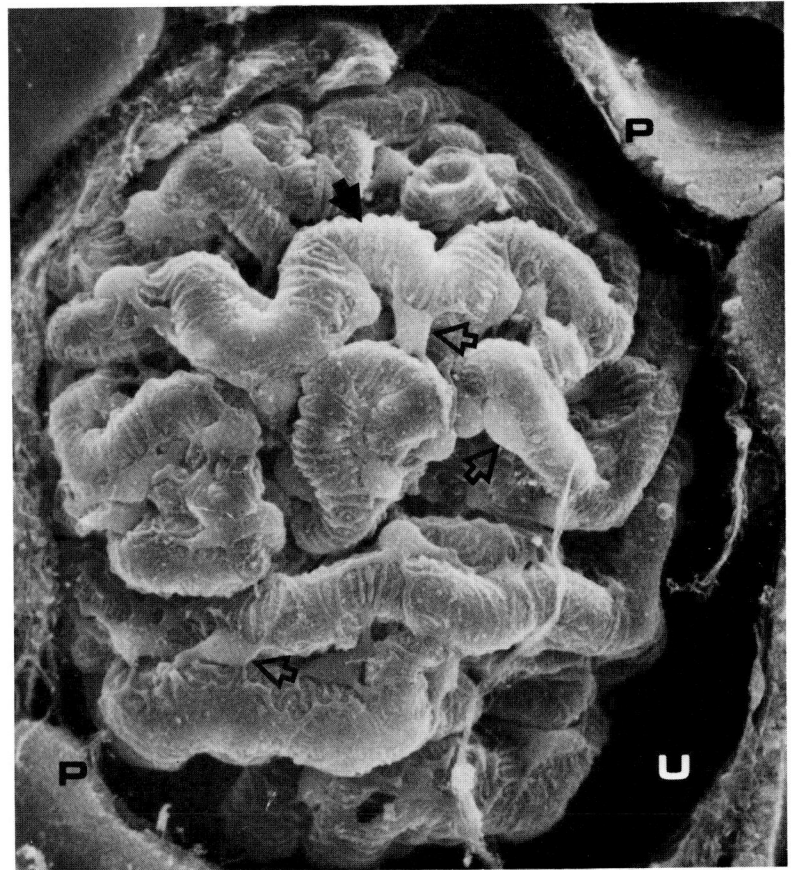

Fig. 20.6 A scanning electron micrograph of a freeze-fractured renal corpuscle of a canine kidney. The renal corpuscle consists of parietal (P) and visceral (*open arrows*) layers of cells separated by a uriniferous space (U). The capillaries (*solid arrow*) form a tuft or glomerulus of vessels. Note the unique morphology of the podocytes (*open arrows*) of the visceral layer of Bowman's capsule. X1000. (Courtesy of D. L. Eisenbrandt).

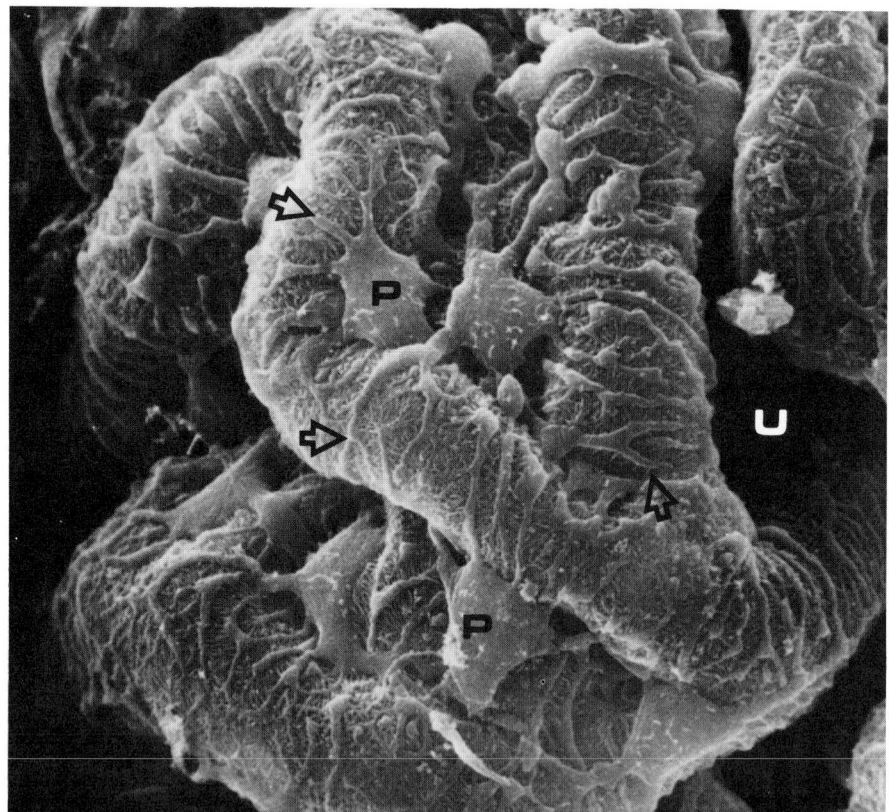

Fig. 20.7 A scanning electron micrograph of a freeze-fractured renal corpuscle of a canine kidney. Podocytes (P) have large or primary foot processes (*open arrows*) that are associated with the capillaries. Smaller foot processes (secondary foot processes) radiate from the primary foot processes and are separated by filtration slits. U, uriniferous space. X2000. (Courtesy of D. L. Eisenbrandt).

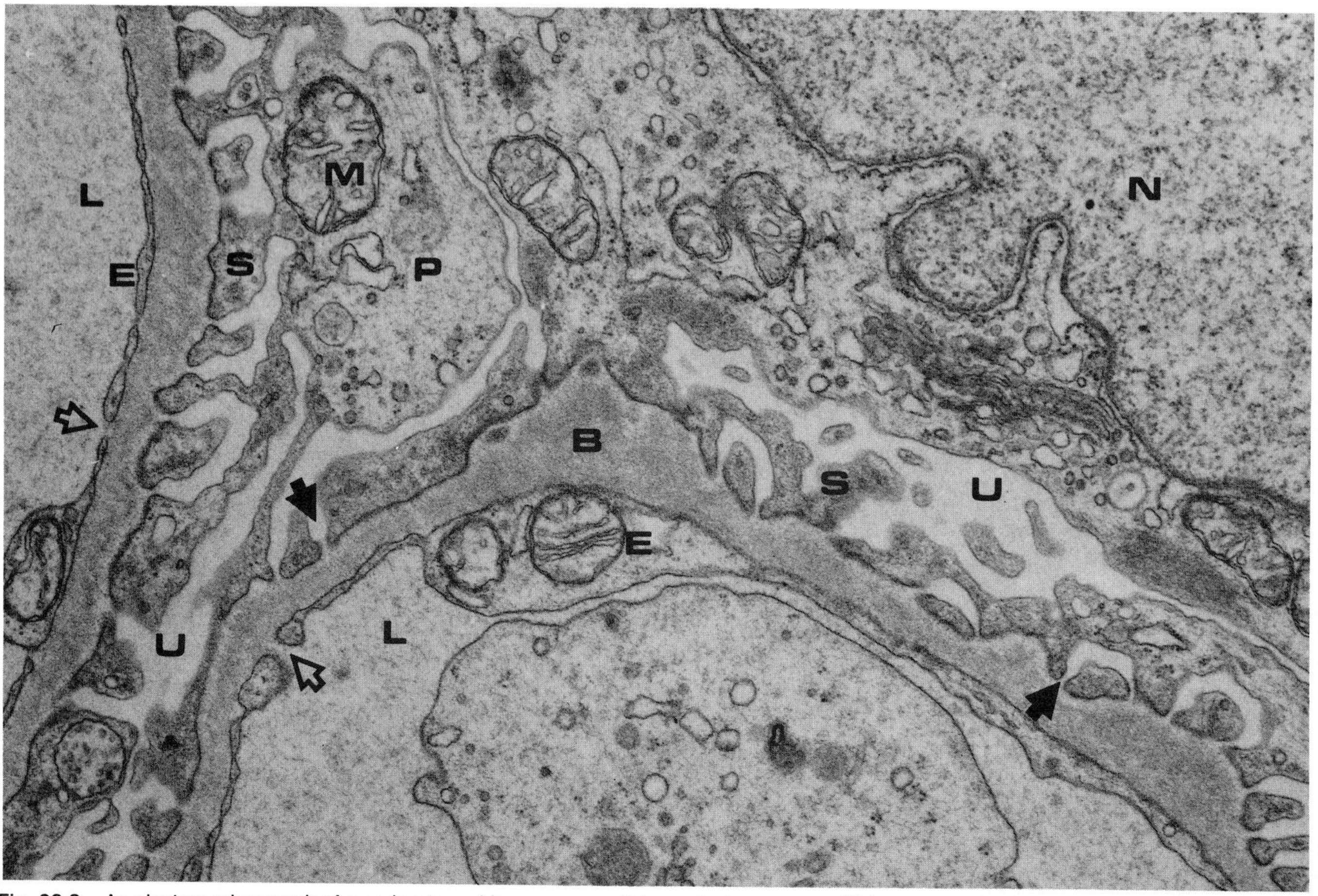

Fig. 20.8 An electron micrograph of a podocyte and its processes. Primary foot processes (P) have secondary foot processes (S) radiating from them. Filtration slits (*solid arrows*) and capillary (E) fenestrations (*open arrows*) are apparent. B, basal lamina; N, nucleus of podocyte; M, mitochondrion; L, capillary lumina; U, uriniferous space. X23,000.

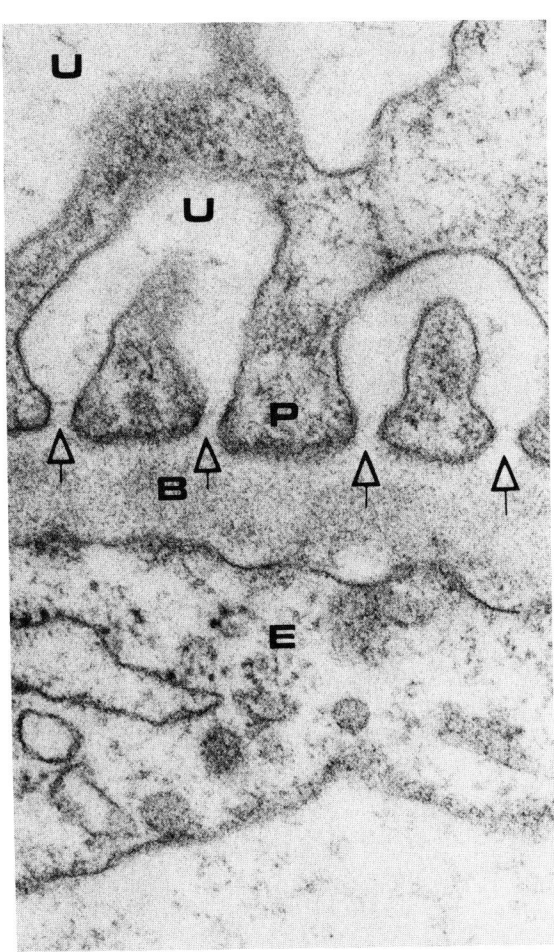

Fig. 20.9   An electron micrograph of podocytic processes. Large foot processes have small pedicels (P) radiating from them. The pedicels contact the basal lamina (B). Filtration slits (*open arrows*) separate adjacent pedicels. Filtration membranes are apparent (*left and right open arrows*). E, endothelium; U, uriniferous space. X77,000.

are distinct. The straight collecting tubules are similar to the arched tubules; however, the epithelium of the straight tubules is taller in the medullary region than their arched counterparts (Fig. 20.14). Straight tubules fuse within the inner zone of the medulla to form papillary ducts. The papillary ductal epithelium is columnar (Fig. 20.15). As the ducts open into the renal pelvis or minor calyses, the *area cribrosa* is formed at the apex of the pyramid or along the renal crest. The ductal epithelium is reflected as the transitional epithelial lining of the intrarenal continuation of the ureter.

Vascular, Lymphatic and Neural Relationships. The blood supply for the kidney is the *renal artery* (Fig. 20.16). Upon entering the hilus of the organ the renal artery divides into smaller *interlobar arteries*. The interlobar arteries, coursing parallel to the long axes of the pyramids, turn parallel to the long axis of the kidney at the corticomedullary junction and are continued as the *arcuate* or *arciform arteries*.

The blood supply to the cortex is achieved through ascending or perpendicular branches of the arcuate artery, the *interlobular arteries*. The interlobular arteries course through the cortical labyrinth giving rise to numerous short lateral branches, the *afferent arterioles*. The afferent arterioles may be considered *intralobular arterioles*. The afferent arterioles enter the vascular pole of Bowman's capsule and divide into large capillary branches, the *glomerulus*. The capillaries of the glomerulus form a loop and reunite as the *efferent arteriole* which exits Bowman's capsule at the vascular pole (Figs. 20.2, 20.10). (*N.B.: The capillary bed of the glomerulus is within the arterial circulation.*) The efferent arteriole then divides into a capillary bed which forms a *peritubular plexus* around the uriniferous tubules of the cortex.

The medullary blood supply is derived from efferent arterioles originating from renal corpuscles close to the medulla. The vessels extending from these efferent arterioles descend into the medulla along straight paths and are called *false straight arterioles* (*arteriolae rectae spuriae*). Vessels originating from the arcuate arteries to supply the medulla are called *true straight arterioles* (*arteriolae rectae verae*). Capillary branches of these arterioles enmesh and surround the medullary uriniferous tubules and form a *peritubular plexus*. The arterioles (*arteriolae rectae*), capillaries and venules (*venae rectae*) comprise the *vasa recta*.

The interlobular arteries continue to the surface and terminate as a capsular plexus.

The venous drainage of the kidney is accomplished through companion vessels to the aforementioned arteries and their branches.

Lymphatic drainage of the kidney is accomplished by two sets of lymph vessels. A superficial set of lymph vessels drains the capsular area, whereas a deeper set of vessels, distributed in an manner similar to the blood vessels, drains the renal interstitium.

The innervation of the kidney is achieved by the autonomic nervous system. Many of the unmyelinated nerves are vasomotor branches of the sympathetic division. The glomerular arterioles are well-innervated. Some branches of the nerves are associated intimately with the tubular epithelial cells. General visceral afferent fibers originate in the capsule, pelvis or calyses and perivascular region. The precise distribution of parasympathetic fibers to and within the kidney has not been determined.

Juxtaglomerular Complex

Histologic Components. The *juxtaglomerular complex* or *apparatus* consists of three components: juxtaglomerular cells, polkissen cells and macula densa (Fig. 20.17). The *juxtaglomerular cells* are myoepithelioid cells that replace the smooth muscle of the wall of the afferent arteriole as the vessel approaches the vascular pole. While *granular juxtaglomerular cells* predominate, some *agranular juxtaglomerular cells* contribute to the myoepithelioid cuff. One pole of the juxtaglomerular cells contacts the basal lamina associated with the endothelial cells of the afferent arterial, whereas the other pole contacts the basal lamina associated with the epithelial cells of the macula densa in the distal convoluted tubule. The *polkissen cells* are extra-glomerular mesangial cells situated between the afferent and efferent arterioles adjacent to the glomerulus. The precise function of the polkissen cells (*lacis cells, polar cushion*) is not understood. The *macula densa* is a part of the distal convoluted tubule characterized by tall epithelial cells crowded together along that portion of the duct adjacent to the vascular pole (Fig. 20.18). The precise functional relationships of the components of the juxtaglomerular complex have not been determined.

Functional Correlates. Despite the uncertainty concerning the integrated functioning of the components of the juxtaglomerular complex, insights about some of the components are available. The granular juxtaglomerular cells secrete the proteolytic enzyme *renin*. Renin converts *angiotensinogen*, a plasma protein in the α_2-globulin fraction, to *angiotensin I*. Activation of angiotensin I to *angiotensin* II occurs in the lungs and

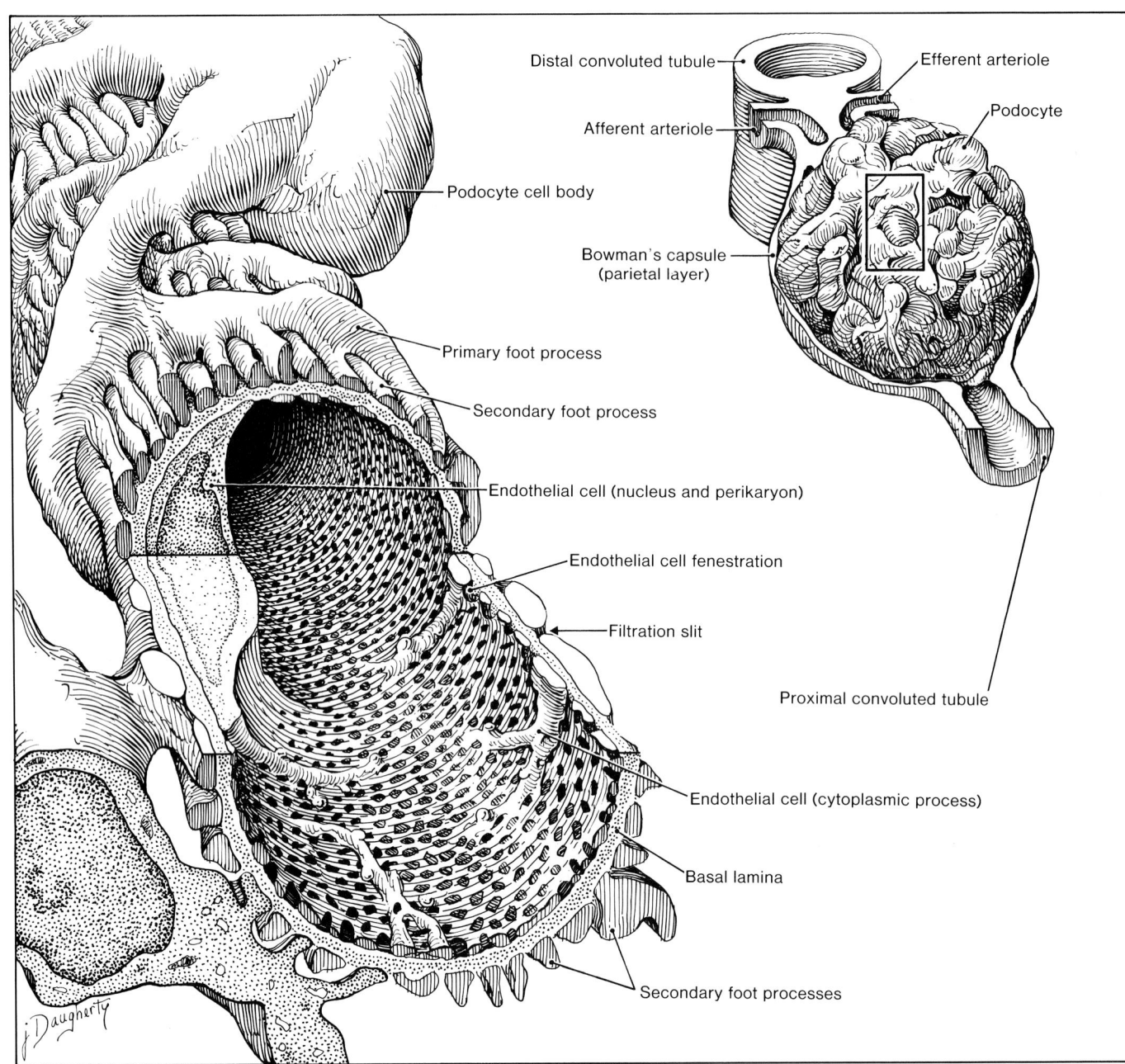

Distal convoluted tubule

Efferent arteriole

Afferent arteriole

Podocyte

Podocyte cell body

Bowman's capsule
(parietal layer)

Primary foot process

Secondary foot process

Endothelial cell (nucleus and perikaryon)

Endothelial cell fenestration

Filtration slit

Proximal convoluted tubule

Endothelial cell (cytoplasmic process)

Basal lamina

Secondary foot processes

J. Daugherty

Fig. 20.10   A diagram of the renal corpuscle and podocytes as visualized with the scanning electron microscope.

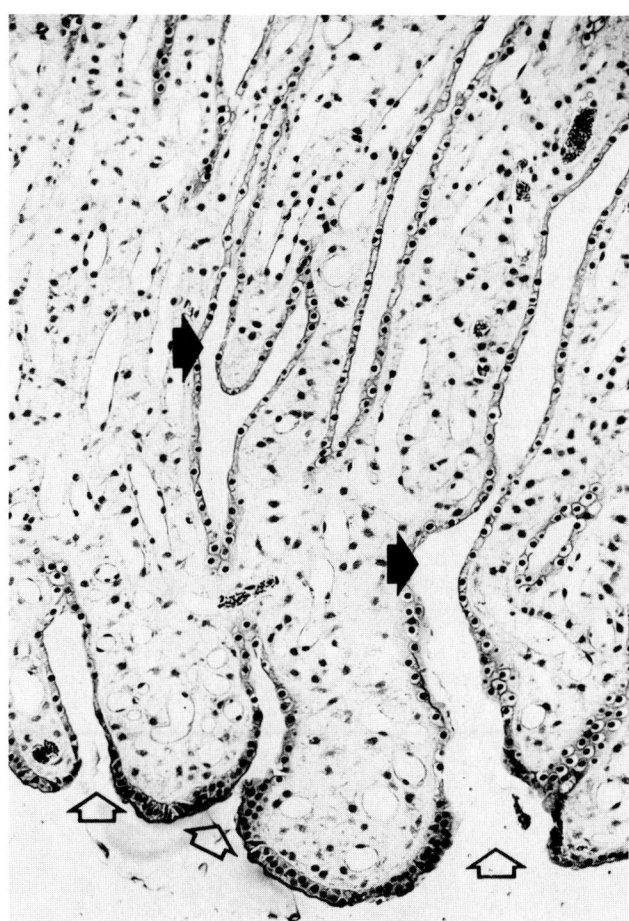

Fig. 20.15   Area cribrosa of the feline kidney. The collecting ducts become confluent as papillary ducts (*solid arrows*). These ducts open into the renal pelvis (*open arrows*) and form an area ribrosa. X40.

active metabolites of vitamin D), an increased GFR increases the clearance of calcium and phosphate. Parathormone also increases calcium reabsorption while blocking phosphate reabsorption in the proximal convoluted tubule. The resulting increased urinary phosphate (*phosphaturia*) excretion enhances the elevation of blood calcium.

The movements of water, ammonia, sodium, chloride, potassium, bicarbonate, urea and hydrogen ions are essential components of countercurrent and/or acid/base mechanisms. Their contributions to these processes is discussed subsequently.

Countercurrent Mechanism. The *countercurrent mechanism* is predicated upon the maintenance of an osmolality gradient that is established from the base of the pyramid to the apex of the pyramid (papilla) (Fig. 20.19). The base of the pyramid (interstitium, tubules and vasa recta) is *isosmolar* compared to blood (300 mOsm), whereas the apex is approximately 4x more concentrated (*hyperosmolar*) or 1200 mOsm. The loop of Henle, the *countercurrent multiplier*, establishes the gradient by virtue of its permeability characteristics, juxtaposition of descending and ascending components and the direction of the flow of urine within the tubules. The inflow in the descending limb runs parallel and counter to the outflow in the ascending limb. The operation of the countercurrent mechanism is explained by various theories: the following satisfies many of the observations made. The descending limb of the loop of Henle, although, relatively impermeable to most solutes, permits the movement of water into the interstitium. The ascending limb of Henle's loop is impermeable to water but allows free movement of sodium into the interstitium. This relationship, alone, establishes an increasing tonicity toward the hairpin loop in the descending limb and interstitium and a decreasing tonicity from the hairpin loop up the ascending limb and interstitium. The transport of sodium, linked to the active transport of chloride in the thick segment of the ascending limb, produces a hypotonic tubular fluid in this segment. Sodium may be actively transported out of the convoluted tubule and collecting duct. Sodium also may be passively transported out of the collecting duct, whereas water moves passively into the interstitium in the distal convoluted tubule and collecting duct.

Urea also contributes to the concentration gradient. Urea reabsorption is dependent upon the rate of urine flow and tubular urine concentration. The concentration of urea increases toward the apex of the loop of Henle, both within the tubules and the medullary interstitium. The gradient is dependent upon the recirculation from the collecting duct into the interstitium and then into the ascending and descending limbs of Henle's loop. The dynamic and constant circulation of urea assures a high concentra-

to the amount filtered because of tubular reabsorption. An increased BUN may indicate abnormal kidney function; however, other factors may cause an increased BUN—increased dietary protein intake, increased protein catabolism, decreased renal perfusion, postrenal obstruction. *Prerenal*, *renal* and *postrenal* problems may result in an elevated BUN.

Urea tends to concentrate in the renal interstitium, and is especially concentrated at the apex of the pyramids. The graded concentration of urea within the medullary pyramids contributes to the ability of the kidney to concentrate other solutes in the urine.

Despite the urine being an ultrafiltrate of plasma, small amounts of low molecular weight *proteins* (albumin) are constituents of the filtrate. Most of the filtered protein is reabsorbed by the tubular epithelial cells. Protein in the urine (*proteinuria*) may result from a decreased capacity of tubular resorption or tubular damage, but most proteinuria is a consequence of altered glomerular filtration.

Tubular Secretion. Tubular secretory mechanisms complement the clearance of substances that are filtered at the glomerulus.

The substances secreted include not only those compounds produced endogenously (creatinine, histamine and metabolic products of hormones) but also exogenously administered compounds and their metabolic products (antibiotics, aspirin, various other drugs). Additionally, water, various cations (H^+, K^+, Na^+) and anions (HCO_3^-, $PO_4^{\equiv}$) pass into the tubular lumen by active or passive mechanisms.

Whereas separate mechanisms are utilized by the kidney for the reabsorption of various substances, only two distinct processes are used for the tubular secretion of organic compounds. Both processes are part of the active transport by the proximal convoluted tubular epithelium. One system secretes *organic acids* and the other system secretes *organic bases*. Each system has a maximal capacity, and compounds within each group compete with each other. Creatinine, having amphoteric properties, is secreted by both mechanisms.

Phosphate ions, reabsorbed by the proximal convoluted tubule, may be resecreted by the distal convoluted tubule under certain physiologic conditions. Under the influence of hypocalcemia and the release of parathormone (and probably some of the

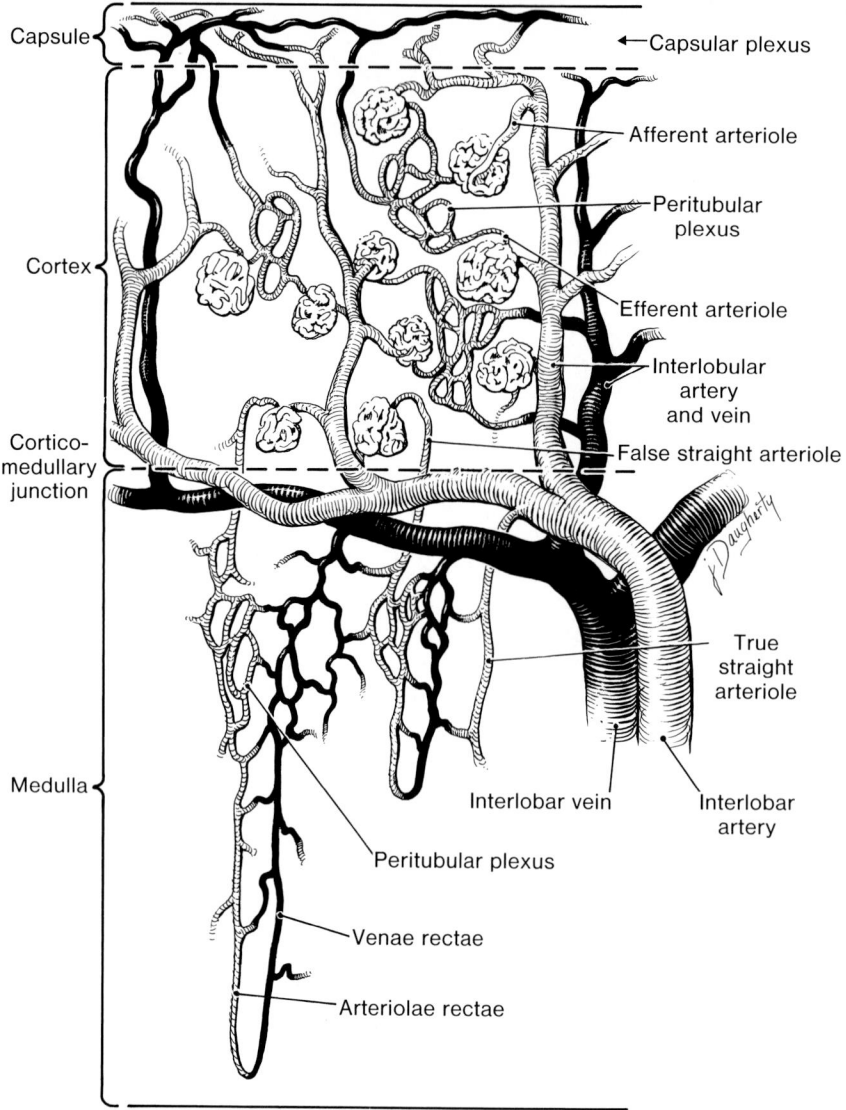

Fig. 20.16 A diagram depicting the vascular supply of the kidney.

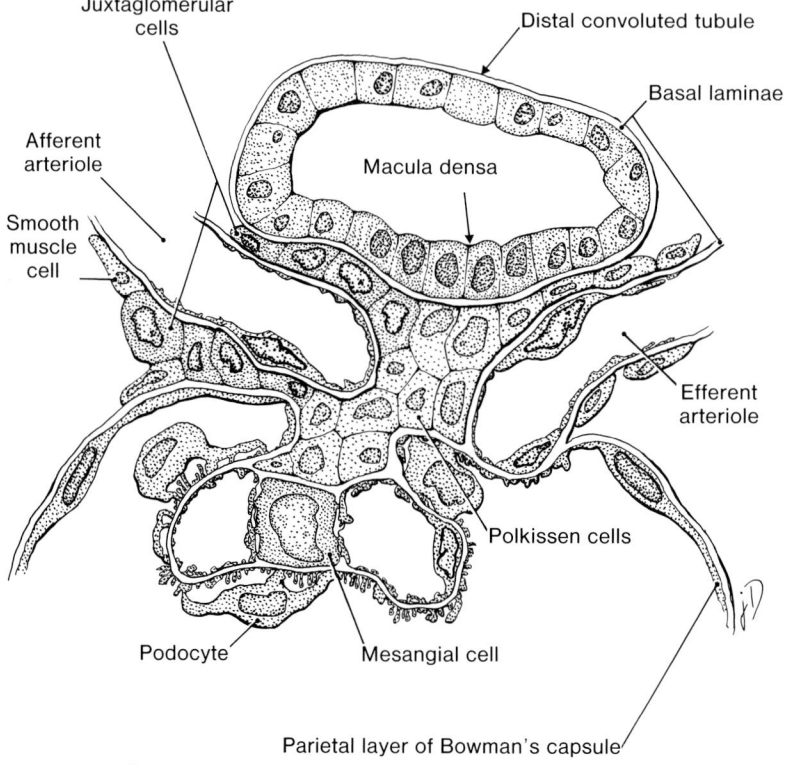

Fig. 20.17 A diagram of the juxtaglomerular apparatus.

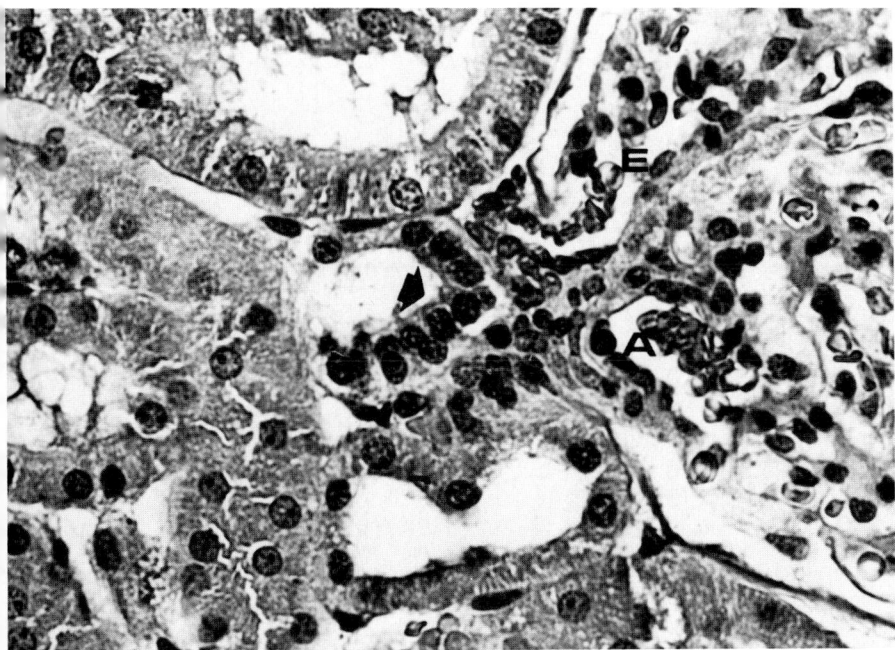

Fig. 20.18 Macula densa of a canine kidney. The macula densa (*arrow*) marks the beginning of the distal convoluted tubule. The macula densa is positioned at the vascular pole in close association with the afferent (A) and efferent (E) arterioles. The cells between the afferent arteriole, efferent arteriole and macula densa are polkissen cells. X160.

tion of the compound in the urine and aids in increasing the sodium and chloride concentrations of the inner medulla.

The vasa recta contribute to the countercurrent mechanism as *countercurrent exchangers*. Water diffuses out of the arteriolae rectae while sodium and urea move down their concentration gradients into the vessels. Conversely, water diffuses into the venae rectae while solutes (sodium, urea) move into the interstitium. The fluids within the tip of the basa recta are in equilibrium with the hairpin loop of Henle and interstitium. The recirculation phenomenon maintains the tubular, vascular and interstitial gradient. The meager and retarded flow of blood through the medulla assists in the maintenance of the gradient.

The establishment of the medullary gradient, a tubular function, occurs passively and is attributed to the selective permeability of the tubular epithelium. Evidence exists that the passive movement of sodium occurs with the active transport of chloride in the ascending thick segment of Henle's loop. The maintenance of the gradient, a vascular function, occurs passively.

The maintenance of proper tissue fluid and blood osmolality is essential for proper cellular function. Hyperosmolar tissue fluid and blood draw fluids from cells, thereby decreasing cellular volume. Hypotonic extracellular fluids cause fluids to move into cells, increasing cellular volume. Both situations impair cellular function. The countercurrent multiplier and exchanger mechanism provides a mechanism to conserve water and sodium. The reabsorption of wa-

ter in the proximal convoluted tubule accounts for approximately 80% of the filtered fluid volume; the loop of Henle reabsorbs about 5%. Another 14% is reabsorbed in the distal convoluted tubule and collecting ducts under the influence of *antidiuretic hormone* (*ADH*). The remaining 1% is the fluid volume of the excreted urine.

The proximal convoluted tubule accounts for the reabsorption of 80% of the filtered sodium, while the loop of Henle reabsorbs 17% of filtered sodium. The remaining 3% is reabsorbed in the distal convoluted tubule and collecting duct under the influence of *aldosterone*.

The tonicity of the urine may be altered by numerous factors. The imbibition of excessive quantities of water increases extracellular fluid volume and results in cellular swelling. Hypothalamic cells (*osmoreceptor cells*) respond to the increased fluid volume by decreasing ADH secretion. In the absence of ADH, the distal convoluted tubule and collecting duct become impermeable to water resulting in the excretion of a dilute (hypotonic) urine. Conversely, a decreased fluid volume, resulting in the release of ADH, is characterized by a low volume and hypertonic urine. Animals with *diabetes insipidus* are unable to produce ADH or proper quantities of the hormone; they characteristically produce large volumes of dilute urine (*polyuria*). To compensate for the urinary fluid loss, they must ingest large quantities of water (*polydipsia*). Polyuria is not always characterized by a hypotonic urine. The retention of osmotically active substances within the tubules causes the re-

tention of water also. Exceeding the glucose threshold, as occurs in *diabetes mellitus*, results in a hypertonic high volume urine. Glucose causes an *osmotic diuresis*, whereas ADH insufficiency results in a *water diuresis*; however, polydipsia is a compensatory mechanism for both.

Acid/Base Balance. The maintenance of the pH of the internal environment is essential for optimal cellular functions. Deviations from normal pH result in altered metabolic processes by accelerating or depressing enzymatic activity. The animal body is exposed to large quantities of acids daily. Carbon dioxide, the primary metabolic product, results in the formation of acid;

$$CO_2 + H_2O \rightleftharpoons H_2CO_3 \rightleftharpoons H^+ + HCO_3^-$$

Other acids are components of the diet or result from metabolism (sulfate, phosphate, lactate, hydrochloric acid, beta-hydroxybutyrate). Various mechanisms are utilized by the body to neutralize excess acids or bases. The lungs, through normal gaseous exchange, rid the body of excess carbon dioxide. Buffer systems (carbonate, phosphate, protein, hemoglobin) serve to neutralize excess acids and bases. Also, the kidney functions to excrete or conserve acids and bases. The normal pH of the urine varies among species and individuals within a species. The normal pH of the urine of carnivores is acidic, whereas that of herbivores is alkaline; the pH of the urine of omnivores (swine, man) may be acidic or alkaline. Numerous factors (diet, metabolism, disease) can alter urinary pH.

Deviations from normal blood pH, which is usually about 7.4, occur under various circumstances. *Hyperventilation*, the excessive loss of carbon dioxide through the lungs, causes a *respiratory alkalosis*, whereas *hypoventilation*, the inadequate elimination of carbon dioxide through the lungs, results in a *respiratory acidosis*. *Metabolic acidosis* may result from various conditions that cause a loss of base (diarrhea, vomiting) or an increased production of acid (ketoacidosis). *Metabolic alkalosis* may result from vomiting in which only gastric contents are lost. Similarly, metabolic alkalosis may result from the sequestration of acids in the stomach as occurs in abomasal displacements and other abomasal disorders. The lungs and kidneys function significantly to compensate acidotic and alkalotic conditions. In acidotic conditions, the kidney compensates by secreting excess hydrogen ion and conserving base (HCO_3^-). In alkalotic conditions, the reverse occurs. However, a *paradoxic aciduria* does accompany some metabolic alkalotic conditions (canine vomiting, bovine abomasal displacements). The need to conserve electrolytes (Na^+, K^+, Cl^-) may be considered a more important renal function than the conservation of H^+ under these circumstances.

The secretion of hydrogen ion is achieved by the epithelium of the proximal and distal

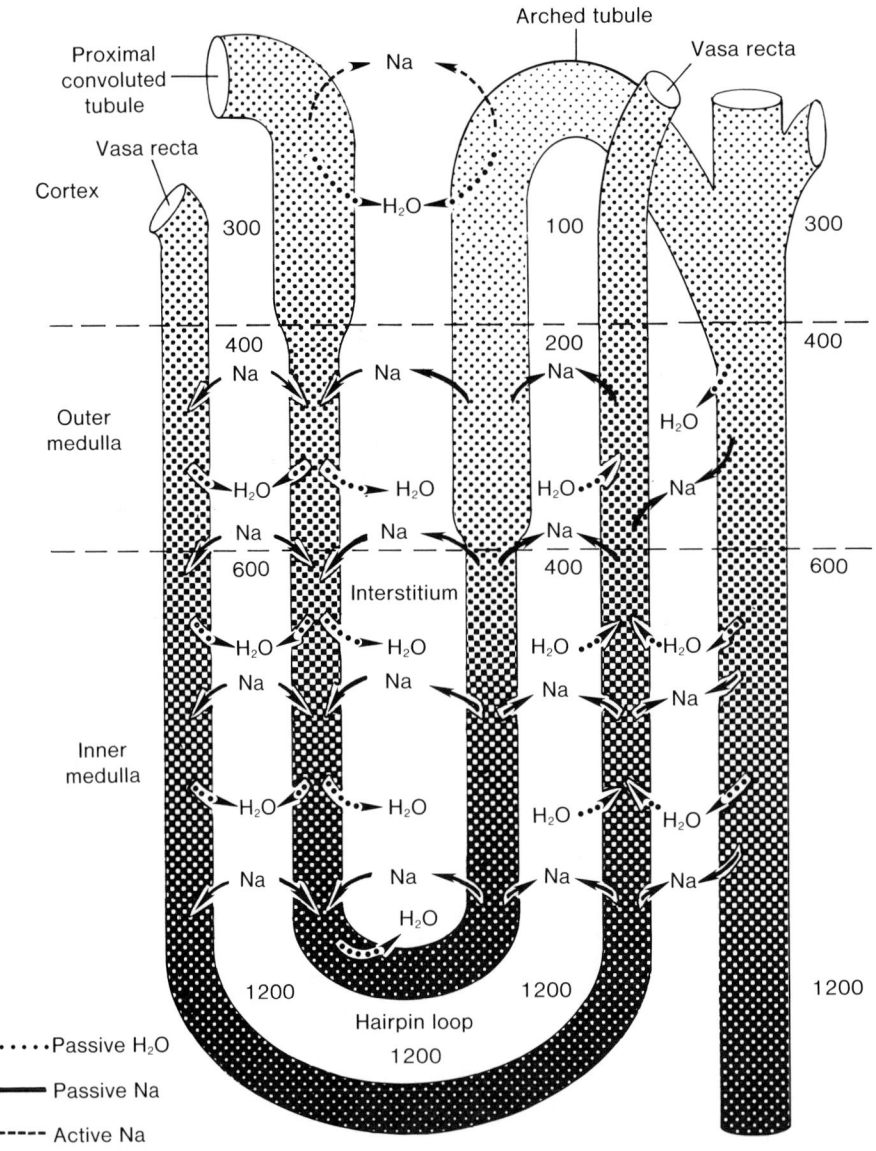

Fig. 20.19   A simplified diagram depicting the movement of water and sodium as it relates to the countercurrent mechanism. The concentration of urine within the collecting tubules, as illustrated, occurs under the influence of ADH. Other solutes, notably urea, contribute to the gradient. The gradient, as depicted, 300–1200 milliosmols, is not the same in all species; however, the relationships are similar. The gradient within the interstitium is similar to that noted for the tubules and vessels. Tubular urine becomes progressively more concentrated toward the hairpin loop, decreases to a hypotonic urine in the thick segment of the ascending limb and becomes hypertonic in the collecting duct system under the influence of ADH.

convoluted tubules in a manner similar to that used by the parietal cell (Fig. 19.42). The active transport (secretion) of H$^+$ is associated with the passive uptake of Na$^+$. The secretion of one H$^+$ is linked to the movement of Na$^+$ into the interstitium and K$^+$ into the cell (Na$^+$–K$^+$ pump); a bicarbonate moves out of the cell into the interstitium also.

Although the transport mechanism for H$^+$ is active, a limiting concentration exists beyond which the transport mechanism does not work. Free hydrogen ions are "removed" from the urine by reacting with HCO$_3^-$, HPO$_4^=$ and NH$_3$ (ammonia). Hydrogen ions react with tubular HCO$_3^-$ to form carbonic acid (H$_2$CO$_3$). Carbonic an-

hydrase on the brush border of the proximal convoluted tubular epithelial cells catalyzes the conversion of H$_2$CO$_3$ to CO$_2$ and H$_2$O, and effectively removes hydrogen from the tubular fluid. Carbon dioxide diffuses into the cell and becomes part of the available CO$_2$ to form more H$_2$CO$_3$. The intercellular dissociation of H$_2$CO$_3$ into HCO$_3^-$ and H$^+$ is facilitated by carbonic anhydrase. The HCO$_3^-$ diffuses into the extracellular fluid and the H$^+$ is secreted actively into the tubular lumen. Combination of H$^+$ with HPO$_4^=$ in the distal convoluted tubules and collecting ducts removes H$^+$ from the tubular urine. Finally, ammonia (NH$_3$) is formed within all of the tubular epithelial cells by the activity of enzymes associated with the

removal of amines from amino acids. The NH$_3$, because of its lipid-solubility, flows freely across the plasmalemmal barrier into the lumina of the tubules. Once within the tubular fluid, NH$_3$ reacts with H$^+$ to form NH$_4^+$ (ammonium ion). Because of its charge, NH$_4^+$ remains in the tubular urine. The amount of NH$_4^+$ in urine depends upon the amount of H$^+$ secreted. Ammonium ion concentration is high in acid urine and virtually zero in alkaline urine. These mechanisms facilitate the secretion of H$^+$ by the kidneys.

Although the mechanisms described previously account for H$^+$ secretion, the reactivity of H$^+$ with HCO$_3^-$, HPO$_4^=$ and NH$_3$ are important mechanisms for base conser-

ation. During periods of excess H⁺ secretion, an increase in detectable (titratable)
urinary acids occurs (H⁺, $H_2PO_4^-$ and
NH_4^+) when the body has a need for more
HCO_3^- to neutralize the excess acidity. The
formation of H_2CO_3 within the tubule, its
conversion to CO_2 and H_2O and subsequent
reabsorption by the tubular cells returns the
base (HCO_3^-) to the somatic pool. The formation of titratable acids also serves to conserve sodium. The ammonium ion replaces
Na⁺ that may be exchanged while a H⁺ is
excreted.

Urinary Passages

Renal Pelvis. The inner surface of the renal
pelvis is continuous with the epithelial lining of the papillary ducts. The epithelium
becomes a thin transitional lining that
becomes thicker toward the pelvis. The lamina propria-tunica submucosa is composed
of areolar connective tissue. In equids,
branched tubuloalveolar mucous glands occur in this region and extend into the ureter.
These glands account for the frothy appearance of the urine of these species. The tunica
muscularis may be composed of three layers
of muscle which are arranged in bundles.
The layers, however, are not always distinct.
The contraction of these muscle bundles
tends to "milk" urine from the kidney.

Ureters. The ureters are lined by a lamina
epithelialis of transitional epithelium (Fig.
20.20). Goblet cells may be present in the
horse. The lamina propria-tunica submucosa consists of areolar connective tissue.
Mucous glands may be present in some
species (Fig. 20.21). The tunica muscularis
is present and three layers of muscle may be
apparent. The tunica adventitia, also, is
present and typical. Part of this structure is
covered by a tunica serosa (peritoneum).

Urinary Bladder. The ureters open obliquely
into the bladder near the neck and the longitudinal coat of the tunica muscularis continues into the bladder wall. There is very
little circularly oriented muscle at this junction. Pressure within the bladder tends to
close the orifice. The contractions of the
ureteral musculature tend to spurt urine into
the bladder.

The mural elements of the bladder are
similar to those of the ureter.

The tunica mucosa of the ureters and the
bladder may be highly folded. At this time,
the lamina epithelialis will be thick (Fig.
20.16). Upon distention of the bladder, the
transitional epithelium is reduced in thickness and the mucosal folds are effaced (Fig.
20.17).

The urethrae are discussed with their respective reproductive systems.

Micturition. *Micturition (urination)*, the passage of urine from the bladder to the exterior
of the body, is a spinal reflex that may be
facilitated and/or inhibited by higher brain
centers. The parasympathetic innervation to

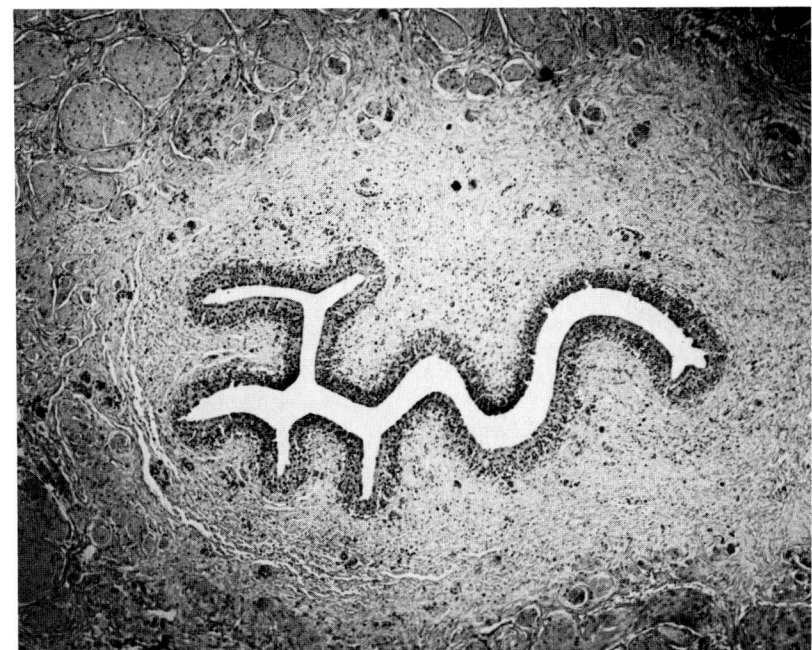

Fig. 20.20 Canine ureter. The ureter is lined by transitional epithelium. The lamina propria-
submucosa is extensive and surrounded by smooth muscle. X4.

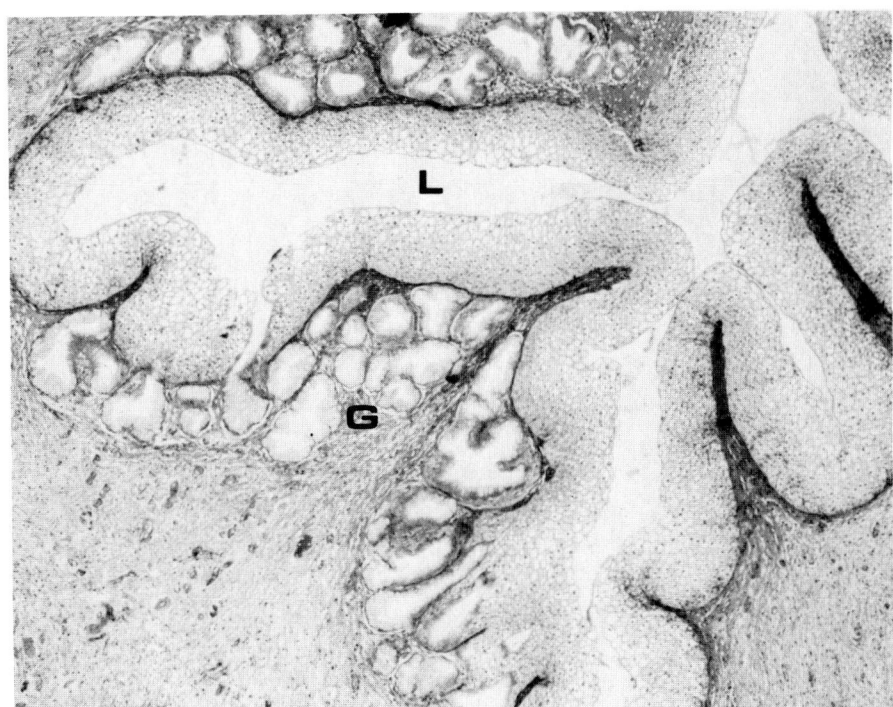

Fig. 20.21 A section of part of an equine ureter. The lumen (L) is lined by transitional epithelium.
Note the mucous glands (G) in the lamina propria. X25.

the smooth muscle of the bladder (GVE) is
derived from neurons the cell bodies of
which are located in the sacral segments (S_1,
S_2) of the spinal cord. Their axons traverse
the pelvic nerve and plexus. The parasympathetic fibers are stimulatory to the smooth

muscle. Sympathetic innervation to the
smooth muscle of the bladder (GVE) is from
the lumbar portion of the spinal cord via the
hypogastric nerve. Sympathetic nerves are
inhibitory to bladder smooth muscle. The
urethral musculature, which is skeletal mus-

cle, is innervated by GSE fibers of the pudendal nerve. General visceral afferent fibers (GVA), with stretch receptor terminals in the wall of the bladder, synapse with sacral lower motor neurons and ascend to higher brain centers to achieve conscious perceptive levels.

Inhibitory sympathetic fibers permit filling of the bladder, whereas conscious inhibition is achieved by contraction of the urethral musculature. After appropriate stimulation of stretch receptors, reflex emptying of the bladder occurs via stimulation by the parasympathetic nerves; however, voluntary inhibition can be achieved by contraction of the urethral musculature.

Damage to the sacral segments of the spinal cord may result in an *autonomous bladder* which is devoid of extrinsic stimulatory innervation and sensation. Voluntary control is lost and urine flow results from bladder overflow. Residual bladder volume is high. An *automatic bladder* results when damage occurs to the nervous system cranial to the sacral spinal segments. The reflex arc remains intact, but voluntary control is lost. Residual bladder volume is low.

References

Andrews, P. M. and Porter, K. R.: A scanning electron microscope study of the nephron. Am. J. Anat. *140:*81, 1974.

Barajas, L.: The ultrastructure of the juxtaglomerular apparatus as disclosed by three dimensional reconstructions from serial sections. J. Ultrastruct. Res. *33:*116, 1970.

Beeuwkes, R. and Bonventre, J. V.: Tubular organization and vascular tubular relations in the dog kidney. Am. J. Physiol. *229:*695, 1975.

Calhoun, M. L.: Comparative histology of the ureters of domestic animals. Anat. Rec. *133:*365, 1959.

Christensen, G. C.: Circulation of blood through the canine kidney. Am. J. Vet. Res. *13:*236, 1952.

Dalton, A. J. and Haguenau, F. (eds.): *Ultrastructure of the Kidney*, Vol. 2. Academic Press, New York, 1967.

Dicker, S. E.: *Mechanisms of Urine Concentration and Dilution in Mammals*. Arnold, London, 1970.

Fisher, E. R.: Lysosomal nature of juxtaglomerular granules. Science. *152:*1752, 1966.

Gans, J. H. and Mercer, P. F.: The kidneys. *In*: Swenson, M. J. (editor) 9th edition. *Duke's Physiology of Domestic Animals*. pp. 463–492, Comstock Publishing, Ithaca, 1977.

Gingerich, D. A. and Murdick, P. W.: Paradoxic aciduria in bovine metabolic acidosis. J. Am. Vet. Med. Assoc. *166:*227, 1975.

Grahame, T.: The pelvis and calyses of the kidneys of some mammals. Brit. Vet. J. *109:*51, 1953.

Jorgensen, F.: Electron microscopic studies of normal visceral epithelial cells. Lab. Invest. *17:*225, 1967.

Kaneko, J. J. and Cornelius, C. E.: *Clinical Biochemistry of Domestic Animals*. Vol. 2. 2nd edition, Academic Press, New York, 1971.

Latta, H.: The glomerular capillary wall. J. Ultrastruct. Res. *32:*526, 1970.

Latta, H., Johnston, W. H. and Stanley, T. M.: Sialoglycoproteins and filtration barriers in the glomerular capillary wall. J. Ultrastruct. Res. *51:*354, 1975.

Monis, B. and Zambrano, D.: Transitional epithelium of urinary tract in normal and dehydrated rats. Z. Zellforsch. *85:*165, 1968.

Osawa, G., Kimmelsteil, P. and Seiling, V.: Thickness of glomerular basement membranes. Amer. J. Clin. Path. *45:*7, 1966.

Osborne, C. A., Low, D. G. and Finco, D. R.: *Canine and Feline Urology*. W. B. Saunders, Philadelphia, 1972.

Pease, D. C.: Electron microscopy of the tubular cells of the kidney cortex. Anat. Rec. *121:*723, 1955.

Woodburne, R. T.: The sphincter mechanism of the urinary bladder and the urethra. Anat. Rec. *141:*11, 1961.

21: Respiratory System

General Characteristics

Form and Function. The respiratory system consists of organs that accomplish the primary functions of *conduction* and *exchange* of gaseous substances. Predicated upon the two primary functions, the respiratory system may be subdivided into three main components: conductive, transitional and exchange components (Fig. 21.1). The *conductive components* of the airways extend from the external nares and include the *nasal cavity, paranasal sinuses, nasopharynx, larynx, trachea, extrapulmonary bronchi, intrapulmonary bronchi* and *bronchioles*. A *transitional component* is present in some animals and consists of *respiratory bronchioles*—structures which conduct and exchange gases. The *exchange component* consists of *alveolar ducts, alveolar sacs* and *alveoli*. Although conduction occurs within the exchange components, the primary function is the exchange of gases.

Numerous ancillary functions are achieved by the respiratory system: *phonation, olfaction, body temperature regulation, excretion.* The lungs are important organs in *acid/base balance.* Also, *blood pressure* is influenced by the activation of angiotensin I to angiotensin II by converting enzyme within the lung and other organs. Numerous active substances (histamine, prostaglandins E and F, kallikrein) are produced by the lungs for release into the circulation. Similarly, other active substances (prostaglandins E and F, serotonin, bradykinin, norepinephrine) are removed from the pulmonary circulation by the lungs. The respiratory system also performs *protective* functions for the body. Inhaled air is humidified by the glandular secretions and cooled or warmed by the erectile tissue of the upper respiratory tract. Hairs trap large foreign particles, whereas those that gain entrance to the respiratory tract are moved to the nasopharynx by the numerous cilia of the epithelium of the upper respiratory tract and lung. Finally, alveolar macrophages are scattered throughout the lung and phagocytize particulate matter that reaches the alveoli.

Respiratory Tract

Conductive Components

General Remarks. The conductive portion of the respiratory tract includes all those structures from the *nares* to the *terminal bronchioles.* Besides the *conduction* of air, this portion of the system is responsible for *cleansing* the air of particulate matter, *hu-*

midifying the air and either *cooling* or *warming* the air. Specific portions of the tract are responsible for *olfaction* and *phonation.*

Nasal Cavity. The nasal cavity is divisible into three histologically distinct regions: *vestibular region, respiratory region* and *olfactory region.*

The extent of the *vestibular region* is species-variable. It does represent, however, the point of reflection of the integument as the mucous membrane of the nasal cavity. The lamina epithelialis is stratified squamous epithelium which is nonkeratinized. Pigment cells may be present. The lamina propria-tunica submucosa is coarse areolar connective tissue that blends with the underlying fascia of muscle or the fibrous layer of the

associated investments of bone or cartilage. Hairs (vibrissae), sweat glands and sebaceous glands occur in the cutaneous part. Branched tubuloalveolar glands (serous and mixed) may also be present. These glands assist in humidifying the inspired air.

The mucous membrane of the vestibular region gradually changes to the mucous membrane of the *respiratory region* (Fig. 21.2). The latter comprises the bulk of the nasal cavity. The lamina epithelialis is a pseudostratified ciliated columnar epithelium which contains goblet cells. Together, these cells both humidify and cleanse the air. The lamina propria-tunica submucosa is areolar connective tissue. Numerous branched tubuloaveolar mixed glands, the

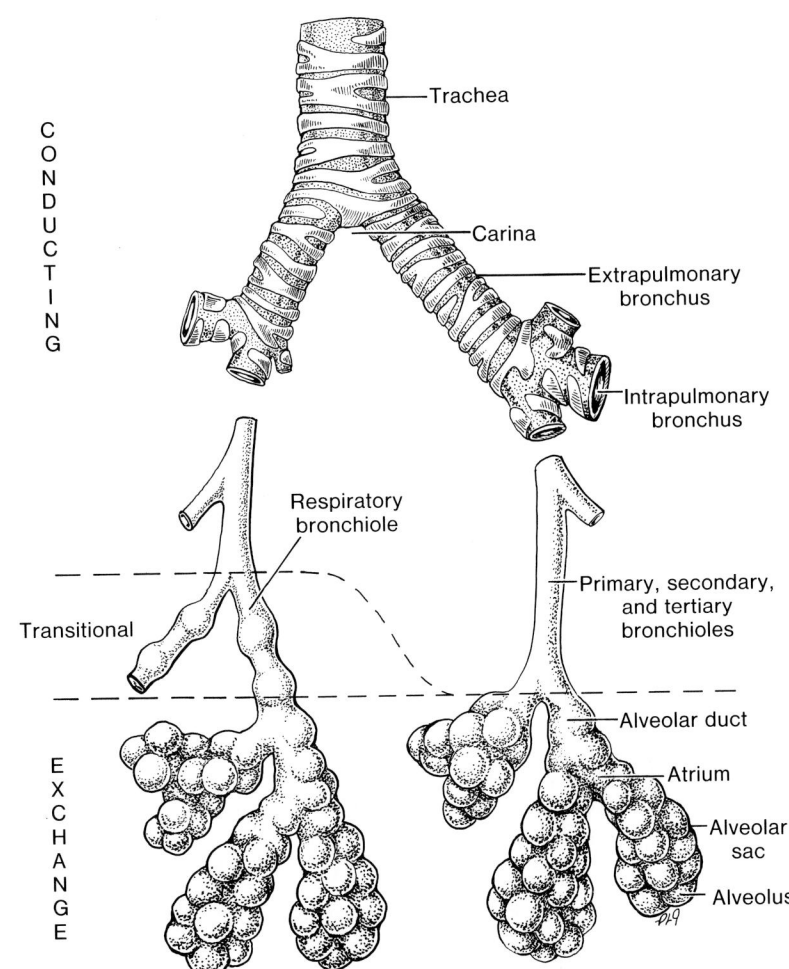

Fig. 21.1 A diagram of airways from the trachea to the alveoli. The transitional zone is not present nor equally developed in all species. All light micrographs are labeled as the magnification with the microscope before photographic enlarging. All electron micrographs are labeled as total magnification, including photographic enlarging.

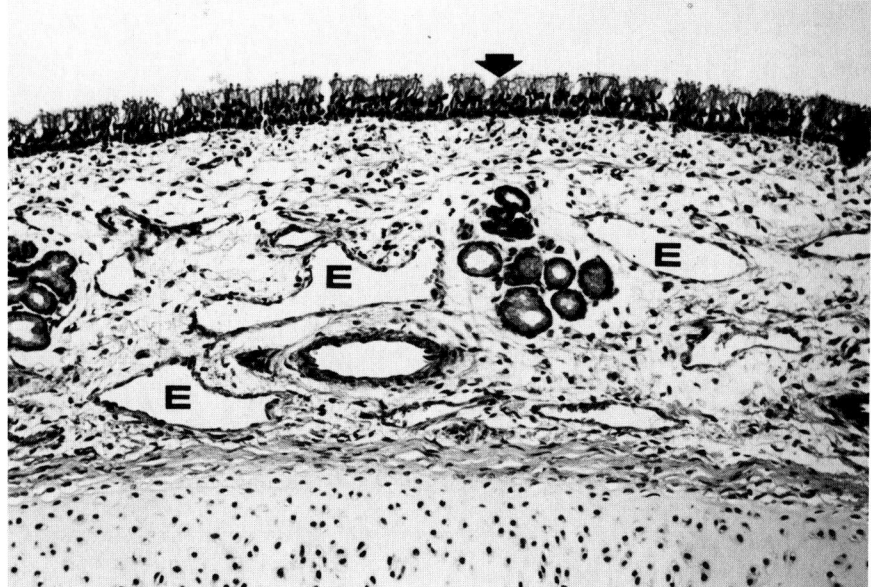

Fig. 21.2 Respiratory mucosa. The lamina epithelialis (*arrow*) is pseudostratified ciliated columnar epithelium with goblet cells. The lamina propria contains serous glands and erectile tissue (E). The connective tissue of the lamina propria is continuous with the fibrous perichondrium of the underlying cartilage. X40.

nasal glands, which are predominantly serous, are scattered throughout this layer. *Erectile tissue* may also be present in this area. Erectile tissue consists of cavities which are lined by endothelium and are continuous with the blood vessels of a particular area. Although they are usually collapsed, they become engorged with blood under proper nervous stimulation. The glandular tissue humidifies the air, whereas the engorged erectile tissue cools or warms it by using the mucous membrane as a heat transfer device. The connective tissue of this region is continuous with the underlying connective tissue associated with the bone or cartilage.

The *paranasal air sinuses* are continuous with the nasal cavity. These are spaces within the maxillary, frontal, ethmoid and sphenoid bones of the skull. The epithelium varies from cuboidal or squamous to thin pseudostratified ciliated columnar. Goblet cells and nasal glands occur less frequently than in the nasal cavity proper. Erectile tissue is not present. The remaining connective tissue and bone relationships are similar to those of the nasal cavity proper. Because of the intimate relationship of the mucosa to the underlying bone, these structures ar referred to collectively as a *mucoperiosteum*.

The *olfactory region* is a specialized area for olfaction that is positioned on the ethmoturbinates, adjacent dorsal turbinates and nasal septum (Fig. 21.3). Grossly, it may be yellow, brown, gray or black due to the accumulation of pigment. The lamina epithelialis consists of nonciliated pseudostratified columnar epithelium. It is a very thick lamina and as many as 15 strata of nuclei may be apparent. This region consists of three cell types: *sustentacular cells, basal*

cells and *olfactory cells*. The *sustentacular cells* are tall cells with broad apices and narrow bases. The oval, vesicular nuclei are positioned toward the apex of the cell. Pigment granules responsible for the color of this region are contained within these cells. The *basal cells* are typical of those that occur in this type of epithelium. The *olfactory cells* are modified neurons, the basal processes of which continue to the brain as axons of the first cranial nerve. The apex of the cell is modified as a bulblike projection, the *olfactory vesicle*, from which modified cilia, *olfactory hairs*, project. The hairs are the receptors for olfactory stimuli. The round, vesicular nucleus is positioned centrally or basally. The underlying lamina propria is typical and contains branched tubuloaveolar serous glands (*Bowman's glands*) (Plate II.8). These are responsible for the cleansing of the olfactory surface, as well as solubilizing odor-producing substances.

Nasopharynx. The *nasopharynx* is that portion of the pharynx above the soft palate. It connects the nasal cavity with the oropharynx.

The lamina epithelialis consists of pseudostratified ciliated columnar epithelium. Goblet cells are present. The lamina propria-tunica submucosa consists of areolar connective tissue with numerous diffuse and aggregated lymphatic tissue and tonsils. Elastic fibers are prominent in the connective tissue space. Branched tubuloalveolar glands (mucous, serous and mixed) occur throughout this region. The tunica muscularis is composed of skeletal muscle in various orientations. The tunica adventitia is continuous with the fascia of this area.

Larynx. The larynx is that portion of the respiratory tract which connects the pharynx

with the trachea. It is an irregularly shape muscular tube which is reinforced with ca tilage (Fig. 21.4).

The lamina epithelialis varies with spe cific foci within the larynx. It may be stra ified squamous or pseudostratified ciliate columnar epithelium. Taste buds may b present in the epiglottic region of some spe cies (carnivores, swine, ruminants, man).

The lamina propria-tunica submucos consists of areolar connective tissue wit various numbers of elastic fibers. Diffus and nodular lymphatic tissue is presen Branched tubuloalveolar glands are pre dominantly mucoid, but serous and mixe glands are present also.

The tunica muscularis does not consi exclusively of striated muscle fibers. Rathe cartilage replaces some of the muscle mas in a specific manner that accounts for th recognition of specific laryngeal cartilage and muscle masses at the gross level c examination. Although hyaline cartilag predominates, elastic cartilage is preser also.

The tunica adventitia is typical loose cor nective tissue.

Trachea. This tubular organ continues fro the larynx and terminates at the primar bronchi (Fig. 21.5).

The lamina epithelialis is composed c pseudostratified ciliated columnar epithe lium with goblet cells. The number an distribution of the latter are subject to spe cies variation.

The lamina propria-tunica submucosa i areolar connective tissue. Elastic fibers ar prominent and are believed to replace th lamina muscularis mucosae in the deepe layers. Mucosal glands of the branchec coiled tubuloalveolar mucous type are pres ent and extend into the depths of the sub mucosal region between and peripheral t the cartilage that is present.

The tunica muscularis is reduced to transversely oriented mass of smooth muscl (*trachealis muscle*) that extends between th open ends of the horseshoe-shaped cartilage The actual attachment of the muscle to th cartilage is species-variable. The smooth muscle mass may also be interrupted by th mucosal glands.

The tunica adventitia is areolar connec tive tissue which blends with the surround ing fascia.

Extrapulmonary Bronchi. The *extrapulmon ary* or *primary bronchi* arise at the bifircatio of the trachea and are structurally similar t it.

Lung

General Remarks. Structurally, the lun may be considered a compound tubuloa veolar gland. Its excretory product, carbo dioxide, is "secreted" across the alveola surface in exchange for the uptake of oxy gen. This exchange is facilitated by the elas tic properties of the lung. An extensive net work of elastic fibers accounts for part of it contractility in response to an alteration i the size of the thoracic cavity. The latter i

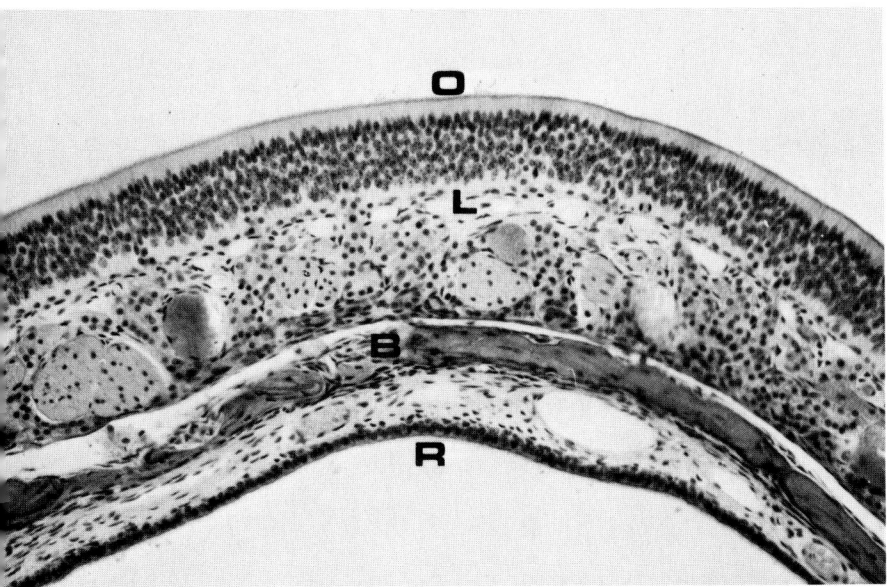

g. 21.3 Olfactory and respiratory mucosal covering of an osseous portion of a turbinate. The factory mucosa (O) is a nonciliated pseudostratified columnar epithelium that is thicker than the spiratory epithelium (R). The lamina propria (L) contains numerous serous glands and bone (B). 40.

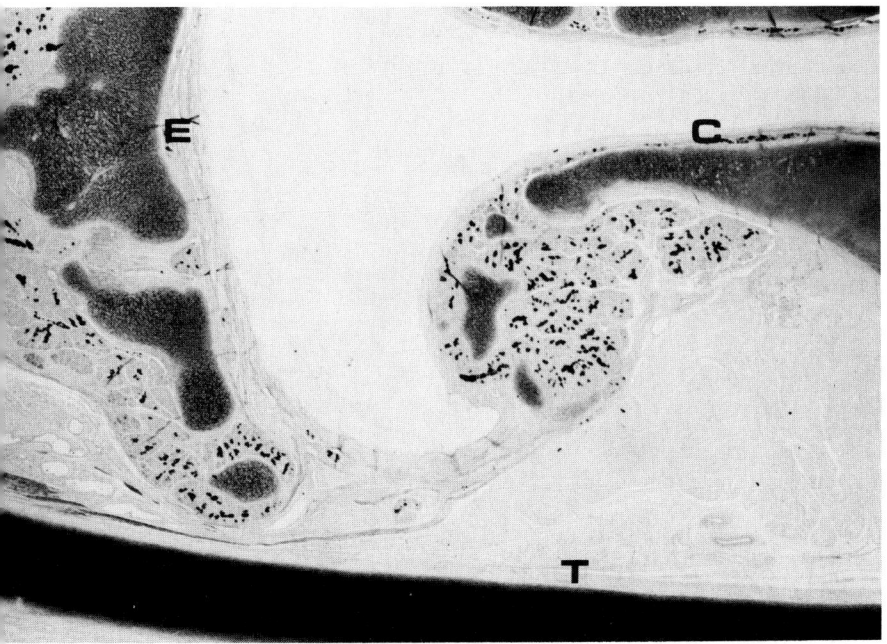

ig. 21.4 A frontal section of a portion of a larynx. The dark-staining tissue is the epiglottic (E), ricoid (C) and thyroid (T) cartilages. X4 (aldehyde fuchsin).

ontrolled by the expansion and contraction f the diaphragm and thoracic cage.

The lung consists of two *half-lungs*. Each alf-lung, often referred to simply as a lung, s subdivided into various numbers of *lobes* species variable). Lobes are subdivided into *obules*. In ruminants and the pig the lobular ubdivisions are readily apparent on the ung surface. In the horse and man the obular subdivisions are less distinct. In the log and cat the lobular subdivisions are not resent.

The lung is covered by a serous membrane (*visceral pleura*). The subserosal connective tissue, often referred to as the capsule of the lung, consists of a thin layer of coarse areolar connective tissue that is rich in elastic fibers (Fig. 21.6). This serous membrane follows the surface contours of the lobes. The interlobular connective tissue is loose connective tissue that is also rich in elastic fibers. The intralobular or interstitial space is occupied by reticular connective tissue. Elastic fibers may also be present.

The embryologic development of the lung requires contributions from the endoderm and mesoderm. The endoderm gives rise to the lining of the conductive and alveolar portions, whereas the mesoderm is responsible for all interstitial elements. There are three distinct but continuous stages of pulmonary development: *glandular, canalicular* and *alveolar* stages. The *glandular stage* is characterized by an extensive arborization of the airways. The *canalicular stage* is characterized by the initial attenuation of the lining cells and the differentiation of two distinct types of lining cells. The *alveolar stage* represents the achievement of the functional blood-air barrier.

Intrapulmonary Bronchi. The intrapulmonary duct system is a modification of the extrapulmonary bronchi. The elastic fibers of extrapulmonary bronchi, positioned in the area normally occupied by the lamina muscularis mucosae, become closely associated with the lamina membrana propria in the intrapulmonary bronchi. The smooth muscle fibers of the trachealis muscle become positioned as the lamina muscularis mucosae. The cartilage, however, remains in the position normally occupied by the tunica muscularis.

Intrapulmonary bronchi may be subdivided into *primary, secondary* and *tertiary bronchi* on the basis of their branching, luminal size and mural constituents. There is a gradual continuum of change from the primary to the tertiary bronchi. The intrapulmonary primary bronchi are continuations of the extrapulmonary primary bronchi. Their mural constituents are similar (Fig. 21.7). The lamina epithelialis is a pseudostratified ciliated columnar epithelium which contains numerous goblet cells. The lamina propria, which is continuous with the connective tissue of the *hilus*, is areolar. It contains numerous elastic fibers. The lamina muscularis mucosae is present and disposed in a manner similar to that of the elastic fibers. The spiral configuration of these components results in a highly folded tunica mucosa. The tunica submucosa also consists of areolar connective tissue and contains branched, coiled tubuloalveolar mucous glands. Usually, these glands diminish in number toward the tertiary bronchi. In the cat, however, they may extend into the primary bronchioles. In some species, they are present only in the extrapulmonary bronchi or may extend only a short distance into the lung. The cartilaginous rings of the larger bronchi diminish in size, become cartilaginous plaques and are missing at the transition to primary bronchioles (Fig. 21.8). The peripheral connective tissue is areolar and is continuous with that of the interstitial space.

Bronchioles. The bronchioles are the smallest divisions of the nonrespiratory or conductive portions of the lung (Fig. 21.9). The lamina epithelialis consists of simple columnar or cuboidal cells and is devoid of goblet cells. The lining cells are ciliated in the *primary bronchioles*. The cilia diminish in

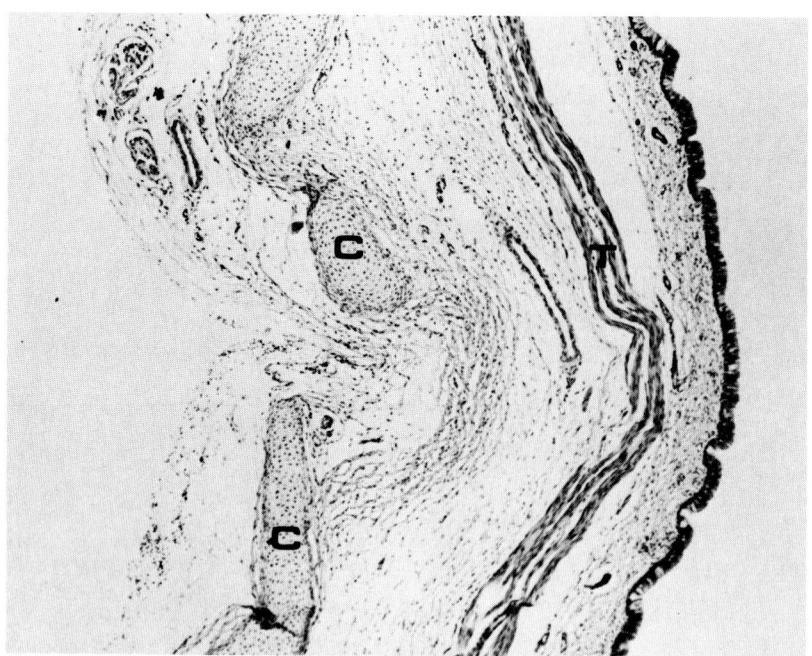

Fig. 21.5 A section of porcine trachea. The cartilage rings (C) are incomplete and connected by connective tissue. The trachealis muscle (T) is internal to the cartilage. The epithelial lining of the mucosa is typical pseudostratified ciliated columnar epithelium with goblet cells. X16.

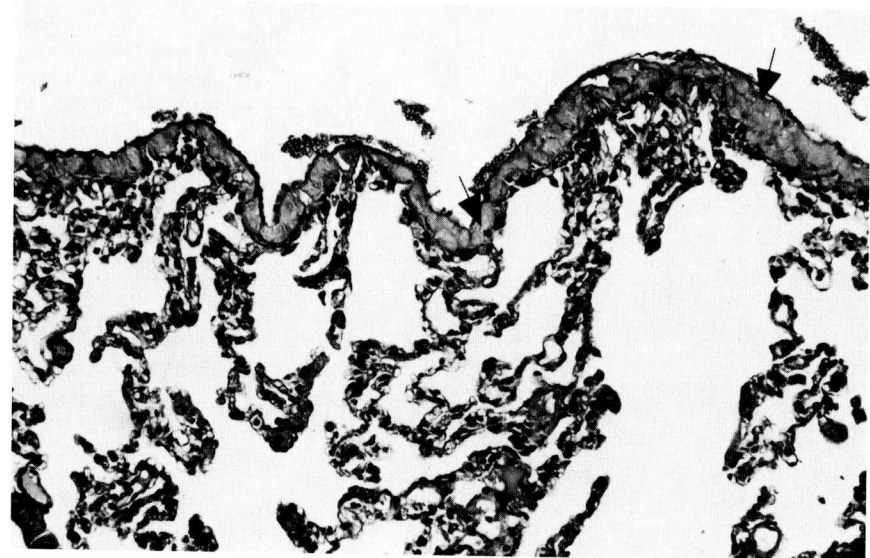

Fig. 21.6 Capsule of the feline lung. The capsule (*arrows*) is covered by a layer of mesothelium—visceral pleura. X40.

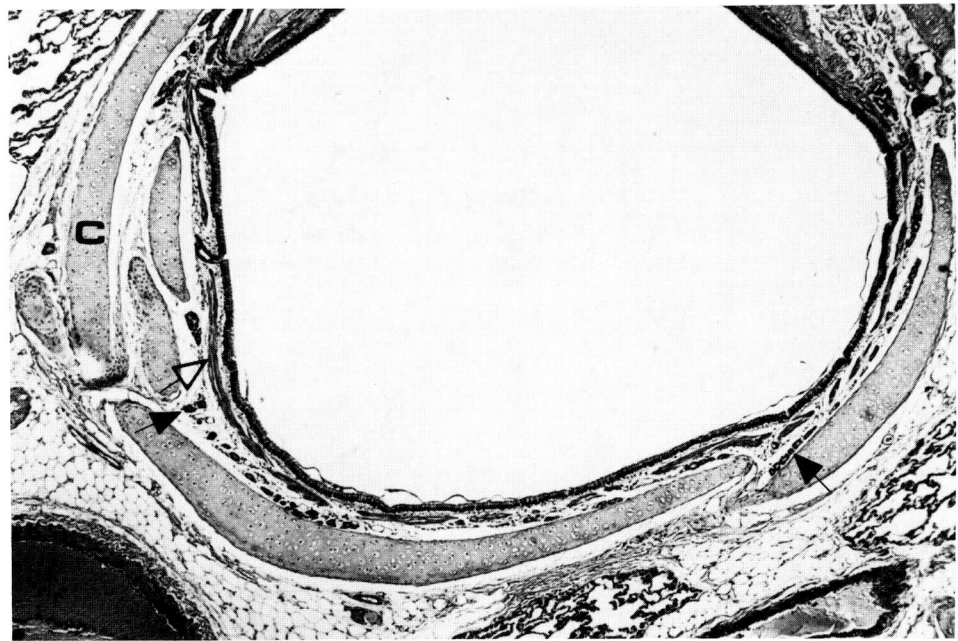

ig. 21.7 Primary bronchus (feline lung). The cartilage (C) is disposed as plates. A lamina muscularis (*open arrow*) and mucous glands (*solid rrows*) are present. X10.

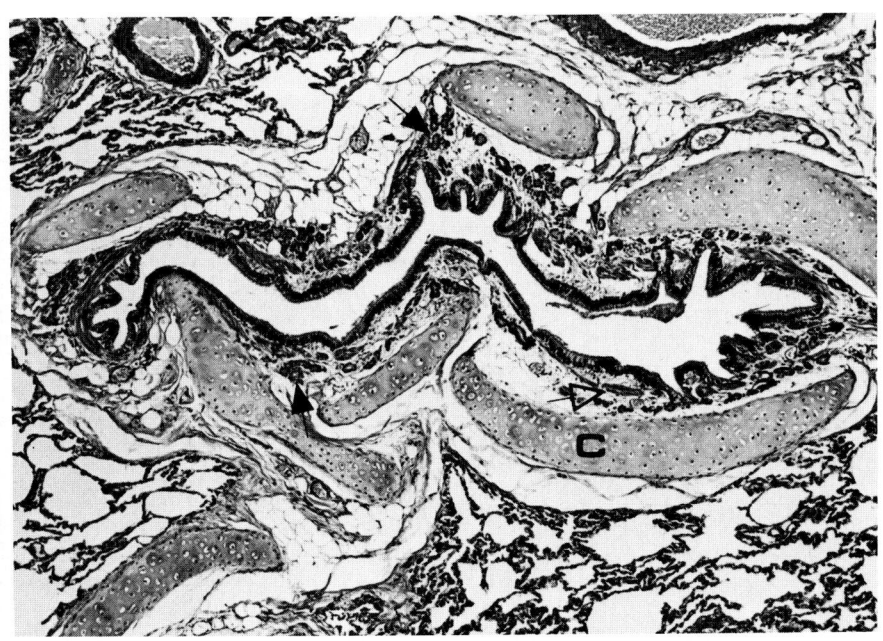

ig. 21.8 Small bronchus (feline lung). Cartilage plates (C), mucous glands (*solid arrow*) and mooth muscle (*open arrow*) are present, but the luminal diameter is reduced. X16.

he more distal bronchioles and are lost in he tertiary bronchioles. Importantly, cilia xtend further down the respiratory tree han do glands. The lamina propria consists f fine collagenous and elastic fibers. The amina muscularis mucosae is present and ontinuous. The peripheral connective tisue is similar to the lamina propria but is ot extensive. No cartilage is present. The ertiary or terminal bronchioles are the primary conducting supply to a secondary loble and divide into several respiratory bronhioles.

Respiratory Bronchioles. The *respiratory bronchioles* are the initial portion of the lung responsible for the exchange of gases (Fig. 21.10). The lamina epithelialis consists of cuboidal cells, some of which may be ciliated (Fig. 21.11). The cuboidal cells are not a continuous lining but are interrupted by alveoli that outpocket from the walls of this bronchiole (Fig. 21.12). The lamina propria is indistinct, but fine collagenous and elastic fibers support the lining cells. Smooth muscle is present, but it is loosely organized beneath the cuboidal epithelium.

Respiratory bronchioles are not equally developed, nor are they present in all species. They are infrequently observed in ruminants and swine, poorly developed in horse and man, well-developed in monkey and carnivores and absent in the mouse. In those species in which they are absent, the terminal bronchioles open directly into several alveolar ducts. The transitional and exchange components of the lung are drawn in Figure 21.13.

Some of the cuboidal cells of these bronchioles, *Clara cells*, have been implicated in the metabolism of *surface-active substance (surfactant)*. Although originally proposed as being responsible for its production, other cells now have been demonstrated as being responsible for the production of surfactant. The role of the Clara cell, therefore, is not clarified.

Alveolar Ducts, Saccules and Atria. The respiratory bronchiole of a lobule or the terminal bronchiole of a lobule, divide into numerous *alveolar ducts* (Fig. 21.14).

These tubules are completely lined by alveoli. Smooth muscle may be present along the luminal border at the apices between adjacent alveoli. Alveolar ducts divide and expand peripherally into *saccules* (sacs) which are completely lined by alveoli (Fig. 21.15). The common opening of the saccules is referred to as the *atrium*.

Pneumonocytes and Alveoli. The lining of the alveoli consists of two types of cells: *membranous pneumonocytes* (*type I pneumonocytes*) and *granular pneumonocytes* (*type II pneumonocytes, alveolar giant cells, dust cells*).

The *membranous (agranular) pneumonocyte* is the primary constituent of the alveolar lining (Fig. 21.16). It is an endothelial-like cell with an attenuated cytoplasm which

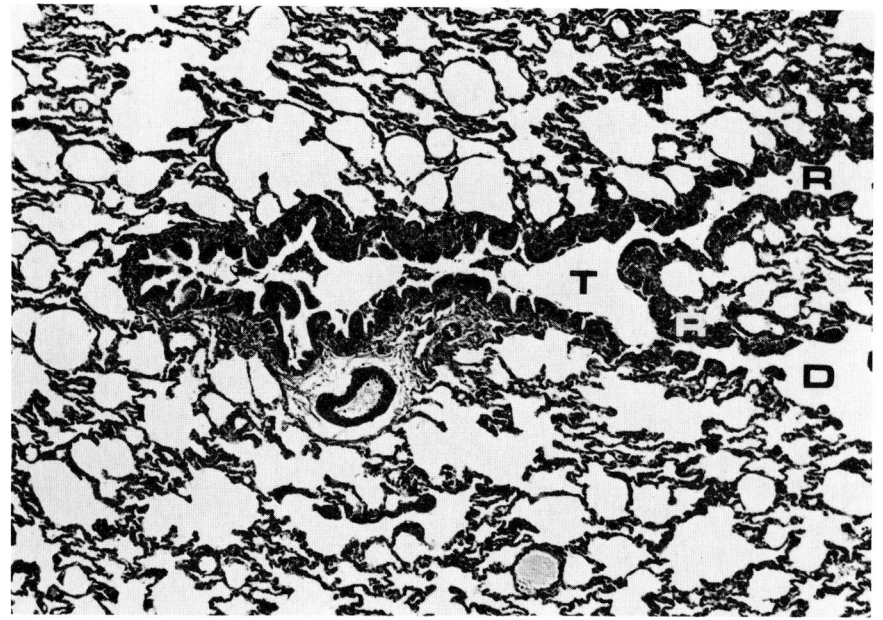

Fig. 21.9 Bronchioles of a feline lung. The walls are devoid of cartilage. The terminal bronchiole (T) has divided into two respiratory bronchioles (R). An alveolar duct (D) is present also. X16.

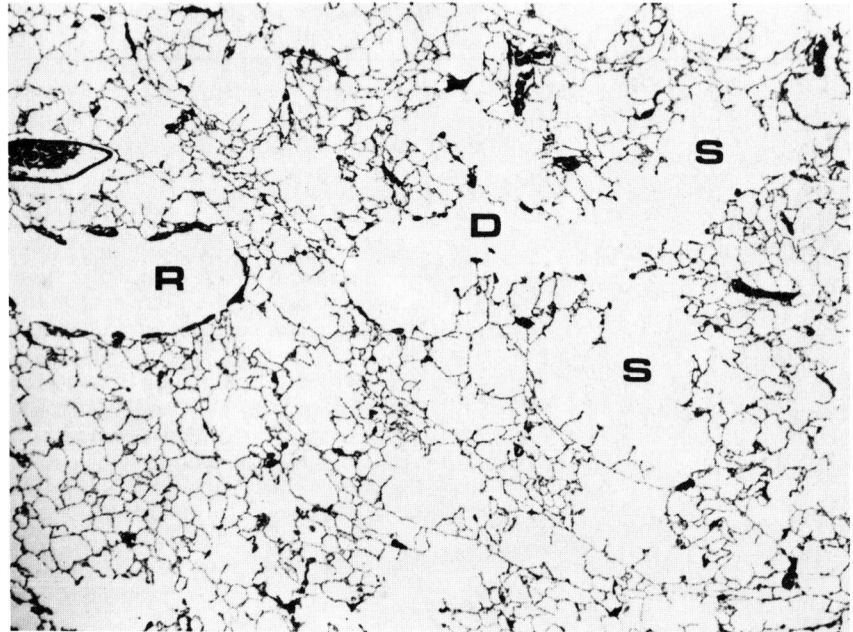

Fig. 21.10 Distal airways of a canine lung. A respiratory bronchiole (R) continues as an alveolar duct (D) which then continues as two alveolar sacs (S). The atrium is the common opening of the alveolar sacs. X40.

is of variable occurrence; the numbers ma vary from one to several per alveolus. Thes are cuboidal or rounded cells which inter mittently line the alveolar surface. Their cel bodies are foamy and project into the alveo lar lumina. Tight junctions connect the cy toplasmic processes of these cells with thos of the membranous pneumonocytes. Osmio philic, *lamellar bodies* are the diagnosti features of these cells at the electron micro scopic level (Fig. 21.19).

A third lining cell, the *alveolar brush cel* has been described in the alveoli of rat This type III pneumonocyte is covered by thin process of the type I cell. The alveola brush cell may function in absorption, che moreception or stretch reception. Althoug this cell constitutes 5–10% of the alveola lining cell population in the rat, it has no been established as a resident cell in othe species.

Adjacent alveoli are sometimes connecte by pores. These pores are believed to dis tribute equally the gases and resulting pres sure among alveoli. They may also serve fo the interalveolar transmission of fluids, par ticulate matter, bacteria and alveolar mac rophages.

Blood-Air Barrier. These cells, both type and type II, are supported by a basal lamin and fine collagenous, reticular and/or elas tic fibers. The proximity of adjacent alveol clearly delimits a distinct, but greatly re duced, interstitial or *septal space*. This spac contains the aforementioned fibers, fibro blasts, macrophages and blood capillaries.

The blood-air barrier (blood-air pathway consists of the following elements: *alveola lining cell, alveolar basal lamina, septal space endothelial-associated basal lamina* and *en dothelial cell* (Fig. 21.20). The thickness o the barrier, however, is variable. Minimally it is composed of the *alveolar lining cel fused basal laminae* and *endothelial cel* (Figs. 21.21). This is the thinnest and mos efficient diffusion pathway. The least effi cient and thickest would involve an expan sion of the septal region.

Because the lung is exposed to inspire foreign materials, various methods are uti lized to cleanse the air—goblet cells, cilia and macrophages. Macrophages are the pri mary mediators of this activity in the lowe portion of the respiratory tree (Fig. 21.22) Transalveolar migration of these cells (his tiocytes) from the septal areas as well a from the blood (monocytes) is probable They may protrude into the alveolar lumin between the lining cells, reside on the linin cells or be free in the lumina. They ar rarely observed as a constituent of the linin in residence upon the basal lamina. Thes and associated cells comprise the *transien alveolar cell population*, whereas the pneu monocytes comprise the *resident alveolar cel population*.

Vascular, Neural and Lymphatic Relation ships. The vascular supply to the lung i achieved by two arterial systems: the *pul*

is reduced to the limit of resolution of the light microscope. Its nucleus is apparent and protrudes into the alveolar lumen. Exami nation of alveoli with the electron micro scope supplied the first conclusive evidence that the alveoli were in fact lined by cells (Fig. 21.17).

The *type II pneumonocyte* has been, until recently, the subject of much controversy. Although the cell was thought originally to

be a macrophage, current evidence supports the secretory role of this cell. It is the cell responsible for the elaboration of *surfactant* material. Surfactant is a detergent-like ma terial which reduces alveolar surface tension and prevents alveolar collapse during expi ration. Despite the numerous synonyms given for this cell, the most precise names for this cell are *type II pneumonocyte* or *granular pneumonocyte* (Fig. 21.18). This cell

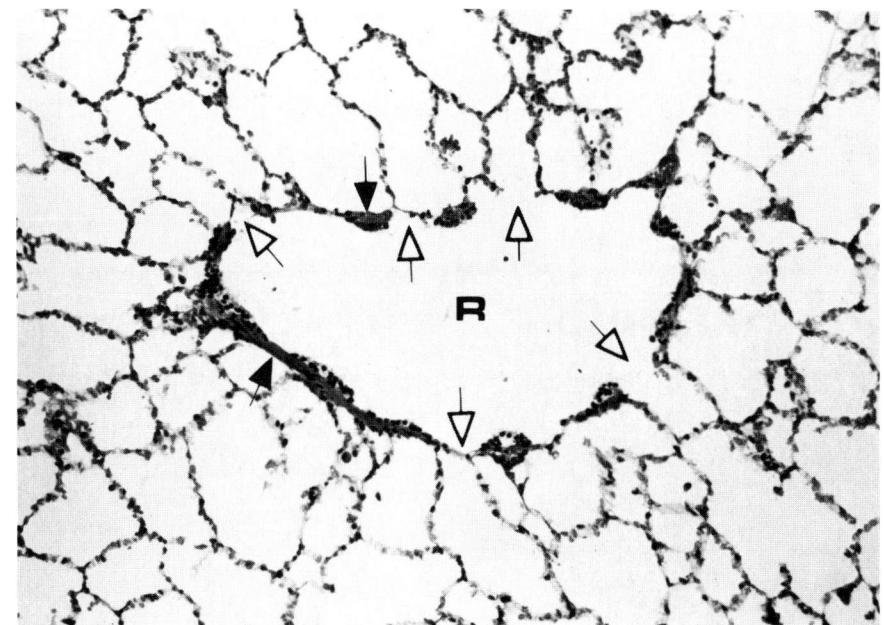

Fig. 21.11 Respiratory bronchiole (R) of a canine lung. The lamina epithelialis is underlaid by smooth muscle (*solid arrows*). The epithelial lining is interrupted by alveoli (*open arrows*). X40.

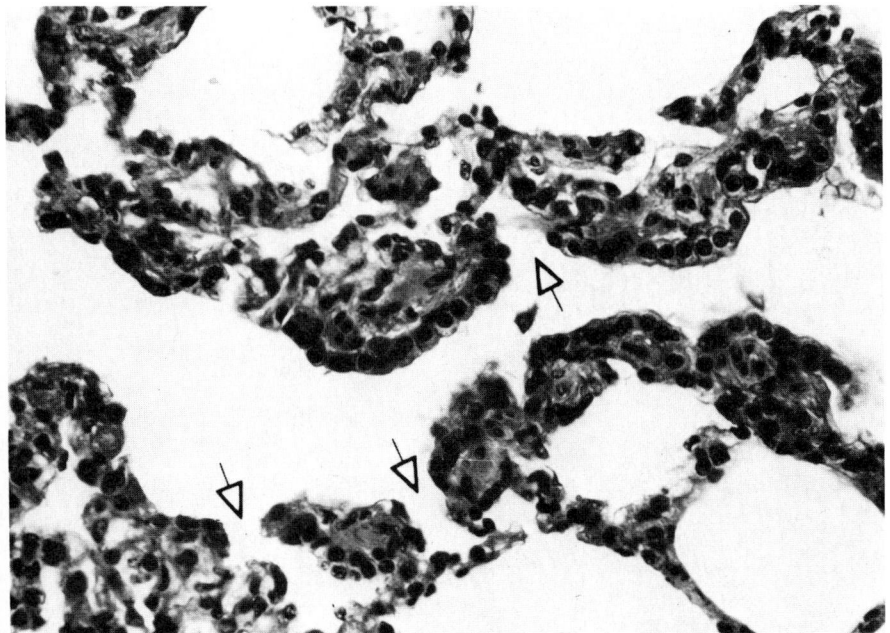

Fig. 21.12 Lining of a feline respiratory bronchiole. The cuboidal epithelium is interrupted by alveoli. X100.

monary artery and *bronchial artery* (Fig. 21.23). This type of dual circulation is not unique to the lung, but it does represent a division of functional and nutritional blood supply, respectively. The pulmonary artery and its peripheral subdivisions follow the distribution of the airways to the level of the respiratory bronchioles at which point they are continued as an extensive capillary bed associated with the alveoli. In carnivores and the monkey, this artery also supplies the pleura. In ruminants, swine, horse and man the bronchial artery supplies the pleura.

The position of the pulmonary veins is species variable. In some species the pulmonary vein is interlobular in position and thus receives blood from adjacent lobules. In others, it is intralobular and requires that each lobule has its own pulmonary vein.

The bronchial arteries, which may supply the pleura (horse, man, ruminants and swine) as well as the alveoli (horse), are the primary blood supply for the walls of the bronchi and bronchioles. Although bronchial veins are present, most of the bronchial arterial blood is returned to the heart via the pulmonary veins. The pulmonary vein of the ox is unique. The tunica media is very thick and disrupted. This imparts a sphincter-like appearance to the vessel when it is cut in cross-section.

Two sets of lymphatic vessels drain the lungs: *superficial vessels* and *deep vessels* (Fig. 21.23). The lymphatic capillaries of the superficial drainage originate in the pleural connective tissue and drain toward the hilus in the interlobular septa. The deep vessels originate at the level of the respiratory bronchioles or terminal bronchioles and follow the path of the bronchial tree to the hilus of the lung. The deep vessels anastomose with the superficial drainage in the interlobular septa. Lymphatic vessels have not been demonstrated in the interalveolar septa.

General visceral efferent fibers from the vagus and thoracic segments of the sympathetic trunk innervate the smooth musculature of the airways. The parasympathetic nerves stimulate *bronchoconstriction*, whereas the sympathetic nerves cause *bronchodilation*. General visceral afferent fibers originate from stretch receptors within the lung substance and from nerve endings within the epithelium that lines the conductive airways.

Histophysiology of the Lung

Exchange of Gases. The delivery of oxygen to the tissues is a function that is achieved by the complementary activity of the cardiovascular and respiratory systems. Oxygen delivered to the blood-air barrier must traverse the barrier, be picked up by the blood and be transported to the tissues. The oxygenation of blood within the pulmonary capillaries is dependent upon varied factors: the amount of oxygen in inspired air; the integrity of the blood air barrier; the amount of blood flowing within the pulmonary circulation; the quantity of O_2 dissolved in the blood, and the amount of hemoglobin as well as its affinity for O_2.

The partial pressure of oxygen (P_{O_2}) in dry air, based upon 20% of 760 mm Hg at sea level, is approximately 150 mm Hg. After the addition of water, the P_{O_2} within alveoli is 100 mm Hg. The P_{O_2} of venous blood (Pv_{O_2}) is approximately 40 mm Hg. Oxygen moves down its pressure gradient, traverses the blood-air barrier and is carried by the blood. Some of the oxygen dissolves in the plasma and is carried to the tissues in this form; however, the amount of dissolved oxygen within the plasma amounts to about 0.3 ml% due to solubility limitations. Most of the oxygen is carried by the hemoglobin of the erythrocytes. Hemoglobin increases the oxygen-carrying capacity of blood about 70 times, to approximately 20 ml%. Each hemoglobin molecule contains 4 porphyrins, *heme*, each with a *ferrous iron atom*. The oxygenation of hemoglobin occurs progres-

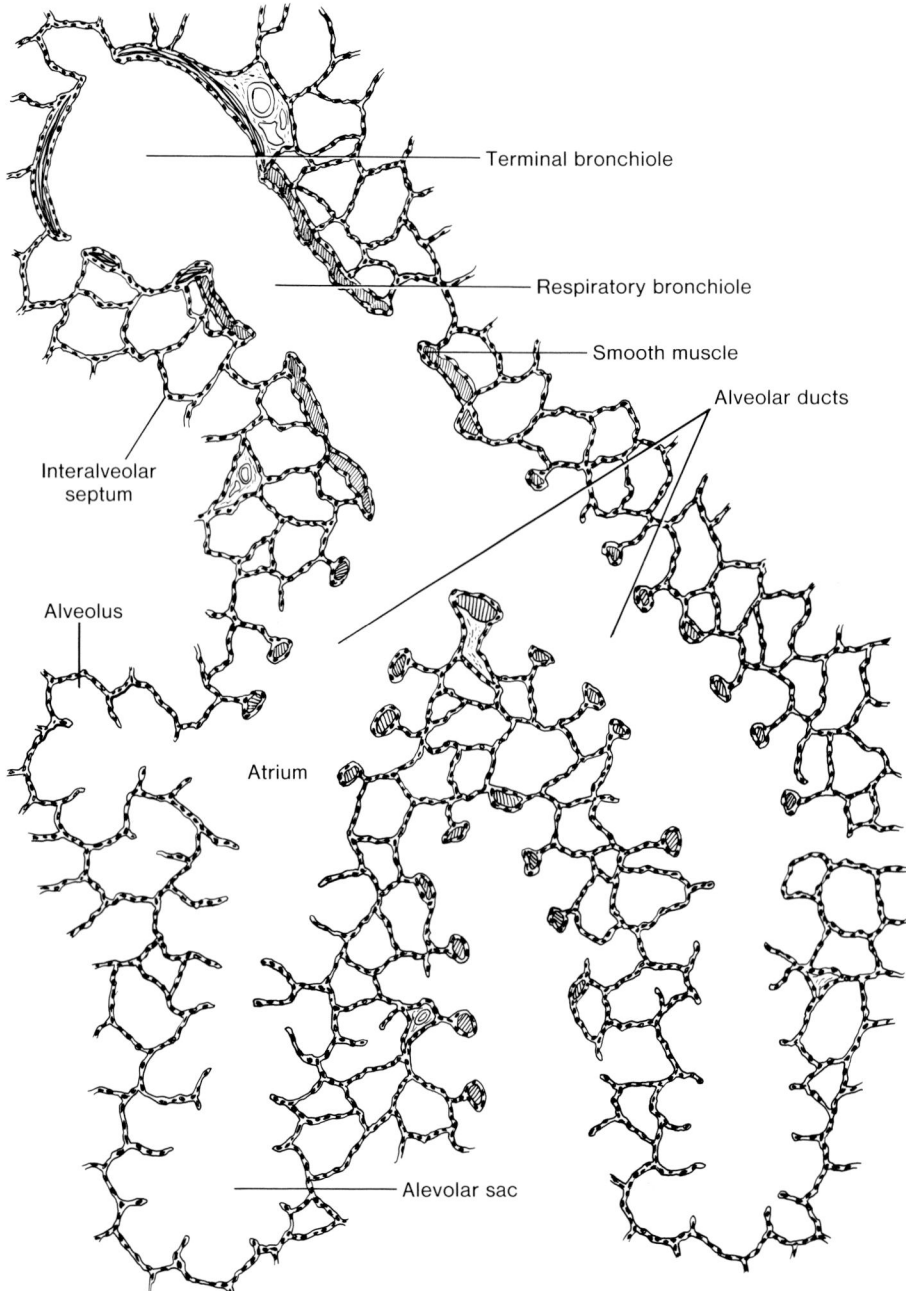

Fig. 21.13 A diagram of the transitional and exchange components of the lung. Respiratory bronchioles do not exist nor are they equally developed in all domestic species.

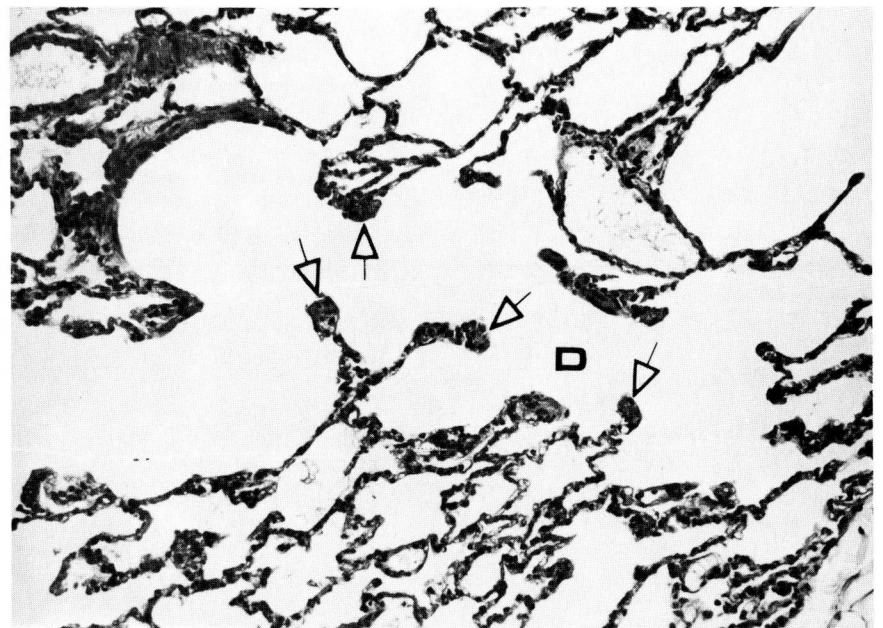

Fig. 21.14 Alveolar duct of the feline lung. The alveolar duct (D) is lined by alveoli. Smooth muscle overlaid with attenuated lining cells (arrows) occupies the apices of septa between adjacent alveoli. X40.

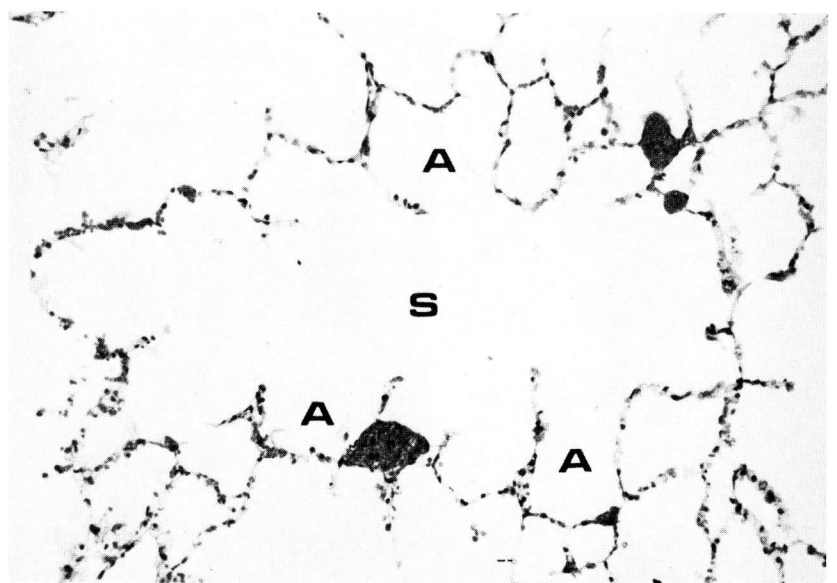

Fig. 21.15 An alveolar sac of the canine lung. The walls of the alveolar sac (S) consist of alveoli (A). The interalveolar septa are devoid of smooth muscle. X40.

30 mm Hg and may be much less than 10 mm Hg, while the P_{O_2} of arterial blood is between 40 and 100 mm Hg. Oxygen then dissociates from the hemoglobin, moves into the plasma and then into the tissues. The dissociation of oxygen from hemoglobin follows a characteristic sigmoid curve (oxygen-hemoglobin dissociation curve) which relates to the varying affinities for oxygen by the heme moieties (Fig. 21.24). At rest, about 27% of the oxygen is released to the tissues; venous blood contains hemoglobin at 70% saturation. Various factors influence the dissociation of oxyhemoglobin: P_{CO_2}, temperature, pH. Active tissues produce more CO_2, elevate local temperature and increase hydrogen ion concentration ([H^+]); more oxygen dissociates from hemoglobin and is available to the tissues. The converse occurs when CO_2, temperature and [H^+] are decreased.

The nature of the oxygen-hemoglobin dissociation curve tells much about hemoglobin and the manner in which O_2 is delivered to tissues. The P_{O_2} of blood is due to the small amount of dissolved O_2 in the plasma, approximately 0.3 ml%. But 70X this amount is carried by the hemoglobin. As more dissolved O_2 leaves the plasma, more O_2 dissociates from hemoglobin. The dissociation and/or saturation of hemoglobin is dependent upon the P_{O_2} of dissolved oxygen in plasma. The shoulder of the curve between a P_{O_2} of 40–100 mm Hg is the normal range of arterial blood. A large change in the P_{O_2} (100–40) is accompanied by a small decrease in percent hemoglobin saturation. In the resting organism, much more oxygen is carried by the blood than is needed by the tissues. The normal P_{O_2} of venous blood is considered to be 40 mm Hg. Metabolically active tissues have high oxygen requirements. As more oxygen diffuses to them, the P_{O_2} of the blood decreases. Hemoglobin is less able to hold its O_2 and dissociation occurs rapidly below 40 mm Hg. A small drop in P_{O_2} below 40 mm Hg delivers a large quantity of O_2 to the tissues from dissociated hemoglobin. The flat portion of the curve between 100–70 mm Hg is associated with a minor change in Hb saturation, from 97 to 93%. Accordingly, animals are able to live at altitudes higher than sea level (P_{O_2} = 150 mm Hg) without reducing markedly the O_2 carrying-capacity of the blood.

The partial pressure of CO_2 (P_{CO_2}) within the tissues is approximately 50 mm Hg, whereas the P_{CO_2} of arterial blood is 40 mm Hg. Carbon dioxide moves down its pressure gradient from the tissues into the blood. Within the blood, the transport of CO_2 is achieved in three ways: dissolved in the plasma (8%); carried in the RBC as a carbaminohemoglobin (27%); carried in the plasma as bicarbonate (65%). Some of the carbon dioxide reacts chemically with reduced hemoglobin to form the carbaminohemoglobin molecule. Most of the CO_2 that

vely in 4 steps and is summarized by the following equation:

$$Hb_4 + 4O_2 \rightleftharpoons Hb_4(O_2)_4$$

The reversible reaction, which proceeds to the right in the pulmonary capillaries, occurs in less than 10 msec within the lungs. Each of the heme moieties has a different affinity for O_2. The affinity increases with each oxygenation, so the last heme has a much greater affinity for O_2 than the first heme. The oxygen-carrying capacity of the blood is maximized at atmospheric pressure,

and most of the oxygen is attached to hemoglobin. Whereas hemoglobin saturation or 100% of its oxygen-carrying capacity may be achieved experimentally, hemoglobin saturation in vivo at an alveolar P_{O_2} of 100 mm Hg is only 97% of saturation. Bronchial venous drainage achieved via the pulmonary veins, dilutes the saturation percentage.

Once carried to the level of the tissues, oxygen must dissociate from the hemoglobin, move across the capillary wall into the tissue fluid and diffuse into the cells. The P_{O_2} within the tissues is generally less than

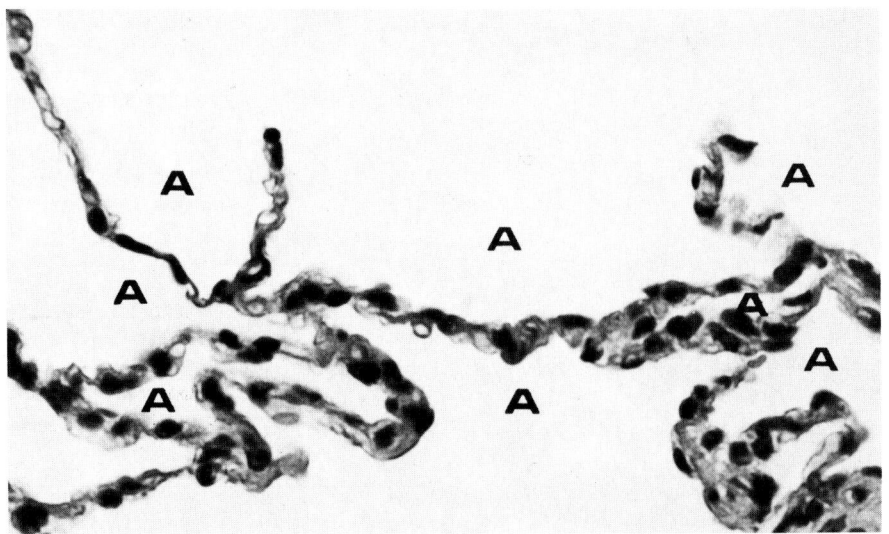

Fig. 21.16 An alveolus of a bovine lung. Alveoli (A) are adjacent to each other and are separated by capillaries and a minimal amount of connective tissue. Some of the alveoli are collapsed from processing. X160.

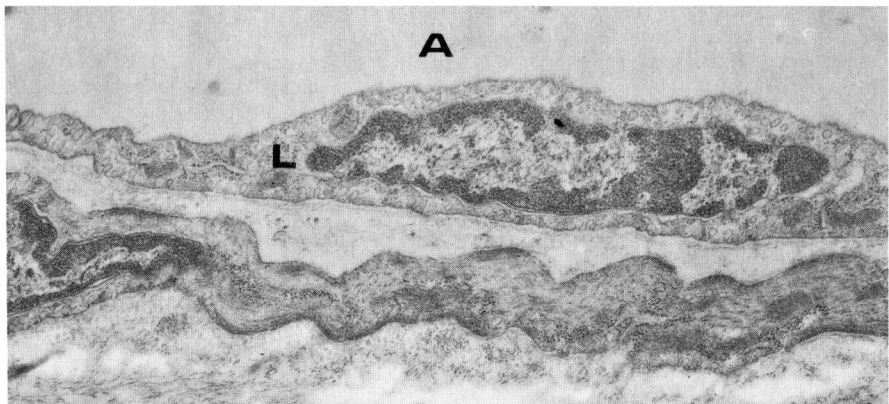

Fig. 21.17 An electron micrograph of a membranous (agranular) pneumonocyte from a bovine lung. The squamous lining cell (L) lines the alveolus (A). A fibroblast is subjacent to the lining cell. X18,000. (Courtesy of G. P. Epling).

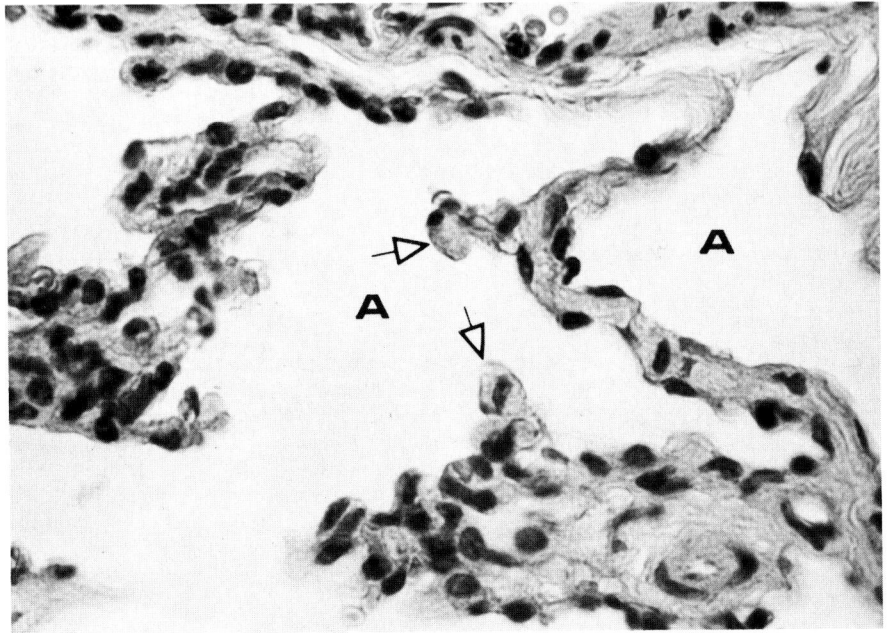

Fig. 21.18 Type II lining cells. The predominant cell of the alveoli (A) is the membranous pneumonocyte. Type II cells (*arrows*) are scattered along the lining. The distinguishing feature of these cells is their vacuolated cytoplasm; however, they are difficult to identify in light microscopic sections. X160.

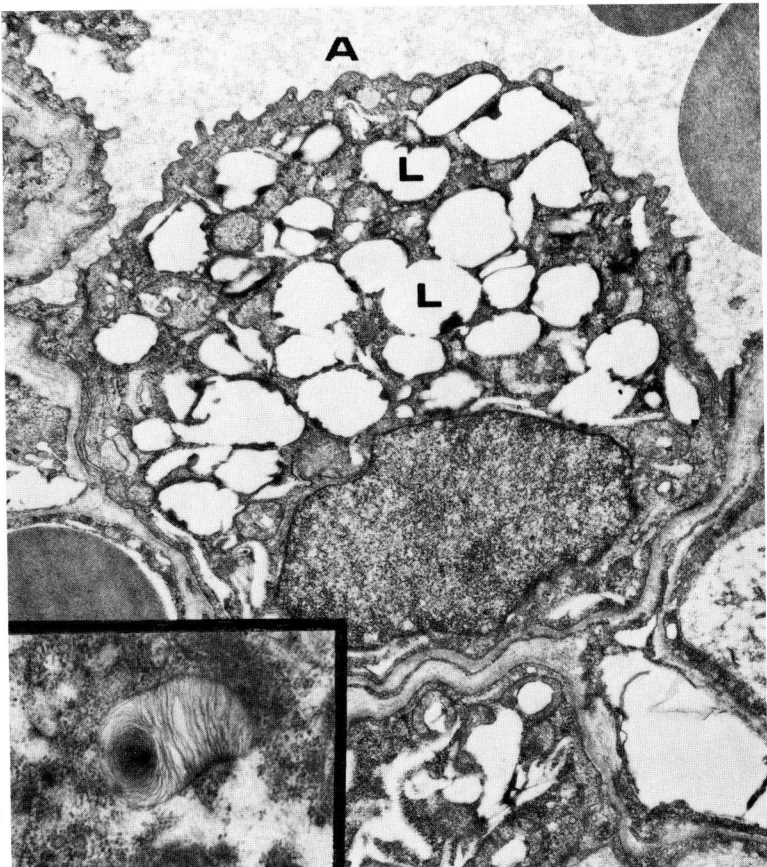

Fig. 21.19 An electron micrograph of a granular pneumonocyte. The cytoplasm protrudes into the alveolus (A). Pale areas (L) are lamellar bodies; their dissolution was a result of the processing. X14,000. (Courtesy of G. P. Epling). *Inset*: A typical lamellar body of a granular pneumonocyte. X17,000.

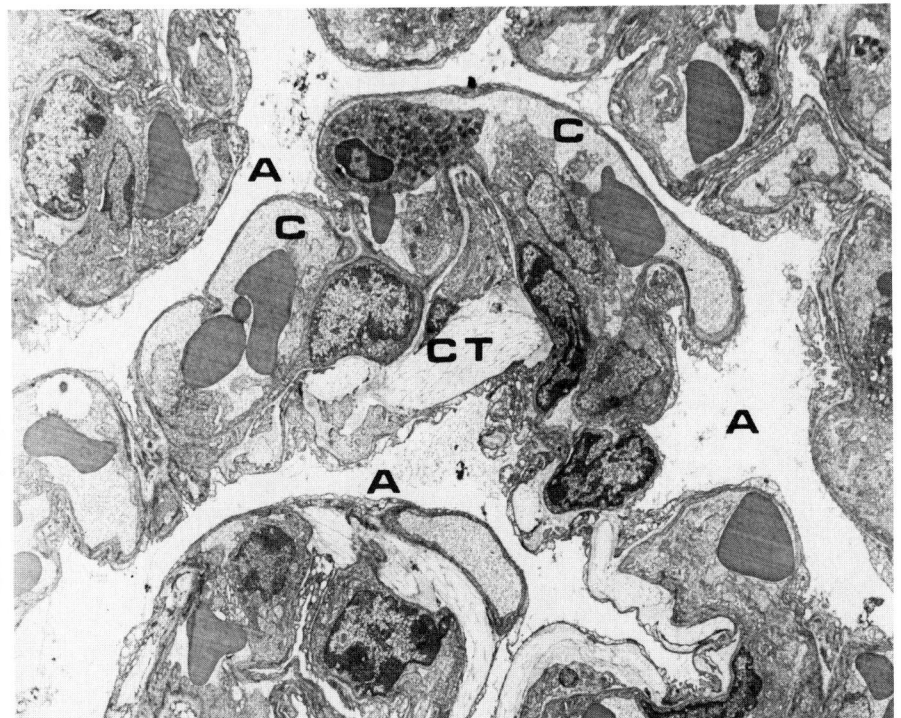

Fig. 21.20 An electron micrograph of a bovine lung. Capillaries (C) are juxtaposed to alveolar lining cells. These components and the interdigitated basal lamina comprise the blood-air barrier. Alveoli (A) are collapsed. Small amounts of connective tissue (CT) comprise the septa areas. X4000. (Courtesy of G. P. Epling).

enters the RBC is converted to carbonic acid (H_2CO_3) by the enzyme carbonic anhydrase. (Some of the plasma-dissolved CO_2 slowly forms HCO_3^- and H^+.) The subsequent dissociation of H_2CO_3 forms HCO_3^- and H^+ within the RBC. The HCO_3^- diffuses out of the RBC into the plasma wherein it is carried for exchange in the pulmonary circulation. The P_{CO_2} of venous blood is approximately 46 mm Hg, whereas that of the alveolar air is 40 mm Hg. Within the pulmonary vessels the reverse reactions occur. Carbon dioxide diffuses down its pressure gradient from the plasma and bicarbonate, diffusing into the RBC, is converted back to CO_2 by carbonic anhydrase. More CO_2 leaves the RBC, enters the plasma and is exchanged. Similarly, the carbamino CO_2 separates from the hemoglobin and is replaced by O_2.

The chemical events of gas exchange are summarized in Figure 21.25.

Acid/Base Balance. The bicarbonate system comprises a significant buffer system for the body. Carbon dioxide produced by the tissues reacts according to the following equation under the catalytic influence of *carbonic anhydrase*:

$$CO_2 + H_2O \rightleftharpoons H_2CO_3 \rightleftharpoons H^+ + HCO_3^-$$

Carbonic acid, a weak acid, dissociates to hydrogen ion and bicarbonate ion, the latter being the conjugate base of carbonic acid. With excess H^+, the equilibrium shifts to the left, whereas in the presence of excess base (OH^-), the equilibrium shifts to the right with the formation of water:

$$H_2CO_3 \leftarrow H^+ + HCO_3^-$$
$$OH^- + H_2CO_3 \rightarrow H_2O + HCO_3^-$$

The function of the carbonate buffer system is not to prevent pH change with excess acid or base but to minimize the change.

The amount of CO_2 in the blood greatly influences these relationships. Increased carbon dioxide shifts the equilibrium to the right:

$$\uparrow CO_2 \therefore CO_2 + H_2O \rightarrow H_2CO_3$$
$$\rightarrow H^+ + HCO_3^-$$

The inability of the lungs to eliminate CO_2, as in *hypoventilation*, results in an increased CO_2 and a decreased pH (increased $[H^+]$) – *respiratory acidosis*. Renal secretion of excess H^+ and conservation of HCO_3^- are compensatory mechanisms—*compensated respiratory acidosis*. A decreased amount of CO_2 shifts the equilibrium to the left:

$$\downarrow CO_2 \therefore CO_2 + H_2O \leftarrow H_2CO_3$$
$$\leftarrow H^+ + HCO_3^-$$

The elimination of too much CO_2, as in *hyperventilation*, causes a decreased CO_2 and an increased pH (decreased $[H^+]$)—*respiratory alkalosis*. *Compensated respiratory alkalosis* results as the kidneys conserve H^+ and excrete HCO_3^-. Respiratory acidosis and alkalosis are not only associated with

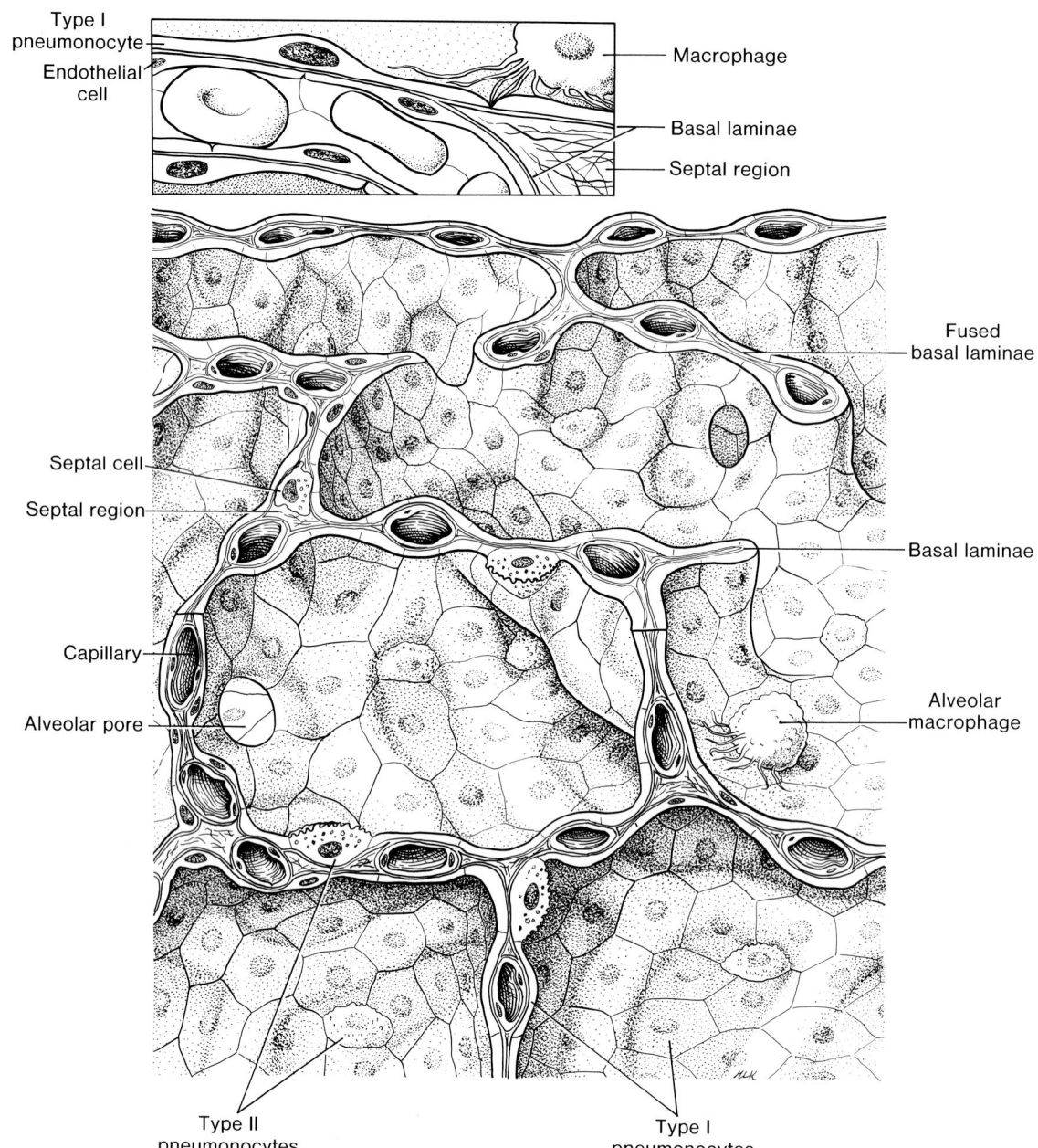

Type I pneumonocyte

Endothelial cell

Macrophage

Basal laminae

Septal region

Fused basal laminae

Septal cell

Septal region

Basal laminae

Capillary

Alveolar pore

Alveolar macrophage

Type II pneumonocytes

Type I pneumonocytes

Fig. 21.21 A diagram of alveoli. The inset is a drawing of the blood-air barrier. The entire lung surface is lined by a continuous layer of epithelial cells.

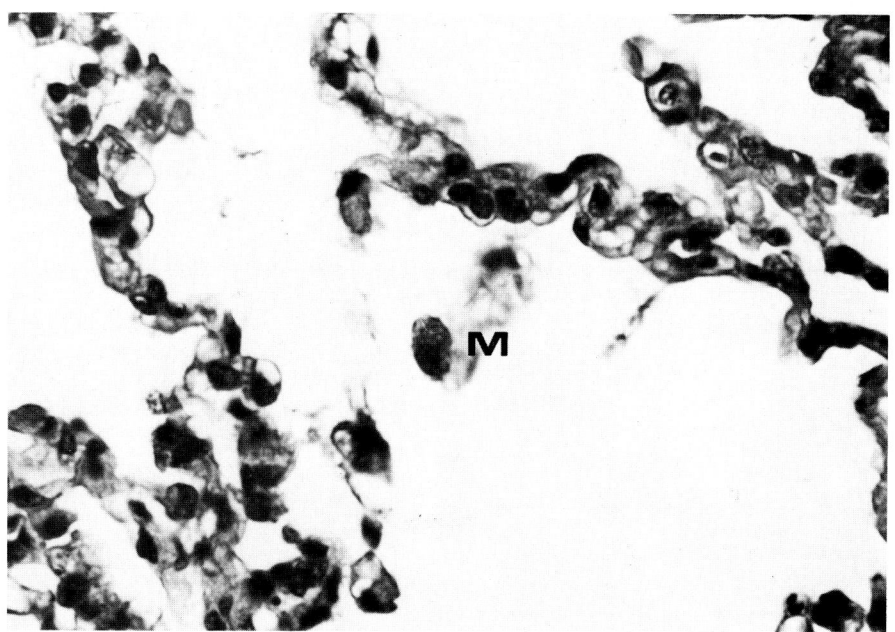

Fig. 21.22 An alveolar macrophage (M) in the alveolar lumen of a canine lung. The transalveolar migration of these cells is a significant protective mechanism. X160.

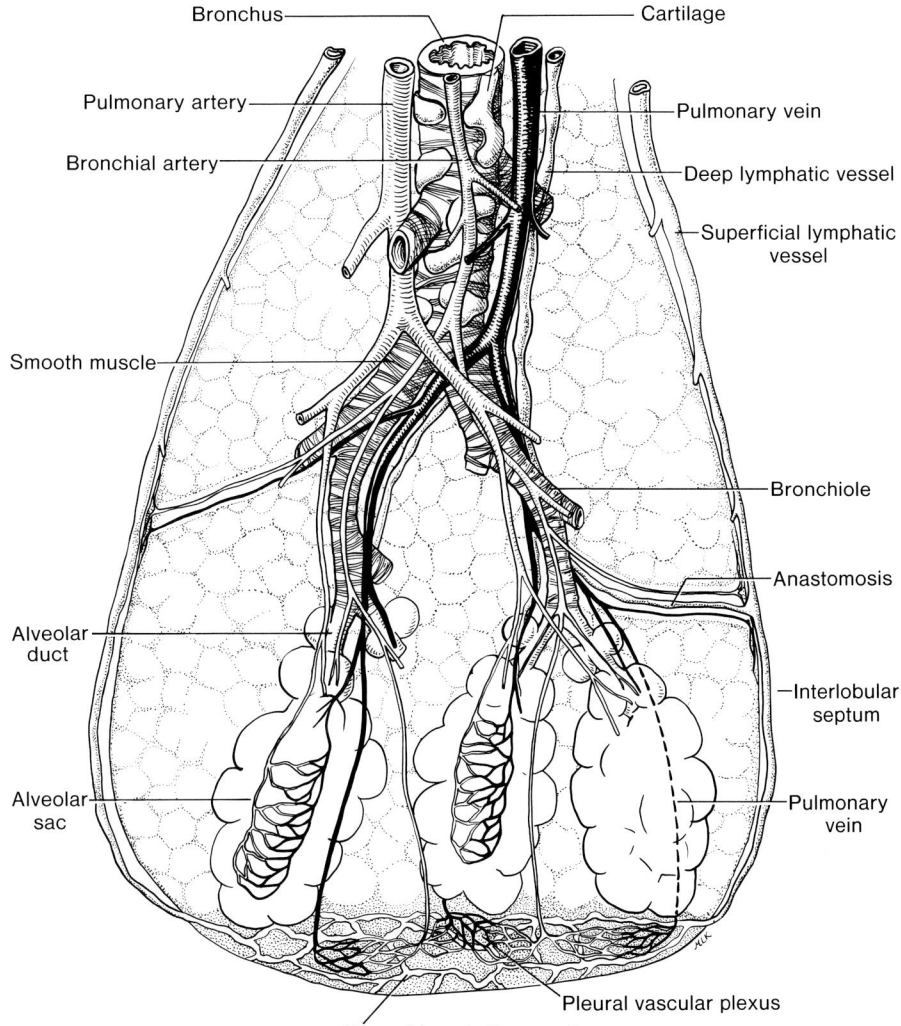

Fig. 21.23 A diagram depicting the relationships of arteries, veins and lymphatics to the distal airway in a bovine lung.

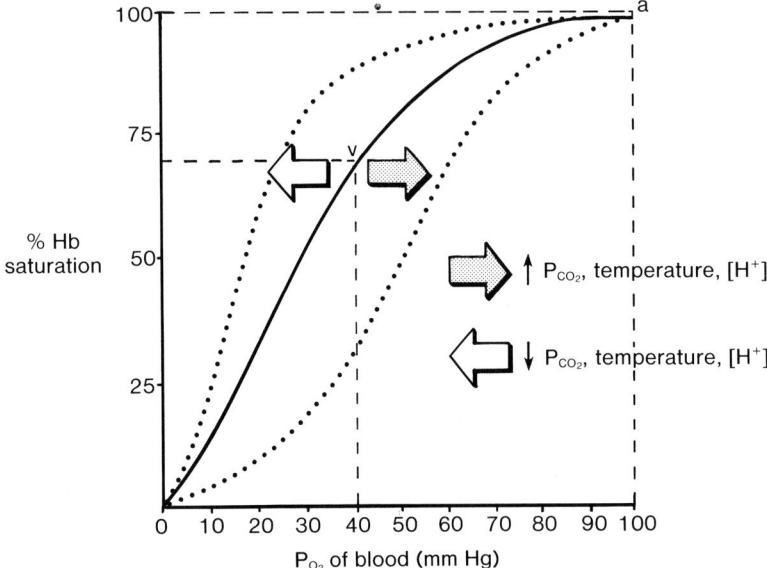

Fig. 21.24 Oxygen-hemoglobin dissociation curve. a, arterial blood; v, venous blood. An alveolar P_{O_2} of 100 mm Hg results in 97% hemoglobin saturation. Arterial blood varies from 100 to 40 mm Hg P_{O_2}. Venous blood has a P_{O_2} of ≤40 mm Hg. Active tissues cause a shift to the right, whereas inactive tissues cause a shift to the left.

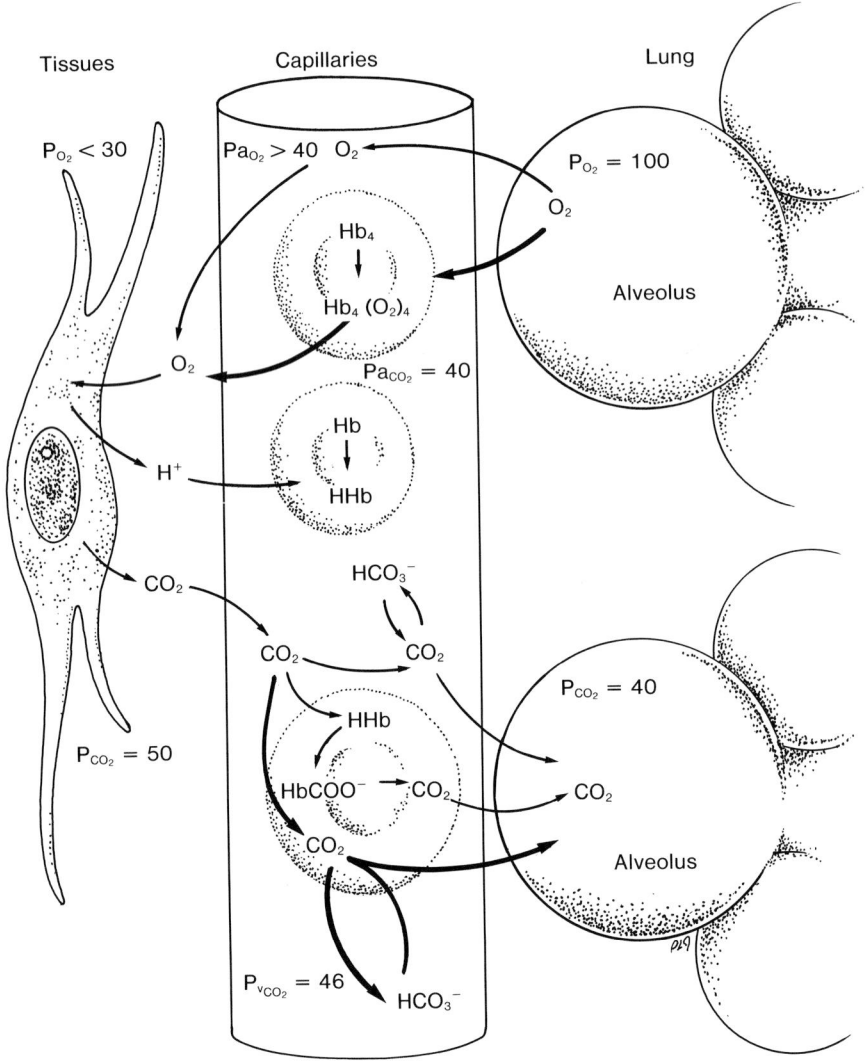

Fig. 21.25 A diagram of the chemical events resulting in the exchange of gases within the lung and somatic tissues.

changes in blood CO_2 but result from these changes.

Ventilation and Perfusion. *Ventilation* is the oxygenation of blood within the pulmonary capillaries, whereas *perfusion* is the movement of blood through the capillaries. The proper exchange of gases occurs at the blood-air barrier when alveolar ventilation ($\dot{V}$) is matched appropriately to pulmonary perfusion ($\dot{Q}$) and is expressed as the $\dot{V}/\dot{Q}$ ratio. The $\dot{V}/\dot{Q}$ ratio for the entire lung averages about 1.0 under normal circumstances; however, not all aveoli have a $\dot{V}/\dot{Q}$ ratio of 1.0. In quadripeds, dorsally-positioned alveoli are usually underperfused and ventrally-positioned alveoli are overperfused. Underperfused alveoli represent wasted ventilation: air is moved (inspired and expired), but exchange either does not occur or is insufficient. An increased amount of pulmonary dead space exists. Overperfusion represents wasted circulation to the lung, because more blood is flowing to the alveoli than air. The $\dot{V}/\dot{Q}$ ratio may be altered by changes in both ventilation and perfusion.

Changes in the $\dot{V}/\dot{Q}$ ratio that affect the entire lung appreciably alter arterial P_{O_2} and P_{CO_2}. A low $\dot{V}/\dot{Q}$ ratio is characterized by a decreased arterial P_{O_2}. *Anoxia* (reduced P_{O_2}) and *cyanosis* (blue mucous membranes) result. Whereas perfusion may be adequate, ventilation is decreased. Various lung problems (asthma, bronchitis, pneumonia) result in low $\dot{V}/\dot{Q}$ ratios. A high $\dot{V}/\dot{Q}$ ratio is characterized by an increased arterial P_{CO_2}, whereas arterial P_{O_2} may not reflect changes. Vascular problems (pulmonary stenosis, pulmonary emboli, right-to-left cardiac shunts) generally account for high $\dot{V}/\dot{Q}$ ratios.

Neural and Chemical Regulation. Numerous mechanisms are utilized to regulate the lungs. Pulmonary regulation is integrated with cardiovascular regulation, because the control of both is essential for appropriate ventilation and perfusion. Metabolic demands are accompanied by alterations in respiratory and cardiovascular activity. Increased metabolic demands require an augmented delivery of O_2 to the tissues as well as an increased ability to remove CO_2. Such metabolic activity is accompanied by increased ventilation and perfusion. The converse is true also.

Breathing (external respiration, inspiration and expiration) is accomplished through the rhythmic activity of neurons located in the brain stem (pons and medulla oblongata). The automatic discharge of specific neuronal pools within the brain stem is modulated by information from conscious centers (cerebrum) and afferent information transmitted to respiratory centers from the periphery. Whereas the central regulatory neuronal pools are referred to as *respiratory centers*, little agreement exists concerning the nature, extent, distribution, location, subdivision and discreteness of the centers. Classically, the region within the medulla oblongata has been called the *respiratory center*, a region consisting of dorsal and ventral neuronal pools that are responsible for rhythmic inspiratory and expiratory activity. The dorsal neuronal pool controls the discharge of the phrenic nerve to the diaphragm, whereas the ventral neuronal pool controls the intercostal and accessory respiratory musculature. Two additional respiratory centers occur within the pons. The *pneumotaxis center*, located in the rostral pontine area prevents apnea (respiratory arrest), while the caudally-positioned *apneustic center* causes apnea. The pontine centers, which respond to afferent information from the periphery, probably mediate their influence upon respiration through the medullary respiratory center.

Chemical alterations of the blood influence respiratory activity. Arterial P_{O_2}, P_{CO_2}, and pH are monitored by central and peripheral chemoreceptors (Chapter 16). The peripheral chemoreceptors (carotid and aortic bodies) are sensitive to altered P_{O_2}, P_{CO_2}, and pH. A decreased arterial P_{O_2}, increased P_{CO_2} and increased $[H^+]$, translated into GVA impulses in the vagus and glossopharyngeal nerves, result in an augmented ventilatory effort. The central chemoreceptors located within the medulla are sensitive to the P_{CO_2}, and $[H^+]$ of cerebrospinal fluid or the fluid within the brain interstitium. The hydration of CO_2 within the CSF or brain interstitium produces H^+. The increased $[H^+]$ causes an increase in respiration.

Although the chemoreceptors respond to P_{CO_2} and P_{O_2}, increased P_{CO_2} (*hypercapnia*) is a stronger influence on respiration than is decreased P_{O_2} (*hypoxia*). Arterial P_{O_2} must decrease to about 60 mm Hg before the hypoxic drive is evident. Also, a decreased P_{O_2} depresses neuronal activity.

Avian Respiratory System

Upper Respiratory Tract. The upper respiratory tract of birds includes all those structures described for mammals with the addition of the syrinx. These organs function in a manner similar to those in mammals.

The *nasal cavity* is lined by the same types of epithelia characteristic of the mammal. The vestibular region is lined by a stratified squamous epithelium which, from surface view, has a beaded appearance. The basal and intermediate cell layers are vertically oriented. They consist of large cells with centrally located nuclei. These rows are covered by a thin double layer of cornified cells. The remaining respiratory and olfactory epithelium is typical. Intraepithelial glands typify the respiratory epithelium (Fig. 5.20). The lamina propria is areolar connective tissue with diffuse and aggregated lymphatic tissue. It is continuous with the underlying connective tissue investments of bone or cartilage.

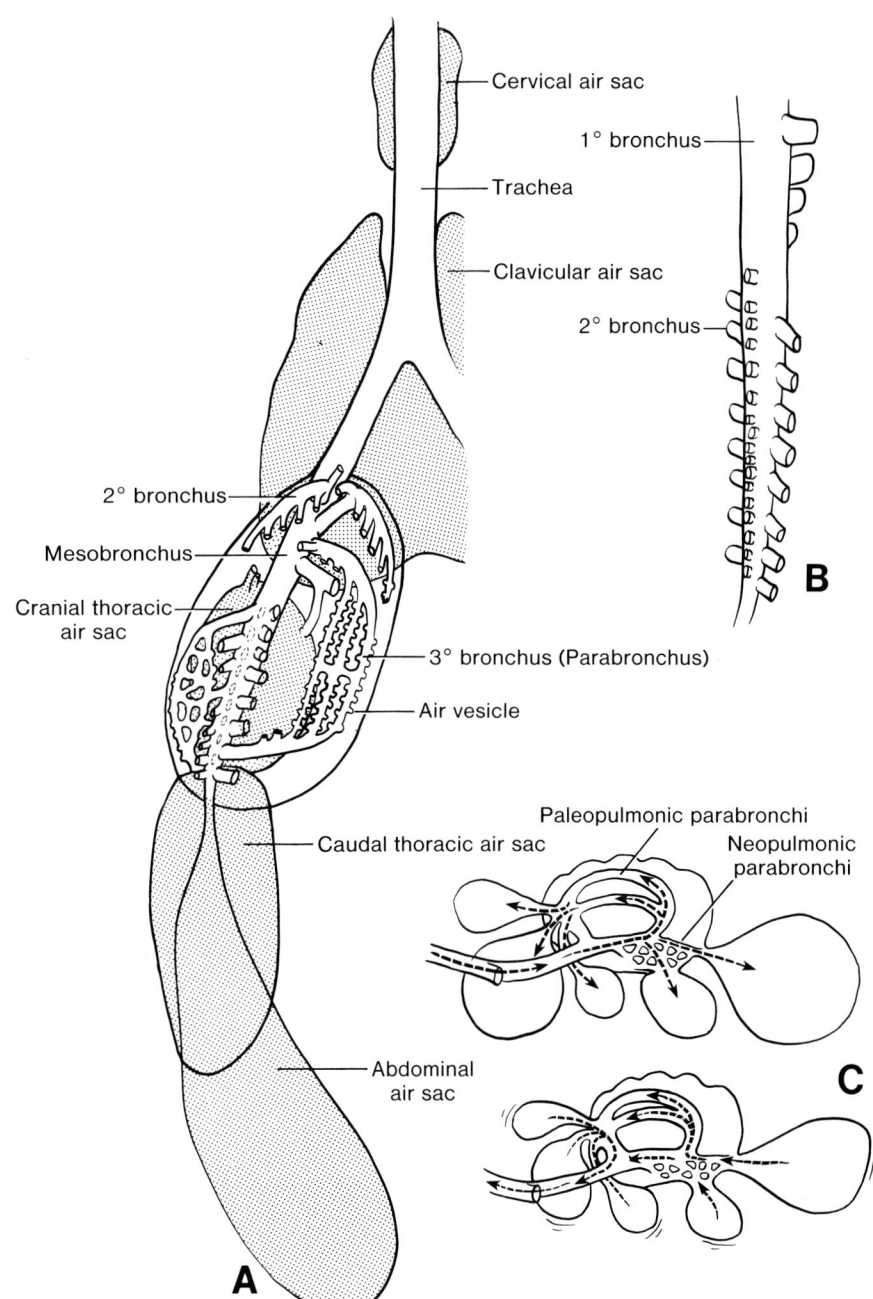

Fig. 21.26 A diagram depicting the major portion of the avian respiratory system. A, The trachea, lung and air sacs are depicted. B, Primary and secondary bronchial relationships are shown. C, The movement of air through the lung and air sacs is shown.

The *trachea* of the bird is similar to that of the mammal. The following differences are apparent. The typical epithelium contains intraepithelial mucous glands that may protrude slightly into the typical lamina propria. Mucosal and submucosal glands are of variable occurrence. The cartilaginous rings are complete and alternate in size. Ossification of these supportive rings is common in some species (goose, duck). Longitudinally oriented striated muscle is located at the periphery of the trachea in a lateral position.

The primary bronchi are similar in structure to the trachea. The cartilaginous rings, however, are gradually replaced by dense white fibrous connective tissue, and smooth muscle may connect the free surfaces of the cartilage.

The *syrinx* is located at the junction of the trachea and bronchi. It is an inverted Y-shaped structure. At the bifurcation of the trachea, a cartilaginous bar with a mucosal-submucosal fold constitutes the *median vocal fold*. By drawing the bronchi toward each other, two *lateral vocal folds* are produced at the level of the median vocal fold. The combination of these folds is responsible for phonation.

The lamina epithelialis of the syrinx consists of either a bistratified squamous or a columnar epithelium. Mucosal glands as well as diffuse and nodular lymphatic tissue are present in the lamina propria.

Lung. The lungs of birds are very different from the lungs of mammals. Compared to the size of the thoracic cavity, the lungs are extremely small. Moreover, they do not change volume during inhalation and exhalation. The structures that do change volume are the air sacs, which are continuous with the duct system of the lung.

The duct system bears no similarity to the one in mammals (Fig. 21.26). The *primary bronchi* enter the lung and expand as the *vestibulum*. This continues through the lung as the *mesobronchus* and is connected to the *abdominal air sac*. Secondary bronchi and air sacs arise from the vestibulum and mesobronchus. Secondary bronchi are described as *dorsal bronchi*, *ventral bronchi* or *lateral bronchi* on the basis of their gross orientation. Secondary bronchi give rise to *tertiary bronchi* (*parabronchi*) that are then continuous with other secondary bronchi. Thus, a complete air-conducting loop is formed. The parabronchi are analogous to the alveolar ducts of mammals. *Air vesicles* (*atria*) project radially from the parabronchi. These atria are continuous with the *air capillaries* (*air cells*). These air capillaries are continuous loops that open back into the atria. These are the moieties responsible for the actual exchange of gases with the closely associated vascular capillaries.

The air sacs associated with the avian lung aid in the movement of air through the lung. They are membranous structures which do not contribute to the exchange of gases. Most birds have nine air sacs: *unpaired cervicals*, *paired claviculars*, *paired cranial thoracics*, *paired caudal thoracics*, *paired abdominals*. The air sacs occur free in the body cavities and send diverticula into the bones with which they are associated. *Recurrent bronchi* extend from the air sacs and attach to the parabronchi. *Recurrent bronchi* are involved in the return of the air from the air sacs to the lung proper.

Histology of the Lung and Associated Structures. The *intrapulmonary primary bronchi* are extensions of the bifurcated trachea and are similar in structure to their extrapulmonary counterparts. The lamina epithelialis consists of pseudostratified ciliated columnar epithelium with goblet cells and intraepithelial mucous glands. The lamina propria is areolar connective tissue with numerous diffuse and aggregated lymphatic tissue. Lymph nodules, however, are rarely present. The lamina muscularis mucosae is disposed primarily as a circularly or spirally oriented mass of muscle with some longitudinal bundles as well. Cartilaginous rings are present in the initial portions of these bronchi but are replaced by plaques of car-

tilage. The latter are lost within the vestibulum. The tunica adventitia blends with the surrounding interstitial connective tissue.

The mural elements of the *vestibulum*, except for the previously mentioned differences in the cartilage, are similar to those of the intrapulmonary primary bronchi. The vestibulum, however, is an enlarged portion of the primary conductive pathway through

the lung which is continued caudally by the *mesobronchus*. The latter is a continuation of the primary conductive pathway. Its morphology is similar to the vestibulum. The luminal diameter of this tubule, however, is smaller than those described previously.

Secondary bronchi, whether they are lateral, dorsal or ventral, have a similar morphology (Fig. 21.27). The lamina epithelialis is composed of columnar or cuboidal cells

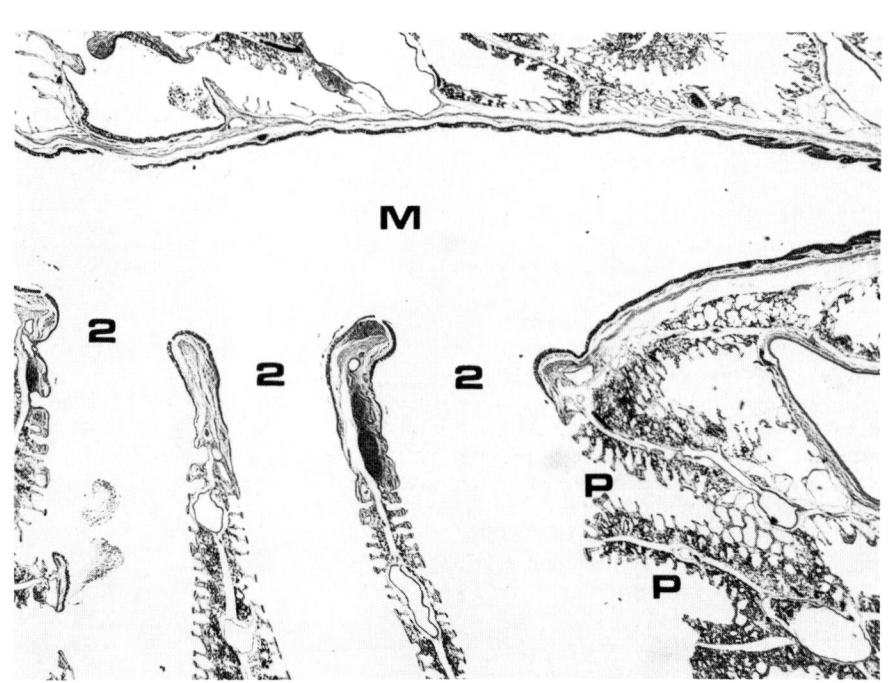

Fig. 22.27   A section of an avian lung. M, mesobronchus; 2, secondary bronchi; P, parabronchi (3° bronchi). X4.

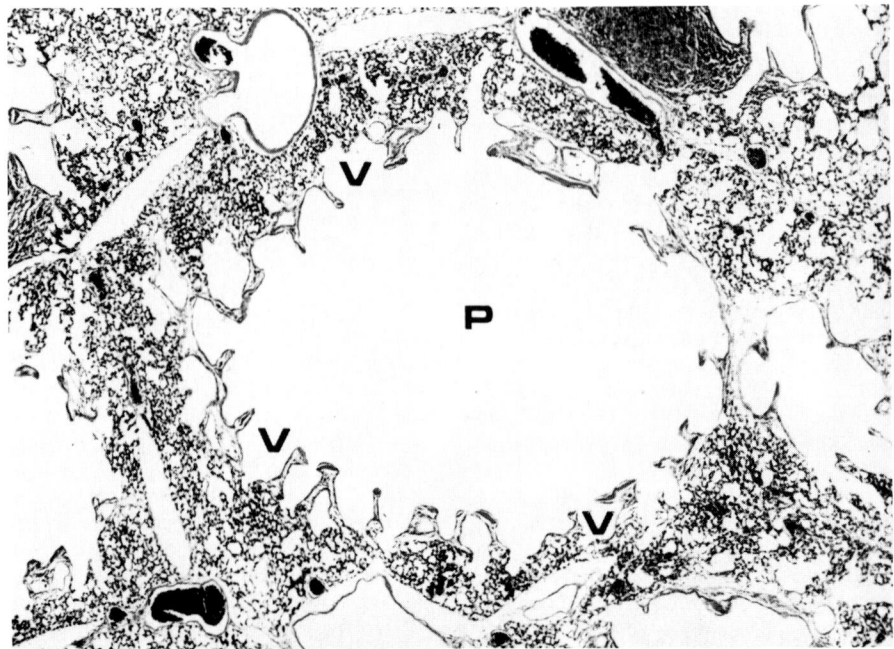

Fig. 21.28   A parabronchus of the avian lung. The parabronchus (P) has numerous air vesicles (V) in its wall. X16.

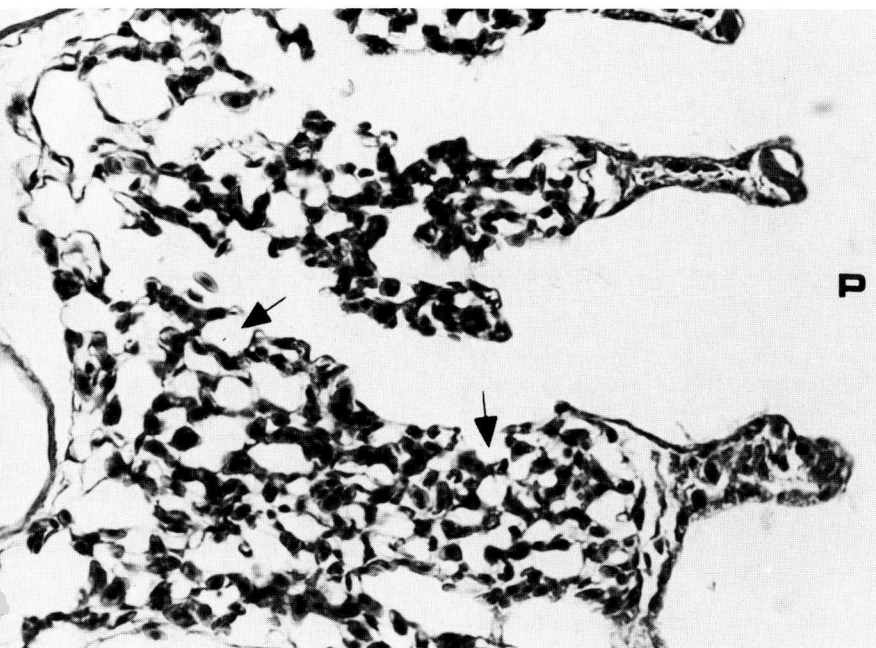

Fig. 21.29 Air vesicles of the avian lung. The air vesicles comprise the walls of the parabronchi. The air vesicles are composed of air capillaries (*arrows*) and blood capillaries. X100.

nd is devoid of goblet cells. The lamina propria is composed of areolar connective tissue which is usually devoid of lymphatic tissue. The lamina muscularis mucosae is interrupted and multidirectionally oriented. Cartilage is not present. Numerous interruptions of the mural elements are commonly encountered due to the occurrence of parabronchi and, in some areas, air vesicles. Because of the latter, portions of the secondary bronchi may be considered analogous to mammalian respiratory bronchioles.

The mucosal lining of *parabronchi* is interrupted by the laterally projecting air vesicles (Fig. 21.28). Between the interruptions, the parabronchi are lined by a cuboidal or squamous epithelium. The reduced lamina propria is composed of a fine areolar connective tissue. The lamina muscularis mucosae is confined to the area beneath the edges of the lamina epithelialis as separate bundles of smooth muscle.

The *air vesicles* are lined by a simple squamous epithelium and are supported by fine interstitial connective tissue (Fig. 21.29). The epithelium of the air vesicles is continuous as a simple squamous lining of the *air capillaries*. The air capillary-blood capillary relationship is similar to that described for mammals.

Ventilation of the Lung. Ventilation of the avian lung is achieved by the air sacs functioning as bellows without any alteration to the volume of the lung. The bird is an abdominal breather. Inspiratory muscle movements increase the size of the air sacs, decrease pressure and cause air to move inwardly. The reverse occurs during expiration. Air movement through the avian lung is unidirectional and bidirectional dur-

ing inspiration and expiration (Fig. 21.26). Air moves in a bidirectional pattern through neopulmonic parabronchi to and from the caudal air sacs during inspiration and expiration. Inspiratory and expiratory effort is characterized by the unidirectional flow of air through the paleopulmonic parabronchi. The ventilation flow pattern through the lung permits the bird to extract more oxygen from a specified volume of inspired air than its mammalian counterparts. The axes of the parabronchi are at right angles to the axes of the blood capillaries within the lung (*cross-current exchanger*). The relationship of these structures permits gas exchange independent of direction of flow. The relationship between the blood capillaries and air capillaries is that of a *countercurrent-type exchanger*. Mixed venous blood enters a blood capillary and flows adjacent and opposite to the flow in an air capillary. The blood flow in the capillary exits at the point in which parabronchial air enters. The relationship may facilitate gaseous exchange and enhance gaseous equilibration between blood and air capillaries.

References

Respiratory Tract—Conductive
Ali, M. Y.: Histology of the human nasopharyngeal mucosa. J. Anat. *99:*657, 1965.
Amoore, J. E., Johnston, J. W. and Rubin, M.: The stereochemical theory of odor. Sci. Amer. *210:*43, 1964.
Arstila, A. and Wersall, J.: The ultrastructure of the olfactory epithelium of the guinea pig. Acta Otolaryngol. *64:*187, 1967.
Baradi, A. F. and Bourne, G. H.: Gustatory and olfactory epithelia. Int. Rev. Cytol. *2:*289, 1953.
Bojsen-Moller, F.: Topography and development of the anterior nasal glands in pigs. J. Anat. *101:*321, 1967.

Frisch, D.: Ultrastructure of mouse olfactory mucosa. Amer. J. Anat. *121:*87, 1967.
Hansell, M. M. and Moretti, R. L.: Ultrastructure of the mouse tracheal epithelium. J. Morph. *128:*159, 1969.
Rhodin, J. and Dalhamn, T.: Electron microscopy of the tracheal ciliated mucosa in rat. Z. Zellforsch. *44:*345, 1956.

Mammalian Lung
Banks, W. J., Jr. and Epling, G. P.: Differentiation and origin of the type II pneumocyte: An ultrastructural study. Acta Anat. *78:*604, 1971.
Bertalanffy, F. D.: Respiratory tissue: structure, histophysiology and cytodynamics. I. Review and basic cytomorphology. Int. Rev. Cytol. *16:*233, 1964.
Bowden, D. H., Adamson, I. Y. R., Grantham, G. and Wyatt, J. P.: Origin of the lung macrophage: Evidence derived from radiation injury. Arch. Pathol. *88:*540, 1969.
Comroe, J. H., Jr.: *Physiology of Respiration: An Introductory Text.* Year Book Medical Publishers, Chicago, 1965a.
Comroe, J. H. et al.: *The Lung: Clinical Physiology and Pulmonary Function Tests.* 2nd edition. Year Book Medical Publishers, Chicago, 1965b.
Epling, G. P.: Electron microscopy of the bovine lungs: Lattice and lamellar structures in the alveolar lumina. Amer. J. Vet. Res. *25:*1424, 1964.
Engel, S.: *Lung Structure.* C. C. Thomas, Springfield, 1962.
Engel, S.: *The Prenatal Lung.* Pergamon Press, New York, 1966.
Karrer, H. E.: The ultrastructure of mouse lung. The alveolar macrophage. J. Biophys. Biochem. Cytol. *4:*693, 1958.
King, R. J.: The surfactant system of the lung. Fed. Proc. *33:*2238, 1974.
Krahl, V. E.: Current concept of the finer structure of the lung. Arch. Intern. Med. (Chicago) *96:*342, 1955.
Krahl, V. E.: Anatomy of the Mammalian Lung. In *Handbook of Physiology. Sect. 3, Respiration.* Vol. 1, Chapter 6, edited by W. O. Fenn and H. Rahn, American Physiological Society, Washington, D.C. Williams & Wilkins, 1964.
Krahl, V. E.: *The Human Lung* (translation of *Die Menschliche Lunge* by H. von Hayek, Springer Verlag, Berlin, 1953). Hafner, New York 1960.
Loosli, C. G. and Porter, E. L.: Pre- and postnatal development of the respiratory portion of the human lung. Amer. Rev. Resp. Dis. *80:*5, 1959.
Low, F. N.: Electron microscopy of the rat lung. Anat. Rec. *113:*437, 1952.
Meyrick, B. and Reid, L.: The alveolar brush cell in rat lung—a third pneumocyte. J. Ultrastruct. Res. *23:*71, 1968.
Miller, W. S.: *The Lung.* 2nd edition. C. C. Thomas, Springfield, 1950.
Sorokin, S. P.: A morphologic and cytochemical study of the great alveolar cell. J. Histochem. Cytochem. *14:*884, 1966.
Tobin, C. E.: Lymphatics of the pulmonary alveoli. Anat. Rec. *120:*625, 1954.
Tyler, W. S., Gillespie, J. R. and Nowell, J. A.: Modern functional morphology of the equine lung. Eq. Vet. J. *3:*84, 1971.

Avian Lung and Associated Structures
Akester, A. R.: The comparative anatomy of the respiratory pathways in the domestic fowl, pigeon and domestic duck. J. Anat. *94:*488, 1960.
Cover, M. S.: The gross and microscopic anatomy of the respiratory system of the turkey. I. The nasal cavity and infraorbital sinus. Amer. J. Vet. Res. *14:*113, 1953.
Cover, M. S.: The gross and microscopic anatomy of the respiratory system of the turkey. II. The larynx, trachea, syrinx, bronchi and lungs. Amer. J. Vet. Res. *14:*230, 1953.
Cover, M. S.: Gross and microscopic anatomy of the respiratory system of the turkey. III. The air sacs. Amer. J. Vet. Res. *14:*239, 1953.
McLeod, W. M. and Wagers, R. P.: The respiratory system of the chicken. J. Amer. Vet. Med. Assoc. *95:*59, 1939.
Sturkie, P. D. (editor): *Avian Physiology.* 3rd edition. Springer-Verlag, New York, 1976.

22: Endocrine System

General Characteristics

Introduction. The glands that comprise the endocrine system are those structures described as *ductless glands* or *glands of internal secretion.* Although they are derived from all the germ layers, they do not maintain anatomical contacts with these layers (Fig. 5.21). Furthermore, the glands may be a distinct organ (pituitary, adrenals, thyroid, etc.) or they may be parts of other organs (islets of Langerhans, interstitial cells of the testes, follicles and corpora lutea of the ovary).

The organization of these glands is simple. They may be encapsulated, lack an extensive stroma, are highly vascularized and possess cells in varied configurations. The configurations may include *single cells, cell clusters, cell cords* or *cell follicles.* Whatever their configuration, they are intimately associated with an extensive vascular supply (capillaries or sinusoids) into which they secrete their products.

The *hormones* that these glands secrete are variable. They may be proteins, glycoproteins, polypeptides, steroids or catecholamines. One gland may secrete one hormone, whereas other glands may secrete several hormones. These hormones may be synthesized and immediately secreted (adrenal cortex), synthesized and temporarily stored as presecretory granules (islets of Langerhans) or synthesized and stored in a follicle (thyroid). Once these products have been secreted into the blood stream, they may have an effect upon the entire organism, selected organs or a specific organ. Although the entire organism may be affected, one organ or group of organs may respond specifically. The latter are termed the *target organ* or *target organs*; i.e., some organs have a sufficiently low threshold to a specific hormonal stimulation that their response is measured readily.

The endocrine system consists of organs with an exclusive endocrine function (pituitary, pineal, thyroid, parathyroid, adrenal), as well as organs with an endocrine and exocrine function (pancreas, gonads, kidneys, liver, stomach, intestines, placenta).

Nature and Function of Hormones. Hormones are chemical substances secreted by endocrine cells into the body fluids exerting an influence upon other cells of the body. Whereas some hormones (secretin, cholecystokinin-pancreozymin, gastrin) exert their influence locally (*local hormones*), others (adrenocorticoids, growth hormone, thyroxine) are transported by the blood and exert their influence throughout the body as *general hormones.* Hormones are regulatory substances that function to alter the rates at which existing reactions occur without contributing mass nor energy to the reaction. These substances are significant contributors to homeostasis, because they influence metabolic reactions, cellular differentiation, as well as developmental, maturation and aging processes. Hormones influence cell function by either activating cyclic AMP within cells or by activating specific genes within cells.

Cyclic AMP is an intracellular mediator of hormonal activity, often called the *second messenger.* The first messenger is the protein or polypeptide hormone that influences the formation of cyclic AMP. The exciting hormone binds with a specific receptor located within the plasma membrane of the target cells. The hormone/receptor complex activates the enzyme *adenylcyclase* which is located within the cell membrane also. Adenylcyclase catalyzes the conversion of cytoplasmic ATP to cyclic AMP. Cyclic AMP causes the initiation of various cellular functions that include alteration of cell membrane permeability to various substances (water, calcium), activation of enzymes, initiation of cellular secretion, augmentation of protein synthesis and initiation of cellular contraction and/or relaxation.

Steroid hormones influence cellular activity by promoting cells to produce proteins. Steroid hormones pass through the cell membrane and attach to a specific cytoplasmic protein receptor molecule. The hormone/protein receptor complex, perhaps altered during its transport or diffusion to the nucleus, becomes an activation factor for the transcription of messenger RNA. Messenger RNA, diffusing into the cytoplasm, affects translation, and the production of enzymes results. The enzymes then mediate altered cell function.

Regulatory Mechanisms. The release of hormones is an adjunctive mechanism in the maintenance of homeostasis. Hormones affect cellular activity and regulate various substances within the body. The activities and substances regulated by specific hormones vary; also, the specific mechanisms utilized in regulation differ. Despite the diversity, some generalizations about the mechanisms are possible. The regulation of a substance (*regulated system*) requires the participation of a receptor, regulator and effector. The *receptor*, perceiving alterations in the level of a particular substance, informs the *regulator.* The regulator sends signals to the *effector*, which initiates the appropriate response; thereby the level of the regulated substance is changed. The most important regulated systems in the animal body are *negative feedback systems* or *loops*—the effector reverses the initiating event. If a controlled substance were to increase, then the effector decreases the substance (Fig. 22.1). The converse is true also. Although the simplified scheme represents the essence of a negative feedback loop, variations exist. The receptor and regulator may be combined; more than one regulator and effector may be involved. Figure 22.2 demonstrates two alterations of the basic pattern of regulation. Others exist and are discussed with the specific hormones.

Positive feedback loops amplify or intensify the initiating event in a regulated system. They are not common in the normal organism; however, such systems may be operational in various disease conditions.

Hypophysis Cerebri

Organization and Development. Figure 22.3 represents the organizational pattern of the hypophysis cerebri (*pituitary gland*). The *pars tuberalis* and *pars distalis* constitute the *anterior lobe* or *anterior pituitary* (Fig. 22.3). The *pars intermedia* and the *infundibular process* constitute the *posterior lobe* or *posterior pituitary.* The *pars tuberalis* and the

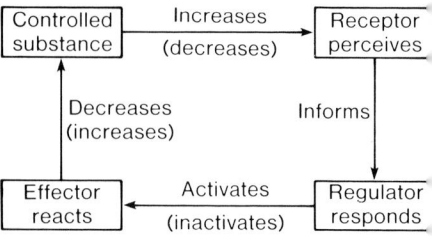

Fig. 22.1 A flow chart that depicts the relationships of the components of a regulated system. A negative feedback loop is the common servomechanism of the body. Alterations of the regulated substance or activity results in a reversal of the initiating event by the effector tissues or organs. If the level of a substance or activity were to increase, then the effectors decrease the level of the substance or activity; the converse occurs also. All light micrographs are labeled as the magnification with the microscope before photographic enlarging. All electron micrographs are labeled as total magnification, including photographic enlarging.

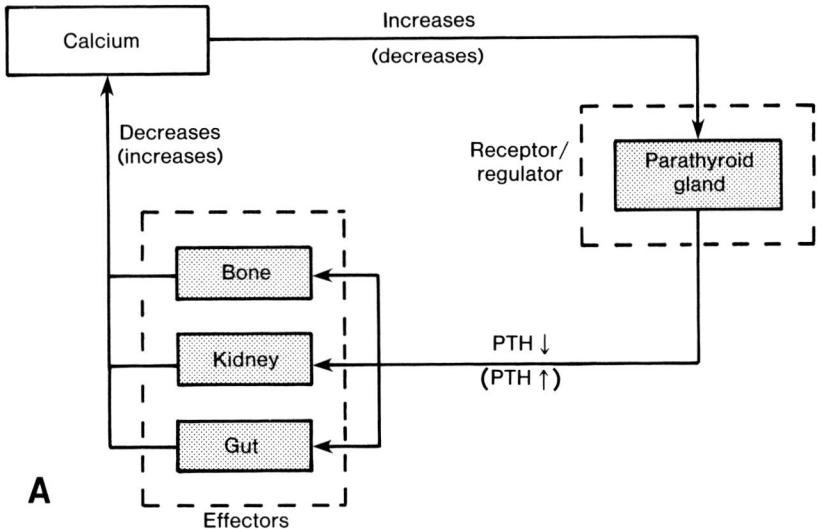

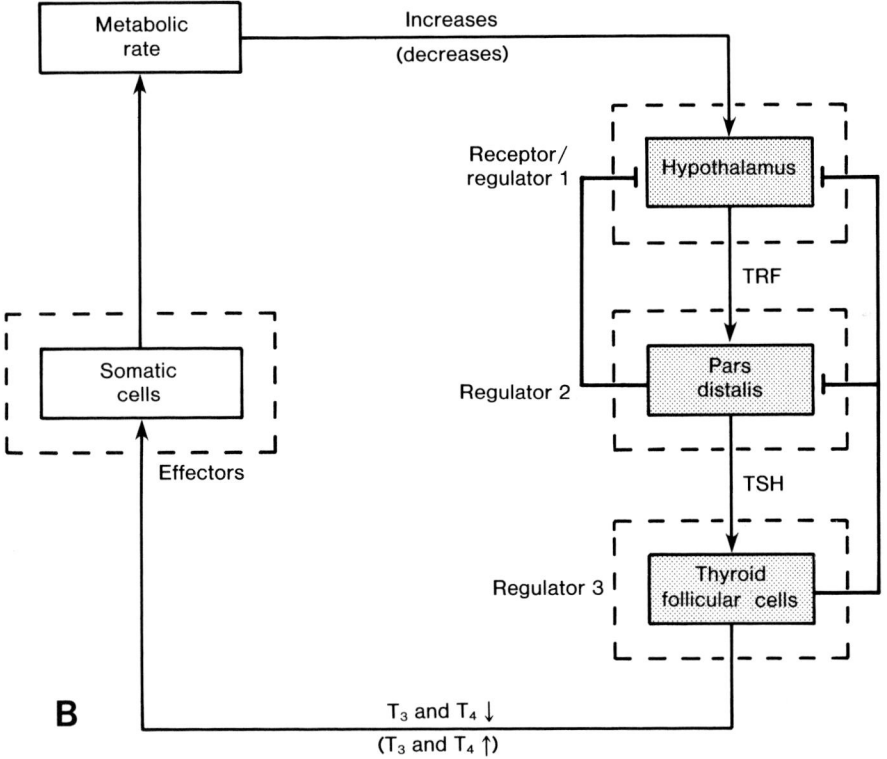

Fig. 22.2   Diagrams depicting two of numerous variations that characterize negative feedback loops in the body. A. One part of the calcium control servomechanism is depicted. Thyrocalcitonin responds to the opposite alterations in levels of calcium and utilizes bone as the effector. Two variations of a servomechanism are evident in this diagram. The receptor and regulator are combined, and more than one effector is involved in the system. The dual control mechanism involving PTH and thyrocalcitonin permits a more precise control than a single control mechanism. B. The servomechanism partially responsible for the regulation of metabolic rate. Four variations of the basic scheme are evident within this system. More than one regulator exists. One of the regulators also serves as the receptor. Two negative feedback loops exist within the overall regulated system (negative feedback loop). Regulator 2 exerts a negative influence on regulator 1; regulator 3 exerts a negative influence on regulator 1 and 2. Finally, numerous cells function as the effectors. The increased number of regulators insures a more precise regulation than a single regulator. TRF, thyroid-releasing factor; TSH, thyroid-stimulating hormone; T_3 and T_4, thyroid hormones; PTH, parathormone.

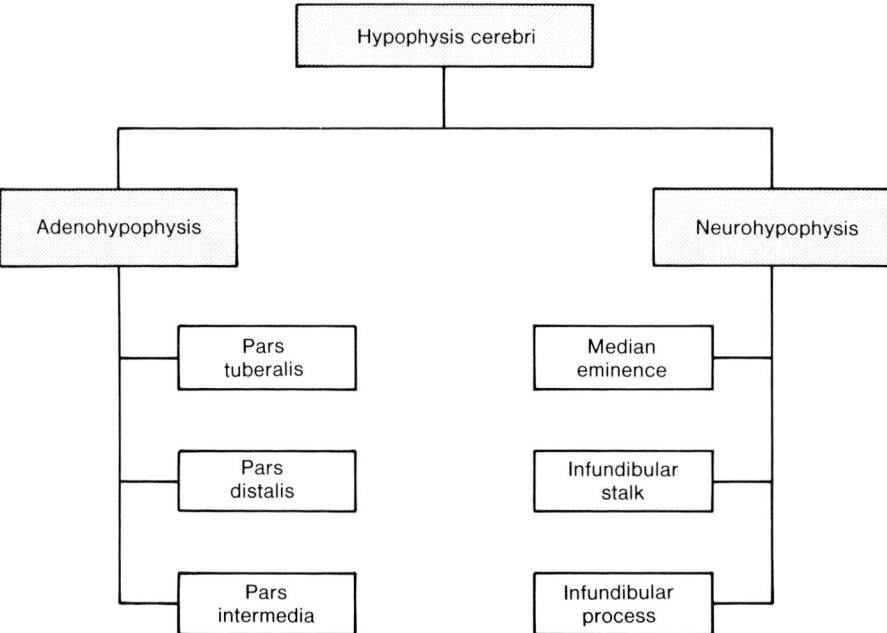

Fig. 22.3   A diagram that depicts the organization of the hypophysis cerebri. The adenohypophysis is the glandular lobe, whereas the neurohypophysis is the neural lobe of the organ.

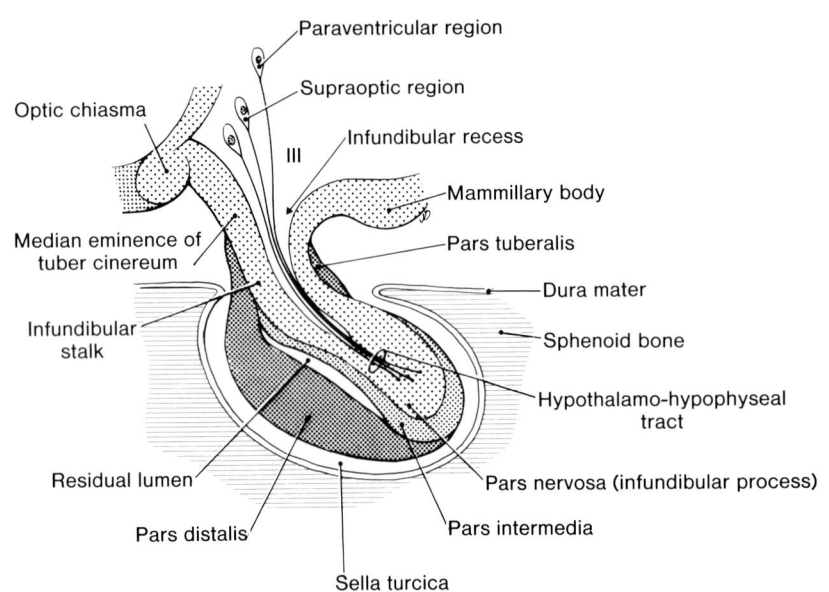

Fig. 22.4   A drawing of the hypophysis cerebri of a pig. The hypophysis cerebri is a ventral evagination of the diencephalon that occupies a recess, the sella turcica, within the sphenoid bone.

The infundibular stalk is an outgrowth of the median eminence. The median eminence is the ventral boundary of the third ventricle in this region. As the infundibular stalk grows, part of the third ventricle is carried with it as the *infundibular recess*. In most species, the recess is confined to the region of continuity of the infundibular stalk with the median eminence (Fig. 22.5). In others (pig and cat especially), the infundibular recess extends into the infundibular process.

Adenohypophysis

The constituents of the adenohypophysis are the *pars distalis, pars intermedia* and *pars tuberalis*.

Pars Distalis

The *pars distalis* comprises the greatest bulk of the adenohypophysis (Fig. 22.6). It is covered by a fibrous capsule of dense white fibrous connective tissue (DWFCT) which is continuous with the reticular fibers that comprise the stroma of the organ. The parenchyma consists of cords or clusters of cells which are intimately associated with sinusoids. The cells of the pars distalis may be divided into two groups: *chromophobic cells* and *chromophilic cells*. The cells of the adenohypophysis and their secretory products are summarized in Table 22.1.

Chromophobic Cells. The *chromophobic cells* are also referred to as *chief cells, principal cells, reserve cells, C cells* or *gamma cells*. These small round cells have little cytoplasm which is usually devoid of granules (Fig. 22.7). As their name chromophobe implies, they have very little affinity for stains. These cells are usually clustered and may form the center of a cord of cells. The exact nature of these cells has not been clarified. They may be reserve cells that are capable of differentiating into chromophilic cells, or they may be cells in the process of degranulation.

Chromophilic Cells—Acidophils. The *chromophils* are initially divisible into *acidophils* and *basophils*. The acidophils include *alpha cells* and *epsilon cells*. These cells contain granules which are periodic acid-Schiff (PAS)-negative but stain with eosin, acid fuchsin, orange G and azocarmine. *Acidophils*, generally, are much larger than chromophobes, possess a granular cytoplasm which is acidophilic and may be polarized (Fig. 22.7). Specific staining techniques permit the subdivision of the acidophils into two distinct groups. The alpha cell has granules about 300 nm in diameter. These granules also stain positively with orange G; thus, they are also referred to as *orangeophils*. The *epsilon cells*, however, have granules which range between 100 and 900 nm. These granules specifically stain with the azocarmine dye. These cells are referred to as *carminophils*.

Chromophilic Cells—Basophils. The *basophils* contain granules which are especially PAS-positive because of the glycoprotein

---

infundibular stalk are referred to as the *hypophyseal stalk*. The terms anterior and posterior pituitary are not totally applicable to all mammalian species (Fig. 22.4). In some species, the posterior pituitary is actually dorsal to the anterior pituitary, whereas in other species the anterior pituitary totally surrounds the posterior pituitary.

The development of the pituitary gland is dependent upon contributions from the buccal cavity (ectoderm) and the floor of the diencephalon (neuroectoderm). *Rathke's pouch*, an outgrowth of the roof of the oral cavity, grows toward the base of the brain.

This pouch is responsible for the differentiation of the *adenohypophysis*. As it grows and contacts the infundibulum from the floor of the diencephalon, its connection with the oral cavity is lost. That portion of Rathke's pouch that contacts the neurohypophysis differentiates into the pars intermedia. The rostral portion becomes the pars distalis, while the dorsal extension of the pars distalis that comes in contact with the infundibular stalk becomes the pars tuberalis. The *residual lumen* of Rathke's pouch may be persistent and separates the anterior from the posterior pituitary.

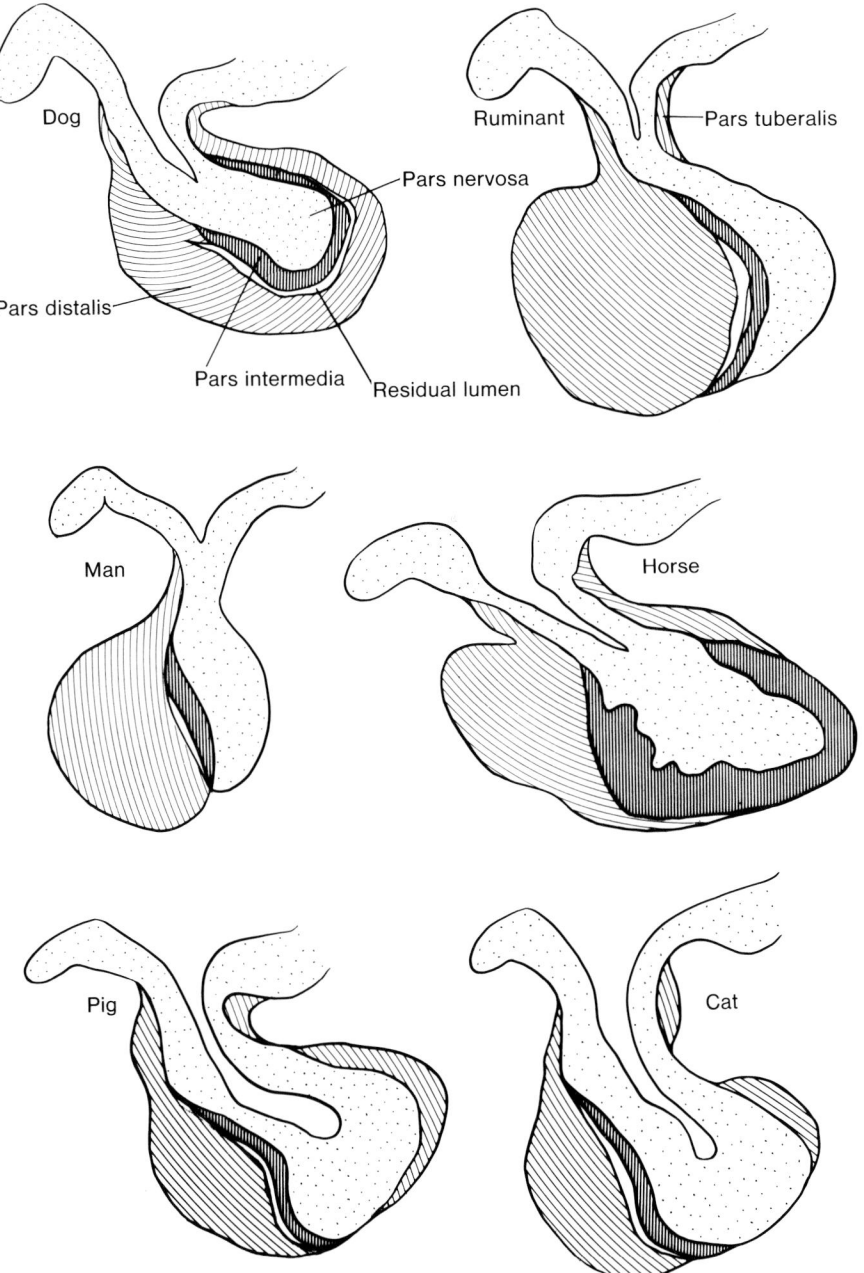

Fig. 22.5   A diagram of the hypophysis cerebri of selected species. The pituitary glands are not drawn to scale.

of the pars tuberalis has not been established.

Pars Intermedia

Form and Function. The *pars intermedia* is not well-developed in man, but it is well-developed in domestic animals (Fig. 22.9). This portion of the pituitary is adjacent to, but separated from, the neurohypophysis by a discontinuous connective tissue sheath. Migration of cells of the pars intermedia into the pars nervosa is common. The predominant cell type of this area is a nonspecific basophil (Fig. 22.10). Although these cells are usually disposed as cords or clusters of cells, follicles are commonly encountered. Cells in the pars intermedia secrete *melanocyte-stimulating hormone (MSH, intermedin)*.

Histophysiology of the Adenohypophysis

Vascular Relationships. The unique blood supply to the adenohypophysis is an essential component of its regulation. Whereas the origin and specific course of the vessels that supply the adenohypophysis vary among the domestic species, the common feature is the formation of the *hypophyseal portal system (hypothalmo-hyopohyseal portal system)*. *Rostral hypophyseal arteries* form an arterial ring around the median eminence and give rise to arterioles that supply the hypothalamus, including the infundibular stalk but do not extend into the infundibular process. The pars distalis is supplied indirectly by the rostral hypophyseal arteries.

Arteriolar branches terminate as *primary capillary loops* within the median eminence and infundibular stalk. *Short primary capillary loops* supply the external portion of the median eminence, whereas *long primary capillary loops* supply the inner portion of the median eminence. The primary capillary loops coalesce to form veins which descend via the pars tuberalis into the pars distalis. The veins divide into a second set of capillaries or sinusoids throughout the pars distalis. The hypophyseal portal system, formed by primary capillary loops, veins and secondary capillary plexuses, comprises the major blood supply to the pars distalis. Small neurosecretory neurons (*parvicellular neurons*) of hypothalamic nuclei influence the activity of the pars distalis by releasing neurosecretory substances into the primary capillary loops of the hypophyseal portal system.

Somatotrophic Hormone. *Somatotrophic hormone (somatotropin, STH, GH, growth hormone)*, produced by the alpha cell population, causes the tissues and cells of the body to increase in size (*hypertrophy*) and number (*hyperplasia*). Although growth hormone may have a direct effect upon some of its target tissues, its influence on many tissues is mediated indirectly by causing the liver (and perhaps other organs) to produce and secrete *somatomedin* and other *growth factors*.

nature of the secretory products (Fig. 22.7). They are larger cells than the acidophils. The granules of the basophils range from 150 to 200 nm in diameter. Although all of the basophilic granules are strongly PAS-positive, the cells are further subdivided on the basis of specific staining reactions accordingly: *beta cells* and *delta cells*. The granules of *beta cells* are alcianophilic and aldehyde fuchsin-positive. The delta cells have granules that are aldehyde fuchsin-negative, alcianophilic and fast green-positive.

With routine staining (hematoxylin and eosin) only three cell types are identifiable:

chromophobe (agranular and unstained), *acidophils* (granules which are eosinophilic) and *basophils* (granules with an affinity for hematoxylin). The proportion of cell types varies according to the age, species, sex, physiologic condition, etc. Generally, 50% are chromophobes 40% are acidophils and 10% are basophils.

Pars Tuberalis

Form and Function. The *pars tuberalis* is composed of cuboidal cells which are weakly basophilic (Fig. 22.8). Granules, if present, are small. The cells are disposed in cords or clusters or as follicles. The function

Metabolic processes are altered by the secretion of growth hormone. Protein synthesis is enhanced by the augmented cellular uptake of amino acids, the decreased catabolism of proteins, the reduced utilization of amino acids as energy sources and the increased formation of RNA. Glucose utilization is decreased, and glycogen storage is enhanced. The increased blood levels of glucose associated with growth hormone secretion are sufficient to identify the hormone as *diabetogenic*. Under stimulation from growth hormone, animals mobilize lipid stores and utilize them as sources of energy. Excessive lipid metabolism may result in the formation of many ketone bodies; therefore, somatotropin is also *ketogenic*.

The precise mechanisms that govern the secretion of growth hormone have not been determined. Cellular protein levels and blood glucose levels influence its release.

The response of skeletal tissues to abnormal somatotropin levels throughout life may be marked by dramatic changes. An oversecretion during adolescence causes *gigantism*, whereas an undersecretion in adolescence causes *dwarfism*. After the closure of the growth plates, an oversecretion of the hormone results in *acromegaly*.

Prolactin. *Prolactin* (*luteotrophic hormone, LTH, lactogenic hormone*) is secreted by the epsilon cells of the pars distalis. Mammary gland development occurs under the combined influence of prolactin, estrogen and progesterone. Prolactin causes the secretion of milk after the development of the mammary gland. Murine and ovine prolactin has luteotrophic activity. In columbiform birds, prolactin is responsible for the secretory activity of the crop associated with the formation of "crop milk."

Adrenocorticotrophic Hormone. Current evidence indicates that *adrenocorticotrophic hormone* (*ACTH, corticotropin*) is secreted by basophils. The primary effects of ACTH are manifested upon the adrenal glands to effect the secretion of *glucocorticoids*. Whereas small amounts of ACTH (permissive effect) are required for the secretion of *mineralocorticoids*, aldosterone secretion is regulated by other mechanisms. As a trophic hormone affecting glucocorticoid release, the effects of ACTH are manifested as those of the glucocorticoids.

The regulated release of ACTH is mediated by circulating levels of glucocorticoids manifesting a negative feedback influence. ACTH release and the subsequent increase in circulating glucocorticoids is affected by emotional and physical stress. Additionally, circulating levels of glucocorticoids are subject to the circadian rhythm of hypothalamic and adenohypophyseal secretion. This circadian activity is manifested as a sine wave-type rhythm in which maximal ACTH and glucocorticoid levels occur in the morning.

Follicle-stimulating Hormone. *Follicle-stimulating hormone* (*FSH*) is the secretory product of specific delta cells (gonadotropes). The hormone is responsible for the growth and development of ovarian follicles. It also activates the testes to produce spermatozoa. The combined activities of FSH and LH (luteinizing hormone) are responsible for the maturation of ova, ovulation and the development of the corpus luteum. The role of FSH in the estrous cycle is discussed in Chapter 24.

Luteinizing hormone. *Luteinizing hormone* (*LH*), also a secretion of delta cells, promotes the conversion of ruptured follicles into corpora lutea. The combined activity of FSH and LH was mentioned previously.

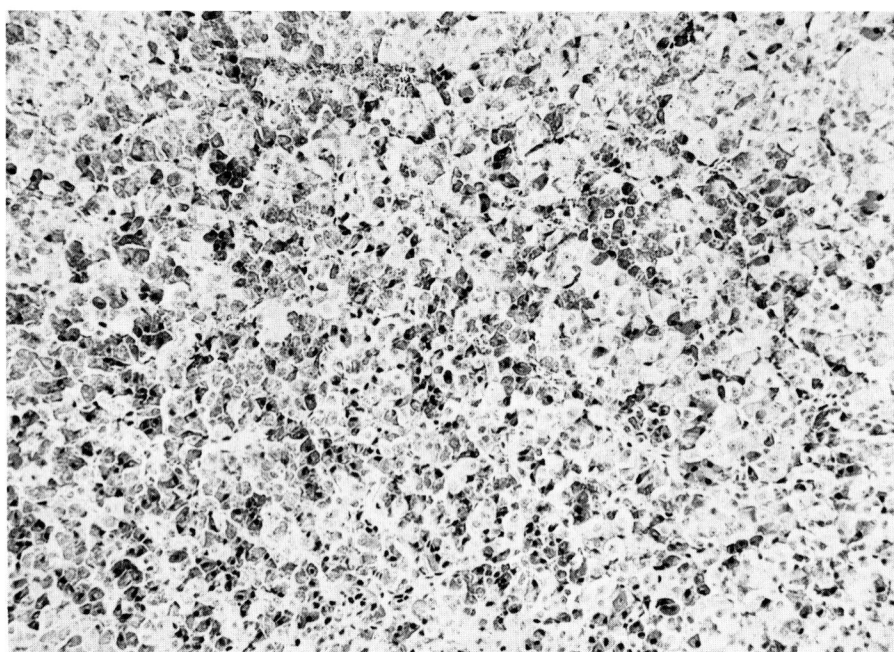

Fig. 22.6 A section of the pars distalis of a feline pituitary gland. Cords and clumps of variously stained cells are associated intimately with sinusoids. X10.

Table 22.1
Cells and Hormones of the Adenohypophysis

Cell Type	Stain Affinity	Synonyms	Hormone
Acidophils	Orange G	Alpha cell Somatotrope	Growth Hormone
	Azocarmine	Epsilon cell Carminophil Mammotrope Prolactin cell Luteotrope	Prolactin
Basophils	Alcian blue PAS + Aldehyde Fuchsin(+)	Beta cell Thyrotrope	Thyroid-Stimulating Hormone
	Alcian blue PAS + Aldehyde Fuchsin(−)	Delta cell* Gonadotrope	Follicle Stimulating Hormone Luteinizing hormone
		Corticotrope**	Adrenocorticotropic Hormone
		Melanotrope**	Melanocyte Stimulating Hormone
Chromophobes†	None	Reserve Cell	Undifferentiated, degranulated

* Separate delta cells for FSH and LH have been identified, but some delta cells may produce both hormones.

** Determined to be basophils by immunocytochemical techniques.

† Function of chromophobes is controversial.

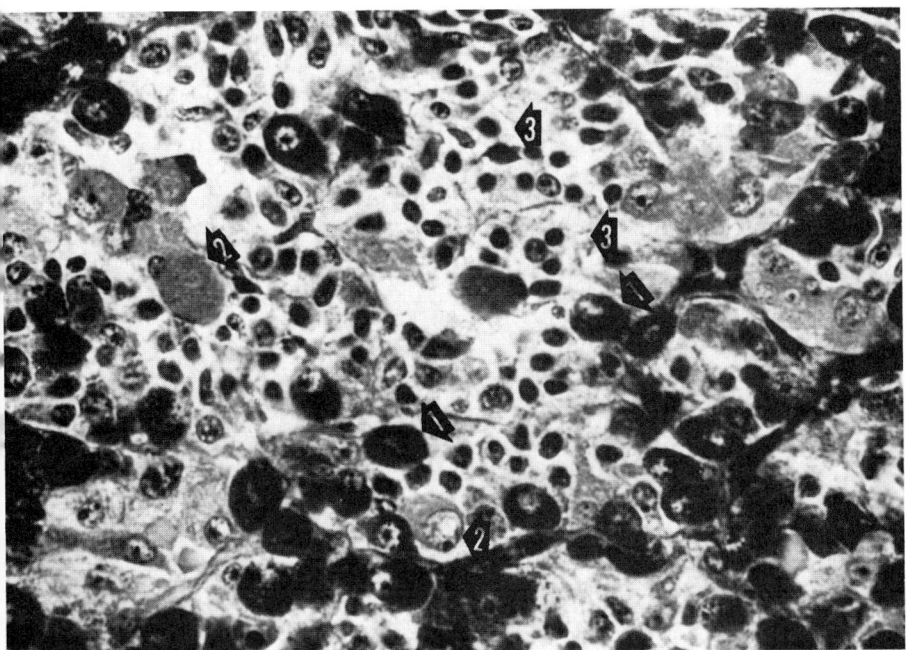

Fig. 22.7 A section of an equine pars distalis. Three different cells are identifiable within this Azan-stained specimen: acidophils (1), basophils (2) and chromophobes (3). Fine connective tissue septa delineate clumps of cells. ×160.

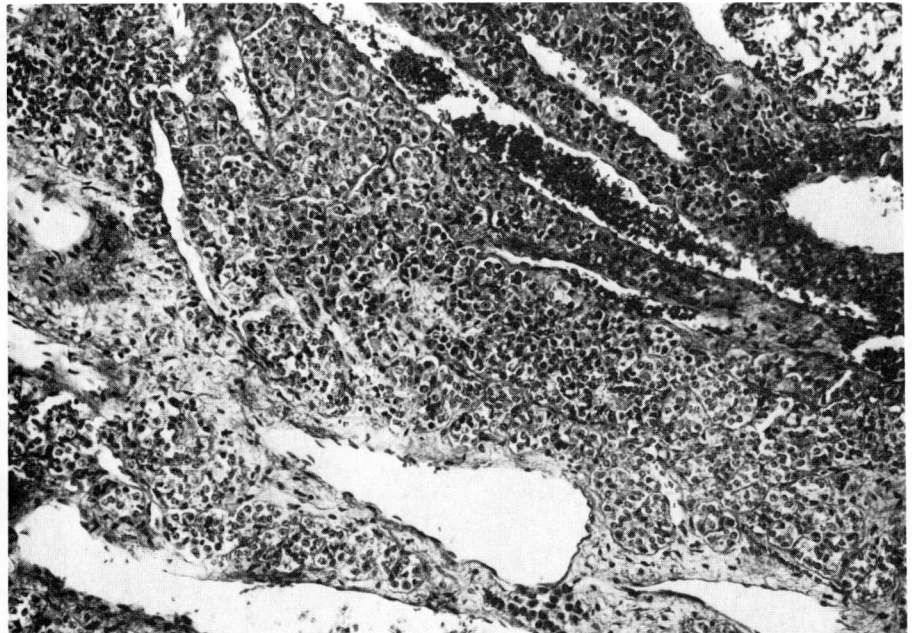

Fig. 22.8 A section of bovine pars tuberalis. The cords of weakly basophilic cells are separated by large vessels. X40.

The role of LH in the estrous cycle is discussed in Chapter 24. In the male, LH is called *ICSH* (*interstitial cell-stimulating hormone*). The hormone stimulates the secretion of testosterone by *testicular interstitial cells* (*cells of Leydig*).

Thyrotrophic Hormone. *Thyrotrophic hormone* (*TSH, thyroid-stimulating hormone*) is responsible for the stimulation and maintenance of the secretory activity of the thyroid gland. The involvement of TSH in the regulated system governing thyroid secretions was demonstrated in Figure 22.2.

Melanocyte-stimulating Hormone. *Melanocyte-stimulating hormone* (*MSH, intermedin*) is a secretory product of the pars intermedia that is responsible for the dispersion of melanin in melanocytes. Although this activity has been well-established in lower vertebrates (amphibians), the precise role of

MSH in mammals has not been documented.

Regulation of the Adenohypophysis. The hypothalamus has been described previously as the control center of autonomic function (Chapter 15). It should not be surprising to find that the hypothalamus, through the activity of different neurosecretory neuronal pools, also regulates the pituitary gland. Adenohypophyseal secretions are regulated by *releasing* and *inhibitory factors* that are secreted by the parvicellular neurons of the hypothalamus. The primary capillary loops of the hypophyseal portal system and the telodendria of the neurons comprise the *neurohemal organs*. Hypothalamic hormones released into the portal system regulate the activity of the secretory cells of the adenohypophysis and include:

> *Growth hormone releasing factor—GHRF*
> *Growth hormone inhibitory factor—GHIF*
> *Prolactin releasing factor—PRF*
> *Prolactin inhibitory factor—PIF*
> *ACTH releasing factor—CRF*
> *FSH releasing factor—FRF*
> *LH releasing factor—LRF*
> *TSH releasing factor—TRF*

Specific excitatory or inhibitory events—body temperature, blood glucose concentration, cellular protein levels, circulating levels of certain general hormones or trophic hormones—exert an influence upon the secretory activity of hypothalamic neurons. The hypothalamic hormones adjust the activity of the adenohypophysis. The trophic hormones, besides mediating their influence upon target organs, may function in a short negative feedback loop to affect the secretion of the hypothalamic cells.

The secretions of the adenohypophysis and the activities of their target organs—endocrine organs or other cells and tissues—are subject to careful regulation. The involvement of more than one regulator generally assures a more precise regulation of a particular substance or event.

Neurohypophysis

Structure. The *neurohypophysis* is a ventral evagination of the hypothalmic region of the diencephalon. It includes the *median eminence* of the *tuber cinereum, infundibular stalk* and *infundibular process* (Fig. 22.11). This region, therefore, is nervous tissue. It includes numerous unmyelinated neurons as part of the *hypothalamohypophyseal tract*. The cell bodies of these fibers are located in the supraoptic and paraventricular nuclei of the hypothalamus. These *magnocellular neurons* are neurosecretory. Their *neurosecretions* move along the axons and accumulate in the nerve fibers as *Herring bodies* (Fig. 22.12). Numerous *pituicytes* and neuroglial elements are scattered among the nerve fibers.

Histophysiology. The secretory products elaborated by the magnocellular neurons of

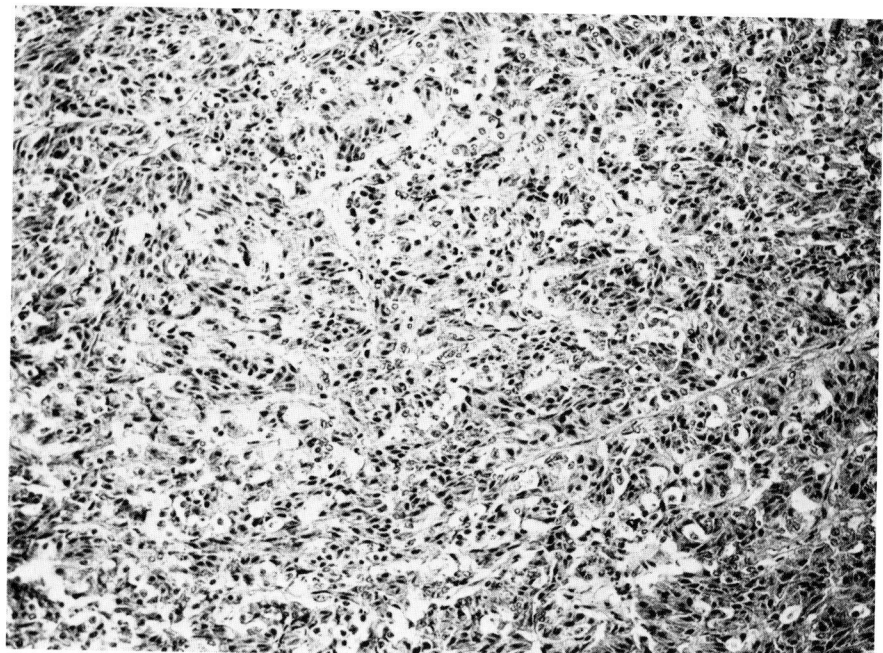

Fig. 22.9 Bovine pars intermedia. The nonspecific basophils are disposed as cords and clumps associated closely with vessels. X40.

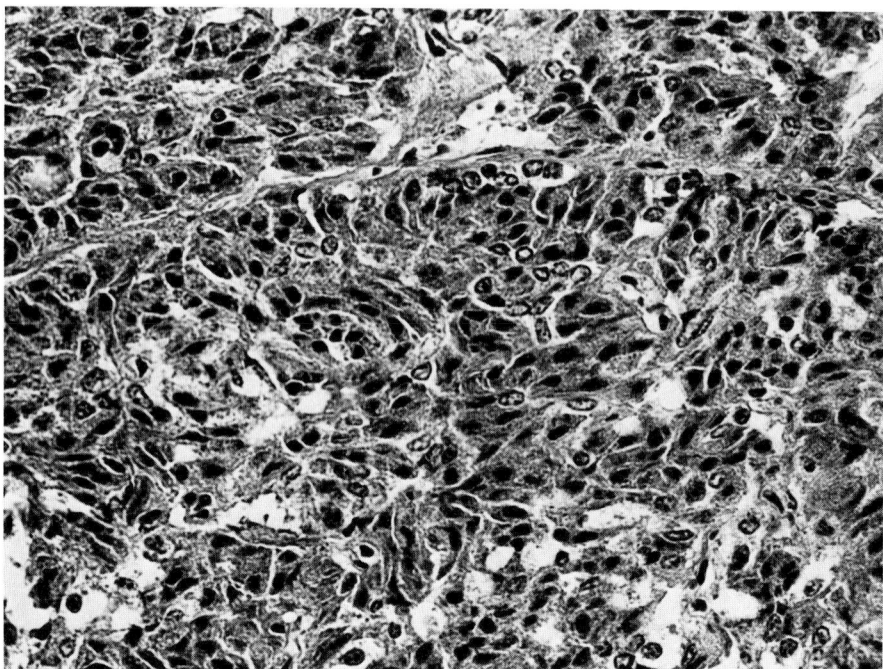

Fig. 22.10 Cells of the bovine pars intermedia. The nonspecific basophils are clumped closely. Although not apparent in this section, follicles may be present. X100.

the supraoptic and paraventricular nuclei include *oxytocin*, *vasopressin* and *neurophysins*. Neurophysins are cystine-rich proteins that function as intracellular carrier molecules for the prohormones. Specific neurophysin for each hormone is packaged into each secretory granule with prohormone and a converting enzyme. The secretory granules move by rapid axoplasmic flow to the nerve terminals of the neurohemal organs. An action potential, triggered by the cell body in response to some excitatory events, causes a change in cell membrane permeability, an increase in intracellular calcium and the exocytotic release of the hormones and neurophysins.

Oxytocin, produced primarily within the paraventricular nucleus, manifests its effects upon the reproductive organs. "Milk letdown" is mediated by oxytocin in response to suckling. The afferent stimulation reaches the hypothalamus, causing the release of the hormone. The hormone has a stimulatory effect upon the myometrium. Oxytocin-induced contractions facilitate the ascent of spermatozoa into the oviduct. During pregnancy, oxytocin is secreted by the maternal hypophysis under the influence of fetal and placental estrogens and prostaglandins. The release of oxytocin stimulates myometrial contractions and accelerates parturition. As the fetus passes through the dilated cervix, point pressure of the fetus upon the vagina stimulates additional oxytocin release and the marked abdominal contractions characterizing labor. These cascading events are irreversible. Oxytocin can be used to induce parturition in the mare.

Antidiuretic hormone (ADH, vasopressin), produced primarily within the supraoptic nucleus, manifests its antidiuretic properties on the lining cells of the distal convoluted tubules and collecting ducts of the kidneys. Blood osmolality and fluid volume are the stimuli for ADH secretion. Osmoreceptors within the hypothalamus respond to the osmolality of the fluid bathing them and influence the magnocellular neurons responsible for ADH secretion. An increased blood osmolality increases the activity of the osmoreceptors and results in the release of ADH. The kidney, responding to ADH by increasing the tubular resorption of water, excretes a low volume, hypertonic urine. The converse is true when blood osmolality decreases.

The extracellular fluid (ECF) volume of the body influences ADH release. An increased ECF volume decreases ADH secretion, whereas a decreased ECF volume increases ADH secretion. Changes in ECF volume effect changes in blood volume. Low pressure, venous baroreceptors located in the great veins of the heart, atria and pulmonary vessels monitor blood volume and influence ADH release. The venous baroreceptors probably influence ADH greater than the high pressure, arterial baroreceptors, because subtle changes in blood volume are not always associated with arterial pressure changes. The marked reduction of blood volume, as resulting from hemorrhage, involves the arterial baroreceptors (carotid and aortic sinuses) in the regulation of ADH release. The attendant fall in blood pressure causes an increased release of ADH.

The vasopressive activity of ADH is manifested by the exogenous administration of the hormone at dosages exceeding physiologic levels. Even after hemorrhage, it is dubious that ADH will manifest sufficient vasopressive activity to alter blood pressure.

Epiphysis Cerebri

Form and Function. This organ is also referred to as the *pineal gland.* It is a dorsal evagination of the roof of the diencephalon.

An understanding of the functional significance of the pineal body has been slow

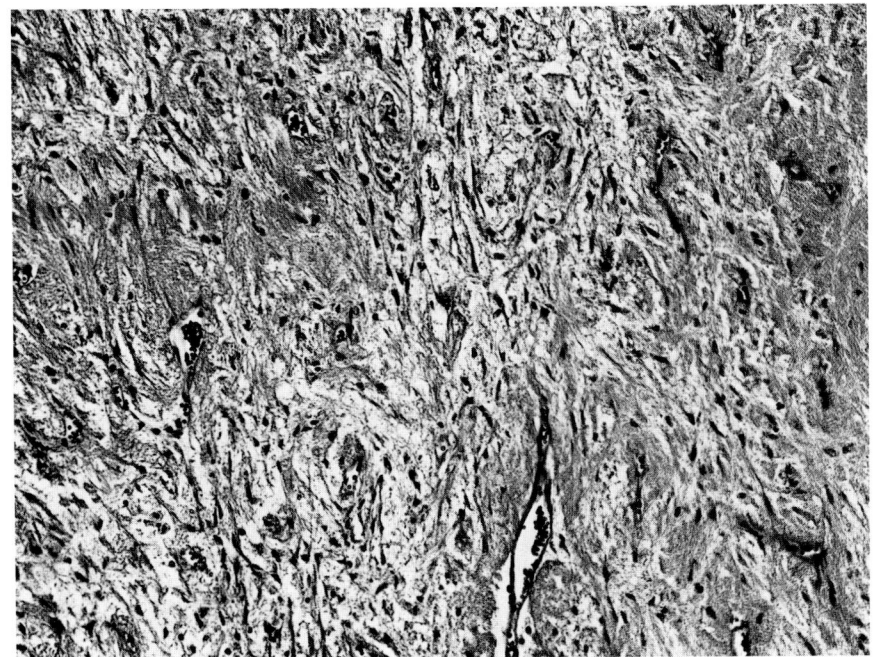

Fig. 22.11 A section of bovine neurohypophysis. It appears as typical nervous tissue. X40.

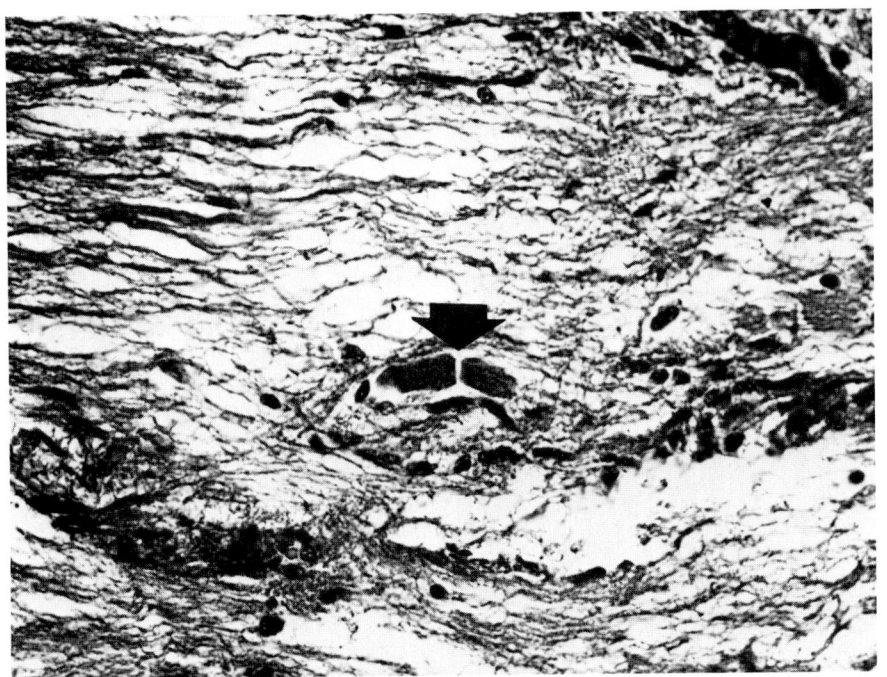

Fig. 22.12 Herring bodies. The neurosecretory products and carrier molecules of specific hypothalamic nuclear regions are transported along axons as Herring bodies (*arrow*). X100.

the hypothalamus (releasing factors), pars distalis, or directly upon the gonads.

The gland is sensitive to indirect stimulation from light and does affect the gonads. It is probably the biological clock which sets circadian rhythms associated with estrous cycles and seasonal breeding characteristics of some species.

Histology. The pineal body is covered by the connective tissue of the pia mater (Fig. 22.13). Septation and lobulation of the organ is accomplished by invasion of the connective tissue elements. The primary cellular components are *astrocytes* and *pinealocytes* (epithelioid cells). Typical connective tissue cells (plasma cells, fibroblasts, mast cells and macrophages) may also be present.

The *pinealocytes (chief cells)* are large cells with a large, round and open nucleus set in an acidophilic cytoplasm (Fig. 22.14). The *astrocytes* are typical and are interdigitated between the vascular supply and the pinealocytes. These are often referred to as *interstitial cells.*

The pineal body gradually undergoes retrogressive changes after puberty which involve the stromal elements. Increased connective tissue and the presence of *acervuli* (*brain sand, corpora arenacea*) are common changes.

Thyroid Gland

Structure

General Remarks. The thyroid gland is an outgrowth from the floor of the buccal cavity which subsequently loses its cellular connection (*thyroglossal duct*) with the pharyngeal endoderm. This glandular mass fuses with cellular masses from each fifth pharyngeal pouch (*ultimobranchial body*). Endodermal evaginations from the third and fourth pharyngeal pouches (parathyroid glands) also become intimately associated with or are embedded within the mass of thyroid tissue. The thyroid gland eventually assumes a dorsolateral relationship with the trachea in the region of the larynx.

Histology. The capsule of the two lobes of the thyroid gland consists of areolar connective tissue. Connective tissue septa of similar tissue support the organ. Perifollicular connective tissue consists of extensive quantities of reticular fibers.

The structural unit of the thyroid gland is the *thyroid follicle* (Fig. 22.15). Follicles are hollow spheres that are variable in size. Individual follicular size is a function of the activity of the lining cells. The center of the follicle is filled with a gel-like material called *colloid.* This is the storage form of the follicular epithelial secretory products. The lining epithelium varies from low cuboidal to high columnar (Fig. 22.16). The height of the cells within a given follicle, however, is uniform.

The thyroid epithelium actually consists of two cell types: *follicular lining cells* that comprise at least 90% of the cellular population and *light cells (parafollicular cells, C cells).* The *follicular lining cells* are acido-

to evolve. In lower vertebrates, it is a photoreceptor organ, the *third eye* or *pineal eye.* Its position in the mammalian cranium, however, would appear to preclude a light-sensitive function. In fact, despite its position in the cranium, it is a light-sensitive organ. Information from the optic system is carried to the midbrain and thence to the thoracic region of the spinal cord wherein sympathetic nerves carry the information to the apex of the pineal body.

Melatonin and *serotonin* have been identified as secretory products of this gland. Under continuous light stimulation, the pineal gland decreases in activity, melatonin production decreases and gonadal activity increases. Melatonin, therefore, has an inhibitory effect on gonadal development. This is consonant with the observation that pineal body tumors result in delayed puberty. It is not clear, however, whether the pineal gland mediates its influence through

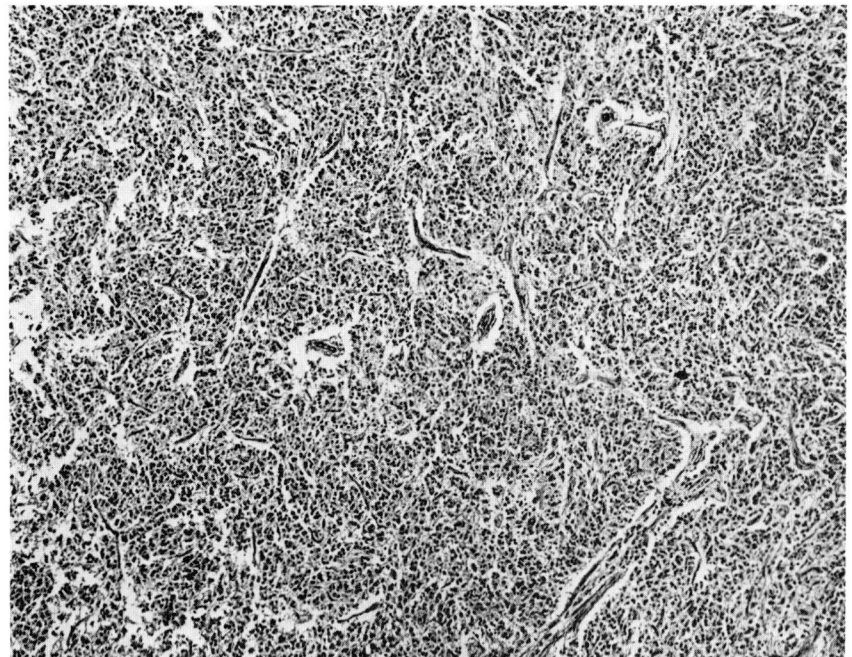

Fig. 22.13 A section of the bovine epiphysis cerebri. The cellular constituents are separated by connective tissue septa. X16.

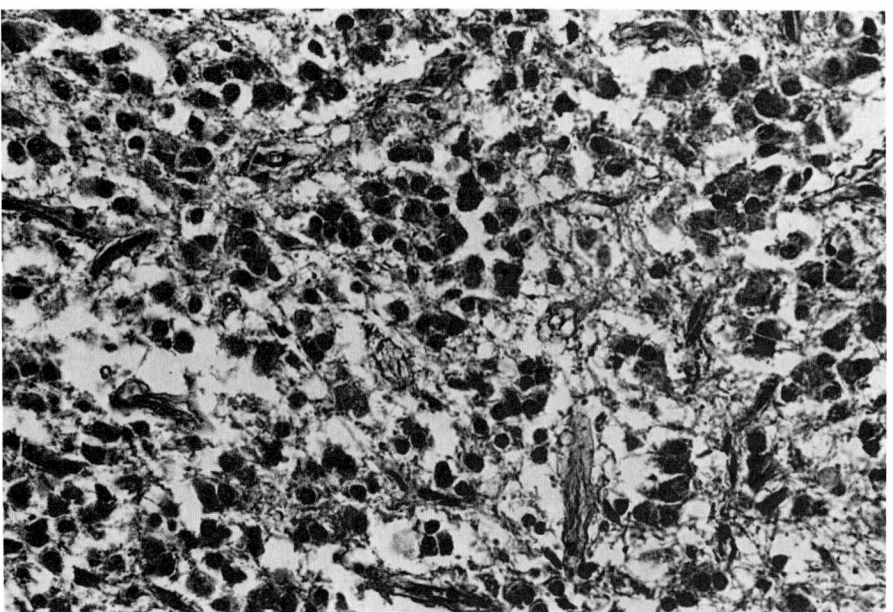

Fig. 22.14 Cellular components of an ovine pineal body. X90.

philic with a basally positioned nucleus (Fig. 22.16). A pale-staining Golgi area may be seen in a supranuclear position. There may be colloid droplets adjacent to the luminal surface. The *parafollicular cells* may occur in a parafollicular position as the name implies, or they may occur within the lining of the follicle wherein they occasionally reach the luminal surface (Fig. 22.17). In either instance, they are surrounded by the basal lamina that delimits the follicle from the connective tissue space. They are cells with a pale-staining cytoplasm. The parafollicu-

lar cells have an entirely different function than the lining cells of the follicle.

Colloid, which contains proteins, glycoproteins and enzymes, is usually acidophilic. The glycoprotein component imparts a strong PAS-positive reaction. In an active follicle, the colloid has peripheral irregularities and vacuoles as well as a strong acidophilia. In an inactive follicle, the colloid is slightly basophilic or even acidophilic. The periphery has a smooth profile and vacuoles are not present. The size of the follicles as well as the height of the epithelium are also

indicators of follicular or glandular activity. The activity of a follicle is approximately inversely proportional to the diameter of the follicle. Small follicles usually have a high epithelium (and the appropriate colloid characteristics) and are active. Large follicles usually have a low epithelium (and the appropriate colloid characteristics) and are less active than small follicles. In inactive follicles, the follicular epithelium may even be squamous.

Histophysiology

Synthesis and Secretion of Thyroid Hormones. The simplicity of thyroid follicular morphology is barely indicative of the complex mechanisms involved in the synthesis, storage, mobilization and subsequent secretion of its hormones—T_4 (*Thyroxine* or *tetraiodothyronine*) and T_3 (*triiodothyronine*). The events that culminate in the secretion of thyroid hormones are illustrated in Figure 22.18.

The synthesis of T_3 and T_4 is dependent upon thyroid-stimulating hormone (TSH) and the availability of iodide. Iodide (I^-) is actively transported across the basal cell membrane under the influence of TSH. The iodide pump permits the concentration of iodide within the thyroid follicular cell. Moving through the epithelial cell to the apical border, iodide is oxidized or activated to its reactive form, iodine (I_2). A *peroxidase* located in the microvilli of the cell may cause the activation of the halogen. Concomitantly, amino acids that enter the cell permit the synthesis of a polypeptide within the rough endoplasmic reticulum. Glycosylation of the polypeptide within the Golgi apparatus results in the formation of a *glycoprotein* contained within a secretory vesicle that is transported across the apical cell border into the colloid. The *iodination* or *organification* of the glycoprotein occurs within or on the apical surface of the cells as the glycoprotein is secreted. Organification results in the formation of *thyroglobulin*, a glycoprotein with a molecular weight in excess of 650,000. Thyroglobulin contains some carbohydrates (galactose, mannose, N-acetylglucosamine, sialic acid) and *iodoamino acids*. The iodoamino acids are 3-monoiodotyrosine (*MIT*), 3,5-diiodotyrosine (*DIT*), 3,5,3'-triiodotyrosine (T_3) and 3,5,3', 5'-tetraiodotyrosine (T_4, *thyroxine*).

The iodination of tyrosyl residues attached to thyroglobulin and the formation of MIT and DIT is the key to the formation of T_3 and T_4. The DIT moieties of adjacent thyroglobulin molecules, probably under the influence of a peroxidase, attach to each other to form T_4. Similarly, DIT and MIT on adjacent thyroglobulin molecules attach to each other to form T_3. The coupling of DIT with DIT and DIT with MIT may occur under the influence of TSH.

The synthesis of thyroglobulin conforms to the typical cellular mechanisms utilized to produce a glycoprotein. The organifica-

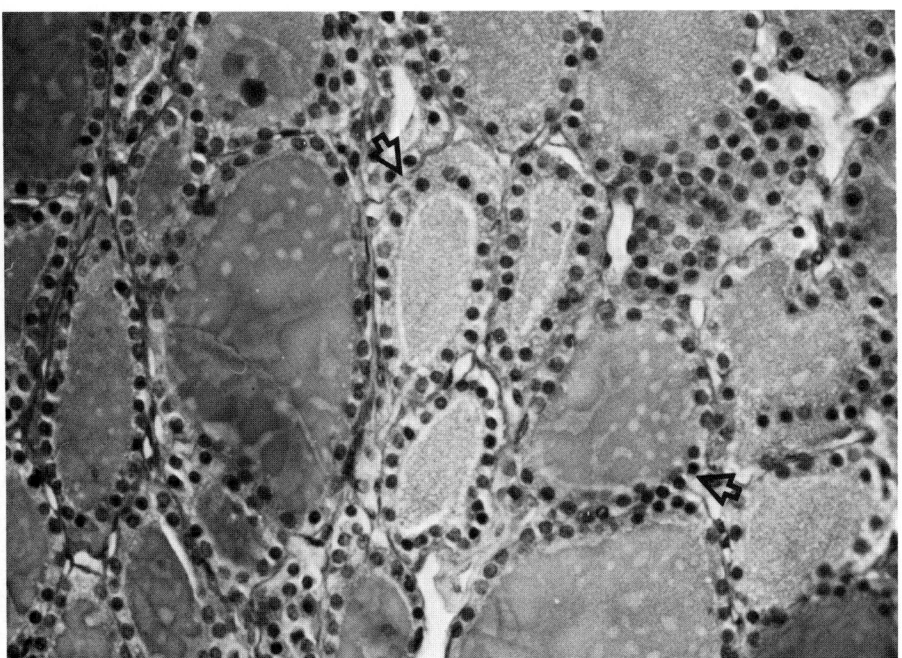

Fig. 22.15 A section of a canine thyroid gland. The parenchyma is disposed as follicles (*arrows*) surrounding colloid, X100 (PAS).

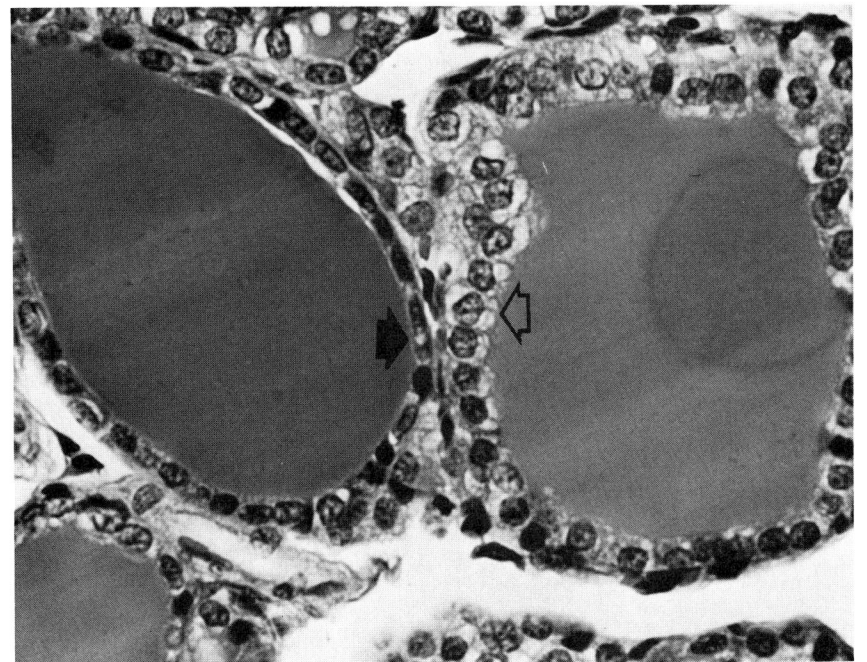

Fig. 22.16 Thyroid follicular epithelial cells and follicles. The lining cells may vary from low cuboidal (*solid arrow*) to columnar (*open arrow*), depending upon the level of activity of the gland and individual follicles. X160.

tion process is a unique feature of thyroid follicular epithelial cells. Moreover, the storage of the secretory products within the thyroglobulin of colloid is a unique feature of this endocrine gland. The mobilization of thyroglobin is essential for the secretion of T_3 and T_4. Thyroglobulin must move back into the cell and be digested before release of T_3 and T_4 is achieved.

After stimulation by TSH, follicular epithelial cells undergo morphologic changes linked to the transport of thyroglobulin back into the cell. The tall columnar epithelial cells increase in height and acquire numerous microvillous projections along their apical borders. The microvilli move in and out of the colloid. The foamy and serrated appearance of the colloid at the apical border/ colloid interface of active cells is indicative of the mobilization of colloid. The endocy-

totic movement of thyroglobulin into the cells is manifested as numerous colloid-containing vesicles within the apical margins of the cells. These vesicles, which may be considered phagosomes, migrate toward the basal border and fuse with a primary lysosome. The secondary lysosome, with its activated complement of hydrolases, digests the thyroglobulin molecule. T_3 and T_4 are secreted across the basal cell border, while MIT and DIT, also released by the protease activity, are re-cycled within the cell as free tyrosyl and iodide. Under normal conditions, thyroglobulin never occurs outside of the thyroid follicle.

Actions and Regulation of Thyroid Hormones. The thyroid hormones manifest numerous effects upon the cells, tissues and organs of the body. Whereas the specific activities of the hormones are diverse, most of them involve energy metabolism, growth and differentiation. The hormones increase the consumption of O_2 by metabolically active tissues and effect the increased production of energy. Because heat is lost during this process, it is often termed the *calorigenic effect*. The thyroid hormones increase the rates of carbohydrate and lipid metaboli.m, effects consistant with a generalized increase in basal metabolism. Increased absorption of glucose from the intestines, gluconeogenesis and glycogenolysis occur under the influence of these hormones. Although the peripheral utilization of glucose is increased, a transitory rise in blood glucose, even to the point of exceeding the renal threshold, may occur in response to T_3 and T_4 secretion. Additionally, the rate of synthesis and secretion of cholesterol, as well as a total body loss of the substance occurs in response to thyroid hormone stimulation. Although the thyroid hormones generally stimulate protein synthesis, protein catabolism may occur when metabolic demands require energy supplementation from gluconeogenesis. Similarly, excessive quantities of the thyroid hormones are accompanied by protein catabolic processes. Numerous other specific effects are manifested by T_3 and T_4 upon other tissues and organs of the body.

The thyroid hormones influence growth and developmental processes. They are essential for the normal development of most organs and systems within the animal body. The nervous system and skeletal system especially manifest altered development and growth in the absence of these hormones. The mechanisms utilized by the thyroid hormones to influence the normal progression of growth and development are not understood.

Some iodine occurs free in the plasma, but most of it occurs as *protein-bound iodine (PBI)*, of which the majority is attributable to T_4 and T_3. Protein binding is achieved primarily by a *thyroxine-binding globulin (TBG)*. The free hormones, in equilibrium with those bound to TBG, diffuse into the tissues to manifest their varied influences

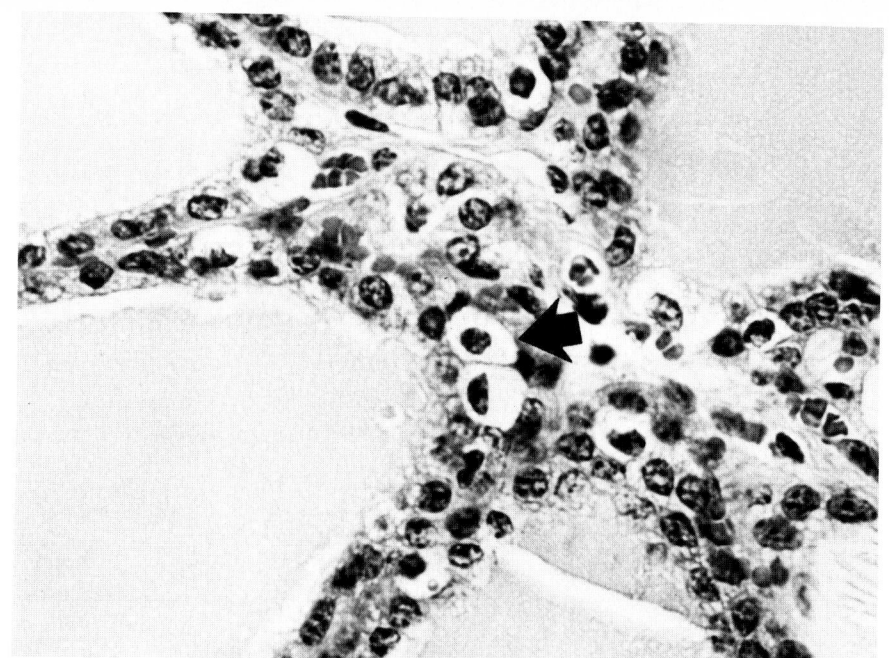

Fig. 22.17 Parafollicular cells. The parafollicular cells (*arrow*) are light-staining cells positioned at the edges of the follicles. X160 (PAS).

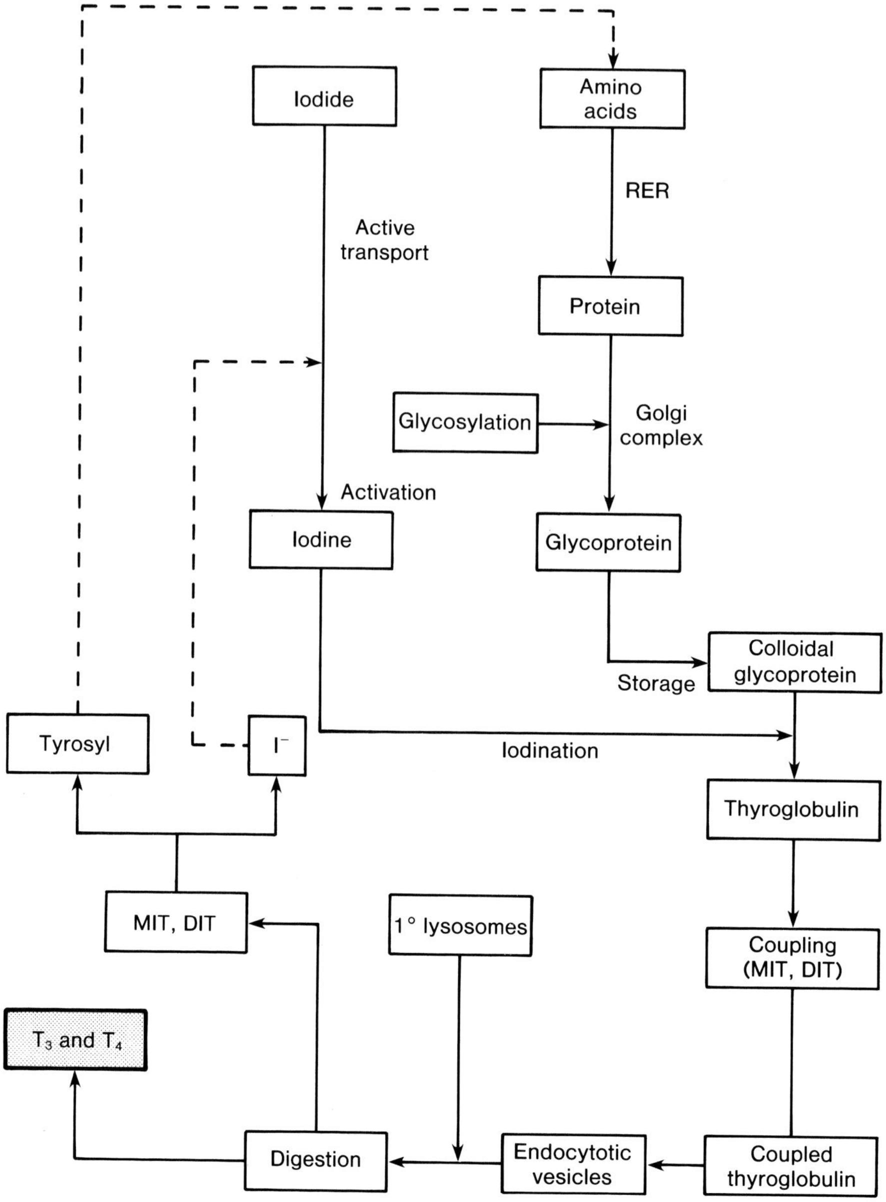

Fig. 22.18 A diagram showing the synthesis, storage and secretion of the thyroid hormones.

466

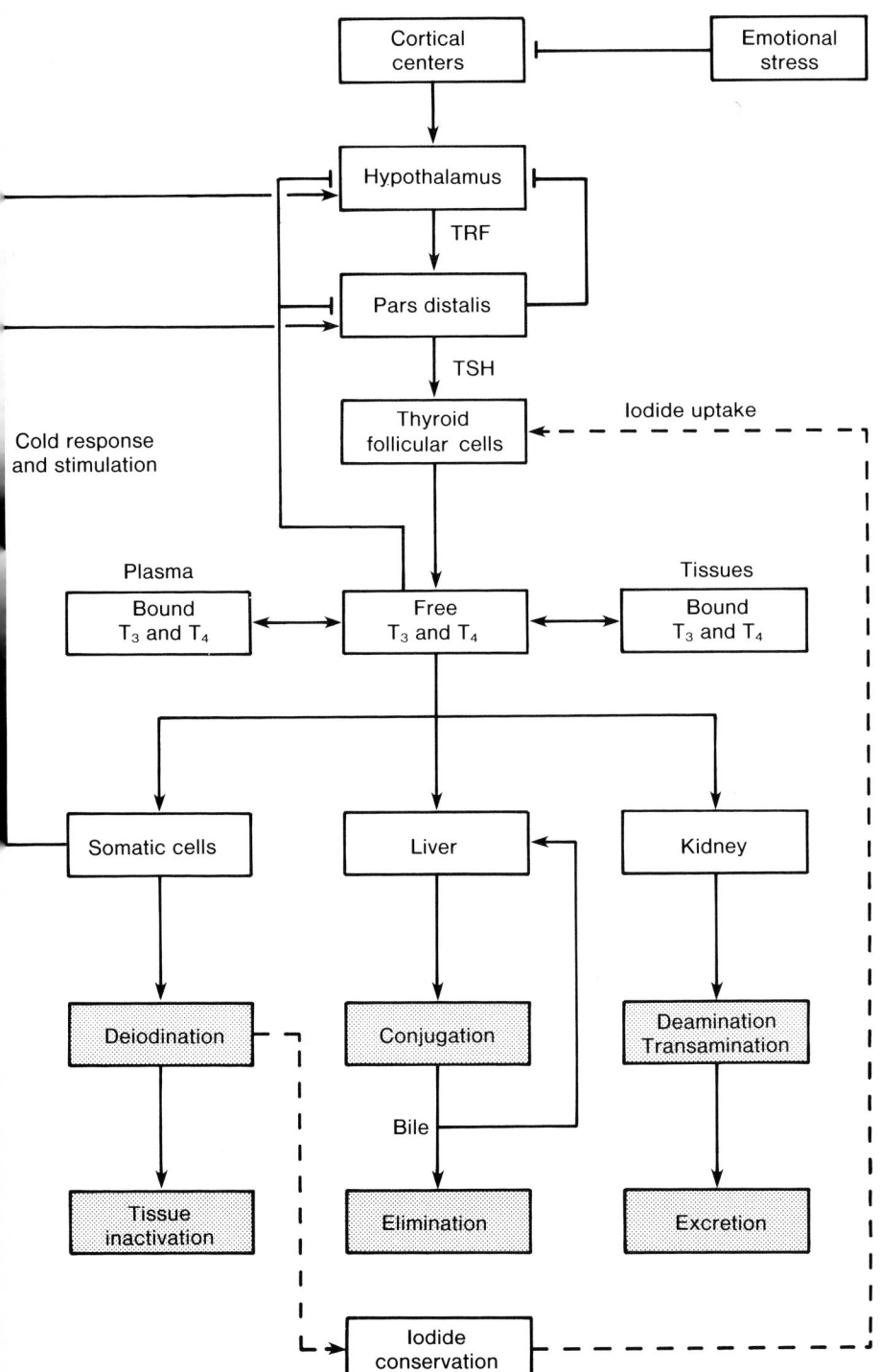

Fig. 22.19 A scheme which shows the regulation, transportation, distribution and inactivation of the thyroid hormones.

deiodination of the hormones within the target cells. The regulation, transportation, distribution and inactivation of T_4 and T_3 are illustrated in Figure 22.19.

The release of T_4 and T_3 by the thyroid gland is regulated by secretion of thyroid-stimulating hormone (TSH) by the pars distalis. TSH release is controlled by the hypothalamic secretion of TSH releasing factor (TRF). The thyroid hormones have a negative feedback influence upon the pars distalis and hypothalamus. Exposure to cold ambient temperatures stimulates the hypothalamus to secrete TRF. Emotional stress also has an effect upon TRF release; however, such stress, usually associated with sympathetic discharge and increased metabolic activity, inhibits the release of TRF.

Alterations in thyroid gland activity may be manifested as a decreased secretory activity (*hypothyroidism*). Hypothyroidism may be manifested as a primary or secondary condition. Primary hypothyroidism, a condition in which the thyroid gland is unable to respond to TSH stimulation and produce appropriate quantities of the thyroid hormones, may result from various disease processes that affect the thyroid gland. Without the appropriate T_3 and T_4 hormones to influence the hypothalamus and pars distalis, the thyroid gland is subjected to constant stimulation by TSH; thyroid enlargement (*goiter*) may result. Iodine-deficient diets manifest this type of change in the thyroid gland. Secondary hypothyroidism is a condition that results from a defect in the hypothalamic or pituitary portion of the control axis. Although the thyroid gland is capable of producing T_3 and T_4, the gland does not have appropriate stimulation. Thyroglobulin, normally sequestered within the follicles of the thyroid gland, may be exposed to immune system components subsequent to damage to the thyroid gland. Upon exposure, thyroglobulin functions as an antigen; an immune-mediated (autoimmune) hypothyroid condition may result. *Hyperthyroidism* may result from excessive stimulation of the gland or from a thyroid tumor.

Parafollicular Cell Activity. The parafollicular cells secrete the hormone *calcitonin* (*thyrocalcitonin*), a polypeptide consisting of 32 amino acids with a molecular weight of 3000. Calcitonin is a *hypocalcemic factor* which reduces blood calcium levels; its release is triggered by *hypercalcemia*, an increase in the concentration of blood calcium. Calcitonin, functioning as an antagonist to parathormone, represents one arm of the dual control system that regulates calcium levels in the blood; parathormone is the other. The parafollicular cells are the receptors and regulators within the regulated scheme of calcium control. Bone is the effector organ. Osteoblastic activity increases, osteoclastic activity decreases and the formation of new osteoclasts is inhibited in response to calcitonin stimulation. The net effect of calcitonin is the removal of

upon metabolic processes. The precise biologic relationships between T_4 and T_3 have not been clarified. T_4 has a greater binding affinity for protein, a more prolonged action and a longer half-life than T_3. Although some investigators believe that both hormones are active, some believe that T_4 is a prohormone that undergoes deiodination to the more rapidly active T_3.

Three mechanisms are used to metabolize the iodothyronines (T_4 and T_3): *conjugation*,

deamination/transamination and *deiodination*. Conjugation with a glucuronide occurs within the liver followed by the excretion of the conjugated hormones in the bile. Hydrolysis of the conjugated product within the intestines may result in the reabsorption of the hormones via the enterohepatic circulation. As amino acids, the iodothyronines are subject to deamination/transamination reactions within the liver and kidneys. The most important deactivation process is the

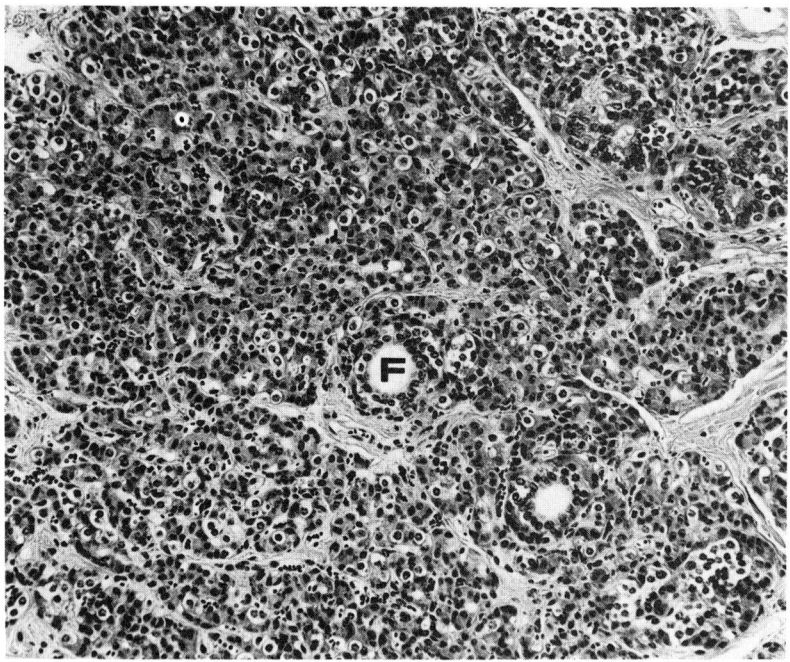

Fig. 22.20 A section of bovine parathyroid gland. Cords or clumps of cells characterize the parenchyma. Follicles (F) may occur also. X40.

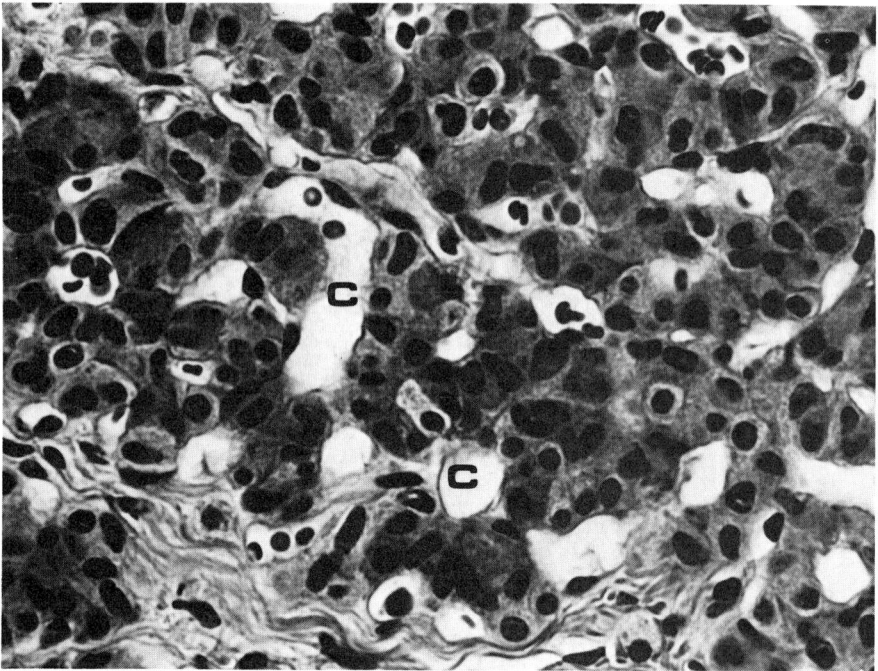

Fig. 22.21 Cells of the bovine parathyroid gland. The cords or clumps of cells are associated closely with capillaries (C). X160.

calcium from the blood with an increased deposition of calcium salts in bone (Chapter 8).

Parathyroid Glands

General Considerations. The parathyroid glands are derived from the third (*external parathyroids*) and fourth (*internal parathyroids*) pharyngeal pouches. The position of the external parathyroids may vary from cranial to the thyroids to the level of the thoracic inlet. The internal parathyroids may be missing (bird, pig) or may be embedded within, upon or close to the thyroid gland.

Histology. The capsule of the external parathyroids is areolar connective tissue that blends with the surrounding fascia. The internal parathyroids do not have a capsule per se but are surrounded by the areolar connective tissue of the interstices of the thyroid gland.

The parenchyma of the organ consists of cords, clusters, strands, sheets or rosettes of secretory cells. Occasionally, follicles may be present (Fig. 22.20). These cells are supported by a fine stromal network of reticular fibers with numerous capillaries in close association with the parenchyma. The primary cell types of the organ include *chief cells* and *oxyphil cells*. The *chief* or *principal cells* may be subdivided into *clear or light chief cells* and *dark chief cells*. Chief cells are more abundant than the oxyphilic cells.

The dark and light chief cells may represent different physiologic states of the same cell. The *light chief cell* is a small cell with a large, vesicular nucleus (Fig. 22.21). Its cytoplasm is acidophilic, agranular and has lipid and glycogen inclusions. The *dark chief cell* has an acidophilic cytoplasm which contains argyrophilic granules. The nucleus is vesicular but smaller than that of the light chief cell. The dark chief cell contains less glycogen and lipid than its lighter counterpart. Dark chief cells produce parathormone.

The *oxyphil cells* occur in the ox, the horse and man, but they do not occur regularly in other domestic species. They are large cells with a granular, acidophilic cytoplasm (Fig. 22.21). Their nuclei are small and dark-staining. These cells usually occur in small clusters. It is presumed that chief cells give rise to these cells. The precise function of these cells has not been determined.

Parathyroid Hormone. The secretory product of the chief cells of the parathyroid glands is the polypeptide hormone, *parathormone*. It is a polypeptide hormone consisting of 84 amino acids with a molecular weight of 9500. This is a *hypercalcemic factor* that is antagonistic to thyrocalcitonin. Calcium levels in the blood are maintained at a homeostatic level of 10 mg/100 ml. A lowering of this level results in the release of parathormone. Although it was thought that this hormone resulted in the differentiation and increased activity of osteoclasts, current experimental evidence indicates otherwise. The delayed differentiation of osteoclasts from exogenous administration of parathormone is too slow to maintain homeostatic calcium levels and preclude the occurrence of tetany from hypocalcemia. It is currently hypothesized that the action of this hormone in the mobilization of mineral from bone is mediated through the combined activity of osteoblasts and osteocytes. The osteoblast/osteocyte axis probably is responsible for the immediate responses associated with homeostatic calcium maintenance, whereas protracted calcium problems involve the activity of the osteoclast.

Parathormone is the hypercalcemic factor which serves as one portion of the dual regulation scheme; calcitonin is its antagonist (chapter 8).

Adrenal Glands

Introduction. The *adrenal glands* or *suprarenal glands* are small organs situated at the cranial poles of the kidneys. Embryologically, the adrenal glands are derived from two germ layers: *mesoderm* and *neural crest ectoderm*. The adrenal cortex develops from a thickening of coelomic mesothelium in close association to the kidneys and gonads. The neural crest ectoderm migrates to this region and invades the cortex as adrenal medullary tissue. In mammals a distinct cortex and medulla are apparent despite the striking interdigitations that may occur (Fig. 22.22). In birds, the cortical and medullary tissue is intermixed (Fig. 22.23). Auxiliary cortical adrenal tissue is a common occurrence in some species. In some rodents, auxiliary adrenal tissue is contained within the epididymis.

The organ is enclosed within a capsule of DWFCT. The trabeculae of areolar connective tissue invade the parenchyma to the level of the medulla. The supportive stroma consists of fine collagenous and reticular fibers.

Vascular, Lymphatic and Neural Relationships. The adrenal glands are highly vascularized organs. The main arteries branch before entry into the gland giving rise to numerous arterioles. Three primary circulation patterns arise from the arteriolar supply. A subcapsular capillary plexus branches throughout the subcapsular region and drains into subcapsular veins. The second pattern is the blood supply to the cortex, which drains through veins into the medulla. Lastly, arterioles traverse the cortex to supply the medulla and drain into medullary veins.

Nerves of the parasympathetic and sympathetic nervous systems innervate the cortex and medulla; however, little information is known about the function of the parasympathetic innervation of the gland. Most of the nerve fibers are preganglionic sympathetic fibers to the adrenal medulla.

Lymph vessels occur in the connective tissue of the capsule and interstitial tissue of the gland.

Adrenal Cortex

Histology. The adrenal cortex consists of polyhedral secretory cells which are organized into cords, usually two cells thick, that are oriented radially from the medullary region (Fig. 22.24). The orientation of the cords and some cytologic differences permit the identification of cortical subdivisions: *zona glomerulosa, zona fasciculata, zona reticularis.*

The *zona glomerulosa* is also referred to as the *zona arcuata* and the *zona multiformis* (Fig. 22.25). This subcapsular zone (Fig. 22.26) consists of curved cords or arcades (horse, carnivores, pig), or clustered groups of glomeruli (ruminants, man). The cells of

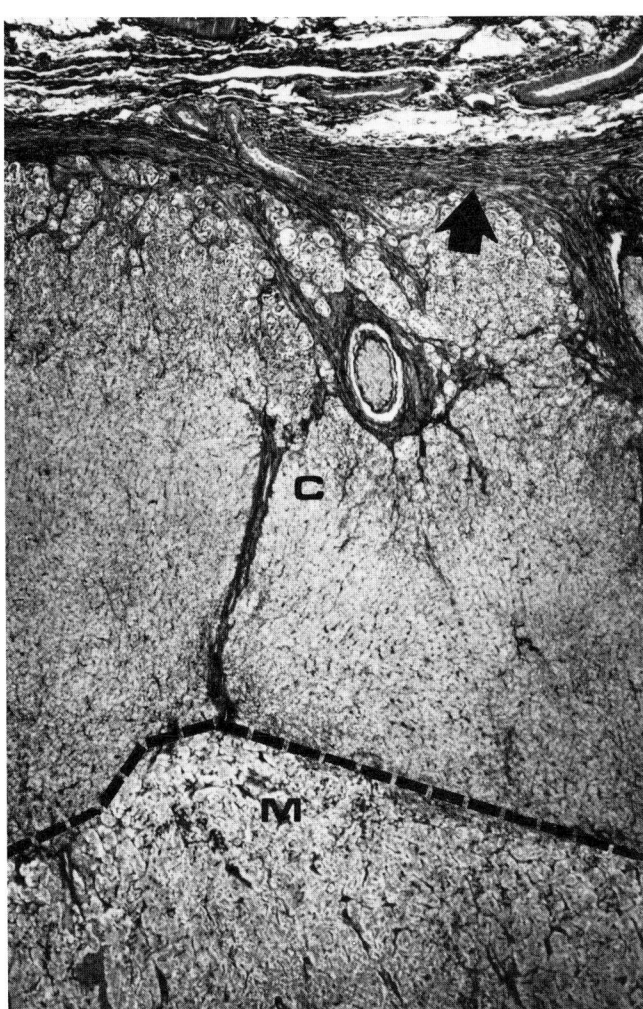

Fig. 22.22 Bovine adrenal gland. The adrenal gland capsule (*arrow*) is continuous with connective tissue septa. The gland is divided into a cortex (C) and medulla (M) which are delimited clearly (*dashed line*). X10 (Azan stain).

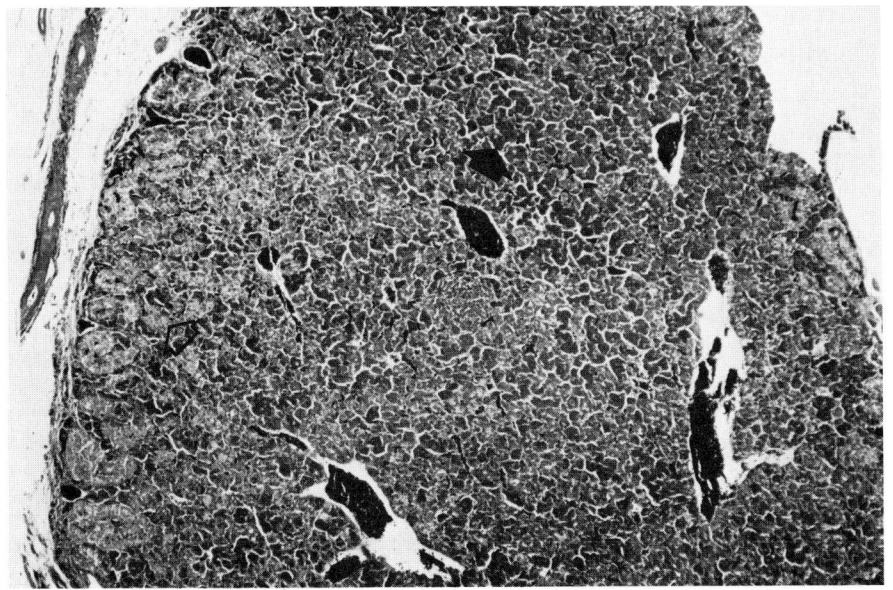

Fig. 22.23 Avian adrenal gland. The gland is not divided into a distinct cortex and medulla. The medullary tissue (*solid arrow*) is dark-staining and is interspersed among the light-staining cortical tissue. X9. (Azan stain).

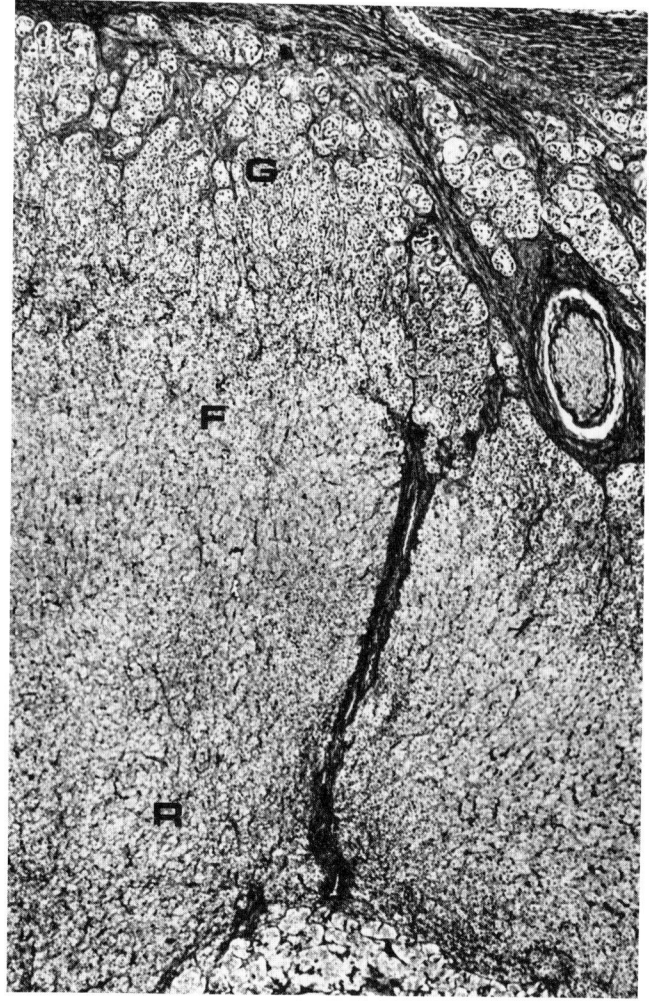

Fig. 22.24 Bovine adrenal cortex. G, zona glomerulosa; F, zona fasciculata; R, zona reticularis. X16. (Azan stain).

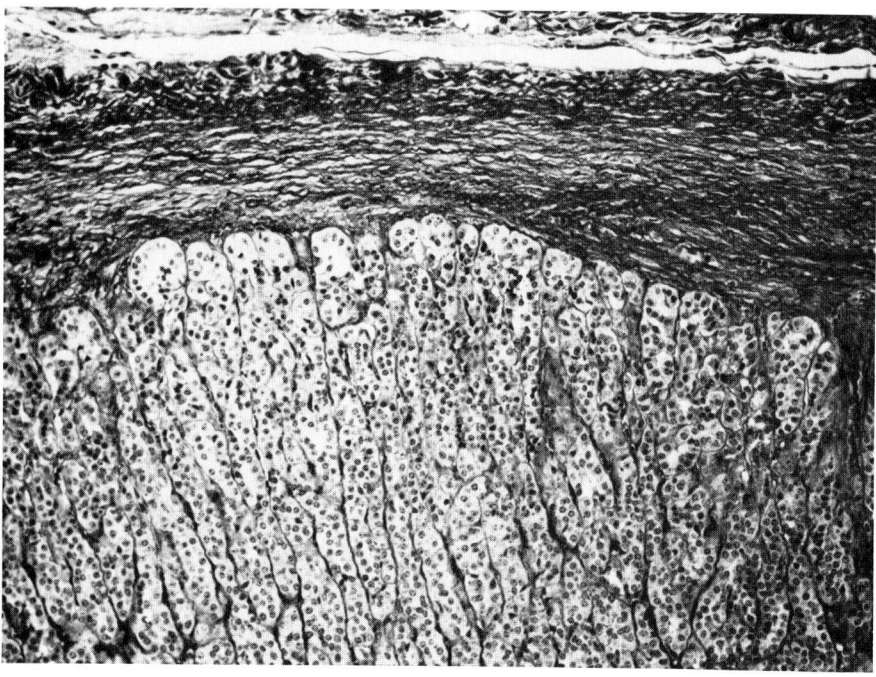

Fig. 22.25 Bovine zona glomerulosa. The cells of this zone are clustered as glomeruli. ×40 (Azan stain).

this zone are columnar (man, horse, carnivores, pig) or polyhedral (other species) (Fig. 22.27). The parenchyma, despite its spatial arrangement, is closely associated with an extensive vascular network. The cytoplasm is more evenly acidophilic and less foamy than the cells of the adjacent zone. The nuclei of the cells of the zona glomerulosa are smaller and darker than those of the adjacent zone. The occurrence of fine lipid inclusions is usually linked with an increased cellular activity. In man and ruminants, basophilic granules may be observed in the cytoplasm.

The *zona fasciculata* is the widest zone of the cortex (Fig. 22.28). It consists of cuboidal or polyhedral cells which are arranged in radial cords. Each cord consists of one or two cells separated from adjacent cords by an extensive sinusoidal network. The large cells of the outer two-thirds of this zone contain a large, vesicular nucleus (binucleations are common) within a very foamy cytoplasm (Plate II. 3). These cells are often referred to as *spongiocytes* (Fig. 22.29). The inner third of this zone contains cells that are free of lipids and have a more basophilic cytoplasm.

The *zona reticularis* consists of cells that are disposed as freely anastomosing cords (Fig. 22.30). The cells are very similar to the cells of the zona fasciculata. The cells contain less lipid than the cells of the peripherally adjacent zone. Their nuclei and cytoplasm are dark-staining. Lipofuscin pigments are commonly encountered.

Initially, it was thought that the zonation of the adrenal cortex represented a centripetal differentiation process. Mitosis occurs in all zones, however.

The aforementioned zonation is predicated upon the organizational pattern of the cells. On the basis of cytologic and cytochemical features, some authors divide the adrenal cortex into five zones: *zona glomerulosa, outer part of the zona fasciculata, inner part of the zona fasciculata, outer part of the zona reticularis* and the *inner part of the zona reticularis* adjacent to the adrenal medulla.

The adrenal cortex is required for life because its hormones influence numerous essential somatic processes. Although numerous steroid hormones have been isolated from the cortical tissues, they are readily grouped accordingly: *mineralocorticoids, glucocorticoids* and *sex hormones*.

Histophysiology—Mineralocorticoids. The *mineralocorticoids* secreted by the adrenal cortex primarily from the activity of the cells of the zona glomerulosa exert a regulatory influence upon extracellular fluid electrolytes—especially sodium and potassium. The most important mineralocorticoid is *aldosterone*; however, other corticosteroids have mineralocorticoid activity (corticosterone, cortisol, desoxycorticosterone). The most important activity of aldosterone is the increased tubular resorption of Na^+ by the kidneys. Aldosterone exerts a similar effect upon the sweat glands, salivary

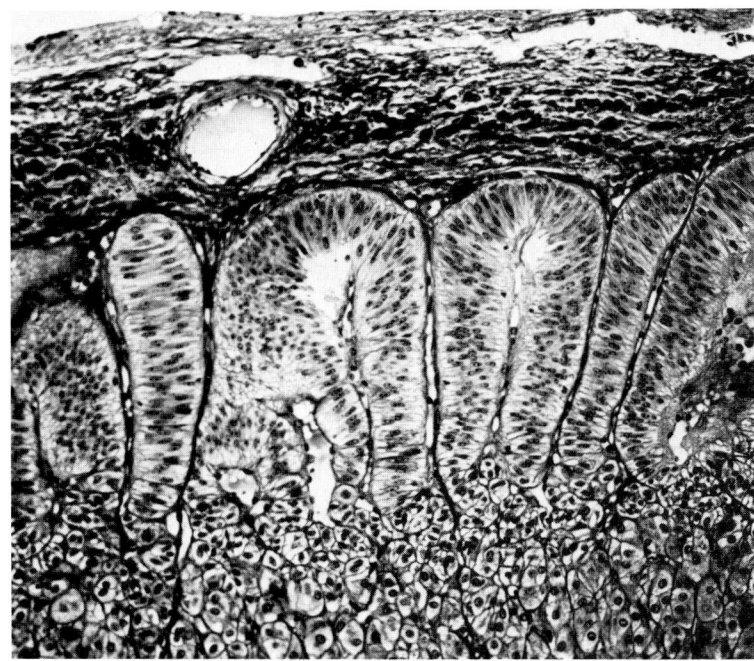

Fig. 22.26 Equine zona arcuata. Arcades of cells characterize the outermost zone in this species. X40 (Azan stain).

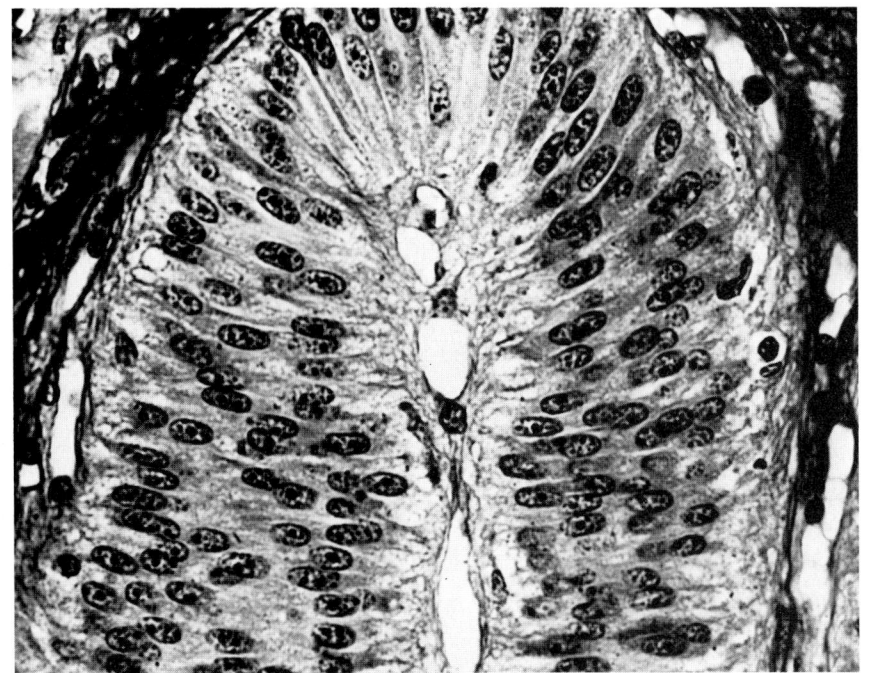

Fig. 22.27 Columnar cells of the zona arcuata of the equine adrenal gland. X160. (Azan stain).

and decreased fluid volume can be anticipated without the proper release of aldosterone. The cardiovascular system is unable to function properly because of the decreased fluid volume (hypovolemia), and cardiac activity decreases in response to the decreased fluid volume and increased levels of K^+. *Hypovolemic shock* (insufficient tissue perfusion) and death can result.

The regulated maintenance of Na^+ and K^+ levels within the body is essential to minimize an increase or decrease of these ions. Aldosterone is essential for this balance. The secretion of aldosterone is regulated by the concentration of K^+ and Na^+ in the extracellular fluid and the renin-angiotensin system. Insufficient adrenocortical secretions of mineralocorticoids (and glucocorticoids) are characteristic of *hypoadrenocorticism (Addison's disease)*. Whereas *Cushing's syndrome (hyperadrenocorticism)* may manifest effects associated with excessive secretions of aldosterone, the primary effects are those manifested by the glucocorticoids. The chemotherapeutic approach to Cushing's syndrome, if not monitored carefully, can produce an Addisonian animal.

Histophysiology—Glucocorticoids. The glucocorticoids are secreted primarily by the zona fasciculata of the adrenal cortex. Although other corticosteroids possess glucocorticoid activity (corticosterone, cortisone), the most important glucocorticoid is *cortisol*. Cortisol transported in the blood bound to a plasma globulin, *transcortin* or *cortisosteroid-binding globulin (CBG)*, has diverse effects upon the tissues of the body. Cortisol causes an increased blood glucose (*hyperglycemia*) and a decreased peripheral utilization of glucose. Glycogenesis and gluconeogenesis complement the increased release of hepatic glucose. Cortisol is diabetogenic. Whereas the glucocorticoids stimulate the synthesis of hepatic proteins, the synthesis of proteins in other tissues is inhibited. The role of cortisol in lipid metabolism is not understood well. Whereas cortisol is lipolytic and causes an increased release of free fatty acids from adipose tissue, excessive quantities of the hormone result in excessive lipid deposition. The stimulation of insulin release by cortisol may account for increased lipid deposition, because insulin promotes lipogenesis and increased amounts of adipose tissue. The anti-inflammatory properties of the glucocorticoids are significant functions. These hormones stabilize lysosomal membranes, decrease collagen synthesis, increase collagen degradation and inhibit the proliferation of fibroblasts. Glucocorticoids exert numerous other effects upon the body that are related to the reduction of peripheral protein synthesis—depressed immunocompetency, delayed wound healing, quantitative osteopenia. Gastric ulceration can result from excessive glucocorticoids; the precise mechanism of parietal cell stimulation is not understood. Glucocorticoids, released in response to

glands and intestines. Numerous secondary effects are related to this Na^+ conservation mechanism under the influence of alsosterone. The reabsorption of Na^+ is linked to the secretion of K^+ and H^+. Potassium wasting and a slight metabolic alkalosis can result. Decreased K^+ levels can result in muscular weakness, muscular paralysis and cardiac arrhythmias. The metabolic alkalosis that results from aldosterone is usually transitory and can be corrected by acid/base

regulating mechanisms. Increased Na^+ retention also increases the retention of water, causing an increased extracellular fluid and blood volume that is compounded by polydipsia. The increased fluid volume increases the amount of work that must be accomplished by the heart. Polyuria also occurs as a compensation for the increased fluid volume. The reverse effects occur in the absence of aldosterone. Hyponatremia (decreased Na^+), hyperkalemia (increased K^+)

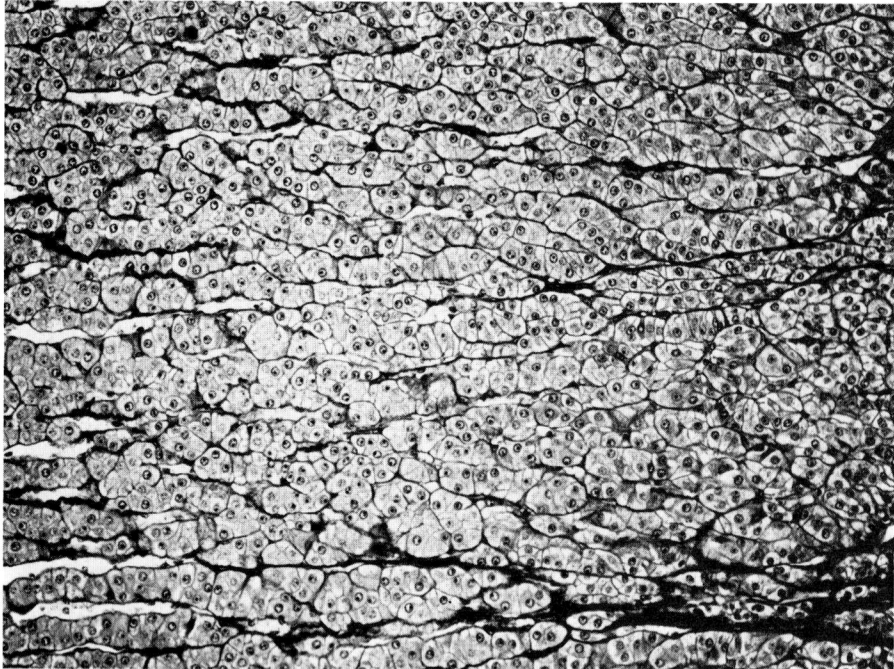

Fig. 22.28 Zona fasciculata of the equine adrenal gland. Polyhedral cells arranged as cords characterize this zone. X40 (Azan stain).

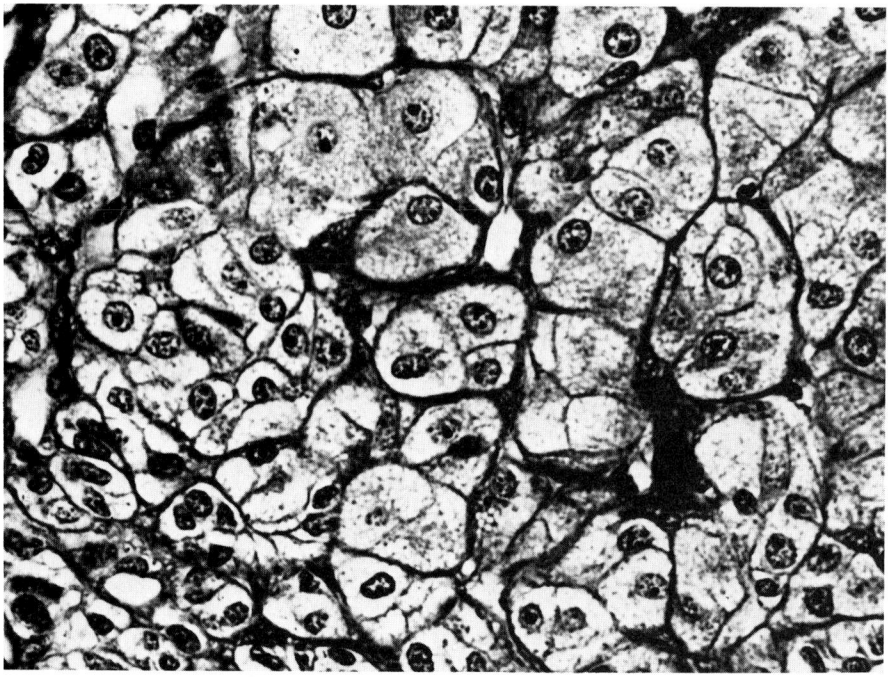

Fig. 22.29 Spongiocytes of the outer zona fasciculata (equine). The large cells have a foamy cytoplasm and vesicular nuclei. X160 (Azan stain).

stress, help to maintain extracellular fluid volume and decrease vasodilatation associated with shock. Cortisol and similar drugs exert an influence on mental status. Mental depression associated with glucocorticoid insufficiency may progress to euphoria after the administration of glucocorticoids. Cortisol also possesses permissive properties that complement the functioning of other

hormones (growth hormone, glucagon, catecholamines). Glucocorticords also manifest antiallergic properties by preventing the release of histamine associated with the type I hypersensitivity reaction.

The synthesis and release of glucocorticoids from the adrenal cortex is regulated by the secretion of ACTH from the pars distalis. The hypothalamic secretion of

ACTH releasing factor controls the activi of the pars distalis. Circulating levels of glucocorticoids exert a negative feedbac influence upon the hypothalamus and pa distalis. Notwithstanding the significance of the servomechanism, other factors influenc glucocorticoid release. The circadian rythi micity of ACTH and glucocorticoid releas is probably influenced by cerebral cortica and limbic system activity. Similarly, th emotional influence upon circulating leve of glucocorticoids is probably mediate through the limbic system. Trauma, perhap triggering activity in the limbic and reticu lar-activating systems, stimulates the in creased release of glucocorticoids. Stress i a significant stimulus of glucocorticoid se cretion.

Adrenal insufficiency (Addison's disease is marked by the inability of the adrena glands to produce mineralocorticoids an glucocorticoids. Cushing's syndrome result from the excessive secretion or administra tion of glucocorticoids.

Sex Hormones. Sex hormones, both andro gens and estrogens, are produced by th adrenal cortex. Whereas the synthesis an secretion of these hormones may be signifi cant in abnormally functioning animal: they are not significant in the normal ani mal.

Adrenal Medulla

Histology. The corticomedullary junctio may be a sharply delineated junction or ma be highly interdigitated (Fig. 22.31). Th primary constituents of the medulla includ *glandular cells, ganglion cells, venules* an *capillaries.* The aforementioned cells are de rived from neural crest ectoderm.

The *glandular cells* are large columnar o polyhedral cells which possess a large, vesic ular nucleus (Fig. 22.32). The cells are po larized: one pole is opposed to a capillary the other is opposed to a venule. The cyto plasm is basophilic and contains fine, chro maffin-positive granules (Fig. 22.33). Th resulting pigments are sometimes referred t as *adrenochromes.* As a result of this chro maffin reactivity, the glandular cells are als called *chromaffin cells* or *pheochrome cell:* This reactivity is due to the presence of th biogenic amines (catecholamines), *epineph rine* and *norepinephrine.* The reaction of th catecholamines with chromic acid produce a brown reaction product. The chromaffir cells secrete one or the other of the cate cholamines. In most species, these cells ar randomly distributed throughout the me dulla. In the ox, however, an outer lamina of epinephrine-producing cells is distinc from an inner lamina of norepinephrine producing cells.

Sympathetic ganglion cells are randoml scattered throughout the medulla.

Histophysiology. The synthesis and releas of norepinephrine and epinephrine i achieved synaptically by the termination o preganglionic fibers on the glandular cells

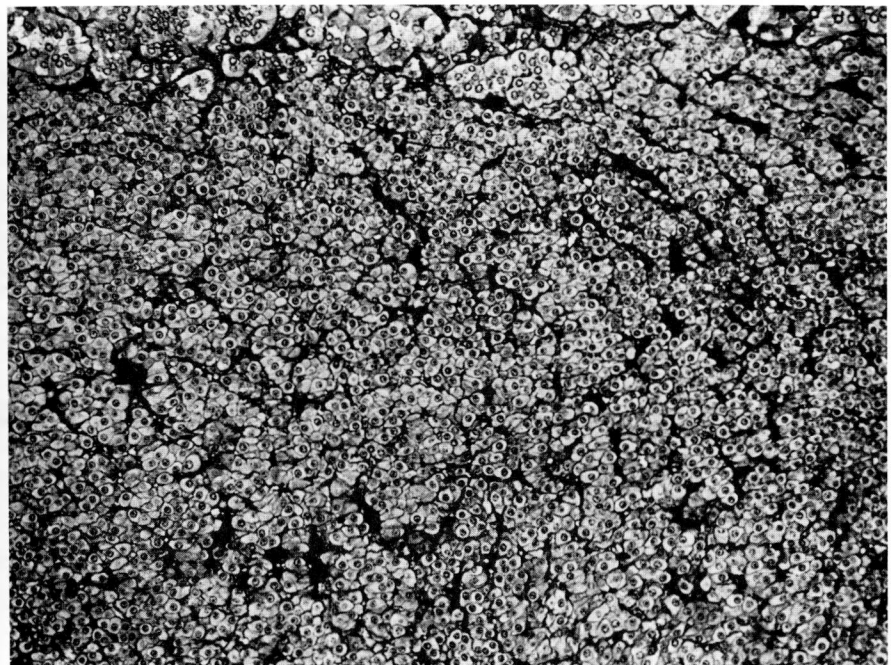

Fig. 22.30 Zona reticularis of the equine adrenal gland. The cells are disposed as freely anastomosing cords. X25 (Azan stain).

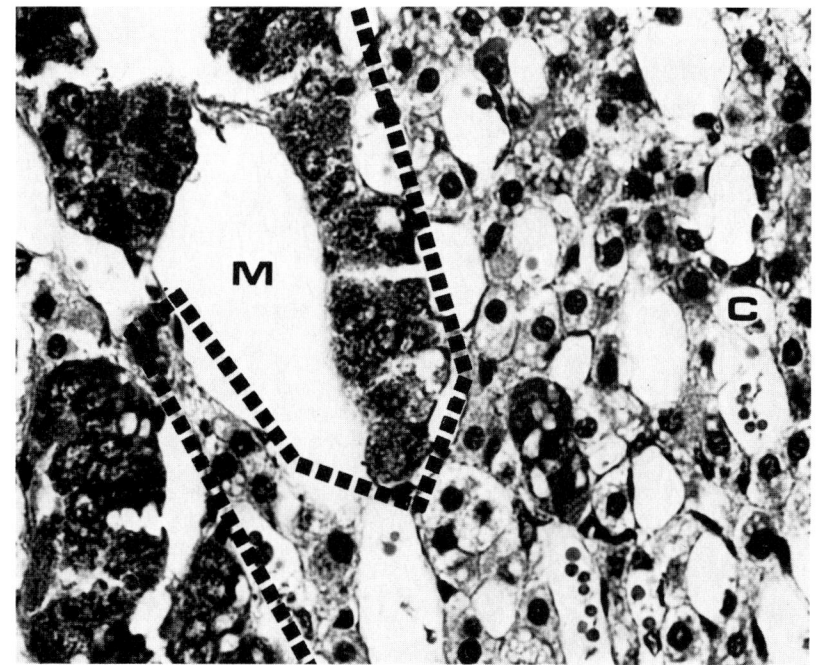

Fig. 22.31 Adrenal medulla and zona reticularis of a porcine adrenal gland. The corticomedullary junction (*dashed line*) is irregular. The medulla (M) consists of dark-staining cells, while the zona reticularis of the cortex (C) consists of light-staining cells. X160 (Chromaffin stain).

Epinephrine has a general somatic effect that includes increased cardiac output, increased cellular respiration and oxygen consumption, glycogenolysis and the release of glucose for increased metabolic needs. Epinephrine, therefore, is the hormone of "fight or flight."

The adrenal medulla is not essential for life. The function of the adrenal medulla and its relationship to the autonomic nervous system were discussed in Chapter 15.

Chromaffin System. Besides the occurrence of chromaffin cells in the adrenal medulla, there are numerous small bodies (*paraganglia*) associated with the abdominal aorta in a retroperitoneal position. The paraganglia include two large bodies, the *glands of Zuckerkandl*. The paraganglia contain chromaffin-positive granules. The paraganglia plus the adrenal medulla comprise the chromaffin system.

Endocrine Pancreas

Structure

General Remarks. The organization of the pancreas reflects its duplicity of function as an exocrine and endocrine organ. The endocrine portions are the *islets of Langerhans* that are randomly scattered throughout the organ. Developmentally, the cells of the islets, as well as those of the acini, were derived from endoderm. The islet cells became detached from the developing duct system and were established as endocrine cells.

Histology. The islets are scattered masses of pale-staining cells which are supported by reticular connective tissue (Fig. 22.33). Large sinusoids separate the cords or clusters of cells. The basic cell types of the islets are *alpha cells* and *beta cells*. C cells and *delta (D) cells* have been identified also.

The *alpha (A) cells* are polygonal cells with a nucleus that has a coarse distribution of heterochromatin. The granules of the alpha cells are insoluble in alcohol, stain pink or red with the Gomori aldehyde fuchsin technique and stain red with the Mallory-Azan stain.

The *beta (B) cells* are structurally similar to the alpha cells. Their granules, however, are soluble in alcohol, stain dark purple with the Gomori aldehyde fuchsin technique and stain orange with the Mallory-Azan stain.

C cells do not contain granules. Delta cells stain blue with the Mallory-Azan technique. Enterochromaffin-like cells also have been identified in the islets.

The B cells are the predominant cells and may comprise more than 75% of the islet cell population in the dog. *B cells secrete insulin, whereas A cells secrete glucagon.* The functional significance of C cells, which have been identified in the guinea pig pancreas, has not been clarified. Some investigators believe that the C cell may be a progenitor of the A cell; others believe that the C cell may be a resting or exhausted A or B cell. The C cells comprise a small percentage of the cell population. Immunofluorescent studies have shown that the D cell produces *somatostatin*. Because somatostatin exerts a potent inhibitory influence upon A and B cell activity, it has been postulated that the D cells may serve as local inhibitors for insulin and glucagon secretion.

Histophysiology

Insulin is the *hypoglycemic factor* secreted by the B cells of the pancreatic islets. *Glucagon*, the *hyperglycemic factor*, is secreted by the A cells.

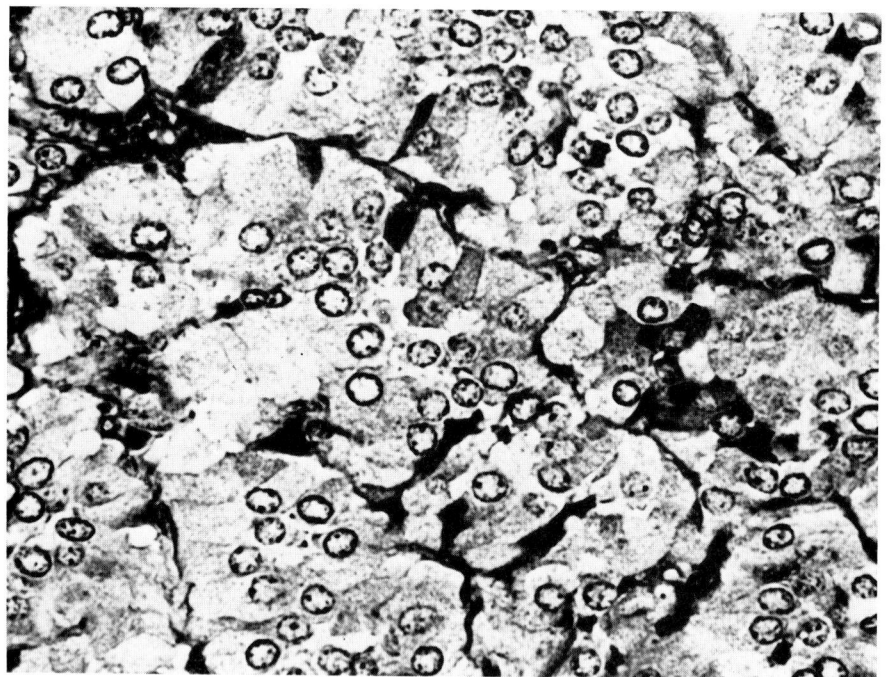

Fig. 22.32 Cells of the bovine adrenal medulla. The large columnar cells are polarized. Their basal borders are associated with capillaries. X160 (Azan stain).

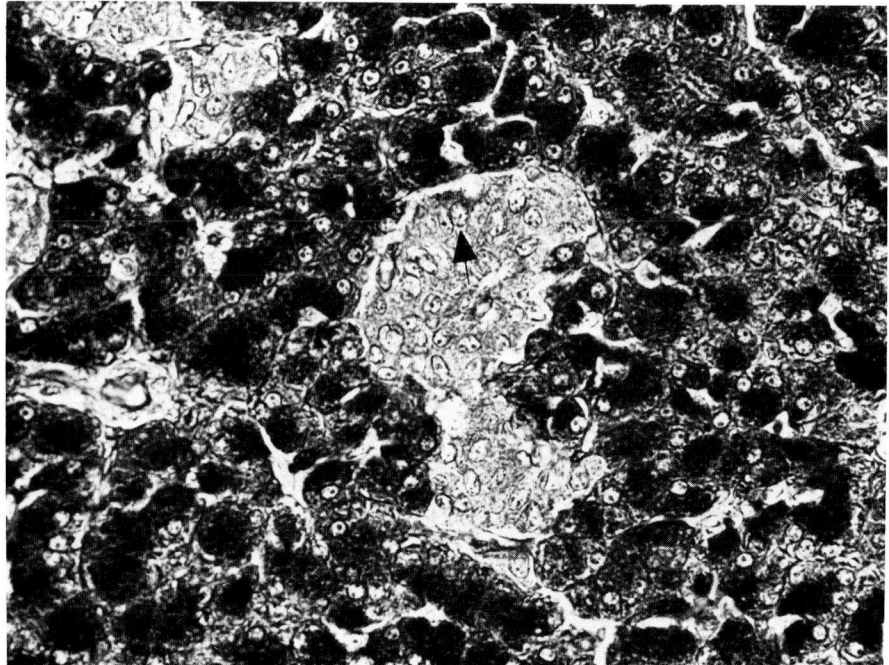

Fig. 22.33 Islets of Langerhans within the canine pancreas. The light-staining cells are alpha cells. The dark-staining cell (*arrow*) is a beta cell. X100 (Gomori aldehyde fuchsin).

Synthesis and Secretion. Proinsulin is synthesized as an inactive, single polypeptide with a molecular weight of approximately 9000. Activation occurs within the secretory granules of the cell during which time proinsulin is cleaved by the action of a trypsin-like enzyme into *insulin* and a cleavage fragment (connecting segment). Insulin is a di-

peptide with a molecular weight of approximately 6000.

Glucagon is a single polypeptide with a molecular weight of approximately 3500. Whereas most of the glucagon is produced by the A cells of the pancreatic islets, some glucagon (*enteroglucagon*) is secreted by cells of the gastrointestinal mucosa. The

functional significance of enteroglucagon is not understood completely.

Insulin and glucagon regulate carbohydrate metabolism within the body. Insulin release is achieved in response to increased levels of blood glucose (*hyperglycemia*), whereas glucagon is secreted in response to decreased blood glucose concentrations (*hypoglycemia*). The A and B cells are the receptors and regulators of the servomechanism that responds to blood glucose levels, whereas numerous tissues of the body serve as effectors to maintain homeostatic levels of blood glucose and insure an ample supply of energy for the body.

Actions of Insulin. Insulin exerts numerous and varied influences upon the cells and tissues of the body. The generalized effect of insulin upon carbohydrate metabolism is the facilitation of cellular uptake of glucose. This effect reduces blood glucose levels while making glucose available for cellular metabolic processes. The brain, liver, proximal convoluted tubules of the kidney, intestinal mucosa and red blood cells do not require insulin for the uptake of glucose.

Muscle metabolism is affected by insulin. Glucose uptake is increased and the metabolism of glucose is enhanced. Glycogenesis and glycolysis are increased. Amino acid uptake is increased and protein synthesis is enhanced, whereas fatty acid utilization is decreased.

Insulin also increases the glucose uptake by adipocytes. The augmented transport of glucose increases the utilization of glucose as a source of energy, enhances the storage of glucose as glycogen and favors lipogenesis from carbohydrates. Blood levels of free fatty acids and triglycerides decrease in response to insulin.

Although insulin does not exert a direct effect upon the uptake of glucose by the liver, the hormone increases hepatocytic metabolism of glucose. Gluconeogenesis decreases under insulin stimulation. Lipogenesis, amino acid uptake and protein synthesis increase within hepatocytes under the influence of insulin.

Insulin is one of the most important anabolic hormones of the body. It facilitates the utilization of glucose as an energy source and enhances the storage of glucose as glycogen for future use. It increases the storage of triglycerides and diminishes their use as an energy source. Moreover, amino acids are incorporated into proteins instead of being used as a source of energy. Insulin also has an effect upon intracellular and extracellular K^+. The uptake of glucose is accompanied by the movement of K^+ into cells.

Insulin is inactivated by a group of enzymes, collectively called *insulinases*, that are present in many cells of the body (liver, kidneys, skeletal muscle). The rapid turnover of insulin—the plasma half-life is approximately 10 minutes—requires the connual secretion of insulin to maintain roper metabolic activities.

The absence or insufficient secretion of nsulin by the B cells causes *diabetes mellitus.* ilucose levels are high and exceed the renal ireshold; therefore, glucosuria is a signifi- ant feature of the disease. The osmotic iuresis from glucose in the urine causes a olyuria accompanied by polydipsia. Ani- aals suffering from diabetes mellitus are iterally "starving in a sea of plenty." Glu- ose levels are high, but the animal is unable) utilize glucose as an energy source. *Com- licated diabetes mellitus* is characterized by etoacidosis. Excessive mobilization of lip- ls overwhelms the metabolic capacity of ie liver and ketone bodies form. The excess elease of H^+ from the dissociation of ketone odies causes an acidosis. Diabetic coma nd death follow if uncorrected. Hypogly- emia occurs under various circumstances; n islet cell tumor (*insuloma*) causes the xcessive and unregulated release of insulin. .ctions of Glucagon. Glucagon, as the an- agonist of insulin, is glycogenolytic, gluco- eogenic and lipolytic. The hormone insures ie availability of glucose as an energy ource. Hepatocytes respond to glucagon timulation by increasing the release of glu- ose, the availability of free fatty acids, the xidation of amino acids and ketone body ormation. Adipocytes release free fatty cids in response to glucagon. Although aost of the effects of glucagon are mani- ested in the liver, the limited effects of this ormone are sufficient to counterbalance

the effects of insulin. Glucagon inactivation results from the enzymatic degradation of the polypeptide; however, little is known of the precise mechanism.

Miscellaneous Endocrine Glands

Numerous cells of the body perform en- docrine functions that may be adjunctive activities of the organs with which they are associated. Although the organs of which these cells are a part may not be considered endocrine organs, the functional signifi- cance of their contribution to endocrine reg- ulatory mechanisms is no less important than the classic endocrine organs.

Reproductive Hormones. The *ovary* and *testes* are responsible primarily for the pro- duction of gametes, but these organs synthe- size and secrete hormones that affect repro- ductive as well as other somatic structures and functions. The ovaries secrete *estrogens* and *progestins* at various stages of the es- trous cycle. *Relaxin* is produced by the ova- ries in those species that require functional ovaries throughout gestation. The testes, through their population of interstitial cells, produce *androgens*. *Estrogens* are produced by the Sertoli cells of the testes, especially in the stallion. The *placenta* is an essential reproductive structure in eutherian mam- mals. Among its numerous functions, it is also an endocrine oxygen. The placentas of many mammals secrete *estrogens, progester- one, placental gonadotropins* and *prostaglan- din* $F_{2\alpha}$.

Gastrointestinal Hormones. Various cells of the mucosal lining of the stomach and in- testine secrete hormones that exert an influ- ence on gastrointestinal function. The hor- mones secreted by these cells are amines and polypeptides. Some of the lining cells do not contain preformed amines but are capable of converting precursors to amines (serotonin, dopamine, histamine) by decar- boxylation. Such cells have been designated *APUD cells* (*A*mine *P*recursor *U*ptake and *D*ecarboxylation cells). Neural crest ecto- derm has been postulated as the source of these cells.

Numerous peptide hormones have been isolated from the gastrointestinal tract and characterized: *gastrin, secretin, cholecystoki- nin-pancreozymin* (*CCK-PZ*), *gastric inhibi- tory peptide* (*GIP*), *vasoactive intestinal pep- tide* (*VIP*), *motilin* and *substance P. Entero- gastrone,* although postulated, has never been isolated and characterized chemically. *Enteroglucagon, somatostatin* and *bulbogas- trone* have been isolated from the gastroin- testinal mucosa. A summary of the physio- logic actions of these hormones is given in Table 22.2.

The cells that secrete gastrointestinal hor- mones may be classified on the manner by which their secretions reach the target or- gans. *Neurocrine cells* secrete a neurotrans- mitter substance across a synapse to achieve excitation of target cells. *Paracrine cells*, se- creting their hormones into the surrounding extracellular fluid, influence target cells by the diffusion of their localized hormones through the extracellular fluid. *Endocrine cells* secrete their generalized hormones into the blood for transport throughout the body.

Although the activity and origin of gas- trointestinal hormones are confined gener- ally to this system, one hormone somatosta- tin, is produced in a number of locations. *Somatostatin (Growth Hormone Inhibitory Factor)* is secreted by the hypothalamus, D cells of the pancreatic islets and gastrointes- tinal mucosa.

Miscellaneous Hormones. Although the pri- mary function of the kidneys is excretion, the organ is involved in endocrine functions also. *Erythrogenin* is essential for the gen- eration of erythropoietin (Chapter 10), whereas *renin* is involved in the generation of angiotensin I (Chapter 20). Some inves- tigators consider *vitamin D* and its active metabolites to be hormones (Chapter 8). If these substances obtain the status of hor- mones, then the liver, integument and kid- neys, by virtue of their involvement in the synthesis and activation of cholecalciferol, have endocrine functions.

The *prostaglandins* (*PG*) are a family of lipid components that serve as hormones. Prostaglandins are synthesized from *arach- idonic* acid, a fatty acid with 20 carbons and 4 unsaturated carbon bonds that is part of the phospholipid component of cell mem- branes. Microenvironmental changes induce alterations in the plasma membrane that

able 22.2
Selected Gastrointestinal Hormones

Hormone	Target	Action
Cholescystokinin-Pancreozymin (CCK-PZ)	Stomach	↑ Motility
	Small Intestine	↑ Motility
	Pancreas—Acini	↑ Secretion
Chymodenin	Pancreas—Acini	↑ Chymotrypsin secretion
Enterogastrone*	Stomach	↓ HCl secretion
		↓ Motility
Gastric Inhibitory Peptide (GIP)	Stomach	↓ HCl secretion
Gastrin	Stomach	↑ HCl secretion
		↑ Enzyme secretion
		↑ Motility
	Small Intestine	↑ Motility
Histamine	Stomach	↑ HCl secretion
Motilin	Stomach	↑ Motility
Secretin	Pancreas—Ducts	↑ HCO_3^- secretion
	Liver	↑ HCO_3^- secretion
	Small Intestine	↓ Motility
Somatostatin	Pancreas—Islets	↓ Insulin secretion
	Pancreas—Acini	↓ Secretion
	Stomach	↓ Gastrin secretion
Substance P	Stomach	↑ Motility
	Small Intestine	↑ Motility
Vasoactive Intestinal Peptide (VIP)	Stomach	↓ HCl secretion
		↓ Enzyme secretion
		↓ Motility
	Pancreas—Ducts	↑ HCO_3^- secretion
	Pancreas—Acini	↑ Enzyme secretion

* Postulated but not isolated.

cause the enzymatic release of arachidonic acid under normal and disease conditions. Subsequent endoperoxidation and hydroxylation produces prostaglandins. Various prostaglandins have been characterized chemically: *prostaglandins A, B, D, E, F, G, H* and *I*. Additionally, a closely related compound, *thromboxane (TXA₂)*, has been isolated and characterized. Although research has afforded numerous insights about the biologic activity of these substances, research is ongoing and continues to clarify their functions.

The biologic effects of prostaglandins are manifested locally, because the liver and lungs rapidly deactivate the substances. The prostaglandins exert their influence upon the organ in which they are produced or downstream upon an organ associated with the venous drainage from the organ or tissue of origin.

PGA_2, PGE_1 and PGE_2 are vasodilators. Bronchodilation, sodium/water diuresis and increased gastrointestinal motility are mediated by PGE_2. Also, PGE_2 may stimulate renin release and inhibit gastric secretion. The vasopressor activity of $PGF_{2\alpha}$ is well-documented. It is also a bronchodilator and luteolytic compound. $PGF_{2\alpha}$ is produced in the endometrium and transported to the ovary by a utero-ovarian vein. The mechanism of transfer to the ovarian artery has not been determined. The regression of the corpus luteum occurs under the influence of $PGF_{2\alpha}$. The luteolytic activity of the compound terminates the luteal phase of the estrous cycle and permits the next wave of follicles to mature. The luteolytic function has been documented in the mare, ewe, cow and sow. *Prostacyclin (PGI₂)* is a vasodilator that also inhibits platelet aggregation (*antithrombotic agent*). *Thromboxane (TXA₂)* is a vasoconstrictor that also stimulates platelet aggregation (*thrombogenic*). The interaction of TXA_2/PGI_2 at the endothelial-blood interface may serve as mediators in the maintenance of vascular homeostasis in health and disease.

References

Pituitary Gland

Brahms, S.: The development of the hypophysis of the cat (*Felis domestica*). Amer. J. Anat. *50:*251, 1932.

Conklin, J. L.: The identification of acidophilic cells in the human pars distalis. Anat. Rec. *156:*347, 1966.

Goldberg, R. C. and Chaikoff, I. L.: On the occurrence of six cell types in the dog anterior pituitary. Anat. Rec. *112:*265, 1953.

Harris, G. W. and Donovan, B. T. (eds.): *The Pituitary Gland*, University of California Press, Berkeley, 1966.

Herlant, M.: The cells of the adenohypophysis and their functional significance. Int. Rev. Cytol. *17:*299, 1964.

Knigge, K. M., Scott, D. E. and Weindl, A. (editors): *Brain Endocrine Interaction. Median Eminence: Structure and Function.* S. Karger, Basal, 1971.

Lederis, K.: An electron microscopical study of the human neurohypophysis. Z. Zellforsch. *68:*847, 1965.

Nakane, P. K.: Classification of anterior pituitary cell types with immunoenzyme histochemistry. J. Histochem. Cytochem. *18:*9, 1970.

Page, R. B., Munger, B. L. and Bergland, R. M.: Scanning microscopy of pituitary vascular casts. Am. J. Anat. *146:*273, 1976.

Share, L. and Grosvenor, C. E.: The neurohypophysis. *In:* Guyton, A. C. and McCann, S. M. (editors). *International Review of Science. Endocrine Physiology.* Series 1, Vol. 5 pp. 1–30. Butterworth & Co., London, 1974.

Zambrano, D.: Ultrastructural changes of the neurohypophysis of the rat after castration. Z. Zellforsch. *86:*14, 1968.

Pineal Body

Anderson, E.: The anatomy of bovine and ovine pineals: Light and electron microscope studies. J. Ultrastruc. Res. Suppl. *8:*1, 1965.

Axelrod, J.: The pineal glands: A neurochemical transducer. Science *184:*1341, 1974.

Herbert, J.: The pineal gland and light-induced oestrus in ferrets. J. Endocr. *43:*625, 1969.

Jordan, H. E.: The histogenesis of the pineal body of the sheep. Amer. J. Anat. *12:*249, 1911.

Wurtman, R. J., Axelrod, J. and Kelly, D. E.: *The Pineal.* Academic Press, New York, 1968.

Thyroid Gland

Ekholm, R.: Thyroglobulin biosynthesis in the rat thyroid. J. Ultrastruct. Res. *20:*103, 1967.

Ekholm, R. and Ericson, L. E.: The ultrastructure of the parafollicular cells of the thyroid gland in the rat. J. Ultrastruct. Res. *23:*378, 1967.

Kingsbury, B. E.: Ultimobranchial body and the thyroid gland in the fetal calf. Amer. J. Anat. *56:*445, 1935.

Klinck, G. H., Oertel, J. E. and Winship, I.: Ultrastructure of normal human thyroid. Lab. Invest. *22:*2, 1970.

Martin, J. B.: Regulation of the pituitary—thyroid axis. *In:* Guyton, A. C. and McCann, S. M. (editors). *International Review of Science. Endocrine Physiology.* Series 1, Vol. 5 pp. 1–30. Butterworth & Co., London, 1974.

Sobel, H. J.: Electron microscopy of I-irradiated thyroid. Arch. Path. *78:*53, 1964.

Welsch, U., Flitney, E. and Pearse, A. G. E.: Comparative studies of the ultrastructure of the thyroid parafollicular C cells. J. Microscop. *89:*83, 1969.

Parathyroid Glands

Capen, C. C. and Rowland, G. N.: The ultrastructure of the parathyroid glands of young cats. Anat. Rec. *162:*327, 1968.

Gaillard, P. J., Talmage, R. V. and Budy, A. M. (eds.): *The Parathyroid Glands.* University of Chicago Press, Chicago, 1965.

Godwin, M. C.: The development of the parathyroids in the dog with emphasis upon the origin of accessory glands. Anat. Rec. *68:*305, 1937.

Gray, T. K., Cooper, C. W. and Munson, P. L.: Parathyroid hormone, thyrocalcitonin and the control of mineral metabolism. *In:* Guyton, A. C. and McCann, S. M. (editors). *International Review of Science. Endocrine Physiology.* Series 1, Vol. 5 pp. 239–278. Butterworth & Co., London, 1974.

Nakagami, K., Yamazaki, Y. and Tsunoda, Y.: An electron microscopic study of the human fetal parathyroid gland. Z. Zellforsch. *85:*89, 1968.

Adrenal Glands

Bloodworth, J. M. B., Jr. and Powers, K. L.: The ultrastructure of the normal dog adrenal. J. Anat. *10:* 457, 1968.

Brenner, R. M.: Fine structure of adrenocortical cells adult male rhesus monkeys. Amer. J. Anat. *119:*42, 1966.

Elfvin, L. G.: The development of the secretory granul in the rat adrenal medulla. J. Ultrastruct. Res. *1:* 45, 1967.

Hopwood, D.: Adrenal medullary basophilia in ox, p and sheep: A histochemical, immunohistochemic and cell fractionation study. Histochemie *11:*26, 1967.

Merklin, R. J.: Suprarenal gland lymphatic drainag Am. J. Anat. *119:*359, 1966.

Mulnix, J. A.: Adrenal cortical disease in dogs. Ve Scope. *19:*12, 1975.

Rhodin, J. A. G.: The ultrastructure of the adrenal corte of the rat under normal and experimental cond tions. J. Ultrastruct. Res. *34:*23, 1971.

Thorn, G. W. (editor): *Steroid Therapy: A Clinical Upda for the 1970's.* Upjohn Company. Kalamazoo, 197

Whitehead, R. H.: The histogenesis of the adrenal in t pig. Amer. J. Anat. *2:*349, 1903.

Wood, J. G.: Identification of and observations on ep nephrine and norepinephrine containing cells in th adrenal medulla. Amer. J. Anat. *112:*285, 1963.

Endocrine Pancreas

Greider, M. H., Howell, S. L. and Lacy, P. E.: Isolatic and properties of secretory granules from rat isle of Langerhans. J. Cell Biol. *41:*162, 1969.

Lacy, P. E.: Electron microscopy of the beta cells of t pancreas. Amer. J. Med. *31:*851, 1961.

Like, A. A.: The ultrastructure of the islets of Langerha in man. Lab. Invest. *16:*937, 1967.

Machino, M.: On the substructure of secretory granul of the chick beta islet cell. J. Ultrastruct. Res. *3* 199, 1970.

Unger, R. H.: The pancreas as a regulator of metabolis In: Guyton, A. C. and McCann, S. M. (editors *International Review of Science.* Endocrine Physic ogy. Series 1, Vol. 5 pp. 179–204. Butterworth Co., London, 1974.

Miscellaneous Hormones

Bell, T. G. et al.: Biologic interaction of prostaglandin thromboxane, and prostacyclin: Potential nonr productive veterinary clinical applications. J. Am Vet. Med. Assoc. *176:*1195, 1980.

Hightower, N. C. and Janowitz, H. D.: Gastrointestina hormones. *In:* Brobeck, J. R. (editor). *Best an Taylor's Physiological Basis of Medical Practice.* 10 edition, pp. 20–23. Williams & Wilkins, Baltimor 1979.

Kindahl, H.: Prostaglandin biosynthesis and metabolis J. Am. Vet. Med. Assoc. *176:*1173, 1980.

Seguin, B. E.: Role of prostaglandins in bovine repr duction. J. Amer. Vet. Med. Assoc. *176:*1178, 198(

Welbourn, R. B. et al.: The APUD cells of the alimenta tract in health and disease. Med. Clin. N. A. *5* 1359, 1974.

23: Male Reproductive System

General Characteristics

Introduction. The male reproductive system consists of the *testes, excretory (genital) ducts, accessory glands* and *penis*. The constituent organs contribute to the primary function—reproduction. The *production* and *transport of spermatozoa, secretion* of fluids and the *placement* of semen in the female tract are necessary reproductive functions. The intermittent copulatory organ also functions to *transport urine* to the external environment. The testes serve as an endocrine organ.

Testes and Associated Structures

General Remarks. These organs are contained within a specialized pouch of the skin, the *scrotum*, which contains the usual epidermal and dermal constituents, as well as smooth muscle (*tunica dartos*), fascia and peritoneum.

The testes are combined exocrine and endocrine organs. The exocrine portion is a compound, coiled tubular gland that produces cells, spermatozoa, as its secretory product. The endocrine portion is represented by the interstitial *cells of Leydig* and the sustentacular *cells of Sertoli*.

Testicular Investments. The testes are enclosed by a capsule, the *tunica albuginea*, which is composed of dense white fibrous connective tissue (DWFCT) (Fig. 23.1). This capsule is covered by mesothelium, the *visceral layer of the tunica vaginalis*, and is separated from the *parietal layer of the tunica vaginalis* by a portion of the peritoneal cavity. Both these membranes are typical serous membranes, but the areolar connective tissue of the visceral layer of the tunica vaginalis blends insensibly with the connective tissue of the tunica albuginea. The retroperitoneal development of the testes within the abdominal cavity and their subsequent migration to the scrotum account for the presence of serous membranes and coelomic space associated with the testes.

A *stratum vasculare*, or vascular layer, is present in the tunica albuginea of most species. It is superficial in the dog and ram, and it is deep in the stallion and boar. Smooth muscle fibers may be present in the tunica albuginea of the horse.

The tunica albuginea is continuous with the areolar connective tissue of the *medias-tinum testis*, in most species, at the anterior pole of the testis (Fig. 23.1). It surrounds the *rete testis*. Although the mediastinum of the stallion is atypical and inconspicuous, it exists as a true mediastinum. The rete testis of the stallion is extratesticular and penetrates the tunica albuginea to unite with the efferent ducts.

The tunica albuginea also gives rise to areolar connective tissue of the *septuli testis* (Fig. 23.1). These septa vary in thickness and completeness, extend from the tunica albuginea to the mediastinum testis and effectively divide the testis into lobules, called *lobuli testis*. The tubules of the lobule, *tubuli contorti* and *tubuli recti*, are surrounded by a delicate network of areolar connective tissue which contains numerous reticular fibers. The interstitial cells of Leydig are located within this connective tissue space.

Seminiferous Tubules. The parenchyma of the organ consists of the lining cells of the seminiferous tubules and their ducts, as well as the *cells of Leydig.*

The *seminiferous tubules (tubuli contorti)* are the exocrine portions of the gland (Fig. 23.2). They radiate from the mediastinum testis as coiled, tubular adenomeres. The tubules are lined by a stratified epithelium which consists of basal, intermediate and superficial zones (Fig. 23.3). The presence as well as the constituents of the zones is dependent upon the spermatogenic activity of the tubules. Although the epithelium is stratified, it is not similar to the stratified epithelia thus far encountered (Fig. 23.4). The stratified cells consist of *spermatogonia, primary spermatocytes, secondary spermatocytes, spermatids* and *spermatozoa.* The developmental sequence of these cells will be presented in a subsequent section on *spermatogenesis.*

The other parenchymatous components of the testes are the *Leydig cells* (Fig. 23.5). These cells are the endocrine portion of the testes and are responsible for the elaboration of *testosterone.* The cells, which are located in the connective tissue between the tubuli contorti, are polyhedral with a large spherical nucleus and a distinct nucleolus. Their acidophilic cytoplasm contains numerous lipid droplets and granules, but these are lost during routine processing (Plate II.1). As a result, they are foamy (similar to the spongiocytes of the zona fasciculata of the adrenal cortex). These cells are especially abundant in the boar and the ox.

Tubuli Recti and Rete Testes. The seminif-

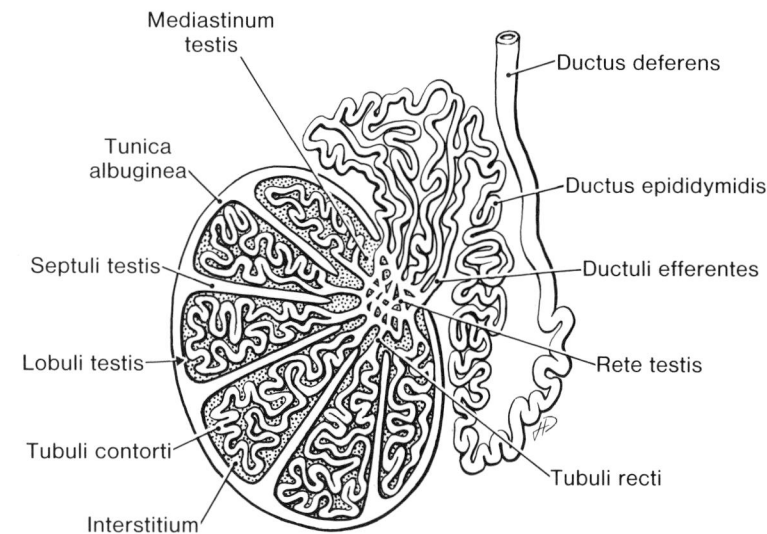

Fig. 23.1   A drawing of the testis and associated structures. The connective tissue investments of the extratesticular ducts are not shown. All light micrographs are labeled as the magnification with the microscope before photographic enlarging. All electron micrographs are labeled as total magnification, including photographic enlarging.

477

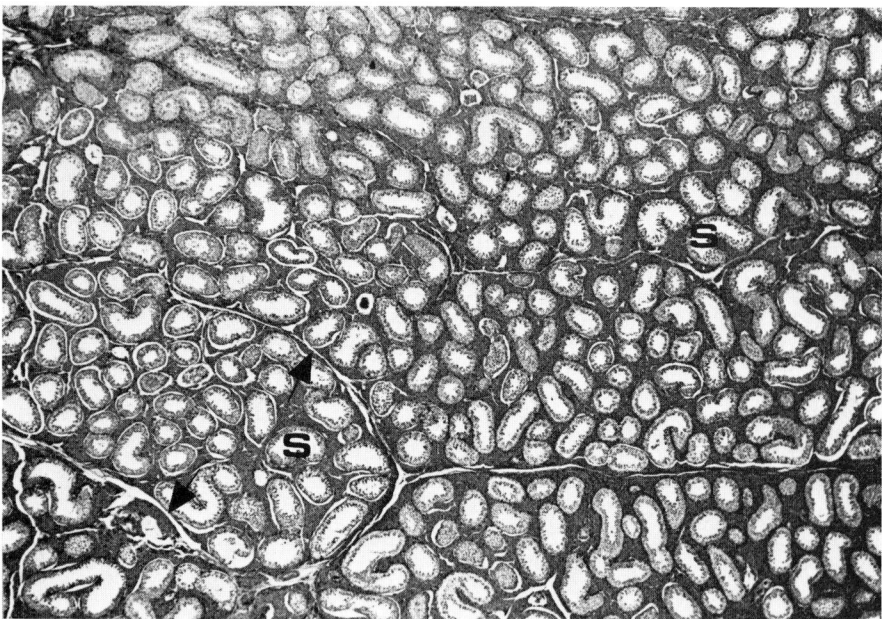

Fig. 23.2 Organization of the testis. The seminiferous tubules (S) occur within lobules which are separated from each other by connective tissue septa (*arrows*). X4.

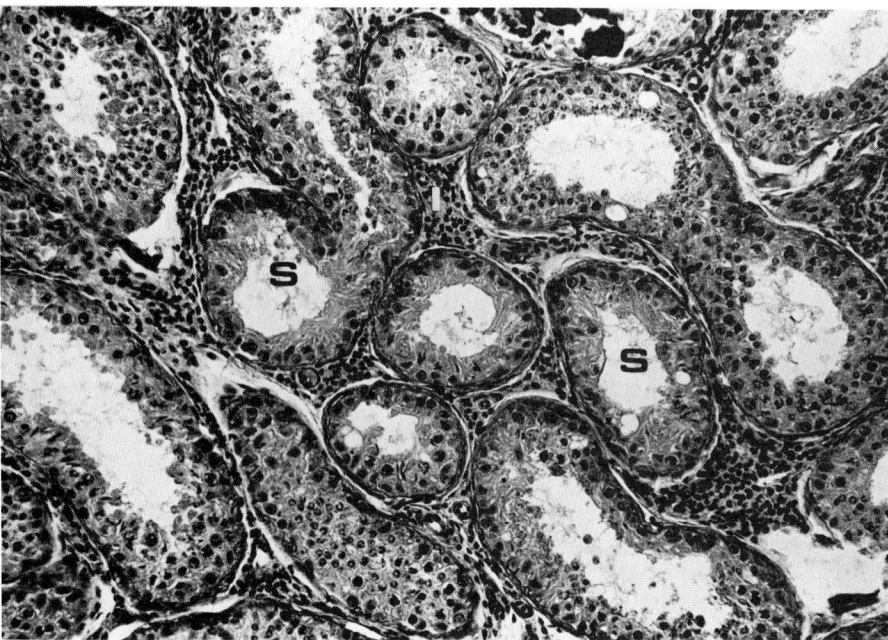

Fig. 23.3 Seminiferous tubules of a cervine testis. The seminiferous tubules (S) are separated by connective tissue and interstitial cells (I). X40.

erous tubules are continuous with the *straight tubules* (*tubuli recti*) and the passages of the *rete testis* (Fig. 23.6). These areas are lined by a squamous, cuboidal or columnar epithelium. In the bull, the rete testis may be lined by a bistratified cuboidal epithelium. These two regions are similar to each other and are best identified by position within the testis. Whereas the tubuli recti are straight tubules, the rete testis consists of randomly anastomotic tubules (Fig. 23.7). In the boar, the apical borders of the lining

cells may possess blebs which have been interpreted as apocrine secretory activity. Some believe that the lining cells of these regions actually represent a continuation of the Sertoli cell population of the tubuli contorti.

Genital Ducts

Ductuli Efferentes. The *ductuli efferentes* connect the rete testis with the ductus epi-

didymidis (Fig. 23.8). The efferent ductule vary from 6 to 20 coiled ducts. These duc tules, on the basis of their tortuous path an increasing diameter, are also referred to a *coni vasculosi*. They are lined by intermit tently kinociliated columnar epithelium (Fig. 23.9). The current created by the move ment of the cilia assists in the movement o spermatozoa toward the larger ducts. Th nonciliated cells possess secretory blebs a their apical surface, but the significance c this secretory product is not understood The surrounding lamina propria blends wit the other connective tissue of the area, an some smooth muscle cells are present. Th widened and tightly convoluted portions c these tubules which connect with the ductu epididymidis constitute the head of the or gan.

Ductus Epididymidis. This is the coiled tub which, with associated connective tissue an muscle, forms the *head*, *body* and *tail* of th epididymis (Fig. 23.10). The latter continue as the ductus deferens.

The lamina epithelialis consists of pseu dostratified stereociliated columnar epithe lium (Fig. 23.11). The basal cells contai lipid droplets, whereas the columnar cell are long and slender, contain lipids an have apical modifications in the form o stereocilia (Fig. 23.12). These processes ar nonmotile and serve to increase the absorp tive and/or secretory surface of the lining They are usually heavily matted together b their secretory products. The nature an significance of these products is not known The lamina propria consists of a highl vascularized areolar connective tissue. Th lamina muscularis is arranged in a circula array and becomes thicker toward the tai of the epididymis. The tunica submucosa i areolar connective tissue centrally an DWFCT peripherally which is continuou with the tunica albuginea. Numerous sper matozoa are stored within the lumen of th ductus epididymidis during which time the mature.

Ductus Deferens. The ductus deferens is th continuation of the ductus epididymidi (Fig. 23.13). The lamina epithelialis consist of a pseudostratified columnar epithelium There is, however, a gradual transition fron the lining epithelium of the ductus epididi ymidis to that of the ductus deferens. Th lamina propria-submucosa consists of areo lar connective tissue. The tunica mucosa submucosa is highly folded. The tunica mus cularis is very thick and varies from two distinct inner and outer layers to intermin gled fibers. The tunica serosa is present an typical.

Spermatogenesis

Introduction. *Spermatogenesis* occurs withir the tubuli contorti and the ductus epididy midis. The former is responsible for the actual production of the male gametes while the latter aids in their maturation

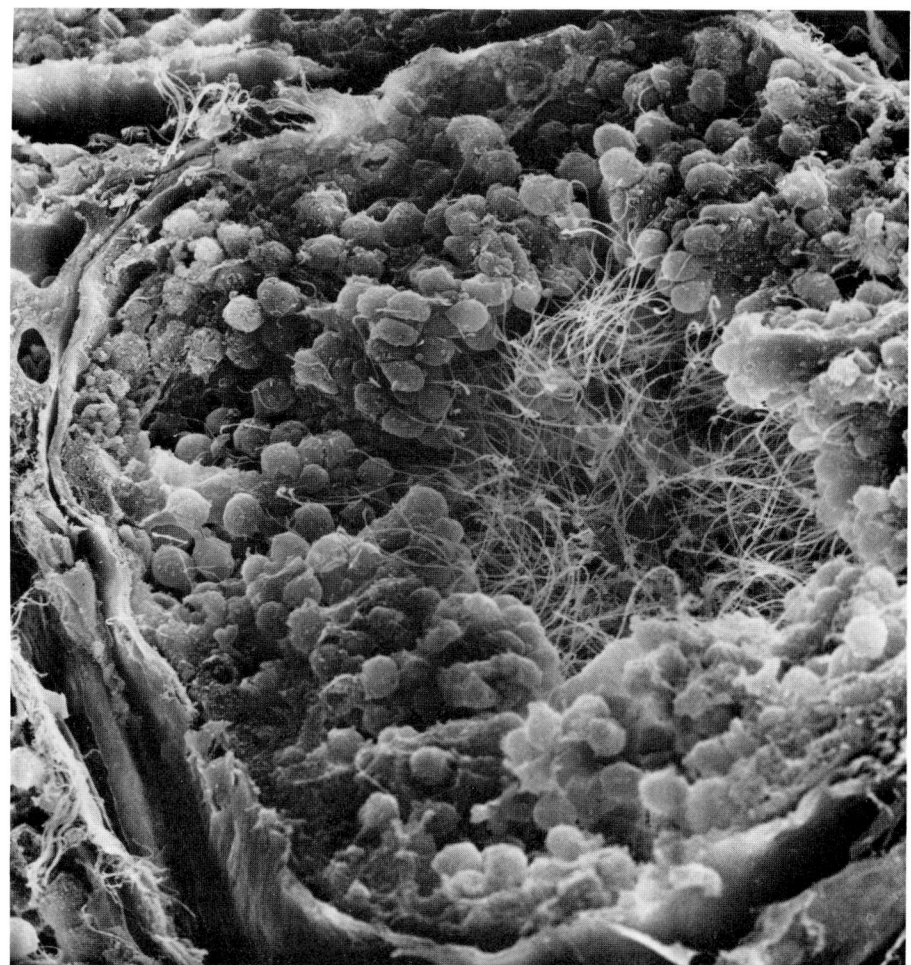

Fig. 23.4   A scanning electron micrograph of a freeze-fractured sample of a canine seminiferous tubule. Numerous cells comprise the stratified epithelium. The tails of developing spermatozoa protrude into the lumen of the tubule. X670 (Courtesy of C. J. Connell).

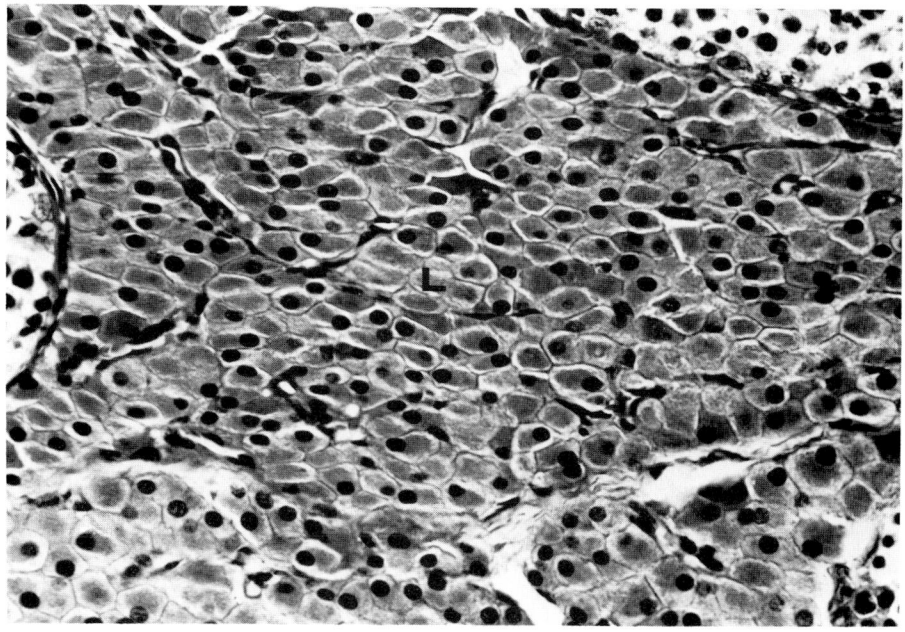

Fig. 23.5   Interstitial cells of a porcine testis. The Leydig cells (L) have an acidophilic and foamy cytoplasm. X100.

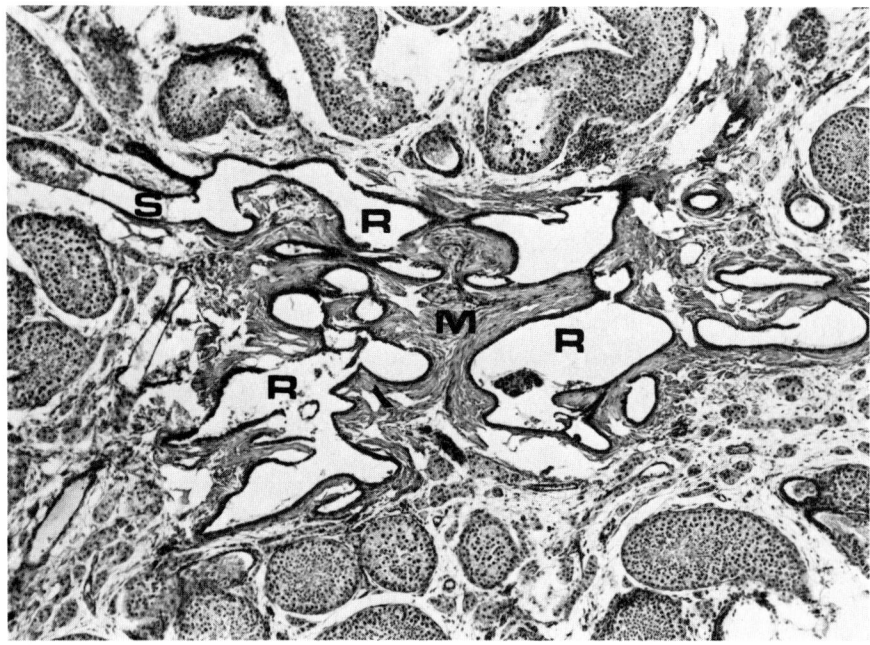

Fig. 23.6 Mediastinum of a feline testis. The mediastinum (M) contains the rete testis (R). Straight tubules (S) connect the rete testis with the seminiferous tubules. X10.

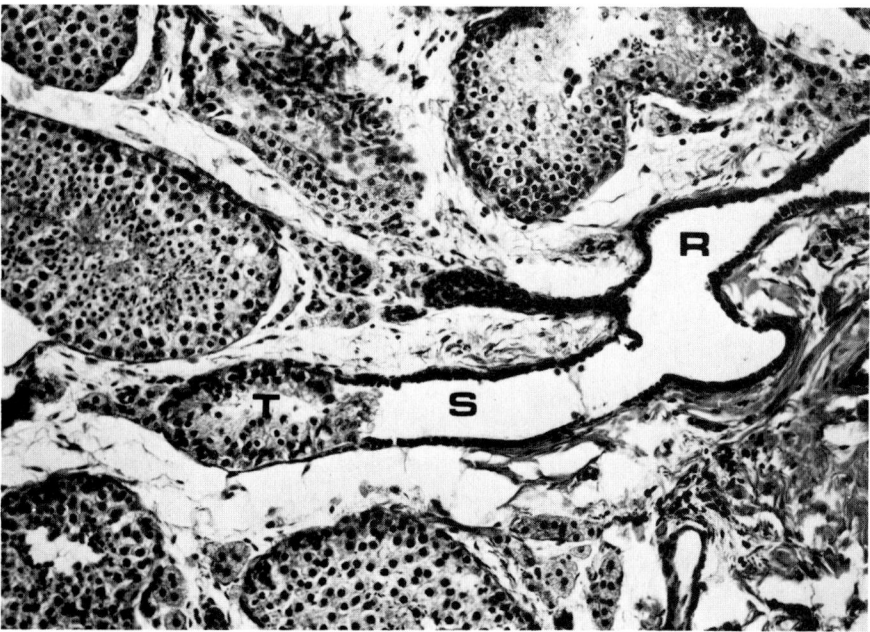

Fig. 23.7 Rete testis and tubuli recti of a feline testis. The tubuli contorti (T) are connected to the rete testis (R) by the tubuli recti (S). X40.

process. The sequence of events involves a series of nuclear and cytoplasmic changes that result in haploid cells that are highly motile and suited to survive for short periods outside the body. The progression begins with *spermatogonia* and terminates with *spermatozoa*. These cells, with *Sertoli cells*, comprise the stratified seminiferous tubular lining. The most primitive cells are located near the periphery of the tubule (near the basement membrane), whereas the more ad-

vanced cells are located on the luminal border. In the case of the spermatozoa, they eventually occur within the lumina.

Three distinct periods are characteristic of the spermatogenic process: *mitotic*, *meiotic* and *metamorphic*. Not all seminiferous tubules will be in the same period of activity, nor will different portions of the same tubule possess cells with the same degree of differentiation. Although there are species variations, the spermatocytogenic

process is described as occurring in helical waves down the tubule contorti to the straight tubules.

Sertoli Cells. The *Sertoli cells* of the seminiferous tubules serve as sustentacular or nurse cells for the developing gametes (Fig. 23.14). Sertoli cells are tall columnar or triangular cells the cytoplasm and cellular margins of which are difficult to distinguish with light microscopy (Plate II.2). Developing gametes appear to be embedded within the Sertoli cell cytoplasm. They are the only cells of the seminiferous tubules that extend from the basal lamina to the tubular lumen. The nuclear morphology is helpful in identifying the cell. The oval nucleus is usually positioned basally. It is vesicular and has a distinct nucleolus. A characteristic longitudinal fold in the nuclear membrane may be visible. Whereas the intimate relationships between Sertoli cells and developing gametes are obvious with light microscopy, electron microscopy was required to clarify the nature of the intimacy. Developing gametes are contained within cytoplasmic depressions along the margins of the Sertoli cells (Fig. 23.15). Although the Sertoli cells surround the developing gametes completely, the gametes are not within the cytoplasm of the nursing cells. Smooth endoplasmic reticular profiles are extensive along the basal border of the cell. The presence of this organelle has been interpreted as a priori evidence of the ability of the Sertoli cell to synthesize steroids. The Golgi apparatus is extensive; protein synthesis and secretion occurs. An *androgen binding protein* (ABP), secreted into the seminiferous tubular lumen, is degraded in the ductus epididymidis. Numerous cytofilaments are scattered throughout the cell. The cytofilaments are obvious especially along the lateral margins of the cell where they are oriented parallel to the long axis of the cell and aggregated in bundles. The movement of developing gametes from the basal border to the apical margin is dependent upon changes in the Sertoli cell probably attributable to alterations in the cytofilaments. Lysosomes in various stages of activity are conspicuous. The presence of lysosomes correlates with the removal, phagocytosis and digestion of residual cytoplasmic droplets from developing spermatozoa. The basilar regions of the lateral cell membranes of adjacent Sertoli cells are joined by tight (occluding) junctions. The tight junctions effectively divide the seminiferous tubule into two distinct regions—basilar and apical compartments. The *basilar compartment*, located peripherally between the tight junctions and the basal lamina, is the location of the spermatogonia. The spermatogonia are influenced by substances that move across the basal lamina from the testicular interstitium. Exchange between the basal border of the Sertoli cell and the surrounding interstitial vasculature is facilitated by the relationship. The *apical compartment*, located be-

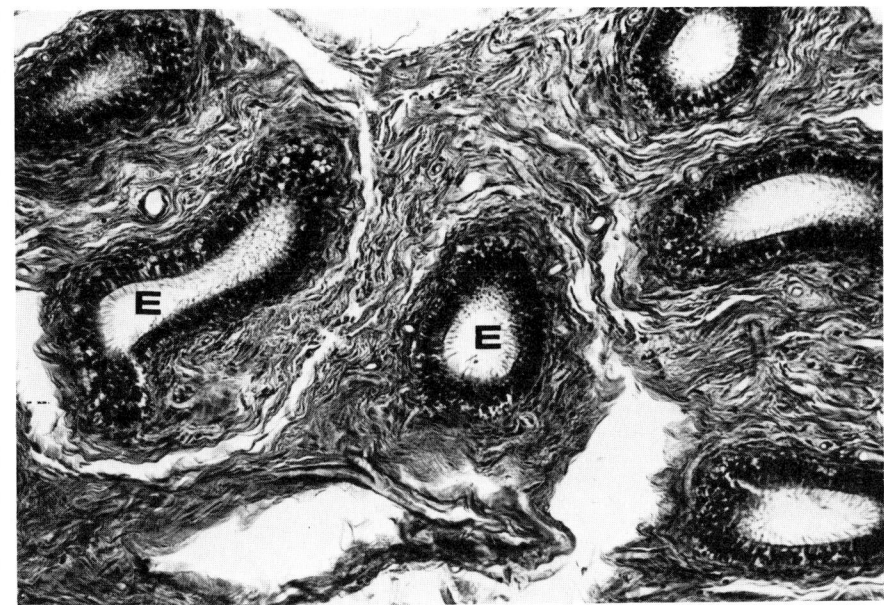

Fig. 23.8 Ductuli efferentes. The tubules (E) connect the rete testis to the ductus epididymidis. X40.

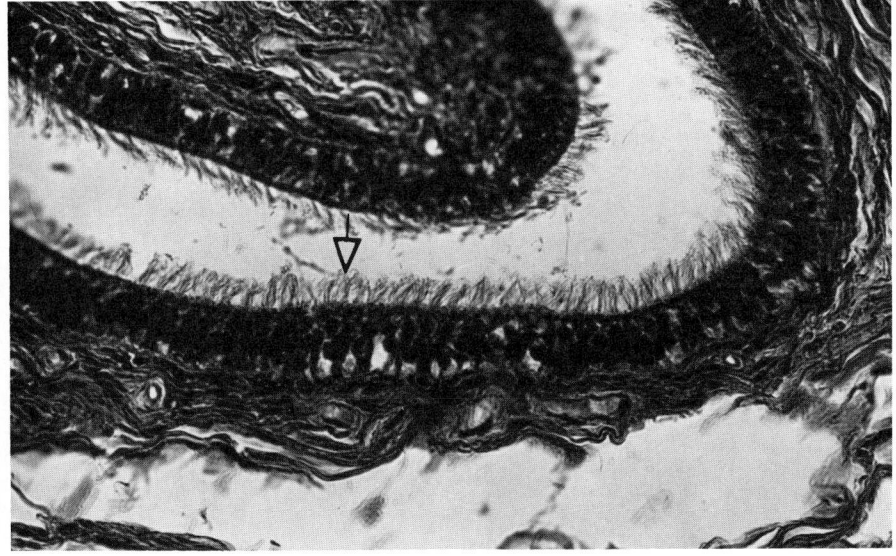

Fig. 23.9 Lining cells of the efferent ducts. The columnar epithelial cells are kinociliated (*arrow*). X100.

Through successive mitotic divisions numerous spermatogonia undergo changes which result in spermatozoa—all derived from one cell. If one spermatogonium differentiated into subsequent cell types, then only four haploid gametes would be produced. As a result of the mitotic stage, the number of spermatogonia is increased greatly. Accordingly, the number of potential spermatozoa increases also. Just as importantly, however, not all spermatogonia differentiate simultaneously. Some are retained as stem cells for future differentiation. If complete differentiation were to occur, it is obvious that the potential for gamete production would diminish rapidly and eventually terminate.

Spermatogonia actually represent many generations of cells. These include: A cells, intermediate cells (I_1 and I_2), and B cells. The *A spermatogonia* are the stem cells for this process. The cell is round with a large, round nucleus that contains finely dispersed chromatin and an eccentrically positioned nucleolus. Upon mitotic division, one cell remains as a stem cell whereas the other divides and its progeny differentiate into *intermediate (I) spermatogonia*. I spermatogonia are oval with an oval nucleus. The nucleus contains peripheral coarsely clumped chromatin and two or three nucleoli. Subsequent divisions of intermediate spermatogonia give rise to *B spermatogonia*. These cells are round and small. The oval nucleus contains coarsely clumped chromatin. Subsequent division of these spermatogonia leads to the differentiation of *primary spermatocytes*. As many as 16 primary spermatocytes are derived from a single A spermatogonium. Incomplete cytokinesis is characteristic of the mitotic process that results in B spermatogonia.

Spermatogonia occur adjacent to the basement membrane, either singly or in clusters. They do not form a complete basal layer and may be difficult to find.

Spermatocytogenesis. This stage of the spermatogenic process involves the *spermatocytes*. These are the largest cells of the spermatogenic epithelium which comprise the intermediate zone. Type B spermatogonia differentiate into *primary spermatocytes*. These cells have rather long lifetimes (approximately 16 days in the bull) and usually are easy to find and identify. Although their interphase nuclei contain a fine chromatin network, they are often observed in the first division of meiosis. They also have a long premeiotic prophase. Therefore, the nucleus may be coarsely granulated or chromosomes may be visible.

The end of the first division of meiosis marks the differentiation of the *secondary spermatocytes*. These cells are still diploid (2N number of chromosomes). These cells are smaller than primary spermatocytes and are difficult to find. Their life-span varies from minutes to one hour. The division of these cells results in the formation of *sper-*

tween the tight junctions and the apical border, contains the developing gametes. Whereas the Sertoli cell is influenced by direct exchange from the surrounding vasculature, the developing gametes are "insulated" from direct influences by the Sertoli cell relationship. The tight junctions and contiguous Sertoli cells form an effective *blood-testis barrier*.

The Sertoli cell provides physical support and protection for the developing gametes. The nutrional requirements of the gametes are probably supplied by the sustentacular cell. The Sertoli cell may participate actively in the centripetal movement, development

and release of the gametes, because alterations in Sertoli cell morphology correlate with events in the spermatogenic cycle. The intimacy of the relationship implies that the Sertoli cell is a metabolic regulator. Additionally, damaged gametes are phagocytized by the Sertoli cells.

The Sertoli cells also secrete estrogens. Sertoli cell tumors, which are common in the dog, may be accompanied by the development of secondary female sex characteristics.

Stage of Multiplication. The *stage of multiplication* or *mitotic stage* is characterized by an increase in the number of spermatogonia.

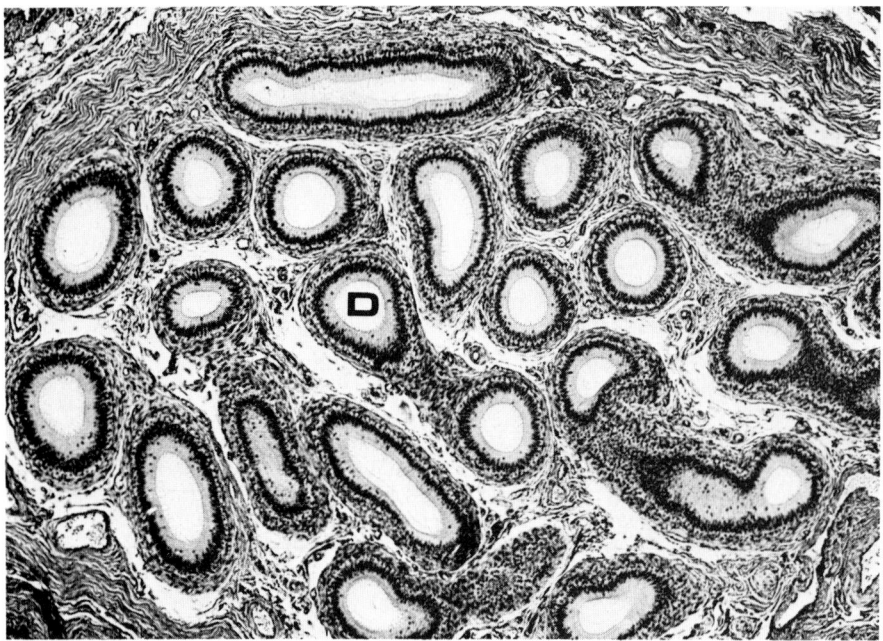

Fig. 23.10 A portion of the epididymis. The ductus epididymidis (D) is the tubular portion of the organ. X20.

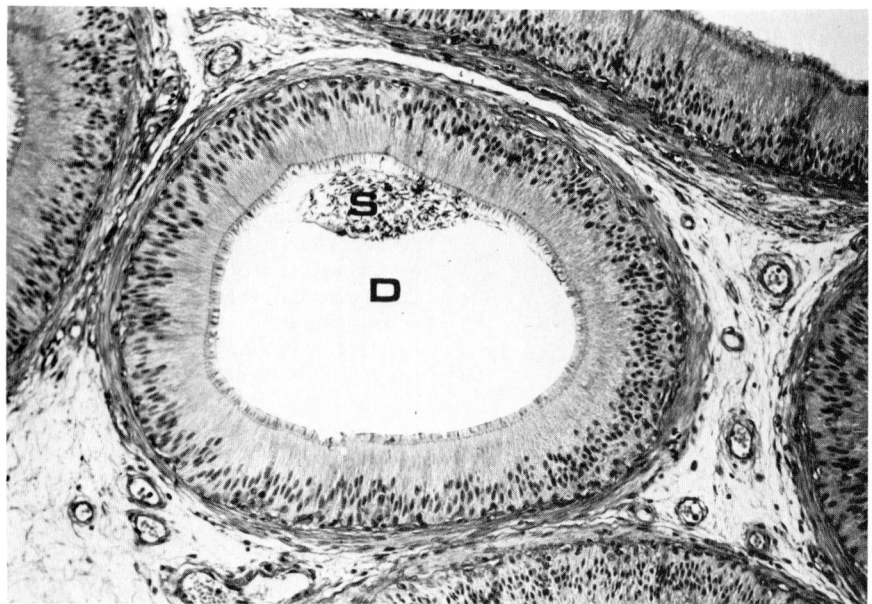

Fig. 23.11 Lining cells of the ductus epididymidis. The tubules (D) contain spermatozoa (S) and are lined by stereociliated epithelium. X10.

matids. Throughout these divisions cytokinesis is incomplete and the cells are joined by numerous intercellular bridges.

Spermiogenesis. The *spermatids* that result from the division of the secondary spermatocytes are haploid (1N number of chromosomes). These cells, spermatids, comprise the most developed, most numerous and largest layer of the seminiferous tubular epithelium. The luminal zone in which they are located is referred to as the *zone of metamorphosis.* The process by which sper-

matids are converted to spermatozoa is referred to as *metamorphosis* or *spermiogenesis.* As spermatogenesis ensues the spermatids move in a centrifugal direction (toward the basement membrane) then in a centripetal direction toward the lumen.

The primary organelles involved in the spermiogenic process are the nucleus, Golgi apparatus and centrioles (Fig. 23.16).

Small granules (*proacrosomal granules*) appear in the vesicles of the Golgi apparatus. These small vesicles coalesce to form a

single large *acrosomal vesicle* that contains the *acrosome.* The acrosome results from a coalescence of proacrosomal vesicles. The acrosomal vesicle migrates to the nucleus and contacts the outer nuclear membrane at the acrosome.

The acrosomal vesicle enlarges and extends itself over half the nucleus and collapses to form the *head cap.* At the same time, the centrioles migrate to the periphery of the cell in a position opposite the acrosome. Residual Golgi apparatus also migrates to this general region.

The acrosome becomes indistinguishable from the head cap. The nucleus becomes dense and begins to elongate. At this time, the centrioles and developing *flagellum* migrate toward and come in contact with the nuclear membrane. A *caudal sheath* or *manchette* develops at the caudal edge of the head cap. This sheath is composed of microtubules. At the same time, the spermatid elongates.

A small dense ring condenses around the proximal centriole. This *annulus* is attached to the inner lamina of the plasmalemma. It slides down the flagellum. At the same time, the mitochondria orient themselves in a helical pattern between the proximal centriole and the annulus. Nine longitudinal fibers develop in a position between the flagellar doublets and the mitochondria. This structure comprises the *middle piece.*

The *principal piece* is composed of a flagellar core, dense fibers and a fibrous sheath.

The irregularly arranged flagellar microtubules comprise the *endpiece.*

As the formation of these entities occurs, the remaining cytoplasm is displaced distad along the tail and eventually lost as the *residual body.*

The mature spermatozoon, therefore, consists of the following: *head, neck, middle piece, principal piece* and *endpiece* (Fig. 23.17). The *head* is covered by the head cap on the rostral and lateral surface and the calyx on the lateral and caudal surface. The *neck* has a depression (fossa) in which the centriole is located. Longitudinally segmented columns connect the head to the tail. The *middle piece* consists of a flagellar core in a 9 + 2 arrangement, fibers which are continuous with those of the neck, a helical arrangement of mitochondria and an annulus that is attached to the plasmalemma. The *principal piece* contains a flagellar core in a 9 + 2 arrangement, fibers of various sizes that end in this segment and a fibrous sheath. The *endpiece* consists of a flagellar 9 + 2 core that terminates in a random fashion. Naturally, the entire spermatozoon is enclosed with a plasmalemma.

Spermatogenic Cycle. As mentioned previously, not all seminiferous tubules or regions of the same tubule are in the same stage of development (Fig. 23.18). The activity is cyclic, may occur in a helical pattern within a seminiferous tubule and is referred to as a *spermatogenic wave.* Various combinations

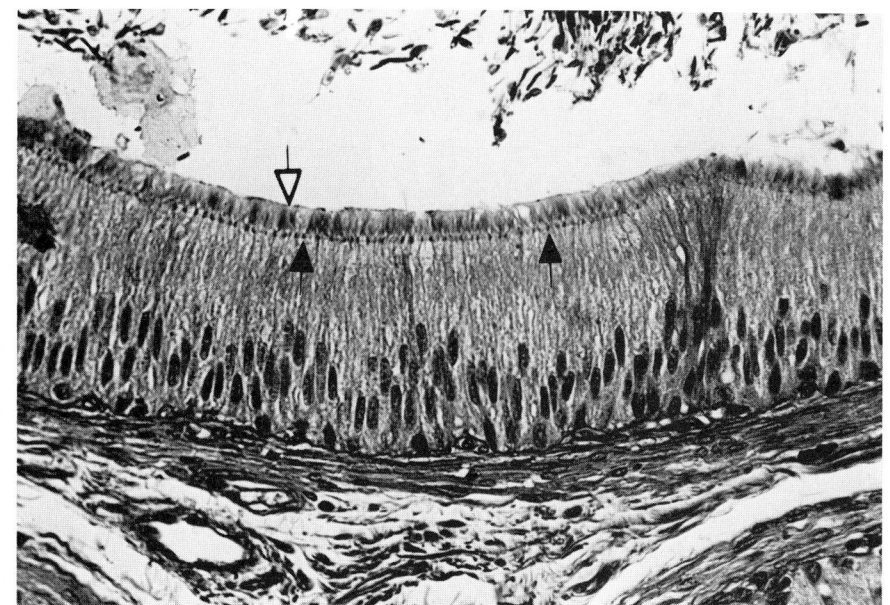

Fig. 23.12 Stereocilia of the ductus epididymidis. The lining cells are stereociliated (*open arrow*). Terminal bars (*solid arrows*) are apparent. X100.

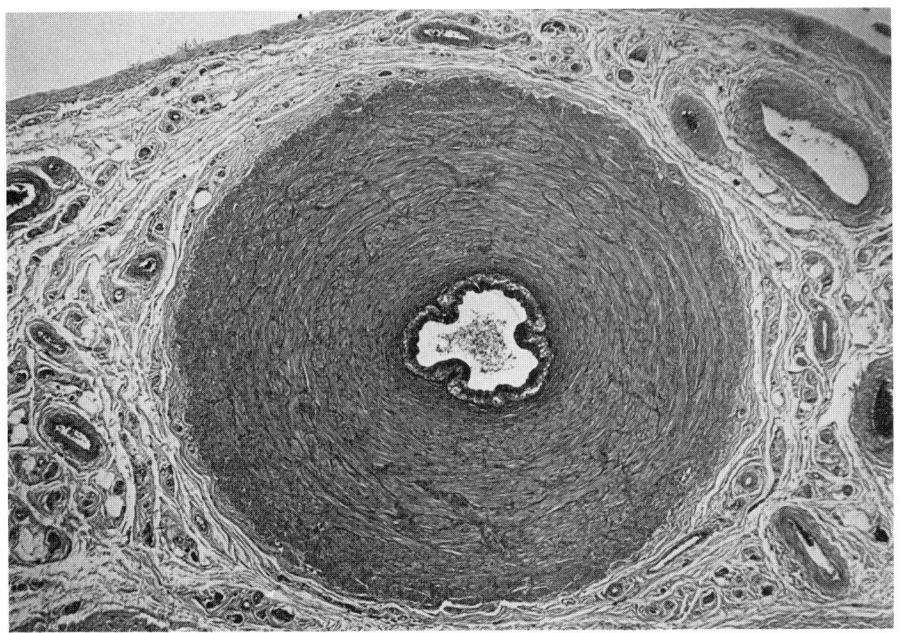

Fig. 23.13 Ductus deferens. The duct is a continuation of the ductus epididymidis. Note the extensive amount of smooth muscle peripheral to the lumen of the organ. The ductus deferens is the tubular portion of the vas deferens. X10.

of cells are always associated with each other during the developmental process. In the bull, for example, eight stages have been identified. Stage 1, from basal to luminal border would include the following: *spermatogonia, pachytene primary spermatocytes* and *round spermatids*. Stage 8, however, would include: *spermatogonia, zygotene primary spermatocytes, secondary spermatocytes, round spermatids* and *spermatozoa*. The six remaining stages involve other permutations of the basic cell types. Various

stages, the number of stages, as well as the overall duration of the stages are species variable. The *spermatogenic wave* or *cycle*, therefore, is the sequence of cellular events that occurs between two successive identical stages (Fig. 23.19).

In some species, from a spermatogenic point of view, the male is always capable of spermiation; i.e., the ejection of viable sperm from the testes. In seasonal breeders, the epithelium of the seminiferous tubules is incapable of producing spermatozoa except

during specific periods of the year, the breeding season (Fig. 23.3). Examination of tubuli contorti during the nonbreeding season would reveal the presence of scattered spermatogonia and Sertoli cells. Few other cells would be present. Also, the tubules would be involuted and replaced by connective tissue.

Testicular Secretions

The testes are responsible for the production of gametes and the elaboration of steroid hormones. Both are secretory functions; gamete secretion is a holocrine-type secretory activity, whereas steroid hormone secretion is an endocrine function. The seminiferous tubules produce the gametes and the interstitial cells of Leydig are responsible primarily for steroid hormone synthesis and secretion. Spermatogenesis and testicular steroidogenesis are integrated and associated activities. Regulation of testicular function is achieved through the hypothalamo-pituitary-gonadal axis. The axis is separated into a hypothalamo-interstitial cell axis and a hypothalamo-tubuli contorti axis for convenience. The functions of both axes are related intimately.

Hypothalamo-Interstitial Cell Axis. The hypothalamus is the first regulator of the axis by virtue of its synthesis and secretion of gonadotropin releasing factors—*luteotropin releasing factor* (*LRF*) and *follicle-stimulating hormone releasing factor* (*FRF*). The secretion of LRF and FRF from the hypothalamus is subject to modulation by external influences. The effects of temperature upon testicular activity may be directed upon the testes or mediated through the hypothalamus. Light is probably the most important influence upon the axis. The seasonal breeding activity of deer, animals that have a rutting season, is responsive to decreasing amounts of light in the photoperiod. Some domestic animals (goat) increase testicular activity with decreasing daylength, whereas others (horse) manifest increased activity with increasing daylength. The tonic activity of the hypothalamus also accounts for the maintenance of testicular activity. Additionally, hypothalamic secretory activity is subject to regulation by the negative feedback influence of testicular hormones.

The secretion of LRF and FRF initiates secretory activity by specific basophilic cells of the pars distalis and the release of *luteinizing hormone* (*LH*) and *follicle-stimulating hormone* (*FSH*). Luteinizing hormone and *interstitial cell-stimulating hormone* (*ICSH*) are identical; the term LH is now used for both the male and female. LH is the tropic hormone which regulates the secretory activity of the Leydig cells. The function of FSH is discussed with the hypothalamo-tubuli contorti axis. *Prolactin* also exerts an influence upon the male reproductive tract by potentiating the effect of LH upon the Leydig cells. Additionally, prolactin and tes-

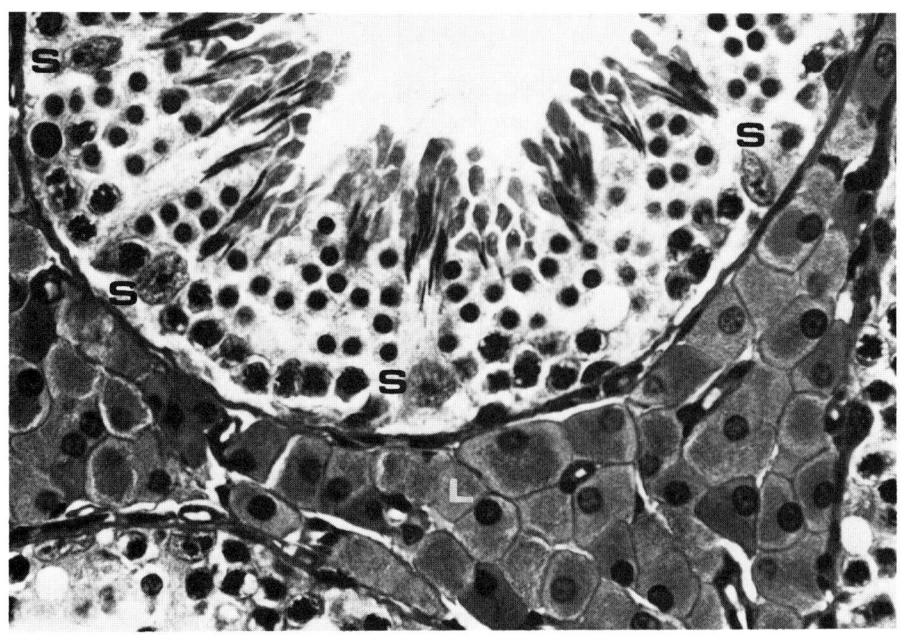

Fig. 23.14 Sertoli cells of the porcine testis. The Sertoli cells (S) are triangular cells with triangular nuclei that are positioned basally. The developing gametes are associated intimately with the Sertoli cells. L, Leydig cells. X160.

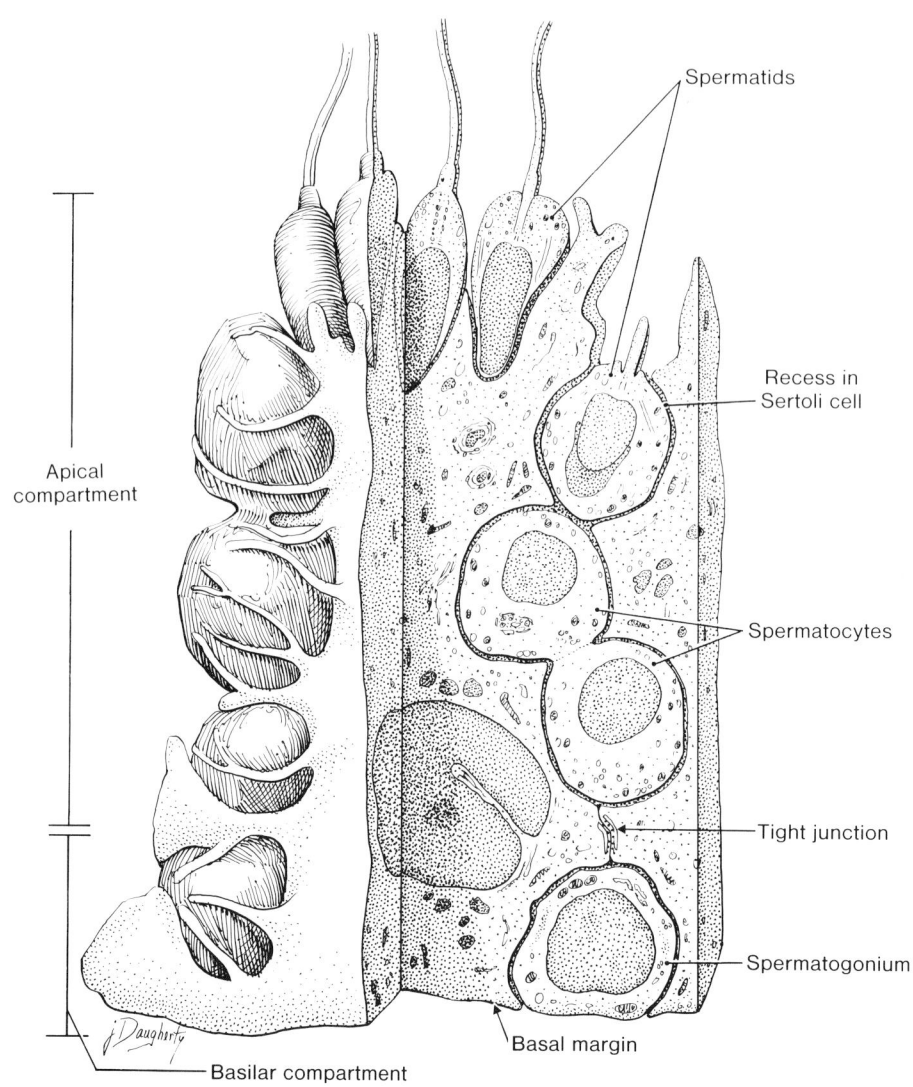

Spermatids

Recess in
Sertoli cell

Apical
compartment

Spermatocytes

Tight junction

Spermatogonium

Basal margin

Basilar compartment

Fig. 23.15 A three-dimensional drawing of the electron microscopic appearance of adjacent Sertoli cells. Spermatogonia occupy the basilar compartment and are exposed directly to influences from the interstitium. Spermatocytes occupy the apical compartment and are insulated from direct influences by the blood-testis barrier.

484

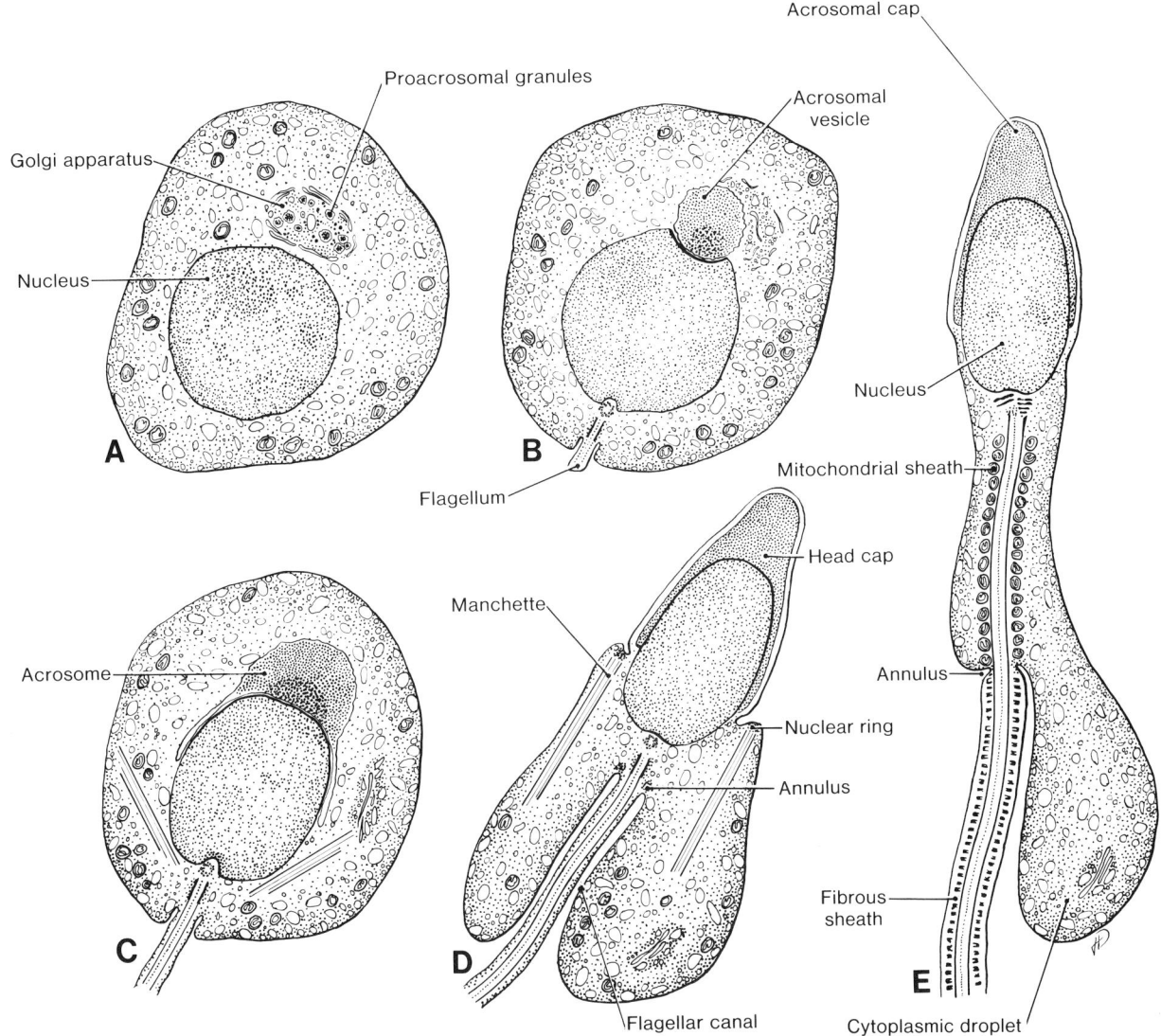

Fig. 23.16 A diagram of the successive stages in the differentiation of a spermatid during spermiogenesis. (Redrawn and modified from Clermont, Y. and Leblond, C. P.: Amer. J. Anat. *96*:229, 1955).

osterone increase the secretory activity of the prostate and vesicular glands. Cells responsive to androgens have membrane receptor sites for prolactin.

Testosterone, the steroid hormone of the Leydig cells, is synthesized from acetate or circulating cholesterol. Although other androgens occur in the male, testosterone is the most important of these hormones. Small amounts of testosterone occur free as active hormones within the blood; however, most of the hormone is bound to a *testosterone-estradiol-binding globulin (TeBG)*, a β globulin distinct from that used for cortisol binding. Upon entry into a cell from the active pool within the blood, testosterone may be converted to a more active form (dihydrotestosterone) or inactivated to metabolites characterized as *17-ketosteroids*. The 17-ketosteroids are the primary excretory products of testosterone, although the liver participates in testosterone inactivation by converting the hormone to sulfates and glucuronides that are secreted in the bile. Other tissues inactivate testosterone by converting it to *estradiol*, a potent estrogen.

Actions of Testosterone. Although testosterone exerts a significant influence upon the gonads, accessory sex glands and those organs responsible for secondary male sex characteristics, the hormone affects almost every cell of the body. During development, the elaboration of testosterone by the forming testes within the genital ridge is responsible for the development of the external genitalia, accessory sex glands and the descent of the testes into the scrotum. The external genitalia and accessory sex glands grow under the influence of this hormone. Secondary sex characteristics also develop in response to testosterone. The effects of testosterone upon the reproductive organs, accessory sex glands and the organs responsible for secondary sex characteristics are the *androgenic effects* of the hormone. The effects upon somatic tissues generally are described as the *anabolic effects* of the hormone.

The anabolic properties of testosterone are expressed in many cells and tissues. Testosterone has a positive influence upon basal metabolic rate, electrolyte balance, red blood cell production, nitrogen retention, skeletal muscle mass, bone development and bone maintenance.

Hypothalamo-Tubuli Contorti Axis. The seminiferous tubules are subject to the regulatory activity of the hypothalamus and pars distalis. The secretion of LH and FSH by the pars distalis, controlled by the secretion of hypothalamic releasing factors, is essential for development of the tubuli contorti. Although FSH manifests a direct effect upon the seminiferous tubules, the effects of LH are manifested through testosterone. Testosterone and FSH stimulate the synthesis of androgen binding protein (ABP) by the Sertoli Cells. FSH initiates spermatogenic events, but testosterone is required for

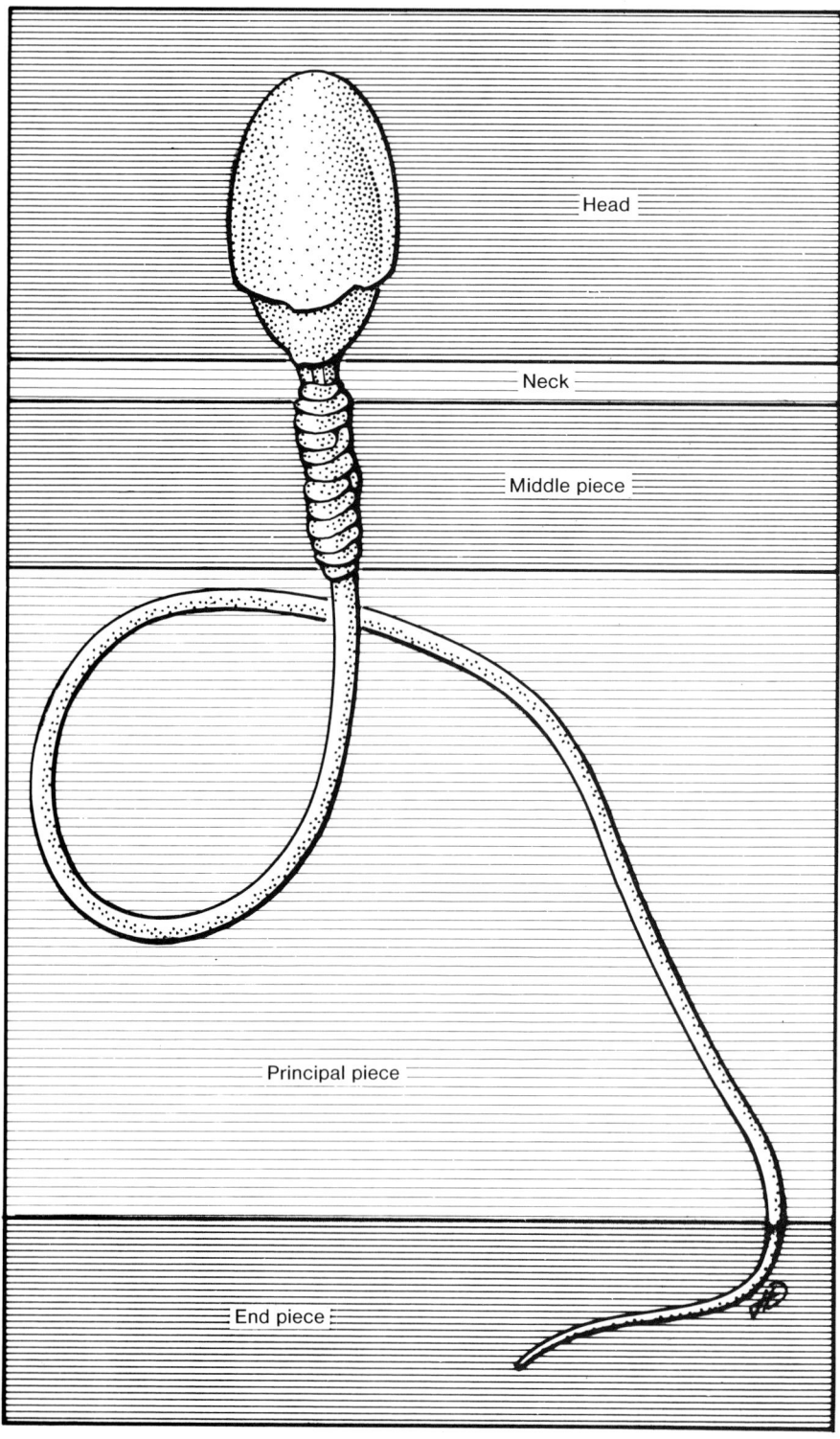

Fig. 23.17 A drawing of a typical spermatozoon.

the maturation of the spermatozoa. The mechanisms that regulate the release of FSH need further clarification. Testosterone does not exert a negative feedback influence upon FSH secretion; however, experimental evidence indicates that steroid-free extracts of testicular tissues suppress FSH secretion. *Inhibin*, a substance probably originating from the Sertoli cells, may be the testicular regulator of FSH secretion.

Accessory Glands

Introduction. The accessory genital glands of the male include *ampullary glands, vesicular glands, prostate gland, bulbourethral glands* and *urethral glands*. They elaborate serous and mucous secretory products that subserve various functions. Together these secretory products may serve to nourish the spermatozoa, activate the spermatozoa,

clear the urethral tract before ejaculation, serve as a vehicle for the transport of the spermatozoa within the female tract, as well as plugging the female organs to help ensure fertilization.

All of the glands are generally described as branched tubular or branched tubuloalveolar glands that are arranged into lobular units. Each lobular unit may drain into a dilated collecting sinus. These sinuses are not present in all the glands of all species, however. They are absent in equine vesicular glands and in porcine and ruminant pars disseminata prostatica. The glandular epithelium and that of the collecting sinus (when present) consist of a simple columnar lining that is continuous with the pseudostratified or transitional epithelium of the excretory ducts. The glands of a given species may be readily distinguished from one another, but extreme care must be taken when making interspecific comparisons. There is much variation among the domestic species.

Ampullary Glands

Histology. The *ampulla* is an enlargement of the terminal portion of the ductus deferens. The glands are branched, tubular structures with saclike dilations (Fig. 23.20). Some authors describe them as branched tubuloalveolar glands. These glands are lined by a simple columnar epithelium (Fig. 23.21). In the bull, basal accumulations of lipid droplets may be apparent. There is no special excretory duct system.

Species Variation. The ampulla, present in the ruminants, horses and dogs, contains typical glands in the lamina propria-submucosa. Glands are absent in the ampulla of the cat, and they are not well developed in the porcine ampulla.

Functional Correlates. The ampullary glands secrete a white serous fluid the precise function of which is unknown. The secretory product is similar to that of the vesicular gland. The large lumen is capable of storing viable spermatozoa.

Vesicular Glands

Histology. The *vesicular glands* are also referred to as the *seminal vesicles* (Fig. 23.22). The glandular epithelium is simple columnar (Fig. 23.23). Infranuclear lipid droplets may be apparent in the bull. The main excretory ducts are lined by a stratified columnar epithelium. The overall configuration of the gland is that of a pinnately arranged structure; i.e., a central duct is present from which radially branching secretory endpieces emanate. Lobular subdivisions are present.

The lamina propria-submucosa consists of areolar connective tissue. The tunica muscularis may consist of inner circular and outer longitudinal layers or may be entirely intermingled. A tunica adventitia or a tunica serosa may be present. They are typical.

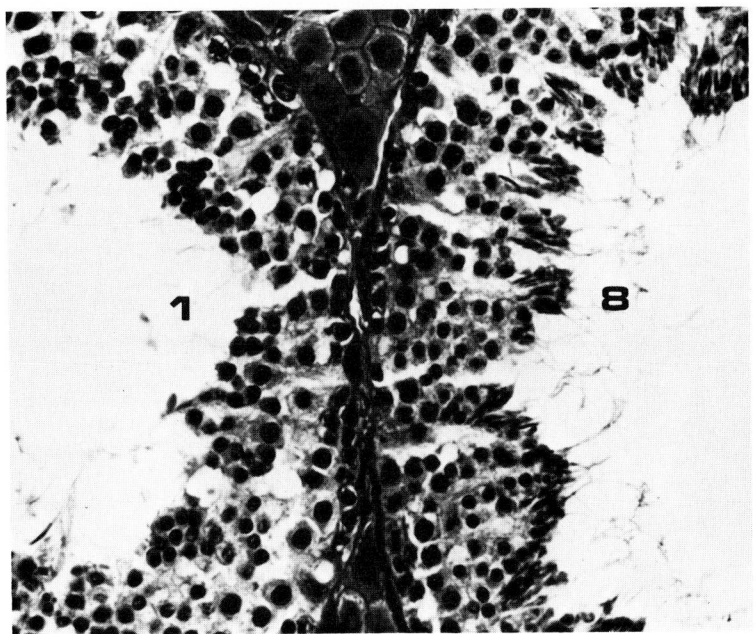

Fig. 23.18 Different developmental stages in adjacent seminiferous tubules. Stages 1 and 8 represent different degrees of development of spermatozoa. X100.

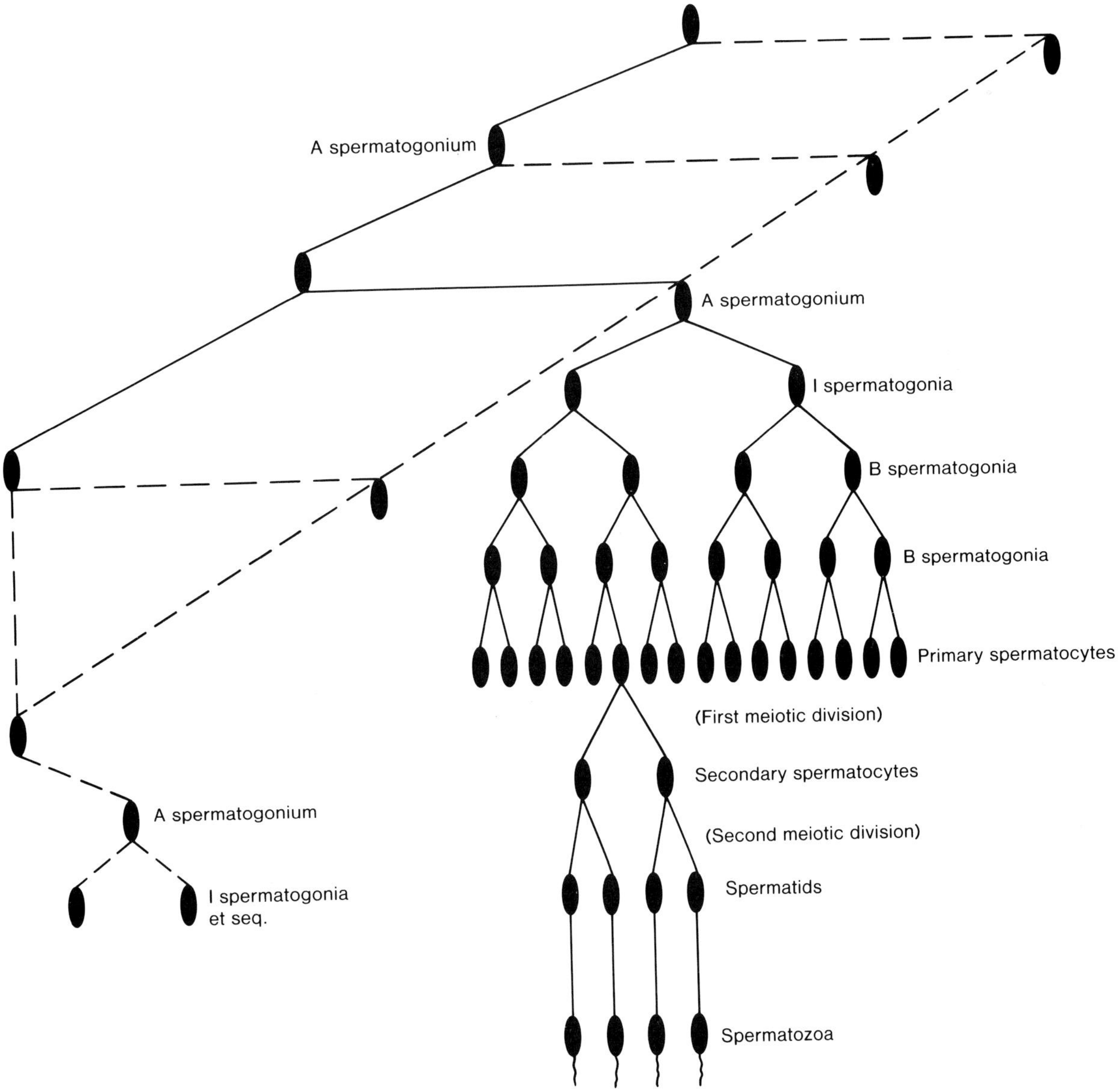

A spermatogonium

A spermatogonium

I spermatogonia

B spermatogonia

B spermatogonia

Primary spermatocytes

(First meiotic division)

Secondary spermatocytes

(Second meiotic division)

Spermatids

Spermatozoa

A spermatogonium

I spermatogonia
et seq.

Fig. 23.19 A diagram of the sequential and repetitive stages of spermatogenesis.

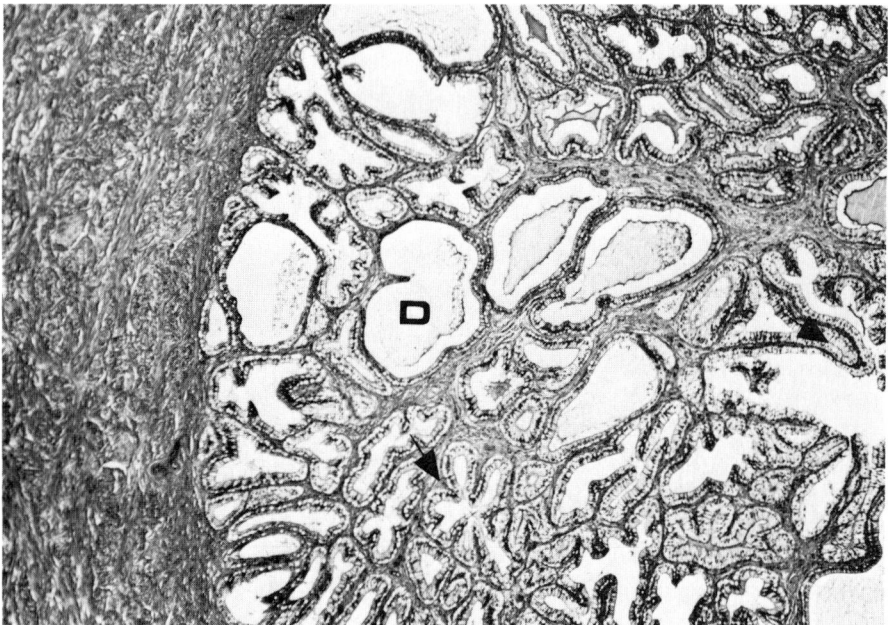

Fig. 23.20 A section of a bovine ampullary gland. The glands are branched (*arrows*), tubular glands which have sac-like dilations (D). X10.

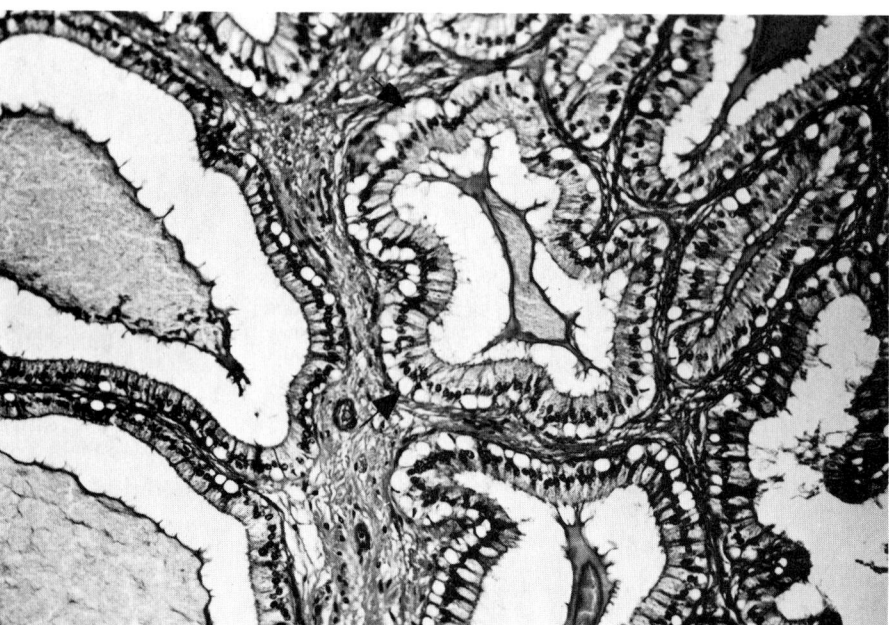

Fig. 23.21 Lining cells of a bovine ampullary gland. Columnar epithelial cells contain basal lipid deposits (*arrows*). X40.

Species Variation. The vesicular glands are absent in carnivores. The glands of the horse are true vesicular outpocketings, whereas those of ruminants and swine are compact glandular structures.

Functional Correlates. Seminal fluid, as well as the secretory products of other accessory sex glands, provide a vehicle for the transport of spermatozoa. The white, gelatinous secretory product aids in the formation of the vaginal plug in some rodents.

The secretory product contains large quantities of fructose that is used as an energy source by ejaculated spermatozoa.

Prostate Gland

Histology. This organ consists of two parts, the *corpus prostatae* and *pars disseminata*. The gland is a compound tubuloalveolar structure which is lined by secretory cells in a cuboidal or low columnar configuration (Figs. 23.24 and 23.25). Secretory cells have apical blebs that indicate an apocrine-type secretory activity. Acidophilic granules and lipid droplets may be present. The duct system, initially lined by a cuboidal or columnar epithelium, is lined by transitional epithelium at the entrance to the urethra.

The body of the gland is surrounded by a capsule of DWFCT that is continuous with the areolar connective tissue of the lamina propria-submucosa in which the adenomeres are located. The disseminate portion is surrounded by the areolar connective tissue of the lamina propria-submucosa.

The pars disseminata is best developed along the dorsal surface of the urethra and extends laterad and ventrad to encompass the urethra totally. The disseminate portion is continuous with both laterally oriented lobes of the body of the gland. Although the disseminate portion is usually confined to the pelvic urethra, *it is not unusual to find isolated portions of the gland in the wall of the penile urethra.*

Species Variation. The body and disseminate portions of the prostate gland are not developed equally in all domestic species. The body of the prostate, which is located peripheral to and surrounds part of the pelvic urethra, is well developed in carnivores and horses. The disseminate portion is better developed than the body in the bull and boar. The ram does not have a distinct corpus prostatae.

Functional Correlates. The gland is basically a serous gland with occasional mucous endpieces. Concretions of these secretory products may be present in the alveoli and duct system. Its secretory activity is known to increase the motility of spermatozoa, as well as contribute to the formation of the vaginal plug. In the bull, the secretory fluid contains high quantities of fructose and citric acid. Little else is known of the functional significance of this secretory product.

Bulbourethral Glands

Histology. These glands are also referred to as *Cowper's glands.* These glands are paired structures that are located dorsolaterally to the pelvic urethra. The bulbourethral glands are compound tubuloalveolar glands (Fig. 23.26). The lining cells of the adenomeres are columnar or pyramidal (Fig. 23.27). They have a basophilic cytoplasm and a basally displaced nucleus which is rounded or flattened. The duct system is lined by columnar, pseudostratified or transitional epithelium.

The capsule of the organ is DWFCT that may contain some smooth muscle. Striated muscle from the bulbocavernosus and urethralis muscle is associated with the capsule. The capsular connective tissue is continuous as septal components (areolar connective tissue) of the lamina propria-submucosa. Diffuse and nodular lymphatic tissue is commonly encountered.

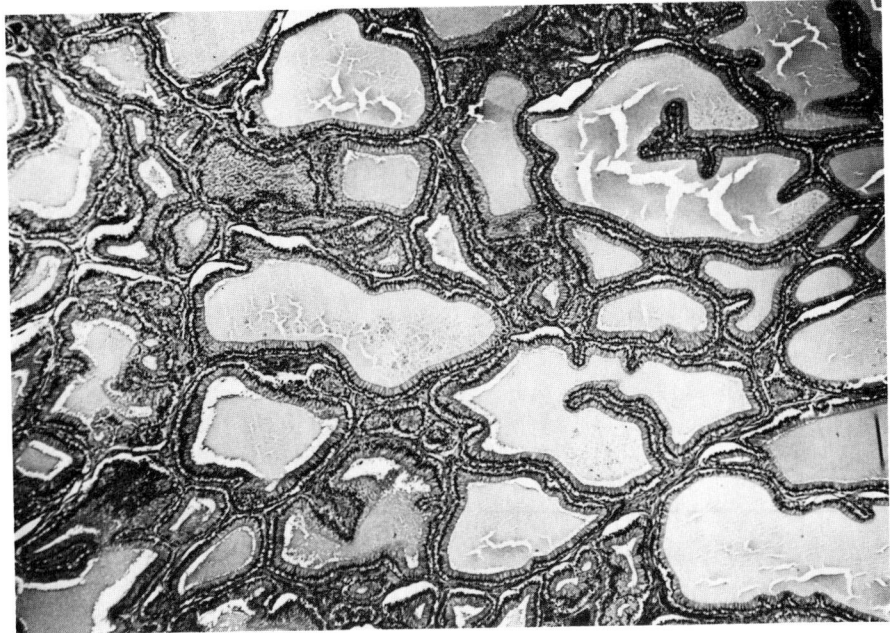

Fig. 23.22 A section of bovine seminal vesicle. X10.

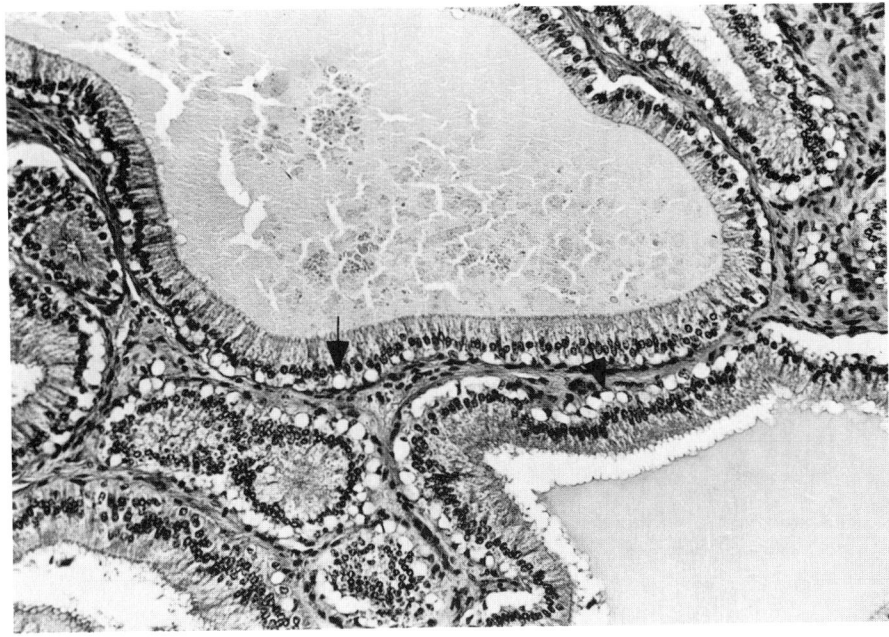

Fig. 23.23 Lining cells of a bovine seminal vesicle. The columnar lining cells have infranuclear lipid deposits (*arrows*). X40.

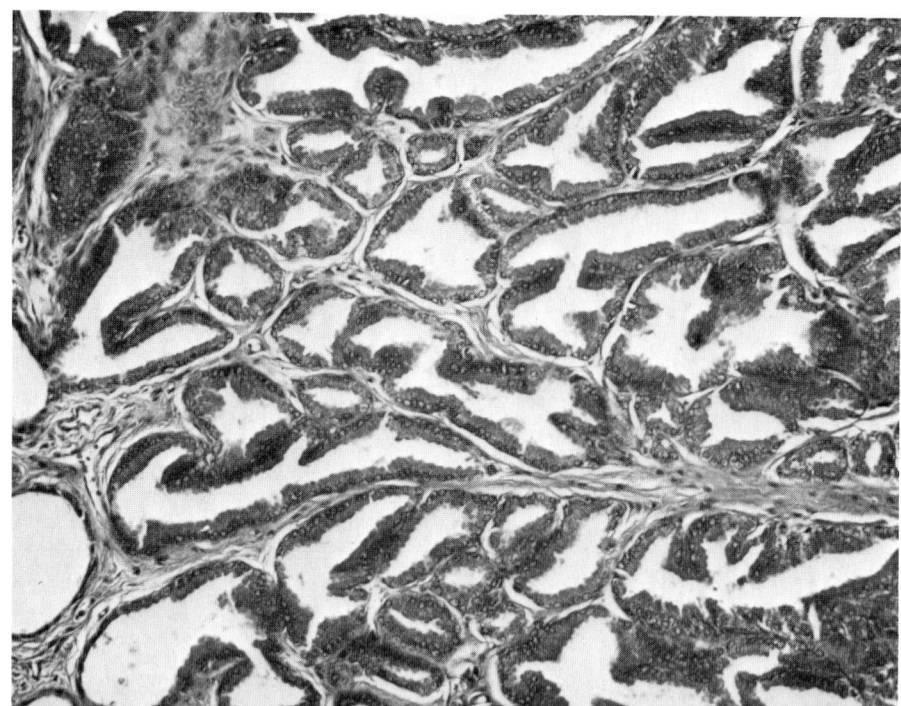

Fig. 23.24   A section of a canine prostate gland. X40.

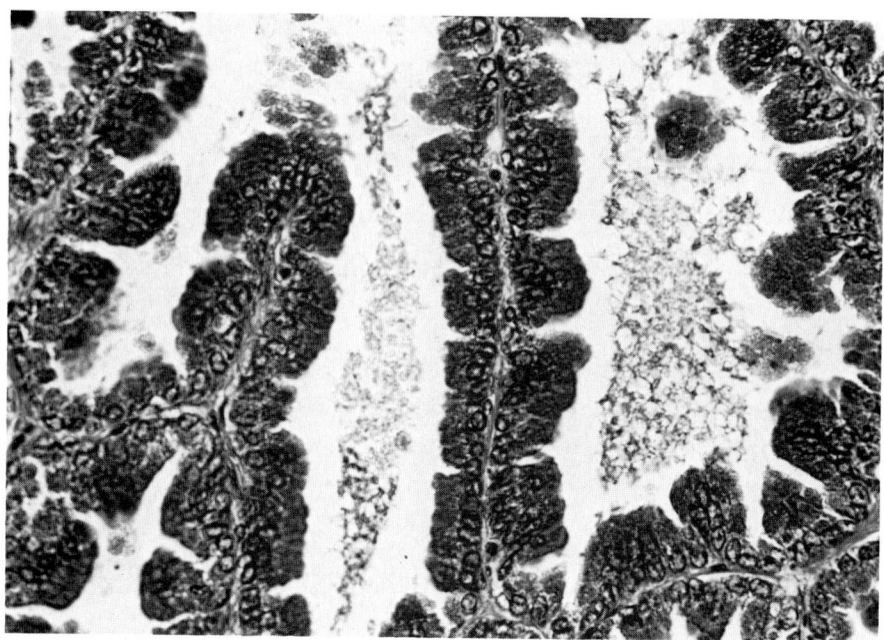

Fig. 23.25   Columnar lining cells of a canine prostate gland. X100.

Species Variation. Bulbourethral glands occur in all domestic species except the dog.

Functional Correlates. The mucus secreted by these glands serves to clear the urethra of urine and to lubricate the urethra and vagina with a pre-ejaculatory fluid. The mucus may serve as a source of energy for ejaculated spermatozoa.

Urethra

General Remarks. The male urethra is the continuation of the duct system that arises at the urinary bladder and opens to the outside. It serves the dual function of transporting urine as well as semen and spermatozoa. Secretory products involved in reproduction gain access to the pelvic urethra at the *colliculus seminalis* that is the apex of the *urethral crest.* It is in this region that the *deferent ducts, vesicular glands* and some *prostatic ducts* gain access to the urethra. The urethra is divided into *pelvic* and *penile portions* that contain erectile tissue along the entire length. The urethra also contains branched tubular mucous glands, *glands of Littré* or *urethral glands,* along its length.

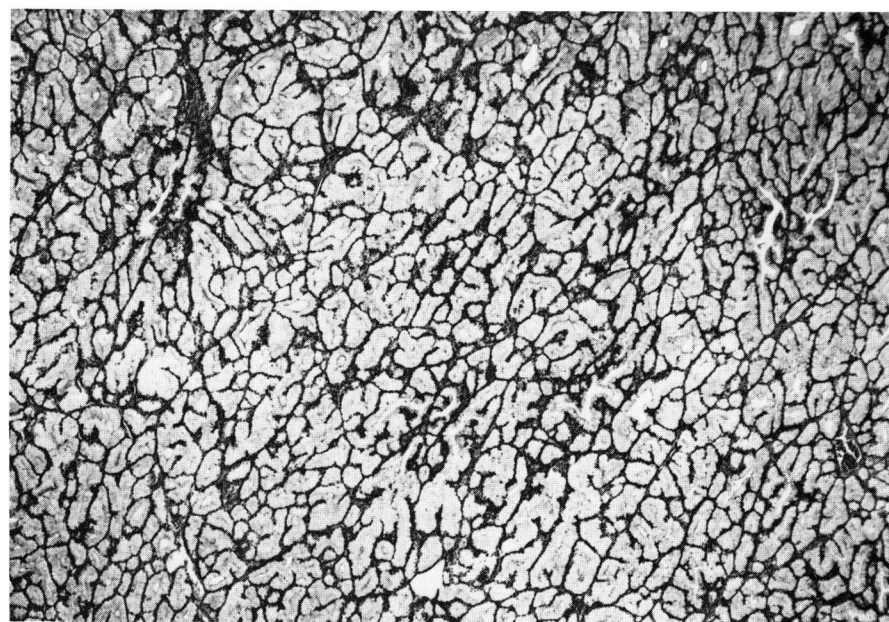

Fig. 23.26 A section of a bovine bulbourethral gland. The compound tubuloalveolar gland secretes mucus. X10.

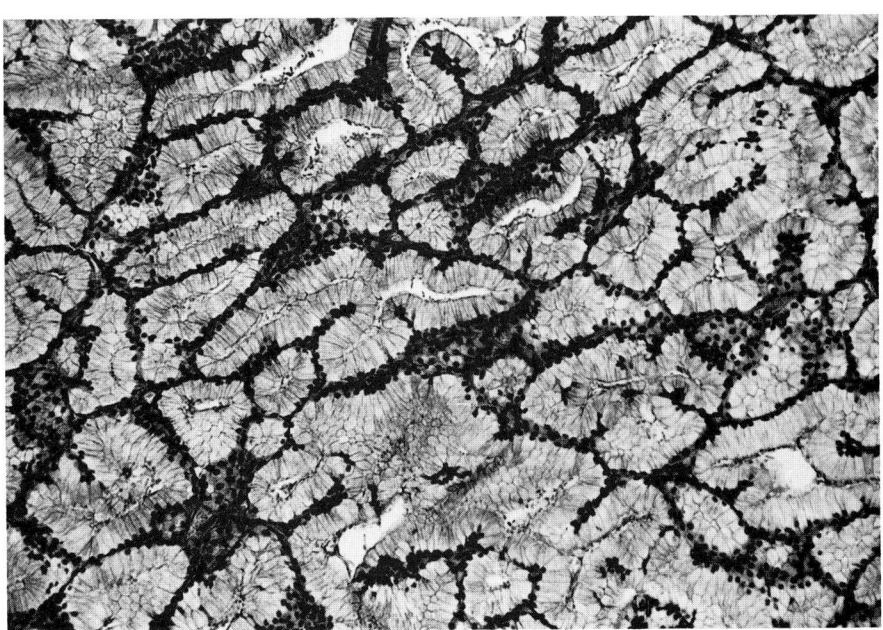

Fig. 23.27 Lining cells of a bovine bulbourethral gland. The lining cells are columnar and basophilic. Nuclei are positioned basally. X40.

The occurrence and distribution of these glands, however, is species-variable. They are obliquely oriented and are especially numerous along the dorsal surface of the urethra.

Pelvic Urethra. The pelvic urethra is lined by a transitional epithelium. The surrounding lamina propria-submucosa consists of areolar connective tissue, numerous glandular elements and erectile tissue (*stratum cavernosum*). A tunica muscularis with three muscle layers is present in the neck of the bladder, but these are rapidly replaced by a striated *urethral muscle*. However, an inner and outer layer (superficial and deep to the musculus urethralis) may be present throughout the extent of the pelvic urethra. A tunica adventitia is present. This portion of the urethra generally has more glands but less erectile tissue than the penile urethra.

Penile Urethra. The penile urethra is lined by a transitional epthelium as well (Fig. 23.28). This, however, may change to stratified squamous epithelium before or at the urethral opening in some species. Glands may be present in the lamina propria-submucosa, especially in the stallion and boar. The tunica muscularis returns to being composed of smooth muscle. Cavernous tissue (*corpus cavernosum urethrae*) is also present in the subepithelial connective tissue space.

Copulatory Organ

Penis. The penis is the organ that serves as the common outlet for urine and the copulatory ejaculate (semen and spermatozoa). It is therefore, a part of the urinary system as well as serving as an intermittent copulatory organ.

Although the histologic components of

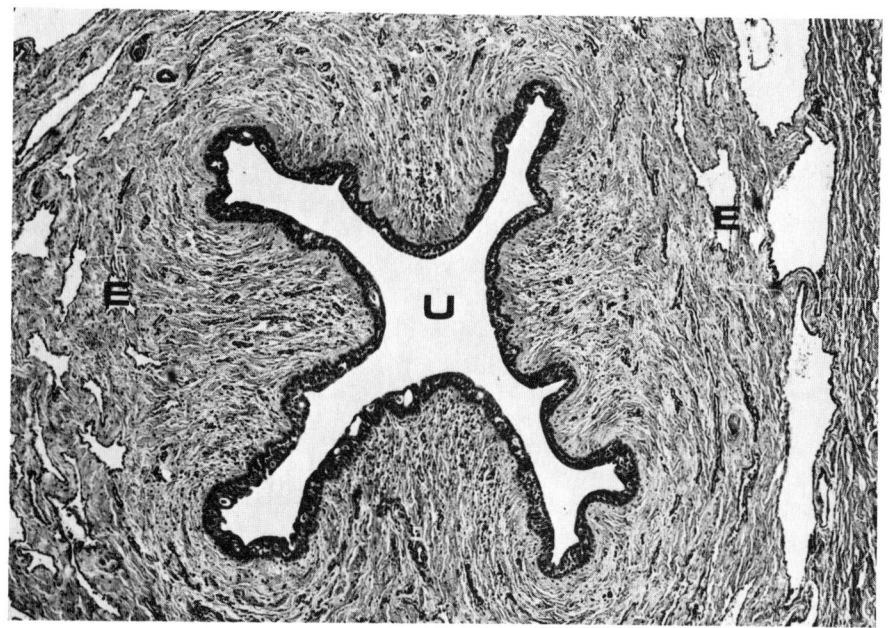

Fig. 23.28 A cross section of a canine penile urethra. The urethra (U) is lined by transitional epithelium. Erectile tissue (E) is peripheral to the lumen of the urethra. X16.

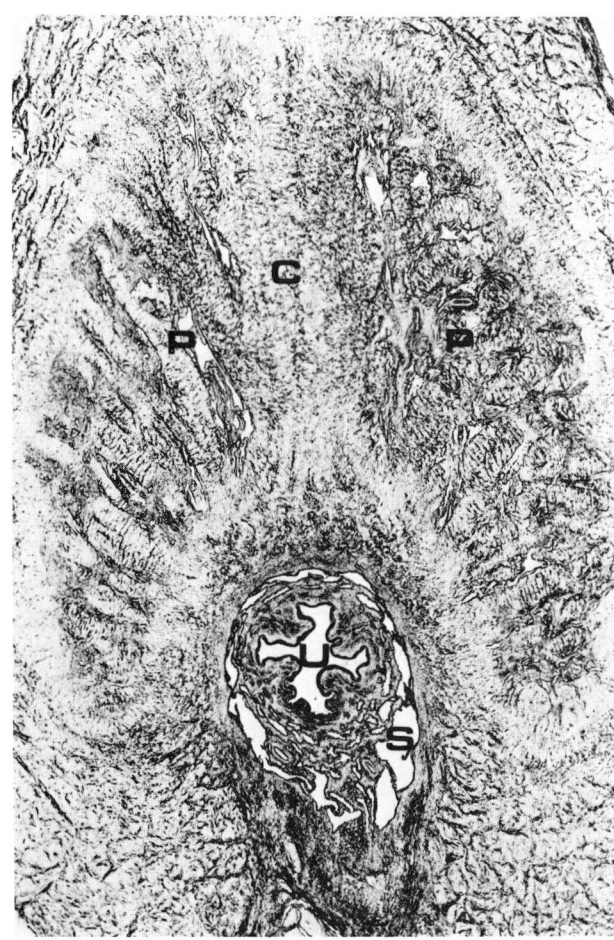

Fig. 23.29 A cross section through a canine penis. The urethra (U) is surrounded by erectile tissue of the corpus spongiosum (S). Dorsally, the two corpora cavernosa penis (P) are separated by connective tissue (C) that is continuous with the peripherally-positioned tunica albuginea. X4.

the penis are similar among most mammalian species, the organizational differences are too numerous to be able to cite a configuration as being absolutely typical. Moreover, a section from one part of the structure may differ appreciably from a section through a different part. This variability is due to the differential distribution of some component parts along the length of the organ.

The following description applies to the general configuration and component parts. The penis is divided into: *roots*, *body* and *glans*. The structure of each root and the body of the penis are similar. The body consists of a capsule, erectile tissue (*corpora cavernosa penis*, *corpus cavernosum urethrae* or *corpus spongiosum*), smooth muscle (*retractor penis muscle*), skeletal muscle (*bulbocavernosus muscle*) and urethra (Fig. 23.29).

The body of the penis is enclosed by the DWFCT of the tunica albuginea that is especially well-developed in those species with a fibrous-type penis (boar, ruminants). Connective tissue septa originate from the capsule and continue as the fibrous coverings of the erectile tissue components. These components may include elastic fibers and smooth muscle.

The erectile tissue consists of DWFCT rich in elastic fibers and sinuses. These are capable of being engorged with blood during erection. In the vascular-type penis (horse, carnivores, man), this erectile tissue is well-developed.

The glans penis is well-developed in primates, the stallion and the dog. It is covered by the penile portion of the prepuce, which is actually a reflection of the integument. The reflected portion is, therefore, a mucous membrane. The glans penis may contain erectile tissue (vascular penis), bone (*os penis* of carnivores), cartilage and DWFCT (bull). The bulk of this portion of the penis consists of highly vascularized areolar connective tissue.

The free portion of the penis is covered by stratified squamous epithelium.

Erectile Mechanism. The primary blood supply of the penis, under erotic stimulation, is directed through *helicine arteries* that open into the cavernous tissue. These vessels, as well as the cavernous tissue, become engorged with blood. The peripherally located, thin-walled veins are occluded against the tunica albuginea. This further enhances rigidity. The cavernous tissue of the corpus spongiosum (corpus cavernosum urethrae) is not as thickly encapsulated as the other cavernous tissue. This permits expansion without occluding the urethra.

During the period of *detumescence*, the helicine arteries contract and regain their initial tone. The resulting diminution of blood supply results in a decreased pressure against the compressed veins. The blood is gradually removed from the erectile tissue and normal blood flow through the penis is resumed.

References

Testes and Associated

Amann, R. P., Johnson, L. and Pickett, B. W.: Connection between the seminiferous tubules and the efferent ducts in the stallion. Amer. J. Vet. Res. *38:*1571, 1977.

Bawa, S. R.: The fine structure of the Sertoli cell of the human testis. J. Ultrastruc. Res. *9:*459, 1963.

Belt, W. D. and Cavazos, L. F.: Fine structure of the interstitial cells of Leydig in the boar. Anat. Rec. *158:*333, 1967.

Christensen, A. K. and Fawcett, D. W.: The fine structure of the interstitial cells of the mouse testis. Amer. J. Anat. 118:551, 1963.

Elftman, H.: Sertoli cells and testis structure. Amer. J. Anat. *113:*25, 1963.

Fawcett, D. W. and Burgos, M. H.: Studies on the fine structure of the mammalian testes. II. The human interstitial tissue. Amer. J. Anat. *107:*245, 1960.

French, F. S. and Ritzén, E. M.: A high affinity androgen binding protein (ABP) in rat testis: Evidence for secretion into efferent duct fluid and absorption by epididymis. Endocrinol. *93:*88, 1973.

Krestser, D. M. D.: The fine structure of the testicular interstitial cells in men of normal androgenic status. Z. Zellforsch. *80:*594, 1967.

Ladman, A. J.: The fine structure of the ductuli efferentes of the opossum. Anat. Rec. *157:*559, 1967.

Nagano, T. and Suzuki, F.: Freeze-fracture observations on the intercellular junctions of Sertoli cells and of Leydig cells in the human testis. Cell Tiss. Res. *166:* 37, 1976.

Roberts, S. J.: *Veterinary Obstetrics and Genital Diseases.* 2nd edition. Edwards Brothers, Ann Arbor, 1971.

Spermatogenesis

Clermont, Y.: The cycle of the seminiferous epithelium in man. Amer. J. Anat. *112:*35, 1963.

Fawcett, D. W. and Ito, S.: The fine structure of bat spermatozoa. Am. J. Anat. *116:*567, 1965.

Goldzvieg, S. A. and Smith, A. U.: The fertility of male rats after moderate and after severe hypothermia. J. Endocr. *14:*40, 1956.

Heller, C. G. and Clermont, Y.: Kinetics of the germinal epithelium in man. Recent Progr. Hormone Res. *20:* 545, 1964.

Kehlstrom, J. E.: A sex cycle in the male. Experientia *22:*630, 1966.

Rattner, J. B. and Brinkley, B. R.: Ultrastructure of spermiogenesis. J. Ultrastruct. Res. *32:*316, 1970.

Roosen-Runge, E. C.: The process of spermatogenesis in mammals. Biol. Rev. *37:*343, 1962.

Steinberger, E.: Hormonal control of mammalian spermatogenesis. Physiol. Rev. *5:*1, 1971.

Swiestra, E. E. and Foote, R. H.: Duration of spermatogenesis and spermatozoan transport in the rabbit based on cytological changes, DNA synthesis and labeling with tritiated thymidine. Amer. J. Anat. *116:*401, 1965.

Accessory Glands

Bharadwaj, M. and Calhoun, M. L.: Histology of the bulbourethral gland of the domestic animals. Anat. Rec. *142:*216, 1962.

Brandes, D.: The fine structure and histochemistry of prostatic glands in relation to sex hormones. Int. Rev. Cytol. *20:*207, 1966.

Fisher, E. R. and Jeffrey, W. Ultrastructure of human normal and neoplastic prostate. Amer. J. Clin. Path. *44:*119, 1965.

Hirsch, E. W.: Comparative anatomy of prostate gland. J. Urol. *25:*669, 1931.

Kainer, R. A., Faulkner, L. C. and Abdel-Raouf, M.: Glands associated with the urethra of the bull. Amer. J. Vet. Res. *30:*963, 1969.

McDonald, L. E.: *Veterinary Endocrinology and Reproduction.* Lea and Febiger, Philadelphia, 1969.

Riva, A.: Fine structure of human seminal vesicle epithelium. J. Anat. *102:*71, 1967.

Young, W. C. (ed.): *Sex and Internal Secretions.* Williams & Wilkins, Baltimore, 1961.

Penis and Associated

Bharadwaj, M. and Calhoun, M. L.: The histology of the urethral epithelium of domestic animals. Amer. J. Vet. Res. *20:*841, 1959.

Bharadwaj, M. B. and Calhoun, M. L.: Mode of formation of the preputial cavity in domestic animals. Amer. J. Vet. Res. *22:*764, 1961.

Hart, B. J. and Kitchell, R. L.: External morphology of the erect glans penis of the dog. Anat. Rec. *152:*193, 1965.

24: Female Reproductive System

General Characteristics

Form and Function. The female reproductive system includes, as its male counterpart, various organs that contribute directly to or complement the primary function of *reproduction*. Among the varied functions are *production* of ova, *transport* of male and female gametes for fertilization, *accommodation* and *nourishment* of the developing organism, *parturition* at the appropriate time and *secretion* of hormones. Portions of the system also complement the function of the urinary system. The organs of the reproductive system include *ovary, oviduct, uterus, vagina* and *vulva*. Although the mammary gland was included with the integument, this gland is also considered part of the reproductive system.

Cyclic activity is an integral part of female reproductive organs. These changes are much more pronounced in the female than the male and have an effect on more organs than in the male. These changes are especially notable in the ovaries, oviducts, uterus and vagina throughout the estrous cycle as well as during pregnancy.

Ovary

General Remarks. The ovaries are paired structures that are the female counterparts of the testes. The ovary performs an endocrine as well as an exocrine function. The former involves the production of estrogen and progesterone, whereas the latter is concerned with the production of the *female gametes*, the *ova*.

Histologic Organization. The ovary is covered by a *surface epithelium* that is a modification of the visceral peritoneal covering of the ovary and is continuous with the *mesovarium* (Fig. 24.1). During early developmental stages of the ovary and oogenesis, the epithelium is cuboidal. It changes with age to a squamous lining. Underlying the germinal epithelium is a capsule of dense white fibrous connective tissue (DWFCT) that may have a lamellar configuration—the *tunica albuginea ovarii*. It is similar to the male counterpart, but it is thinner than that associated with the testis.

The ovaries of most animals, the mare excepted, consist of two distinct zones: an outer *cortex* or *zona parenchymatosa* and the inner *medulla* or *zona vasculosa* (Fig. 24.2). In the mare, the cortex and medulla are reversed. The cortex is confined to the deep zone of the ovary and only reaches the surface at the *ovulation fossa* (Fig. 24.3). The

surface epithelial covering of the ovulation fossa continues over the rest of the ovary as a typical tunica serosa.

The cortex contains numerous *follicles* in various stages of development, *corpora lutea* as well as interstitial cells and stromal elements. Although the connective tissue fibers of the tunica albuginea are continuous with the stromal connective tissue, the connective tissue of the cortex must be considered a specialized tissue. Various cells typical of areolar connective tissue are present. However, this tissue is very cellular and dense aggregates of "fibroblasts" are present. They may be parallel to the surface or in an orderly arrangement around the follicles or vessels with which they are associated. The fibroblasts of this region are not ordinary fibroblasts. They are extremely adaptive and pleomorphic. They are readily converted to macrophages and even assume epithelioid characteristics as follicular sheath cells in association with developing follicles. In the latter instance, they perform a nutritive and secretory function. These epithelioid cells are readily converted back to stromal fibroblasts.

The *medulla* is characterized by large vessels, lymphatics, nerves and some embryonic remnants. It is an areolar connective tissue that is rich in elastic and reticular fibers. The medullary constituents are continuous with the mesovarial attachment. The embry-

onic remnants are parts of the *rete ovarii*, the female homologue of the rete testis. They are short, solid cords of epithelial cells.

Vascular, Neural and Lymphatic Relationships. The ovarian artery, the vascular supply for the ovary, enters the organ at the hilus and is distributed to the medulla. Branches of the vessel continue to the corticomedullary junction and form an extensive plexus from which vessels that supply the cortex arise. The cortical vessels supply stromal elements, the thecae of developing and growing follicles and corpora lutea. Capillaries form a complete spherical network around developing follicles. As corpora lutea develop, nascent branches from the peripherally positioned capillary bed form an extensive vascular network within the corpora lutea. Blood is shunted readily within the cortex. The venous drainage from the cortex is similar to the arterial supply. An extensive medullary venous plexus may form prior to the exit of the vessels at the hilus.

The cortex contains numerous lymphatic vessels that are associated intimately with the theca externa of developing follicles. The vessels coalesce, pass radially through the medulla, exit at the hilus and drain through the lumbar lymph nodes.

The majority of the unmyelinated nerves of the ovary are vasomotor nerves; however, some sensory nerves have been observed.

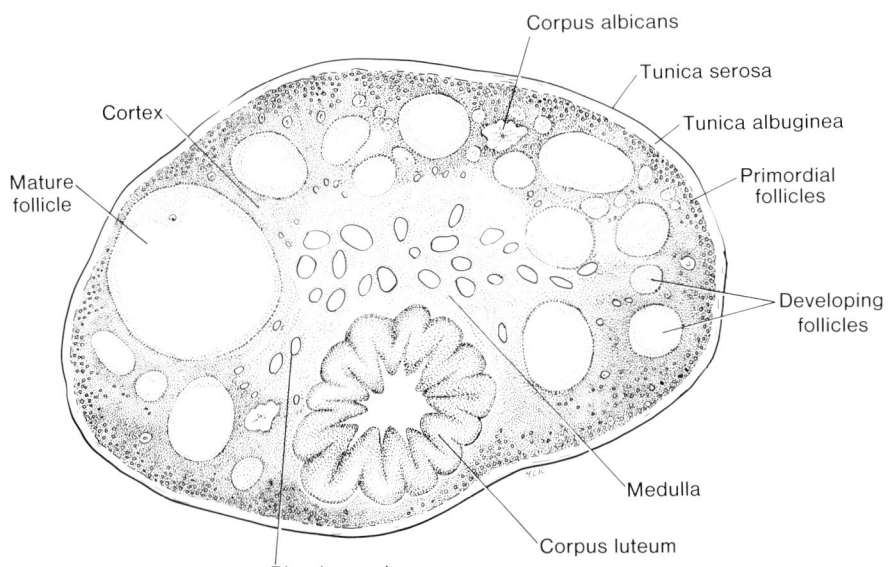

Fig. 24.1 A drawing of a canine ovary. All light micrographs are labeled as the magnification with the microscope before photographic enlarging. All electron micrographs are labeled as total magnification, including photographic enlarging.

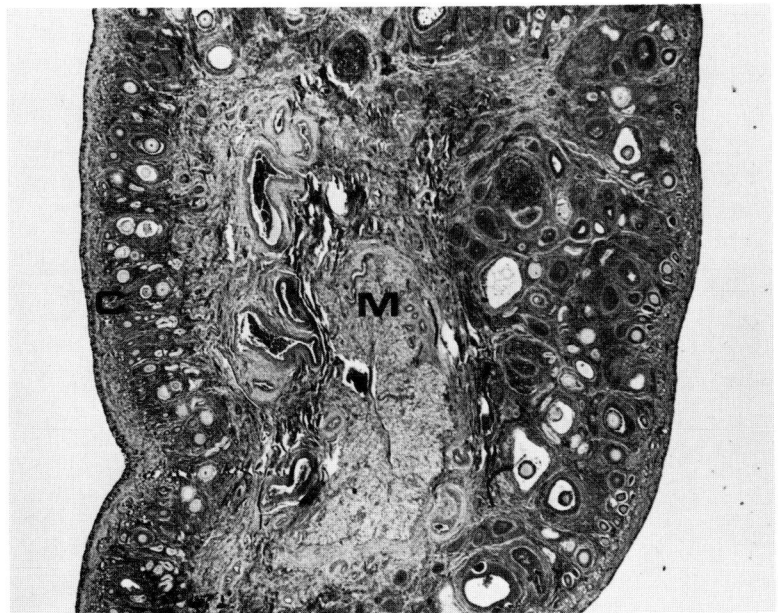

Fig. 24.2   A section of a canine ovary. The ovary has a distinct cortex (C) and medulla (M). X4.

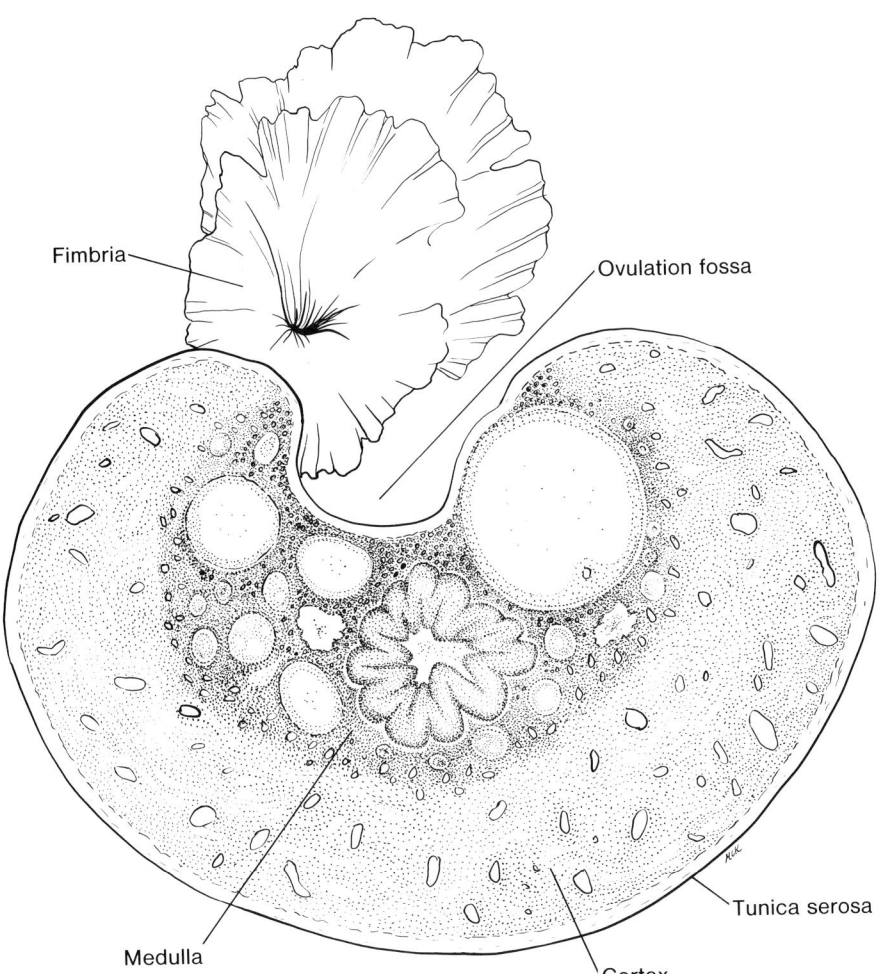

Fig. 24.3   A diagram of the mare's ovary. The cortex and medulla are reversed. An ovulation fossa is apparent. All other structures are the same as those labeled in Figure 24.1.

Whereas ganglion cells have been noted within the medulla of the organ, the precise relationships of the parasympathetic nervous system to the ovary are obscure.

Ovarian Cycle

Regulation. The ovary undergoes cyclic changes that are influenced by the effects of trophic hormones secreted by the pars distalis. Activity of the pars distalis, as in the male, is regulated by hypothalamic releasing factors—*luteinizing hormone releasing factor* (*LRF*) and *follicle-stimulating hormone releasing factor* (*FRF*). Control of hypothalamic activity is subject to regulatory influences similar to those manifested in the male. Optic and olfactory stimuli modulate activity within the *hypothalamo-ovarian axis*. Induced ovulators (cat, mink, lagomorphs) respond to the mechanical stimulation of coitus by ovulating approximately 24–48 post-coitus. Tonic secretory activity of the hypothalamus and negative feedback from ovarian hormones influence the cyclic reproductive activity of the female.

The release of FSH and LH from the pars distalis is the specific regulator of ovarian activity. FSH causes the growth and maturation of ovarian follicles as well as being responsible for the secretion of estrogens by these structures. Ovarian follicle rupture, ovulation and the development of corpora lutea occur under the influence of LH. Some LH may be necessary for FSH to manifest its trophic influence upon the follicles. Prolactin manifests luteotrophic properties upon the ovary in rodents and sheep.

The combined influence of FSH and LH (and prolactin in some species) regulates the cyclic activity of the ovary. The cyclic activities include *differentiation of ova, development of follicles, ovulation, formation of the corpus luteum, degeneration of follicles* and *degeneration of the corpus luteum.*

Oogenesis. *Oogenesis* is the formation and development of the ova. The differentiation of ova occurs in two stages that are similar to the development of male gametes: *stage of mitosis* and *stage of meiosis*. During the stage of mitosis or multiplication, *oogonia* proliferate from *primordial germ cells* that had migrated to the germinal ridges from the yolk sac endoderm (Fig. 24.4). The oogonia divide and give rise to several generations of identical cells. In some species, the differentiation and multiplication of oogonia occur within the developing fetus long before parturition occurs (ruminants, rodents, swine, man). In others (carnivores, lagomorphs), the differentiation is prolonged into the immediate postnatal period. Oogonia, entering into the prophase of the first meiotic division, become primary oocytes before or shortly after birth in most species. *Primary oocytes* are arrested in prophase until sexual maturity is achieved. Further development of primary oocytes is synchronized with the development and matu-

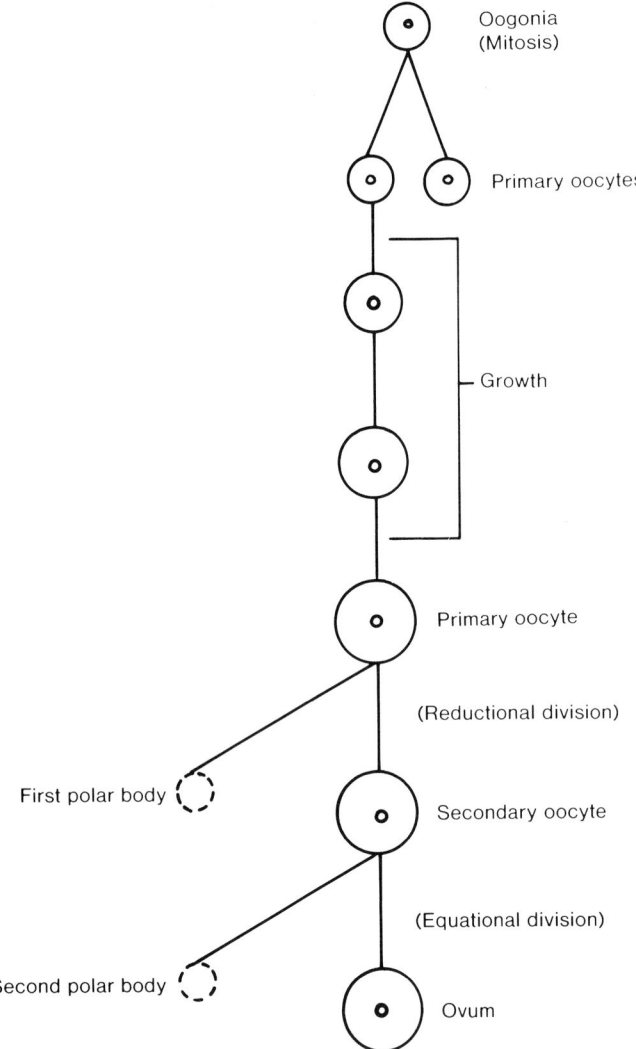

Fig. 24.4 A diagram showing the events of oogenesis. Compare this process to spermatogenesis in Figure 23.19.

ration of follicles. The *first meiotic division (reductional division)*, with the consequent conversion of a primary oocyte to a *secondary oocyte*, occurs just before ovulation in most species and is accompanied by the formation and expulsion of the *first polar body*. In the horse and dog, secondary oocyte formation occurs post-ovulation and may be delayed for 48 hours in the canid. In most species, other than the horse and dog, the *second meiotic division (equational division)* is accomplished when a spermatazoon penetrates the zona pellucida and "activates" the secondary oocyte. The *second polar body* is extruded at this time.

Follicular Development. An *ovarian follicle* is a spherical aggregation of cells that contains the developing gamete. The growth and development of follicles is accompanied by changes in the associated gametes. The cyclic continuum of follicular development is characterized by the identification of specific follicles—*primordial follicle, primary follicle, secondary follicle, mature follicle*

(Fig. 24.5). Follicular growth and maturation occurs under the influence of gonadotropins from the pars distalis (Plates I.6, I.7).

Concomitant with the differentiation of primary oocytes, a single layer of flattened mesodermal cells, *follicular cells*, surrounds the primary oocyte. At this stage, the complex is referred to as a primordial follicle. A *primordial follicle*, therefore, contains a *primary oocyte*. These are also referred to as *quiescent follicles* (Fig. 24.6). They are located in the periphery of the cortex in clusters or evenly distributed.

The activation of the primordial follicle results in a *primary follicle* (Fig.24.6). This activation involves alterations in the primary oocyte, follicular cells and other stromal elements. An accumulation of yolk granules is noted within the primary oocyte. The follicular cells become cuboidal. The *primary follicle still contains a primary oocyte.*

The *secondary follicle* is identified by an increase in the follicular cell population as-

sociated with the primary oocyte and the development of a zona pellucida between the primary oocyte and follicular cells (Figs. 24.7, 24.8). The follicular cells are active mitotically and are now referred to as the *membrana granulosa.* They are separated from the primary oocyte by a periodic acid-Schiff-positive, amorphous material, the *zona pellucida.* This is actually a very thick basal lamina. Stromal cells differentiate into two layers: *theca folliculi interna* and *theca folliculi externa.* The thecal cells are separated from the membrana granulosa cells by a basement membrane, the *glassy membrane.* The theca folliculi interna consists of large, epithelioid cells and an extensive vascular network. The theca folliculi externa is a fibroblastic layer of cells.

The development of a *secondary follicle (vesicular follicle)* results from the secretory activity of the granulosa cells (Fig. 24.9). Intercellular clefts develop, become confluent and form the *follicular antrum* filled with *liquor folliculi.* This is accompanied by the continued growth of the follicle. The primary oocyte is still surrounded, however, by a cluster of granulosa cells that is continuous with the peripherally displaced membrana granulosa. The mound of cells is referred to as the *cumulus oophorus.* Granulosa cells of the cumulus oophorus immediately adjacent to the primary oocyte comprise the *corona radiata.* These cells have cytoplasmic processes which penetrate the zona pellucida and contact microvilli from the ovum. *Despite the development of a vesicular follicle, it still contains a primary oocyte arrested in the first meiotic prophase.*

The *mature follicle (Graafian follicle)* is a greatly enlarged structure (Fig. 24.10). It extends from a protrusion at the surface to the depths of the cortex. The antrum is large and its attenuated wall still consists of the previously mentioned cellular and intercellular components.

Ovulation. *Ovulation* is the rupture of the follicle and the release of the oocyte. Whereas the precise mechanism of ovulation has not been determined, deterioration of the follicular wall through the enzymatic hydrolysis of connective tissue components by an LH-induced *collagenase* may be contributory. An increased intrafollicular fluid pressure is not associated with the ovulatory process. The liquor folliculi released upon ovulation probably assists in the trasport of the oocyte from the ovarian surface to the infundibulum.

The oocyte upon ovulation is surrounded by the zona pellucida and the *corona radiata.* The corona radiata is several layers of cells intimately associated with the oocyte that comprised the innermost zones of the cumulus oophorus. The oocyte and its associated cells may provide a sufficient mass that can be picked up by the fimbria.

Follicular Atresia. Not all of the developing follicles terminate in ovulation. Many follicles undergo *follicular atresia* (degenera-

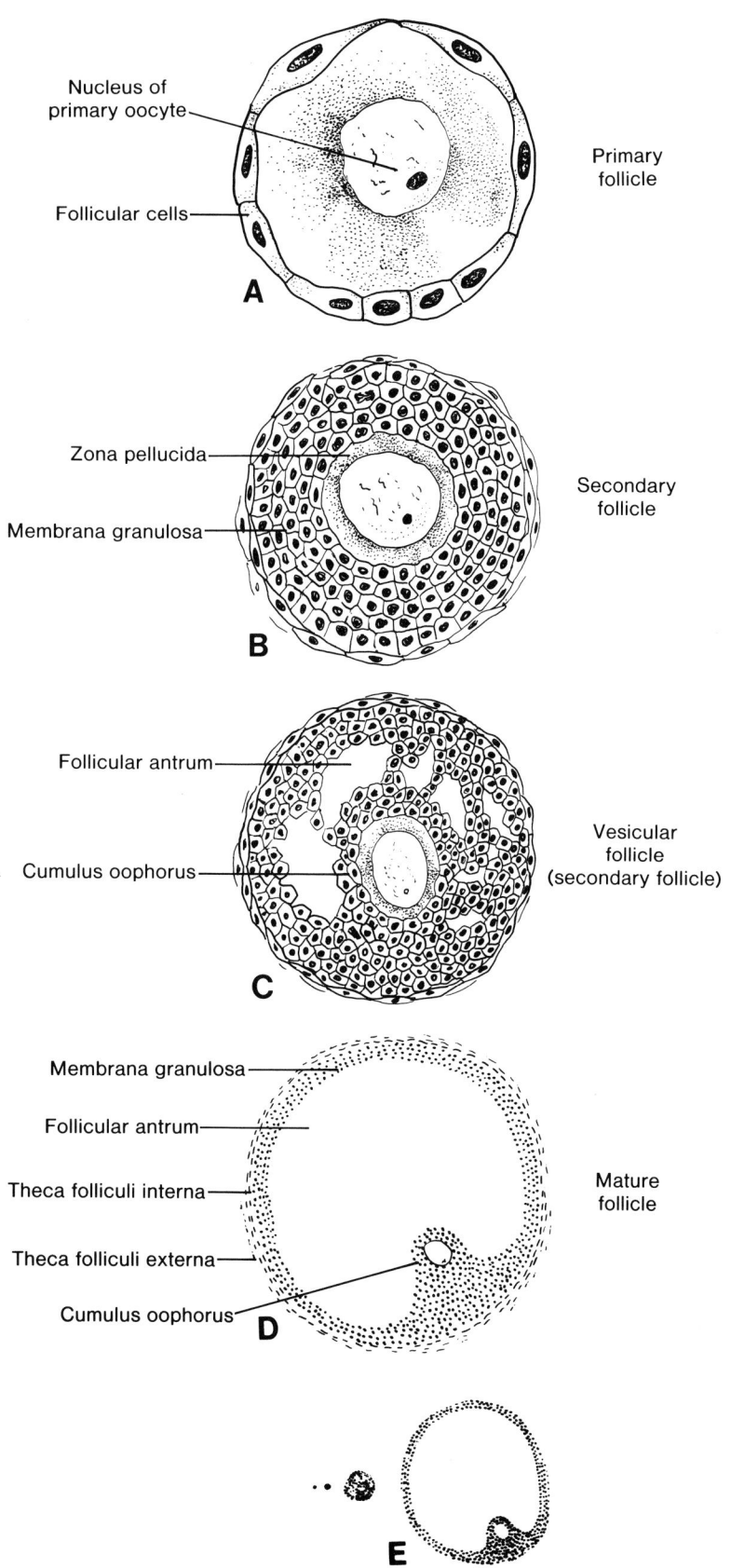

Nucleus of
primary oocyte

Follicular cells

A

Primary
follicle

Zona pellucida

Membrana granulosa

B

Secondary
follicle

Follicular antrum

Cumulus oophorus

C

Vesicular
follicle
(secondary follicle)

Membrana granulosa

Follicular antrum

Theca folliculi interna

Theca folliculi externa

Cumulus oophorus

D

Mature
follicle

E

Fig. 24.5 A diagram of the stages of folliculogenesis from primary to mature follicle formation. Drawings A, B, C and D are not drawn to scale. The approximate scale is indicated in E.

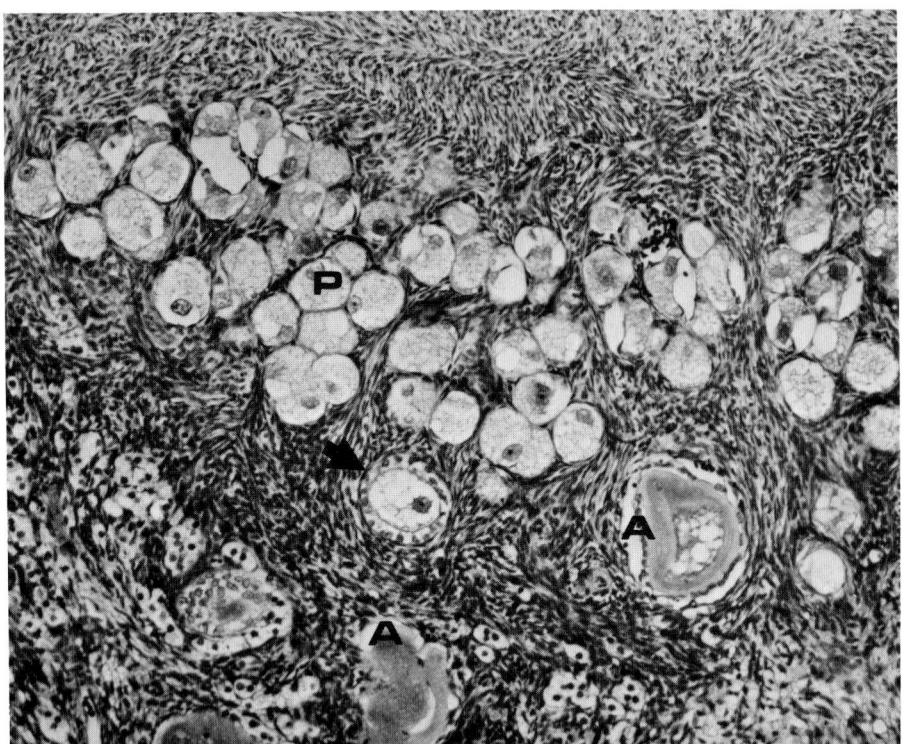

Fig. 24.6 Immature follicles of a feline ovary. Primordial (P) and primary follicles (*solid arrow*) are present. Atretic follicles (A) are apparent also. Note the high cellularity of the interstitial connective tissue. X40.

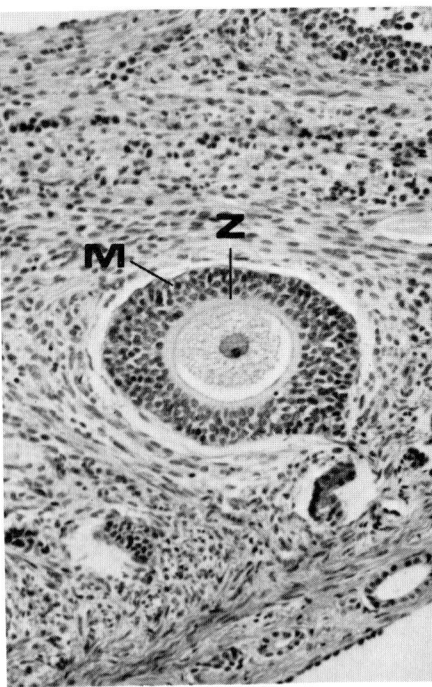

Fig. 24.7 A small secondary follicle from a canine ovary. The follicular cells have proliferated and are called the membrana granulosa (M) at this stage of development. A zona pellucida (Z) separates them from the primary oocyte. X40.

tion). The degeneration of follicles may occur at any point in their developmental sequence (Fig 24.11). During the primordial follicular stage, the dissolution of the ovum and granulosa cells is not characterized by remaining scar tissue. It simply disintegrates. Polyoocytic follicles are common and are invariably destined to become atretic.

In the more advanced stages of follicular development, cystic degeneration results and is followed by the formation of a scar, the *corpus atreticum*. The degenerative process begins with the oocyte and proceeds peripherally. The oocyte liquefies, while the zona pellucida becomes thickened and folded. The membrana granulosa cells degenerate and the walls of the follicle collapse. This is accompanied by a connective tissue and vascular invasion of the follicular antrum. The glassy membrane thickens and the cells of the theca folliculi interna may hypertrophy and undergo changes similar to their conversion to theca lutein cells (see corpus luteum). At this stage the atretic follicle may be considered a temporary gland. The follicular cells are arranged as cords around the degenerating ovum. Phagocytic activity from associated histiocytes and fibrotic activity from fibroblasts completes the transition to a corpus atreticum.

Corpus Luteum. After the rupture of the ovarian wall and associated mural elements of the follicle, the ovum is ejected and passes into the oviduct. The remaining portions of the follicle do not degenerate but undergo pronounced changes which lead to the formation of the corpus luteum (Fig. 24.12).

The follicular walls collapse upon themselves and the granulosa cells protrude into the residual lumen. The hemorrhage that accompanies ovulation eventually clots and the resulting transitory structure is referred to as a *corpus hemorrhagicum*. This structure doesn't occur in the dog. The granulosa cells proliferate, hypertrophy and are transformed into *granulosa lutein cells* (Fig. 24.13). In the mare, cow, bitch, queen and human, the accumulation of a yellow lipid pigment (*lutein*) and other lipids marks the transition to granulosa lutein cells. Although lutein does not accumulate in the ewe and sow, the accumulation of other lipids marks the transition from membrana granulosa cells to granulosa lutein cells.

The invasion of this region by stromal cells and vasculature removes the clot, results in reticular fiber deposition and converts this area into a highly vascularized gland.

The cells of the theca folliculi interna are also converted to lipid-producing cells, the *theca lutein cells*. These cells are smaller than the granulosa lutein cells and are dispersed peripherally or as septal-like clusters intimately associated with the other cell type which is predominant. In some species (ox), two types of lutein cells cannot be distinguished. The process by which granulosa and theca cells are converted to luteal cells is called *luteinization*. Hypertrophy and hy-

perplasia are essential factors in the process.

Whether lutein is present or absent, the resulting structure is referred to as the *corpus luteum* (*yellow body*).

The fate of the corpus luteum is dependent upon the reproductive success or failure of the individual.

If fertilization does not occur, the *corpus luteum spurium* slowly degenerates and is replaced by connective tissue. It is, therefore, converted to a *corpus albicans* or *corpus fibrosum*.

If fertilization does occur, the *corpus luteum verum* is persistent and active for a variable amount of time throughout the pregnancy. Retrogressive changes similar to the aforementioned characterize the degeneration of this structure. In some species, the corpus luteum verum is required throughout the entire pregnancy. In others, it may be removed at various time periods without any detrimental effects upon the gravid uterus.

Ovarian Hormones. The steroid hormones produced by the ovary are estrogens and progesterone. The cells responsible for the production of estrogens is a controversial subject. The membrana granulosa cells probably are the source of *17β-estradiol* and *estrone*, while the theca interna cells probably secrete androgens. Secretion occurs under the influence of follicle-stimulating hormone. *Progesterone* is produced by the lutein cells of the corpus luteum. A nonsteroidal hormone, *relaxin*, may be produced by

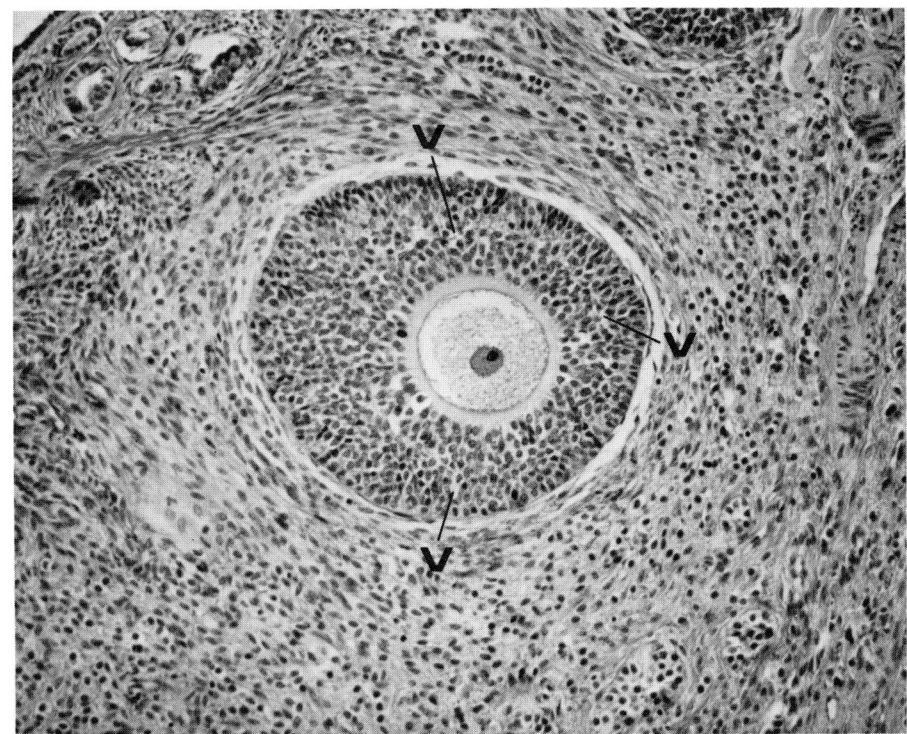

Fig. 24.8   A large secondary follicle from a canine ovary. Small intercellular vesiculations (V) have begun to form. They will coalesce to form the antrum. X40.

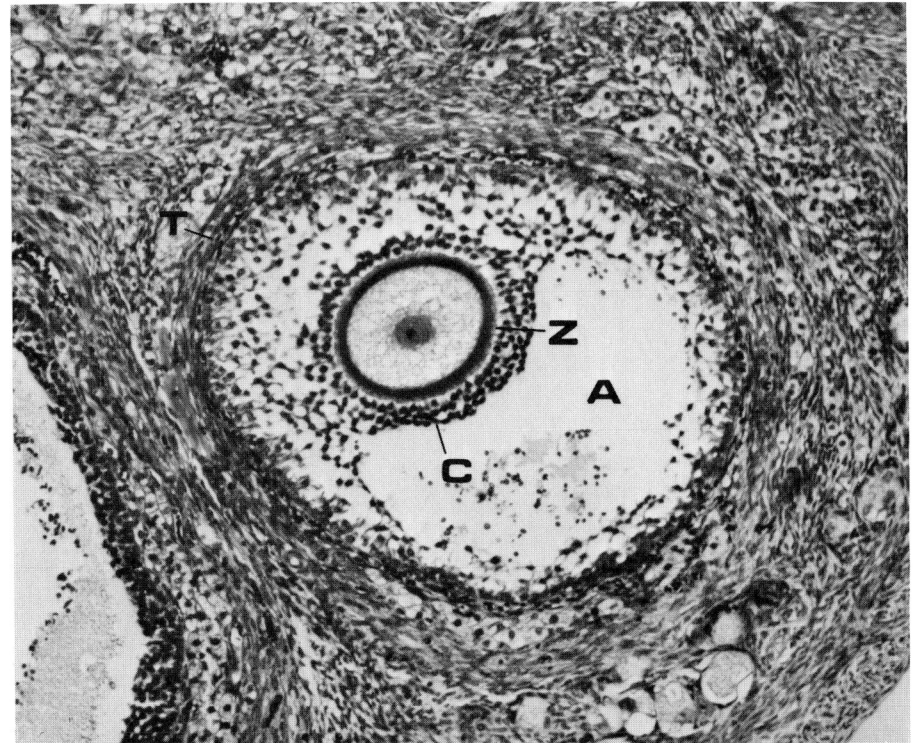

Fig. 24.9   A vesicular follicle from a feline ovary. The follicular antrum (A) has formed. C, cumulus oophorus; Z, zona pellucida; T, thecal cells. X40. (Lendrum's phloxine-tartrazine stain).

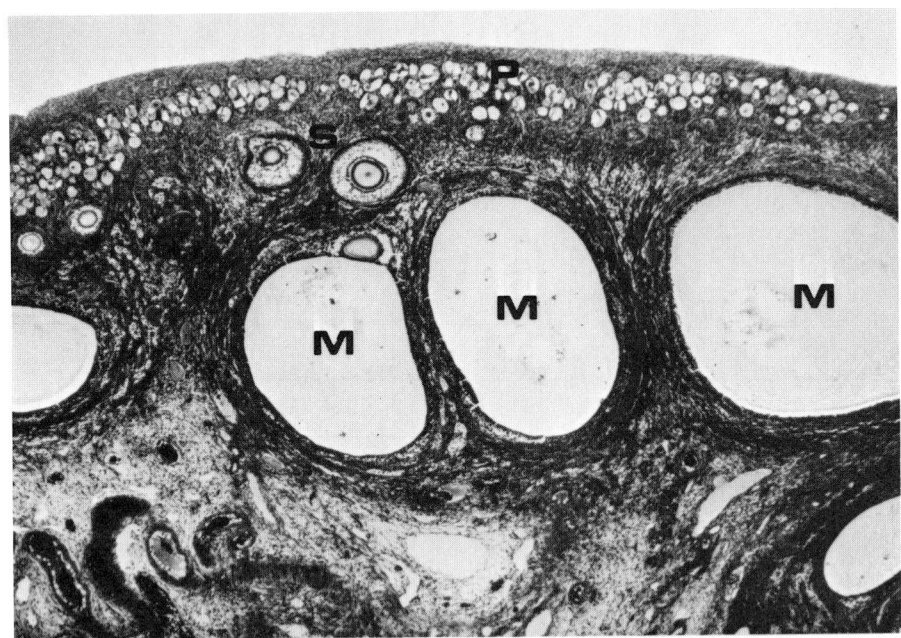

Fig. 24.10 A section of a feline ovary. P, primordial follicles; S, secondary follicles; M, maturing vesicular follicles. Note the size difference. X10 (Lendrum's phloxine-tartrazine).

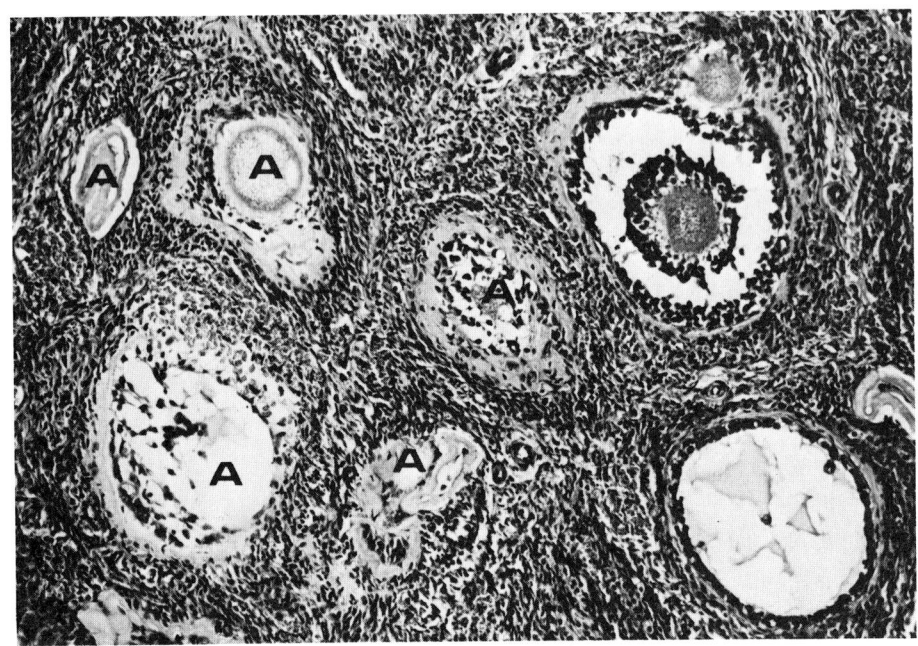

Fig. 24.11 Atretic follicles from a canine ovary. Not all follicles reach maturity. Many undergo atresia (A). X40.

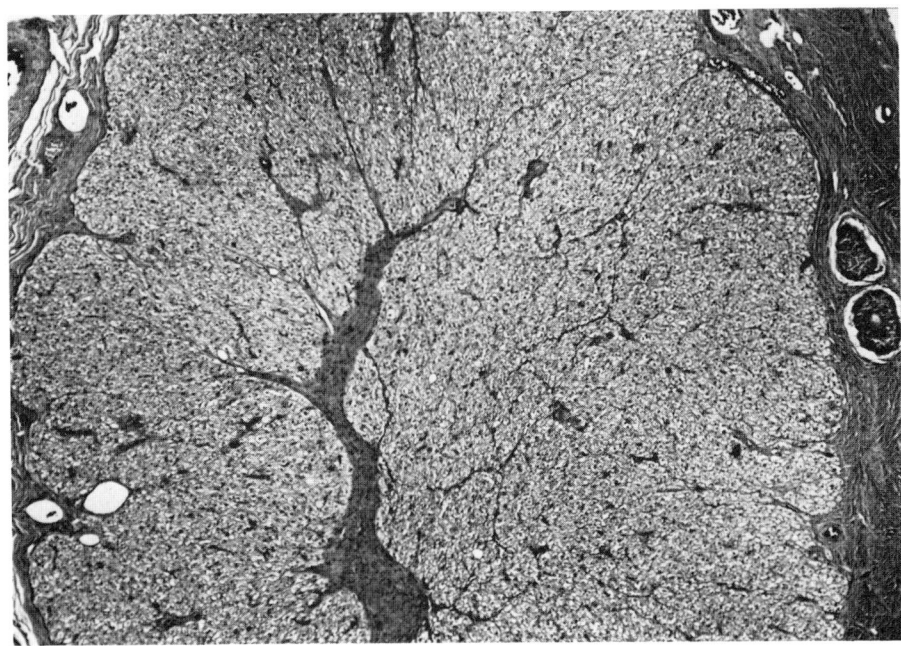

Fig. 24.12 A section of a corpus luteum of a canine ovary. The cellular mass results from the transformation of membrana granulosa and theca interna cells. X10.

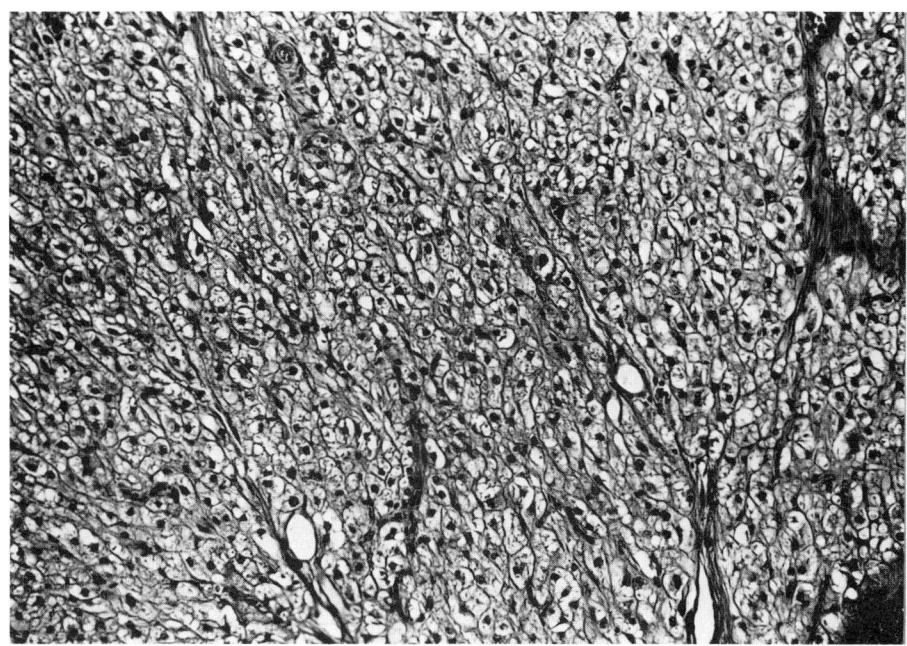

Fig. 24.13 Cells of the corpus luteum. The large clear cells are granulosa lutein cells.X40.

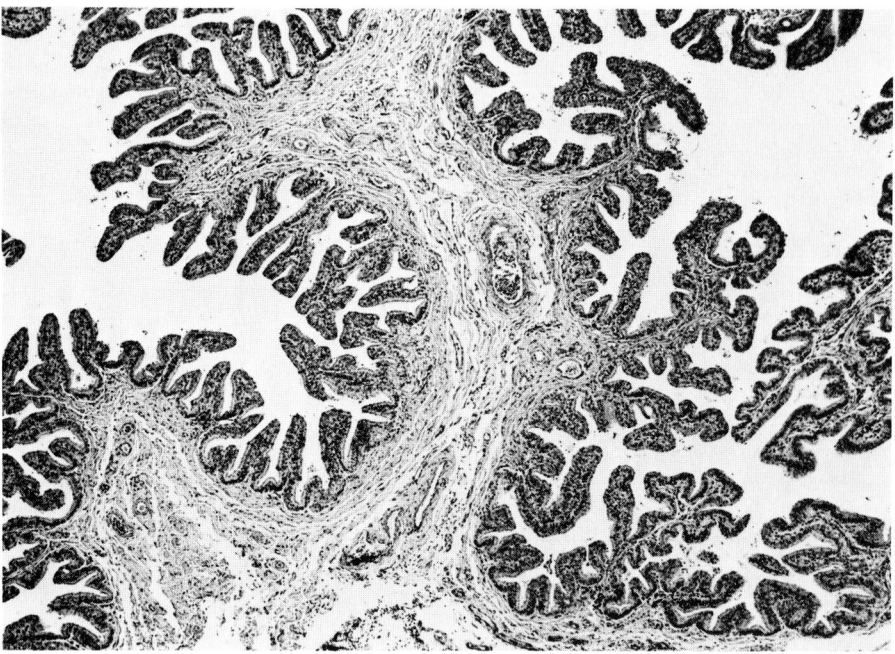

Fig. 24.14 A section of an equine oviduct. The lining consists of intermittently ciliated columnar epithelium. X16.

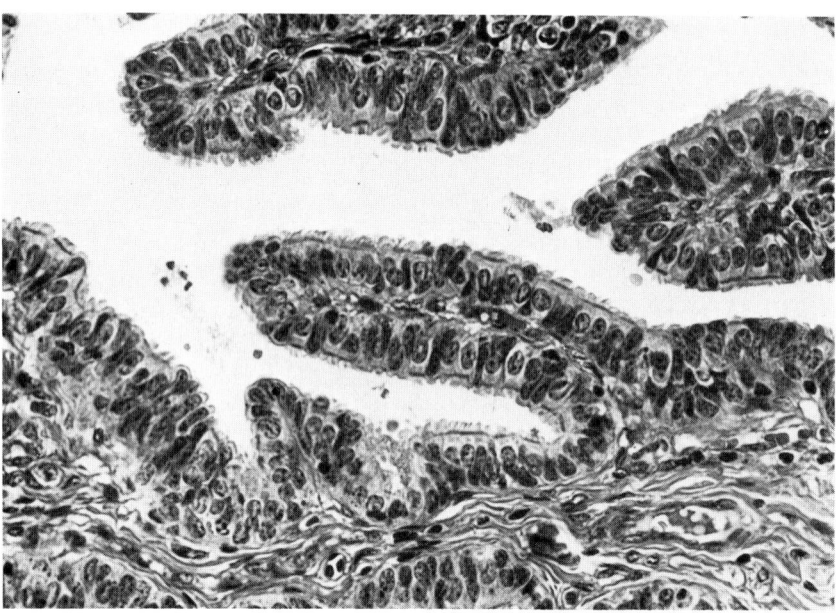

Fig. 24.15 Lining cells of a section of the infundibular portion of the equine oviduct. X100.

the corpus luteum; however, the precise origin of the hormone has not been determined. It functions to relax the ligaments associated with the birth canal before parturition.

The steroidal hormones, responding to the influence of the gonadotropins upon the ovary, are synthesized, released and exert a negative feedback influence upon the hypothalamus and pars distalis. Estrogens are responsible for the receptive behavior of the female during estrus. The development of female secondary sex characteristics is due partially to estrogens. Mammary gland development is influenced by this hormone

also. The normal development and function of the female reproductive tract are dependent upon estrogens. Estrogens also potentiate the effects of oxytocin and prostaglandins upon uterine smooth muscle contraction. Estrogens influence various functions of the body beside those associated with reproduction—skeletal growth, bone maintenance, sebaceous gland activity, electrolyte balance, calcium and phosphate retention, fat deposition. Estrogens are anabolic steroids.

Progesterone is the primary ovarian hormone of the luteal stage of ovarian activity. The main source of the hormone is the

corpus luteum. Progesterone assists estrogens in eliciting the characteristic sexual behavior associated with estrus. The hormone inhibits uterine smooth muscular contraction while promoting uterine gland development; progesterone is required for maintenance of pregnancy. The hormone exerts a negative feedback influence on the hypothalamus and pars distalis. Progesterone also enhances the development of the secretory and excretory portions of the mammary gland. Additionally, progesterone exerts a minor catabolic influence upon somatic proteins and may influence electrolyte balance.

Uterine Tubes

General Remarks. The uterine tubes are extensions of the uterus that serve for the transport of the male and female gametes. Fertilization occurs within the oviducts. Grossly, this structure is subdivided into *infundibulum, ampulla* and *isthmus.*

Histology of the Oviduct. The lamina epithelialis consists of intermittently ciliated columnar cells in most species (Fig. 24.14). In the sow and cow, however, it may be pseudostratified intermittently ciliated columnar epithelium. Kinocilia are especially prominent in the cranial portion of the oviduct wherein they assist in the movement of ova along the highly folded tunica mucosa (Fig. 24.15). Some of the lining cells, *peg cells,* are devoid of cilia. Ciliogenosis occurs in response to circulating levels of estrogen. The secretory cells may nourish the ova as well as capacitate the spermatozoa for fertilization.

The lamina propria-submucosa consists of areolar connective tissue and is devoid of glands. The tunica muscularis is best developed in the isthmus wherein it consists of inner longitudinal, middle circular and outer longitudinal layers. Craniad, it is typical. The tunica serosa is present and typical.

Uterus

General Remarks. The *uterus* performs functions that are essential to reproduction. In the horse, semen is deposited in the uterus; in swine, semen is deposited in the cervix. In other species (ruminants, cat, dog, lagomorphs, man), insemination is vaginal. Uterine contractions are essential for transport of the spermatozoa. Finally, the uterus is the site of development for the embryo and fetus. The uterus consists of a *body* (*corpus uteri*), *uterine horns* (*cornua uteri*) and *cervix* (*neck, cervix uteri*).

The form of the uterus is species-variable. Most domestic species have a *bicornuate uterus,* a uterus with a body and two prominent horns with a single cervix. Primates have a *simplex uterus,* an organ with a prominent body, two small uterine horns and a single cervix. Lagomorphs, monotremes and marsupials have a *duplex uterus.*

Capacitation, a process by which the sper-

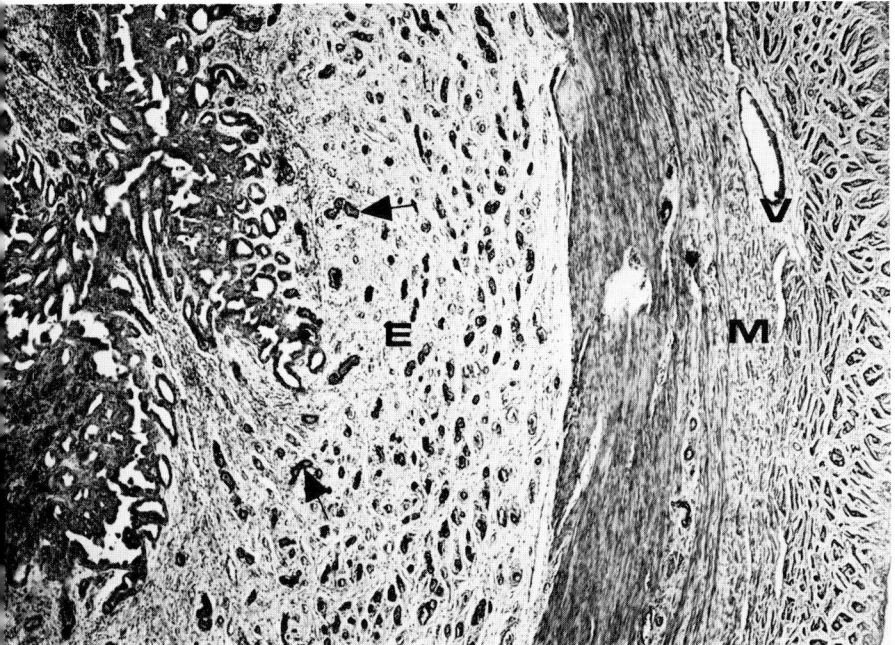

Fig. 24.16 A section of a gravid canine uterus. The tubular glands (*arrows*) are branched and coiled. E, endometrium; M, myometrium; V, vessels of the stratum vasculare. X40.

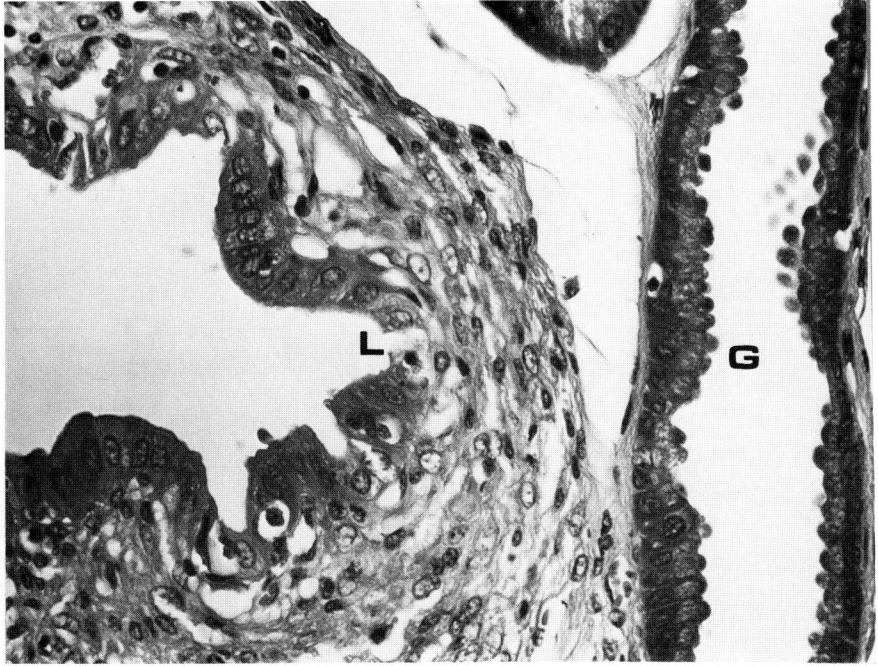

Fig. 24.17 Lining and glandular cells of a bovine metestrous uterus. The lining cells (L) are columnar. The glandular cells (G) are columnar and have apical blebs. X100.

cycle. A general description of the uterus follows; the changes associated with the estrous cycle are discussed subsequently.

Endometrium. The *endometrium* includes the tunica mucosa (Fig 24.17). The lamina epithelialis mucosae is simple columnar epithelium. Patches of pseudostratified columnar epithelium may be encountered in the sow and cow. Isolated foci of cuboidal epithelium may occur also. *Uterine glands* are simple or branched tubular glands (Fig. 24.18). Their distal ends have a variable degree of coiling that is species-dependent. The secretory products of the lining and glandular epithelia include mucus, lipids, glycogen and proteins. These glands extend into the lamina propria.

The lamina propria is a very cellular areolar connective tissue. In ruminants, an area of the lamina propria is highly vascularized and devoid of glands. These *caruncles* are devoid of uterine glands and are the eventual sites at which the maternal tissues make contact with the extraembryonic membranes (Fig. 24.19). Although there is no tunica submucosa, the peripheral connective tissue is less cellular than that which is subepithelial.

The endometrium is subject to changes during the estrous cycle.

Myometrium. The *myometrium* consists of a thick inner circular and thinner, outer longitudinally oriented coat which continues into the mesometrium (Fig. 24.16). A *stratum vasculare* occurs between the two layers of smooth muscle.

Perimetrium. The *perimetrium* or tunica serosa is typical, although a large number of lymphatic vessels may be present (Figs. 24.22, 24.25).

Cervix. The *cervix uteri* serves as a valve to close off the uterine lumen from the vagina. In the bitch, it may possess glands similar to those which occur in the uterus. In other domestic species, it is usually glandless. In the sow, it is a thin-walled structure, whereas in the cow it is extremely well-developed. The lining cells of the cervix of the cow are highly glandular. Their secretory activity varies with the stages of the estrous cycle and pregnancy. A clear mucus is secreted during estrus and a thick cervical seal is produced during pregnancy. Numerous longitudinal folds impart the impression that it is glandular.

The lamina epithelialis mucosae of the endocervical canal is composed primarily of goblet-like cells, but some kinociliated columnar cells may be present. The lamina propria-submucosa varies from loose connective tissue to DWFCT during various stages of the estrous cycle. The tunica muscularis is well-developed and rich in elastic fibers.

Vagina

The lamina epithelialis mucosae is a stratified squamous lining which is usually non-

matozoa achieve the ability to penetrate the corona radiata and zona pellucida to accomplish fertilization, occurs after exposure of the spermatozoa to the female reproductive tract. The uterus and oviducts play a role in the process. The need for capacitation has been determined in a few species but is suspected in others.

The wall of the uterus is divided into three distinct regions: *endometrium, myometrium* and *perimetrium* (Figs. 24.16, 24.17, 24.25). Although the terminology applied to the mural elements of this tubular visceral organ differs from that presented in Chapter 13, the mural elements and their organization is similar to those that occur in other tubular viscera. The morphology of the uterus changes in synchrony with the estrous

glandular (Fig. 24.20). In the cow, isolated foci of goblet cells are present in the cranial portion of the organ. In the bitch, intraepithelial glands have been observed during estrus. The tunica mucosa and tunica submucosa are highly folded.

The underlying DWFCT of the lamina propria-submucosa possess scattered lymphatic nodules.

The tunica muscularis consists of two or three layers: an inner longitudinal (variable), middle circular and an outer longitudinal. A tunica serosa is present cranially and is continued caudad as a tunica adventitia. Some smooth muscle (*muscularis serosae*), as a continuation of that of the broad ligament, may also be observed in the subserosal space.

Vulva

The vulva consists of the *vestibule* and *labia*. The *clitoris* is part of the vestibule and the *urethra* opens into the vestibule.

Vestibule. The structure of the *vestibule* is similar to the caudal portion of the vagina. There is nonkeratinized stratified squamous epithelium with an extensive lymphocytic infiltration. The lamina propria-submucosa consists of loose and dense connective tissue which is rich in elastic fibers. *Vestibular glands* (compound tubuloalveolar mucous glands) are present. *Major vestibular glands* (ewe, cow, queen) are embedded within the constrictor vestibuli muscle. *Minor vestibular glands* (queen, bitch, ewe, sow and mare) are scattered throughout the vestibule. In the cow, they are concentrated near the clitoris.

The tunica muscularis consists of an inner longitudinal and outer circular layer. The outer layer comprises two distinct muscles, *constrictor vestibuli* and *constrictor vulvae*. The tunica adventitia is typical.

Clitoris. The *clitoris* is homologous to the male penis. It consists of a body, glans and preputial covering. The body or *corpus clitoridis* contains cavernous tissue, adipose tissue and smooth muscle which is surrounded by a sheath of DWFCT. The *glans clitoridis* may contain cavernous tissue (bitch, mare) or areolar connective tissue which is highly vascularized. The *preputial* covering is an aglandular and hairless reflection of the cutaneous mucous membrane of the vestibule which is rich in sensory nerve endings.

Urethra. The female *urethra* is lined by transitional epithelium that is continuous with the mucous membrane of the vestibule. Branched tubular mucous glands, *glands of Littré*, may be present. The lamina propria-submucosa is areolar connective tissue that contains cavernous sinuses. The tunica muscularis is composed of two or three layers of smooth muscle.

Labia. The *labia* are folds of the integument that are comprised of typical integumentary structures.

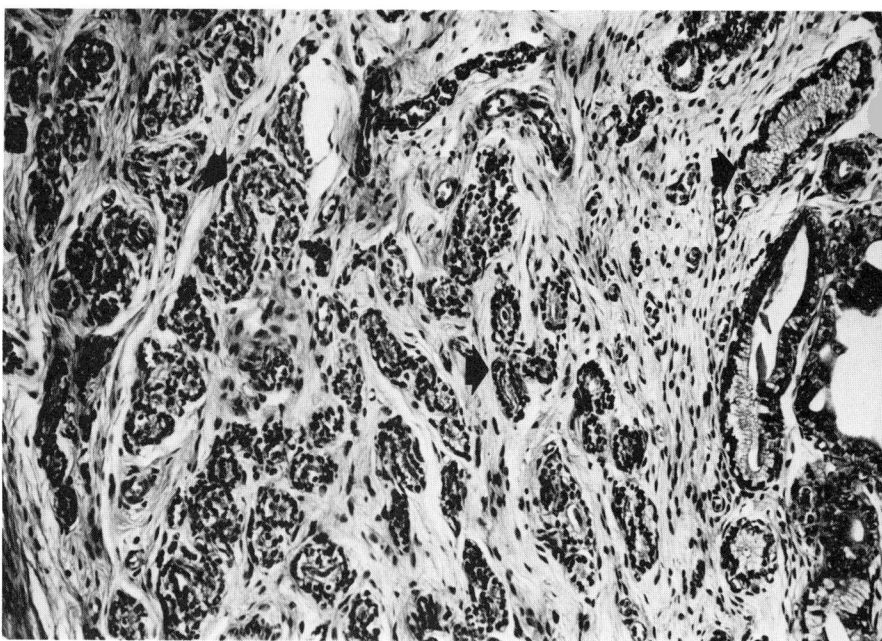

Fig. 24.18 A section of the endometrium of a gravid canine uterus. Tubular glands (*arrows*) are branched and coiled. X40.

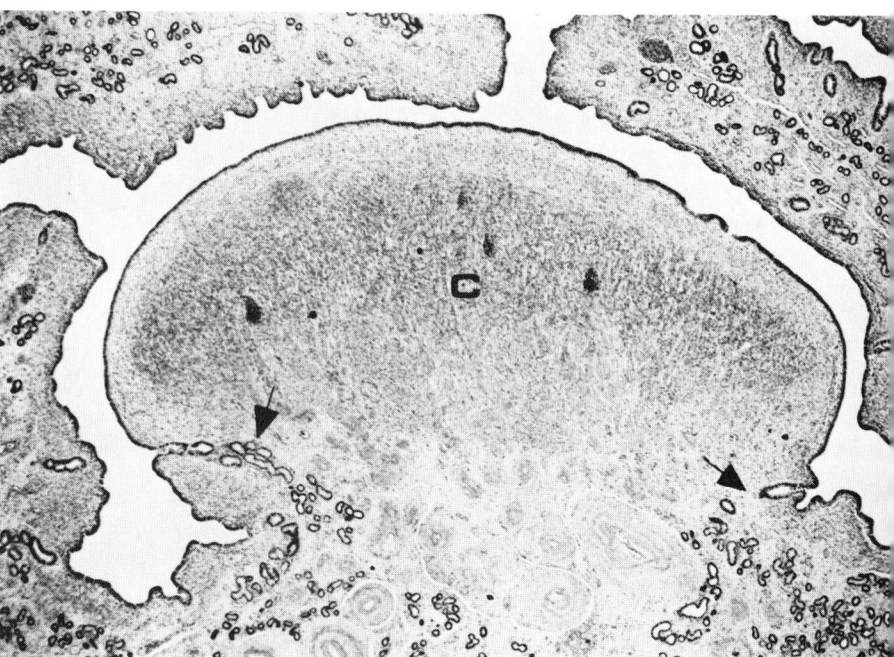

Fig. 24.19 A section of a bovine caruncle. The caruncle (C) is devoid of uterine glands (*arrows*). X5.

Cyclic Changes of the System

Introduction. The female reproductive tract is subject to greater periodic changes than that associated with the male. Moreover, female cyclic activity is manifested microscopically and grossly, as well as behaviorally. These various states of morphology, function and behavior are directly related with the estrous cycle. The estrous cycle, or period of varying reproductive activity, is under the influence of the trophic hormones of the adenhypophysis. This cycle is subdivided into five distinct but continuous stages: *proestrus, estrus, metestrus, diestrus* and *anestrus. Proestrus* is that period of the cycle characterized by the acceleration of follicular growth under the influence of FSH. The follicles begin to secrete estrogen which in turn influences the genital organs. The increasing levels of estrogen suppress the declining levels of progesterone. *Estrus* is marked by the genital organs being under the full influence of estrogen. This is the period of *heat* in which the female will accept the male. *Metestrus* is a transitional stage in which the declining levels of estrogen are counterbalanced by the increasing levels of progesterone. *Diestrus* is that period of the cycle that is under the sole influence of progesterone. Fertilization of the ova and subsequent pregnancy results in a prolonged diestrus. If fertilization is not accomplished, the anestrus period may follow. This is a period of variable length in which the reproductive organs are relatively quiescent.

Species Differences. The stages of the estrous cycle are of varying lengths in domestic species. Table 24.1 summarizes the characteristics of the estrous cycle of selected domestic animals. Animals are either *monestrous* or *polyestrous*. In monestrous species (dog), one estrous cycle (proestrus, estrus, metestrus, diestrus) is followed by a long period of anestrus. In polyestrous animals (cow, sow, rodents) one estrous cycle terminates in a period of diestrus that merges as the proestrus in the succeeding estrous cycle. In seasonally polyestrous animals (mare, queen, ewe), the terminal diestrus continues as a period of anestrus before the next estrous cycle. The anestrous period in these animals is appreciably shorter than that which occurs in monestrous animals.

Blood hormone levels vary throughout the length of the estrous cycle. The levels of hormones at various stages of the reproductive cycle are subject to species variation also. The hormone levels of the cow, mare and bitch are compared non-parametrically in Figure 24.21. Cyclic changes in the ovaries, uterus and vagina are synchronized with the cyclic secretion of gonadotropins and ovarian hormones.

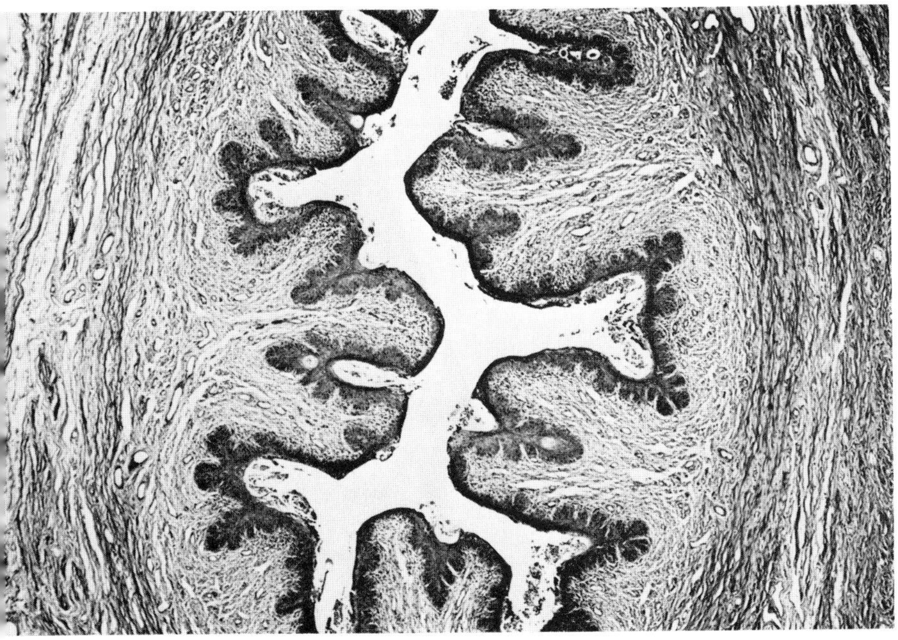

Ovarian Changes. During *proestrus*, the ovaries are influenced by the gonadotrophin, FSH. This results in the rapid growth of the follicles and the initiation of estrogen secretory activity.

During *estrus*, the follicle (or follicles) reaches maturity and estrogen secretory activity is maximal. FSH secretion begins to drop while LH secretion is initiated. This results in ovulation. Ovulation may be considered a transitory period between estrus and metestrus or part of the metestrous stage.

During *metestrus*, the development of the corpus luteum occurs and the secretion of progesterone is initiated.

The *diestrus* is characterized by a maximal development of the corpus luteum and a maximal productivity of progesterone. If pregnancy is not achieved, the latter part of diestrus is characterized by an involution of the corpus luteum spurium and its conversion into a corpus albicans. If pregnancy does occur, the corpus luteum continues its maximal secretory activity.

In *anestrus*, the ovary is relatively quiescent. The corpus luteum continues its involution and follicular development is arrested.

Uterine Changes. During *proestrus* the lining epithelium hypertrophies while the uterine glands remain relatively straight (Fig. 24.22). There is an increasing vascularity and congestion in the connective tissue space, as well as occasional hemorrhage. Heterophils begin to invade the epithelial lining.

During *estrus* the epithelial and glandular proliferation is continued and is more apparent (Fig. 24.23). Secretory activity of the cells is marked, whereas agranulocytic infiltration of the epithelium continues. The connective tissue space is marked by maximal congestion, edema and hemorrhage.

Metestrus is characterized by a continuation of glandular hyperplasia through which the coiling of glands is achieved (Fig. 24.24). The high secretory activity continues, whereas the edema of the connective tissue space declines or disappears.

In *diestrus* maximal glandular hyperplasia is achieved and the glands are extensively coiled. If fertilization occurs, maximal secretory activity is maintained. If fertilization does not occur, the vascularity decreases, the secretory activity is arrested and the lining cells and glands involute.

During *anestrus* the endometrium is thin and lined by a simple cuboidal epithelium (Fig. 24.25). Uterine glands are sparse and assume a simple or branched tubular configuration.

Vaginal Changes. The vaginal changes associated with the estrous cycle are discussed in Chapter 26.

Fig. 24.20 A section of a feline vagina. The tunica mucosa is highly folded and lined by stratified squamous epithelium. X10.

Table 24.1
Reproductive Cycle of Selected Domestic Animals*

Animal	Type of Cycle	Length of Cycle	Duration of Estrous Stage	Time of Ovulation	Pregnancy Length
Cow	Polyestrous (non-seasonal)	21 d	16 hrs	13 hrs postestrus	285 d
Ewe	Polyestrous (seasonal)	17 d	1 d	end of estrus	145 d
Mare	Polyestrous (seasonal)	21 d	6 d	d 5 of estrus	335 d
Sow	Polyestrous (non-seasonal)	21 d	2–3 d	d 2 or 3 of estrus	113 d
Bitch	Monestrous	7–8 mon	4–14 d	d 2 or 3 of estrus	63 d
Queen	Polyestrous (seasonal)	15–21 d	10–14 d**	induced	63 d

* The averages and ranges included are subject to individual and breed variation.

** If mating is achieved, then the duration is reduced to 4–6 d.

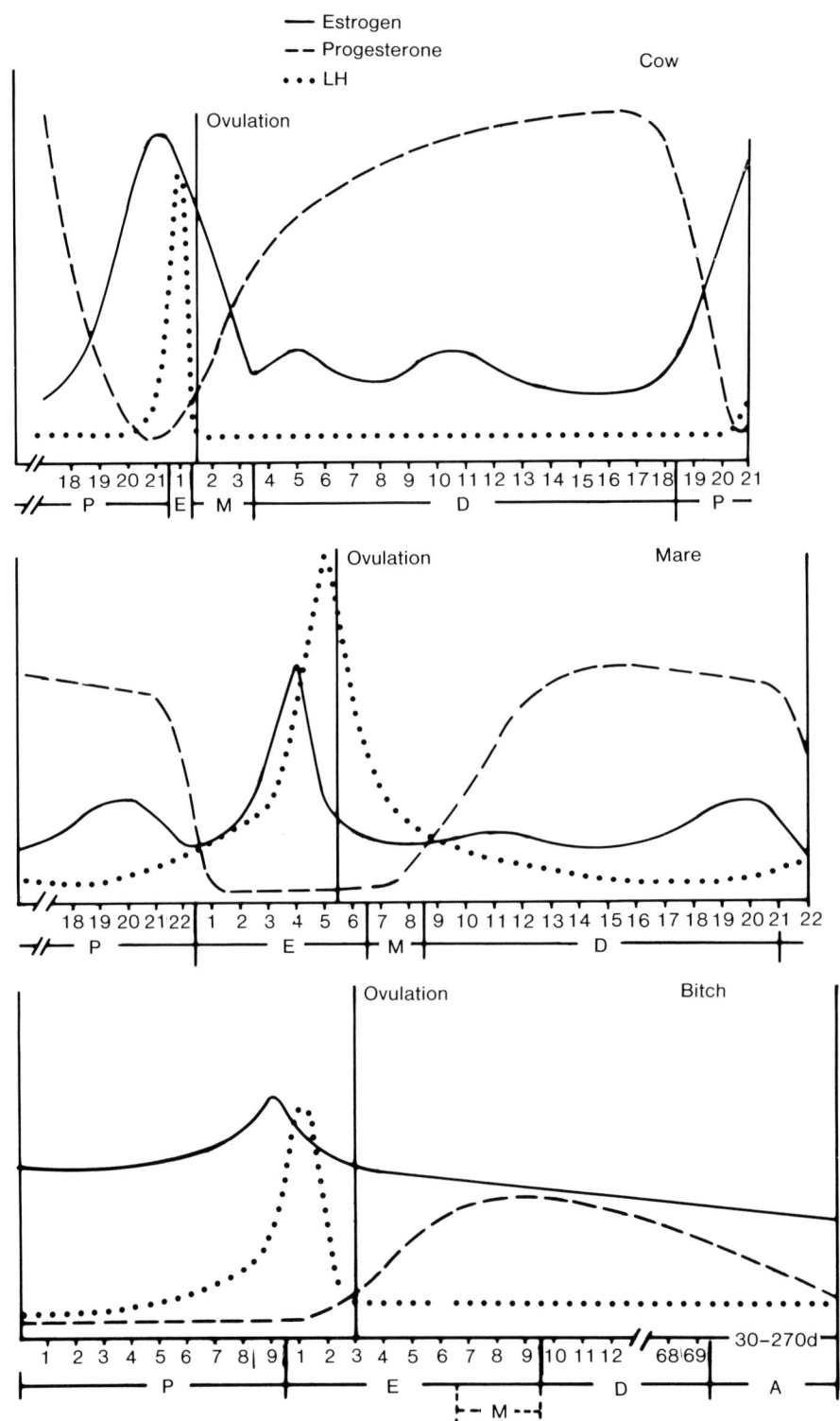

Fig. 24.21 Diagrams of the comparative estrous cycles of the cow, mare and bitch. A prolonged anestrus is a unique feature of the canine estrous cycle.

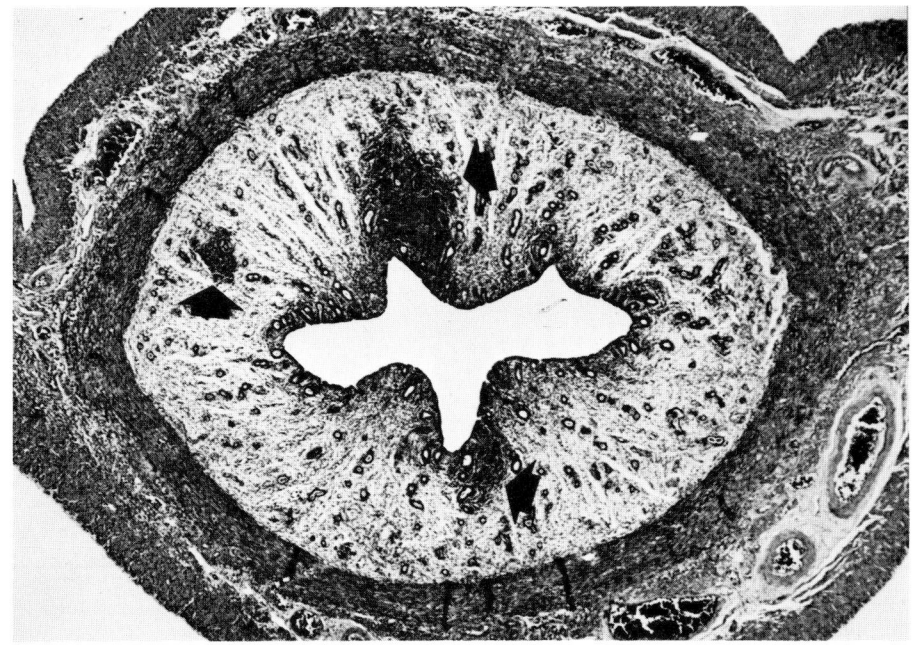

Fig. 24.22 A cross section of a canine proestrous uterus. The uterine glands are straight and hemorrhage is apparent (*arrows*) in the lamina propria. X10. (Note: the magnifications of Figures 24.20, 24.22, 24.23, 24.24 and 24.25 are the same).

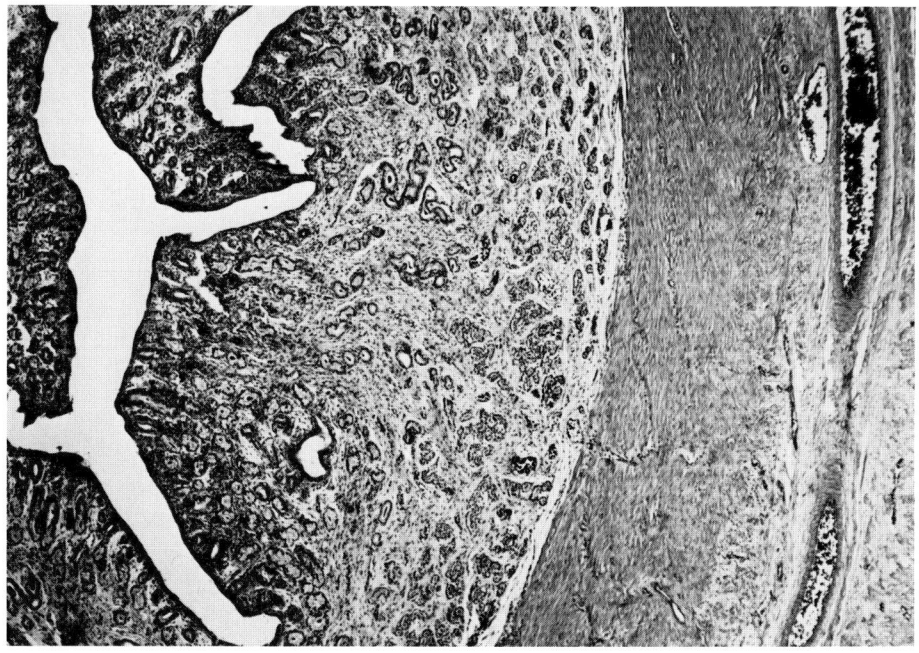

Fig. 24.23 A cross section of a canine estrous uterus. Glandular proliferation and general enlargement of the uterus are apparent. X10.

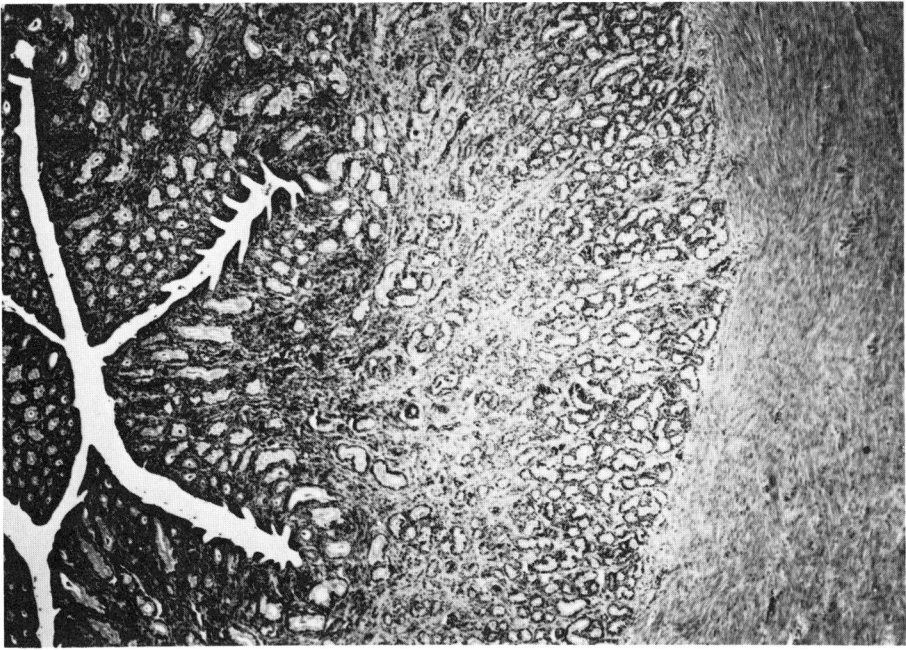

Fig. 24.24 A cross section of a canine metestrous uterus. The uterine glands and uterus are larger than the estrous uterus. X10.

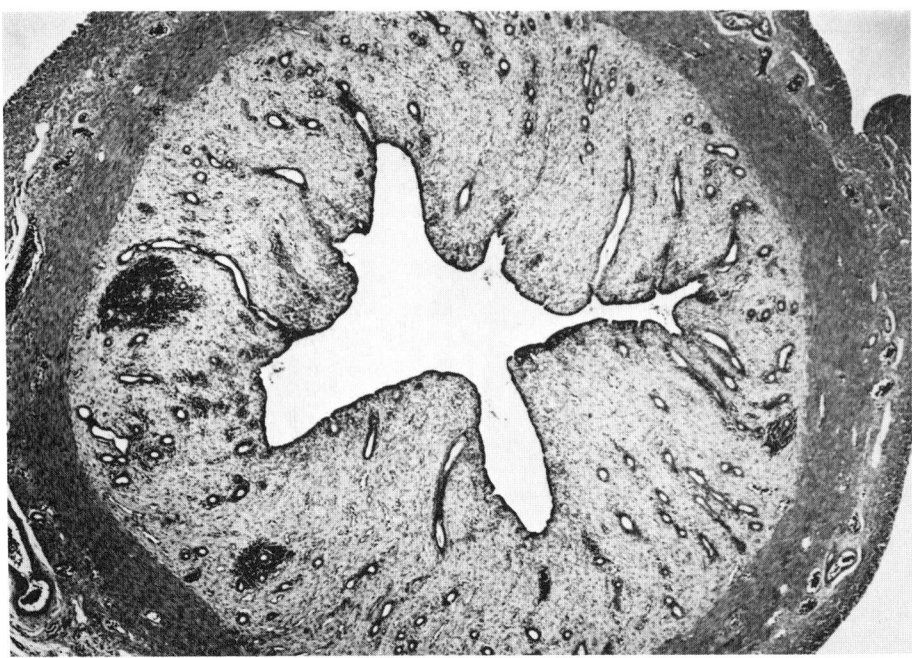

Fig. 24.25 A cross section of a canine anestrous uterus. The uterine glands are reduced in number and the endometrium is reduced in size. X10.

Menstrual Cycle Compared. The menstrual cycle of primates includes two phases: *follicular phase, luteal phase* (Fig. 24.26).

The *follicular phase* is characterized by those events that occur in proestrus and estrus in other species. The phase is under the influence of FSH and estrogen. It is sometimes referred to as the proliferative phase.

The *luteal phase* is also referred to as the *progestational* or *secretory phase*. The events are similar to those of metestrus and diestrus.

Changes associated with the endometrium are referred to as the *ischemic* or *premenstrual phase* and *menstrual phase*. Necrotic endometrial changes occur under the declining influence of progesterone and culminate with hemorrhage and the loss of part of the endometrium. Endometrial repair is

achieved through proliferation of epithelium from the uterine glands and stromal elements of the lamina propria.

Comparative Placentology

Introduction. The female reproductive tract of mammals is designed to facilitate internal fertilization. Subsequent to that, the system permits the development of the fertilized egg within the uterus. Complex relationships are developed within the uterus between fetal and maternal tissues that ensure nutrition, respiration, removal of waste materials and protection. Besides the important aforementioned functions, the placenta is also an endocrine organ that is responsible for the production of progesterone and relaxin. These functions are ensured by the formation of the *placenta*, a complex structure formed by the union of fetal membranes with the endometrium.

The endometrium was prepared for pregnancy during the metestral and diestral stages of the estrous cycle.

Not all mammals, however, are placental. Nor do all mammals bear live young. The classification of mammals is predicted upon the nature of fetal and maternal relationships. The *prototherian mammals* or *monotremes* include the platypus and echidna. These are egg-laying mammals. The *methatherian mammals* or *marsupials* include such animals as the kangaroo and opossum. These animals form a transitory "yolk sac placenta." However, there is no intimate contact between the fetal membranes and the uterine mucosa. They, in fact, do not form a true placenta.

The remaining extant mammals comprise the *eutherian* subclass. These are the true *placental mammals*. The fetal membranes (chorion, amnion, yolk sac and allantois) and the endometrium contribute to the formation of the placenta. This is accomplished individually or in specified combinations.

Classification. Various means have been devised to classify or characterize certain placental characteristics. These include the distribution of contact, the contributing extraembryonic membranes, the degree of implantation, the configuration of the chorionic attachment and the combination of fetal and maternal tissues that comprise the placenta. These classifications are not mutually exclusive. Rather, they may be used in combination to describe the placenta of a particular species.

Distribution of Chorionic Villi

General Remarks. The chorion is in close contact with the uterine mucosa. Highly vascularized regions, *villi*, project from this extraembryonic membrane and form intimate contact with the endometrium. These projections may occur singly or in groups. The subsequent descriptions refer to the chorioallantoic type of placenta.

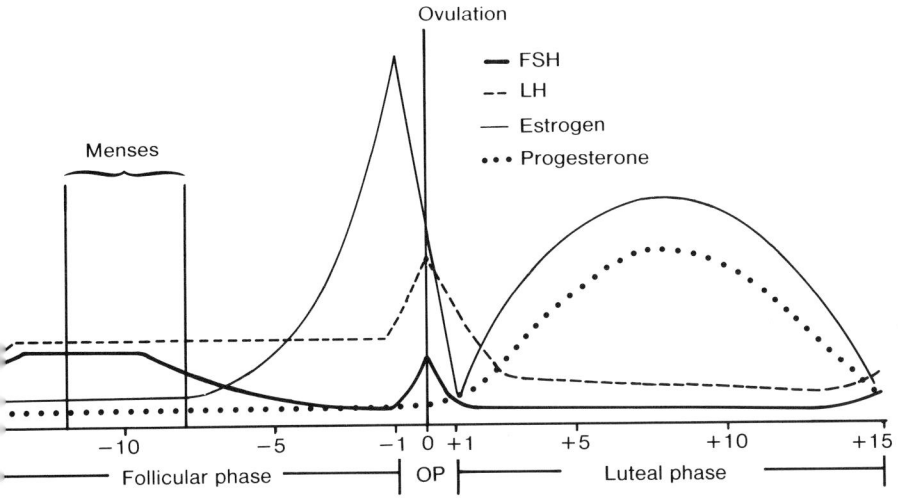

A diagram of the primate menstrual cycle. OP, short ovulatory phase between the vo major phases of the menstrual cycle.

iffuse Placentation. In the *diffuse placenta* e chorionic villi are present over the entire urface of this membrane. The entire chorion, therefore, is attached to the endomeium. This type of placenta is typical of the are and sow.

otyledonary Placentation. The *cotyledonry placenta* or *placenta multiplex* is a mulple structure. The villi are grouped as coledons, while the intercotyledonary space smooth (devoid of villi). The cotyledons ttach themselves to the *caruncles* of the ndometrium. The *fetal cotyledon* and the aternal caruncle comprise the *placentome*. his type of placenta is typical of the cow, we, and doe.

onary Placentation. In the *zonary placenta* e villi are grouped in an area that circumcribes the midportion of the chorion. This ype of placenta is characteristic of the dog nd cat.

iscoidal Placentation. The *discoidal placenta* is characterized by villi being grouped n one or two disc-shaped regions. This placentation is characteristic of rodents and rimates.

xtraembryonic Membrane Contribuions

horionic Placenta. The *trophoblast* is the uter layer of the blastocyst. During *nidaon*, this layer invades the uterine mucosa nd serves as a nonvascularized point of ttachment. This layer serves to nourish the lastocyst by obtaining nutrients from the terus until the definitive placenta is ormed.

horiovitelline Placenta. There are two ypes of yolk sac placenta: *nonvascularized* nd *vascularized*. In the *yolk sac, nonvascuarized placenta*, the differentiated *yolk sac* ndoderm and the *trophoderm* (the tropholast following the differentiation of the erm layers, chorion) fuse. These layers erve to transport nutrients to the embryo rom the uterine mucosa.

In the *yolk sac, vascularized placenta*, the yolk sac endoderm and trophoderm are separated by a layer of mesoderm which contains blood vessels. This is a transitory method of utilizing the embryonic circulation for physiologic exchange between fetal and maternal tissues. It is a transitory structure in most eutherian mammals but persists for some time in the horse. This type of exchange organ is the definitive placenta of metatherian mammals.

Chorioallantoic Placenta. The *chorioallantoic placenta* is the definitive or "true" placenta of eutherian mammals. It is formed by the fusion of the *allantoic mesoderm* with the *chorionic mesoderm*. A vascular invasion accompanies the allantoic mesoderm, while the allantoic vesicle may be extensively large or vestigial in size.

Degree of Implantation

General Remarks. The degree of implantation generally defines the extent of the relationship between the fetal and maternal tissues. Through the relationships so established, the shedding or nonshedding of maternal tissues at parturition is established. In those placentas in which a minimal amount of tissue is eroded during the formation of the organ, the placenta is nondeciduate. In those in which an extensive erosion of tissues accompanies the implantation, the placenta is termed deciduate. Maternal tissues are not shed at parturition in a nondeciduate placenta as they are in a deciduate placenta.

Nondeciduate Placenta. The terms *nondeciduate placenta, apposed placenta, semiplacenta* and *superficial nidation* are used synonymously. The fetal and maternal tissues may be interdigitated and are fused or in apposition to one another. There is, therefore, minimal erosion of the contributing tissues. At parturition, no uterine mucosal elements are lost.

Deciduate Placenta. The *deciduate placenta* is also referred to as a *conjoined placenta* or

a *placenta vera. Interstitial nidation* also refers to the formation of this type of placenta. In the formation of this type of placenta, the uterine mucosa and chorion are eroded to varying degrees and subsequently fuse. At parturition, therefore, some maternal tissue is lost.

Decidual Cells. These are multinucleated, round giant cells. They accumulate lipids and glycogen. These cells first appear in the uterine mucosa after the invasion of it by the trophoblast. *The presence or absence of these cells does not imply that a placenta is deciduate or nondeciduate.* The precise function of these cells is not known. They may serve a nutritive function, delineate a cleavage zone at parturition, protect the uterine mucosa against the invading trophoblast or

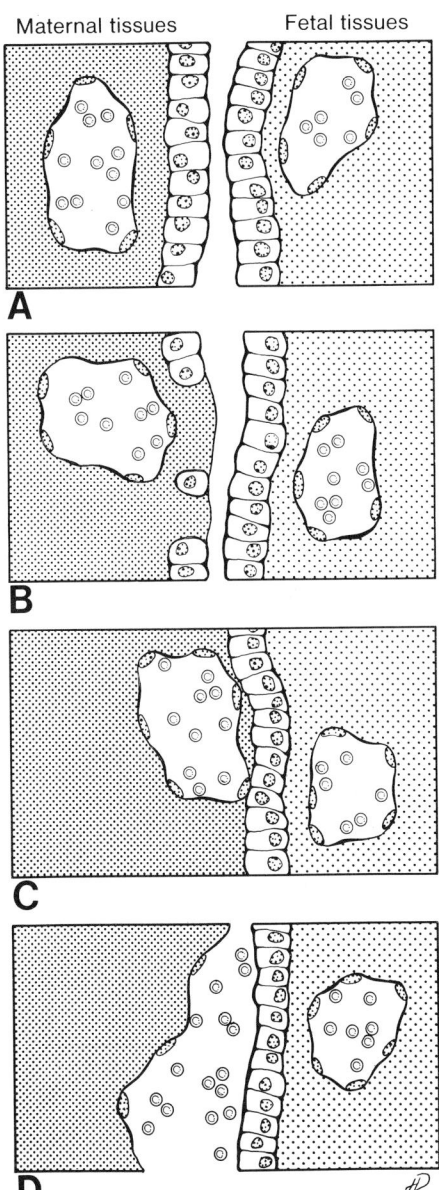

Fig. 24.27 A diagram of four types of placentation. The fetal tissues remain intact in the placental relationships depicted. A, epitheliochorial; B, syndesmochorial; C, endotheliochorial; D, hemochorial.

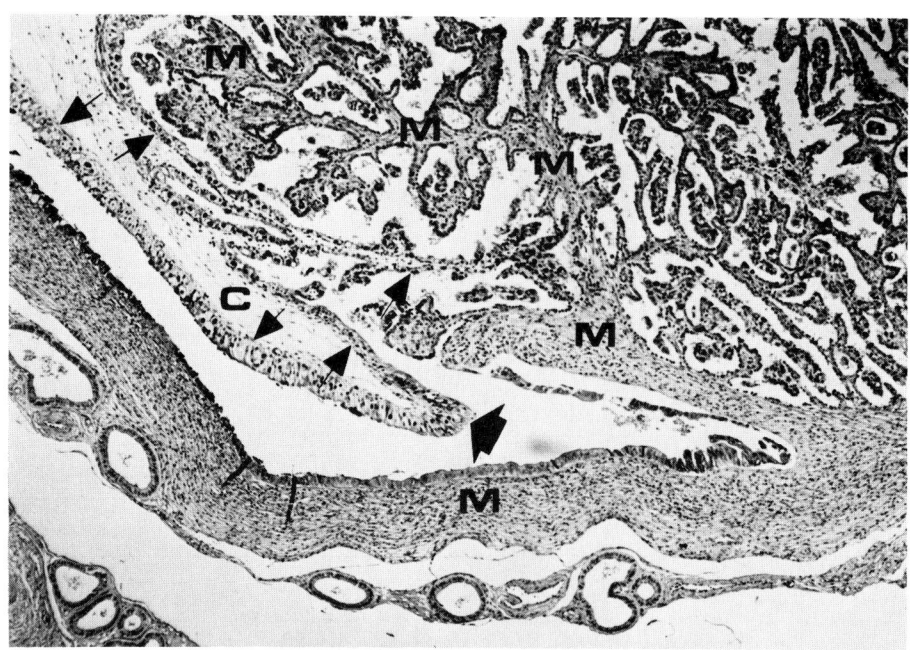

Fig. 24.28 A section of a bovine epitheliochorial placenta. The chorioallantois (C) of the fetus (*small arrows*) interdigitates with the maternal vil (M). The fetal membrane is reflected away from the placentome (*large arrow*). X13.

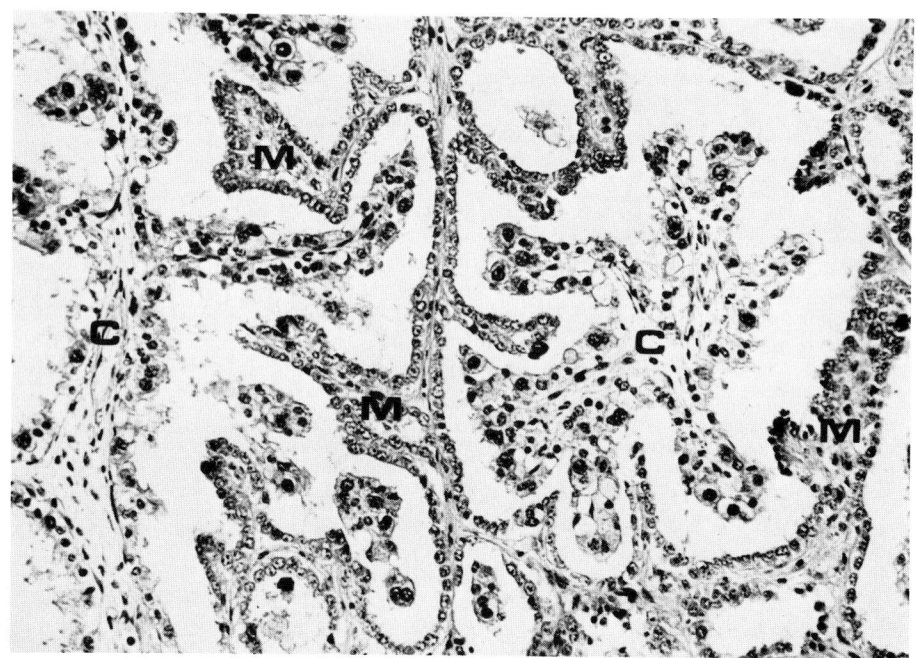

Fig. 24.29 Fetal and maternal tissue relationships in a bovine placentome. The maternal tissue (M) is lined by uterine epithelium. The chorioallantois (C) of the fetus is lined by trophoblastic cells. The separation between the tissues is artifact. X50.

form placental gonadotrophins. These cells are typical of most eutherian mammals but occur minimally or not at all in carnivores and ungulates.

In the mare, masses of cells very similar to decidual cells develop from the mucosa in an interglandular position. These *endometrial cups* may be responsible for the production of gonadotrophins. They regress as gestation progresses.

Configuration of Chorionic Attachments

Folded, Villous and Labyrinthine Attachments. The fetal and maternal tissues are opposed, fused or intimately interdigitated to facilitate physiologic exchange. Three types of fetal and maternal contact are defined: folded, villar, labyrinthine. In the *folded type*, undulations of both contributing

tissues are interdigitated. In the *villous*, chorionic protrusions interdigitate with corresponding maternal crypts. The *labyrinthine placenta* represents a fusion of chorionic villi.

Fetal and Maternal Contributions

General Remarks. When considering the barriers across which physiologic exchange must occur, all the components between the

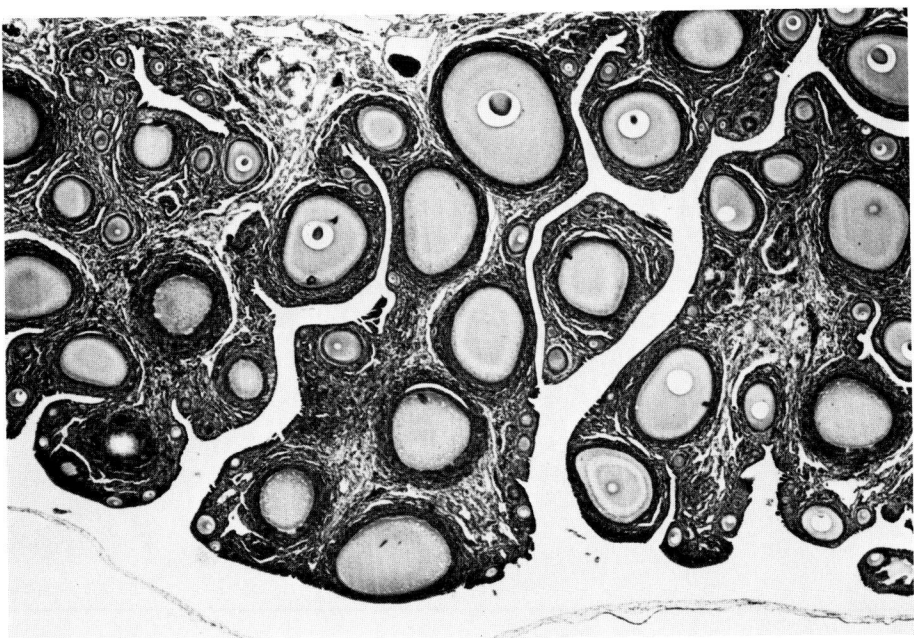

Fig. 24.30   A section of an avian ovary. The ovary is a pendulous structure suspended from the abdominal wall. X10.

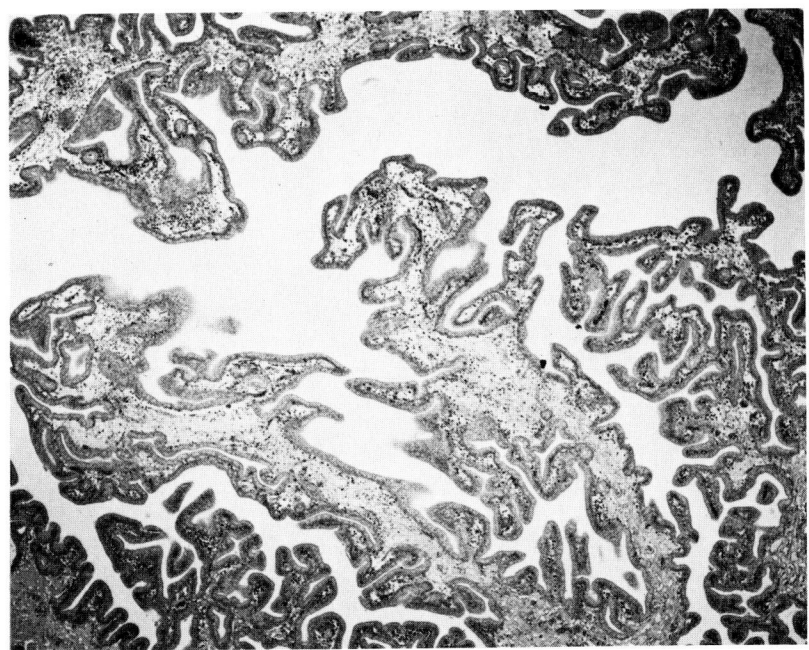

Fig. 24.31   A section of the infundibular portion of an avian oviduct. The tunica mucosa is highly folded and devoid of glands. X10.

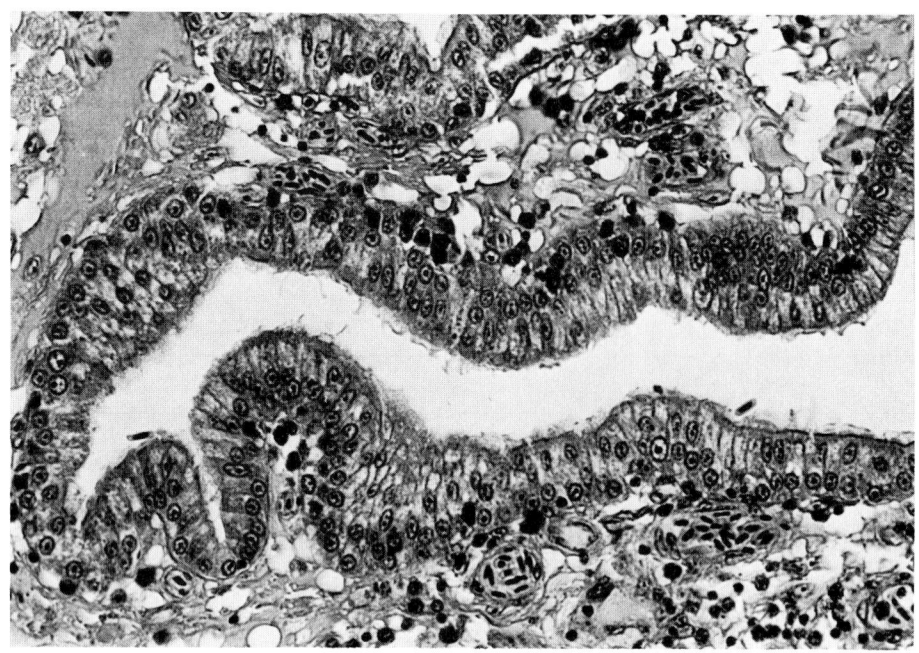

Fig. 24.32 Lining epithelium of an avian infundibulum. The lining epithelium is pseudostratified cilliated. Goblet cells may be present, but multicellular glands are absent. X125.

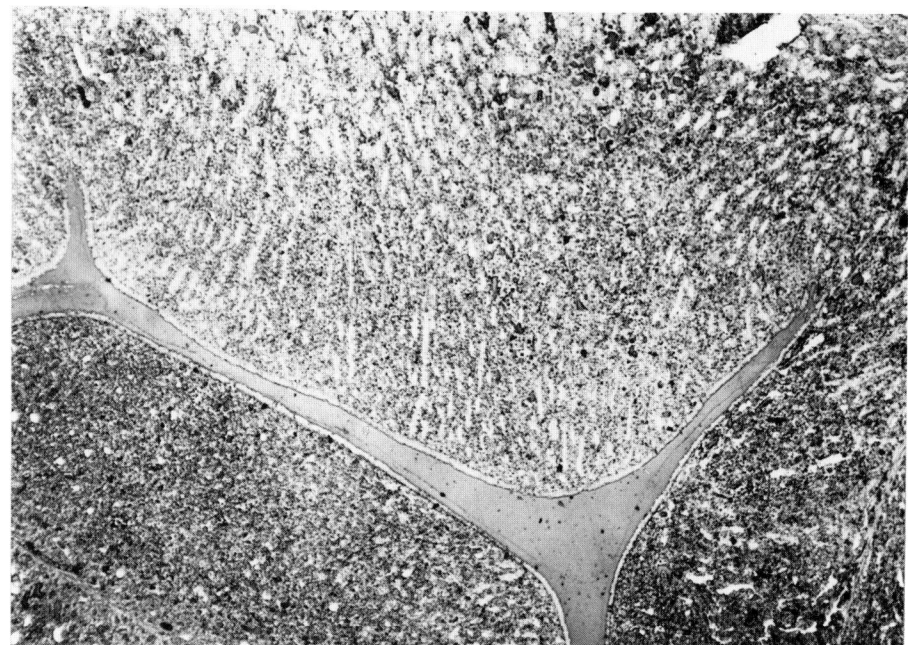

Fig. 24.33 Magnum of the avian oviduct. The tunica mucosa has pronounced folds and numerous branched tubular glands. X10.

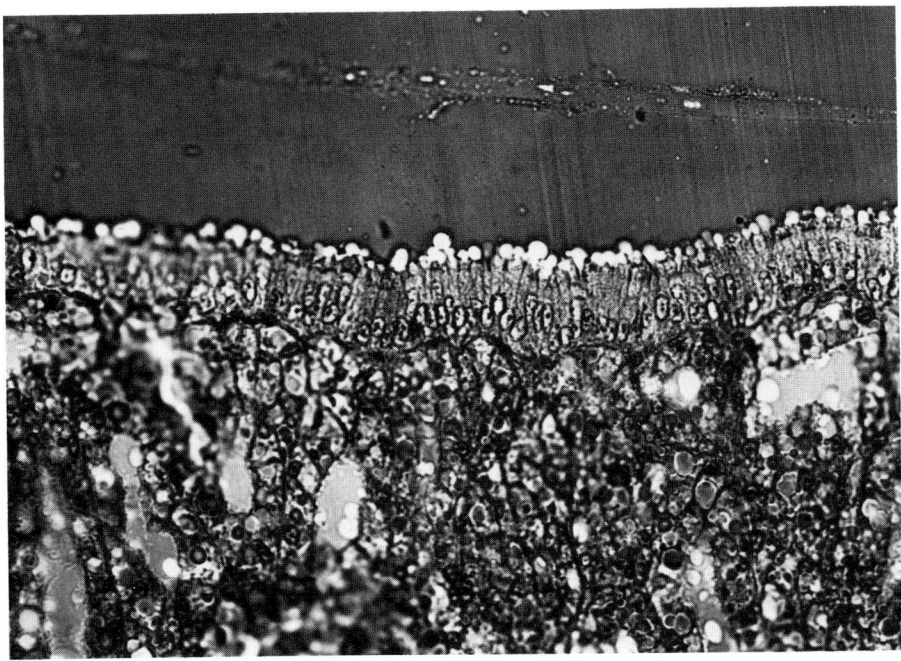

Fig. 24.34 Lining cells of the avian magnum. The lumen is filled with a proteinaceous secretory product. The lamina epithelialis consists of ciliated columnar cells. X125.

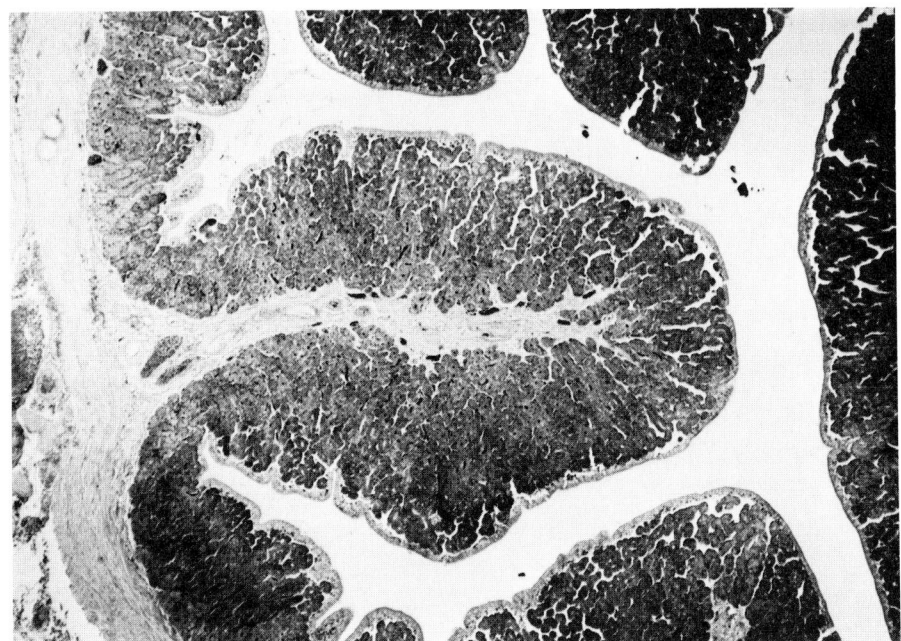

Fig. 24.35 Isthmus of the avian oviduct. The tunica mucosa has pronounced folds. Numerous mucosal glands (*dark areas*) comprise part of the tunica mucosa. X10.

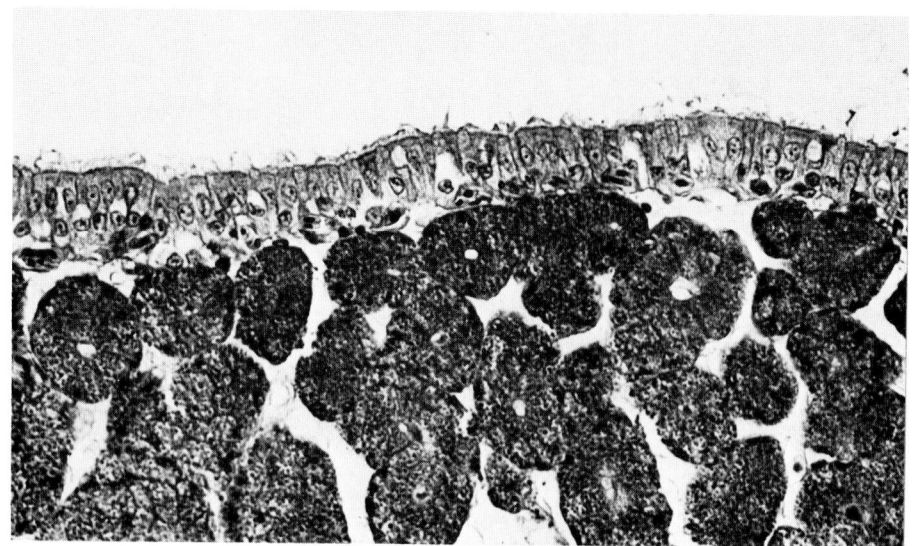

Fig. 24.36 Lining and glandular epithelium of the avian isthmus. Ciliated columnar epithelial cells line the lumen of the organ. Mucosal glands (*dark areas*) are branched and tubular. X100.

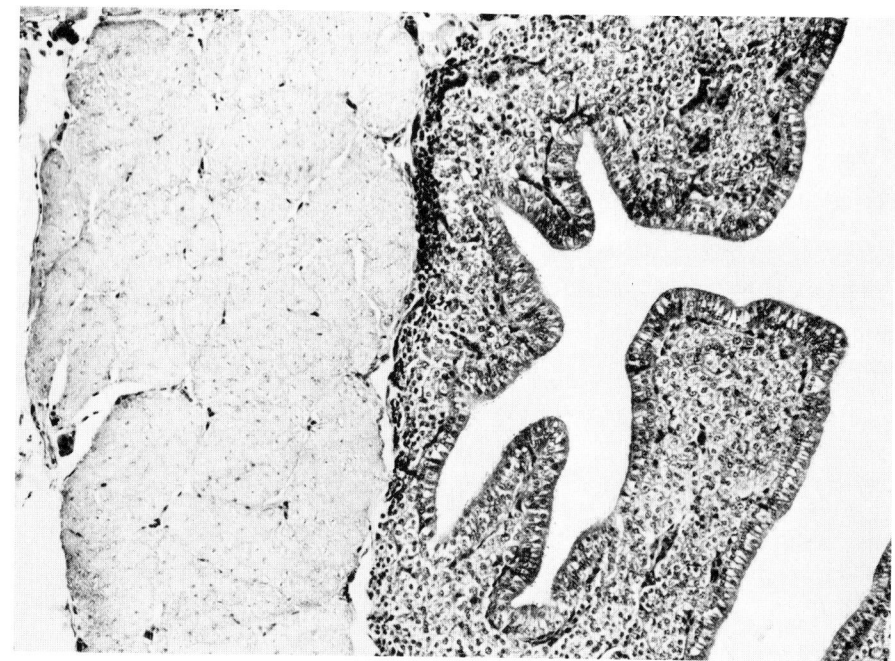

Fig. 24.37 A section of the avian uterus. The tunica mucosa is highly folded. This organ produces the shell of the egg. X50.

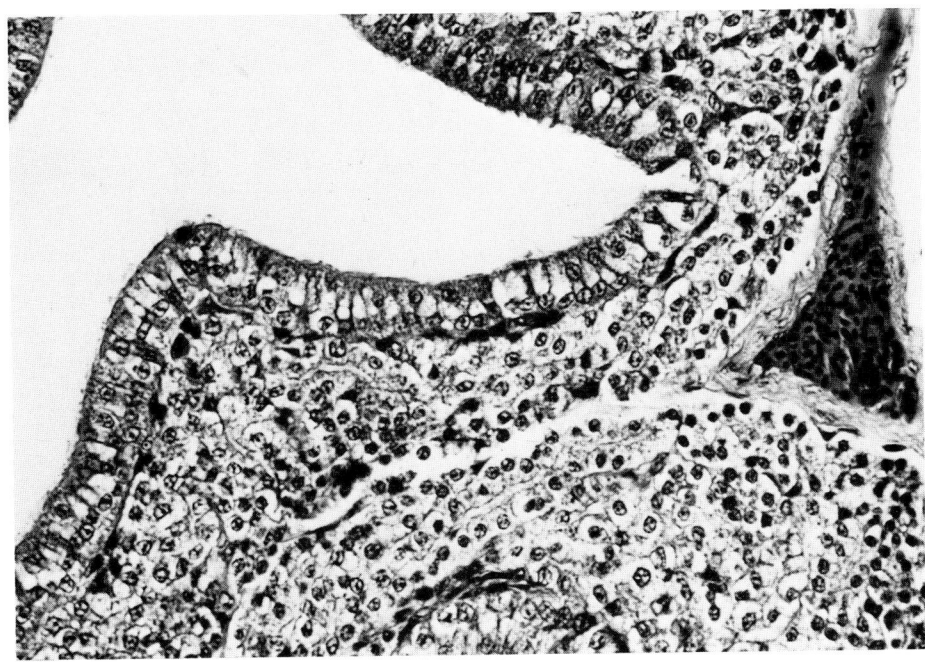

Fig. 24.38 Lining cells of the avian uterus. The lamina epithelialis consists of pseudostratified intermittently ciliated columnar epithelium. X125.

fetal and maternal capillaries must be included. The maximal barrier would include the following: *uterine endothelium, uterine connective tissue, uterine epithelium, chorionic epithelium, chorioallantoic connective tissue* and *allantoic endothelium*. Various placentas are formed by the intact relationship of these components or by the deletion of one or more of these components. On this basis, the following types of placenta are recognized: *epitheliochorial, syndesmochorial, endotheliochorial, hemochorial* and *hemoendothelial* (Fig. 24.27). In the formation of these compound terms, the first term refers to the maternal component, whereas the second term refers to the fetal component.

Epitheliochorial Placenta. In this type of placenta all six layers are present (Fig. 24.28). The chorionic and uterine epithelia are in contact with one another (Fig. 24.29). This configuration is nondeciduate and is typical of the sow, mare, cow and ewe.

Syndesmochorial Placenta. In this type of placenta the chorionic epithelium is in direct contact with the uterine connective tissue, the uterine epithelium having been eroded. This configuration is also nondeciduate. Although this type of placentation has been described in the ewe, current evidence is contrary to this.

Endotheliochorial Placenta. This type of placentation is characterized by the intimate contact of the chorionic epithelium with the uterine capillaries. Therefore, the uterine epithelium and connective tissue have been eroded. This is a deciduate type of placentation characteristic of carnivores.

Hemochorial Placenta. In hemochorial placentation, the chorionic epithelium is in direct contact with the maternal blood. This is achieved by the erosion of the uterine epithelium, connective tissue and endothelium. Further subdivision of this type of placentation is predicated upon the number of cell layers of the trophoderm in contact with the maternal blood. Thus, *hemomonochorial, hemodichorial* and *hemotrichorial* placentation is recognized.

Hemochorial placentation occurs in primates and rodents.

Hemoendothelial Placenta. This placentation is characterized by the endothelium of the fetal tissues being in direct contact with the maternal blood. It requires, therefore, that all three maternal components, as well as fetal epithelium and connective tissue, have been eroded.

It was believed that certain rodents possessed this type of placentation. Its existence, however, has been questioned.

Species Differences.

The following unified classification is based upon the previously discussed characteristics:

Swine: diffusely folded, epitheliochorial, nondeciduate.

Horse: diffusely villous, epitheliochorial, nondeciduate.

Ruminants: cotyledonary villous, epitheliochorial, nondeciduate.

Carnivores: zonary labyrinthine, endotheliochorial, deciduate.

Man: discoidal villous, hemochorial, deciduate.

Avian Reproductive System

General Remarks. The avian reproductive system is designed to facilitate internal fertilization as in the mammal. The oviduct and uterus, however, are modified to ensure the survival and development of the offspring outside the body. These structures, therefore, supply the necessary nutrients and enclose the offspring within a protective shell.

Only the left ovary and oviduct are retained in the adult as functional entities.

Ovary. The ovaries of birds are not as compact as those in mammals. Rather, the ovary consists of finger-like projections which are suspended pendulously from the abdominal wall by the mesovarium (Fig. 24.30). A cortex and medulla are distinguishable, but the latter is not well-developed and is diffuse. The cortex consists of "follicles" in various stages of development. Actually, the term follicle is a misnomer because an antrum does not develop. The oocytes and accompanying cells are extremely large structures. The follicle contains a primary oocyte, a single layer of membrana granulosa cells, a theca folliculi interna and a theca folliculi externa. The primary oocyte reaches a diameter, in some domesticated species, of approximately 30 mm. Ovulation is not followed by the development of a corpus luteum.

Oviduct. The avian oviduct is divided into five regions: *infundibulum, magnum, isthmus, shell gland* (uterus) and *vagina*.

The *infundibulum* is the funnel-like cranial extension of the oviduct (Fig. 24.31). The tunica mucosa is highly folded and vascularized. The lamina epithelialis mucosae consists of pseudostratified ciliated columnar epithelium with occasional goblet cells (Fig. 24.32). The lamina propria-submucosa is areolar connective tissue. Diffuse lymphatic tissue is commonly encountered. The tunica muscularis and tunica serosa are typical. This portion of the oviduct receives the ova, propels it toward the caudal part of the organ and facilitates fertilization.

The *magnum* is responsible for the deposition of the majority of the egg white (Fig. 24.33). The lamina epithelialis mucosae consists of ciliated columnar cells (Fig. 24.34). The lamina propria contains numerous branched tubular glands that are lined by a cuboidal or columnar epithelium. Secretory granules are present along the apical border. The connective tissue of the lamina propria-submucosa is areolar with much diffuse lymphatic tissue. The tunica muscularis and tunica serosa are typical.

The *isthmus* is lined by a ciliated columnar epithelium (Fig. 24.35). Numerous branched tubular glands extend into the lamina propria (Fig. 24.36). The glandular lining cells have basally displaced nuclei and lining cells have basally displaced nuclei and apically positioned granules. The remaining layers are similar to those of the magnum. This portion of the oviduct is responsible for the formation of the shell membranes. It may be responsible for the secretion of albuminoids also.

Unlike the mammalian uterus, the avian *uterus* is not designed for the implantation of the fertilized ova. Rather, the avian uterus is the *shell gland* (Fig. 24.37). Its secretory activity is responsible for the formation of the egg shell, as well as for the dilution of the albuminoids.

The lamina epithelialis mucosae consists of pseudostratified intermittently ciliated columnar epithelium (Fig. 24.38). Coiled tubular glands project into the underlying connective tissue. The glandular cells have a centrally placed nucleus, whereas the cytoplasm may contain apically positioned granules or vacuoles. The remaining portions of the wall are similar to the aforementioned structures.

The *vagina* is the region that follows the shell gland. It is devoid of glands and has a thick muscular tunic. It functions to propel the completed egg to the cloaca for expulsion to the outside environment.

References

Ovary

Amsterdam, A., Linder, H. and Gröschel-Stewart, U.: Localization of actin and myosin in the rat oocyte and follicular wall by immunofluorescence. Anat. Rec. *187*:311, 1977.

Anderson, E. and Albertini, D.: Gap junctions between the oocyte and companion follicle cells in the mammalian ovary. J. Cell Biol. *71*:680, 1976.

Baca, M. and Zamboni, L.: The fine structure of human follicular oocytes. J. Ultrastruct. Res. *19*:354, 1967.

Bjersing, L.: On the ultrastructure of the granulosa lutein cells in porcine corpus luteum. Z. Zellforsch. *82*:187, 1967.

Blanchette, E. J.: Ovarian steroid cells. II. The lutein cell. J. Cell. Biol. *31*:517, 1966.

Grandy, H. G. and Smith, D. E. (editors): *The Ovary*. Williams & Wilkins, Baltimore, 1963.

Hadek, R.: Morphological and histochemical study on the ovary of the sheep. Amer. J. Vet. Res. *19*:873, 1958.

Hope, J.: The fine structure of the developing follicle of the Rhesus ovary. J. Ultrastruct. Res. *12*:592, 1965.

Phemister, R. D., et al.: Time of ovulation in the Beagle bitch. Biol. Reprod. *8*:74, 1973.

Richardson, G. S.: Ovarian physiology. N. Engl. J. Med. *274*:1008, 1966.

Seguin, B. E.: Role of prostaglandins in bovine reproduction. J. Amer. Vet. Med. Assoc. *176*:1178, 1980.

Weakley, B. C.: Differentiation of the surface epithelium of the hamster ovary. An electron microscopic study. J. Anat. *105*:129, 1969.

Uterus and Associated Structures

Abdalla, O.: Observations on the morphology and histochemistry of the oviducts of the sheep. J. Anat. *102*:333, 1968.

Archibald, L. F., Baker, B. A., Clooney, L. L. and Godke, R. A.: A surgical method for collecting canine embryos after induction of estrus and ovulation with exogenous gonadotropins. Vet. Med. Sm. An. Clin. *75*:228, 1980.

Bal, H. S. and Getty, R.: Changing morphology of the uterine tubes of the domestic pig. (*Sus scrofa domesticus*) with age. J. Geront. *25*:347, 1970.

Dessouky, D. A.: Electron microscopic studies of the myometrium of the guinea pig. Amer. J. Obstet. Gynec. *100*:30, 1968.

Ferenczy, A., Richart, R. M., Agate, F. J., Jr., Purkerson, M. L. and Dempsey, E. W.: Scanning electron microscopy of the human fallopian tube. Science *175*:783, 1972.

Ginther, O. J.: Utero-ovarian relationships in cattle. Physiological aspects. J. Amer. Vet. Med. Assoc. *153*:1656, 1968.

Hook, S. J. and Hafez, E. S. E.: A comparative anatomical study of the mammalian uterotubal junction. J. Morph. *125*:159, 1968.

Pineda, M. H., Kainer, R. A. and Faulkner, L. C.: Dorsal median postcervical fold in the canine vagina. J. Amer. Vet. Med. Assoc. *34*:1487, 1973.

Schultz, R. H., Burcalow, H. B. and Fahning, M. L.: A karyometric study of epithelial cells lining the glands of the bovine endometrium. J. Reprod. Fertil. *19*:169, 1969.

Younes, M. S., Robertson, E. M. and Bencosme, S. A.: Electron microscope observations on Langerhans cells in the cervix. Amer. J. Obstet. Gynec. *102*:397, 1968.

Cyclic Changes in the System

Adams, E. C. and Hertig, A. T.: Studies on the human corpus luteum. I. Observations on the ultrastructure of development and regression of the luteal cells during the menstrual cycle. J. Cell. Biol. *41*:696, 1969.

Adams, E. C. and Hertig, A. T.: Studies on the human corpus luteum. II. Observations on the ultrastructure of luteal cells during pregnancy. J. Cell Biol. *41*:716, 1969.

Akins, E. L. and Morrissette, M. C.: Gross ovarian changes during estrous cycle of swine. Amer. J. Vet. Res. *29*:1953, 1968.

Fowler, E. H., Feldman, M. K. and Loeb, W. F.: Comparison of histologic features of ovarian and uterine tissues with vaginal smears of the bitch. Amer. J. Vet. Res. *32*:327, 1971.

Fowler, E. H., Loeb, W. F. and Wilson, G. P.: Vaginal cytologic examination of intact and ovariohysterectomized bitches with mammary neoplasia. Amer. J. Vet. Res. *31*:51, 1970.

Hatch, R. D.: Anatomic changes in the bovine uterus during pregnancy. Amer. J. Vet. Res. *2*:411, 1941.

Holst, P. A. and Phemister, R. D.: Onset of diestrus in the Beagle bitch: Definition and significance. Ame J. Vet. Res. *35*:401, 1974.

Johnston, S. D.: Diagnostic and therapeutic approach infertility in the bitch. J. Amer. Vet. Med. Asso *176*:1335, 1980.

McDonald, L. E.: *Veterinary Endocrinology and Repr duction*. Lea and Febiger, Philadelphia, 1969.

Peters, H. and Levy, E.: Cell dynamics of the ovaria cycle. J. Reprod. Fertil. *11*:227, 1966.

Sanger, V. L., Engle, P. H. and Bell, D. S.: The vagin cytology of the ewe during the estrous cycle. Ame J. Vet. Res. *19*:283, 1958.

Schutte, A. P.: Canine vaginal cytology. II. Cycli changes. J. Small Anim. Pract. *8*:307, 1967.

Wagner, W.: Bovine parturition. Compend. Cont. Ed Pract. Vet. *11*:517, 1980.

Comparative Placentology

Allen, W. R., Hamilton, D. W. and Moor, R. M.: Th origin of equine endometrial cup: Anat. Red. *177* 485, 1973.

Amoroso, E. C.: Histology of the placenta, foetal an neonatal physiology, Brit. Med. Bull. *17*:2, 1961.

Anderson, J. W.: Ultrastructure of the placenta and fet membranes of the dog. I. The placenta labyrinth Anat. Rec. *165*:5, 1969.

Ashley, C. A.: Study of the human placenta with th electron microscope. Arch. Path. Chicago *80*:377 1965.

Bjorkman, N.: The fine structure of the ovine placen tome. J. Anat. *99*:283, 1965.

Bjorkman, N.: Fine structure of the fetal-maternal are of exchange in the epitheliochorial and endotheli ochonial types of placentation. Acta. Anat. Suppl 1, *86*:1, 1973.

Bjorkman, N. H.: Fine structure of cryptal and tropho blastic giant cells in the bovine placentome. J. Ul trastruc. Res. *24*:249, 1968.

Bjorkman, N. H.: Light and electron microscopic studie on cellular alterations in the normal bovine placen tome. Anat. Rec. *163*:17, 1969.

Bjorkman, N. H.: *An Atlas of Placental Fine Structure* Williams & Wilkins Company, Baltimore, 1970.

Davies, J. and Glasser, S. R.: Histological and fin structural observations on the placenta of the rat Acta Anat. *69*:542, 1968.

Enders, A. C.: A comparative study of the fine structur of the trophoblast in several hemochorial placentas Amer. J. Anat. *116*:29, 1965.

Wimsatt, W. A.: Some aspects of the comparative anat omy of mammalian placentome. Amer. J. Obstet. *84*:11, Part 2, 1962.

Avian Reproductive Tract

Brambell, F. W. R.: The oogenesis of the fowl (*Gallus bankiva*). Phil. Trans. Royal Soc. (B). *214*:113, 1926.

Fell, H. F.: Histological studies of the gonads of the Fowl. II. The histogenesis of the so-called "luteal" cells in the ovary. Brit. J. Exp. Biol. *1*:293, 1924.

Fertuck, H. C. and Newstead. J. D.: Fine structural observations on magnum mucosa in quail and hen oviducts. Z. Zellforsch. *103*:447, 1970.

Hewitt, E. A.: The physiology of the reproductive system of the fowl. J. Amer. Vet. Med. Assoc. *95*:201, 1939.

Kohler, P. O., Grimley, P. M. and O'Malley, B. W.: Estrogen-induced cytodifferentiation of the ovalbu min-secreting glands of the chick oviduct. J. Cell Biol. *40*:8, 1969.

Narbaitz, R. and DeRobertis, R. M., Jr.: Postnatal evo lution of steriodogenic cells in the chick ovary. Histochemie *15*:187, 1968.

Nevalainen, T. J.: Electron microscope observations on the shell gland mucosa of calcium-deficient hens (*Gallus domesticus*). Anat. Rec. *164*:127, 1969.

Sturkie, P. D. and Mueller, W. J.: Reproduction in the female and egg production. *In*: Sturkie, P. D. (editor): *Avian Physiology*. 3rd edition, pp. 302–330, Springer-Verlag, New York, 1976.

25: Eye and Ear

General Characteristics

Introduction. The response of the organism to varied internal and external stimuli is dependent upon the distribution of different sensory receptors scattered throughout the body. A group of receptors or receptor organs that are classified apart from most of the somatic receptors comprise the *special sensory system*. The special sensory system is subdivided into general and visceral components. The special somatic afferent (SSA) system includes the eye and ear. The SSA receptors are responsive to visual (*eye*) and auditory (*cochlea*) information. The vestibular apparatus (*semicircular canals* and *saccules*) is considered to be part of the SSA system by some authors. It is a special proprioceptive apparatus that responds to linear and angular acceleration. The special visceral afferent (SVA) system consists of receptors that are responsible for gustatory and olfactory sensations (Chapters 19 and 21).

Eye

Anatomic Features

General remarks. The eyeball (*bulbus oculi*) is a globe-shaped structure that is flattened slightly along the optic (rostral-caudal) axis. Light enters the globe through the rostrally positioned, transparent *cornea*. The light continues through the aperture (*pupil*), the peripheral margins of which are defined by an adjustable diaphragm, the *iris*. Light then passes through a biconvex *lens* that is suspended from the *ciliary body*. Focusing of light upon the *retina* is accomplished usually by changing the curvature of the lens through the contraction and relaxation of *ciliary muscles*. Photosensitive cells (*rods* and *cones*) located within the retina transduce the photon energy into useable information by the body. Neural activity resulting from photoreceptor cell responsiveness is processed by the central nervous system as vision.

Development. The eye is a complex organ that is associated intimately with the central nervous system. The structural relationships within the eye and its relationship to the central nervous system can best be appreciated through an understanding of normal eye development. An understanding of the organogenesis of this structure simplifies the complexity, establishes a framework for evaluation of developmental anomalies and provides a basis for understanding the alteration of structure subsequent to ocular injury.

The embryonic components that contribute to the structure of the eye are derived from *ectoderm, neurectoderm* and *mesoderm*. After closure of the neural tube, lateral evaginations of the diencephalon, *optic vesicles*, grow toward and make contact with the ectoderm of the surface or presumptive skin (Fig. 25.1). The optic vesicle maintains its continuity with the neurectoderm of the diencephalon through an *optic stalk*. The optic stalk and vesicle are hollow structures. The continued growth of the optic vesicle causes an elongation of the optic stalk. The optic stalk serves as a guide for the ingrowing nerve fibers of the retina that form the optic nerve. The optic vesicle grows and invaginates to form a double-layered *optic cup* (Fig. 25.2). The invagination continues along the ventral border of the optic stalk as the *choroid fissure* (*optic fissure*). The inner and outer layers of the wall of the optic cup are separated by a space, *intraretinal space*. The outer layer develops into the *pigment epithelium* of the retina, whereas the inner layer becomes the *neural retina*.

While optic cup development progresses, the portion of the optic cup in contact with the surface ectoderm continues to grow and induces the formation of a *lens placode* in the surface ectoderm (Fig. 25.1). The lens placode invaginates, grows and pinches away from the surface ectoderm as a *lens vesicle* (Fig. 25.2). The lens vesicle, located within the "mouth" of optic cup, is separated from the inner wall of the optic cup by mesoderm. The space is destined to become the *vitreous body* (Fig. 25.3). The lens vesicle is separated from the surface ectoderm by mesoderm (Fig. 25.3). A cavitation that develops in this mesodermal space is lined by epithelial cells (*mesenchymal epithelium*). The mesenchymal epithelium forms the *iridopupillary membrane* and the rostral lining of the iris. Note that the iris consists of three layers of epithelial cells. The rostral mesenchymal epithelium is separated by mesoderm (connective tissue) from the pigmented and nonpigmented epithelium derived from the inner (neural) and outer (pigmented) layers of the optic cup.

The *sclera* is derived from the mesoderm peripheral to the developing eye and is homologous to the *dura mater* (Fig. 25.3). The sclera is dense connective tissue that encircles the eye and is continuous with the *stroma* or *substantia propria* of the *cornea*. The cornea from without inward consists of epithelium (surface ectoderm), substantia propria and mesenchymal epithelium that is reflected from the rostral surface of the iris

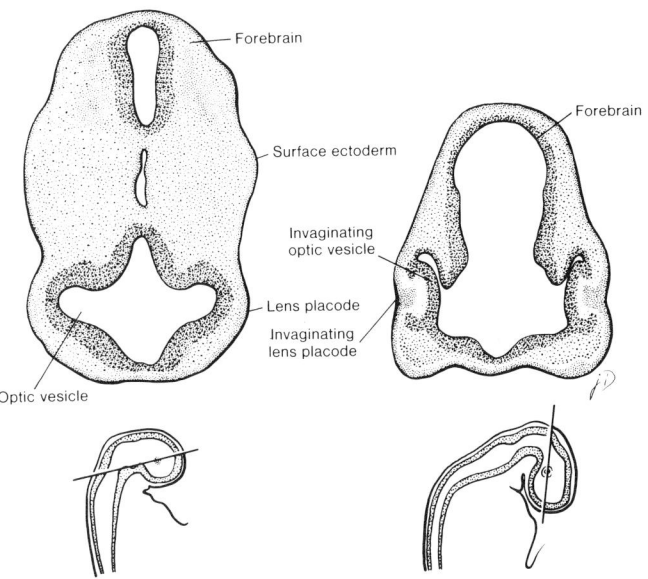

Fig. 25.1 Formation of the eye during the early somite stage of development. The optic vesicle evaginates from the neural tube, contacts the surface ectoderm and then begins to invaginate. All light micrographs are labeled as the magnification with the microscope before photographic enlarging. All electron micrographs are labeled as total magnification, including photographic enlarging.

(Fig. 25.3). The cavity between the caudal surface of the cornea and the rostral surface of the iris is the *anterior chamber*. It is continuous through the *pupil* with the *posterior chamber*, the space between the caudal surface of the iris and the rostral surface of the lens.

The mesoderm between the developing sclera and the outer wall of the developing eye is homologous to the *leptomeninges*. This mesoderm develops into the *vascular coat* or *uveal tract* of the eye. The components of the uveal tract include the *choroid, ciliary body* and *iridial stroma*. The choroid is associated intimately with the pigment epithelium. The ciliary part of the retina, the pigment epithelium and nonpigmented epithelium cover the ciliary body. The iridial part of the retina, two layers of pigmented cells, covers the caudal surface of the iris. The lens is suspended from the ciliary body by the delicate *suspensory ligament*.

The optic retina, (*pars optica retinae*) derived from the inner and outer walls of the optic cup, undergoes differential growth. The outer wall remains a single layer of cells, the *pigment epithelium*, separated by the *intra-retinal space* (*cavity of the optic cup, opticoel*) from the inner wall or *neural retina*. The neural retina grows and differentiates into a structure characterized by numerous layers of cells. The photoreceptor cells are the outermost portion of the inner layer. They and the pigment epithelium are homologous to *ependyma*. The remaining cellular layers of the neural retina are homologous to the *mantle* and *marginal layers* of the neural tube. The neural retina and pigment epithelium are "attached" to each other as nerve fibers from the neural retina emerge from the caudal pole at the *optic disc*. They are also attached to each other at the junction with the ciliary retina, the *ora ciliaris retinae*.

The innermost portion of the neural retina is adjacent to the *hyaloid membrane*, the peripheral lining of the vitreous body. A remnant of the *hyaloid artery*, the blood supply to the caudal aspect of the lens, may be apparent within a fold of the hyaloid membrane in the mature eyes in some species, notably the ox. The hyaloid artery gained access to the vitreous body and caudal aspect of the lens during the formation of the *choroid* or *optic fissure*. The portion of the hyaloid artery within the optic nerve is retained as the *central artery of the retina*.

Retinal detachment is related to the development of the pigmented and neural components of the retina. The intra-retinal space, obliterated in the mature eye, is a potential space that may reappear post trauma. *Persistent iridopupillary membranes* may remain as a complete covering over the pupil; however, they are observed most commonly as fibrous strands attached to the rostral surface of the lens and/or iris. A colobome, a cleft-like defect, may occur in any part of the eye along the tract of the choroid fissure. A cleft may occur in the iris, ciliary body, retina, choroid and optic nerve from the incomplete closure of the choroid fissure. Colobomas of the iris (*coloboma iridis*), optic nerve and optic disc are observed readily upon ophthalmic examination.

Organization. The wall of the eye is composed of three layers (tunics) that surround and enclose the refractive or dioptric components (Fig. 25.4). The three tunics of the globe are the *fibrous layer, vascular layer* and *nervous layer*. The outermost fibrous layer consists of the *sclera* over most of the eye and the *cornea* rostrally. The vascular layer or uveal tract is comprised of the *choroid, ciliary body* and *iris*. The innermost layer, *nervous tunic*, consists of the *retina*. The pigment epithelium and non-neural epithelium of the neural portion of the retina contribute to the formation of the ciliary body (*pars ciliaris retinae*) and iris (*pars iridica retinae*).

The *dioptric media* of the eye include the *cornea, aqueous humor, lens, vitreous body* and *retina*.

The eye is divisible into an *anterior compartment*, positioned rostrally between the lens and cornea, and a *posterior compartment* occupied by the vitreous body. The anterior compartment is divided into an *anterior chamber* and *posterior chamber*. The anterior chamber occurs between the cornea and iris. The point at which the iris and cornea are in contact is the *filtration angle*. The posterior chamber is the space between the lens and iris. The posterior chamber communicates with the anterior chamber through the pupil.

Fibrous Tunic

The fibrous tunic consists of the *sclera* and *cornea*.

Sclera

The *sclera* is composed of dense white fibrous connective tissue (DWFCT) that is rich in elastic fibers (Fig. 25.5). It is divisible into three zones: *episcleral zone, sclera proper* and *lamina fusca*.

Episclera. The outermost *episclera* (*episcleral zone* or *layer*) is a transparent fibroelastic connective tissue that is attached

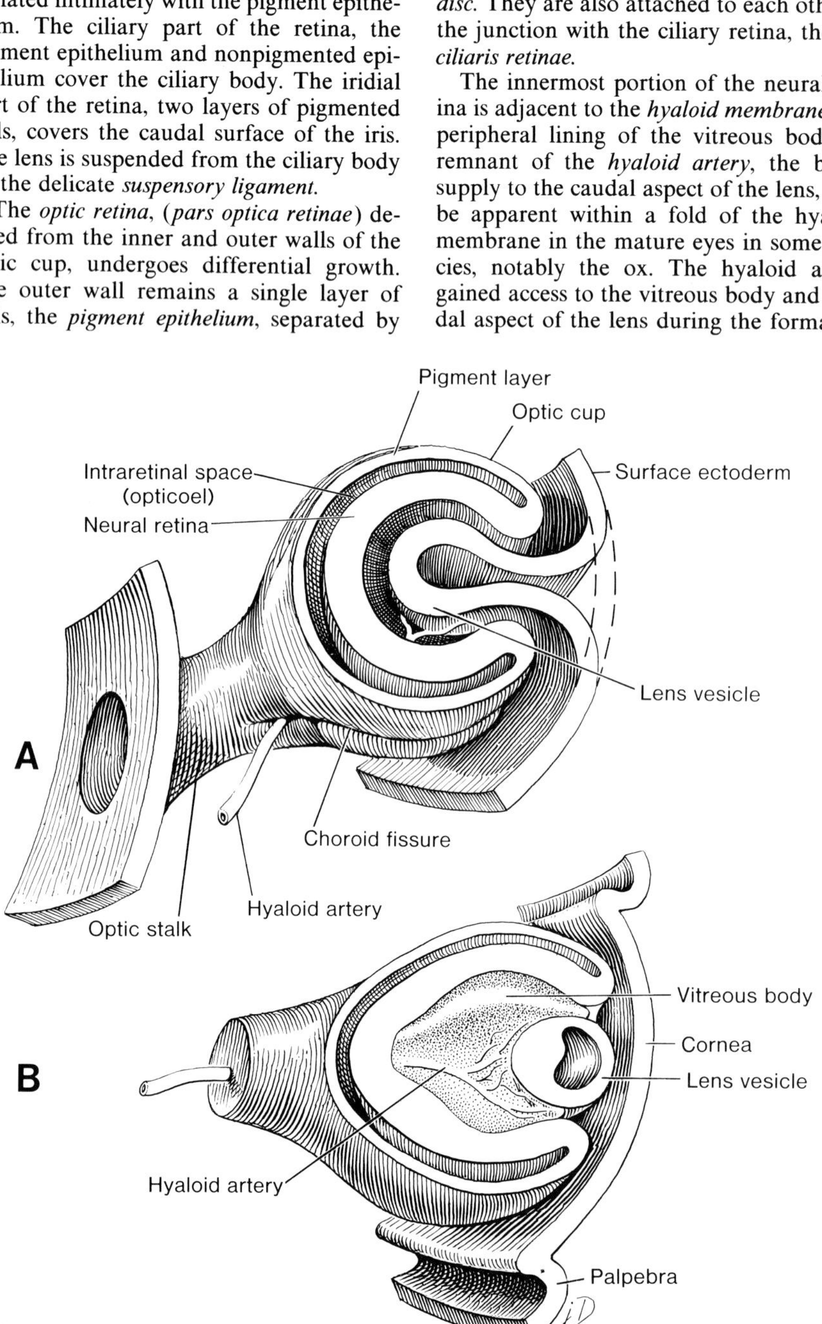

Fig. 25.2 Progression in the development of the eye. A. The optic cup has formed and is joined to the diencephalon by the optic stalk. The lens placode has invaginated to form a lens vesicle. The hyaloid artery has become associated with the choroid fissure. B. The lens vesicle has separated from the surface ectoderm.

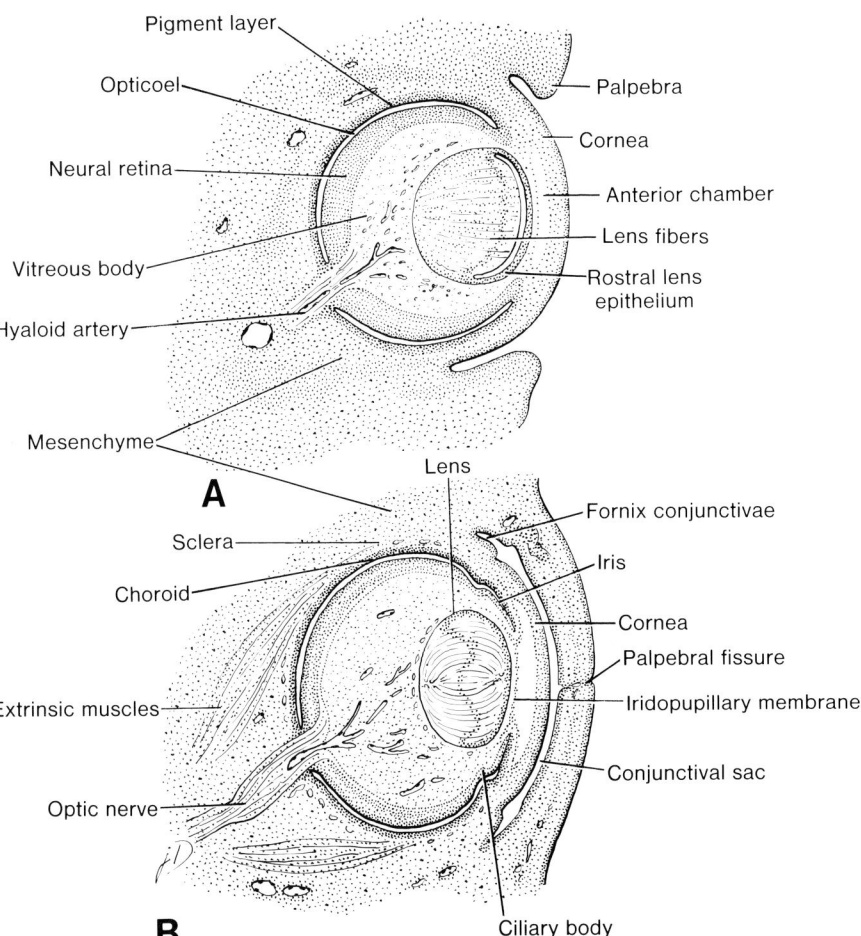

Fig. 25.3 Continued development of the eye. A. The lens is contained within the optic cup and the entire bulb is enclosed by mesenchyme. B. Anterior chamber has formed and the iridopupillary membrane is apparent. The fibrous and vascular tunics have begun to differentiate.

loosely to the sclera proper. The episcleral blood vessels supply the outer, relatively avascular portion of the sclera proper. The episclera, which unites with the sclera and cornea in the rostral portion of the eye, is adjacent to but separated from a peripherally positioned thin layer of dense fibrous connective tissue, *Tenon's capsule*, by *Tenon's space*. Tenon's capsule is the fascial covering of the globe (*fascia bulbi*). It is difficult to visualize grossly.

Sclera proper. The *middle portion* or *sclera proper* is a dense fibroelastic connective tissue that is vascularized minimally. It is continued rostrally into the connective tissue of the cornea. This point of transition is termed the *corneoscleral junction* and contains blood vessels and lymphatics. The edge of the cornea at this junction is termed the *limbus*.

The fibrous components of the sclera, collagen and elastin, comprise successive layers of flattened laminae that are wider than they are thick (Fig. 25.5). The laminae radiate in all directions around the globe and interlace with each other. Rostrally, the fibers are oriented in a circular direction around the optical axis, affording firm at-

tachment points for the insertion of the extraocular muscles.

Lamina fusca. The *inner portion* or *lamina fusca* is a fibroelastic connective tissue that is especially rich in elastic fibers. The presence of pigment cells that probably migrated to the sclera from the juxtaposed choroid imparts a brown coloration to the lamina fusca.

Cornea

The *cornea* is the transparent extension of the sclera. The transition from opaque sclera to transparent cornea occurs crisply at the *corneoscleral junction (limbus)*. The corneal edge of the junction is overlapped by the sclera. The scleral vessels extend to the limbus but do not cross the corneoscleral junction normally.

The cornea consists generally of five layers: *epithelium*, *Bowman's membrane*, *substantia propria*, *Descemet's membrane* and *mesenchymal epithelium* (*endothelium*) (Fig. 25.6).

Epithelial layer. The *rostral epithelial covering of the cornea* is a nonkeratinized stratified squamous epithelium. The epithelial covering of the cornea is continuous with

the *bulbar conjunctival epithelium*. It continues as the *palpebral conjunctival epithelium* at the *fornix conjunctivae*. The bulbar conjunctival epithelium and its associated connective tissue comprise a mucous membrane called the *bulbar conjunctiva*. The *palpebral conjunctiva* is constituted similarly.

The corneal epithelium varies in thickness but contains basal, intermediate and superficial cells. The epithelium is richly endowed with numerous naked nerve endings.

Bowman's membrane. *Bowman's membrane* or the *rostral limiting membrane* is a combination of the basement membrane and a feltwork of fine collagenous fibers. It is most clearly evident in primates but is defined vaguely in other species.

Substantia Propria. The *substantia propria* forms the bulk of the cornea. It consists of collagenous fibers disposed in platelike configurations. Flattened fibroblasts (*keratoblasts*) are contained within the interfibrillar spaces. The ground substance consists of *mucosubstances* (chondroitin sulfate, keratan sulfate, hyaluronic acid) that are essential for the maintenance of proper corneal hydration. Numerous unmyelinated nerve fibers are present, but the substantia propria is devoid of blood vessels.

Caudal Limiting Membrane. The *caudal limiting membrane* or *Descemet's membrane* separates the substantia propria from the endothelium. Although considered to be a basal lamina, electron microscopic investigations have revealed it to be an ordered, three-dimensional array of atypical collagen.

Mesenchymal Epithelium. The covering of the caudal border of the cornea is achieved by *mesenchymal epithelium*. The mesenchymal epithelial lining of the cornea as well as the lining of the rostral iridial surface is commonly termed *endothelium*. These cells are not similar morphologically to true endothelial lining cells of blood and lymphatic vessels. The corneal endothelium consists of large squamous or low cuboidal cells that form a tightly interdigitated cellular covering over the caudal margin of the cornea, separating the cornea proper from the aqueous humor of the anterior chamber. However, the endothelium of the anterior chamber is continuous with the endothelial lining cells of the venous plexus through which aqueous humor is returned to the circulation. Being aware of the synonymous use of mesenchymal epithelium and endothelium precludes confusion.

Functional Correlates. Various structural modifications of the cornea are characteristic among domestic animals. The size of the cornea varies. Nocturnal animals have relatively larger corneas than their diurnal counterparts. The cornea of nocturnal animals may comprise 35% of the surface of the globe. The relative surface area of the cornea of domestic animals ranges from 17–30%. The thickness of the cornea is species variable, and individual corneas, except in

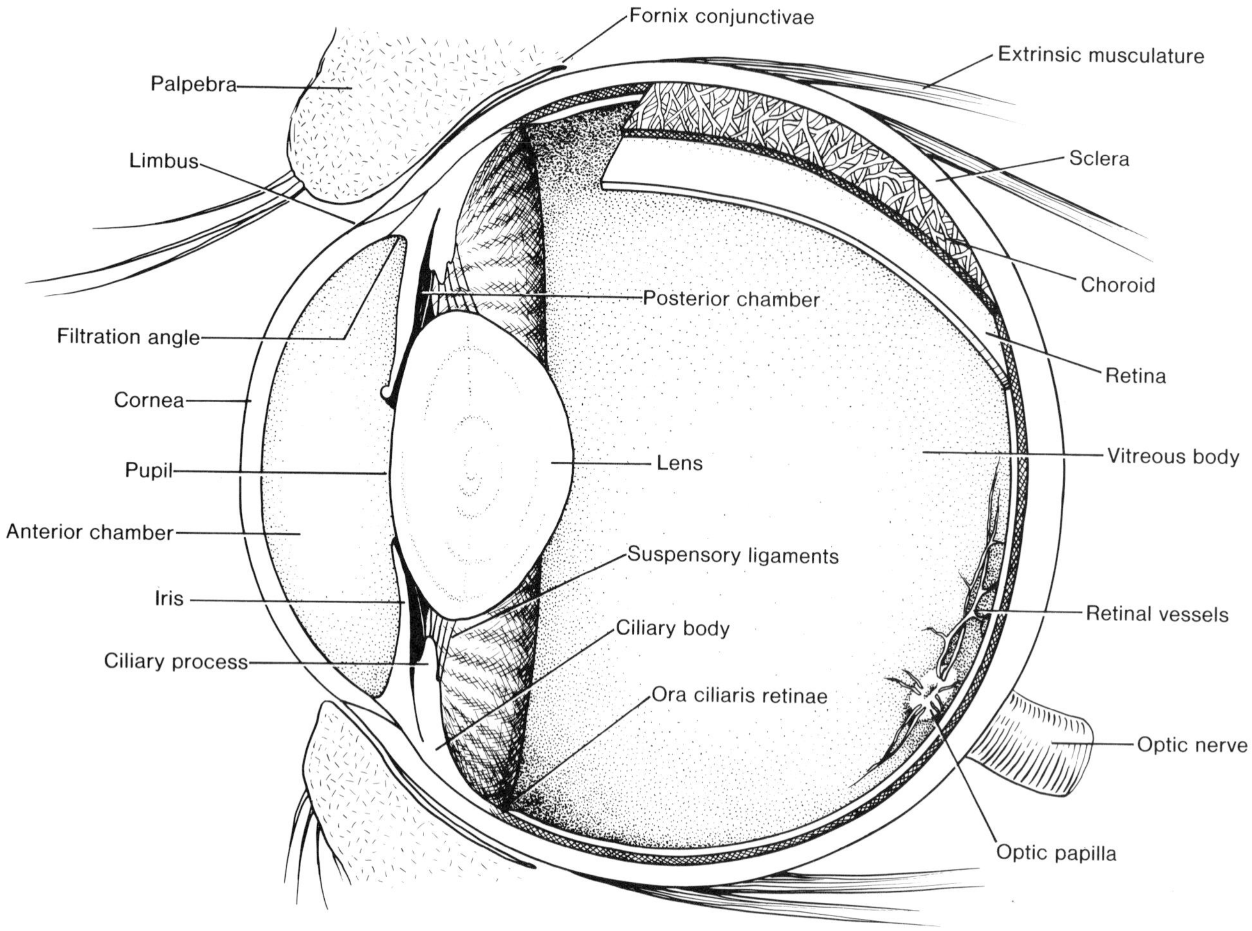

Fornix conjunctivae

Palpebra

Extrinsic musculature

Limbus

Sclera

Choroid

Filtration angle

Posterior chamber

Cornea

Retina

Pupil

Lens

Vitreous body

Anterior chamber

Iris

Suspensory ligaments

Retinal vessels

Ciliary process

Ciliary body

Ora ciliaris retinae

Optic nerve

Optic papilla

Fig. 25.4 A diagram of a parasagittal section of a bovine eye.

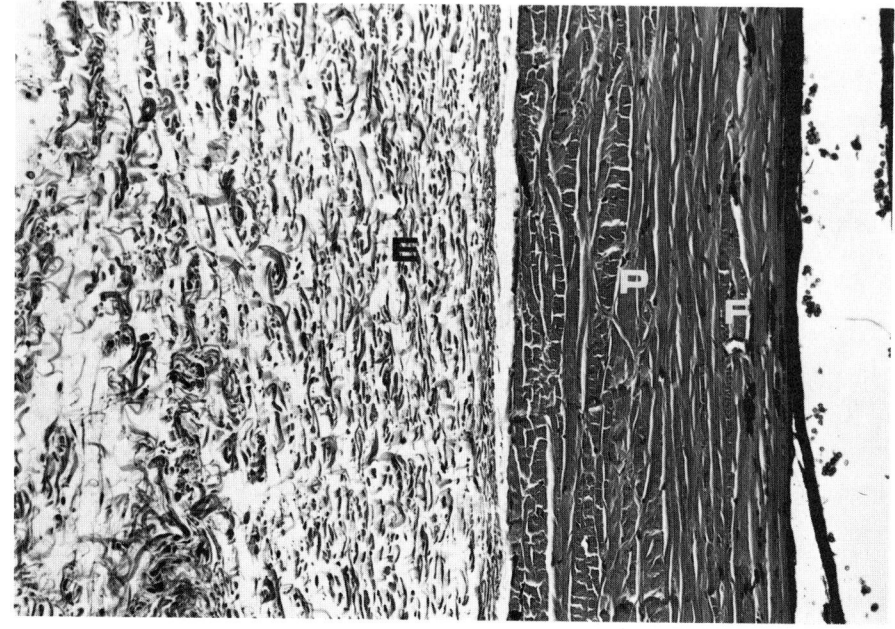

Fig. 25.5 Sclera of a canine eye. The episclera (E) is fibroelastic tissue. The sclera proper (P) is dense fibroelastic tissue that is vascularized minimally. The lamina fusca (F) is fibroelastic tissue which is pigmented. X40.

man, are not a uniform thickness. The thickness of the cornea of most domestic animals ranges between 0.56 to 1.0 mm. The centers of the bovine, canine, feline and porcine corneas are thicker than the periphery, whereas the reverse occurs in the horse.

Transparency is the essential property of normal corneal function. The transparency of the cornea is attributable to the orderly arrangement of its constituent collagenous fibers. Collagenous fibers are arranged in laminae that parallel the corneal surface. Intralaminal fibers are parallel to each other, but the laminae are oriented in different direction as they parallel the surface. By comparison, the random arrangement of collagenous fibers in the sclera contributes to its opacity. The amount of water (hydration) within the substantia propria also contributes to corneal transparency. Edema of the cornea is characterized by various degrees of corneal opacity that range from a minor opacity (*nebula*), light gray opacity (*macula*) to a dense white opacity (*leukoma*). The intact and normally functioning stratified squamous epithelium and mesenchymal endothelium are essential barriers that

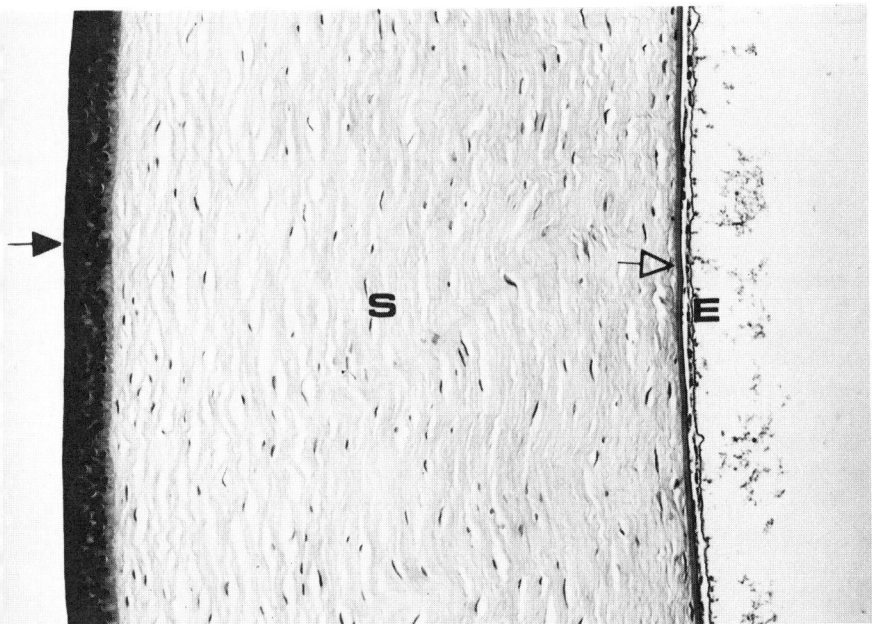

Fig. 25.6 Cornea of a canine eye. The rostral epithelium (*solid arrow*), substantia propria (S), Descemet's membrane (*open arrow*) and endothelium (E) are indicated. Bowman's membrane, a light microscopic structural feature of primate eyes, is not apparent. The endothelium is artifactually displaced from the cornea. X40.

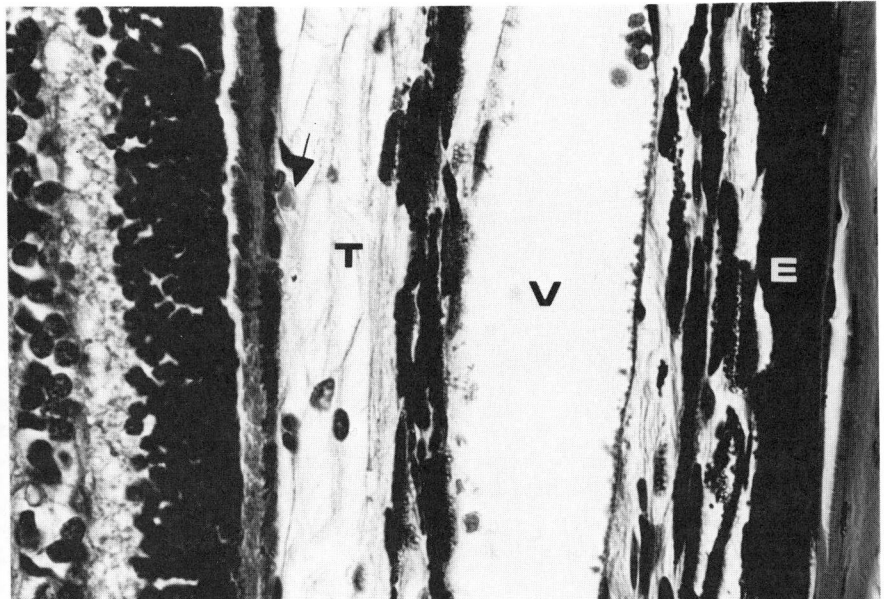

Fig. 25.7 Choroid of a canine eye. The epichoroid (E), lamina vasculosa (V), cellular tapetum (T) and choriocapillary layer (*solid arrow*) are indicated. X160.

by cellular migration without mitosis. *Deep wounds* into the substantia propria are characterized by inflammation. The cornea, devoid of its superficial epithelial lining, swells and becomes cloudy. Migration and mitosis of basal epithelial cells accounts for epithelial repair. Because the formation of the basement membrane occurs at a slower rate than epithelial cell replacement, new lining cells are attached loosely to the cornea and are sensitive to reinjury. Neovascularization from the limbic blood vessels occurs within 3–6 days of injury. Fibroblasts which accompany the nascent blood vessels and regenerating keratoblasts deposit collagen randomly, accounting for the resulting corneal scar. Complete resolution of the repair process may result in minimal scarring and a loss of the neovascularization. *Penetrating wounds* into the anterior chamber disrupt all corneal components, including the endothelium. Fibrin originating from the aqueous humor plugs the defect. The repair of such a wound requires the resolution of the fibrin clot, regeneration of the endothelium and the other events described previously.

Species differences characterize the susceptibility of the cornea to injury and the repair of the cornea subsequent to injury. Ruminant corneas are the least sensitive to injury and heal rapidly. Feline corneas are not characterized by extensive neovascularization and heal slowly with minimal scarring. Conversely, canine corneas develop extensive neovascularization. The equine cornea is the most sensitive cornea, reacts severely to injury, heals slowly and culminates in extensive cicatrization.

Allographic corneal transplant is an effective method of repair of certain types of corneal injuries. The cornea, devoid of blood and lymphatic vessels is a "privileged site" that may protect the transplant from the host's immunologic response.

Corneoscleral Junction. The *corneoscleral junction*, the transition from opaque sclera to transparent cornea, is an important anatomic landmark during an ophthalmic examination. Scleral blood vessels terminate at this point and the region contains the apparatus for the return of aqueous humor to the general circulation. The limbus is the point of gradual transition from rostral corneal epithelium to bulbar conjunctival epithelium. Bowman's membrane terminates at the limbus. The conjunctival stroma, interdigitated between the conjunctival epithelium and rostral attachment of Tenon's capsule, contributes to the *limbic conjunctiva*. The limbic conjunctiva continues as the *palpebral conjunctiva*.

Vascular Tunic

The *vascular tunic* or *uveal tract* consists of the *choroid coat, ciliary body* and *iris*. The uveal tract is not continued rostrally adjacent to the cornea but is reflected as the ciliary body and iris.

prevent the imbibition of water and resultant corneal opacity.

The avascular cornea is dependent upon diffusion of metabolites, including O₂, from three sources: peripherally positioned limbic capillaries, aqueous humor and tear film. Although the tear film may not be a primary source of metabolites, it is a major source of dissolved O₂.

Repair. The cornea, as evidenced by its developmental origin, is modified skin. The most common congenital lesion of the cornea is a *dermoid growth* (*choristoma*)—the development of long (ox, dog) or short (horse) hairs and some adipose tissue within the cornea. Since the cornea is modified skin, the principles governing the repair of the integument apply.

Superficial wounds involving the rostral lining epithelium heal rapidly by epithelial basal cell migration and subsequent mitosis; however, a simple, *superficial scratch* heals

Choroid

The choroid coat is subdivided into five layers: *epichoroid, lamina vasculosa, tapetum, lamina choriocapillaris, lamina elastica choroidea* (Fig. 25.7).

Epichoroid. The *epichoroid* layer is also referred to as the *suprachoroid* layer. This layer is separated from the lamina fusca by a *perichoroidal* or *suprachoroidal* space. However, collagenous fibers pass through this space and attach the tunics to each other. This avascular layer consists of a loose array of collagenous fibers, chromatophores and fibroblasts.

Lamina Vasculosa. The *lamina vasculosa* consists of large vessels embedded within a loose connective tissue that contains some chromatophores.

Tapetum. The *tapetum (tapetum lucidum)* is a fibrous or cellular layer of the choroid coat positioned between the lamina vasculosa and choriocapillary layer. The tapetum, often described as a light-reflective surface or "ocular mirror," ostensibly reflects light back to the photoreceptors in the retina to enhance dark-adapted *(scotopic)* vision—vision that occurs under conditions of poor illumination. The shape, size, color and distribution of the tapetum along the ocular fundus is species-variable. The tapetum is responsible for the "eyeshine" that is obvious when light enters the eye under dark circumstances—at night or under reduced illumination during a fundic examination with an ophthalmoscope.

A *fibrous tapetum*, characteristic of many ungulates, consists of interdigitated layers of collagenous fibers and fibroblasts. A *cellular tapetum* is characteristic of carnivores (Fig. 25.7). It consists of various layers of elongated, flattened polygonal cells *(fibroblasts)* that have characteristic crystalline structures containing zinc. The cells of each layer are arranged in tandem, and their long axes are oriented parallel to the retina. The highly pigmented, nonreflective portion of the fundus is the *nontapetal region* of the eye. A tapetum lucidum does not occur in the eyes of swine and man.

Choriocapillary layer. The *choriocapillary layer (lamina capillarium)* is a layer that is rich in capillaries. These are the vascular supply that provide nourishment for the outer part of the tunica nervosa.

Elastic Membrane. The *elastic membrane* is an accumulation of elastic fibers adjacent to the basal lamina of the pigmented epithelium. It is also referred to as *Bruch's membrane.*

Ciliary Body

The *ciliary body* is the anterior continuation of the choroid (Fig. 25.8). It consists of contributions from the choroid and retina. The ciliary body begins at the *ora ciliaris retinae*, the point at which the nervous portion of the retina stops (Fig. 25.9). The pigmented epithelium and a nonnervous columnar cell continuation of the retina continue rostrally to cover the ciliary body.

Histologic Organization. The bulk of the ciliary body consists of areolar connective tissue rich in elastic fibers, an extensive capillary network and smooth muscle (Fig. 25.10). The smooth muscle, *ciliary muscle*, consists of three layers that arise from the ciliary tendon that is attached to the sclera. Ciliary muscles of domestic animals are generally not well developed and result in poor accommodation potential.

The mass of smooth muscle, areolar connective tissue and vasculature is bounded by an *elastic lamina*. This is the anterior continuation of *Bruch's membrane*. Internal to this membrane is the *basal lamina* of the *pigmented epithelium* of the retina that is continued rostrally. Internal to this cellular layer is the *ciliary epithelium*. This layer of columnar cells is the rostral continuation of nonnervous and nonpigmented cells that began at the *ora ciliaris retinae*. This bilayered sheet of cells comprises the *pars ciliaris retinae* (Fig. 25.11). The *internal limiting membrane* is a peripheral fibrillar condensation of the vitreous body. It covers the retina and ciliary body, continues rostra[l] and blends with the fibers that extend fro[m] the ciliary process to the lens.

Ciliary Process. The *ciliary process* is t[he] most rostral extension of the ciliary body [at] the base of the iris. Zonular fibers exte[nd] from it as suspensory fibers of the lens. T[he] extensive capillary network of the cilia[ry] process and associated epithelium are [re]sponsible for the elaboration of aqueo[us] humor into the posterior chamber of t[he] anterior compartment.

Functional Correlates. Contraction of t[he] ciliary musculature does not stretch the le[ns] and accommodate it for distant visio[n.] Rather, contraction of the muscle fibe[rs] causes the sclera to indent slightly. Th[is] relieves the tension on the suspensory fibe[rs] that causes the lens to thicken for clo[se] vision. When these muscle fibers are relaxe[d] the elasticity of the supporting coat flatte[ns] the lens for distant vision.

The ciliary muscles are innervated b[y] postganglionic fibers of the parasympathet[ic] nervous system. The preganglionic fiber[s] originating in the parasympathetic nucle[us] (Edinger-Westphal nucleus) of the oculo[-]

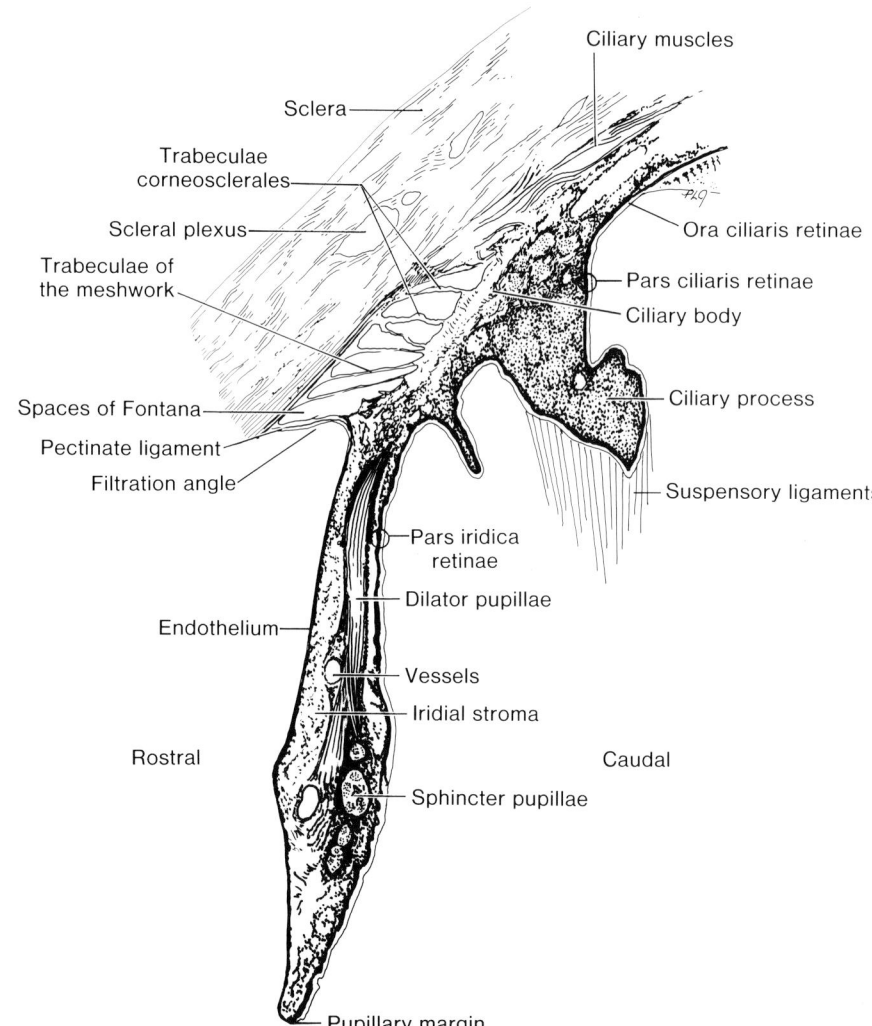

Fig. 25.8 An idealized drawing of the anterior uvea (iris and ciliary body) and associate[d] structures of a canine eye.

Labels in figure:
Ciliary muscles
Sclera
Trabeculae corneosclerales
Scleral plexus
Trabeculae of the meshwork
Spaces of Fontana
Pectinate ligament
Filtration angle
Endothelium
Rostral
Pars iridica retinae
Dilator pupillae
Vessels
Iridial stroma
Sphincter pupillae
Pupillary margin
Ora ciliaris retinae
Pars ciliaris retinae
Ciliary body
Ciliary process
Suspensory ligaments
Caudal

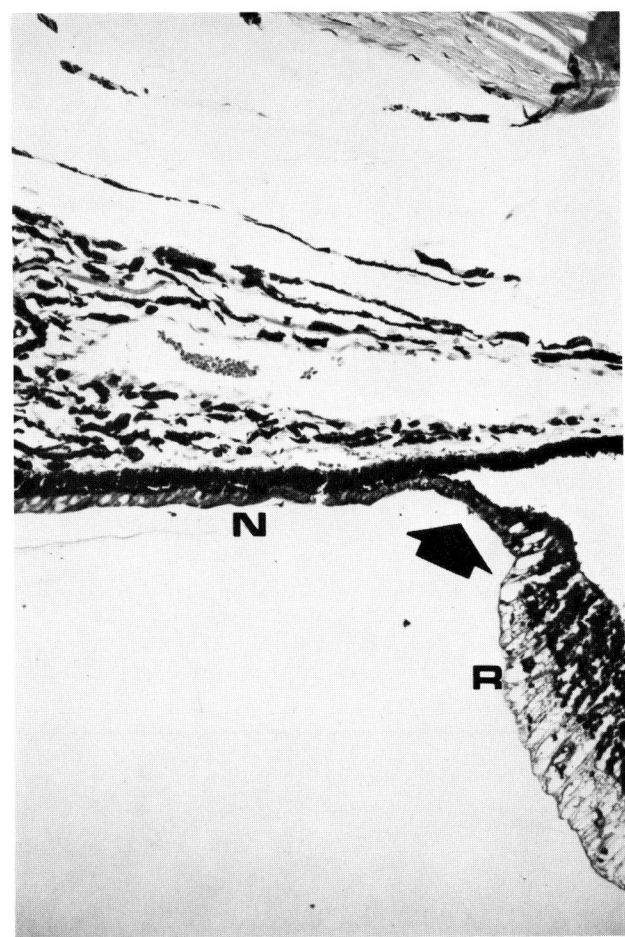

ig. 25.9   Ora ciliaris retinae of the canine eye. The ora ciliaris retinae (*arrow*) is the rostral ontinuation of the nonneural retina (N) as the double-layered epithelial covering of the ciliary ɔdy, ciliary processes and caudal aspect of the iris. R, *pars optica retinae*. X40.

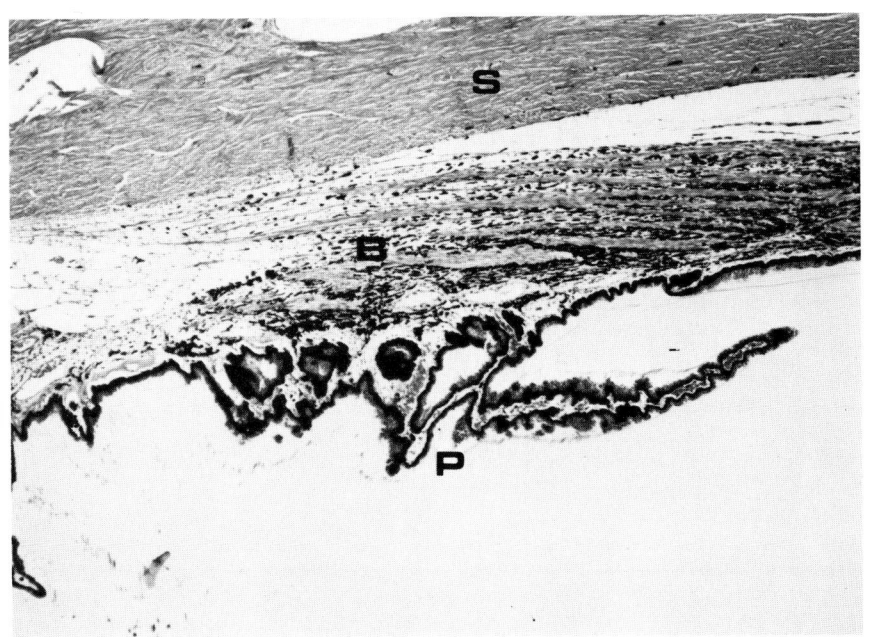

ig. 25.10   Ciliary body and processes of a canine eye. The ciliary body (B) and processes (P) ʳe internal to the sclera (S). The ciliary body and processes are part of the anterior uveal tract. he choroid comprises the posterior uvea. X10.

motor nerve, reach the ciliary ganglion, synapse with the parasympathetic ganglion cells and emerge as *short ciliary nerves* (postganglionic fibers) to the globe.

Iris

The *iris* is the extension of the choroid coat into the anterior compartment (Fig. 25.8, 25.12).

Histologic Organization. The iris is oriented radially and its distal margin defines the *pupil*. The rostral border of the iris is covered by *endothelial cells* (*mesenchymal epithelium*) that are reflected from the posterior lining of the cornea. These cells reside on the *rostral limiting layer* that consists of basal lamina, pigmented cells as well as collagenous and reticular fibers. The *iridial stroma* consists of areolar connective tissue, blood vessels, chromatophores and smooth muscle. The *pupillary sphincter* consists of a mass of circumferentially oriented smooth muscle fibers along the pupillary border of the iris. The *pupillary dilator* consists of radially oriented fibers along the caudal border of the iris.

The caudal border of the iris is covered by the same cells as the ciliary body. The cells include the anterior extension of the pigmented epithelium of the retina and the ciliary epithelial cells. These cells form the *pars iridica retinae*.

Corpora nigra (*iridial granules*) occur along the pupillary margin of the iris in horses and ruminants (Fig. 25.12). Iridial granules are well vascularized and proliferative extensions of the iridial stroma and pigment epithelium (Fig. 25.13). The cyst-like structures vary in size among ungulates and are most prominent along the dorsal border of the equine pupillary opening. The corpora nigra of ruminants may be of equal size along the dorsal and ventral margin of the pupil. The iridial granules may function in the elaboration of aqueous humor, as well as occluding the central portion of the pupil when the pupillary sphincter contracts.

Functional Correlates. The iris and ciliary body comprise the *anterior uvea*. (The choroid is the *posterior uvea*.) Inflammatory changes of one of the components of the anterior uvea (*anterior uveitis*) usually affects the other because of their intimate relationship to each other.

The iris lies in direct contact with the lens, and alterations of lens curvature or position are reflected as altered iridial curvatures. Iridial pigmentation differences are characteristic of domestic animals. The distribution of iridial pigment in the dog normally imparts a two-toned (*heterochromia*) distribution of brown pigment. The feline iris is usually a single color or mixture of pigment without pigmentary zonation. The irides of ungulates are characterized by an even distribution of pigment. Hyperpigmentary changes in the iris are suggestive of chronic inflammation. Hypopigmentation of the iris is apparent in subalbinotic and albinotic animals.

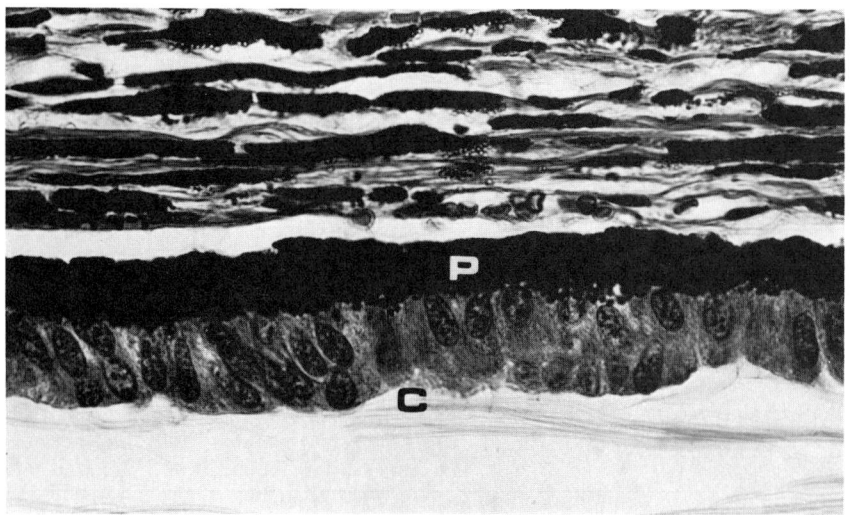

Fig. 25.11   Pars ciliaris retinae of a canine eye. This double layer of cells consists of pigment epithelium (P) and the nonneural epithelial continuation (C) of the neural retina. X160.

surrounded by a basement membrane upon which endothelial cells reside. The trabecular meshwork is continuous peripherally with a fine meshwork of trabeculae called the *trabeculae corneosclerales,* which are subjacent to the inner surface of the sclera. Adjacent to the anterior chamber, the trabecular meshwork coalesces as *pectinate ligaments.* The pectinate ligaments of the horse are visible at the filtration angle by direct examination, because the corneoscleral junction does not completely overlap the filtration angle. In other species, a special optical device, a goniolens, is necessary to visualize the pectinate ligaments and filtration angle. Gonioscopy is an important adjunctive procedure used to evaluate the filtration angle, especially in cases of glaucoma.

Aqueous humor passes from the anterior chamber through the spaces between the pectinate ligaments into the spaces of the trabecular meshwork. The fluid continues through the spaces associated with the trabeculae corneosclerales to a scleral venous

Because of the method of development of the anterior chamber, varying degrees of *persistent pupillary membranes* may be observed (Fig. 25.14). Although complete obliteration of the pupil may occur, most commonly fibrous strands originating from the iris may project into the anterior chamber or attach to the iris, lens and/or cornea.

The smooth muscle of the iris is innervated by postganglionic fibers of the autonomic nervous system. The pupillary sphincter receives its innervation from the parasympathetic fibers originating in the Edinger-Westphal nucleus of the oculomotor nerve. The pupillary dilator receives its sympathetic innervation from postganglionic fibers originating in the cranial cervical ganglion of the sympathetic trunk. The integrity of the innervation of the two muscle masses is essential for maintaining proper muscle tone and pupillary diameter. The sympathetic innervation of the eye and periorbita is responsible for the smooth muscle tone of the periorbita, pupillary dilator, tarsus and third eyelid (cat). The normal smooth muscle tone is manifested as normal eyeball protrusion, pupillary dilation, width of the palpebral fissure and third eyelid retraction, respectively. Disruption of the sympathetic innervation of the eye and periorbita (*Horner's Syndrome*) may be manifested as a sunken eyeball (enophthalmus), drooping superior palpebra (ptosis), small pupil (miosis) and protrusion of the third eyelid, respectively.

The parasympathetic fibers of the oculomotor nerve innervate the pupillary sphincter and are the efferent limb of a II–III reflex called the *pupillary reflex* (Fig. 25.15). The pupillary aperture decreases in size in response to light stimulation. Because of the cross-over of optic nerve fibers in the optic chiasma, the cross-over of fibers between the pretectal nuclei and the cross-over of fibers within the parasympathetic nucleus of the oculomotor nerve, the reflex contraction of the pupillary sphincter is manifested as a

direct and *indirect* (*concensual*) response to light stimulation. The stimulation of one eye with light results in the contraction of the pupillary sphincter in both eyes. An evaluation of the pupillary reflex is a useful diagnostic tool in determining the integrity of the afferent and efferent limbs of the reflex in both eyes.

Compartments of the Eye

The eye is divided into an *anterior* and *posterior compartment* by the lens, suspensory ligament and ciliary process.

Anterior Compartment

Anterior and Posterior Chambers. The anterior compartment is bounded by the lens, suspensory ligaments, ciliary processes, ciliary body, iris and cornea (Fig. 25.4). The anterior compartment is subdivided into *anterior* and *posterior chambers*. The posterior chamber, the region into which aqueous humor is "secreted," is bounded by the iris rostrally and the lens and its associated structures caudally. The posterior chamber communicates with the anterior chamber through the pupil. The anterior chamber, the chamber through which aqueous humor must pass before being returned to the circulation at the *filtration angle*, is bounded by the iris and cornea.

Iridial Angle. The *iridial angle* (*iris angle, filtration angle, iridocorneal angle*) is the peripheral margin of the anterior chamber at the region of the limbus (Fig. 25.16). The filtration angle, formed between the base of the ciliary body and iris as well as the initial caudal portion of the cornea, is filled by a triangular mass of spongy tissue, the *meshwork of the iridial angle* (Fig. 25.17). The meshwork is comprised of solid trabeculae separated by fluid spaces, the *spaces of Fontana*. The trabeculae of the meshwork consist of cores of collagenous and elastic fibers

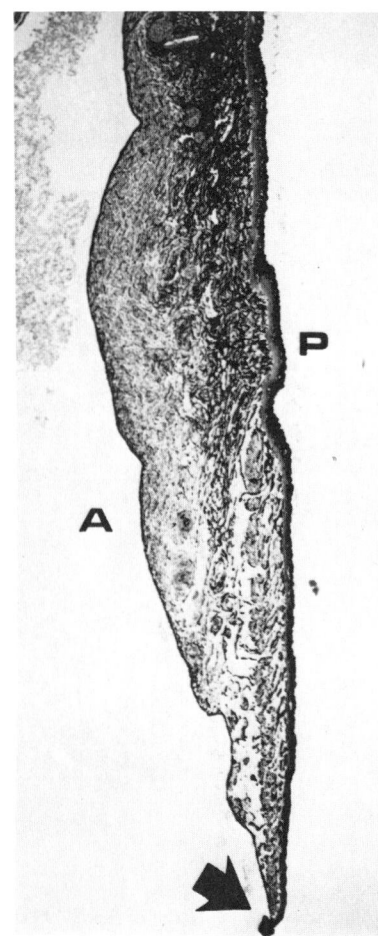

Fig. 25.12   Iris of an ovine eye. The pars ciliaris retinae is continued on the caudal surface of the iris as the pars iridica retinae. A corpus nigrum (*arrow*) is obvious along the pupillary margin of the iris. A, anterior chamber; P, posterior chamber. X10.

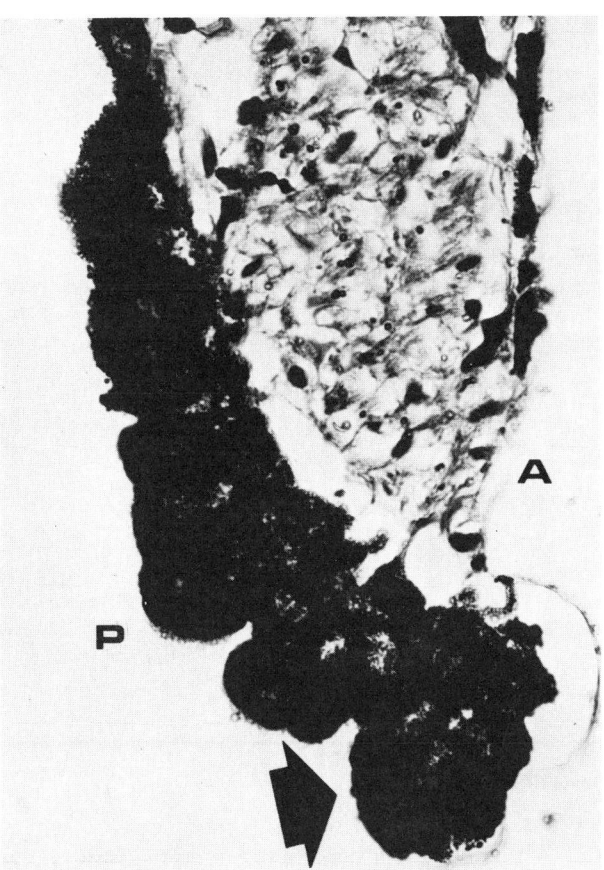

Fig. 25.13 Corpus nigrum of an ovine iris. The corpus nigrum (*arrow*) is a proliferative mass of pigment epithelium and iridial stroma along the pupillary margin of the iris. A, anterior chamber; P, posterior chamber. x160.

plexus and exists the eye via the scleral veins. The *canal of Schlemm* is a modified vein in the filtration angle that is part of the outflow tract for aqueous humor. The canal occurs in the ox and man.

Whereas aqueous humor passes freely through the filtration angle, particulate matter is trapped within the trabecular meshwork. Plugging of the meshwork with debris, as can occur in inflammation, may retard or stop the egress of aqueous humor and result in an increased intraocular pressure—*glaucoma*.

Aqueous Humor—Blood/Aqueous Barrier. The aqueous humor carries nutrients and oxygen to the lens, cornea and retina as well as being the medium through which metabolic waste is removed from the intraocular spaces. Also, aqueous humor is the means by which intraocular pressure is maintained to insure proper spatial relationships of ocular components. The fluid is formed by the ciliary body as an ultrafiltrate of the blood. The Starling-Landis principles are applicable, in part, to aqueous humor formation; however, the lining cells of the ciliary body utilize active transport mechanisms to secrete certain substances. The clear, watery and slightly alkaline fluid has a chemical composition similar to cerebrospinal fluid. The mechanisms involved in aqueous humor formation are similar to those utilized in CSF formation. Because of the selective nature of the epithelial lining of the ciliary body in forming a fluid that differs from plasma, the boundary is called the *blood-aqueous barrier*. The actual barrier is probably comprised by the epithelial cells and their tight junctions.

The rate of formation of aqueous humor is balanced with the rate of egress of aqueous humor at the filtration angle. Increased rates of formation or decreased rates of return result in increased intraocular pressure—*glaucoma*.

Posterior Compartment

Vitreous Body. The *vitreous body* (*vitreous humor*) occupies the space between the lens and the retina (Fig. 25.4). The posterior compartment is filled by the vitreous body. (The posterior compartment and posterior chamber are not synonymous.) The vitreous body consists of water, some hyaluronic acid and collagenous fibers that impart a gelatinous consistency. Despite its gelatinous nature, aqueous humor freely percolates through the vitreous body. The peripheral limit of the vitreous body is defined by the inner limiting membrane of the retina. This membrane, actually the basal lamina of the supportive cells of the retina, has collage-

nous fibers and fibroblast-like cells (*hyalocytes*) adjacent to it. The hyalocytes may be responsible for the synthesis of vitreous body components.

The vitreous body adheres tightly to the *optic papilla, ora ciliaris retinae, orbicularis ciliaris* (darkly pigmented and ridged portion of the ciliary body) and posterior lens capsule. A hyaloid canal passing through the vitreous body somewhat parallel to the optical axis is the remnant of the hyloid artery.

Lens

The lens is one of the *dioptric* or *refractive media* of the eye. The dioptric media include all entities through which incoming light rays must pass to reach the photoreceptor cells—cornea, aqueous humor, lens, vitreous body and retina. The cornea and lens are the most important refractive media and exert the greatest influence upon incoming light rays. The lens is responsible for focusing light rays on the retina. The components of the lens are the *capsule, lens epithelium* and *lens fibers*.

Capsule. The *lens capsule* completely envelopes the lens and consists of a basement membrane and fine reticular fibers (Fig. 25.18). The transparent capsule does not have a uniform thickness; it is thicker near the equator and thin at the rostral and caudal poles. The caudal part of the capsule is thinner than the rostral component. The capsule, as the site of insertion of the suspensory ligaments, influences the shape of the lens. Metabolites must pass through the capsule as they move between the lens and the aqueous humor.

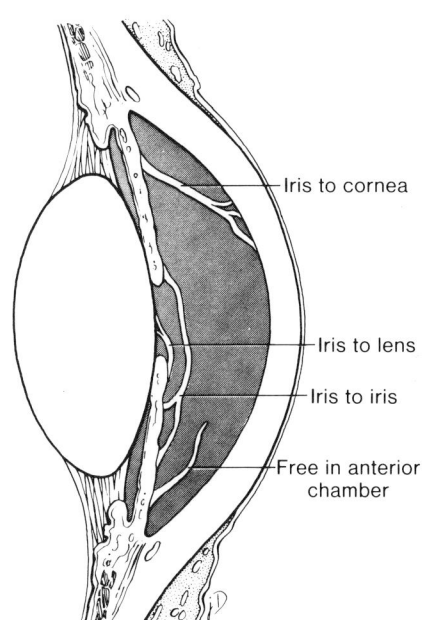

Fig. 25.14 A drawing depicting the types of residual iridopupillary membranes that may persist in the adult eye as persistent pupillary membranes.

Iris to cornea

Iris to lens

Iris to iris

Free in anterior chamber

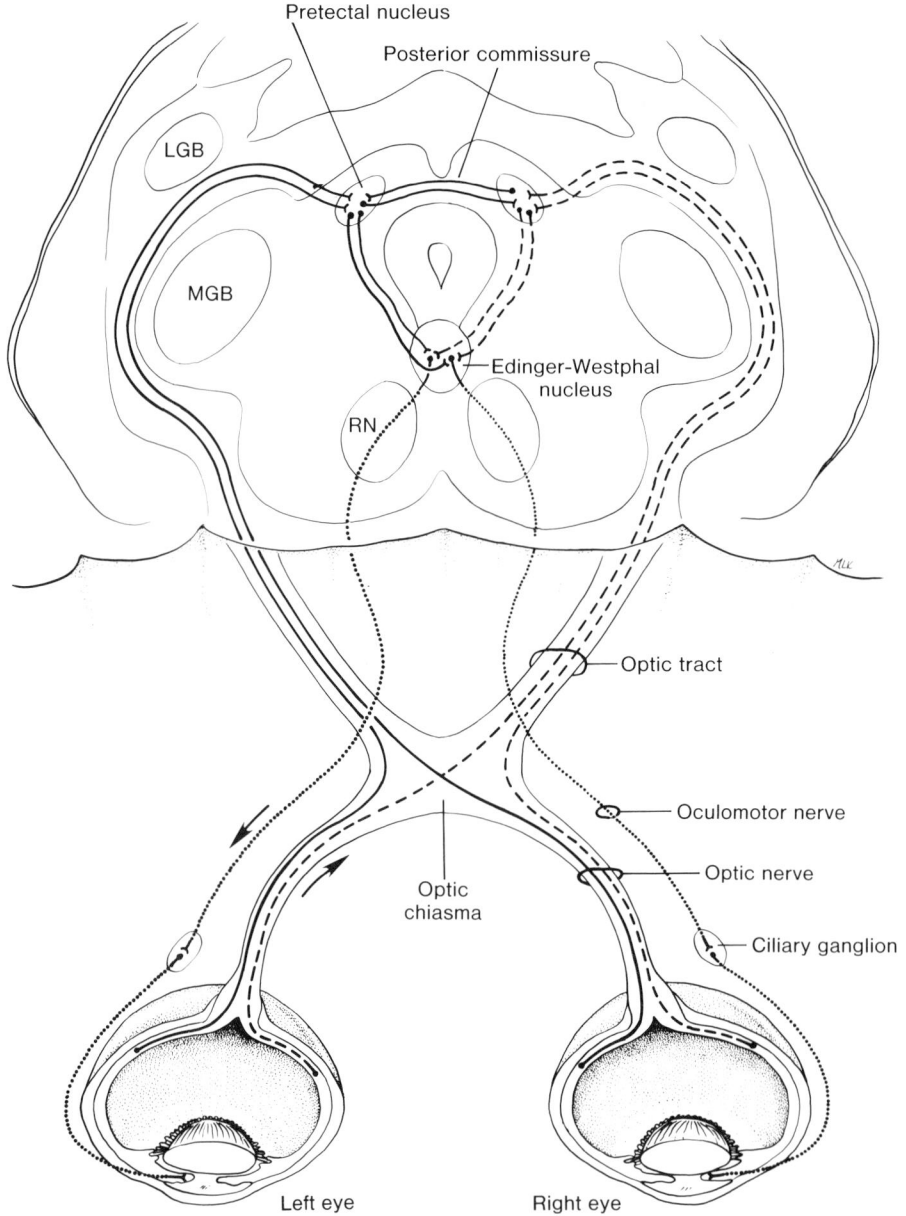

Fig. 25.15   A diagram of the pathways of the pupillary reflex in the dog. The brain stem is shown in cross section and the eyes are shown in frontal section. LGB, lateral geniculate body; MGB, medial geniculate body; RN, red nucleus.

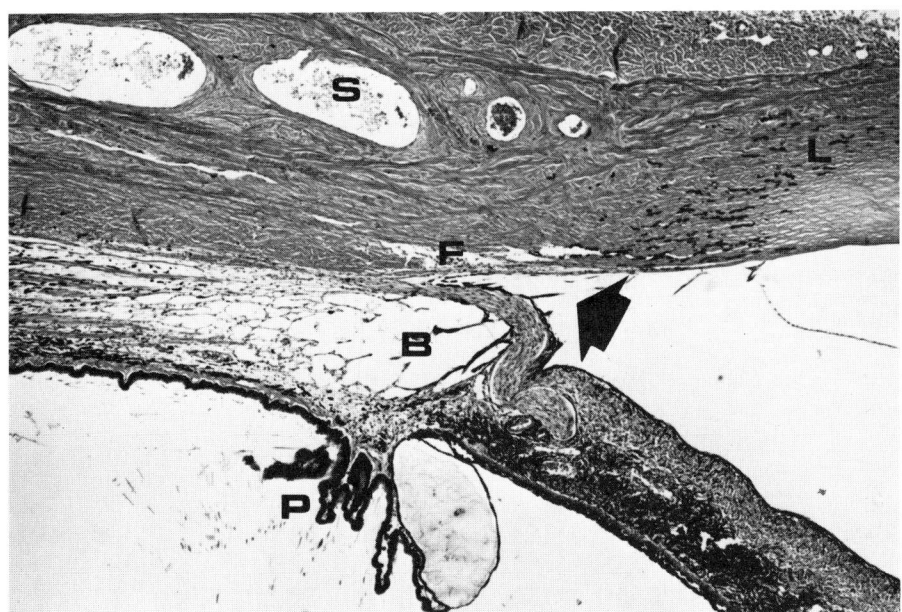

Fig. 25.16 Filtration angle of a canine eye. The filtration angle (*arrow*) is located at the angle formed by the junction of the cornea, iris and ciliary body (B). The spaces of Fontana (F) are continuous with the scleral plexus (S). L, limbus; P, ciliary processes. X10.

Epithelium. The lens epithelium of the adult lens is confined to the rostral surface beneath the capsule. The caudal lens epithelium, present during development, was converted to lens fibers during early lens development. The rostral epithelium is cuboidal at the pole and becomes elongated at the equator forming the *lens bow* as the cells are converted to *lens fibers*. The lens fibers are elongated, modified cells that are oriented meridionally in concentric laminae around the lens. The most primitive lens fibers, located at the periphery in the lens *cortex*, contain nuclei. Progressive differentiation results in their conversion to typical anucleated fibers. The inner portions of the lens is called the *nucleus*. Fetal, juvenile and adult nuclei may be evident as concentric zones of lens fibers. Older fibers are more dense, less transparent and less elastic than younger fibers. The rostral and caudal apices of the elongated lens fibers contact each other at points called *sutures* (Fig. 25.19). The sutures, often called *lens stars*, are Y-shaped regions of lens fiber contact. An amorphous cementing substance binds the hexagonal-shaped lens fibers together. The amorphous material and the interdigitations of lens fibers at the rostral and caudal pole account for the formation of visible sutures.

Functional Correlates. The lens capsule is semipermeable and helps to regulate the low, glucose-based metabolism of the lens. Most of the metabolism of the lens is anaerobic and is limited to the rostral epithelium and cortical lens fibers.

The posterior lens capsule is tightly adherent to the vitreous body (dog, horse). The adherent relationship between these two structures precludes the possibility of intracapsular delivery of a lens. In man, the limited attachment of the lens to the vitreous body via the ring-like *hyaloideocapsular ligament* permits the intracapsular removal of the lens.

The transparency of the lens is achieved through the registration and tight packing of the constituent lens fibers. The gradual hardening of nuclear lens fibers is a characteristic aging change called *nuclear sclerosis*. Other disruptions to lens fiber orientation and relationships—vacuolation, lens protein precipitation—result in a loss of transparency called *cataracts*.

Nervous Tunic

Organization of the Retina.

The *retina* or *nervous tunic* is responsible for the reception and transduction of light stimuli and the transmission of these signals in the form of nerve impulses to the appropriate portions of the brain. Cells of the retina are not confined to the photosensitive retina. The retina continues as a nonnervous (nonphotosensitive) layer of epithelial cells and pigment epithelium associated with the ciliary body and iris. The point of transition from retina to nonphotosensitive epithelial cells is called the *ora ciliaris retinae* in domestic animals and the *ora serrata* in man. At this point the nonphotosensitive epithelial cells and pigment cells of the retina are juxtaposed as a cellular bilayer. The rostral continuation of the cellular bilayer in association with the ciliary body is called the *pars ciliaris retinae*, whereas the cellular bi-

layer in association with the caudal iridial surface comprises the *pars iridica retinae*. An understanding of the developmental relationships within the eye serves to clarify these relationships. The inner and outer walls of the optic vesicle were monolayers of cells. The inner wall caudal to the ora ciliaris retinae proliferated to produce the characteristic cellular stratification of the retina. The inner wall, rostral to the ora ciliaris retinae, remained a cellular monolayer. The outer wall, rostral and caudal to the ora ciliaris retinae retained its monolayer characteristics as the pigment epithelium. The intimate juxtaposition of these two monolayers of cells forms the characteristic bilayers rostral to the ora ciliaris retinae. The subsequent discussion is confined to the photosensitive portion of the retina.

The retina (*pars optica retinae*) is divisible into ten distinct layers: *pigmented epithelium, photoreceptor cell layer, external limiting membrane, outer nuclear layer, outer plexiform layer, inner nuclear layer, inner plexiform layer, ganglionic cell layer, optic nerve fiber layer* and *inner limiting membrane* (Figs. 25.20 and 25.21).

Pigment Epithelium. The *pigment epithelium* resides on a basal lamina adjacent to the elastic membrane of the choroid. These cells are cuboidal with a paracentrally positioned nucleus and centrally disposed pigment granules. Long cellular processes extend between the photoreceptors. Under high illumination, pigment moves into the cellular processes and prevents diffusion of the light to adjacent receptors. The intimate contact of the pigmented cells with the photorecep-

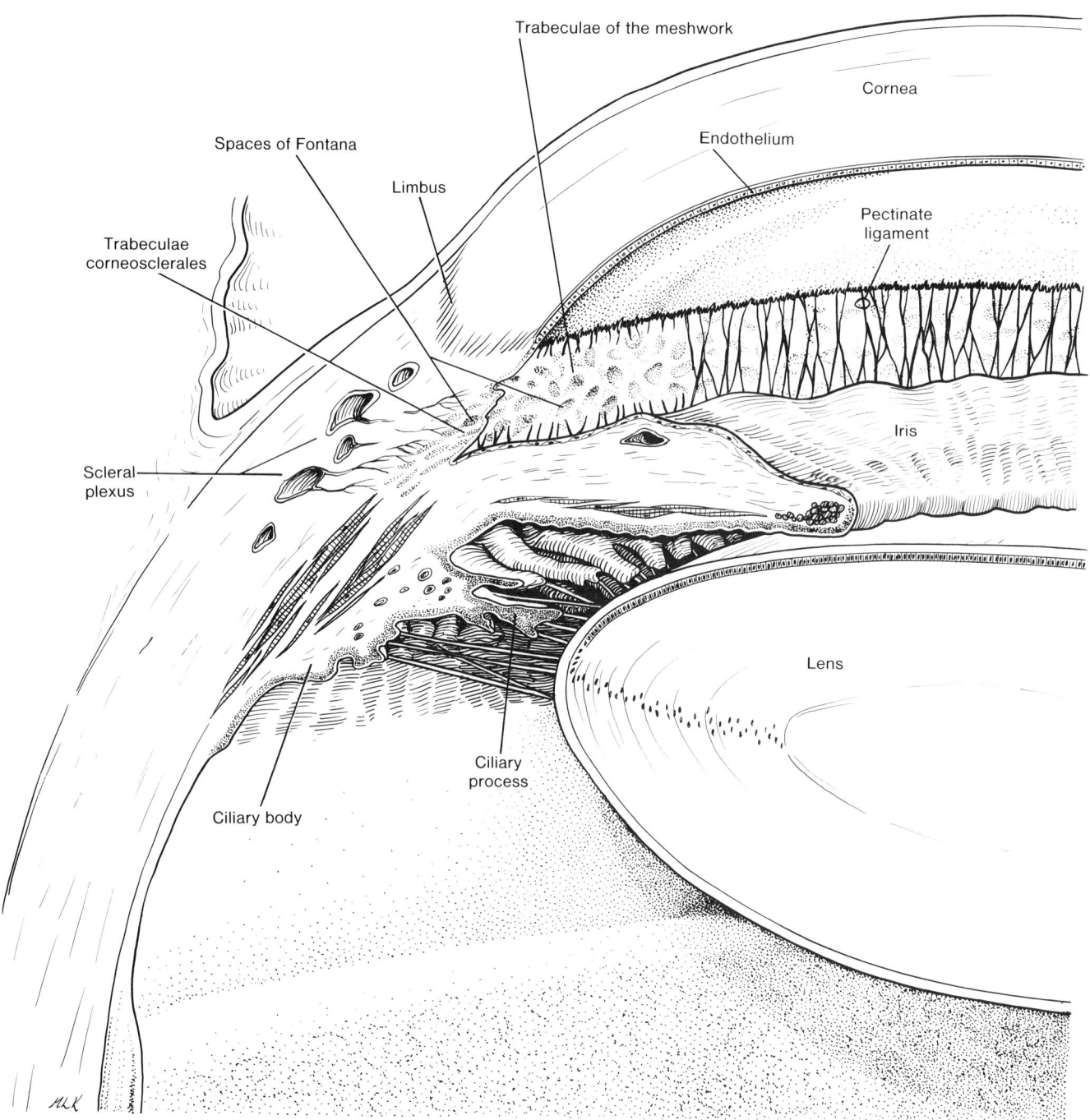

Fig. 25.17 A three-dimensional drawing of the filtration angle and associated structures.

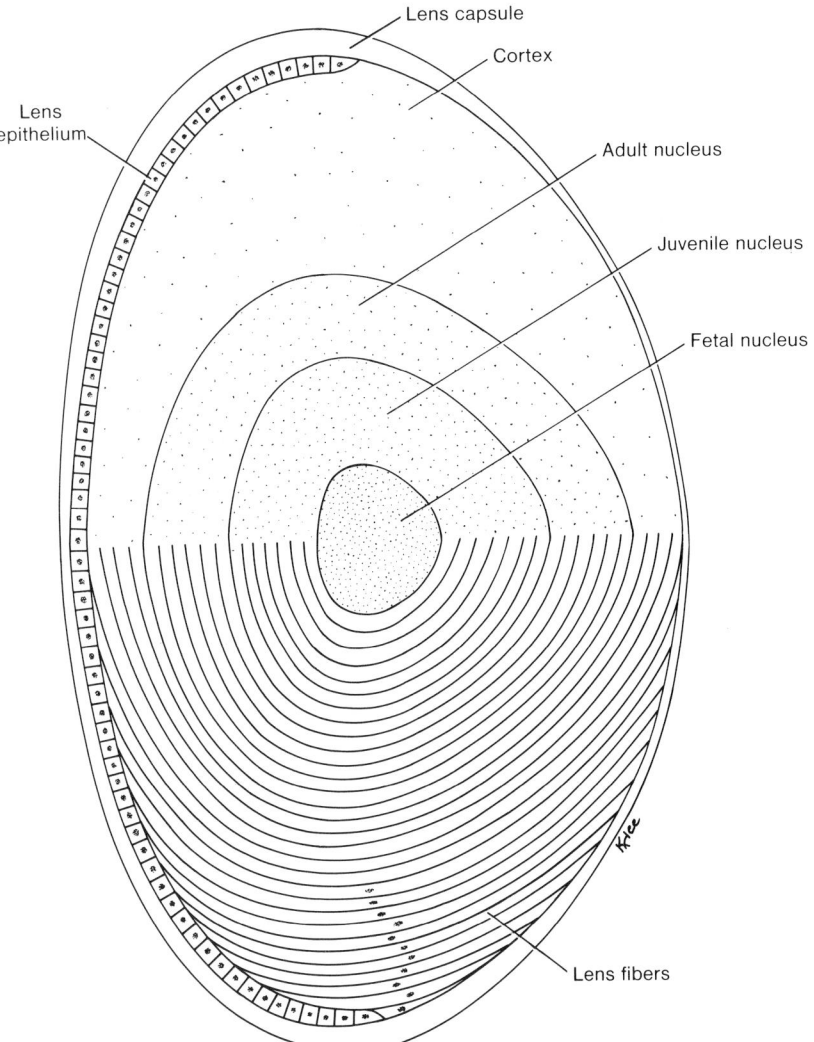

Fig. 25.18   A diagram of a section through an adult canine lens.

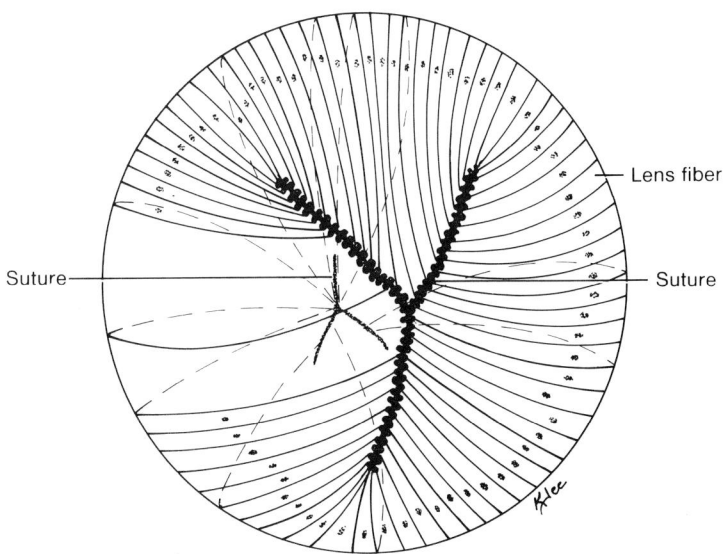

Fig. 25.19   A diagram illustrating the relationship of the lens fibers to the rostral and caudal sutures.

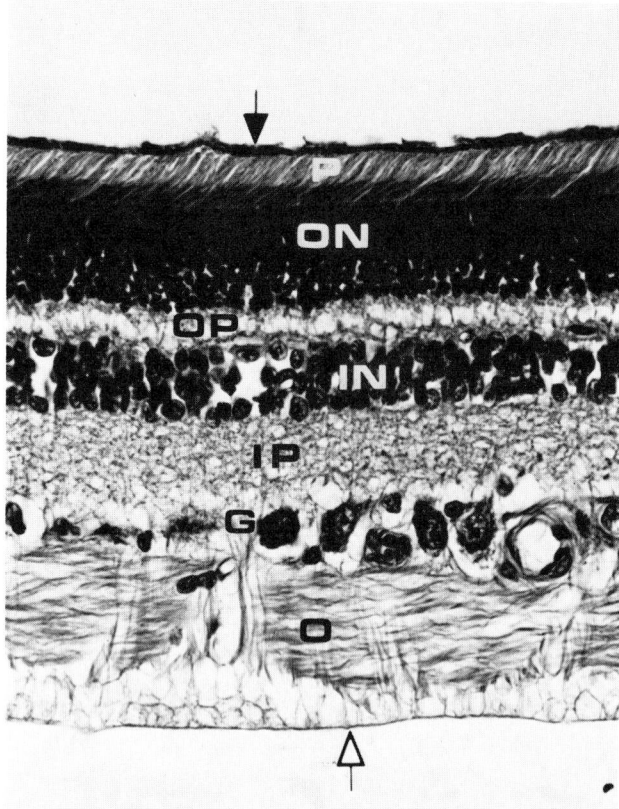

Fig. 25.20   Retina of a canine eye. *Solid arrow,* pigment epithelium; P, photoreceptor cell layer; ON, outer nuclear layer; OP, outer plexiform layer; IN, inner nuclear layer; IP, inner plexiform layer; G, ganglion cell layer; O, optic nerve fiber layer; *Open arrow,* inner limiting membrane. The outer limiting membrane is not apparent. X100. (N.B.: The photoreceptor cell layer is positioned away from incoming light rays.)

tors is apparently necessary for visual pigment synthesis. Current evidence suggests that the pigment epithelial cells may be a storage site for vitamin A. Additionally, the pigment epithelial cells phagocytize the continually growing and shedding outer segments of the rods and cones.

Photoreceptor Layer. The *photoreceptor layer* consists of the rods and cones. These are modified neuronal processes of the photoreceptor rod and cone cells that will be described in detail after the description of the retinal layers.

Outer Nuclear Layer. The *outer nuclear layer* is comprised of the nuclei of the photoreceptor cells.

Outer Plexiform Layer. The *outer plexiform layer* consists of axons of the photoreceptor cells, the dendrites of the subjacent bipolar neurons, as well as the fibers from association neurons located in this zone or the periphery of the subjacent nuclear zone.

Inner Nuclear Layer. The *inner nuclear layer* contains the cell bodies of bipolar neurons and association neurons.

Inner Plexiform Layer. The *inner plexiform layer* consists of axons of the bipolar neu-

rons, the dendrites of subjacent ganglionic cells and the processes of association neurons.

Ganglionic Cell Layer. The *ganglionic cell layer* consists of the cell bodies of the ganglion cells.

Optic Nerve Fiber Layer. The *optic nerve fiber layer* consists of axonal processes of the ganglion cells that are directed toward the *optic papilla* (*blind spot*) and emerge from the eye as the optic nerve (Fig. 25.22).

Limiting Membranes. The *internal limiting membrane* consists of fibrillar material (basal lamina) and the conjoined processes of the supporting Müller cells. The *outer limiting membrane,* located just peripheral to the outer nuclear layer, is an incomplete structure formed by the processes of Müller cells forming junctions with the cell bodies of the photoreceptor cells. The cell bodies of these cells are located in the inner nuclear area. The peripheral processes form the external or outer limiting membrane, whereas their internal processes abut on the outer surface of the inner limiting membrane.

Despite the apparent complexity of the retina, it may be simplified by recognizing

that it consists of three neurons in succession with intervening regions of synapses. Also, light must pass through the retina in order to stimulate the photoreceptor cells.

Ocular Fundus. The area of most acute vision in domestic animals is the *area centralis retinae.* Cone cells, bipolar neurons and ganglion cells are increased in number in this area. Although a depression (*fovea centralis*) does not occur in domestic species, this macular region is comparable to that which occurs in man.

The retina of most species is regularly curved along the posterior portion of the globe of the eye. The horse, however, has a *ramp retina.* The retina in these animals is irregularly curved along the posterior surface in such a manner as to permit different axial lengths associated with near and far vision. A rotation of the eye for near vision results in a long focal distance.

Photoreceptor Cells

The cells that comprise the retina include *pigment epithelium, photoreceptor cells, bipolar neurons, ganglionic cells, association neurons* and *neuroglial elements.*

The *photoreceptor cells* are neuroepithelial cells modified for the reception, transduction and transmission of visual stimuli. The cells are the *rod cells* and *cone cells.*

Rod Cells. The *rods* consist of an *outer segment, connecting cilium, inner segment, outer rod fiber, perikaryon, inner rod fiber* and *rod spherule* (Fig. 25.23). The outer segment is an elongated process of the cell that contains numerous double-membraned lamellae and the visual pigment, *rhodopsin.* Nine doublets of microtubules (devoid of a central pair) continue through the *connecting cilium* to terminate in a typical basal body within the expanded inner segment. The inner segment narrows as the outer rod fiber. This is continuous with the perikaryon. The inner rod fiber or axon terminates in a swelling, the *rod spherule,* and synapses with the dendrite of a bipolar neuron.

Cone Cells. The *cones* are similar to the rods (Fig. 25.23). The lamellae of the outer segment are often continuous with the plasmalemma. This segment, which is larger than that of the rods, contains *iodopsin.* The connecting cilium is not constricted. The inner and outer segments, therefore, have a conelike appearance. The nucleus of the cones does not contain as much dense chromatin as that of the rods. Also, the cell bodies are located in the outer portion of the outer nuclear layer.

The rods are generally distributed throughout the retina, whereas the cones are the predominant or only type of photoreceptor in the *area centralis retinae.* This is the region for bright light vision and is the area of most acute vision. The remaining portion of the retina, rich in rods, is for dark-

Caudal

Pigment epithelium

Photoreceptor cell layer

Outer limiting membrane

Outer nuclear layer

Müller cell

Outer plexiform layer

Association neuron

Inner nuclear layer

Inner plexiform layer

Ganglion cell layer

Optic nerve fiber layer
Inner limiting membrane

Rostral

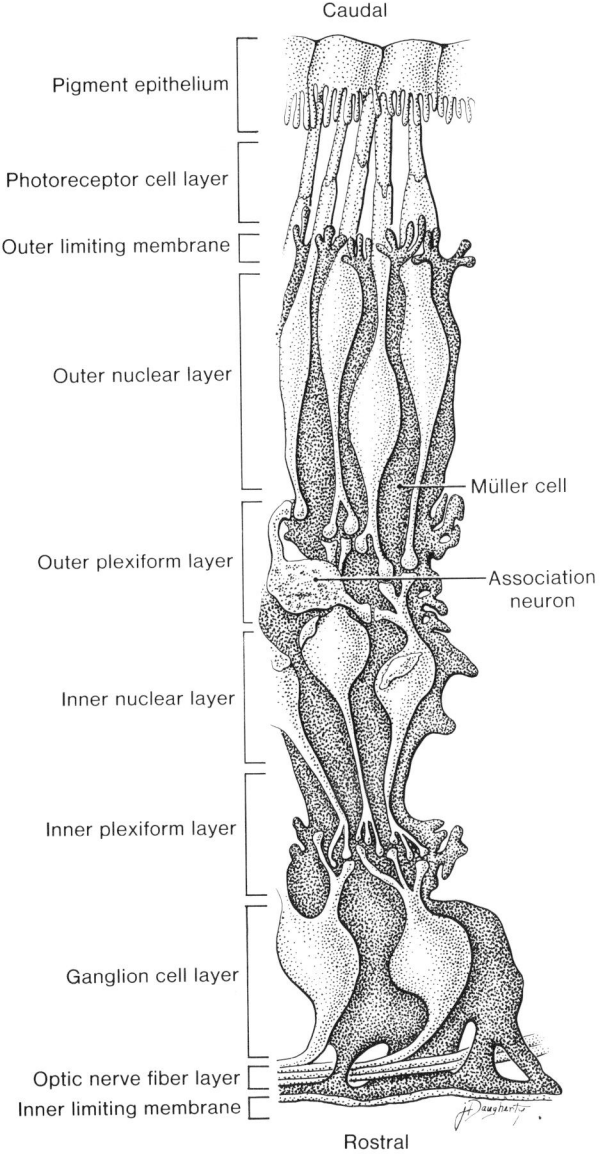

Fig. 25.21 A stylized three-dimensional drawing of the retina.

Ocular Adnexa

Eyelids. The eyelids (*palpebrae*) are folds of skin which cover the anterior surface of the eye (Fig. 25.24).

The external surface is covered with stratified squamous epithelium and underlaid by the dermis. Fine hairs, sweat glands and sebaceous glands are present. The glands are especially well-developed in the pig. The margin of the upper eyelid is characterized by thick hairs. Sweat and sebaceous glands are associated with them. Occasionally, sinus hairs may be present. Hairs are either small or absent (dog, pig) along the margin of the lower eyelid.

At the margin of the eyelids the skin is continued by a mucous membrane (*palpebral conjunctiva*). The lamina epithelialis of the internal surface (*conjunctiva*) varies throughout its distribution. It may be stratified columnar or stratified squamous with goblet cells. At the point of reflection on to the surface of the cornea, it is stratified squamous.

The DWFCT of the dermis and lamina propria fuse centrally as the *tarsus*. The tarsus consists of laminae of collagenous fibers. The extent of the tarsus corresponds to the shape of the eyeball covered by the palpebra. Anterior to the tarsus are bundles of striated muscle fibers of the *orbicularis oculi* and the *levator palpebrae superioris*. Smooth muscle is present also.

The *tarsal glands* (*glands of Meibom*) are modified sebaceous glands that open at the margin of the eyelid (Fig. 25.24). Sweat and sebaceous glands of this region are associated with hairs, glands of *Moll* and *Zeiss*, respectively. Serous and/or seromucoid *glands of Krause* and *Wolfring* are accessory lacrimal glands that may be present in the palpebral conjunctiva. Glands of Krause are usually located at the fornix conjunctivae. Intraepithelial mucous *glands of Manz* may occur within the palpebral conjunctiva.

Nictitating Membrane. The *nictitating membrane* or *third eyelid* (*palpebra tertia*) is a fold of conjunctiva that contains hyaline cartilage (ruminants, dog) or elastic cartilage (horse, pig, cat). The areolar connective tissue may contain some smooth muscle fibers (cat). Lymphatic nodules are extensive along the bulbar surface (Fig. 25.25).

The *superficial glands* of this organ surround the cartilaginous plate (Fig. 25.26). Their secretion is serous (horse, cat), seromucoid (dog, ruminants) and mucoid (pig). The *deep gland* (*gland of Harder*) is a mixed gland which occurs in the pig and ox (Fig. 25.27).

Lacrimal Apparatus. The lacrimal apparatus consists of the *lacrimal glands*, the *conjunctival sac* and the *lacrimal passages*.

The *lacrimal glands* are located at the dorsolateral margins of the orbit. (Figs. 25.28 and 25.29). In the pig, the glands are mucoid.

The secretion of these glands serves to

adapted vision. There is wide species variation in the distribution of the type of photoreceptor cells.

Müller cells are neuroglial elements unique to the retina. *Astrocytes, oligodendroliocytes* and *microgliocytes* are present and typical. *Amacrine cells* and *horizontal cells* are association neurons within the retina which serve to modify the visual stimuli from other cells of the retina. The *horizontal cells* are in contact with groups of rods. The amacrine cells are in contact with bipolar cells, ganglion cells and other amacrine cells.

Retinal Blood Supply

Outer Layers. The outermost layers of the retina—pigment epithelium through outer plexiform layer—are devoid of blood vessels. The vessels of the choriocapillaris are the blood supply for the outermost regions of the retina.

Retinal Artery. The retinal artery is the viable remnant of the hyaloid artery. The intimate relationship of the artery to the optic nerve was established during the development of the choroid fissure. The central artery of the optic nerve is the source of the retinal artery and its branches. The retinal artery and its branches supply those portions of the retina not nourished by the choriocapillaris. The distribution of retinal vessels varies among the domestic species. Most of the domestic animals (ruminants, swine, carnivores) have a *holoangiotic* vascular pattern characterized by major retinal vessels emanating from the optic papilla. The horse has a *paurangiotic* vascular pattern characterized by a few small vessels restricted to the area of the optic papilla. A *merangiotic* vascular pattern (rabbit) is one in which only a limited portion of the retina has obvious vessels emerging from the optic papilla. The fundus of avian species is devoid of obvious vessels (*anangiotic*).

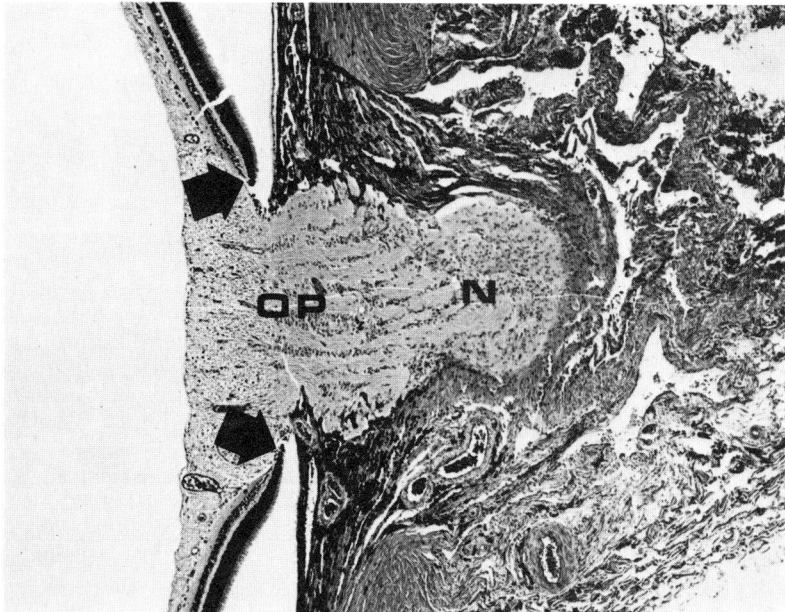

Fig. 25.22 Optic papilla of a canine eye. The neural retina stops (*arrows*) and the optic nerve fibers continue into the optic papilla (OP). The fibers continue as the optic nerve (N). X10.

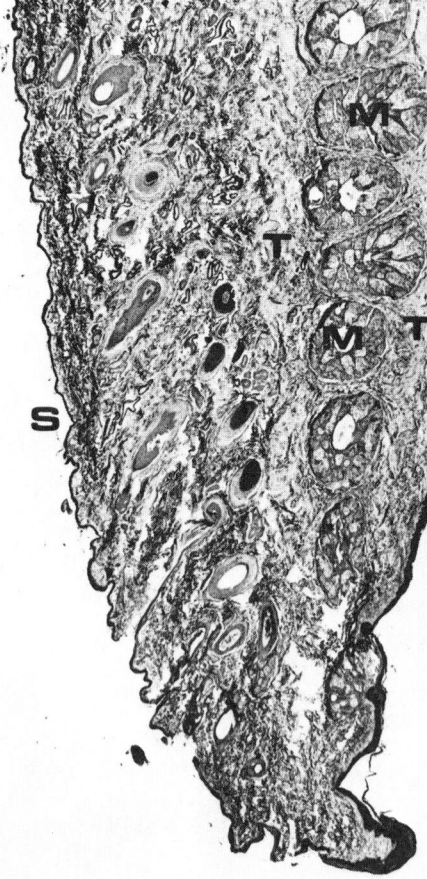

Fig. 25.24 A section of a palpebra. The skin (S) is reflected at the margin of the lid as the palpebral conjunctiva (C). The palpebra contains Meibomian glands (M) within a core of DWFCT, the tarsus (T). X4.

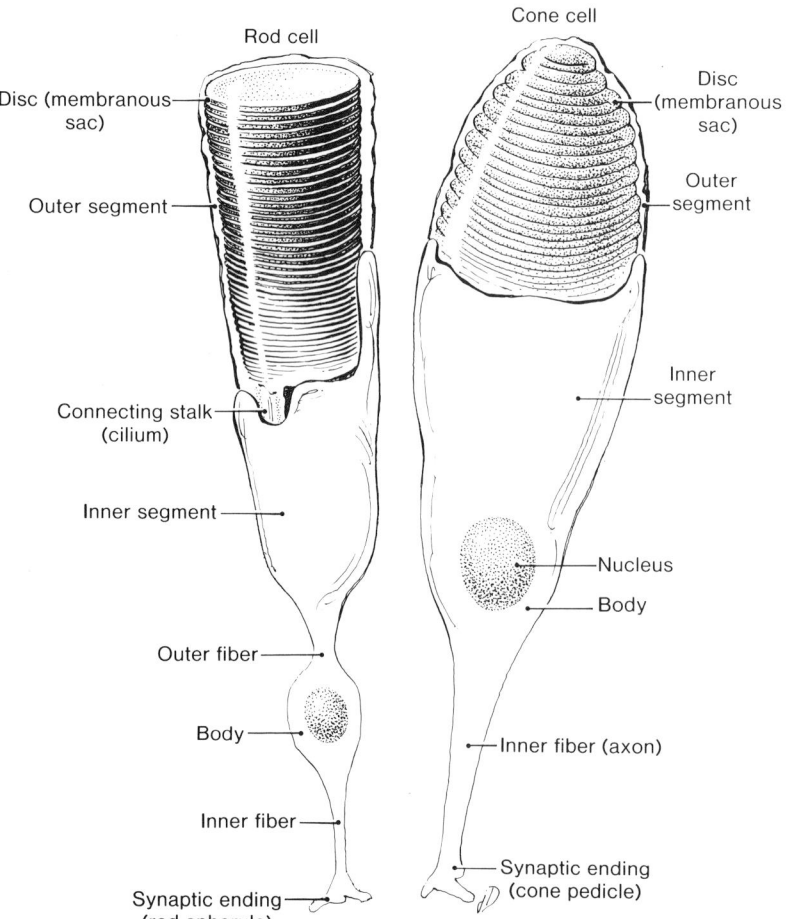

Rod cell

Cone cell

Disc (membranous sac)

Disc (membranous sac)

Outer segment

Outer segment

Connecting stalk (cilium)

Inner segment

Inner segment

Nucleus

Body

Outer fiber

Body

Inner fiber (axon)

Inner fiber

Synaptic ending (cone pedicle)

Synaptic ending (rod spherule)

Fig. 25.23 A stylized three-dimensional drawing of rod and cone cells. The discs are folds of membranes that contain the visual pigments rhodopsin (rods) and iodopsin (cones) and are formed at the base of the outer segment. The discs of rods lose contact with the plasmalemma, whereas those of the cones remain attached to the plasma membrane of the outer segment.

moisten the conjunctiva, while evaporative water loss is diminished by the mucoid secretion of the palpebral glands and the oily secretion of the glands of Meibom.

The fluids of the *conjunctival sac* accumulate in the medial widening of the sac, *lacus lacrimalis*, enter the *lacrimal canaliculi* through the *puncta lacrimalia* and continue to the *lacrimal sac* and thence to the *nasolacrimal duct*. The luminal surfaces of the lacrimal sac and duct are lined by a squamous or columnar epithelium (horse).

Ear

General Remarks. The ear is responsible for the reception of auditory stimuli, mechanical transduction of the stimuli and the transmission of nerve impulses to appropriate portions of the central nervous system. To accomplish these functions, the ear consists of various components: *auricle, auditory meatus, tympanic membrane, tympanic cavity with ossicles, cochlea* and *organ of Corti*.

The ear also functions, however, as an organ of balance. The components of the vestibular portion of the inner ear include *semicircular canals, utriculus* and *sacculus*.

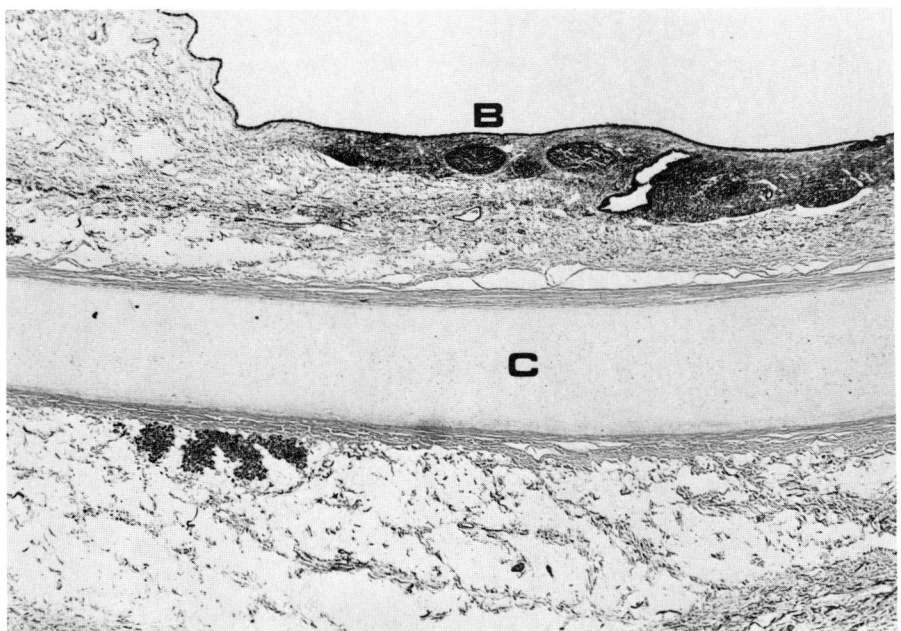

Fig. 25.25 A portion of a bovine nictitating membrane. The bulbar surface (B) has lymphatic nodules associated with it. The core of the structure is hyaline cartilage (C). X4.

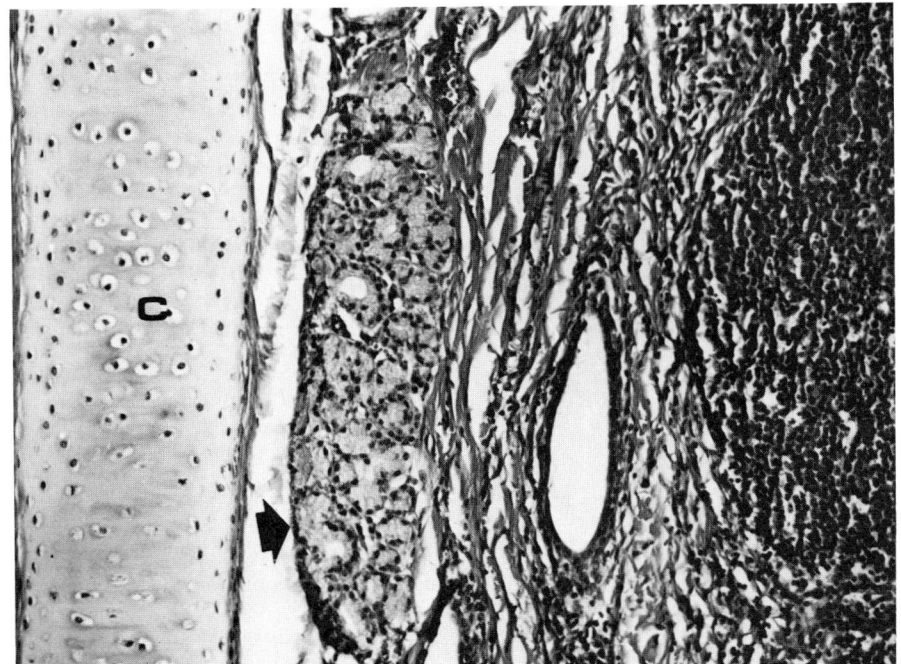

Fig. 25.26 Canine nictitating membrane. The cartilage (C) is closely associated with superficial glands of the organ (*arrow*). These are seromucoid glands. X40.

External Ear.

The external ear includes the *auricle* and *external auditory meatus.*

Pinna. The *auricle* or *pinna* is a sac of typical skin that contains hairs and associated glands. On the anterior surface (concave side), sebaceous glands are numerous and the frequency of hairs diminishes toward the external auditory meatus. The dermal tissue contained within the sac is typical and

contains supportive structures composed of hyaline or elastic cartilage. Striated muscle associated with the movement of the ear is also contained with the fold of integument.

The pinna is the "antenna" of the auditory apparatus. In most species, it also serves the important function of "directional finding."

External Auditory Meatus. The *external auditory meatus* or canal is the tubular extension of the auricle. The surface lining of the meatus is typical skin with some hairs and numerous sebaceous and *ceruminous glands.* Ceruminous glands are modified apocrine tubular sweat glands. The combined product of the ceruminous glands and the sebaceous glands, *cerumen,* is a brown waxy material that protects the canal and keeps the tympanic membrane moist and pliable.

The underlying dermis is typical and blends with the periosteum or perichondrium of the supportive bone or cartilage.

Middle Ear.

The middle ear includes the *tympanic membrane, tympanic cavity, ear ossicles* and the *internal auditory meatus.* Within the middle ear, the vibrations of the air are transduced to mechanical movement of the ossicles. These, in turn, produce waves in the perilymph of the inner ear via vibrations of the membranous *oval window.*

Tympanic Membrane. The *tympanic membrane* consists of an outer and inner epithelium that covers a core of collagenous fibers. The *outer epithelium* is a reflection of the epithelial lining of the external auditory meatus. It is, however, hairless and glandless. The core of connective tissue consists of outer radial and inner circular fibers. The *inner epithelium* is a simple squamous or cuboidal lining that is continuous with that which lines the tympanic cavity.

Tympanic Cavity. The *tympanic cavity* is lined by a squamous or cuboidal epithelium. At the opening of the *auditory tube (internal auditory meatus),* ciliated columnar cells are present. The cavity contains three *auditory ossicles: malleus (hammer), incus (anvil)* and *stapes (stirrup).* These bones are covered by a periosteum and are connected to each other by two diarthrodial joints. The handle of the malleus is embedded in the tympanic membrane, whereas the stapes is attached to the oval window by a fibrous joint. Two muscles are associated with these ossicles, the *tensor tympani* and *stapedius* muscles. These are striated muscles that serve to dampen the effects of high-frequency vibrations.

Auditory Tube. The *auditory tube (Eustachian tube, internal auditory meatus, pharyngotympanic tube)* connects the tympanic cavity with the nasopharynx. It is lined by respiratory epithelium—pseudostratified ciliated columnar epithelium. The lamina propria-submucosa consists of areolar connective tissue with diffuse lymphatic tissue and numerous serous and mixed glands. The connective tissue is continuous with the periosteum or perichondrium of the bone and cartilage that lines the canal. During deglutition (swallowing), the tube is opened and the air pressure within the tympanic cavity is equalized with the air pressure in the external auditory meatus.

The *guttural pouches* of the horse are lined by a pseudostratified ciliated columnar epithelium with goblet cells. The supportive lamina propria is rich in smooth muscle

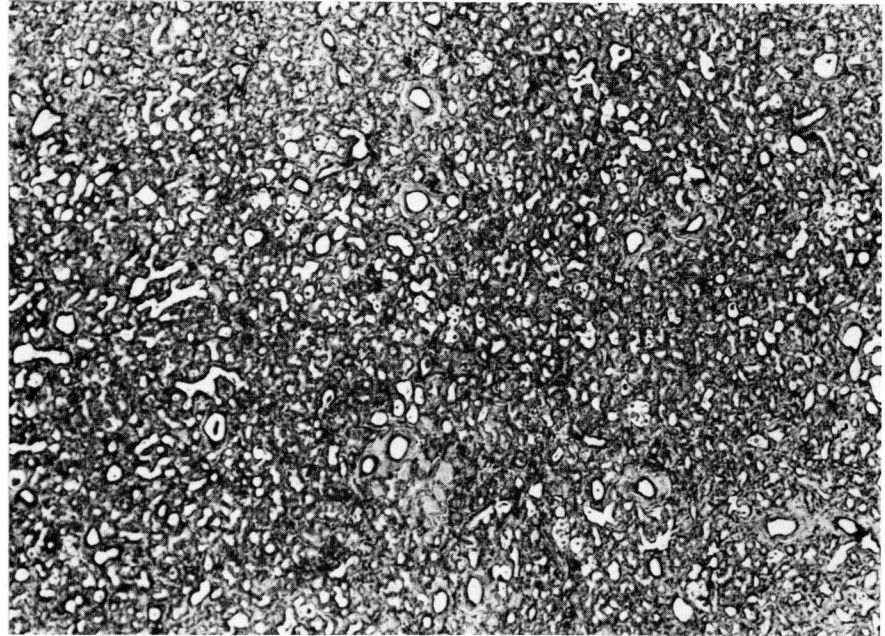

Fig. 25.27 Bovine gland of Harder. This gland is seromucoid. X16.

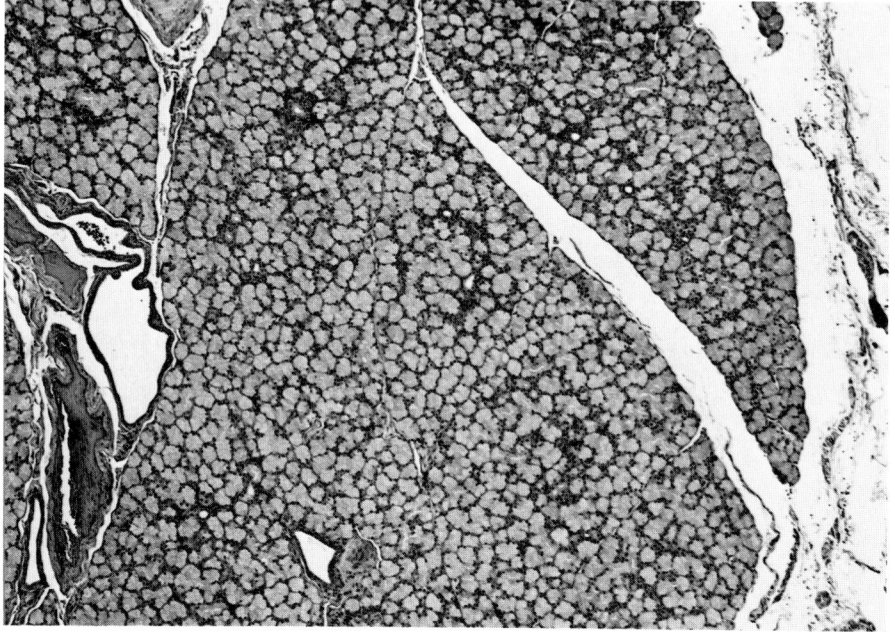

Fig. 25.28 Equine lacrimal gland. These are serous glands. X16.

fibers, elastic and collagenous fibers, serous and mucous glands, and lymph nodules.

Inner Ear

Osseous Labyrinth. The inner ear is located within the petrous portion of the temporal bone. The bone forms the *osseous labyrinth.*
Membranous Labyrinth. A *membranous labyrinth* is contained within the osseous chamber. Its shape conforms to that of the osseous labyrinth and consists of squamous epithelium throughout most of its distribution. The membranous labyrinth contains *endo-lymph* and is surrounded by *perilymph.* It was believed that endolymph is derived from cerebrospinal fluid, because the endolymphatic sac is close to the dura mater near the posterior margin of the petrous temporal bone. However, other areas (*stria vascularis*) have been implicated in the production of endolymph. It is more probable that endolymph is returned to the cerebrospinal fluid via the endolymphatic sac. Perilymph is probably tissue fluid.

The form of the membranous labyrinth is complex, for it is divided into numerous sacs and canals that are interconnected and sep-arated by bone. The subdivisions of the membranous labyrinth include *utriculus, sacculus, endolymphatic duct, endolymphatic sac, semicircular canals, ductus reuniens* and the *ductus cochlearis* (Fig. 25.30). The latter is involved with auditory sensations, while the saccule, utricle and semicircular canals are involved in balance.

Vestibular Apparatus

General Remarks. The vestibular apparatus is that special sensory organ that is concerned with awareness of the position of the body. Two types of sensations are involved in this sense: *static sensation* and *kinetic sensation.* Special sensory regions of the sac-culus and utriculus (*macula sacculi* and *macula utriculi*) contain substances that respond constantly to gravity. Other sensory areas (*cristae ampullares*) of the semicircular canals respond to movement of endolymphatic fluid and are responsible for the kinetic sensations of angular acceleration.

Utriculus and Sacculus. These portions of the membranous labyrinth are lined by a squamous or cuboidal epithelium, except in the sensory areas. The sensory areas are similar to each other, but their orientation is different. They are oriented perpendicular to one another.

The *macula utriculi* and the *macula sacculi* are responsible for the static sensations associated with balance. The epithelium of these sensory areas consists of sensory cells and sustentacular cells (Fig. 25.31). There are two types of sensory cells in the maculae (Fig. 25.32). One type (type I) is a goblet-shaped cell that does not reach the basal surface. Its apical border has numerous stereocilia and one kinocilium. The other type (type II) is a columnar cell with a similar apical morphology. The stereocilia (hairs) and kinocilia of both of these cells are not free in the endolymph. Rather, they are embedded in a gelatinous matrix that contains *otoconia* or *otoliths.* These are concretions of calcium carbonate and protein that move in response to gravity as the position of the head changes. The gelatinous material and otoliths are referred to as the *otolithic membrane.*

The *sustentacular cells* are nonciliated columnar cells. They support and nurture the other cells with which they are associated.

The basal margins of the sensory cells are surrounded by nerve endings that arise from the vestibular branch of the auditory nerve.
Semicircular Canals. The semicircular canals are tubules that arise from the utriculus. The three canals are oriented perpendicular to each other. There are three sensory areas, *cristae ampullares,* located at the bulbous enlargements (ampullae) of the canals close to the point of contact with the utriculus (Figs. 25.31 and 25.33).

The lining of the semicircular canals is simple squamous or cuboidal. In the sensory areas, the epithelium is thickened and a mound of cells is formed (Fig. 25.34). The constituent cells are similar to those described with the maculae. However, the otoliths are not present and the kinocilia and stereocilia project into the conical mass of gelatinous material, the *cupula*.

The currents of the endolymph during movement distort the cupula and embedded hairs, thus accounting for kinesthetic sensation.

Auditory Apparatus

General Remarks. The auditory apparatus is responsible for the reception of auditory stimuli, the transduction of the mechanical signal, the transmission of nerve impulses to the central nervous system and the dissipation of the energy of the auditory signal. This is accomplished through the *ductus cochlearis, scala vestibuli* and *scala tympani*.

The cochlear duct is part of the membranous labyrinth and is connected to the vestibular apparatus by the *ductus reuniens*. The scala vestibuli and scala tympani are perilymphatic spaces that surround the cochlear duct. The scala vestibuli is continuous with the scala tympani at the *helicotrema*. This is the apex of the spirally arranged organ.

The movement of the stapes causes a corresponding movement in the oval window. In turn, this causes waves to move through the perilymph of the scala vestibuli. These waves ascend in the scala vestibuli, communicate with the scala tympani at the helicotrema, descend within the perilymph of the scala tympani and dissipate at the *round window*. The latter is a fibrous covering in the wall of the tympanic cavity.

Cochlea. The cochlear duct, scala vestibuli and scala tympani are disposed in a spiral manner within the osseous labyrinth of the petrous portion of the temporal bone (Fig. 25.35). A central core of bone, the *modiolus,* and its lateral projections, the *bony spiral lamina,* support the membranous subdivisions of the *cochlea*. Fibrous connective tissue extends from the *spiral lamina* to the outer wall of the osseous labyrinth forming the *basilar membrane*. Another fibrous sheath extends from the spiral lamina and passes obliquely to the outer wall of the osseous labyrinth forming the vestibular membrane. The osseous labyrinth, therefore, is subdivided into three membranous compartments (Fig. 25.36). The dorsal compartment, *scala vestibuli*, is lined by a squamous epithelium. The middle compartment, *cochlear duct*, is lined by various epithelial types. Adjacent to the scala vestibuli, the lining is squamous. Thus, the *vestibular membrane* consists of two laminae of squamous cells and a thin central core of collagenous fibers. The lining of the ventral duct, the *scala tympani*, is similar to that of the scala vestibuli.

Nerve fibers of the auditory nerve ascend through the osseous modiolus and pass lat-erally to the *organ of Corti* which is contained within the cochlear duct.

Cochlear Duct and Organ of Corti. The cochlear duct, as mentioned previously, is an endolymphatic space continuous with the vestibular apparatus through the ductus reuniens (Fig. 25.37). The squamous cells adjacent to the scala vestibuli aid in the formation of the vestibular membrane (*Reissner's membrane).* The lateral or outer wall of the cochlear duct is composed of a bistratified layer of cuboidal or columnar cells. This region is referred to as the *stria vascularis.* It is underlaid by connective tissue, the *spiral ligament,* which is highly vascularized. The stria vascularis is believed to be responsible for the production of endolymph. The basal cells of this region con-

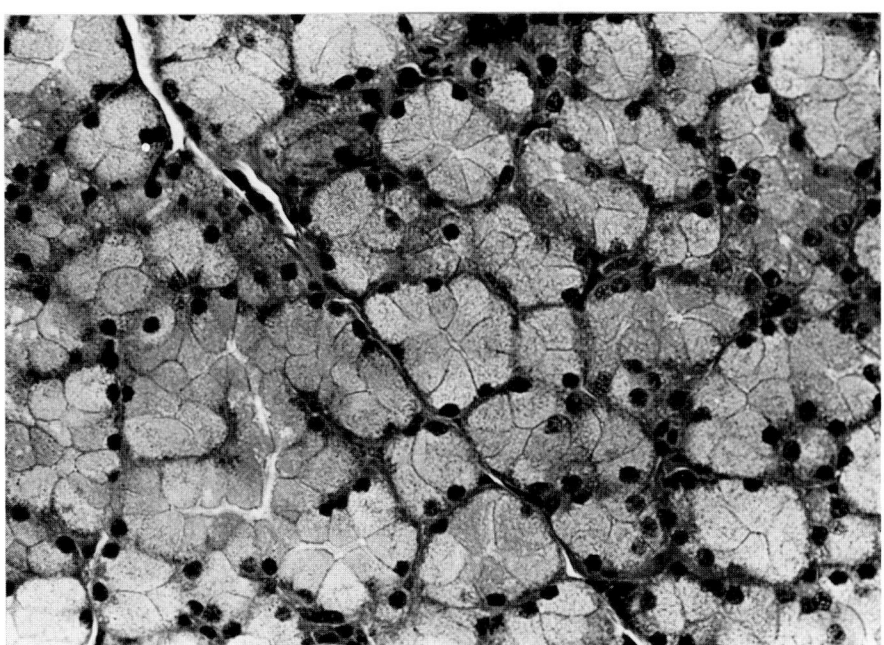

Fig. 25.29   Serous lining cells of an equine lacrimal gland. X100.

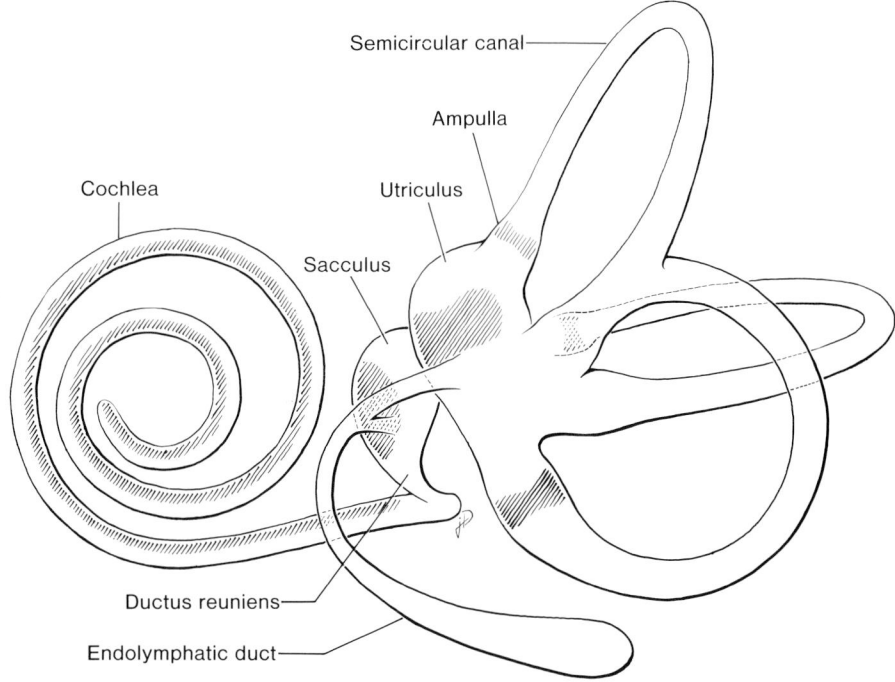

Semicircular canal

Ampulla

Cochlea

Utriculus

Sacculus

Ductus reuniens

Endolymphatic duct

Fig. 25.30   A diagram of the membranous labyrinth of the inner ear. The *hatched areas* are locations of sensory receptors.

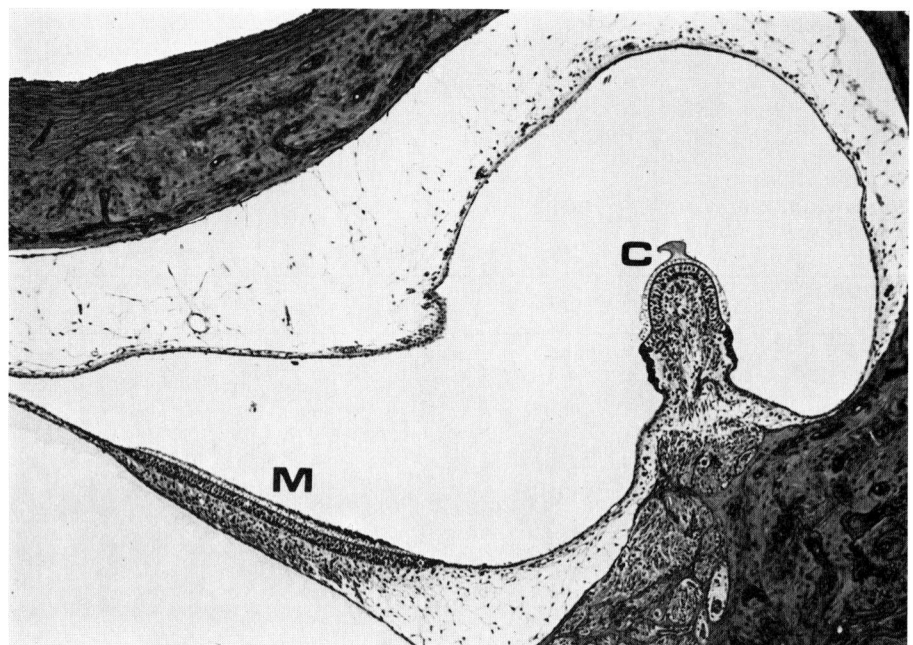

Fig. 25.31   A semicircular canal and utriculus. The macula utriculus (M) and one of the three cristae ampullares (C) are apparent. X16.

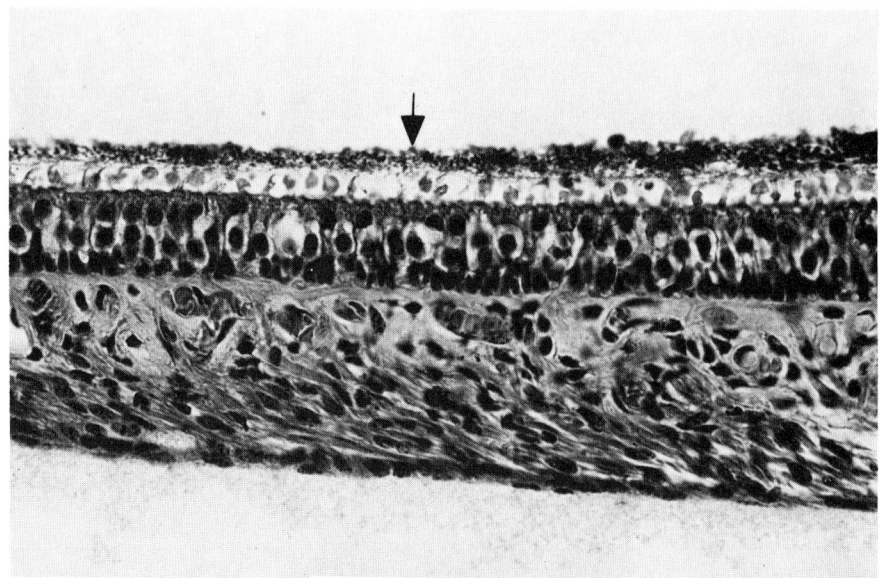

Fig. 25.32   Macula utriculus. Otoconia (*arrow*) are positioned above the cells. The otoliths are embedded within a gelatinous material. X100.

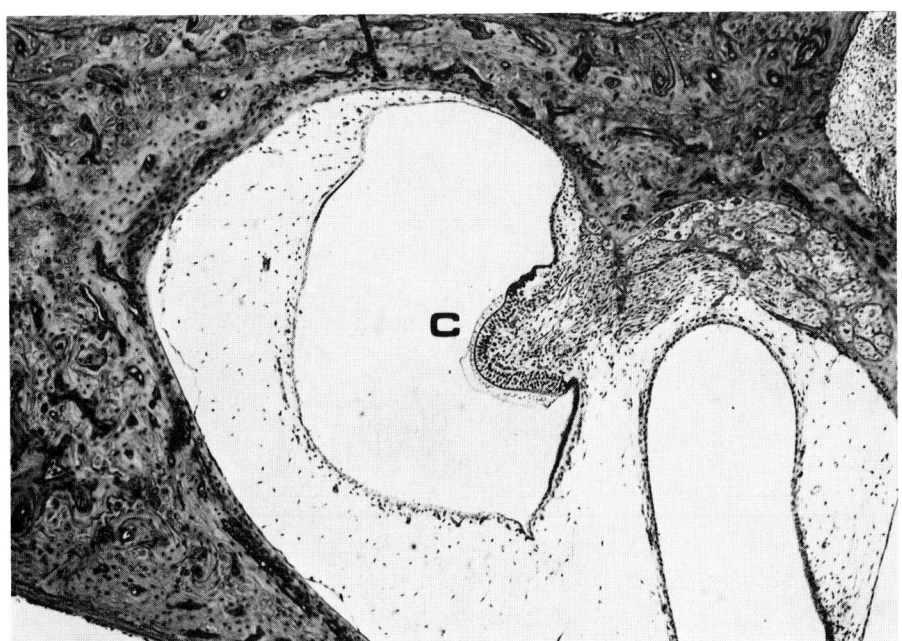

Fig. 25.33   Semicircular canal. One of the cristae ampullares (C) protrudes into the endolymphatic space of the canal. X16.

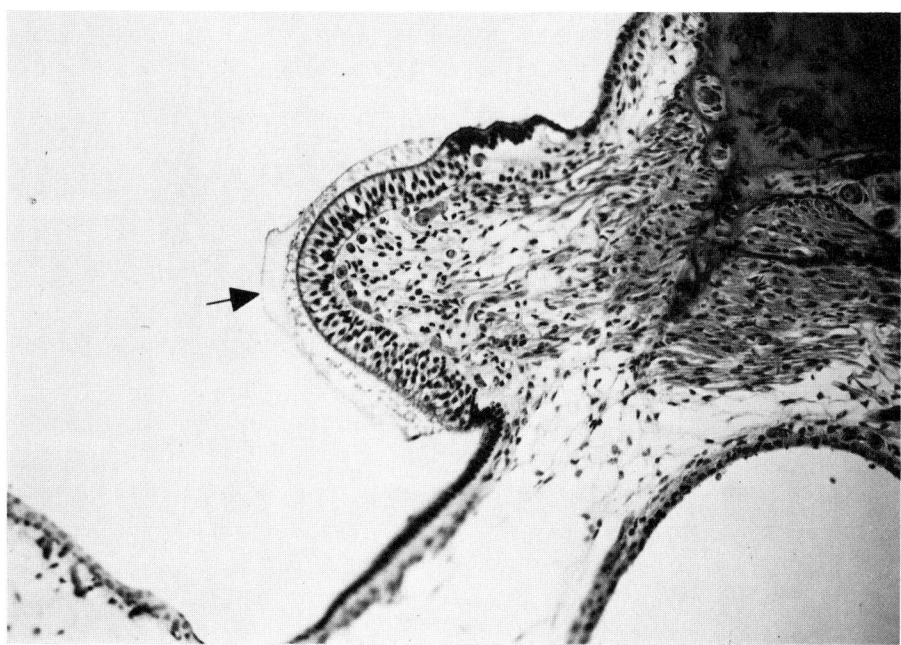

Fig. 25.34   The cupula (*arrow*) is a gelatinous mass devoid of otoliths. X40.

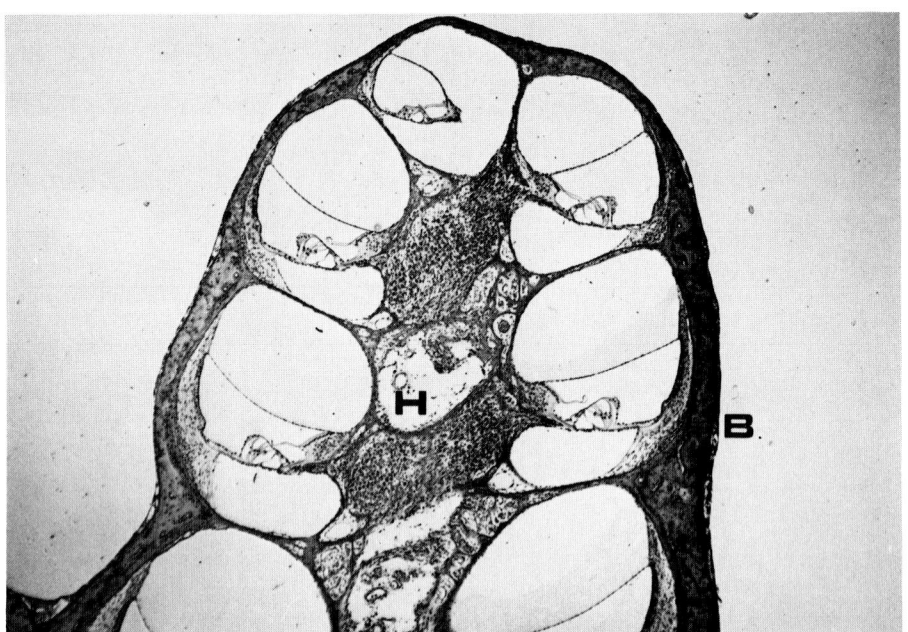

Fig. 25.35 The auditory apparatus. The cochlea is embedded within the bone (B) of the petrous portion of the temporal bone. The modiolus (H) is the central core of supporting bone. X10.

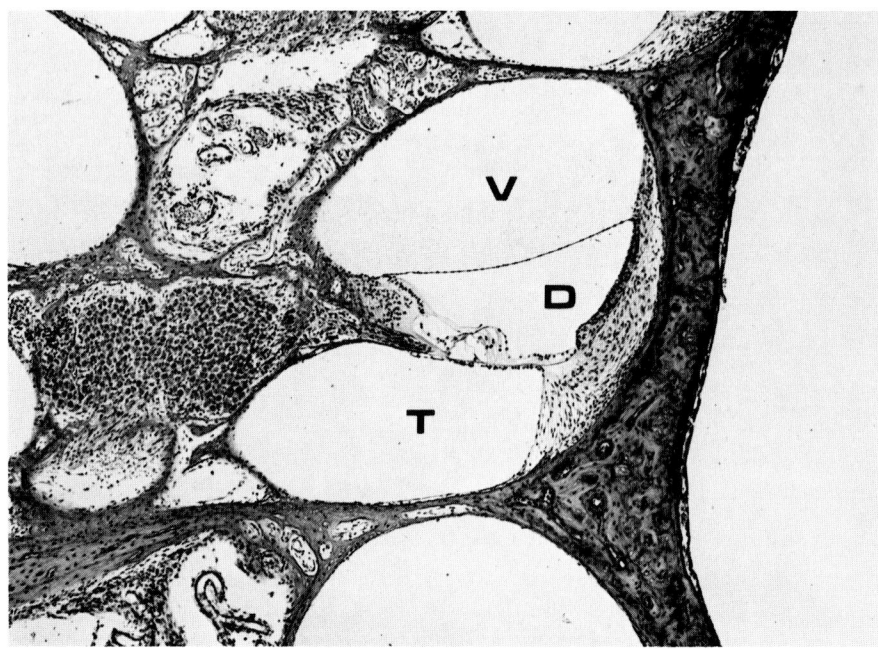

Fig. 25.36 The cochlea. The cochlea is divided into compartments. V, scala vestibuli; D, cochlear duct; T, scala tympani. X16.

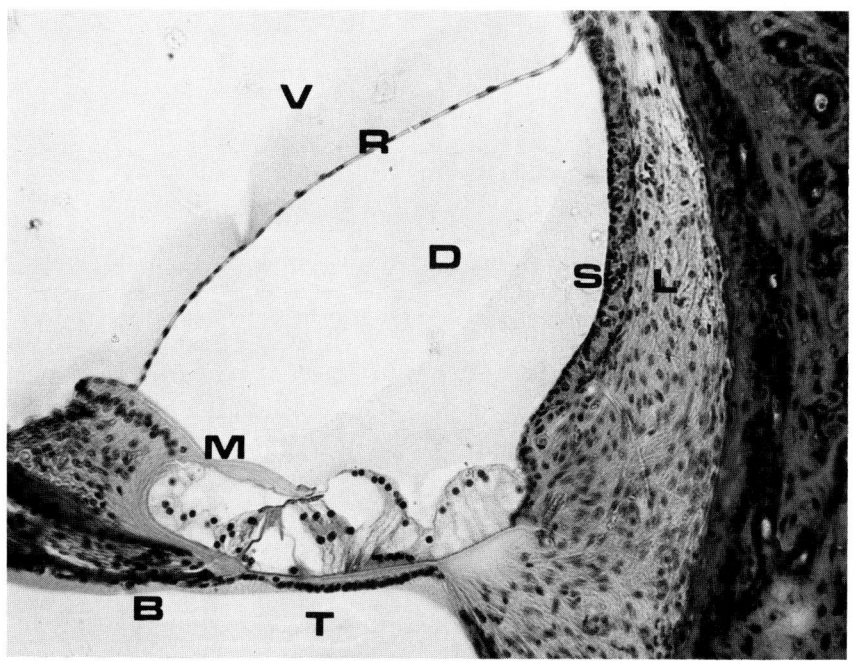

Fig. 25.37   The cochlear duct. D, cochlear duct; V, scala vestibuli; R, Reissner's membrane; T, scala tympani; B, basilar membrane; S, stria vascularis; L, spiral ligament; M, tectorial membrane. X40.

nue as the *spiral prominence* and are continuous with the cuboidal lining cells of the basilar membrane.

The *basilar membrane* is the supportive structure for the *organ of Corti*. The organ of Corti consists of *sensory (hair) cells, sustentacular cells* and a *tectorial membrane*. The hair cells have numerous stereocilia projecting from them arranged in a V pattern. In young organisms a central kinocilium is usually present at the base of the V. It is usually lost in adults. The sustentacular cells are numerous and varied. They, in conjunction with the hair cells, account for the complex morphology of the organ of Corti. The *tectorial membrane* is a fibrous and gelatinous, tonguelike structure that rests upon the hair cells. It is believed to be a secretory product of specific supportive cells, the *interdental cells*.

The following disposition of sensory and sustentacular cells accounts for the complexity of this organ. Besides the neuroepithelial cells, the organ includes: *inner* and *outer pillar cells, inner* and *outer phalangeal cells, interdental cells, border cells, cells of Hensen* and *cells of Claudius*. Other structures include the *tectorial membrane*, the *outer tunnel (tunnel of Corti)* and the *spiral tunnel* (Figs. 25.37 and 25.38).

The *inner* and *outer pillar* cells are narrow triangular cells with broad bases and narrow apices. Microtubules are prominent in these cells. These cells are joined at their apices and delimit the *inner tunnel.*

The *inner phalangeal cells* are medial to the inner pillar cells. They are columnar cells with a cuplike depression that almost totally surrounds the *inner hair cell*. The inner hair cell is a goblet-like cell. Nerve terminals are associated with it in the space between the hair cell and the inner phalangeal cell. The inner phalangeal cells gradually diminish in size and are transformed into squamous *border cells* which, with the tectorial membrane and inner phalangeal cells, define the spiral tunnel.

The border cells are continuous with columnar cells, *interdental cells*, which probably secrete the tectorial membrane.

The *outer phalangeal cells* are adjacent to the outer pillar cells. They are columnar cells with a cup-shaped depression which supports the outer hair cells. A cytoplasmic process of the outer phalangeal cells reaches the apex of the columnar outer hair cells. Microtubules extend from the base to the apex of the outer phalangeal cells. A smooth border is formed, therefore, above which the stereocilia of the hair cells project to touch the tectorial membrane.

Columnar and polygonal cells, the *cells of Hensen*, are lateral to the outer phalangeal cells. There is a space, the *outer tunnel*, between these cells. Toward the *spiral prominence* the cells are reduced in size to cuboidal cells, the *cells of Claudius*.

Vibrations of the perilymph within the scala vestibuli are transmitted to the vestibular membrane. This causes the endolymph to vibrate. The basilar membrane vibrates accordingly. These vibrations cause a distortion of the hairs that are resting against the tectorial membrane. This distortion results in the transduction of the stimulus and the generation of a nerve impulse. This is carried via the auditory branch of the eighth cranial nerve to the spiral ganglia, which are contained within the osseous labyrinth, and then to appropriate centers in the brain.

References

Eye

Aguirre, G. D. and Gross, S. L.: Ocular manifestations of selected systemic diseases. Compend. Cont. Ed. Pract. Vet. *11*:144, 1980.

Bedford, P. G. C.: Gonioscopy in the dog. J. Sm. An. Pract. *18*:615, 1977.

Bok, D. and Young, R. W.: The renewal of diffusely distributed protein in the outer segments of rods and cones. Vision Res. *12*:161, 1972.

deLahunta, A.: *Veterinary Neuroanatomy and Clinical Neurology*. W. B. Saunders, Philadelphia, 1977.

Jakus, M. A.: *Ocular Fine Structure*. Churchill, Ltd., London, 1964.

Pedler, C. M. H. and Tilly, R.: The fine structure of photoreceptor discs. Vision Res. *7*:829, 1967.

Prince, J. H., Diesem, C. D., Eglitis, I. and Ruskell, G. L.: *Anatomy and Histology of the Eye and Orbit in Domestic Animals*. C. C Thomas, Springfield, Il., 1960.

Shively, J. N. and Epling, G. P.: Fine structure of the canine eye: Cornea. Am. J. Vet. Res. *31*:713, 1970.

Tripathi, R. C.: Ultrastructure of Schlemm's canal in relation to aqueous outflow. Exp. Eye Res. *7*:335, 1968.

Villegas, G. M.: The ultrastructure of the human retina. J. Anat. *98*:501, 1964.

Young, R. W.: The renewal of photoreceptor cell outer segments. J. Cell Biol. *33*:61, 1967.

Young, R. W.: Visual cells and the concept of renewal. Invest. Ophthalmol. *15*:700, 1976.

Ear

Bredberg, G., Lindemann, H. H., Ades, H. W. and West, R.: Scanning electron microscopy of the organ of Corti. Science *170*:861, 1970.

Hinojosa, R. and Rodriguez-Echandia, E. L.: The fine structure of the stria vascularis of the cat inner ear. Amer. J. Anat. *188*:631, 1966.

Iurta, S.: *Submicroscopic Structure of the Inner Ear*. Pergamon Press, Oxford, 1967.

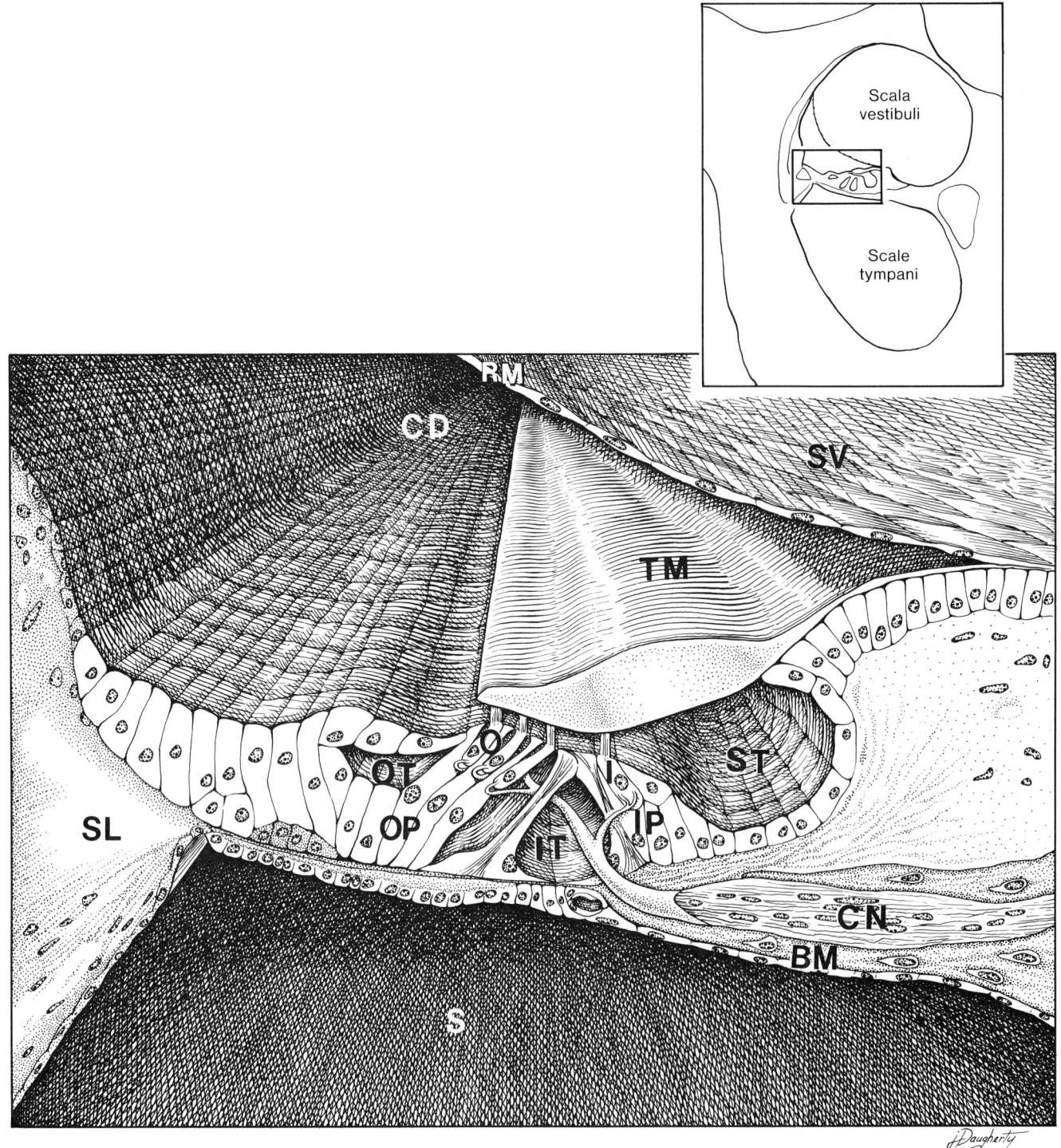

Fig. 25.38   A three-dimensional drawing of the cochlea. CD, cochlear duct; RM, Reissner's membrane; ST, spiral tunnel; SV, scala vestibuli; TM, tectorial membrane; O, outer hair cells; I, inner hair cells; OT, outer tunnel; OP, outer phalangeal cells; SL, spiral ligament; IT, inner tunnel; BM, basilar membrane; CN, cochlear nerve; IP, inner phalangeal cells; S, scala tympani.

SECTION V:

EXFOLIATIVE CYTOLOGY

26: Introduction to Clinical Cytology

Introduction

General Considerations. Cytology is the study of individual cells without regard to the architectural patterns of the tissues of origin of the cells examined. Although cytologic biopsy techniques do not replace incisional or excisional biopsies, they provide a rapid and simple means of diagnosis that occasionally preclude the need for a histopathologic examination. Cytology may be superior to histopathology in the evaluation of bone marrow and certain types of tumors. Cytologic examination requires exfoliated cells. Some cells spontaneously exfoliate into body cavities or are components of inflammatory exudates; others have to be exfoliated mechanically by techniques such as scraping, aspirating, or washing. Organ systems ideally suited to cytologic evaluation include the nervous, hemic-lymphatic, integumentary, digestive, urogenital and respiratory systems. Understanding pathologic cytology is predicated upon an understanding of normal cytologic structure and function.

This chapter emphasizes the cytologic characteristics of normal tissues and organs. Techniques are discussed to broaden the overall perspective of the cytologic approach to evaluation. Abnormal cytology associated with various disease processes is included as a means of comparison with normal cytology. The cellular descriptions are based upon staining properties seen with Romanowsky stains.

Techniques. A major advantage of cytologic examination of tissues is that a small amount of equipment and supplies is necessary: plastic disposable syringes (5–20 ml), 20–25 gauge needles, clean glass microscope slides, cover slips, immersion oil, xylene, a microscope with an oil immersion objective and various stains. Suitable stains include new methylene blue, Romanowsky stains and Papanicolaou stain.

Cells to be examined should be smeared soon after collection, especially those in low protein fluids such as cerebrospinal fluid, because they degenerate rapidly. Cells in a fluid medium are prepared as a blood smear. The feathered edge should be retained as an examinable part of the slide, because larger cells tend to accumulate in this portion of the smear. If the material to be smeared is thick, then decreasing the speed of the

pusher slide facilitates the preparation. Alternatively, the material may be placed as a drop between two slides which are then drawn apart, making two preparations.

The cells of cell-poor fluids may be concentrated by sedimentation, centrifugation or filtration. A direct smear at the time of collection is recommended as an ancillary procedure, because artifacts may be induced by the concentrating techniques.

Cytologic samples are obtained from solid tissue masses by aspirating the masses with a needle and syringe. Aspirated materials may not appear in the barrel of the syringe but will be present in the needle. Releasing the negative pressure before removing the needle from the tissue completes the sampling and precludes the loss of the sample into the barrel of the syringe. The material in the needle is expressed onto a glass slide and smeared immediately. Cells aspirated from tissue masses such as lymph nodes are usually suspended in a fluid medium and can be prepared in a manner similar to a peripheral blood smear. Impression smears or "touch preparations" are made from excised tissue samples by blotting a freshly cut surface with absorbent paper and then touching the tissue gently to a glass slide. The sample should not be smeared on the slide, because shearing forces rupture nuclear membranes, resulting in broken strands of nuclear material. Because tissues with a dense stoma do not exfoliate cells readily, scraping the tissue with a cutting blade may be necessary. The scraped material is applied to a slide and spread thinly, forming a cellular monolayer. Tissues from which impression smears are made must not be allowed to dry. If the sample must set for more than a few minutes before making smears, then it should be wrapped in gauze moistened with saline and refrigerated.

Cytologic preparations on slides to be stained with new methylene blue, Wright's stain, Giemsa stain or Gram stain are allowed to air dry. They can be stained immediately or can be stored for several days before staining is necessary. Unfixed smears must not contact formalin fumes nor be subjected to high relative humidity, since both will alter staining affinity.

New methylene blue is a water-soluble stain that provides good nuclear detail. A drop of stain, added to an air dried film, is coverslipped. Excess stain is removed, and

the slide is examined as a wet mount; however, the wet mount is not a permanent preparation. Romanowsky stains are adequate for most cytologic preparations. Smears to be Papanicolaou-stained must be fixed in 95% ethanol while wet.

Smears should be examined with low power and oil immersion objectives. Wright's-stained smears are often retained for future references following their examination with the oil immersion lens. Oil should not be removed from the slide with a paper, because cells are removed and broken. Rather, the oil-covered slide is placed in xylene to remove the oil and then allowed to air dry. The quality of the smear is not altered by this procedure.

Cytology of Selected Organs and Systems

Nervous System

General Considerations. Examination of cells in cerebrospinal fluid (*CSF*) is often a useful aid in obtaining a neurologic diagnosis. Additionally, total cell counts and quantitative protein determinations are helpful. Cells in CSF degenerate rapidly; consequently, total cell counts should be performed immediately after sampling. Normal cerebrospinal fluid contains less than five cells per cubic millimeter. Cell concentration techniques such as membrane filtration or cytocentrifugation are utilized to facilitate evaluation.

Cytology. The cells in normal CSF are primarily small lymphocytes and other occasional mononuclear cells (Figs. 10.22, 10.23, 10.24, 10.25). The blood cells observed approximate the morphologic and staining characteristics of those observed in a peripheral blood smear. An increase in the number of nucleated cells (*pleocytosis*) in CSF occurs with many neurologic diseases. The pleocytosis of viral infections is due to an increase in lymphocytes and some plasma cells. Bacterial and mycotic infections are characterized by an increase in neutrophils (Figs. 10.14, 10.15). Macrophages occur in viral and bacterial infections. In animals with central nervous system trauma, a slight increase in neutrophils and occasional macrophages may be noted. Numerous erythrophagocytes and macrophages containing hemosiderin pigment may be seen in animals with hemorrhage in the central nervous system (Plate VII.6). Tumor cells and inflammatory cells (neutrophils, macrophages) may be present in animals with central nervous system neoplastic diseases.

Hemic-Lymphatic System

The cytology of blood, bone marrow, lymph nodes and related structures is a valuable diagnostic procedure, because tissue architecture is less important in these organs than in many other structures.

Bone Marrow Aspiration Biopsy. *Aspiration biopsy* is indicated when it is impossible to confirm a diagnosis by the history, physical examination and careful examination of the peripheral blood. Cases of unexplained nonregenerative anemias, leukocytic dyscrasias, thrombocytopenias, myeloproliferative disorders, lymphosarcomas and abnormalities of immunoproteins are justifications for aspiration biopsies. *Punch biopsy* is indicated when attempts to obtain an aspirate have been unsuccessful. Abnormalities of the structural architecture of bone marrow may be evaluated by punch biopsy. A bone marrow biopsy is generally contraindicated when an animal is sufficiently ill or anemic that restraint further endangers its life.

The most common sites for bone marrow biopsy in the cat and dog are the iliac crest and the proximal end of the femur (Figs. 26.1, 26.2). The ribs or sternabrae are preferred sites in the horse and cow.

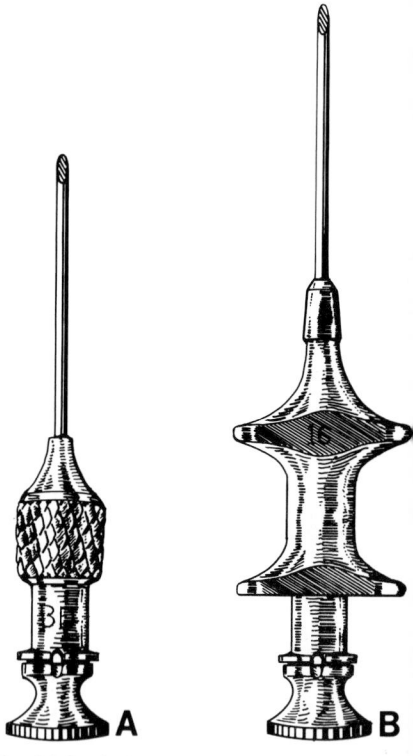

Fig. 26.2 A drawing of two types of needle that are used for bone marrow biopsies. The are designed with a heavy hub and removabl stylet. A, Osgood biopsy needle; B, Rosenth biopsy needle.

Lymph Node Aspiration Biopsy. Selectio of a lymph node for biopsy should be mad on the basis of clinical findings. Lymp node enlargement, whether localized or ger eralized, is an indication for lymph nod aspiration biopsy.

Cytology of Lymph Nodes. Cytologic eval uation of excised lymph nodes can be pe formed by gently touching a cut surface a node to a dry microscope slide. Cell type encountered in normal lymph nodes includ mature lymphocytes, lymphoblasts, neutro phils, macrophages, plasma cells and mas cells.

Mature *lymphocytes* are similar to the ma ture lymphocytes of the peripheral bloo (Plate VII.7). The nuclear chromatin coarsely clumped. The cytoplasm, generall scant, is a narrow rim around the nucleu The mature lymphocyte is the primary ce type of normal and hyperplastic nodes.

The nuclear chromatin in *lymphoblasts* fine and diffuse (Fig. 26.3). A nucleolus ma be seen. Lymphoblasts are approximatel 1½ to 3 times the size of the mature lym phocyte, and may possess a broad or narro rim of cytoplasm. Lymphoblasts are presen in normal and hyperplastic lymph nodes bu usually do not exceed 15% of the total cel population.

Any lymph node involved in inflamma tory processes contains many neutrophils These may appear healthy and intact if th inflammatory process is nonseptic (Fig 26.4). Degenerative changes in the nucleu

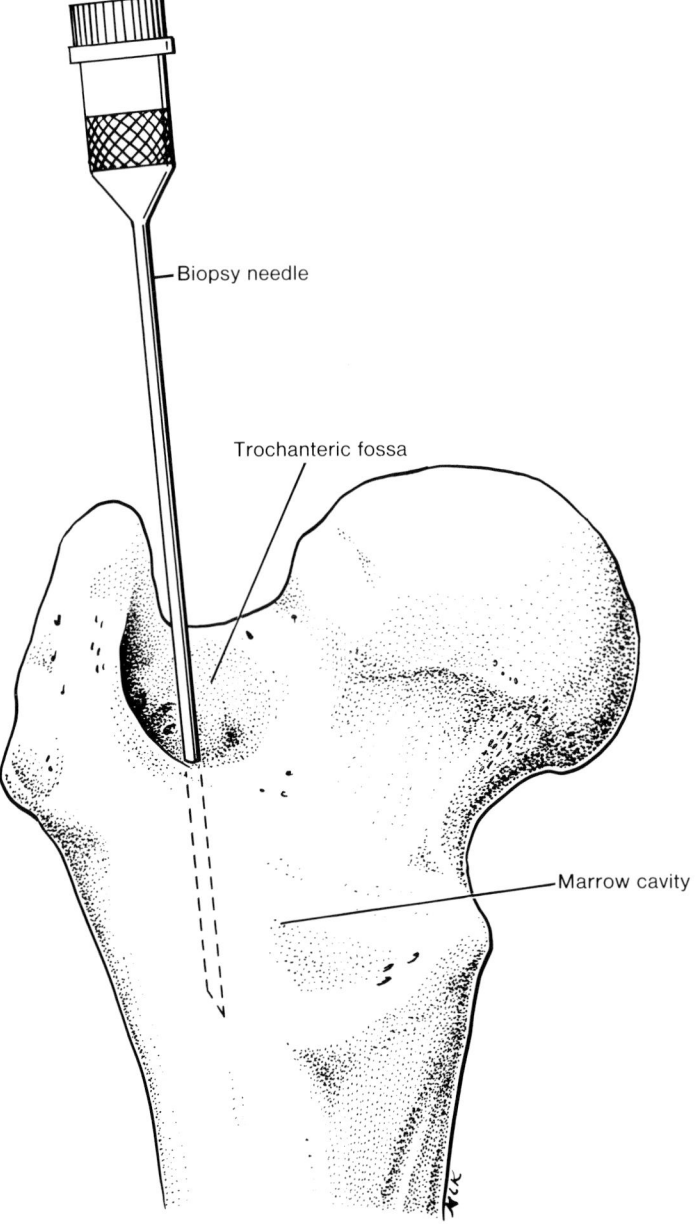

Fig. 26.1 A diagram depicting the site and placement of a bone marrow biopsy needle in the trochanteric fossa of a dog. All light micrographs are labeled as the magnification with the microscope before photographic enlarging. All electron micrographs are labeled as total magnification, including photographic enlarging.

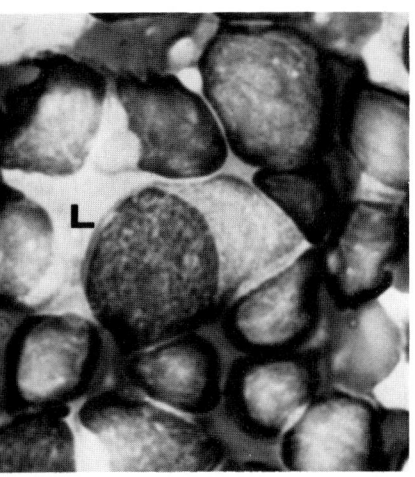

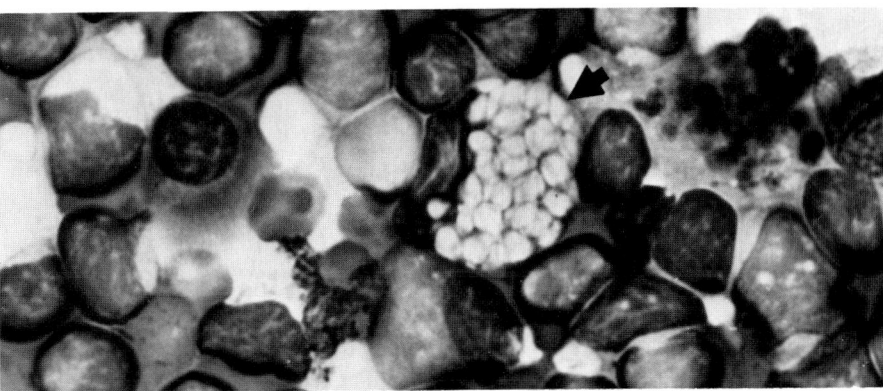

Fig. 26.6   A Mott cell (*arrow*) within a canine lymph node. The large inclusions, Russell bodies, contain packets of immunoglobulins. X400.

ig. 26.3   A lymphoblast from a normal canine ymph node. The lymphoblast (L) is surrounded y distorted lymphocytes. Note the fine chroatin pattern and extensive cytoplasm. X400.

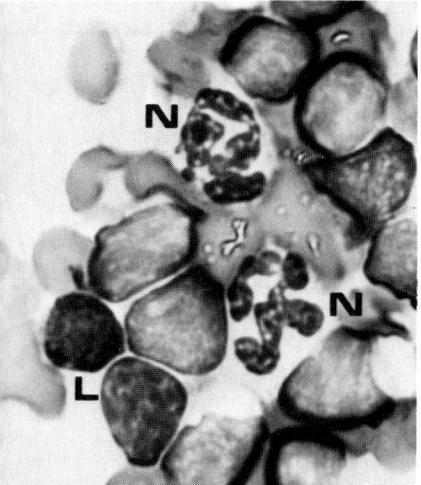

ig. 26.4   Small lymphocytes (L) and normal eutrophils (N) within a canine lymph node. X400.

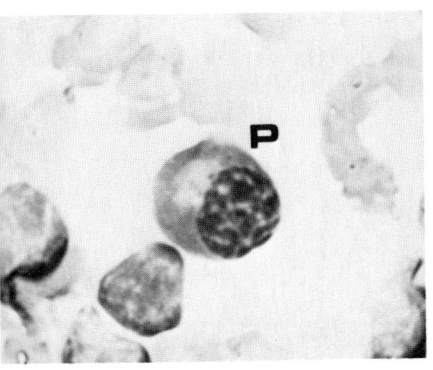

Fig. 26.5   A plasma cell (P) within a canine lymph node. The negative Golgi zone and eccentrically positioned nucleus are identifying features. X400.

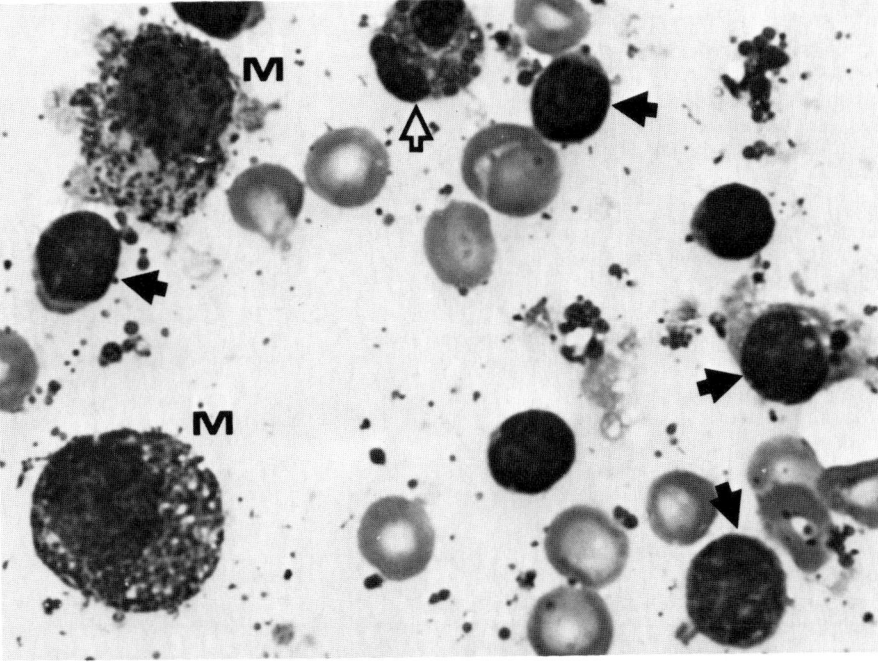

Fig. 26.7   Cells of a mast cell tumor within an aspirate of a canine popliteal lymph node. The mast cells (M) had metastasized to the lymph node. Particulate matter scattered throughout the aspirate are granules from ruptured mast cells. *Solid arrows*, lymphocytes; *open arrow*, eosinophil. ×400.

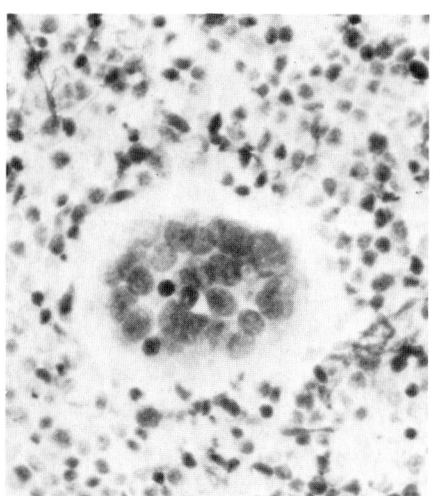

Fig. 26.8 A metastatic mammary gland carcinoma within an inguinal lymph node of a dog. The carcinoma is recognizable as a cluster of epipthelial cells. X100.

(karyolysis, karyorrhexus) of the neutrophil indicate septic inflammation. Bacteria may be observed within the cytoplasm of the neutrophils. Monocytes and macrophages, observed in certain chronic inflammatory conditions, may contain cellular debris. Plasma cells may be present (Fig. 26.5). Plasma cells containing packets of immunoglobulin, *Mott cells*, may be observed in antigen-stimulated lymph nodes (Fig. 26.6, Plate VII.7). A few mast cells occur in all lymph node aspirates; however, increased numbers may indicate mast cell neoplasia with metastatic involvement of the lymph node (Fig. 26.7).

Neoplastic cells, such as carcinoma cells, may be present in lymph nodes involved in metastatic processes (Fig. 26.8). The presence of cells that are not part of the normal cell population of the lymph node should be obvious. (Be certain that a structure such as a salivary gland was not aspirated inadvertently.) Malignant cells are usually pleomorphic with an increased nuclear/cytoplasmic ratio. The nuclei, varying in size and shape, often contain prominent multiple nucleoli. Many mitotic figures and multinucleated cells may be observed. Cytoplasmic vacuolation may be obvious. Malignant cells commonly stain more deeply basophilic than other cells.

Small flakes of cytoplasm may be intermixed with the cells of a lymph node sample. The flakes of cytoplasm, *lymphoglandular bodies*, are characteristic features of lymphoid tissue aspirates (Fig. 26.9).

The cytologic classification of lymph nodes is normal node, inflammatory node (purulent), immunologically reactive node (benign lymphoid hyperplasia), inflammatory and reactive node (mixed), primary neoplastic and metastatic neoplastic nodes (Plate VII.8).

Mature lymphocytes are the predominant cell type in *normal lymph nodes*. Lympho-

blasts do not exceed 15% of the population, while plasma cells and inflammatory cells are observed rarely. *Benign lymphoid hyperplasia* is characterized by increased numbers of immature and mature plasma cells (Plate VII.7).

Cytology of the Spleen. Fine needle aspiration biopsy of the spleen is a commonly rewarding diagnostic procedure; however, aspiration of unruptured hemangiosarcoma is contraindicated. Splenic aspirates are always rich in blood. The tissue cells in the normal spleen are lymphoid cells, endothelial cells, monocytes and macrophages.

Cytology of the Tonsil. The cytology of the normal tonsil consists of a mixture of lymphocytes and squamous epithelial cells o the buccal or pharyngeal mucosa. Cytolog of reactive, inflamed and neoplastic tonsil is very similar to findings in other lymphati tissue aspirates. Primary neoplasia of the tonsils are lymphosarcoma and squamou cell carcinoma.

Integumentary System

General Considerations. The cytologic sam ple of normal integument consists of super ficial epithelial cells containing keratin. I aspirates of the full thickness skin are made

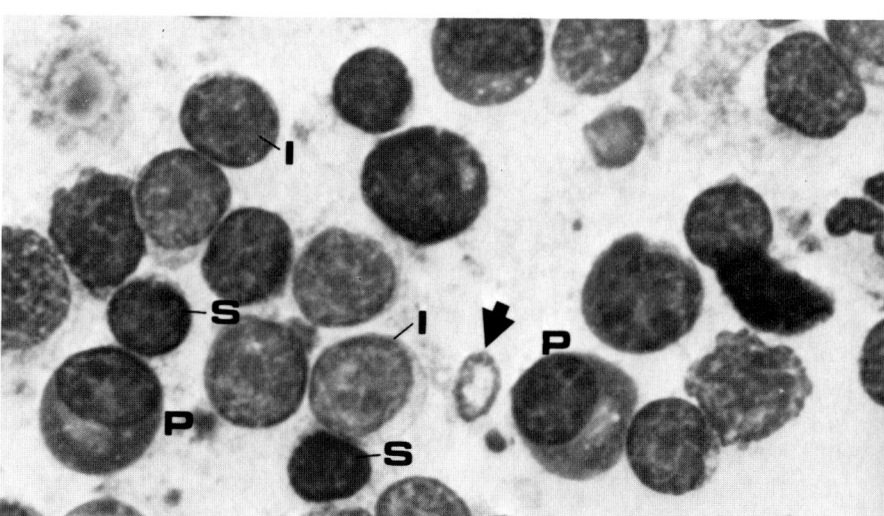

Fig. 26.9 Lymphogranular body (*solid arrow*) within a reactive canine lymph node. S, sma lymphocytes; I, intermediate lymphocytes. P, plasma cell. X400.

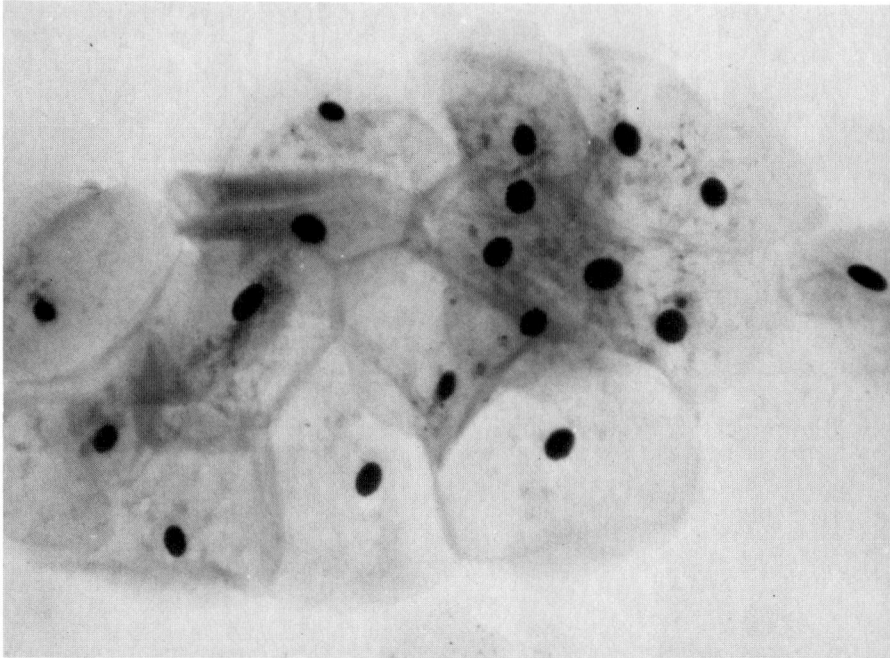

Fig. 26.10 Cells from a scraping of the buccal cavity of a dog. The surface cells of the stratified squamous epithelium contain pyknotic nuclei. X100.

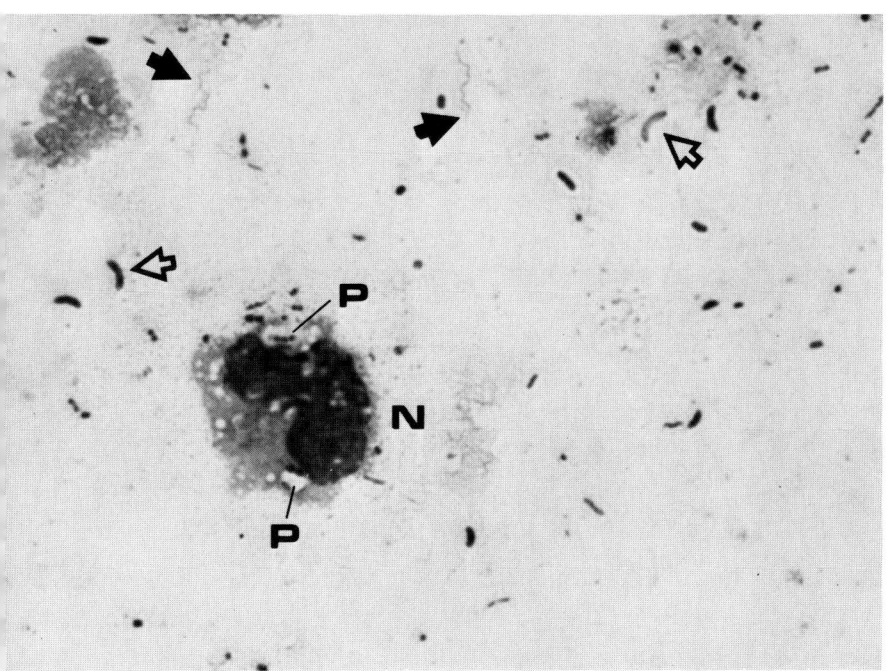

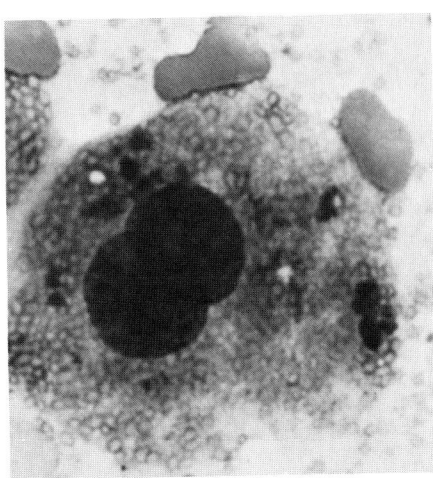

Fig. 26.12 Hepatocyte from a biopsy of a canine liver. The large cell is binucleated, and the cytoplasm contains dark granules of bile pigment. X400.

ig. 26.11 A scraping of the buccal cavity of a cat with gingivitis. Spirochetes (*solid arrows*), ɹsiform bacteria (*open arrows*) and bacilli are scattered throughout the smear. A toxic neutrophil N) contains phagocytized bacteria (P). X400.

ien basilar epithelial cells or glandular ep-helial cells from adnexal structures may be resent. Dermal lesions are some of the most ɔccessible lesions for cytologic examination. nflammatory (neutrophils, macrophages), ystic (sebaceous gland lining cells) and neo-lastic (melanocytes, mast cells) compo-ents involving the integument are identi-ied readily by cytology. Parasites of the kin may be observed while examining cy-ɔlogic specimens.

Digestive System

General Considerations. Impression smears ɔf the oral cavity and esophagus of normal ɪnimals consists of squamous epithelial cells n various stages of maturation and a mixed ɔopulation of bacteria (Fig. 26.10). Neutro-hils may be present also. Inflammatory esions of the mouth usually contain large ɪumbers of neutrophils and bacteria (Fig. ɪ6.11). Neoplastic lesions of the buccal cav-ty contain characteristic cells.

Gastric impression smears or washings ɔonsist of columnar epithelial and goblet ɔells. In the horse, squamous epithelial cells nay be present. Chief cells may be seen ɔccasionally. They contain metachromatic ɟranules and resemble columnar epithelial ɔells.

Rectal swabs from normal animals consist ɔf columnar epithelial cells, goblet cells and ɔacteria. Aspirates of intestinal contents nay consist of large numbers of various ypes of bacteria. Degenerating epithelial ɔells may be seen also.

Impression smears or aspirates may be obtained from the liver. Normal liver cells have round nuclei that contain one or two nucleoli. The abundant lavender cytoplasm may contain bile pigment (Fig. 26.12). Numerous binucleate cells may be present.

Urinary System

General Considerations. The cytologic evaluation of urine sediment is a useful procedure to determine the state of health or disease of the urinary system. The urinary bladder may be evaluated by cytologic examination of urine sediment. Transitional epithelial cells which line the urinary bladder are encountered frequently in normal urine sediment. The cells are variable in size, have round to oval vesicular nuclei with one or two nucleoli (Plate VII.9). The abundant cytoplasm is lavender. Multinucleated cells are encountered frequently (Fig. 26.13). Renal epithelial cells may occur in urine sediment when renal disease is present. Desquamated renal epithelial cells may occur as components of *renal casts*. Renal casts are proteinaceous models of renal tubules. As renal epithelial cell casts degenerate, they progress from *granular casts* to *waxy casts*. Granular casts contain particles that are derived from the disintegrating renal epithelial cells (Fig. 26.14). Waxy casts are refractile yellow casts with broken ends.

Respiratory System

General Considerations. Transtracheal aspiration is a useful method for obtaining cells from the respiratory tract for cytologic

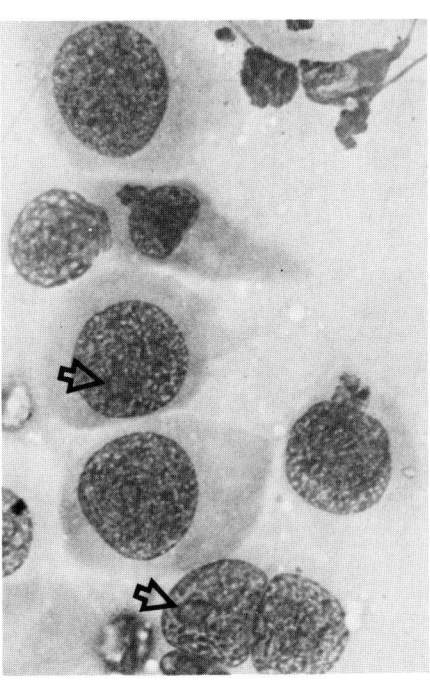

Fig. 26.13 Transitional epithelial cells from the urinary bladder of a normal dog. The large nuclei contain a fine chromatin network. Nucleoli (*arrows*) are evident in some of the cells. X250.

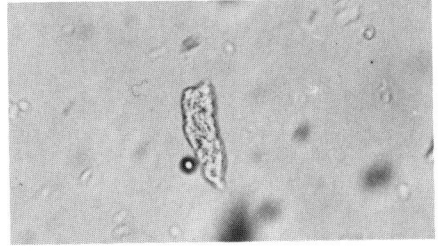

Fig. 26.14 A granular cast from the urinary sediment of a dog. X100.

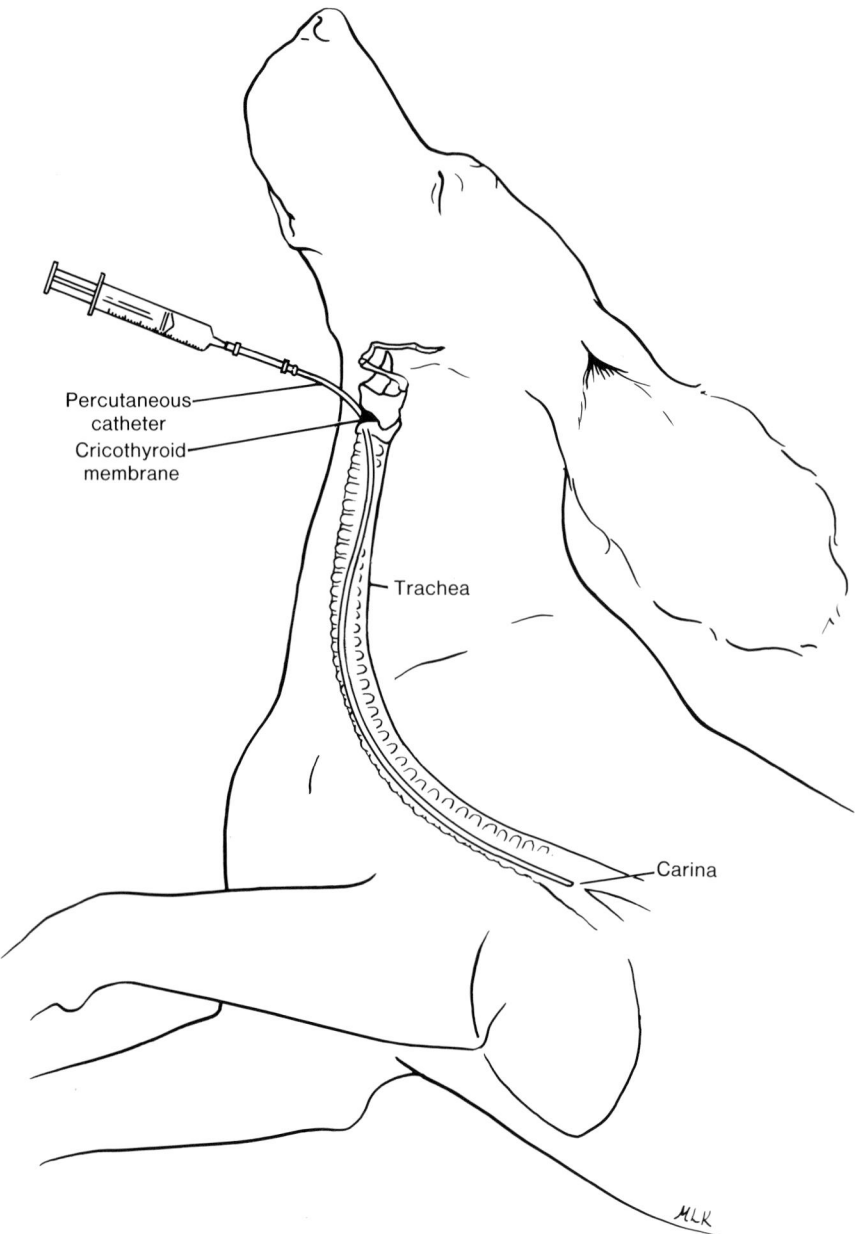

Percutaneous catheter

Cricothyroid membrane

Trachea

Carina

MLK

Fig. 26.15 A diagram depicting the percutaneous passage of a catheter to the level of the carina in order to obtain a tracheal wash.

valuation. Methods that bypass the mouth ₍nd oropharynx, avoiding normal flora that ₍ould be confused with pathogens, are best. These techniques require the percutaneous ₍assage of a catheter that enters the trachea ₍hrough the cricothyroid membrane and is ₍assed to the carina (Fig. 26.15). The instil-₍ation and immediate aspiration of fluid ₍ompletes the sampling.

Cytology. Tracheobronchial epithelial cells ₍nay be ciliated columnar or cuboidal (Fig. ₍6.16). Epithelial cells occur in aspirates ₍rom normal and diseased patients (Plate ₍II.10). Mucus-producing goblet cells may ₍e seen also.

Neutrophils are the predominant cell type ₍n inflammatory conditions (Plate VII.11). The appearance of the neutrophils varies ₍vith the length of time the cells were in the ₍rachea or bronchi and depends on the de-₍ree of sepsis. If neutrophils appear toxic ₍nuclear swelling, nuclear membrane rup-₍ure), then bacteria may be present in the ₍ytoplasm. If bacteria are seen, then an ad-₍itional smear should be gram-stained for ₍acterial characterization. *Eosinophils* occur ₍n varying numbers in animals with allergic ₍ulmonary conditions and dirofilariasis ₍Fig. 26.17). *Lymphocytes* and *plasma cells* ₍re present in viral infections. Their num-₍ers are increased also in other chronic in-₍lammatory conditions. *Macrophages* are ₍resent in numerous types of inflammatory ₍onditions (Figs. 26.18, 26.19). They may ₍ontain phagocytized red blood cells, cellu-₍ar debris, lipids and anthracotic pigment. Macrophages may originate as alveolar ₍hagocytes (histiocytes) or blood mono-₍ytes. *Mucus* is increased in most inflam-₍natory conditions. It appears as a diffuse, ₍light blue-staining and homogeneous back-₍ground. *Fibrin* and other proteins may be ₍present in inflammatory conditions. Fibrin ₍stains pink and appears as fine whorled ₍strands. It should not be confused with de-₍generating nuclear debris. *Fungal* elements ₍hyphae, spores) may be present in pulmo-₍nary mycoses. Fungal contaminants, such as ₍*Alternaria sp.*, are common in aspirates from ₍large animals. *Viral inclusion bodies* may be ₍seen within epithelial cells. Canine distem-₍per viral inclusions and canine adenoviral ₍inclusions have been observed in tracheal ₍aspirations.

Glandular Organs

Thyroid Gland. The cells of the normal thy-₍roid gland are follicular epithelial cells that ₍form pseudosyncytia in which cytoplasmic ₍borders are indistinct (Fig. 26.20). The cy-₍toplasm of thyroid follicular epithelial cells ₍disrupts easily, resulting in the presence of ₍many "naked nuclei" (Plate VII.12). The ₍nuclei are round with small inconspicuous ₍nucleoli, whereas the cytoplasm is baso-₍philic. A few cells may contain vacuoles or ₍blue-black granules within the cytoplasm ₍Plate VIII.1).

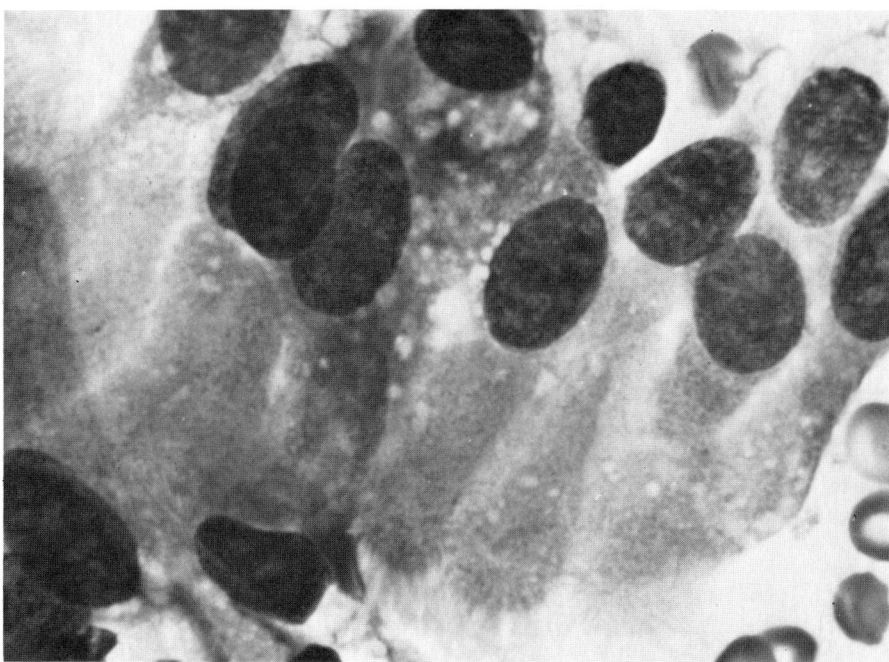

Fig. 26.16 Columnar ciliated cells obtained from a tracheal wash of a normal dog. X400.

Salivary Gland. Aspirates of normal salivary glands contain large (25 mm), foamy, glandular epithelial cells with small dense nuclei and a lavender cytoplasm filled with uniform small vacuoles (Plate VIII.2).

Reproductive System

Introduction. Cytologic techniques are useful aids for evaluation of the male and female reproductive system. The utility is not confined to the diagnosis of disease. Cytology is a significant evaluative technique used to determine the reproductive potential of the male (semen evaluation) and the stage of the estrous cycle in dogs and cats. Various techniques are employed and include ejaculation, massage, washes, aspiration biopsy and scrapings.

Cytology of the Prostate Gland. Prostatic fluid may be obtained by prostatic massage or fine-needle aspiration biopsy (Fig. 26.21). Based upon cytologic findings, prostatic disease can be differentiated into five categories: benign prostatic hyperplasia, prostatic cyst formation, prostatic inflammation (prostatitis or abscessation), prostatic neoplasia and squamous metaplasia.

The normal prostate has clusters of uniform cuboidal or columnar epithelial cells which vary from 10–15 μm in diameter. Nuclei are round to oval and are basilar in the columnar cells. Nucleoli are small and inconspicuous. The cytoplasm is finely granular and basophilic (Plate VIII.3). These cells can be differentiated easily from transitional epithelial cells which are larger and lighter staining than prostatic cells.

Benign prostatic hyperplasia (Plate VIII.4), prostatic cysts, prostatitis (Fig. 26.22), prostatic abscess and prostatic ad-

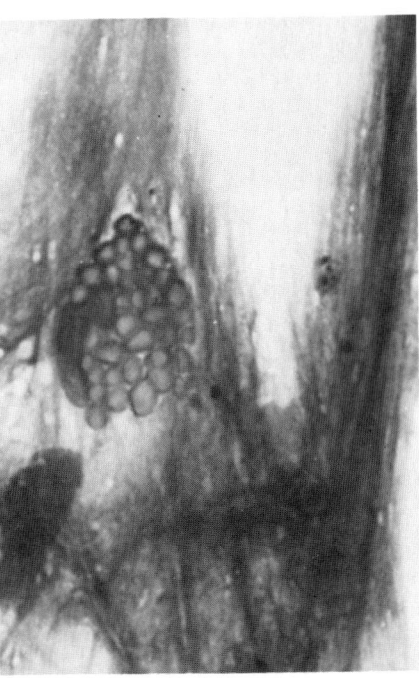

Fig. 26.17 An eosinophil from an equine tracheal wash. The dark-staining background material is mucin. X400.

enocarcinoma (Plate VIII.5) may be identified on the basis of the characteristics of the aspirate. Similarly, squamous metaplasia of prostatic epithelial cells may be identified (Plate VIII.6).

Vaginal Cytology. Examination of cells from the vagina of dogs and cats is a valuable aid in evaluating the stage of the estrous cycle, as well as diagnosing uterine and vaginal disease. The following descriptions refer to the dog specifically. The wall of the anestral

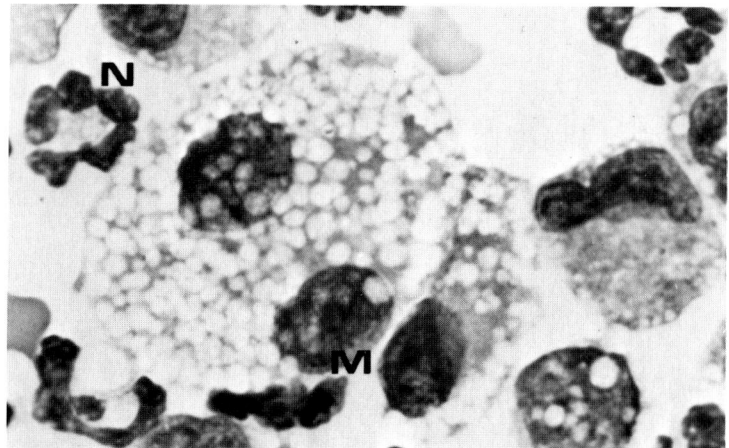

Fig. 26.18 A tracheal wash from a dog with chronic bronchitis. Macrophages (M) and neutrophils (N) are apparent. X400.

vagina normally is lined by epithelium that consists of 2 to 4 cell layers. As estrogen levels increase, the vaginal lining increases in thickness to about 40 cells. The increased thickening of the stratified squamous epithelium is the basis of cytologic changes that are observed in the vaginal smear. Epithelial cells progress from noncornified to cornified as the thickening occurs. Neutrophils disappear during proestrus and estrus because the thickened epithelium does not allow their passage to the lumen of the vagina. Red blood cells from the uterus appear in the vaginal discharge during proestrus and estrus.

The *anestrous* vagina has many noncornified, round to oval epithelial cells which contain large, distinct and unifrom nuclei (Fig. 26.23). A few neutrophils may be present. Minimal cellular debris is present.

The *proestrous* vagina is characterized by cornifying superficial epithelial cells. They constitute a major portion of all epithelial cells by the third day. The rounded cytoplasmic borders are replaced by straight edges. The nuclei become pyknotic and may disappear. Leukocytes are absent by the middle of proestrus. Erythrocytes may be numerous as a result of diapedesis from the underlying vascular bed. Various types of bacteria may be free, on or within epithelial cells.

The *estrous* vagina has epithelial cells that are cornified with straight cytoplasmic borders and pyknotic nuclei (Fig. 26.24) (Plate VIII.7). Late estrus is characterized by epithelial cells without nuclei. The number of erythrocytes is reduced. Various types of bacteria are present. As the epithelial cells begin to disintegrate, cellular debris becomes abundant (Fig. 26.25). Neutrophils reappear one or two days before diestrus.

In *diestrus*, neutrophils are abundant and small, round, noncornified epithelial cells reappear. Neutrophils may occur within epithelial cells (Plate VIII.8). Debris and erythrocytes usually disappear. As diestrus progresses, neutrophils are reduced in number. Late diestrus appears cytologically similar to anestrus.

Large number of neutrophils with phagocytized bacteria are present in *vaginitis* and *pyometra*. The neutrophils may be more degenerate in pyometra than in vaginitis. A white blood cell count on a peripheral blood sample will usually differentiate these two conditions.

Post-partum vaginal secretions contain large numbers of neutrophils, erythrocytes and debris for approximately two weeks. Foamy endometrial epithelial cells may be present. If puppies are undergoing maceration in the uterus, muscle fibers may be present (Fig. 26.26).

Body Cavities

General Remarks. In the normal horse and ox, fluid can be aspirated from the thoracic and abdominal cavities. In the normal dog and cat, the quantity of fluid present in the abdominal cavity is so small that attempts at sampling are usually futile. If four-quadrant paracentesis is unsuccessful, then peritoneal lavage with physiologic saline may be attempted. Unfortunately, saline distorts the cells. Many abnormal conditions are characterized by fluid accumulation. The normal equine thoracic fluid usually contains approximately 4800 nucleated cells/ mm^3, the majority of which are healthy neutrophils with some large mononucleated cells and lymphocytes.

Body Cavity Effusions. Body cavity effusions are generally classified as either *transudates* or *exudates*. Transudates are capillary filtrates that accumulate in the extravascular compartment. The most common causes for the formation of *transudative effusions* are *hypoproteinemia* and *venous stasis*. Low serum albumin (< 1–2 gm/dl) results in low colloid osmotic pressure and a subsequent accumulation of extravascular fluid. Hypoproteinemia may result from inadequate protein intake (starvation, inadequate protein digestion, malabsorption, par-

asitism), inadequate protein synthesis due t chronic liver disease (cirrhosis, congestiv heart failure, portocaval shunts, neoplasia or excessive protein loss (protein-losin glomerulonephropathy, protein-losing en teropathy, hemorrhage, massive exudativ lesions). Venous stasis may be a result o heart failure or venous or lymphatic ob struction. Venous or lymphatic obstructio may occur in disease processes such a thromboembolic disorders, neoplasia an hepatopathies. Pure *transudates* are cause by hypoalbuminemia. They are usuall

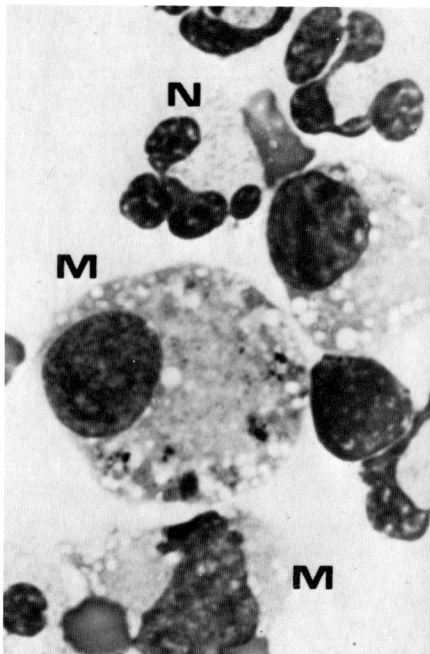

Fig. 26.19 Macrophages (M) and neutrophils (N) from a canine tracheal wash. The dark material within the macrophage is hemosiderin X400.

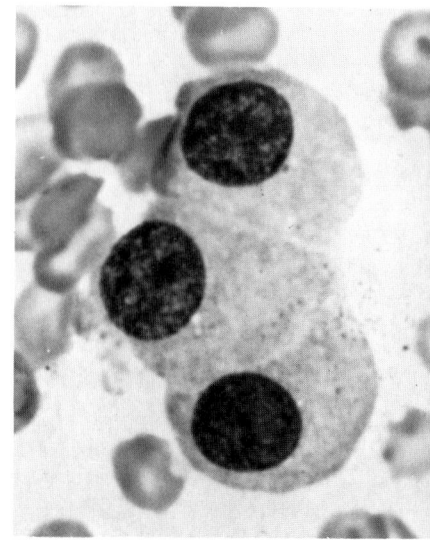

Fig. 26.20 Thyroid follicular cells from a normal dog. X400.

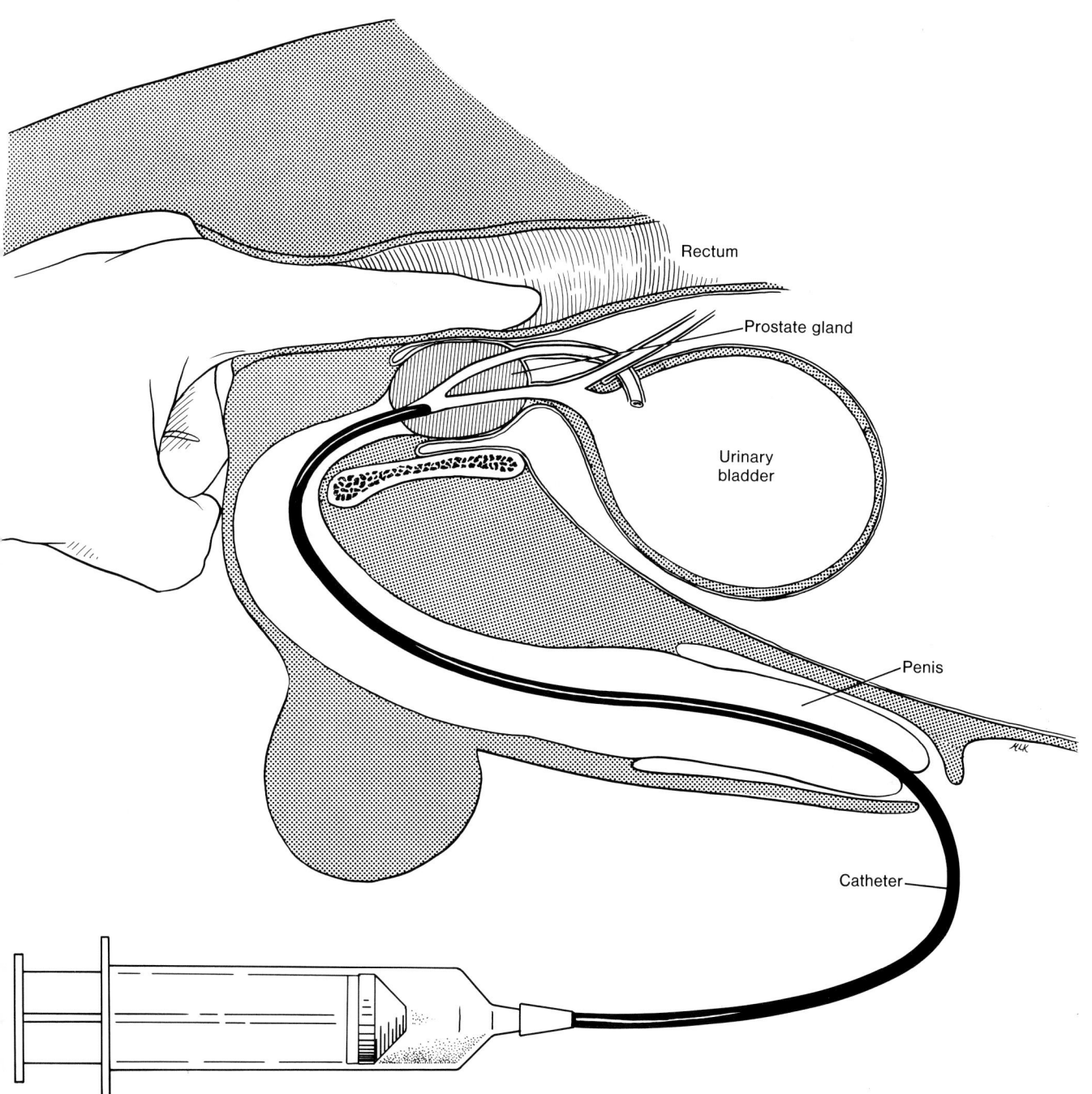

Rectum

Prostate gland

Urinary
bladder

Penis

Catheter

Fig. 26.21 A diagram depicting the method of obtaining a prostatic sample by massaging the prostate per rectum.

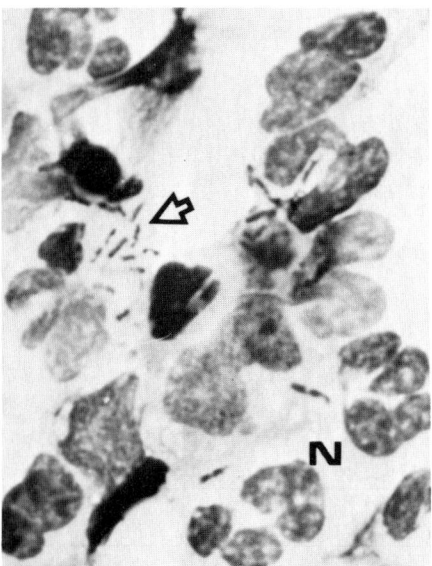

Fig. 26.22 A smear of cells obtained from the urinary tract by a prostatic massage per rectum. Numerous toxic neutrophils (N) and bacteria (*arrow*) are present. X400.

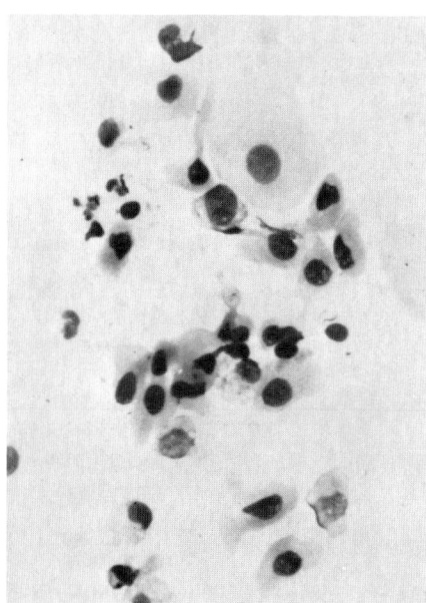

Fig. 26.23 A vaginal smear from a dog in anestrus. X100.

colorless and clear, have a total protein of less than 1.5 gm/dl and contain fewer than 500 cells/μl.

A *modified transudate* is a transudative-type fluid that has been modified by the addition of protein and/or cells. In general, this type of fluid accumulates in patients that have venous stasis or impaired lymphatic drainage (congestive heart failure, passive congestion of the liver, neoplasia). Modified transudates contain 2–3.5 gm/dl of protein and usually less than 5000 cells/μl.

Exudates are formed in conditions in which there is increased capillary permeability, resulting in fluid, protein and cells leaving the capillaries at an increased rate. Increased capillary permeability is a result of an inflammatory process. The inflammation may or may not be due to a bacterial infection. *Nonspecific exudates* contain no bacteria and form in conditions such as gall bladder or urinary bladder rupture, pancreatitis, presence of sterile foreign bodies,

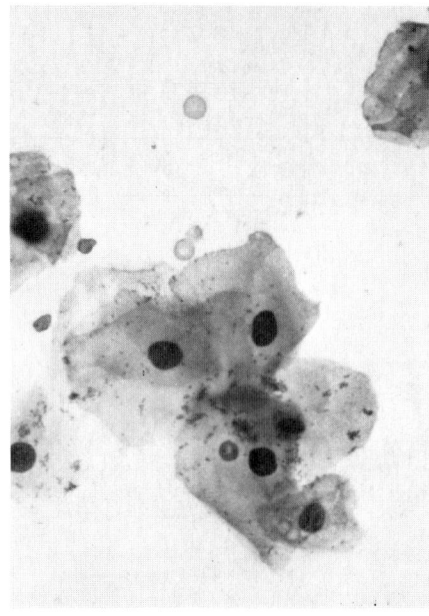

Fig. 26.24 A vaginal smear from a dog in early estrus. Some erythrocytes are present. The straight edges of cytoplasmic borders of the epithelial cells are indicative of cornification. X100.

feline infectious peritonitis, neoplasia and long-standing modified transudates. The latter may eventually initiate an inflammatory response itself. *Septic exudates* are caused by a wide variety of microorganisms.

Hemorrhagic effusions, usually caused by trauma, neoplasia, surgery or infarction of the intestines, consist primarily of blood.

Although a clear cut division between a transudate and an exudate does not exist, fluids are usually classified as transudates or exudates on the basis of several criteria (Table 26.1).

Physical and Chemical Evaluation. Numerous properties of fluids should be determined: volume, color, transparency, clot formation, odor, protein concentration, and occult blood (or RBC count or packed cell volume). The presence of RBC's, WBC's, lipid and bilirubin alters the color and transparency of the fluids. Other tests, such as those for bilirubin, glucose, urea, creatinine and amylase may facilitate a specific diagnosis.

Cytologic Evaluation. A *total nucleated cell count* may be performed with an automatic counter or hemocytometer. A direct smear may be used to evaluate cellularity instead of using a nucleated cell count. *Differential cell counts* are helpful, because various types of cells occur in effusions. In cell poor fluids, samples should be centrifuged and a smear made of the sediment. The feathered edge of the smear should always be examined; the larger cells travel to this area. Generally, smears are air dried routinely and stained with Romanowsky stains; whereas some prefer to stain slides with Papanicolaou stain. A Gram stain is indicated if bacteria are present. *Mesothelial cells* line the pleural, pericardial and peritoneal cavities (Fig.

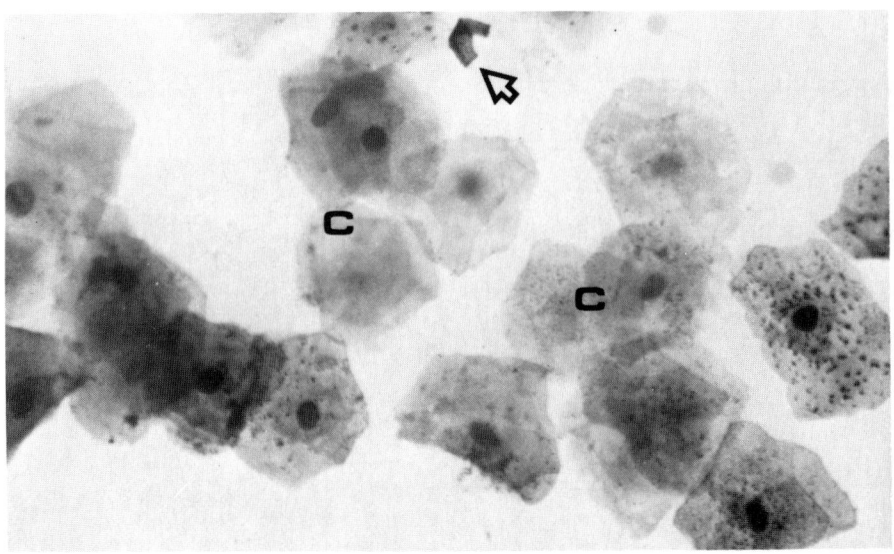

Fig. 26.25 A vaginal smear from a dog in estrus. The dark granules are bacteria. Some cells (C) are devoid of nuclei, while some cells have disintegrated (*arrow*). The nuclei are pyknotic. X100.

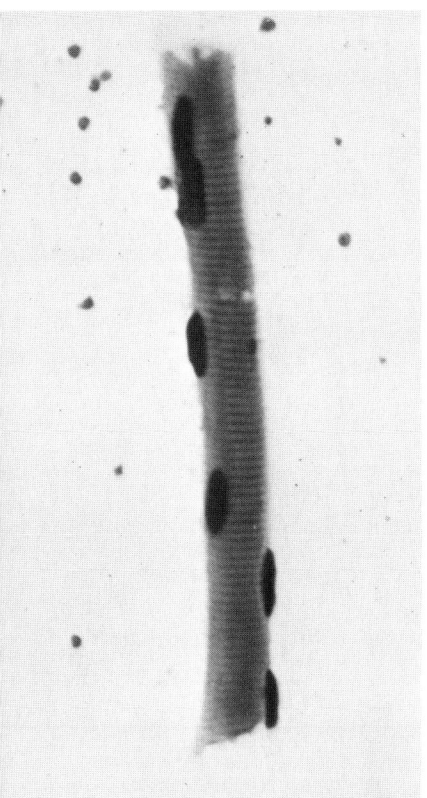

Fig. 26.26 A skeletal muscle fiber within a vaginal smear from a bitch with a puppy undergoing maceration in utero. X160.

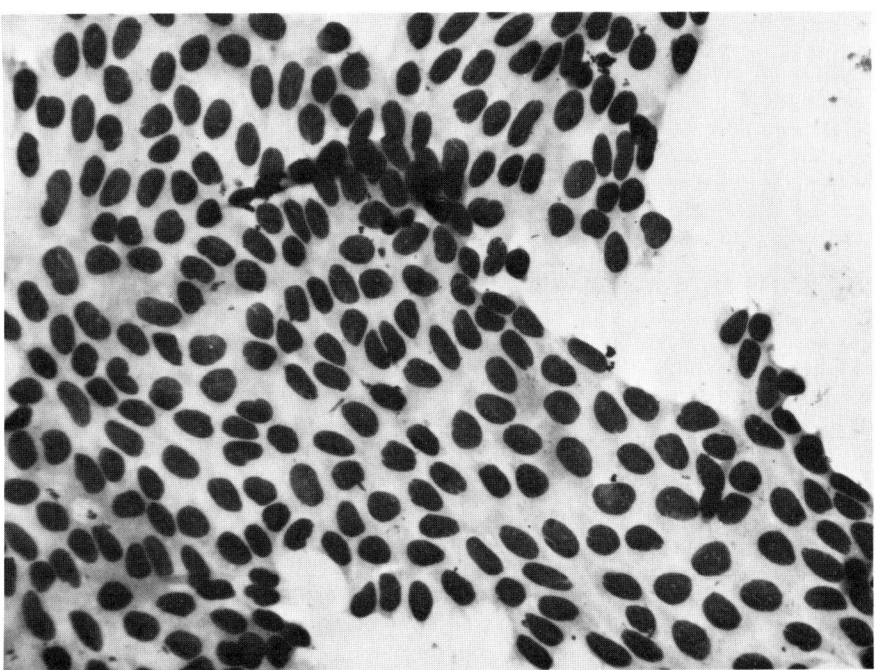

Fig. 26.27 A sheet of mesothelial cells from the abdominal cavity of an ox. X100.

Table 26.1
Effusion Characteristics

Property	Transudate	Exudate
Appearance	Clear	Usually cloudy
Specific Gravity	1.018	1.018
Protein	<3 gm/dl	>3 gm/dl
Clot	No	Yes
Cell count	Usually low	Usually high

26.27). When fluid accumulates in body cavities these cells undergo hypertrophy and hyperplasia and eventually exfoliate into the fluid. The cells may continue to multiply after exfoliation. Mesothelial cells may appear singly or in clusters of 2, 4, 8, 16, 32 or 64 cells (Fig. 26.28). Mesothelial cells are large (12–30 μm) and have a light to dark blue cytoplasm. The nuclear-cytoplasmic ratio is high (Plate VIII.9). The nuclei are single or multiple, round to oval with one or more nucleoli. The nucleoli are generally 3 μm in diameter. Cells in mitosis may be observed. Reactive mesothelial cells should be uniform in size without nuclear molding.

Macrophages vary in diameter from 10 to 50 μm, possess one or more round to oval nuclei that may contain visible nucleoli, and have a light blue, vacuolated cytoplasm (Plate VIII.10). Macrophages phagocytize

neutrophils, red blood cells, lipids, cellular debris, foreign material and certain microorganism; however, it is unusual to observe bacteria within phagocytic vacuoles of macrophages.

Neutrophils, scarce in noninflammatory conditions, are present in large numbers in inflammatory effusions. The state of preservation of the neutrophils is an important determinant. Neutrophils in nonseptic effusions are well preserved and appear much as they do in peripheral blood, with intact nuclear membranes and dense chromatin. As neutrophils age, they become hypersegmented and eventually pyknotic. In septic effusions, neutrophils are affected by bacterial toxins and undergo rapid degeneration and eventual rupture. Nuclear lobes become swollen, karyolysis occurs and the chromatin becomes light pink and smudged (*chromatolysis*). The cytoplasm becomes basophilic, vacuolated and cytoplasmic membranes commonly rupture. Careful examination in thin smeared areas near the feathered edge usually reveals the presence of bacteria within the cytoplasm of the neutrophils or free in the exudate. Bacteria (all of which stain blue with Romanowsky stains) are usually discrete uniform structures that should not be confused with background protein or stain precipitate, both of which appear somewhat amorphous and dark purple. Background protein is a fine granular material seen between cells in high protein fluids. Precipitated stain, resulting from inadequate rinsing of the slide, is extremely variable in size and shape.

Other cells found in effusions include lymphocytes, plasma cells, eosinophils, mast cells and red blood cells.

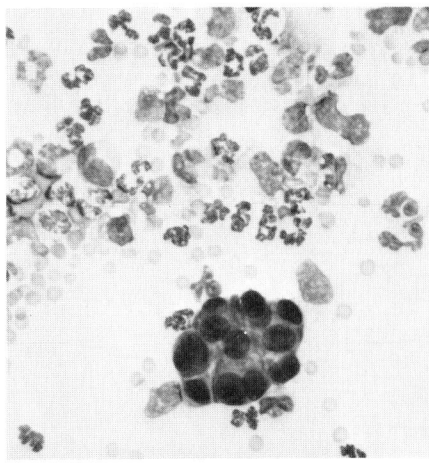

Fig. 26.28 A cluster of mesothelial cells from the abdominal cavity of a horse. Macrophages (M) and neutrophils are apparent. X100.

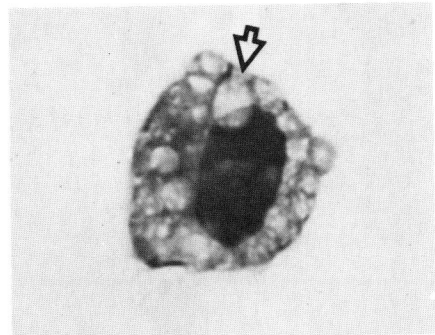

Fig. 26.29 A macrophage from the joint fluid of a dog with phagocytized red bloods within the cytoplasm (*arrow*).

Neoplastic cells may be observed in effusions resulting from a neoplastic process in a body cavity. Neoplastic cells are usually large and pleomorphic with a high nuclear-cytoplasmic ratio. Variability in nuclear size (*anisokaryosis*), nuclear molding, multinucleation, abnormal mitotic figures and large prominent multiple nucleoli are usually obvious. The cytoplasm usually stains quite basophilic. Incomplete cytoplasmic and nuclear division is observed commonly ("indian filing"). The most common neoplastic cells seen are lymphoblasts (lymphosarcoma) and carcinoma cells (malignant tumors of epithelial origin). Sarcoma cells (malignant tumors of connective tissue origin) rarely exfoliate into body cavity effusions.

Cytology of the Eye

The microscopic examination of conjunctival scrapings is a valuable aid in the diagnosis of external eye diseases. Samples are obtained from the central palpebral conjunctiva.

Cytology. The description is based upon staining of a normal conjunctiva. Conjunctival epithelial cells occur in sheets. Deeper scrapings contain parabasal cells that are round and dark-staining (Plate VIII.11). Cells from the intermediate and superficial layers are flatter, appear to have more cytoplasm and are paler staining than deeper cells. The cytoplasm is pale blue and the purple-staining nucleus is round to oval. Cytoplasmic melanin granules stain dark green to black. In some individuals, most epithelial cells contain melanin. Epithelial cells that are keratinizing have a pale lavender cytoplasm with a degenerating pyknotic nucleus. (The eyelid margin normally contains keratinized cells and care should be exercised to avoid sampling this surface, because keratinized cells are atypical in the conjunctival sac). Goblet cells may be identified by the large amount of mucinogen in the cytoplasm (Plate VIII.12). The nucleus is displaced to the periphery of the cell by the inclusion droplet. The mucus precursor is represented by a clear area or may stain very light blue. Goblet cells are found normally in the fornix conjunctivae. Occasional bacteria may be present on the surface of epithelial cells. Neutrophils may be observed rarely. Inflammation of the conjunctiva may be characterized by the presence of numerous neutrophils and macrophages.

Cytology of the Musculoskeletal System

Synovial Fluid. Synovial fluid analysis is of value in determining underlying causes of arthritis. Synovial fluid is a dialysate of plasma and is rich in mucosubstances. Normal synovial fluid of most species contains less than 3000 nucleated cells. Approximately 90% of these cells are lymphocytes and monocytes (Fig. 26.29). The remainder are healthy neutrophils. A large amount of background protein is obvious in joint fluid smears. Various arthritides result in an increase in inflammatory cells. Viral and chlamydial infections are characterized by increased numbers of mononucleated cells, whereas bacterial infections are characterized by an increased number of neutrophils.

The mononucleated and polymorphonu cleated cells are typical.

References

Bach, L. G. and Ricketts, S. W.: Paracentesis as an ai to the diagnosis of abdominal disease in the hors Eq. Vet. J. *6:*116, 1974.

Beech, J.: Cytology of tracheobronchial aspirates i horses. Vet. Pathol. *12:*157, 1975.

Benjamin, M. M.: *Outline of Veterinary Clinical Patho ogy,* 3rd ed. Iowa State Univ. Press, Ames, Iow 1978.

Coles, E. H.: *Veterinary Clinical Pathology,* 3rd ed., V B. Saunders, Philadelphia, 1980.

Creighton, S. R. and Wilkins, R. J.: Evaluation of an mals using transtracheal aspiration biopsy. JAAH *10:*219, 1974.

Crowe, D. T. and Crane, S. W.: Diagnostic abdomin paracentesis and lavage in the evaluation of abdom inal injuries in dogs and cats: Clinical and experi mental investigations. J. Amer. Vet. Med. Asso *168:*700, 1976.

Lavach, J. D., Thrall, M. A., Benjamin, M. M. ar Severin, G. A.: Cytology of normal and inflamme conjunctivas in dogs and cats. JAVMA, *170:*72 1977.

Miller, J. B., Puman, V., Osborne, C. A. Hammer, R. and Gambardella P. C.: Synovial fluid analysis i canine arthritis. JAAHA, Vol. *10:*392, 1974.

Rebar, A. H.: *Handbook of Veterinary Cytology.* Ralsto Purina Company, 1979.

Soderstom, N.: *Fine Needle Aspiration Biopsy,* Grune ar Stratton, New York, 1966.

Spriggs, A. I. and Boddington, M.: *The Cytology Effusions,* 2nd ed. Grune and Stratton, Inc., Ne York, 1968.

Van Pelt, R. W.: Interpretation of synovial fluid findin in the horse. JAVMA, *165:*91, 1974.

Van Pelt, R. W., Oldon, D. P. and Gallagher, K. F Chronic gonitis in cattle: Clinicopathologic finding and treatment. JAVMA, *163:*1378, 1973.

Vandevelde, M. and Spano, J.: Cerebrospinal fluid c tology in canine neurologic disease, Am. J. Ve Res., *38:*1827, 1977.

Zinkl, J. L. and Keeton, K. S.: Lymph node cytolog Calif. Vet. Vol. *33:*9, 1979.